THE ELBOW
AND ITS DISORDERS

THE ELBOW
AND ITS DISORDERS

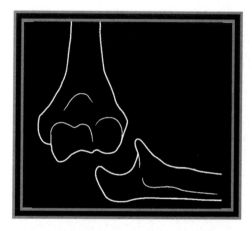

THIRD EDITION

BERNARD F. MORREY, M.D.

Professor of Orthopedic Surgery
Mayo Medical School
Department of Orthopedic Surgery
Mayo Clinic
Rochester, Minnesota

SAUNDERS
An Imprint of Elsevier

SAUNDERS
An Imprint of Elsevier

The Curtis Center
Independence Square West
Philadelphia, PA 19106

Library of Congress Cataloging-in-Publication Data

The elbow and its disorders / [edited by] Bernard F. Morrey.—3rd ed.

p.   cm.

Includes bibliographical references and index.

ISBN 0–7216–7752–5

1. Elbow—Surgery.   2. Elbow—Diseases.   3. Elbow—Fractures.
I. Morrey, Bernard F.   [DNLM: 1. Elbow Joint—injuries.   2. Joint Diseases.
WE 820 E383 2000]

RD558.E43 2000   617.5′74—dc21

DNLM/DLC   99–33416

Editor: Richard Lampert
Editorial Assistant: Beth LoGiudice
Designer: Paul Fry
Production Manager: Natalie Ware
Manuscript Editor: Gina Scala
Illustration Coordinator: Rita Martello

THE ELBOW AND ITS DISORDERS   ISBN 0–7216–7752–5

Permissions may be sought directly from Elsevier's Health Sciences Rights Department in Philadelphia, USA: phone: (+1)215-238-7869, fax: (+1)215-238-2239, email: healthpermissions@elsevier.com. You may also complete your request on-line via the Elsevier Science homepage (http://www.elsevier.com), by selecting 'Customer Support' and then 'Obtaining Permissions'.

Printed in the United States of America.

Last digit is the print number: 9   8   7   6   5

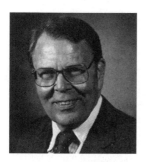

In Memoriam

Richard S. Bryan, M.D.

The second edition of the Elbow Book was dedicated to my longtime friend and mentor, Doctor Richard S. Bryan. Sadly, since the second edition went to print, Doctor Bryan died suddenly and unexpectedly, leaving an unfilled void in our personal and professional lives. The contributions that Doctor Bryan has made to the orthopedic community during his professional career at Mayo are well recognized and span several disciplines, not just those involving the elbow but also the hip and knee. But, as so often is the case, the true legacy of this exceptional person rests in his capacity as a role model and mentor. He has taught us to question accepted dogma, on the one hand, and to commit to sharing our individual knowledge and insights, on the other. I personally am tremendously indebted to this kind and gentle man's insight, tutelage, encouragement, and friendship. Dick will be severely missed not only by his family and his colleagues at Mayo but also by the orthopedic community.

· CONTRIBUTORS ·

Robert A. Adams, M.A., O.P.A.-C.
Department of Orthopedics, Mayo Clinic,
Rochester, Minnesota
*Total Elbow Arthroplasty in Patients with
Rheumatoid Arthritis; Total Elbow
Arthroplasty for Primary Osteoarthritis*

Peter C. Amadio, M.D.
Professor of Orthopedic Surgery, Mayo
Clinic, Rochester, Minnesota
Congenital Abnormalities of the Elbow

Kai-Nan An, Ph.D.
Professor of Bioengineering, Mayo Medical
School; Chair, Division of Orthopedic
Research, Mayo Clinic, Rochester,
Minnesota
*Biomechanics of the Elbow; Functional
Evaluation of the Elbow*

Robert D. Beckenbaugh, M.D.
Professor of Orthopedic Surgery, Hand
Division, Mayo Medical School/Mayo
Foundation, Mayo Clinic; Orthopedic
Hand Surgeon, Rochester Methodist
Hospital, Saint Mary's Hospital,
Rochester, Minnesota
Arthrodesis

James B. Bennett, M.D.
Clinical Professor of Hand Surgery,
Department of Orthopedic Surgery,
University of Texas Medical School at
Houston; Chief of Staff, Texas Orthopedic
Hospital, Houston, Texas
Articular Injuries in the Athlete

Richard A. Berger, M.D., Ph.D.
Associate Professor, Departments of
Orthopedic Surgery and Anatomy, Mayo
Graduate School of Medicine; Consultant,
Division of Hand Surgery, Department of
Orthopedic Surgery, Mayo Clinic/Mayo
Foundation, Rochester, Minnesota
Overuse Syndrome

Thomas H. Berquist, M.D., F.A.C.R.
Professor of Diagnostic Radiology, Mayo
Medical School, Rochester, Minnesota;
Consultant, Diagnostic Radiology, Mayo
Clinic Jacksonville, Jacksonville, Florida
Diagnostic Imaging of the Elbow

Allen T. Bishop, M.D.
Associate Professor of Orthopedic Surgery,
Mayo Medical School; Consultant,
Department of Orthopedic Surgery,
Division of Hand Surgery and
Microvascular Surgery, Mayo Clinic,
Rochester, Minnesota
Soft Tissue Coverage of the Elbow

Mark E. Bolander, M.D.
Professor of Orthopedic Surgery, Mayo
Medical School; Consultant, Department
of Orthopedic Surgery, Mayo Clinic,
Rochester, Minnesota
Hematologic Arthritis

David A. Boone, M.D., M.P.H.
Director, Prosthetics Research Study, Seattle,
Washington
Amputation

Ernest M. Burgess, M.D., L.H.D. (Hon.)
Clinical Professor of Orthopedic Surgery,
University of Washington School of
Medicine; President and Founder of
Prosthetic Outreach Foundation and
Consultant and Advisor to Prosthetic
Research Foundation, Seattle, Washington
Amputation

Kenneth P. Butters, M.D.
Clinical Assistant Professor of Orthopedics,
University of Oregon Health Sciences
Center, Portland; Upper Extremity
Surgeon, Sacred Heart Hospital, Eugene,
Oregon
Septic Arthritis

Miguel E. Cabanela, M.D.
Professor of Orthopedic Surgery, Mayo
Medical School; Consultant, Department
of Orthopedics, Mayo Clinic, Rochester,
Minnesota
Fractures of the Olecranon

Patrick M. Connor, M.D.
Clinical Faculty, Shoulder and Elbow
Surgery, Sports Medicine, and
Orthopaedic Trauma Surgery; Orthopaedic
Surgery Residency Program, Department

of Orthopaedic Surgery, Carolinas Medical
Center, Charlotte, North Carolina
*Total Elbow Arthroplasty for Juvenile
Rheumatoid Arthritis*

William P. Cooney, M.D.
Professor of Orthopedics, Mayo Medical
School, Mayo Graduate School of
Medicine, Department of Orthopedic
Surgery, Rochester, Minnesota
*Elbow Arthroplasty: Historical Perspective
and Current Concepts*

Ralph W. Coonrad, M.D.
Associate Clinical Professor of Orthopedic
Surgery, Duke University School of
Medicine, and Duke University Hospital
and Medical Center; Medical Director and
Chief Surgeon, Lenox Baker Children's
Hospital; Attending Orthopedic Surgeon,
Durham Regional Hospital, Durham,
North Carolina
*Nonunion of the Olecranon and Proximal
Ulna*

**Roger Dee, M.D., Ph.D., F.R.C.S.(Eng),
F.A.A.O.S.**
Professor of Orthopedics, Department of
Orthopedics, School of Medicine, State
University of New York at Stony Brook,
Stony Brook; Chairman of Orthopedics,
Winthrop University Hospital, Mineola,
New York
*Nonimplantation Salvage of Failed
Reconstructive Procedures of the Elbow*

James H. Dobyns, M.D.
Professor of Orthopedic Surgery Emeritus,
Mayo Clinic, University of Texas Health
Science Center San Antonio, San Antonio,
Texas; Mayo Graduate School of
Medicine, Rochester, Minnesota; Honorary
Staff Consultant, Bexar County Medical
District and University Hospital
(UTHSCSA), Baptist Medical Services,
San Antonio, Texas
Congenital Abnormalities of the Elbow

Evan F. Ekman, M.D.
Assistant Professor of Orthopedic Surgery,
University of South Carolina School of
Medicine; Director, University of South
Carolina Sports Medicine Center,
Columbia, South Carolina
Arthroscopy: Débridement

Neal S. ElAttrache, M.D.
Assistant Clinical Professor, Department of
Orthopaedic Surgery, University of
Southern California School of Medicine;
Associate, Kerlan-Jobe Orthopaedic
Clinic, Los Angeles, California
Arthroscopy: Débridement; Diagnosis and

*Treatment of Ulnar Collateral Ligament
Injuries in Athletes*

Donald C. Ferlic, M.D.
Associate Clinical Professor, University of
Colorado Health Sciences Center, Denver,
Colorado
Evaluation of the Problem Elbow

Larry D. Field, M.D.
Clinical Instructor, Department of
Orthopaedic Surgery, University of
Mississippi School of Medicine; Co-
Director, Upper Extremity Service,
Mississippi Sports Medicine and
Orthopaedic Center, Jackson, Mississippi
*Arthroscopy: Portals in Elbow Arthroscopy;
Arthroscopy: Arthroscopic Capsular
Release*

Avrum I. Froimson, M.D.
Clinical Professor of Orthopaedics;
Consultant, Department of Orthopaedics,
Cleveland Clinic Foundation, Cleveland,
Ohio
Interposition Arthroplasty of the Elbow

Gerard T. Gabel, M.D.
Clinical Associate Professor, Baylor College
of Medicine, Houston, Texas
Medial Epicondylitis

Douglas E. Garland, M.D.
Clinical Professor of Orthopedic Surgery,
University of Southern California; Chief,
Neurotrauma, Rancho Los Amigos
Medical Center, Downey, California
Spastic Dysfunction of the Elbow

Gerald S. Gilchrist, M.D.
Helen C. Levitt Professor, Department of
Pediatric and Adolescent Medicine, Mayo
Medical School; Consultant, Pediatric
Hematology and Oncology; Director,
Mayo Comprehensive Hemophilia Center,
Mayo Clinic and Foundation, Rochester,
Minnesota
Hematologic Arthritis

David R. J. Gill, M.D., Ch.B., F.R.A.C.S.
Consultant Orthopaedic Surgeon, Department
of Orthopaedic Surgery, Middlemore
Hospital, Otahuhu, Auckland, New
Zealand
*Total Elbow Arthroplasty in Patients with
Rheumatoid Arthritis*

Hymie Gordon, M.D., F.R.C.P. (Deceased)
Emeritus Professor of Medical Genetics,
Mayo Medical School; Former Chairman,
Department of Medical Genetics, Mayo
Clinic, Rochester, Minnesota
Embryology and Phylogeny: Embryology

E. Richard Graviss, M.D.
Professor of Radiology and Associate
  Professor of Pediatrics, St. Louis
  University Medical Center; Director,
  Diagnostic Imaging, Cardinal Glennon
  Children's Hospital, St. Louis, Missouri
Imaging of the Pediatric Elbow

M. Mark Hoffer, M.D.
Lowman Professor of Pediatric
  Orthopaedics, Orthopaedic Hospital, Los
  Angeles, California
Spastic Dysfunction of the Elbow

Alan D. Hoffman, M.D.
Associate Professor, Mayo Medical School;
  Staff Consultant, Diagnostic Radiology,
  Mayo Clinic, Rochester, Minnesota
Imaging of the Pediatric Elbow

Robert N. Hotchkiss, M.D.
Associate Professor, Clinical Surgery
  (Orthopaedics), Weill Medical College of
  Cornell University; Chief, Hand Service at
  the Hospital for Special Surgery; Director,
  Alberto Vilar Center for Research of the
  Hand and Upper Extremity, New York,
  New York
*Extrinsic Contracture: "The Column
  Procedure," Lateral and Medial Capsular
  Releases; External Fixators of the Elbow*

Frank W. Jobe, M.D.
Clinical Professor, Department of
  Orthopaedic Surgery, University of
  Southern California School of Medicine;
  Associate, Kerlan-Jobe Orthopaedic
  Clinic, and Orthopaedic Consultant, Los
  Angeles Dodgers and PGA Tour and
  Senior PGA Tour, Los Angeles, California
*Diagnosis and Treatment of Ulnar Collateral
  Ligament Injuries in Athletes*

Jesse B. Jupiter, M.D.
Professor of Orthopaedic Surgery, Harvard
  Medical School; Director, Orthopaedic
  Hand Service, Massachusetts General
  Hospital, Boston, Massachusetts
Fractures of the Distal Humerus in Adults

Graham J. King, M.D., M.Sc., F.R.C.S.C.
Associate Professor, Orthopedic Surgery,
  University of Western Ontario; Consultant,
  Hand and Upper Limb Surgery, St. Joseph
  Health Centre, London, Ontario, Canada
Revision of Failed Total Elbow Arthroplasty

Rudolph A. Klassen, M.D.
Consultant in Pediatric Orthopedics, Mayo
  Clinic, Rochester, Minnesota
*Supracondylar Fractures of the Elbow in
  Children*

Tomasz K. W. Kozak, F.R.A.C.S.
Institute of Orthopaedic Specialities,
  Shadyside Medical Center, Pittsburgh,
  Pennsylvania
*Total Elbow Arthroplasty for Primary
  Osteoarthritis*

Susan G. Larson, Ph.D.
Professor of Anatomy, Department of
  Anatomical Sciences, School of Medicine,
  State University of New York at Stony
  Brook, Stony Brook, New York
Embryology and Phylogeny: Phylogeny

Brian P. H. Lee, M.D.
Consultant Orthopaedic Surgeon, Adult
  Reconstruction Service, Department of
  Orthopaedic Surgery, Singapore General
  Hospital, Singapore, Singapore
Synovectomy of the Elbow

Robert L. Lennon, M.D.
Associate Professor of Anesthesiology, Mayo
  Medical School, Rochester, Minnesota;
  Staff, Anesthesiology, Anesthesia and Pain
  Management, Presbyterian Hospitals,
  Charlotte, North Carolina
Continuous Axial Brachial Plexus Catheters

**R. Merv Letts, M.D., M.Sc., F.R.C.S.C.,
F.A.C.S.**
Professor of Surgery, University of Ottawa;
  Head of Surgery, Children's Hospital of
  Eastern Ontario, Ottawa, Ontario, Canada
Dislocations of the Child's Elbow

Ronald L. Linscheid, M.D.
Emeritus Professor of Orthopedic Surgery,
  Mayo Medical School, Rochester,
  Minnesota
*Resurfacing Elbow Replacement
  Arthroplasty: Rationale, Technique, and
  Results*

Harvinder S. Luthra, M.D.
John F. Finn Minnesota Arthritis Foundation
  Professor, and Chair, Division of
  Rheumatology, Mayo Medical School,
  Rochester, Minnesota
Rheumatoid Arthritis

Pierre Mansat, M.D.
Clinical Assistant of Orthopedic Surgery,
  University Hospital of Toulouse-Purpan,
  Toulouse, France
*Extrinsic Contracture: "The Column
  Procedure," Lateral and Medial Capsular
  Releases*

Thomas L. Mehlhoff, M.D.
Clinical Assistant Professor of Orthopedic
Surgery, Baylor College of Medicine;
Team Physician, Houston Astros, and
Staff, Texas Orthopedic Hospital,
Houston, Texas
Articular Injuries in the Athlete

Bernard F. Morrey, M.D.
Professor of Orthopedic Surgery, Mayo
Medical School; Consultant, Department
of Orthopedic Surgery, Mayo Clinic,
Rochester, Minnesota
*Anatomy of the Elbow Joint; Biomechanics
of the Elbow; Physical Examination of the
Elbow; Functional Evaluation of the
Elbow; Evaluation of the Problem Elbow;
Surgical Exposures of the Elbow;
Rehabilitation; Splints and Bracing at the
Elbow; Proximal Ulnar Fractures in
Children; Post-Traumatic Elbow Stiffness
in Children; Fractures of the Distal
Humerus in Adults; Nonunion and
Delayed Union of Distal Humeral
Fractures; Radial Head Fracture;
Fractures of the Olecranon; Nonunion of
the Olecranon and Proximal Ulna;
Coronoid Process and Monteggia
Fractures; Complex Instability of the
Elbow; Chronic Unreduced Elbow
Dislocation; Ectopic Ossification About
the Elbow; Extrinsic Contracture: "The
Column Procedure," Lateral and Medial
Capsular Releases; External Fixators of
the Elbow; Injury of the Flexors of the
Elbow: Biceps in Tendon Injury; Rupture
of the Triceps Tendon; Arthroscopy:
Complications of Elbow Arthroscopy;
Medial Epicondylitis; Surgical Failure of
Tennis Elbow; Lateral Collateral
Ligament Injury; Semiconstrained Elbow
Replacement Arthroplasty: Rationale and
Surgical Technique; Total Elbow
Arthroplasty in Patients with Rheumatoid
Arthritis; Total Elbow Arthroplasty for
Juvenile Rheumatoid Arthritis;
Semiconstrained Elbow Replacement:
Results in Traumatic Conditions; Total
Elbow Arthroplasty for Nonunion and
Dysfunctional Instability; Total Elbow
Arthroplasty for Primary Osteoarthritis;
Complications of Elbow Replacement
Surgery; Treatment of the Infected Total
Elbow Arthroplasty; Revision of Failed
Total Elbow Arthroplasty; Synovectomy of
the Elbow; Interposition Arthroplasty of
the Elbow; Primary Degenerative Arthritis
of the Elbow: Ulnohumeral Arthroplasty;
Septic Arthritis; Loose Bodies; Bursitis;
The Elbow in Metabolic Disease*

Scott J. Mubarak, M.D.
Clinical Professor, Department of
Orthopedics, University of California, San
Diego; Director of Orthopedic Program at
Children's Hospital, Children's Hospital
and Health Center, San Diego, California
*Complications of Supracondylar Fractures of
the Elbow*

Robert P. Nirschl, M.D.
Associate Professor of Orthopedic Surgery,
Georgetown University School of
Medicine, Washington, D.C.; Director,
Orthopedic Sports Medicine Fellowship
Program, Nirschl Orthopedic Clinic,
Arlington Hospital, Arlington, Virginia
*Rehabilitation; Muscle and Tendon Trauma:
Tennis Elbow Tendinosis*

Eugene T. O'Brien, M.D.
Clinical Professor of Orthopaedic Surgery,
University of Texas Health Sciences
Center; Chief, Orthopaedic Surgery,
Methodist Hospital, San Antonio, Texas
Flaccid Dysfunction of the Elbow

**Shawn W. O'Driscoll, M.D., Ph.D.,
F.R.C.S.(C)**
Professor of Orthopedic Surgery, Mayo
Clinic, Rochester, Minnesota
*Continuous Passive Motion; Elbow
Dislocations; Complex Instability of the
Elbow; Arthroscopy: Elbow Arthroscopy:
Loose Bodies; Arthroscopy: Elbow
Arthroscopy: The Future; Lateral
Collateral Ligament Injury*

Panayiotis J. Papagelopoulos, M.D., D.Sc.
Consultant, Department of Orthopedics,
Athens University Medical School, KAT
Hospital; Consultant in Orthopedic
Surgery, Hygeia Athens Medical Center,
Athens, Greece
*Nonunion of the Olecranon and Proximal
Ulna*

**Hamlet A. Peterson, M.D.,
M.S. (Orthopedics)**
Emeritus Professor of Orthopedic Surgery,
Mayo Medical School; Emeritus
Consultant in Orthopedic Surgery, Mayo
Clinic, Rochester, Minnesota
Physeal Fractures of the Elbow

Douglas J. Pritchard, M.D.
Professor of Orthopedic Surgery and
Oncology, Mayo Medical School;
Consultant, Department of Orthopedics,
Mayo Clinic, Rochester, Minnesota
Neoplasms of the Elbow

Matthew L. Ramsey, M.D.
Assistant Professor of Orthopaedic Surgery,
  Shoulder and Elbow Service, University
  of Pennsylvania School of Medicine,
  Philadelphia, Pennsylvania
*Total Elbow Arthroplasty for Nonunion and
  Dysfunctional Instability*

William D. Regan, M.D., F.R.C.S.(C)
Assistant Professor of Orthopaedics,
  University of British Columbia,
  Vancouver, British Columbia, Canada
*Physical Examination of the Elbow;
  Coronoid Process and Monteggia
  Fractures*

Felix H. Savoie, III, M.D.
Co-Director, Upper Extremity Service,
  Mississippi Sports Medicine and
  Orthopaedic Center, Jackson, Mississippi
*Arthroscopy: Portals in Elbow Arthroscopy;
  Arthroscopy: Arthroscopic Capsular
  Release*

Alberto G. Schneeberger, M.D.
Assistant Professor of Orthopedic Surgery
  and Consultant, Department of
  Orthopedics, University of Zurich, Zurich,
  Switzerland
*Semiconstrained Elbow Replacement: Results
  in Traumatic Conditions*

William J. Shaughnessy, M.S., M.D.
Assistant Professor of Orthopedics, Mayo
  Medical School; Consultant, Department
  of Orthopedics, Mayo Clinic, Rochester,
  Minnesota
Osteochondritis Dissecans

Franklin H. Sim, M.D.
Professor of Orthopedic Surgery, Mayo
  Medical School; Consultant, Department
  of Orthopedic Surgery and Subsection of
  Orthopedic Oncology, Mayo Clinic,
  Rochester, Minnesota
*Nonunion and Delayed Union of Distal
  Humeral Fractures*

Morton Spinner, M.D.
Clinical Professor, Orthopaedic Surgery,
  Albert Einstein College of Medicine,
  Bronx, New York
Nerve Entrapment Syndromes

Robert J. Spinner, M.D.
Chief Resident, Department of Neurologic
  Surgery, Mayo Clinic/Mayo Foundation,
  Rochester, Minnesota
Nerve Entrapment Syndromes

David Stanley, M.B., B.S., B.Sc., F.R.C.S.
Honorary Lecturer, University of Sheffield;
  Consultant Orthopaedic, Trauma and
  Upper Limb Surgeon, Northern General
  Hospital, Sheffield, United Kingdom
*Resurfacing Elbow Replacement
  Arthroplasty: The Kudo Total Elbow
  Replacement*

John K. Stanley, M.Ch.Orth., F.R.C.S.Ed.
Professor of Hand Surgery, Wrightington
  Hospital, Wigan, Lancashire, United
  Kingdom
*Resurfacing Elbow Replacement
  Arthroplasty: Souter-Strathclyde Elbow
  Arthroplasty*

Anthony A. Stans, M.D.
Instructor, Mayo Graduate School of
  Medicine, Mayo Clinic, Rochester,
  Minnesota
*Supracondylar Fractures of the Elbow in
  Children; Fractures of the Neck of the
  Radius in Children; Proximal Ulnar
  Fractures in Children; Post-Traumatic
  Elbow Stiffness in Children*

J. Clarke Stevens, M.D.
Professor and Chair, Department of
  Neurology, Mayo Clinic Arizona,
  Scottsdale, Arizona
Neurotrophic Arthritis

Lawrence W. Stinson, Jr., M.D.
Pain Fellowship, Department of Anesthesia,
  University of Arizona, Tucson, Arizona
Continuous Axial Brachial Plexus Catheters

Richard B. Tompkins, M.D., M.S.
Assistant Professor of Medicine, Mayo
  Medical School; Consultant,
  Rheumatology and Internal Medicine, St.
  Mary's Hospital and Methodist Hospital,
  Rochester, Minnesota
Nonrheumatoid Inflammatory Arthritis

Ian A. Trail, M.D., F.R.C.S.
Consultant in Hand and Upper Limb
  Surgery, Wrightington Hospital, Wigan,
  Lancashire, United Kingdom
*Resurfacing Elbow Replacement
  Arthroplasty: Souter-Strathclyde Elbow
  Arthroplasty*

Stephen D. Trigg, M.D.
Assistant Professor of Orthopedics, Mayo
  Medical School, Rochester, Minnesota;
  Consultant in Hand Surgery and Director,
  Orthopedic Residency Program, Mayo
  Clinic Jacksonville, Jacksonville, Florida
Pain Dysfunction Syndrome

K. Krishnan Unni, M.B., B.S.
Professor of Orthopedics and Pathology,
    Mayo Medical School; Consultant,
    Division of Anatomic Pathology, Mayo
    Clinic, Rochester, Minnesota
Neoplasms of the Elbow

C. Douglas Wallace, M.D.
Clinical Instructor, University of California,
    San Diego, La Jolla; Director of
    Orthopedic Trauma, Children's Hospital
    and Health Center, San Diego, California
*Complications of Supracondylar Fractures of
    the Elbow*

Robert L. Waters, M.D.
Clinical Professor of Orthopedic Surgery,
    University of Southern California; Medical
    Director, Rancho Los Amigos National
    Rehabilitation Center, Downey, California
Spastic Dysfunction of the Elbow

John H. Wedge, M.D., F.R.C.S.C.
Rose S. McLaughlin Professor and Chair,
    Department of Surgery, University of
    Toronto, Faculty of Medicine; Surgeon-in-
    Chief, The Hospital for Sick Children,
    Toronto, Ontario, Canada
*Fractures of the Neck of the Radius in
    Children*

Michael B. Wood, M.D.
Professor of Orthopedic Surgery, Mayo
    Graduate School of Medicine; CEO and
    President, Mayo Foundation; Consultant,
    Orthopedic Surgery, Mayo Clinic,
    Rochester, Minnesota
Replantation About the Elbow

Phillip E. Wright, II, M.D.
Professor, Orthopaedic Surgery, University
    of Tennessee College of Medicine;
    Director, Hand Surgery Fellowship,
    University of Tennessee-Campbell Clinic,
    Memphis; Active Staff, Campbell Clinic,
    Baptist Memorial Hospitals, Regional
    Medical Center at Memphis; Courtesy
    Staff, Methodist Hospital, Germantown;
    LeBonheur Children's Hospital, Memphis,
    Tennessee
Interposition Arthroplasty of the Elbow

Ken Yamaguchi, M.D.
Assistant Professor, Department of
    Orthopaedic Surgery, Washington
    University School of Medicine; Chief,
    Shoulder and Elbow Service, Barnes-
    Jewish Hospital, St. Louis, Missouri
*Treatment of the Infected Total Elbow
    Arthroplasty*

· FOREWORD ·

The elbow is a frontier in orthopedic surgery that has been discovered during our professional careers. In retrospect, it was unlikely that the surgeon involved in general adult reconstructive surgery or in surgery of the hand would choose this area as a central focus for study and development. It has been exciting to be a participating observer as the science and practice in this anatomic region have evolved over the last quarter century. This development, of course, is due to many factors—but, quite importantly, the intellect, organization, focused energy, and persistence of the editor of this textbook. The changes in this area have been profound. The first edition was the first definitive textbook on the elbow, and the second, and now the third edition, expand upon the contributions of new knowledge and changes in practice that have occurred during this dynamic period in the treatment of the elbow.

Bernard F. Morrey, with an engineering bent, has consistently participated with Drs. Andrew An and Edward Chao and co-workers in biomechanical investigations at Mayo. They have approached the elbow in a very fundamental way, defining the anatomy, assessing the motion, determining the forces, and understanding the elements contributing to joint stability. Investigations in these areas led directly to improved surgical approaches, including arthroscopic techniques, functional evaluation of the joint, a rationale for better understanding fractures and dislocations, and insight into the design of prosthetic implants. The continually evolving team of active, on-site contributors includes other orthopedic surgical staff, notably Shawn O'Driscoll with his creativeness, residents, fellows, and collaborating visiting physicians. The environment is charged in our clinic, in the operating rooms, and in the conferences, including the weekly shoulder and elbow conference. The output of scholarly activity related to the elbow has never been greater.

Heightening the value of this textbook are the large and impressive number of expert contributors. Consider any area, be it from embryology and phylogeny, pediatric disorders, overuse problems, neuromuscular impairments, sports medicine, or musculoskeletal oncology—a breadth of topics that can be addressed only by focused experts—and it is a part of this text.

So, if the reader is searching for comprehensiveness, a reference source, new information about the old, technical direction, original concepts, or, most importantly, insight, he or she is likely to find it here.

ROBERT H. COFIELD, M.D.
Frank R. and Shari Caywood Professor of
Orthopedics, Mayo Medical School; Chair,
Department of Orthopedic Surgery, Mayo Clinic
Rochester; Past-President, American Shoulder and
Elbow Surgeons; Former Editor-in-Chief, *Journal of
Shoulder and Elbow Surgery*

· PREFACE ·

Encouraged by the support for and favorable reception of the first two editions of the "Elbow Book," I undertook preparation of the third edition with three sentiments: appreciation, responsibility, and excitement.

Appreciation. As in the past, I continue to be very much indebted to my colleagues, particularly at the Mayo Clinic but also around the country and even worldwide, who have shared their experiences, observations, and interesting cases with me. These experiences hopefully are reflected in this third edition, and in some instances they are specifically referenced in the text.

Responsibility. It follows then that a sense of responsibility to sustain and enhance the value of this endeavor would further motivate the preparation of the current volume. This sense of responsibility is reinforced by the recognition of the role this book has played in the management of so many patients, especially those with difficult diagnostic or therapeutic considerations.

Excitement. The growing interest, increased treatment options, and improved outcomes all are sources not only of great satisfaction but also of excitement for the future. The experience with joint replacement arthroplasty has shown marked improvement over the last decade and even since publication of the last edition. Our understanding of sports medicine and the management of the athlete has been complemented by advances in arthroscopy and surgical techniques.

This volume is thus dedicated to the two individuals who have greatly assisted and encouraged me in my understanding of these areas, and both of whom have uniquely contributed in these areas to the orthopedic community: Doctors Frank Jobe and Ralph Coonrad. The burden now, of course, is to expand on their legacy, to remain as objective as possible in assessing outcomes. In the future, careful scrutiny of the impact of intervention, in order to build an evidence-based approach to our management and judgment, is the ultimate requirement and obligation.

BERNARD F. MORREY, M.D.

· ACKNOWLEDGMENTS ·

As in the past, I must continue to express appreciation to my wife, Carla, who has patiently allowed and encouraged me to pursue my interests and commitment to my profession, and specifically in the preparation of this text. Although all four of our children, Michael, Matthew, Mark, and Maggie, are now grown, I continue to appreciate their past and ongoing support for my professional career and activity. A special thanks also goes to my secretaries, Sherry Koperski and Donna Riemersma, who have provided superb expertise in the preparation of the manuscript and in maintaining the correspondence and communication associated with the book. Much of the clinical material from my personal practice could not have been recalled and updated without the assistance of Mary Kessler, who manages our Joint Replacement Database, and of my physician assistant colleague for more than 20 years, Bob Adams. A special note of appreciation goes to all of my colleagues at the Mayo Clinic and to the national and international contributors to this Third Edition. And finally, I would particularly like to recognize Matthew Morrey, a certified medical illustrator, who designed the cover for this third edition. All these efforts and contributions are sincerely appreciated by me and also, I am sure, by our past and future patients.

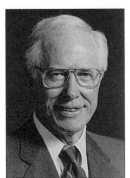

Frank W. Jobe, M.D.

Doctor Frank Jobe is appropriately recognized as one of the most significant contributors to our understanding of sports injuries of the upper extremities. As the future of elbow care continues to develop with regard to the management of the athletic elbow, this entire initiative is, to a large measure, based on the innovative contributions of Doctor Jobe. However, I wish to especially recognize Doctor Jobe not just for the substantive contributions he has made to the sports community, but particularly for the friendship, support, and mentoring that he has provided me throughout the years. This edition is dedicated to Doctor Jobe, a very special person whom I am proud to call friend and colleague.

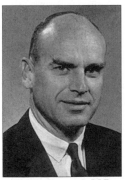

Ralph Coonrad, M.D.

During the development of the first edition of the Elbow Book, I decided to invite other contributors, and Doctor Coonrad was the first author contacted. His enthusiastic willingness to help with this project and his encouragement and support inspired me to enlist other prominent individuals in this effort. As reconstructive elbow surgery continues to evolve, particularly that of joint replacement, the orthopedic community, in general, and I, in particular, owe a significant debt of gratitude to Doctor Coonrad for his pioneering efforts. However, I especially wish to recognize Doctor Coonrad not only for these contributions, which are well recognized by all, but also specifically for the kindness, encouragement, and friendship that he has shown me throughout the years. I am proud to consider him a friend and colleague.

· CONTENTS ·

Fundamentals and General Considerations

• CHAPTER 1 •

Embryology and Phylogeny

• HYMIE GORDON† and SUSAN LARSON

Embryology

• HYMIE GORDON†

THE PRELIMINARY STAGE

During the third week after ovulation, the cells of the paraxial mesoderm (at the sides of the neural tube) condense and segment into blocks, called somites. Within each somite, the mesodermal cells differentiate into a dorsolateral dermatome, an intermediate myotome, and a ventromedial sclerotome.

The dermatome is the precursor of the dermis. The myotome is the precursor of muscles. The sclerotome initially consists of young connective tissue cells (mesenchyme) that will differentiate into fibroblasts, chondroblasts, and osteoblasts (Fig. 1–1).

THE CHRONOLOGY OF THE DEVELOPMENT OF THE UPPER LIMBS[1–2, 5, 6, 9, 11–13]

This account of the chronology of development is selectively biased to emphasize what is known about the development of the elbow. The stages of development are given in days after ovulation and in the crown-rump length of the developing person. For each stage, a brief description of the external appearance of the upper limb is given,

---

†Deceased.

followed by an account of the internal structures of nerves, blood vessels, muscles, bones, and joints.

Days 26–28; 3–6 mm

The upper limb buds appear as small lateral elevations opposite somites C3–8 and T1–2. These elevations are pockets of ectoderm containing mesenchymal cells from the paraxial mesoderm. On the 28th day, a few thin-walled blood vessels are present.

Days 28–32; 5–7 mm

The limb buds now are rounded protuberances that curve ventromedially and taper distally (Figs. 1–2 and 1–3). The ectoderm at the apex of the bud is thickened to form the apical ectodermal ridge. A marginal blood vessel is forming beneath this ridge. Spinal nerves C4–8 and T1 have appeared just proximal to the root of the bud.

Day 33; 7–9 mm

The distal end of the bud expands to form the hand plate. The spinal nerves penetrate into the root of the bud. The mesenchyme along the central axis of the bud begins to condense the first visible sign of the bones of the upper limb.

Days 34–40; 8–11 mm

The condensation of the central mesenchyme has advanced to a stage in which the humerus, radius, and ulna can be discerned. Chondrification begins in the humerus. The brachial plexus has formed. In the proximal part of the bud, nerve fibers aggregate to form the peripheral nerve trunks; the dorsal fibers form the radial nerve; the ventral fibers form the median and ulnar nerves. These nerves reach as far as the level of the future elbow.

Days 41–43; 11–14 mm

Finger rays, which are indicative of longitudinal condensation of the mesenchyme, are visible on the dorsal surface of the hand plate (Fig. 1–3). Discrete muscle masses can now be discerned. The radius, ulna, and metacarpals begin to chondrify, and the radial, median, and ulnar nerves extend down to the hand plate.

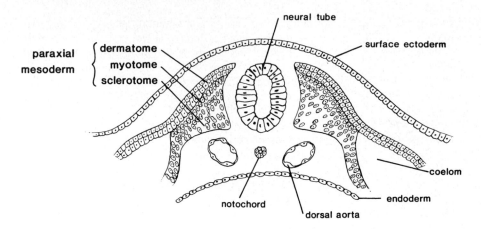

FIGURE 1–1 • Diagrammatic cross-section of an embryo 15 to 21 days after ovulation, showing the antecedents of the constituents of the future limb buds.

Days 44–47; 13–17 mm

Finger rays are clearly visible and interdigital notches have appeared. The elbow is now visible. Most of the large muscles are identifiable, including the trapezius, pectoralis major and minor, deltoid, biceps, triceps, coracobrachialis, brachialis, and brachioradialis. The joints are beginning to form. At the same time, the mesenchyme around the interzones is condensing to initiate the formation of the ligaments and capsules of joints.

Days 48–50; 16–18 mm

The fingers are separated except for interdigital webs of skin. The upper limbs project forward, and their preaxial borders are cranial; that is, the thumbs are uppermost and the right and left palms face each other. Some of the components of the elbow joints are more clearly delineated. Homogeneous interzones have appeared between the ends of the bones. With increasing chondrification, the modeling of the distal ends of the bones has progressed to where the shapes of the olecranon and the humeral epicondyles can be recognized.

Day 51; 18–22 mm

The interdigital webs are breaking down, beginning the separation of the fingers. Mesenchymal consensation and differentiation around the joints are progressing rapidly: the flexor retinaculum, the collateral ligaments of the wrist, and the carpal, metacarpal, and proximal interphalangeal ligaments are present. The annular ligament of the radius has appeared.

Days 52–53; 22–24 mm

The fingers have now separated. Active movements of the upper limb are now beginning and will promote the development of the joints. All the muscles of the upper limb are now in place, and each muscle has an appropriate

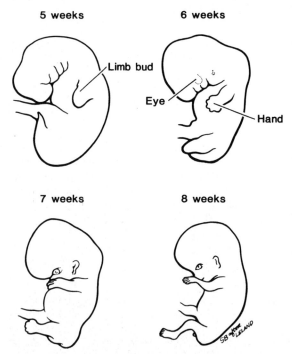

FIGURE 1–3 • Embryonic development from 5 to 8 weeks (not drawn to scale), showing the external appearances of the upper limb. Note that by the eighth week, the position of the limb has changed so that the palms face downward and the elbows point caudally.

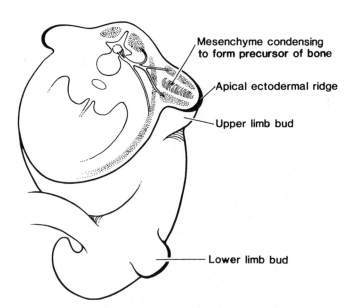

FIGURE 1–2 • Diagram of cross-sectioned embryo at 32 days.

supply of nerves and blood vessels. The humerus and, to a lesser extent, the radius are beginning to ossify.

Days 54–57; 23–31 mm

Growth, passive torsion, and active movements are turning the palms downward and pointing the elbows caudally. The coronoid process of the ulna has chondrified; elsewhere, the ulna is beginning to ossify. The head of the radius has assumed its concave form. The radial tuberosity is visible but has not yet chondrified.

Cavitation now begins in the elbow, shoulder, and radioscaphoid joints. At the elbow, cavitation is seen first in the radiohumeral joint, then in the ulnohumeral and radio-ulnar joints. It begins in the center of the interzones and extends peripherally until all three cavities become confluent. Blood vessels enter the loose mesenchyme adjacent to the interzones to form the primitive synovium of the elbow and other joints.

Summary of Initial Events

O'Rahilly and Gardner have neatly summarized what has been accomplished by the end of the eighth week after ovulation: ". . . all the major skeletal, articular, muscular, neural, and vascular elements of the limbs are present in a form and arrangement closely resembling those of the adult. Most ligaments are discernible, cavitation is frequently beginning in the larger joints, some bursae may be present, and the periosteal ossification has begun in certain skeletal components."[10] All this has happened during a period of 30 days in which the developing human has grown from 3 to 31 mm.

THE ELBOW JOINT

The primary development of the elbow itself takes place in even less time, just 1 week. On the 50th day, the cartilaginized olecranon and humeral epicondyles are visible, and a homogeneous interzone forms between the ends of the skeletal precursors. The annular ligament of the radius appears on the 51st day. Active movements of the elbow begin on the 52nd day. By the 56th day, the position of the upper limbs has changed so that the elbows point caudally. On the 57th day, the joint cavity appears, with collateral ligaments and joint capsule in place and a blood supply to the primitive synovium.

THE DEVELOPMENT OF THE SYNOVIAL JOINT

Between the 48th and 50th days, after chondrification of the humerus, radius, and ulna, the space between the ends of these three bones is occupied by a broad interzone of homogeneous mesenchyme, consisting of tightly packed cells with round or oval nuclei and scanty cytoplasm. This homogeneous interzone merges with the cartilaginous ends of the bones.

During the next 2 or 3 days, the peripheral mesenchyme at the sides of the interzone condenses further to form the capsule and the ligaments, including the annular ligament of the radius. The cells lining the inside of the capsule and the ends of the bones become vascularized to form the primitive synovial membrane (Fig. 1–4). Blood vessels do not penetrate into the center of the interzone. With increasing movement of the joint, the synovium over the ends of the bones will disappear.

The cells in the center are now more loosely packed, and they stain metachromatically. This metachromasia becomes progressively more intense, indicating the accumulation of acid mucopolysaccharides (glycosaminoglycans) (specifically, chondroitin sulfate) in the cells and ground substance of the interzone.[1] This accumulation is at its peak on about the 55th day and is soon followed by cavitation (a nonnecrotic loss of cells) in the center of the interzone. Cavita-

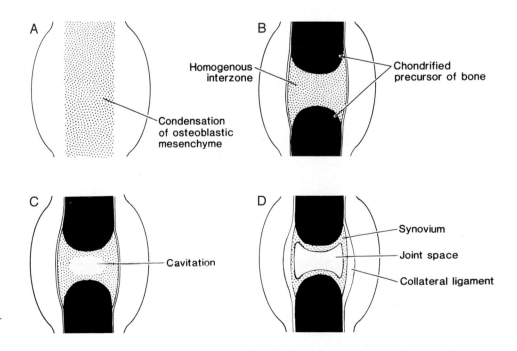

FIGURE 1–4 • Schematic representation of the embryologic development of a typical synovial joint.

tion usually appears first in the radiohumeral joint, then in the ulnohumeral and the radioulnar joints. As the cavities expand, they coalesce so that by about the 57th day only one joint cavity is present. It is lined by the primitive vascularized synovium and is supported by the capsule and ligaments.

MOLECULAR CONTROL OF CELL DIFFERENTIATION

Throughout this discussion, the word *differentiate* has been frequently used. How does a mesenchymal cell become a chondroblast? "It differentiates." In recent years, embryologists have sought to explain what cellular differentiation really means by studying the process at the histochemical and the molecular levels. Some progress has been made, for instance, in understanding how the mesenchymal cells of the limb buds differentiate. One approach has been to investigate the chemical changes associated with differentiation.

In the experimental animal, the chick, the mesenchymal cells of the limb bud are pluripotent until day 4: they can differentiate into muscle or into cartilage cells. After day 4, a particular mesenchymal cell is committed to become either a muscle cell or a cartilage cell, but not both. This phenotypic commitment is determined by the relative positions of the mesenchymal cells in the limb bud and, hence, by their extracellular environment.

The more peripheral mesenchymal cells receive a richer nourishment from the primitive vascular system.[4] During the time when the mesenchymal cells are committing themselves to their future form, a sharp increase occurs in the intracellular concentration of polyadenylic-diphosphoribose (polyADP-ribose). This unusual nucleic acid is derived from NAD. It binds covalently with the histone and nonhistone nucleoproteins. These are the proteins that are associated with the nuclear DNA and play important roles in controlling the genetic activity of DNA: the uncoiling of the double helix, the accessibility of exogenous inducers to DNA, the rate of transcription of the genetic code, and so on. In the case of histone, NAD binds preferentially with the basic amino acids, especially lysine and arginine, which are abundant at the carboxy- and amino-terminals of the histone molecules. Such polyADP-ribosylation of histone probably disrupts its interaction with DNA, thus promoting the transcription of messenger RNA.[3]

Morphogenesis is the process by which cells multiply and differentiate before being organized into specific and consistent forms and relationships to produce tissues, organs, joints, and so on. Progress is being made in understanding the genetic control of morphogenesis, that is, the nuclear-molecular processes that direct this growth, differentiation, and organization of cells. Recent work has implicated a nuclear factor regulating expression of κ light-chain immunoglobin (NF-κB) as being responsible for the "twist" that occurs in the proximal limb bud.[8] When the

activity of NF-κB is blocked, abnormalities of limb development are absent.[3]

As a general concept, it is therefore reasonable to assume that the activities of each of the hundreds of "little" genes involved in the formation of a part are not regulated individually; rather, it is much more likely that the "little" genes are organized into groups ("hierarchies") with related functions and that each group is under the control of a "major" gene. Even these "major" genes have to act in a coordinated fashion, as noted earlier. Current investigations have begun to provide glimpses of how this genetic coordination is achieved.

The principle on which these investigations are based is homeosis, from the Greek *homoiomeros*, "having the same parts." In the present context, it is the process that makes an elbow look like an elbow and function like an elbow. A homeotic complex is a tightly linked cluster of genes that regulates the specific development of a part, such as an elbow.

A number of these homeotic genes have been identified, and their DNA sequences have been determined. A remarkable feature is their evolutionary conservatism. When some of these homeotic genes were analyzed in yeast, fruit flies, mice, and humans, their DNA sequences were found to be not exactly the same but remarkably similar. These "conserved" sequences are referred to as homeoboxes. In fact, this evolutionary conservatism is the most compelling evidence available for the assumption that the homeoboxes play a fundamental role in morphogenesis.[7]

The idea is that very early in embryogenesis a still unidentified signal activates a particular homeobox to transcribe a messenger RNA that specifies the synthesis of a specific nuclear-DNA-binding protein. This protein will activate one or more of the genes in the homeotic complex. The protein products of these genes must be produced in properly coordinated sequences to direct the local morphogenesis of the elbow or some other part of the body.

The postulated protein products of the homeotic genes are now referred to as morphogens. One such morphogen that is being intensely scrutinized is retinoic acid. When retinoic acid is applied experimentally to the tip of the limb bud, it acts locally to promote the development of the digits. Retinoic acid also is known to have morphogenic activity in the development of the neural tube. Its possible role in the development of the elbow has not yet been investigated.

Retinoic acid will probably prove to be just the first of a long list of locally acting morphogens. It is hoped that sooner rather than later, the intense interest that morphogeneticists are now focusing on the limb bud and on the neural tube also will be directed to the elbow. This should give us a much better understanding of the normal and abnormal development of this important part of the body. Consequently, it should become possible to understand the processes that lead to the usually normal but sometimes abnormal development of the elbow, and, in the future, we might be led to the investigation of the possible prevention of these developmental anomalies by rational periconceptional treatment.

Phylogeny

• SUSAN G. LARSON

The human elbow is a link between the shoulder and the hand, acting both to enhance flexibility in hand placement and to transmit generated forces. The anatomy of the elbow reflects this dual function: The circular radial head and spherical capitulum contribute to a wide pronation-supination range, whereas the "tongue and groove" configuration of the humeroulnar joint plus collateral ligaments creates a very stable structure. Most of the characteristic features of the human elbow significantly predate the appearance of modern *Homo sapiens*. In fact, current evidence suggests that this morphology can be traced back to the common ancestor of humans and apes, extant about 15 to 20 million years ago (mya).

EVOLUTION OF THE VERTEBRATE ELBOW

The distal humerus of pelycosaurs, the late Paleozoic (255 to 235 mya) reptiles that probably gave rise to more advanced mammal-like reptiles, possessed a bulbous capitulum laterally and medially. The articulation with the ulna was formed by two distinct surfaces: a slightly concave ventral surface and a more flat dorsal surface (Fig. 1–5).[8] The proximal articular surface of the ulna was similarly divided into two surfaces separated by a low ridge. Reconstruction of the forelimb of these reptiles suggests that they walked with limbs splayed out to the side. The humerus was held more or less horizontal, and the elbow was flexed so that the forearm was sagittally oriented. Forward motion was brought about by rotation of the humerus around its long axis and straightening of the forearm to become more vertical. Therefore, elbow flexion and extension probably were useful only in side-to-side motions. The ulnohumeral joint, with its dual articular surfaces, seems to have been designed to resist the torsional stresses produced by hu-

PHYLOGENY

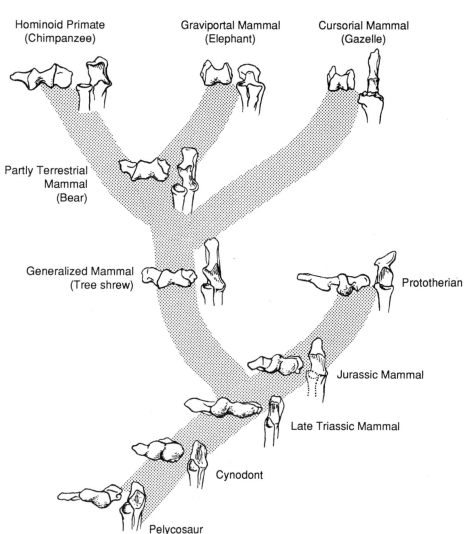

FIGURE 1–5 • The major evolutionary stages in the development of the elbow joint from pelycosaurs to advanced mammals. The distal ends of the humeri are shown on the left, and the corresponding radius and ulna are on the right. The form of the pelycosaur elbow was designed to maximize stability. Subsequent evolutionary stages show accommodations to increasing mobility. (Adapted from Jenkins, F. A. Jr.: The functional anatomy and evolution of the mammalian humeroulnar articulation. Am. J. Anat. **137**:281, 1973.)

meral rotation. In addition, the proximal end of the radius was flat and triangular, indicating an absence of pronation-supination. It appears, therefore, that stability rather than mobility was the major functional characteristic of the elbow of these late Paleozoic reptiles.

The more immediate ancestor of mammals, cynodonts, a group of mammal-like reptiles from the Permo-Triassic period (235 to 160 mya), had begun to bring their limbs underneath their bodies. The distal humeral articular surface consisted of radial and ulnar condyles separated by a shallow groove (see Fig. 1–5). The proximal ulnar articular surface was an elongate spoon shape for articulation with the humeroulnar condyle. The lateral flange on the ulna for articulation with the radius was separated from this surface by a low ridge. This ridge articulated with the groove between the radial and ulnar condyles and represents, therefore, an early stage in the evolution of the "tongue and groove" type of humeroulnar articulation characteristic of many modern mammals.

Early mammals from the Triassic (210 to 160 mya) and Jurassic (160 to 130 mya) periods still retained radial and ulnar condyles. However, the radial condyle was more protuberant than the ulnar, and the ulnar condyle was more linear and obliquely oriented (Fig. 1–5). The two condyles were separated by an intercondylar groove. The ulnar notch had articular surfaces for both the ulnar and the radial condyles, each matching the configuration of the corresponding humeral surface. The oblique orientation of the humeroulnar joint helped to keep the forearm in a sagittal plane as the humerus underwent a complex motion involving adduction, elevation, and rotation during locomotion.

The development of a trochleariform distal humeral articular surface in modern mammals came about largely by widening of the intercondylar groove and the development of a ridge within it (see Fig. 1–5, bear). The articular surface on the proximal ulna is also oblique in orientation, and the distal half retains an articulation with the ulnar condyle. During locomotion, the configuration of the humeroulnar joint provides stability and serves to adjust the rotatory movement of the ulna relative to the humerus so that forearm extension is confined to a sagittal plane as the humerus undergoes adduction, elevation, and rotation.

Most small noncursorial mammals have maintained the spiral configuration of the trochlear articular surface observed in early mammals. In larger and more cursorial mammals, the trochlea displays various ridges and is more narrow to improve stability, although at the expense of joint mobility. Only in the hominoid primates, which include humans, chimpanzees, gorillas, orangutans, and gibbons, is the medial aspect of the distal humeral articular surface truly trochleariform. In the next section, I discuss the functional significance of the unique aspects of the hominoid elbow joint.

COMPARATIVE PRIMATE ANATOMY OF THE ELBOW REGION

Much of what follows is taken from the detailed studies of Rose.[15, 16] The humeral trochlea may be cylindrical, conical, or trochleariform in nonhuman primates.[16] The trochlea is conical in some prosimians, but a cylindrical trochlea

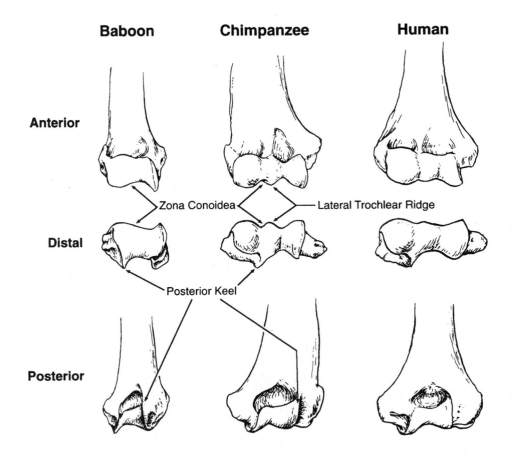

FIGURE 1–6 • Distal humeri of a baboon, a chimpanzee, and a human from anterior, distal, and posterior aspects. The lateral trochlear ridge is well developed in both the human and the chimpanzee, but is largely nonexistent in the baboon. The baboon humerus displays prominent flanges anteromedially and posterolaterally. The lateral epicondyle is placed higher in the chimpanzee than in the human and displays a more strongly developed supracondylar crest.

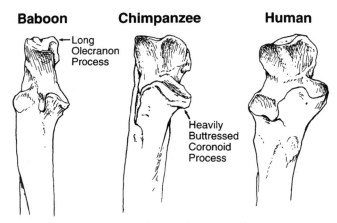

FIGURE 1−7 • Proximal ulnae of a baboon, a chimpanzee, and a human. The trochlear notch is wider in the chimpanzee and the human and displays a prominent ridge for articulation with the trochlear groove. In addition, the radial notch faces laterally in the chimp and human, unlike in the baboon, in which it faces more anteriorly.

seems to be the most common shape and is observed in most prosimians and New World monkeys. The trochlea is also cylindrical in most Old World monkeys but with a pronounced medial flange or keel that is best developed anterodistally (Fig. 1–6). Only in apes and humans is the trochlea truly trochleariform, possessing medial and lateral ridges all around the trochlear margins.[8, 15] In most species, the articular surface of the trochlea expands posteriorly to the area behind the capitulum. In larger monkeys, the lateral edge of the posterior trochlear surface projects to form a keel that extends up the lateral wall of the olecranon fossa (see Fig. 1–6). In hominoids, this keel is a continuation of the lateral trochlear ridge and helps form a sharp lateral margin of the olecranon fossa.[15, 16]

The trochlear notch of the ulna generally mirrors the shape of the humeral trochlea. In humans and apes, the notch has medial and lateral surfaces separated by a ridge that articulates with the trochlear groove (Fig. 1–7).[15, 16]

The differences seen in the configuration of the humeroulnar joint across primate species reflect contrasting requirements for stabilization with different forms of limb use. In most monkeys, the humeroulnar joint is in its most stable configuration in a partially flexed position owing to the development of the medial trochlear keel anterodistally and the lateral keel posteriorly.[15]

It is not surprising that this position of maximum stability is the one assumed by the forelimb during the weight-bearing phase of quadrupedal locomotion. The anterior orientation of the trochlear notch is a direct adaptation to weight bearing with a partially flexed limb. However, such an orientation does limit elbow extension to some degree.

The great apes (chimpanzees, gorillas, and orangutans) and the lesser apes (gibbons) move about in a much less stereotypical fashion than do monkeys. To accommodate this more varied form of limb use, the hominoid humeroulnar joint, with its deeply socketed articular surfaces and well-developed medial and lateral trochlear ridges all around the joint margins, is designed to provide maximum stability throughout the flexion-extension range.[15–17] The use of overhead suspensory postures and locomotion in apes has led to the evolution of the capacity for complete

elbow extension. Apes even keep their elbows extended during quadrupedal locomotion. The ideal joint configuration for resistance of transarticular stress with fully extended elbows would be to have a trochlear notch that was proximally directed. It could then act as a cradle to support the humerus during locomotion. However, a proximal orientation of the trochlear notch would severely limit elbow flexion by the anterior border to the trochlear notch abutting against the distal humerus. The anteroproximal orientation of the trochlear notch in apes thus represents a compromise that safely supports the humerus on the ulna in extended elbow positions during locomotion without unduly sacrificing elbow flexion.[1]

On the lateral side of the elbow, the articular surface on the capitulum extends farther posteriorly in apes and humans than in monkeys, allowing the radius to move with the ulna into full extension of the elbow. In addition, the capitulum of apes and humans is uniformly rounded, reflecting versatility rather than stereotypy in forelimb usage (Fig. 1–8).

The region between the trochlea and capitulum (the zona conoidea) is a relatively flat plane that terminates distally in most monkeys. In the hominoids, it continues posteriorly (see Fig. 1–5).[15, 16] The zona conoidea articulates with the rim of the radial head, and differences in its configuration reflect differences in the shape of the radial head.

The radial head of hominoid primates is nearly circular, and the peripheral rim is symmetrical and beveled all around the circumference of the radial head for articulation with the gutter-like zona conoidea (Fig. 1–9). This configuration provides good contact to resist dislocation of the radial head from the humerus under the varied loading regimes experienced by the hominoid elbow and can stabilize the radial head in all positions of supination or pronation.[15, 16]

In most monkeys and prosimians, the articular surface on the side of the radial head for the radioulnar joint is restricted to the anterior and medial surfaces (Fig. 1–10). In apes and humans, on the other hand, the articular surface on the side of the radial head extends almost all the way around the head.[15] The radial notch of the ulna in most

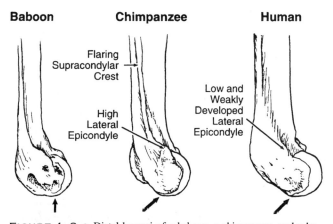

FIGURE 1−8 • Distal humeri of a baboon, a chimpanzee, and a human from the lateral aspect. The articular surface of the capitulum extends further onto the posterior surface of the bone (*small arrows*) in humans and chimpanzees to permit full extension at the humeroradial joint.

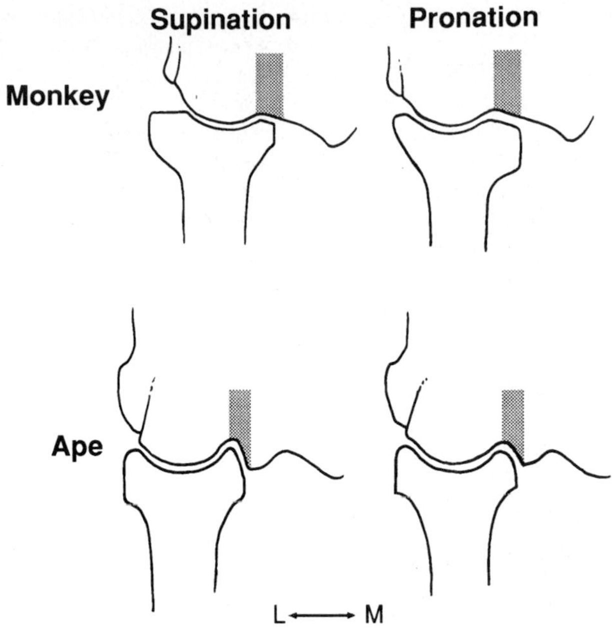

Supination **Pronation**

Monkey

Ape

L ←→ M

FIGURE 1–9 • Diagrammatic anterior views of the left humeroradial joints of a monkey and an ape in the prone and supine positions. In the monkey, the lateral lip of the radial head comes into maximum congruence with the zona conoidea (hatched area) in the prone position, thereby creating a maximally stable joint configuration. In the ape, the rim of the more symmetrical radial head maintains good contact with the recessed zona conoidea in all positions of supination and pronation. This contributes to a configuration emphasizing universal stability at the ape elbow rather than a position of particular stability, as seen in the monkey. (Adapted from Rose, M. D.: Another look at the anthropoid elbow. J. Hum. Evol. **17**:193, 1988.)

monkeys and prosimians faces either anterolaterally or directly anteriorly, whereas in hominoids it faces more laterally.[15, 16] The configuration observed in apes and humans emphasizes a broad range of supination and pronation with a nearly equal degree of stability in all positions.[15, 16]

In general terms, most of the differences in elbow joint morphology between quadrupedal monkeys and the apes can be related to the development of a position of particular stability in monkeys versus more universal stability in apes.

A few additional features of the human elbow can be traced to our hominoid ancestry. Humans, like apes, possess a relatively long radial neck for their body size.[16] In apes, this is probably related to the demands for powerful elbow flexion to raise the center of mass of the body during climbing and suspensory postures and locomotion. Although the radial tuberosity faces more or less anteriorly in most primates, it faces more medially in apes and humans, reflecting their greater range of supination.[14] Extreme supination is an important component of suspensory locomotion in apes.[11] Apes and humans share a relatively short olecranon process compared with that of most other primates. The short olecranon in apes generally is attributed to the demands for rapid elbow extension during suspensory locomotion. Finally, apes and humans are distinguished from other primate species in possessing a biomechanical carrying angle at the elbow. Sarmiento[17] has argued that the evolution of a carrying angle in apes is related to the need to bring the center of mass of the body beneath the supporting hand during suspensory locomotion in a manner

similar to that in which the valgus knee of humans brings the foot nearer the center of mass of the body during the single limb support phase of walking (Fig. 1–11).

All of these features have been retained in humans because of their continued advantage for a limb involved in tool use and a wide variety of other behaviors. Powerful flexion is clearly important. The continued importance of the carrying angle is perhaps less obvious, but one advantage that it does offer is that flexion of the elbow is accompanied by adduction of the forearm, thus bringing the hands more in front of the body, where most manipulatory activities are undertaken.

The morphology of the modern human elbow is not identical to that of the ape elbow, however. In some cases, the differences are simply a matter of degree. For example, although both apes and humans are distinguished from other primates in the medial orientation of the radial tuberosity, it is more extreme in position in the ape; in the human it is typically slightly anterior to true medial. In addition, although the olecranon is short in both humans and apes compared with most monkeys, it is slightly longer in humans than in apes.

Other differences between the elbow morphology of humans and that of apes can be related to the elimination of a locomotor role for the human forearm. These differences include a less robust coronoid process and a relatively narrower trochlear notch in humans. The more pronounced development of these features in the great apes can be related to the need to support the weight of the body during

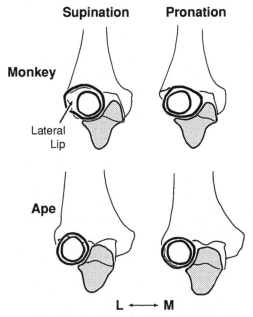

Supination   **Pronation**

Monkey

Lateral
Lip

Ape

L ←→ M

FIGURE 1–10 • Diagrammatic view of the radioulnar joint in pronation and supination in a monkey and an ape. A section through the radius and ulna in the region of the radial notch is superimposed on an outline of the distal humerus. In the monkey, the radial notch faces anterolaterally, whereas in the ape, it faces more directly laterally. The radial head of the monkey with its lateral lip comes into maximum congruence in the pronated position, conferring maximum stability in this position. The ape radioulnar joint, on the other hand, displays no such position of particular stability and instead emphasizes mobility. (Adapted from Rose, M. D.: Another look at the anthropoid elbow. J. Hum. Evol. **17**:193, 1988.)

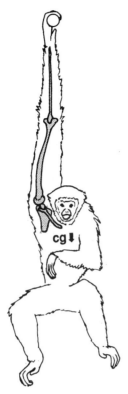

FIGURE 1–11 • Frontal view of an arm-swinging gibbon showing the skeletal structure of the forelimb. The carrying angle of the elbow brings the center of mass (i.e., center of gravity [cg]) more nearly directly under the supporting hand. (Adapted from Sarmiento, E. E.: Functional Differences in the Skeleton of Wild and Captive Orang-Utans and Their Adaptive Significance. Ph.D. Thesis, New York University, 1985.)

quadrupedal locomotion.[1, 10] Humans possess a smaller and more distally placed lateral epicondyle and a less well developed supracondylar crest than is seen in the apes, reflecting diminished leverage of the wrist extensors and brachioradialis.[18–20] Humans also have lost the bowing of both the radius and the ulna observed in apes that is related to enhancing the leverage of the forearm pronators and supinators.[1] Finally, a diminution in the prominence of the trochlear ridges and steep lateral margin of the olecranon fossa in humans can be related to the overall reduction in stresses at the human elbow and the concomitant relaxation on the demands for strong stabilization in all positions.[15, 16]

When exactly did the basic pattern for the hominoid elbow arise, and how old is the morphology of the modern human elbow? For answers to these questions we must turn to the fossil record.

FOSSIL EVIDENCE

Because of the patchy and incomplete nature of the fossil record, it is not clear which, if any, of the currently known Miocene (23 to 5 mya) species of fossil apes was the common ancestor of all the extant hominoids, and many uncertainties remain concerning the individual evolutionary histories of gibbons, orangutans, chimpanzees, gorillas, and humans.[2, 5] It is therefore not possible, with the currently available evidence, to precisely trace the evolutionary history of the hominoid elbow region.

Dendropithecus macinnesi, Limnopithecus legetet, and *Proconsul heseloni* (all from Africa) are among the hominoid species from the early part of the Miocene epoch (23 to 16 mya) for which postcranial material is known. Overall, the distal humeri of the first two of these forms resemble generalized New World monkeys such as *Cebus* (capuchin monkeys). The trochlea does not display a prominent lateral ridge, and the zona conoidea is relatively flat. The trochlear notch faces anteriorly, and the head of the radius is oval in outline with a well-developed lateral lip. These features generally are considered to be primitive for higher primates (monkeys, apes, and humans).[5, 6, 15]

P. heseloni, on the other hand, does display some features characteristic of extant hominoids. It has a globular capitulum, well-developed medial and lateral trochlear ridges, and a deep zona conoidea forming the medial wall of a recessed gutter between the capitulum and trochlea.[15] In general, the elbow region of *Proconsul* resembles that of extant hominoids in features related to general stability and range of pronation-supination; yet full pronation remained a position of particular stability.[15]

The limited fossil material that is available from the late Miocene epoch (16–5 mya) suggests that many hominoid species, including members of the genera *Dryopithecus* (from Europe), *Sivapithecus* (from Europe and Asia), and *Oreopithecus* (from Europe), displayed the features characteristic of the modern hominoid elbow. Although it is possible that these features arose in parallel in different genera, the more parsimonious explanation is that they inherited this morphology from an early to middle Miocene common ancestor, possibly similar to *P. heseloni*.[13, 23, 25] Assuming that the characteristic features of the hominoid elbow are shared derived traits, that is, traits inherited from a single common ancestor, we can say that the elbow morphology of modern apes and humans can be dated to roughly 15 to 20 mya.

The majority of paleoanthropologists agree that humans are most closely related to the African apes (chimpanzees and gorillas) and that the two lineages developed in the late Miocene or earliest Pliocene period (between 10 and 4 mya).[5] The earliest known fossils of the human lineage (hominids) date from the early Pliocenc era, approximately 4 to 5 mya. There are three genera of these earliest hominids currently recognized, *Ardipithecus, Paranthropus,* and *Australopithecus.* The latter is the best known and most widespread genus, and includes the famous "Lucy" skeleton from Hadar, Ethiopia (*A. afarensis*).[9] The genus *Homo,* to which our own species belongs, first appeared about 2.5 to 2 mya in East Africa. The earliest member is a species known as *Homo habilis.* This species is believed to be ancestral to *Homo erectus,* which arose about 1.6 mya.[5] *H. erectus,* in turn, generally is considered to be ancestral to all later hominids, including *Homo sapiens.*

All of the early hominids from the Pliocene period were bipedal, although some probably spent significant time climbing trees.[18–22] Stone tools first appeared at about the same time as *H. habilis,* although there is debate about which species of early hominid was responsible for making them.[24]

Several distal humeri are known from these early hominid species. All of the early hominid distal humeri lack the steep lateral margin of the olecranon fossa that is

PHYLOGENY

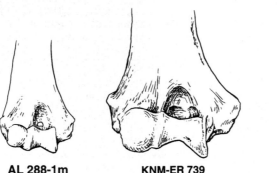

AL 288-1m   **KNM-ER 739**   **Gombore IB 7594**

FIGURE 1-12 • Distal humeri of Plio-Pleistocene hominids. Gombore IB 7594 represents early *Homo* on the basis of the moderate development of the lateral trochlear ridge and low position of the lateral epicondyle. AL 288-1m (part of the "Lucy" skeleton, *Australopithecus afarensis*) displays a more prominent lateral trochlear ridge, a recessed, gutter-like zona conoidea, a high position of the lateral epicondyle, and a well-developed supracondylar crest. It therefore resembles living apes in many features of its elbow morphology. KNM-ER 739 has been attributed to *Paranthropus boisei* and, like AL 288-1m, has a lateral epicondyle that is positioned above the articular surfaces. However, it is more like *Homo*, with the moderate development of the lateral trochlear ridge.

characteristic of chimpanzees and gorillas. However, they do show a considerable amount of morphologic variation in other characteristics (Fig. 1-12). On the basis of the contour of the distal end of the humeral shaft, the placement of the epicondyles, and the configuration of the articular surface, the fossil distal humeri have been divided into two groups. The first group is characterized by a weakly projecting lateral epicondyle that is placed low, at about the level of the capitulum, and by a moderately developed lateral trochlear ridge.[18, 19] These are features shared with modern humans, and consequently, this group generally is referred to as early *Homo*. The second group includes the *Australopithecus* and *Paranthropus* species and is characterized by a well-developed lateral epicondyle that is high relative to the capitulum. These features are similar to those of modern apes.

A number of fragments of early hominid proximal radii have been recovered representing each of the currently recognized species. The proximal radial fragments that have been attributed to early *Homo* display a much narrower rim around the capitular fovea than that of the modern apes. This provides for articulation with a more shallow zona conoidea and a more vertical and uniformly wide surface on the side of the head for articulation with the ulna. The morphologic structure of the radial head of early *Homo*, therefore, resembles that seen in modern humans.

A nearly complete ulna is known from the Omo Basin in southern Ethiopia and has been attributed to *Paranthropus boisei*.[7] This specimen differs from modern human ulnae in a number of features. The shaft is longer and more curved than in modern humans, it lacks a prominent interosseous border, and the head is less convex than in modern humans. However, unlike in modern apes, the trochlear notch of the fossil is anteriorly rather than anteroproximally oriented, and the coronoid process is not heavily buttressed.[1, 7]

Other fragments of ulnae that have been recovered are similar to the Omo ulna[3, 12] or are more like that of modern humans in having a prominent interosseous border, a supi-

nator crest, and a well-marked hollow for the play of the tuberosity of the radius.[3, 4] The latter ulnae have been attributed to early *Homo*. It appears, therefore, that nearly all of the characteristics that distinguish the human elbow from that of the ape can be found in the earliest members of our genus.

In overview, the combination of comparative anatomy and the fossil record indicates that the modern human elbow owes its beginnings to our hominoid ancestry. Current evidence suggests that many of the characteristic features of the human distal humerus and proximal radius and ulna can be projected back approximately 15 to 20 mya to a common ancestor of extant apes and humans. Functional analysis suggests that this morphologic structure arose in hominoid primates in response to the need for stabilization throughout the flexion-extension and pronation-supination ranges of motion to permit a more versatile form of forelimb use. This morphology was still largely intact following the evolution of upright posture and bipedal locomotion in the earliest known hominids. However, as the forelimb became less and less involved in locomotion, the hominid elbow underwent additional modifications, relaxing some of the emphasis on stabilization in all positions. The fossil record indicates that the distinct form of the modern human elbow probably first appeared about 2 mya in our ancestor *H. habilis*. This morphology has remained essentially unchanged during all subsequent stages of human evolution.

ACKNOWLEDGMENTS • I would like to thank Jack Stern and John Fleagle for helpful comments on this paper and Luci Betti for the preparation of figures. This material is based on work supported by the National Science Foundation under Grant No. BNS 8905476 and BCS 9806291.

REFERENCES

• EMBRYOLOGY

1. Andersen, H.: Histochemical studies of the histiogenesis of the human elbow joint. Acta Anat. **51**:60, 1962.
2. Bardeen, C. R., and Lewis, W. H.: Development of the limbs, body-wall and back in man. Am. J. Anat. **1**:1960.

3. Bushdid, P. B., Brantley, D. M., Yull, F. E., Blaeuer, G. L., Hoffman, L. H., Niswander, L., and Kerr, L. D.: Inhibition of Nf-κB activity results in disruption of the apical ectodermal ridge and aberrant limb morphogenesis. Nature **392**:615–618, 1998.

4. Caplan, A. I.: The molecular basis for limb morphogenesis. *In* Littlefield, J. W., and de Groucy, J. (eds.): Birth Defects. Proceedings of the Fifth International Conference. Amsterdam, Oxford, Excerpta Medica, 1978.

5. Gardner, E.: Osteogenesis in the human embryo and fetus. *In* Bourne, G. H. (ed.): The Biochemistry and Physiology of Bone, 2nd ed. New York, Academic Press, 1971, pp. 77.

6. Gehring, W. J.: The molecular bases of development. Sci. Am., **253**:152B, 1985.

7. Gray, D. J., and Gardner, E.: Prenatal development of the human elbow joint. Am. J. Anat. **88**:429, 1951.

8. Kanegae, Y., Tavares, A. T., Izpisua, Belmonte, J. C., and Verma, J. M.: Role of Rel/NF-κB transcription factors during the outgrowth of the vertebrate limb. Nature **392**:611–614, 1998.

9. Lewis, W. H.: The development of the arm in man. Am. J. Anat. **1**:145, 1902.

10. O'Rahilly, R., and Gardner, E.: The initial appearance of ossification in staged human embryos. Am. J. Anat. **134**:291, 1972.

11. O'Rahilly, R., and Gardner, E.: The timing and sequence of events in the development of the limbs in the human embryo. Anat. Embryol. **148**:1, 1975.

12. Windle, W. F.: Genesis of somatic motor function in mammalian embryos: a synthesizing article. Physiol. Zool. **17**:247, 1944.

13. Zwilling, E.: Limb morphogenesis. Adv. Morphogens. **1**:301, 1944.

• PHYLOGENY

1. Aiello, L. C., and Dean, M. C.: An Introduction to Human Evolutionary Anatomy. London, Academic Press, 1990.

2. Conroy, G. C.: Primate Evolution. New York, W. W. Norton & Co., 1990.

3. Day, M. H.: Functional interpretations of the morphology of postcranial remains of early African hominids. *In* Jolly, C. J. (ed): Early Hominids of Africa. London, Duckworth, 1978, pp. 311–345.

4. Day, M. H., and Leakey, R. E. F.: New evidence for the genus Homo from East Rudolf, Kenya (III). Am. J. Phys. Anthropol. **39**:367, 1974.

5. Fleagle, J. G.: Primate Adaptation and Evolution, 2nd ed. New York, Academic Press, 1999.

6. Harrison, T.: The phylogenetic relationships of the early catarrhine primates: a review of the current evidence. J. Hum. Evol. **16**:41, 1987.

7. Howell, F. C., and Wood, B. A.: Early hominid ulna from the Omo Basin, Ethiopia. Nature **249**:174, 1974.

8. Jenkins, F. A. Jr.: The functional anatomy and evolution of the mammalian humeroulnar articulation. Am. J. Anat. **137**:281, 1973.

9. Johanson, D. C., et al.: Morphology of the Pliocene partial hominid skeleton (A.L. 288–1) from the Hadar Formation, Ethiopia. Am. J. Phys. Anthropol. **57**:403, 1982.

10. Knussmann, R.: Humerus, Ulna and Radius der Simiae. Bibliotheca Primatologica, Vol. 5. Basel, S. Karger, 1967.

11. Larson, S. G.: Subscapularis function in gibbons and chimpanzees: implications for interpretation of humeral head torsion in hominoids. Am. J. Phys. Anthropol. **76**:449, 1988.

12. Leakey, R. E. F.: Further evidence of lower Pleistocene hominids from East Rudolf, Northern Kenya. Nature **237**:264, 1972.

13. Martin, L., and Andrews, P.: Cladistic relationships of extant and fossil hominoids. J. Hum. Evol. **16**:101, 1987.

14. O'Connor, B. L., and Rarey, K. E.: Normal amplitudes of radioulnar pronation and supination in several genera of anthropoid primates. Am. J. Phys. Anthropol. **51**:39, 1979.

15. Rose, M. D.: Another look at the anthropoid elbow. J. Hum. Evol. **17**:193, 1988.

16. Rose, M. D.: Functional anatomy of the elbow and forearm in primates. *In* Gebo, D. (ed.): Postcranial Adaptation in Nonhuman Primates. DeKalb, Northern Illinois Press, 1993, pp. 70–95.

17. Sarmiento, E. E.: Functional Differences in the Skeleton of Wild and Captive Orang-Utans and Their Adaptive Significance. Ph.D. Thesis, New York University, 1985.

18. Senut, B.: Outlines of the distal humerus in hominoid primates: application to some Plio-Pleistocene hominids. *In* Chiarelli A. B., and Corruccini, R. (eds.): Primate Evolutionary Biology. Berlin, Springer Verlag, 1981, pp. 81–92.

19. Senut, B.: Humeral outlines in some hominoid primates and in Plio-Pleistocene hominids. Am. J. Phys. Anthropol. **56**:275, 1981.

20. Senut, B., and Tardieu, C.: Functional aspects of Plio-Pleistocene hominid limb bones: implications for taxonomy and phylogeny. *In* Delson, E. (ed.): Ancestors: The Hard Evidence. New York, A. Liss, 1985, pp. 193–201.

21. Stern, J. T. Jr., and Susman, R. L.: The locomotor anatomy of Australopithecus afarensis. Am. J. Phys. Anthropol. **60**:279, 1983.

22. Susman, R. L., Stern, J. T. Jr., and Jungers, W. L.: Arboreality and bipedality in Hadar hominids. Folia Primatol. **43**:113, 1984.

23. Szalay, F. S., and Delson, E.: Evolutionary History of the Primates. New York, Academic Press, 1979.

24. Susman, R. L.: Fossil evidence for early hominid tool use. Science **265**:1570, 1994.

25. Ward, C. V., Walker, A., and Teaford, M. F.: Proconsul did not have a tail. J. Hum. Evol. **21**:215, 1991.

•CHAPTER 2•

Anatomy of the Elbow Joint

• BERNARD F. MORREY

This chapter discusses the normal anatomy of the elbow region. Abnormal and surgical anatomy is discussed in later chapters of this book dealing with the pertinent condition.

TOPICAL ANATOMY AND GENERAL SURVEY

The contours of the biceps muscle and antecubital fossa are easily observed anteriorly. Laterally, the avascular interval between the brachioradialis and the triceps is an important palpable landmark for surgical exposures (Fig. 2–1). Laterally, the tip of the olecranon, the lateral epicondyle, and the radial head also form an equilateral triangle and provide an important landmark for joint aspiration (see Chapter 4). The flexion crease of the elbow is on a line with the medial and lateral epicondyles and thus is actually 1 to 2 cm proximal to the joint line when the elbow is extended (Fig. 2–2). The inverted triangular depression on the anterior aspect of the extremity distal to the epicondyles is called the cubital (or antecubital) fossa.

The superficial cephalic and basilic veins are the most prominent superficial major contributions of the anterior venous system and communicate by way of the median cephalic and median basilic veins to form an M pattern over the cubital fossa (Fig. 2–3).

The extensor forearm musculature originates from the lateral epicondyle and was termed the *mobile wad* by Henry.[35] This forms the lateral margin of the antecubital fossa and the lateral contour of the forearm and comprises the brachioradialis and the extensor carpi radialis longus and brevis muscles. The muscles making up the contour of the medial anterior forearm include the pronator teres, flexor carpi radialis, palmaris longus, and flexor carpi ulnaris. Henry has demonstrated that their relationship and location can be approximated by placing the opposing thumb and the index, long, and ring fingers over the anterior medial forearm. The dorsum of the forearm is contoured by the extensor musculature, consisting of the anconeus, extensor carpi ulnaris, extensor digitorum quinti, and extensor digitorum communis.

The cutaneous innervation of the upper extremity is variable. In general, the skin about the proximal elbow is innervated by the lower lateral cutaneous (C5, C6) and medial cutaneous (radial nerve, C8, T1, and T2) nerves of the arm. The forearm skin is innervated by the medial (C8, T1), lateral (musculocutaneous, C5, C6), and posterior (radial nerve, C6–8) cutaneous nerves of the forearm (Fig. 2–4).

OSTEOLOGY

Humerus

The distal humerus consists of two condyles, forming the articular surfaces of the trochlea and capitellum (Fig. 2–5).

Proximal to the trochlea, the prominent medial epicondyle serves as a source of attachment of the ulnar collateral ligament and the flexor-pronator group of muscles. Laterally, the lateral epicondyle is located just above the capitellum and is much less prominent than the medial epicondyle. The lateral collateral ligament and the supinator-extensor muscle group originate from the flat, irregular surface of the lateral epicondyle.

Anteriorly, the radial and coronoid fossae accommodate the radial head and coronoid during flexion. Posteriorly, the olecranon fossa receives the tip of the olecranon.

A thin membrane of bone separates the olecranon and coronoid fossae in about 90 percent of individuals (Fig. 2–6).[88] The difference in size of the lateral and medial supracondylar columns explains the vulnerability of the medial column to fracture with trauma and some surgical procedures.[56] The posterior aspect of the lateral supracondylar column is flat, allowing ease of application of contoured plates (see Chapter 23). The prominent lateral supracondylar ridge is the site of attachment of the brachioradialis and extensor carpi radialis longus anteriorly and the triceps posteriorly. This serves as an important landmark for many lateral surgical approaches and for the "column procedure" (see Chapter 33).

Proximal to the medial epicondyle, about 5 to 7 cm along the medial intramuscular septum, a supracondylar process is observed in 1 to 3 percent of individuals (Fig. 2–7).[43, 47, 81] A fibrous band termed the ligament of Strothers may originate from this process and attach to the medial epicondyle.[36] When present, this spur serves as an anomalous insertion of the coracobrachialis muscle and an origin of the pronator teres muscle.[31, 47] Various pathologic processes have been associated with the supracondylar process, including fracture[43] and median[4] and ulnar nerve[36] entrapment (see Chapter 71).

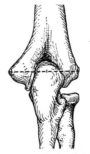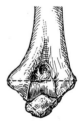

FIGURE 2–1 • The palpable landmarks of the tip of the olecranon and the medial and lateral epicondyles form an inverted triangle posteriorly when the elbow is flexed 90 degrees but are collinear when the elbow is fully extended. (From Anson, B. J., and McVay, C. B.: Surgical Anatomy. Vol. 2, 5th ed. Philadelphia, W. B. Saunders Co., 1971.)

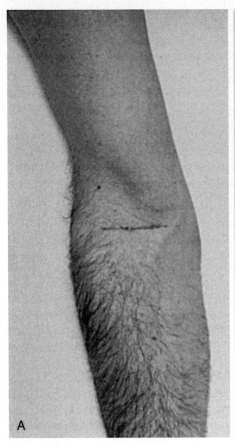

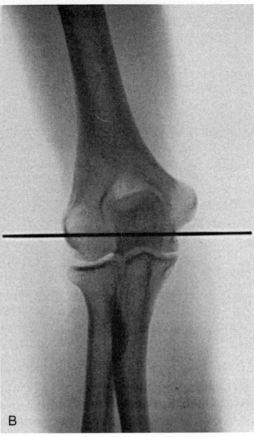

FIGURE 2–2 • A line placed over the flexion crease *(A)* is actually situated about 1 cm above the elbow joint line *(B)*.

Fascia brachii

V. cephalica humeri

M. biceps brachii

V. basilica humeri

N. cutaneus

Lacertus fibrosus

V. mediana cephalica

M. pronator teres

M. flexor carpi radialis

V. mediana basilica

N. cutaneus antibrachii lateralis

V. mediana antibrachii

V. cephalica antibrachii

M. pronator teres

V. basilica antibrachii

Ramus anastomoticus

M. flexor carpi radialis

Fascia antibrachii

FIGURE 2–3 • The superficial venous pattern of the anterior aspect of the elbow demonstrates a rather characteristic inverted **M** pattern formed by the median cephalic and median basilic veins. (From Anson, B. J., and McVay, C. B.: Surgical Anatomy. Vol. 2, 5th ed. Philadelphia, W. B. Saunders Co., 1971.)

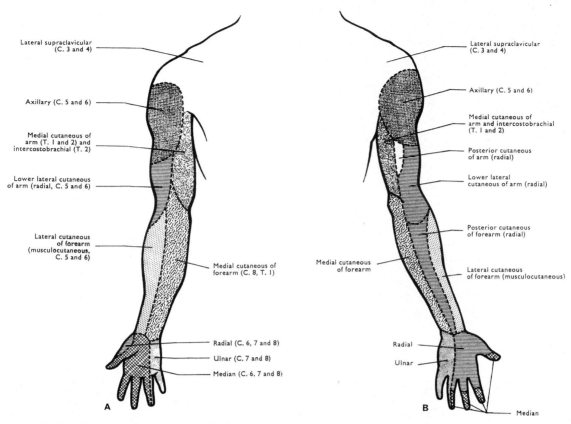

FIGURE 2–4 • Typical distribution of the cutaneous nerves of the anterior *(A)* and posterior *(B)* aspects of the upper limb. (From Cunningham, D. J.: Textbook of Anatomy. 12th ed., Romanes, G. J., ed. New York, Oxford University Press, 1981.)

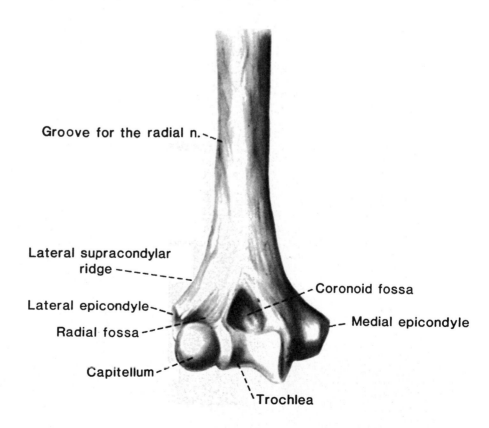

FIGURE 2–5 • The bony landmarks of the anterior aspect of the distal humerus.

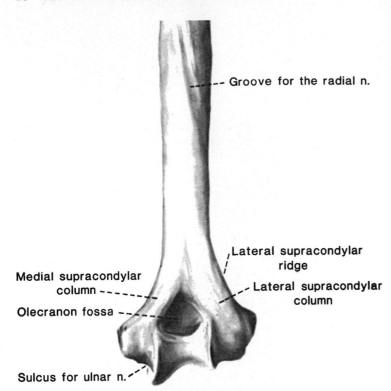

Groove for the radial n.

Lateral supracondylar ridge

Medial supracondylar column

Lateral supracondylar column

Olecranon fossa

Sulcus for ulnar n.

FIGURE 2–6 • The prominent medial and lateral supracondylar bony columns as well as other landmarks of the posterior aspect of the distal humerus.

Radius

The proximal radius includes the radial head, which articulates with the capitellum and exhibits a cylindrical shape with a depression in the midportion to accommodate the capitellum. The disc-shaped head is secured to the ulna by the annular ligament (Fig. 2–8). Distal to the radial head,

the bone tapers to form the radial neck. The head and neck angular relationship has been implicated in the mechanism of head and neck fracture.[83] The radial tuberosity marks the distal aspect of the neck and has two distinct parts. The anterior surface is covered by a bicipitoradial bursa protecting the tendon during full pronation (Fig. 2–9). However, it is the rough posterior aspect that provides the site of attachment of the biceps tendon. The dorsal position of the tuberosity during full pronation allows repair of a ruptured biceps tendon through a posterior approach[12] (see Chapter 35) and may be used as a means of determining axial alignment of radial fractures.[23]

Ulna

The proximal ulna provides the major articulation of the elbow that is responsible for its inherent stability. The

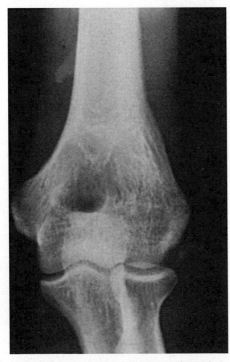

FIGURE 2–7 • Typical supracondylar process located approximately 5 cm proximal to the medial epicondyle with its characteristic configuration.

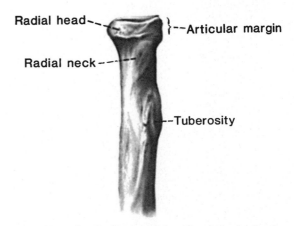

Radial head

Articular margin

Radial neck

Tuberosity

FIGURE 2–8 • Proximal aspect of the radius demonstrating the articular margin for articulation with the olecranon, the radial neck, and tuberosity.

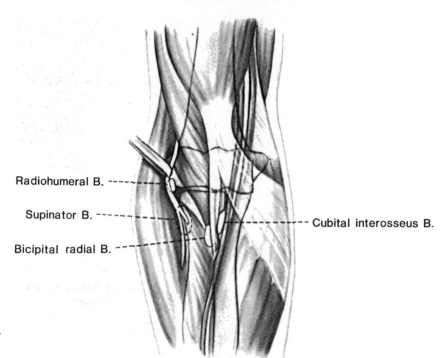

Radiohumeral B. -----

Supinator B. ------

Bicipital radial B. ----

------ Cubital interosseus B.

FIGURE 2–9 • A deep view of the anterior aspect of the joint revealing the submuscular bursa present about the elbow joint.

broad, thick, proximal aspect of the ulna consists of the greater sigmoid notch (incisura semilunaris), which articulates with the trochlea of the humerus (Fig. 2–10). The cortical surface of the coronoid process serves as the site of insertion of the brachialis muscle and of the oblique cord. The olecranon provides the posterior articulation of the humeroulnar joint and as the site of attachment for the triceps tendon.

On the lateral aspect of the coronoid process, the lesser semilunar or radial notch articulates with the radial head and is oriented roughly perpendicular to the long axis of the bone. On the lateral aspect of the proximal ulna a

tuberosity, the crista supinatoris, is the site of insertion of the lateral ulnar collateral ligament. This stabilizes the humeroulnar joint to resist varus stress.[50, 56, 62] The medial aspect of the coronoid process serves as the site of attachment of the anterior portion of the medial collateral ligament.

ELBOW JOINT STRUCTURE

Articulation

The elbow joint consists of two types of articulations. The ulnohumeral joint resembles a hinge (ginglymus), allowing

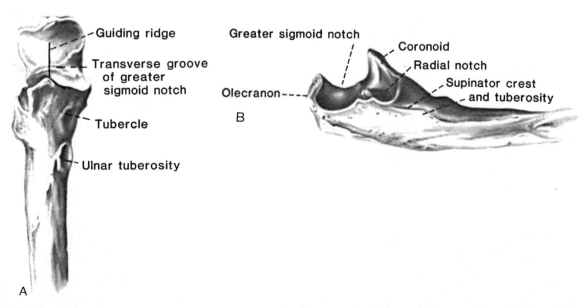

Guiding ridge

Transverse groove
of greater
sigmoid notch

Tubercle

Ulnar tuberosity

A

Greater sigmoid notch

Coronoid

Radial notch

Supinator crest
and tuberosity

Olecranon----

B

FIGURE 2–1O • A, Anterior aspect of the proximal ulna demonstrating the greater sigmoid fossa with the central groove. B, Lateral view with landmarks.

ANATOMY OF THE ELBOW JOINT

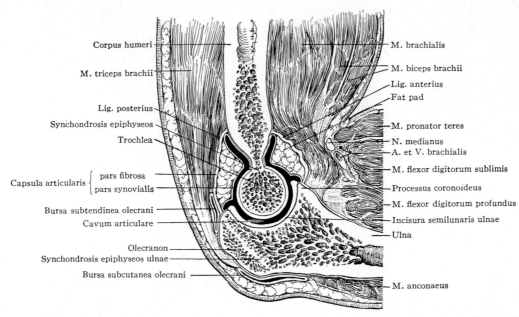

Corpus humeri
M. triceps brachii

Lig. posterius
Synchondrosis epiphyseos
Trochlea

Capsula articularis { pars fibrosa
                      pars synovialis

Bursa subtendinea olecrani
Cavum articulare

Olecranon
Synchondrosis epiphyseos ulnae
Bursa subcutanea olecrani

M. brachialis
M. biceps brachii
Lig. anterius
Fat pad

M. pronator teres
N. medianus
A. et V. brachialis
M. flexor digitorum sublimis
Processus coronoïdeus
M. flexor digitorum profundus
Incisura semilunaris ulnae
Ulna

M. anconaeus

FIGURE 2–11 • Sagittal section through the elbow region, demonstrating the high degree of congruity. (From Anson, B. J., and McVay, C. B.: Surgical Anatomy. Vol. 2, 5th ed. Philadelphia, W. B. Saunders Co., 1971.)

flexion and extension. The radiohumeral and proximal radioulnar joint allows axial rotation or a pivoting (trochoid) type of motion. Technically, therefore, the joint articulation is classified as a trochoginglymoid joint and is one of the most congruous joints of the body.[73, 77]

HUMERUS

The trochlea is the hyperbolic, pulley-like surface that articulates with the semilunar notch of the ulna covered by articular cartilage over an arc of 300 degrees (Fig. 2–11).[40, 72, 77] The medial lip is larger and projects more distally than does the lateral margin (Fig. 2–12). The two surfaces are separated by a groove that courses in a helical manner from an anterolateral to a posteromedial direction.

The capitellum is almost spheroidal in shape and is covered with hyaline cartilage, which is about 2 mm thick anteriorly. The posterior medial limit of the capitellum is marked by a prominent tubercle.[65] A groove separates the capitellum from the trochlea, and the rim of the radial head

articulates with this groove throughout the arc of flexion and during pronation and supination.

In the lateral plane, the orientation of the articular surface of the distal humerus is rotated anteriorly about 30 degrees with respect to the long axis of the humerus (Fig. 2–13). The center of the concentric arc formed by the trochlea and capitellum is on a line that is coplanar with

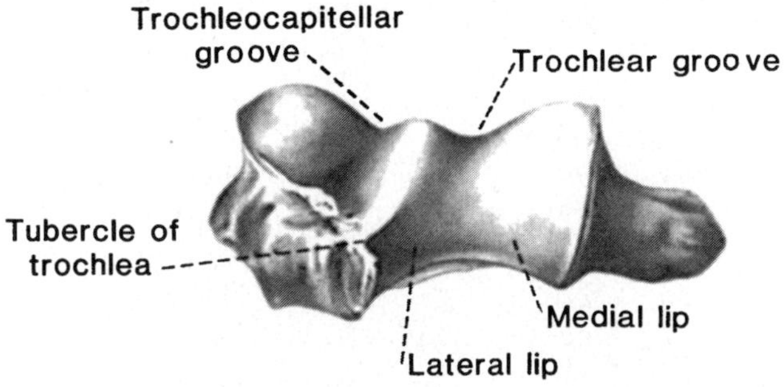

Trochleocapitellar
groove

Trochlear groove

Tubercle of
trochlea

Medial lip

Lateral lip

FIGURE 2–12 • Axial view of the distal humerus shows the isometric trochlea as well as the anterior position of the capitellum. The trochlear capitellar groove separates the trochlea from the capitellum.

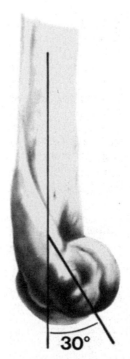

30°

FIGURE 2–13 • Lateral view of the humerus shows the 30-degree anterior rotation of the articular condyles with respect to the long axis of the humerus.

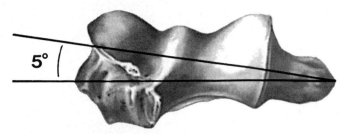

FIGURE 2–14 • Axial view of the distal humerus demonstrates the 5- to 7-degree internal rotation of the articulation in reference to the line connecting the midportions of the epicondyles.

the anterior distal cortex of the humerus.[55] In the transverse plane, the articular surface is rotated inward approximately 5 degrees (Fig. 2–14), and in the frontal plane it is tilted approximately 6 degrees in valgus (Fig. 2–15).[41, 45, 80]

PROXIMAL RADIUS

Hyaline cartilage covers the depression of the radial head, which has an angular value of about 40 degrees,[77] as well as approximately 240 degrees of the outside circumference that articulates with the ulna (Fig. 2–16). The lesser sigmoid fossa forms an arc of approximately 60 to 80 degrees,[40, 77] leaving an excursion of about 180 degrees for pronation and supination. The anterolateral third of the circumference of the radial head is void of cartilage. This part of the radial head lacks subchondral bone and thus is not as strong as the part that supports the articular cartilage; this part has been demonstrated to be the portion most often fractured.[83] The head and neck are not colinear with the rest of the bone and form an angle of approximately 15 degrees, with the shaft of the radius opposite the radial tuberosity (Fig. 2–17).[23]

PROXIMAL ULNA

In most individuals, a transverse portion composed of fatty tissue divides the sigmoid notch into an anterior portion

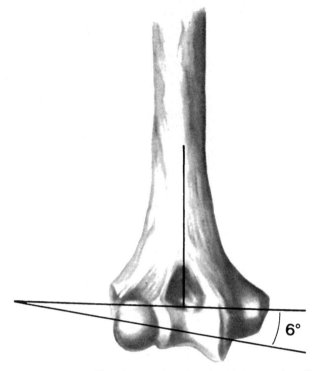

FIGURE 2–15 • There is approximately a 6- to 8-degree valgus tilt of the distal humeral articulation with respect to the long axis of the humerus.

made up of the coronoid and the posterior olecranon (Fig. 2–18).

In the lateral plane, the sigmoid notch forms an arc of about 190 degrees (Fig. 2–19).[74] The contour is not a true semicircle but rather is ellipsoid. This explains the articular void in the midportion (see Fig. 2–18).[85]

The opening of the sigmoid notch is oriented approximately 30 degrees posterior to the long axis of the bone (see Fig. 2–19). This matches the 30 degrees of inferior angulation of the distal humerus, providing stability in full extension (see Chapter 3). In the frontal plane, the shaft is angulated from about 1 to 6 degrees[41, 45, 72] lateral to the

FIGURE 2–16 • Hyaline cartilage covers approximately 240 degrees of the outside circumference of the radial head, allowing its articulation with the proximal ulna at the radial notch of the ulna. (From Langman, J., and Woerdeman, M. W.: Atlas of Medical Anatomy. Philadelphia, W. B. Saunders Co., 1976.)

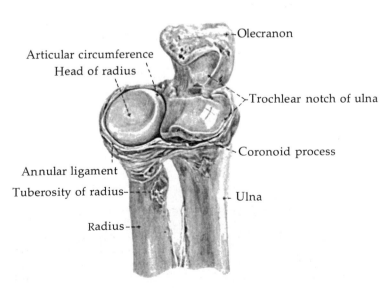

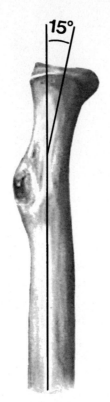

FIGURE 2–17 • The neck of the radius makes an angle of approximately 15 degrees with the long axis of the proximal radius.

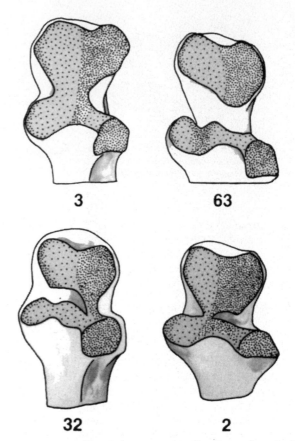

FIGURE 2–18 • The relative percentage of hyaline cartilage distribution at the proximal ulna. (Redrawn from Tillmann, B.: A Contribution to the Function Morphology of Articular Surfaces. Translated by Konorza, G. Stuttgart, George Thieme, Publishers; P. S. G. Publishing Co., Littleton, Mass., 1978.)

articulation (Fig. 2–20). This angle contributes, in part, to the formation of the carrying angle, which is discussed in Chapter 3.

The lesser sigmoid notch consists of a depression with an arc of about 70 degrees and is situated just distal to the lateral aspect of the coronoid and articulates with the radial head.[89]

Carrying Angle

The so-called carrying angle is the angle formed by the long axes of the humerus and the ulna with the elbow fully extended (Fig. 2–21). In the male, the mean carrying angle is 11 to 14 degrees, and in the female, it is 13 to 16 degrees,[3, 41] but Beals measured an angle of 17.8 degrees in adults, with no difference between male and female.[9] This is discussed in detail in Chapter 4.

Joint Capsule

The anterior capsule inserts proximally above the coronoid and radial fossae (Fig. 2–22). Distally, the capsule attaches to the anterior margin of the coronoid medially as well as to the annular ligament laterally. Posteriorly, the capsule attaches just above the olecranon fossa, distally along the supracondylar bony columns, and then down along the medial and lateral margins of the trochlea. Distally, attachment is along the medial and lateral articular margin of the sigmoid notch, and laterally, it occurs along the lateral aspect of the sigmoid notch and blends with the annular ligament.

The anterior capsule is normally a thin transparent structure that allows visualization of the prominences of the articular condyles when the elbow is extended. Significant strength is provided by transverse and obliquely directed fibrous bands (Fig. 2–23).[20, 51] The anterior capsule is, of course, taut in extension but becomes lax in flexion, the

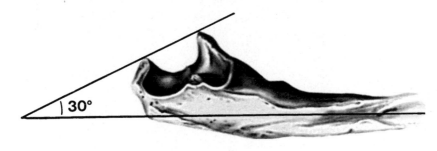

FIGURE 2–19 • The greater sigmoid notch opens posteriorly with respect to the long axis of the ulna. This matches the 30-degree anterior rotation of the distal humerus, as shown in Figure 3–16.

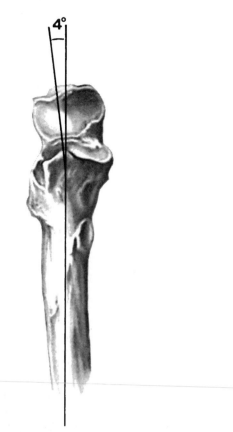

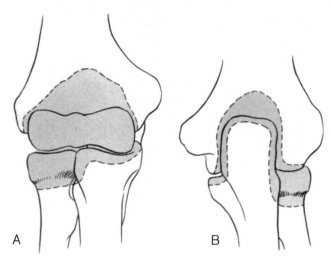

FIGURE 2–22 • Distribution of the synovial membrane from the posterior aspect, demonstrating the presence of the synovial recess under the annular ligament and about the proximal ulna. (From Hollinshead, W. H.: The back and limbs. *In* Anatomy for Surgeons, Vol. 3. New York, Harper & Row, 1969, p. 379.)

FIGURE 2–20 • There is a slight (approximately 4 degrees) valgus angulation of the shaft of the ulna with respect to the greater sigmoid notch.

tions and relative contributions have been carefully documented by Gardner.[27]

Ligaments

The ligaments of the elbow consist of specialized thickenings of the medial and lateral capsules that form medial and lateral collateral ligament complexes.

MEDIAL COLLATERAL LIGAMENT COMPLEX

The medial collateral ligament consists of three parts: anterior, posterior, and transverse segments (Fig. 2–25). The anterior bundle is the most discrete component, the poste-

greatest capacity occurring at about 80 degrees of flexion.[39, 68] The normal capacity of the fully distended joint is 25 to 30 ml.[60] The joint capsule is innervated by branches from all major nerves crossing the joint, including the contribution from the musculoskeletal nerve (Fig. 2–24). The varia-

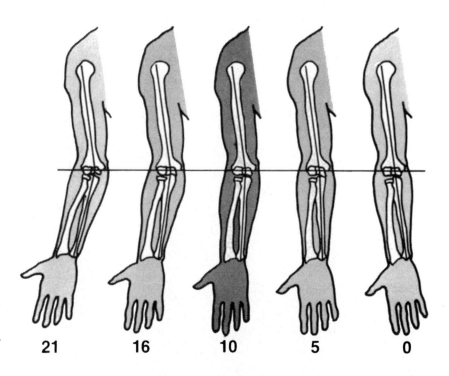

FIGURE 2–21 • The carrying angle is formed by the variable relationship of the orientation of the humeral articulation referable to the long axis of the humerus and the valgus angular relationship of the greater sigmoid fossa referable to the long axis of the ulna. (From Lanz, T., and Wachsmuth, W.: Praktische Anatomie. ARM, Berlin, Springer, 1959.)

21   16   10   5   0

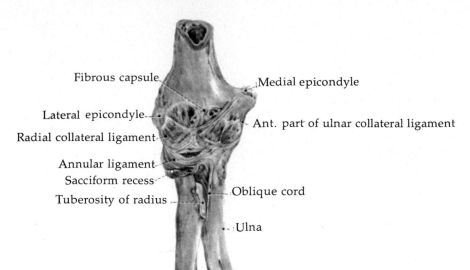

Fibrous capsule

Medial epicondyle

Lateral epicondyle

Ant. part of ulnar collateral ligament

Radial collateral ligament

Annular ligament

Sacciform recess

Oblique cord

Tuberosity of radius

Ulna

FIGURE 2–23 • There is a cruciate orientation of the fibers of the anterior capsule that provides a good deal of its strength. (From Langman, J., and Woerdeman, M. W.: Atlas of Medical Anatomy. Philadelphia, W. B. Saunders Co., 1978.)

rior portion being a thickening of the posterior capsule, and is well defined only in about 90 degrees of flexion. The transverse component (ligament of Cooper) appears to contribute little or nothing to elbow stability.

The precise locus of the origin of the medial collateral ligament has been studied recently to define the relationship of the humeral origin of the medial collateral ligament, the medial epicondyle, and the ulnar nerve.[26, 61] The ligament originates from a broad anteroinferior surface of the epicondyle but not from the condylar element of the trochlea. The ulnar nerve rests on the posterior aspect of the medial epicondyle but is not intimately related to the fibers of the anterior bundle of the medial collateral ligament itself. This has obvious implications with regard to the treatment of ulnar nerve decompression by medial epicondylar ostectomy. A more obliquely oriented excision might be most appropriate to both decompress the ulnar nerve and preserve the collateral ligament origin (Fig. 2–26). On the lateral projection, the origin of the anterior bundle of the medial collateral ligament is just inferior to the axis of rotation (Fig. 2–27), whereas the anterior portion is along

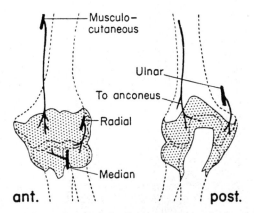

FIGURE 2–24 • A typical distribution of the contributions of the musculocutaneous, radial, median, and ulnar nerves to the joint capsule. (From O'Driscoll, S. W., Morrey, B. F., and An, K. N.: Intraarticular pressure and capacity of the elbow. Arthroscopy 6:100, 1990.)

the medial aspect of the coronoid process. The posterior bundle inserts along the midportion of the medial margin of the semilunar notch. The width of the anterior bundle is approximately 4 to 5 mm compared with 5 to 6 mm at the midportion of the fan-shaped posterior segment.[56]

The function of the ligamentous structures is discussed in detail subsequently (see Chapter 3). Clinically and experimentally, the anterior bundle is clearly the major portion of the medial ligament complex.[32, 58, 71]

LATERAL LIGAMENT COMPLEX

Unlike the medial collateral ligament complex, with its rather consistent pattern, the lateral ligaments of the elbow joint are less discrete, and some individual variation is common.[28, 29, 39, 75] Our investigation has suggested that several components make up the lateral ligament complex: (1) the radial collateral ligament, (2) the annular ligament, (3) a variably present accessory lateral collateral ligament, and (4) the lateral ulnar collateral ligament. These observations have now been confirmed by others.

Radial Collateral Ligament. This structure originates from the lateral epicondyle and terminates indistinguishably in the annular ligament (Fig. 2–28). Its superficial aspect provides a source of origin for a portion of the supinator muscle. The length averages approximately 20 mm with a width of approximately 8 mm. This portion of the ligament is almost uniformly taut throughout the normal range of flexion and extension, indicating that the origin of the ligament is very near the axis of (see Fig. 2–27).

Annular Ligament. A strong band of tissue originating and inserting on the anterior and posterior margins of the lesser sigmoid notch forms the annular ligament and maintains the radial head in contact with the ulna. The ligament is tapered distally to give the shape of a funnel and contributes about four-fifths of the fibro-osseous ring (Fig. 2–29).[50] The structure may not be as simple as it appears. A synovial reflection extends distal to the lower margin of the annular ligament, forming the sacciform recess. The radial head is not a pure circular disc[76]; thus, it has been observed that the anterior insertion becomes

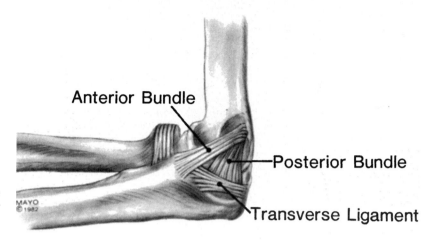

Anterior Bundle

Posterior Bundle

Transverse Ligament

FIGURE 2–25 • The classic orientation of the medial collateral ligament, including the anterior and posterior bundles, and the transverse ligament. This last structure contributes relatively little to elbow stability.

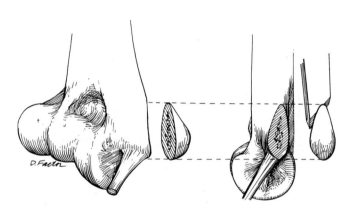

FIGURE 2–26 • An oblique epicondylectomy would be effective at both decompressing the nerve and preserving the integrity of the ligament. (From O'Driscoll, S. W., Horii, E., and Morrey, B. F.: Anatomy of the attachment of the medial ulnar collateral ligament. J. Hand Surg. 17:164, 1992.)

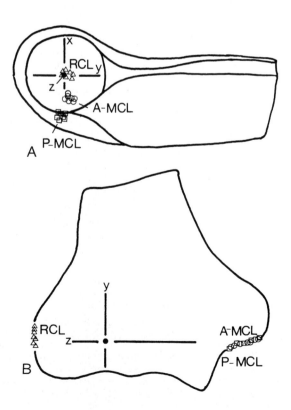

FIGURE 2–27 • A, Lateral view of the distal aspect of the humerus demonstrating the locus of the medial and radial collateral ligaments referable to the axis of rotation, z. B, Frontal projection of the distal humerus showing the locus of the origin of the radial medial collateral ligaments. Note that of these various components, only the radial collateral ligament lies in the axis of rotation z, thereby explaining the length-tension relationship of these ligaments. (From Morrey, B. F., and An, K. N.: Functional anatomy of the elbow ligaments. Clin. Orthop. 201:84, 1985.)

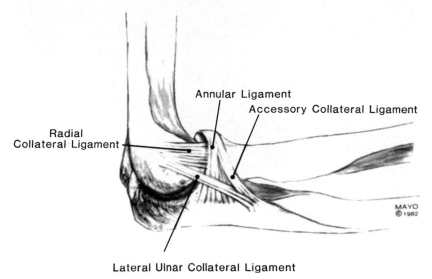

FIGURE 2–28 • More detailed representation of the radial collateral ligament complex showing a portion termed the radial collateral ligament that extends from the humerus to the annular ligament. This is the portion that is most commonly meant when referring to the radial or lateral collateral ligament.

taut during supination and the posterior aspect becomes taut during extremes of pronation.[76]

Lateral Ulnar Collateral Ligament. Although Martin described "additional fibers inserting from the tubercle of the supinator crest to the humerus," Morrey and An first described the so-called lateral ulnar collateral ligament in 1985.[56] This structure subsequently has been demonstrated to be invariably present, originating from the lateral epicondyle and blending with the fibers of the annular ligament but arching superficial and distal to it.[62] The insertion is to the tubercle of the crest of the supinator on the ulna. Although the origin blends with the origin of the lateral collateral ligament complex occupying the posterior portion, the insertion is more discrete at the tubercle (Fig. 2–30). The function of this ligament is to provide stability to the ulnohumeral joint and was shown to be deficient in posterolateral rotatory instability of the joint.[64] That this ligament represents the primary lateral stabilizer of the elbow and is taut in flexion and extension (Fig. 2–31) has been confirmed by several recent investigations.

Accessory Lateral Collateral Ligament. This definition has been applied by Martin to the ulnar insertion of discrete fibers on the tubercle of the supinator, as described previously, but without a demonstrable contribution to the posterior portion of the radial collateral ligament. This pattern was noted in 4 of 10 specimens examined in our laboratory. Proximally, the fibers tend to blend with the inferior margin of the annular ligament (see Fig. 2–31). Its function is to further stabilize the annular ligament during varus stress.

Quadrate Ligament. A thin, fibrous layer covering the capsule between the inferior margin and the annular ligament and the ulna is referred to as the quadrate ligament[18, 59] or the ligament of Denucè.[76] Spinner and Kaplan[76] have demonstrated a functional role for the structure, describing the anterior part as a stabilizer of the proximal radial ulnar joint during full supination. The weaker posterior attachment stabilizes the joint in full pronation.

Oblique Cord. The oblique cord is a small and incon-

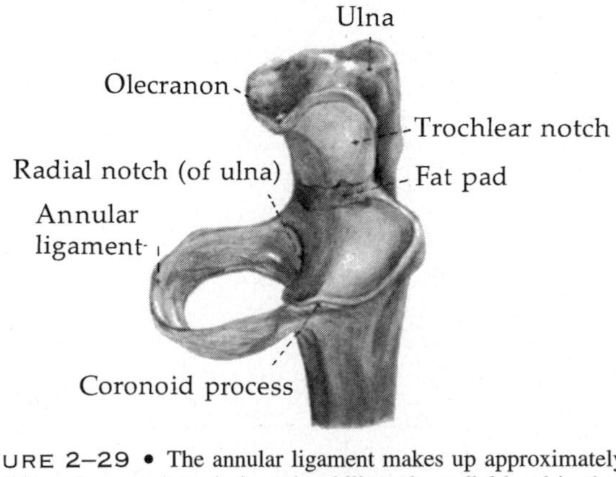

FIGURE 2–29 • The annular ligament makes up approximately four-fifths of a complete circle and stabilizes the radial head in the radial notch of the ulna. (From Langman, J., and Woerdeman, M. W.: Atlas of Medical Anatomy. Philadelphia, W. B. Saunders Co., 1976.)

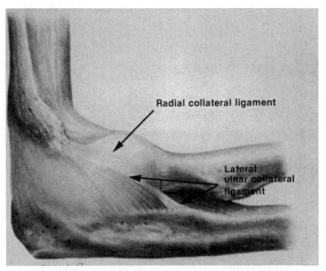

FIGURE 2–30 • Artist's rendition of lateral collateral complex noting the thickening of the lateral ulnar collateral ligament with a more discrete insertion at the tubercle of the supinator. In life, the supinator origin obscures the ligament, making it unnoticeable unless the supinator muscle has been removed. (From Pede.)

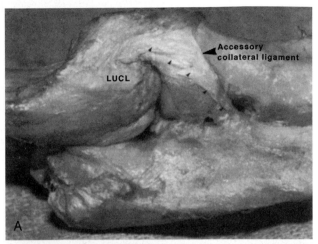

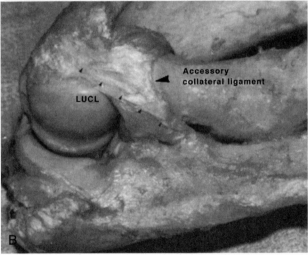

FIGURE 2–31 • Lateral ulnar collateral ligament (LUCL) complex has origin at the axis of rotation and thus is isometric, being taut in both extension *(A)* and flexion *(B)*. Note presence of accessory ligament.

stant bundle of fibrous tissue formed by the fascia overlying the deep head of the supinator and extending from the lateral side of the tuberosity of the ulna to the radius just below the radial tuberosity (see Fig. 2–23). Although the morphologic significance is debatable[51, 76] and the structure is not considered to be of great functional consequence,[29] it has been noted to become taut in full supination, and contracture of the oblique cord has been implicated in the etiology of idiopathic limitation of forearm supination.[10]

Bursae

First detailed by Monro in 1788, several bursae have been described at the elbow joint.[54] Lanz[45] recognized seven bursae, including three associated with the triceps. On the posterior aspect of the elbow, the superficial olecranon bursa between the olecranon process and the subcutaneous tissue is well known (Fig. 2–32).[30] The first appearance of this bursa is at age 7 years. This provides some evidence of its functional demands (see Chapter 75).[16] A very frequent deep intratendinous bursa is present in the substance of the triceps tendon as it inserts on the tip of the olecranon, and an occasional deep subtendinous bursa is likewise

present between the tendon and the tip of the olecranon. A bursa has been described deep to the anconeus muscle in about 12 percent of subjects by Henle,[34] but we have not appreciated such a structure during more than 500 exposures of this region. On the medial and lateral aspects of the joint, the subcutaneous medial epicondylar bursa is frequently present, and the lateral subcutaneous epicondylar bursa occasionally has been observed. The radiohumeral bursa lies deep to the common extensor tendon, below the extensor carpi radialis brevis and superficial to the radiohumeral joint capsule. This entity has been implicated by several authors[15, 66] in the etiology of lateral epicondylitis. The constant bicipitoradial bursa separates the biceps tendon from the tuberosity of the radius (see Fig. 2–9). Less commonly appreciated is the deep cubital interosseous bursa lying between the lateral aspect of the biceps tendon and the ulna, brachialis, and supinator fascia. This bursa is said to be present in about 20 percent of individuals.[75] Finally, the uncommon occurrence of a bursa between the ulnar nerve and the medial epicondyle and margin of the triceps muscle has been mentioned by Hollinshead.[36] The clinical significance of the bursae about the elbow is described in Chapter 75.

VESSELS

Brachial Artery and Its Branches

The cross-sectional relationship of the vessels, nerves, muscles, and bones is shown in Figure 2–33. The brachial artery descends in the arm, crossing in front of the intramuscular septum to lie anterior to the medial aspect of the brachialis muscle. The median nerve crosses in front of and medial to the artery at this point, near the middle of the arm (Fig. 2–34). The artery continues distally at the medial margin of the biceps muscle and enters the antecubital space medial to the biceps tendon and lateral to the nerve (Fig. 2–35). At the level of the radial head, it gives off its terminal branches, the ulnar and radial arteries, which continue into the forearm.

The brachial artery usually is accompanied by medial and lateral brachial veins. Proximally, in addition to its numerous muscular and cutaneous branches, the large, deep brachial artery courses posteriorly and laterally to bifurcate into the medial and radial collateral arteries. The medial collateral artery continues posteriorly, supplying the medial head of the triceps and ultimately anastomosing with the interosseous recurrent artery at the posterior aspect of the elbow. The radial collateral artery penetrates the lateral intermuscular septum and accompanies the radial nerve into the antecubital space, where it anastomoses with the radial recurrent artery at the level of the lateral epicondyle.

The detailed vascular anatomy of the elbow region was recently nicely described in great detail by Yamagucci and colleagues.[91] The major branches of the brachial artery are the superior and inferior ulnar collateral arteries, which originate medial and distal to the profunda brachial artery. The superior ulnar collateral artery is given off just distal to the midportion of the brachium, penetrates the medial intermuscular septum, and accompanies the ulnar nerve to the medial epicondyle, where it terminates by anastomosing

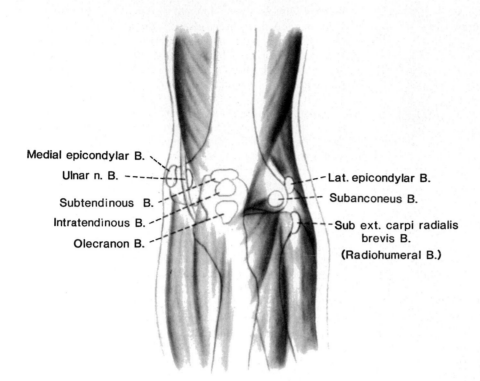

Medial epicondylar B.
Ulnar n. B.
Subtendinous B.
Intratendinous B.
Olecranon B.

Lat. epicondylar B.
Subanconeus B.
Sub ext. carpi radialis
brevis B.
(Radiohumeral B.)

FIGURE 2–32 • Posterior view of the elbow demonstrating the superficial and deep bursae that are present about this joint.

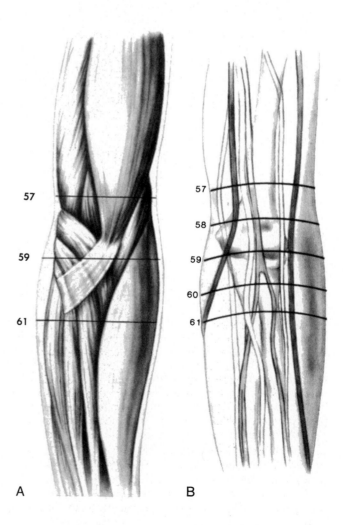

57
59
61

57
58
59
60
61

FIGURE 2–33 • *A* and *B*, Cross-sectional relationships of the muscles *(A)* and the neurovascular bundles *(B)*.

A

B

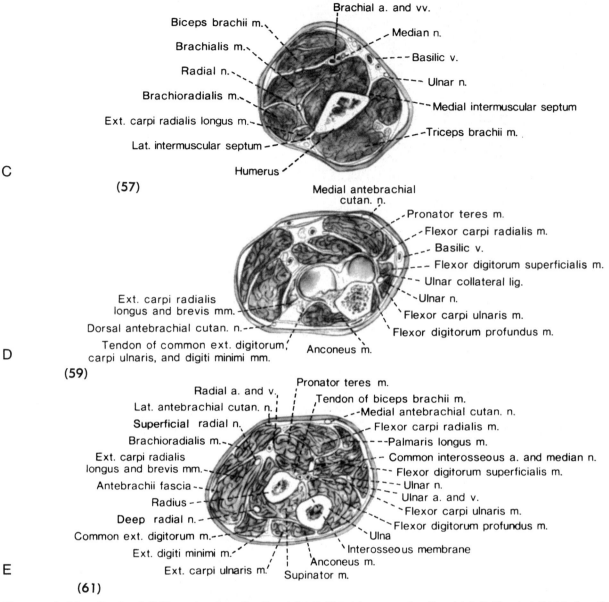

Biceps brachii m.
Brachialis m.
Radial n.
Brachioradialis m.
Ext. carpi radialis longus m.
Lat. intermuscular septum
Humerus

Brachial a. and vv.
Median n.
Basilic v.
Ulnar n.
Medial intermuscular septum
Triceps brachii m.

C
(57)

Medial antebrachial cutan. n.

Ext. carpi radialis longus and brevis mm.
Dorsal antebrachial cutan. n.
Tendon of common ext. digitorum, carpi ulnaris, and digiti minimi mm.

Pronator teres m.
Flexor carpi radialis m.
Basilic v.
Flexor digitorum superficialis m.
Ulnar collateral lig.
Ulnar n.
Flexor carpi ulnaris m.
Flexor digitorum profundus m.
Anconeus m.

D
(59)

Radial a. and v.
Lat. antebrachial cutan. n.
Superficial radial n.
Brachioradialis m.
Ext. carpi radialis longus and brevis mm.
Antebrachii fascia
Radius
Deep radial n.
Common ext. digitorum m.
Ext. digiti minimi m.
Ext. carpi ulnaris m.

Pronator teres m.
Tendon of biceps brachii m.
Medial antebrachial cutan. n.
Flexor carpi radialis m.
Palmaris longus m.
Common interosseous a. and median n.
Flexor digitorum superficialis m.
Ulnar n.
Ulnar a. and v.
Flexor carpi ulnaris m.
Flexor digitorum profundus m.
Ulna
Interosseous membrane
Anconeus m.
Supinator m.

E
(61)

FIGURE 2–33 • *Continued. C,* The region above the elbow joint. *D,* View taken across the elbow joint. *E,* View just distal to the articulation. (Redrawn from Eycleshymer, A. C., and Schoemaker, D. M.: A Cross-Section Anatomy. New York, D. Appleton and Co., 1930.)

with the posterior ulnar recurrent artery and variably with the inferior ulnar collateral artery (Fig. 2–36).

The inferior ulnar collateral artery arises from the medial aspect of the brachial artery about 4 cm proximal to the medial epicondyle. It continues distally for a short course, dividing into and anastomosing with branches of the anterior ulnar recurrent artery, and it supplies a portion of the pronator teres muscle.

Radial Artery

In most instances, the radial artery originates at the level of the radial head, emerges from the antecubital space between the brachioradialis and the pronator teres muscle, and continues down the forearm under the brachioradialis muscle. A more proximal origin occurs in up to 15 percent of individuals.[53] The radial recurrent artery originates later-

ally from the radial artery just distal to its origin. It ascends laterally on the supinator muscle to anastomose with the radial collateral artery at the level of the lateral epicondyle, to which it provides circulation. The radial recurrent artery sometimes is sacrificed with the anterior elbow exposure if distal visualization is required.

Ulnar Artery

The ulnar artery is the larger of the two terminal branches of the brachial artery. There is relatively little variation in its origin, which is usually at the level of the radial head. The artery traverses the pronator teres between its two heads and continues distally and medially behind the flexor digitorum superficialis muscle. It emerges medially to continue down the medial aspect of the forearm under the cover of the flexor carpi ulnaris. Two recurrent branches

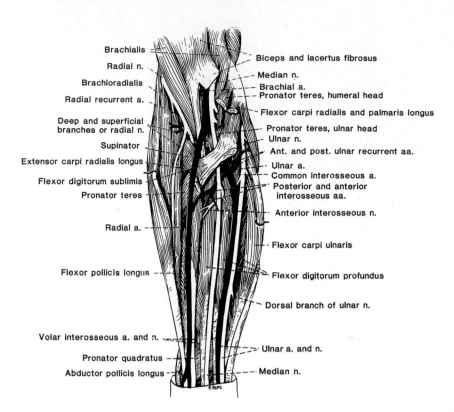

Brachialis
Radial n.
Brachioradialis
Radial recurrent a.
Deep and superficial branches or radial n.
Supinator
Extensor carpi radialis longus
Flexor digitorum sublimis
Pronator teres
Radial a.
Flexor pollicis longus
Volar interosseous a. and n.
Pronator quadratus
Abductor pollicis longus

Biceps and lacertus fibrosus
Median n.
Brachial a.
Pronator teres, humeral head
Flexor carpi radialis and palmaris longus
Pronator teres, ulnar head
Ulnar n.
Ant. and post. ulnar recurrent aa.
Ulnar a.
Common interosseous a.
Posterior and anterior interosseous aa.
Anterior interosseous n.
Flexor carpi ulnaris
Flexor digitorum profundus
Dorsal branch of ulnar n.
Ulnar a. and n.
Median n.

FIGURE 2–34 • Anterior aspect of the elbow region demonstrating the intricate relationships between the muscles, nerves, and vessels. (From Hollinshead, W. H.: The back and limbs. *In* Anatomy for Surgeons. Vol. 3. New York, Harper & Row, 1969, p. 379.)

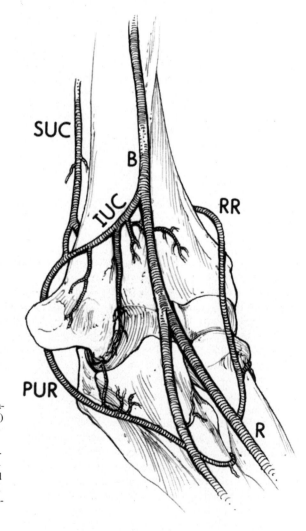

FIGURE 2–35 • Illustration of the anterior extraosseous vascular anatomy demonstrating the medial arcade and the relationship of the radial recurrent artery (RR) to the proximal aspect of the radius. The inferior ulnar collateral artery (IUC) provides perforators to the supracondylar region, medial aspect of the trochlea, and medial epicondyle before it courses posteriorly to anastomose with the superior ulnar collateral (SUC) and posterior ulnar recurrent (PUR) arteries. The radial recurrent artery provides an osseous perforator to the radius as it travels proximally and posterior. B = brachial artery; R = radial artery. (From Yamaguchi, K., Sweet, F. A., Bindra, R., Morrey, B. F., and Gelberman, R. H.: The extraosseous and intraosseous arterial anatomy of the adult elbow. J. Bone Joint Surg. **79A**:1654, 1997.)

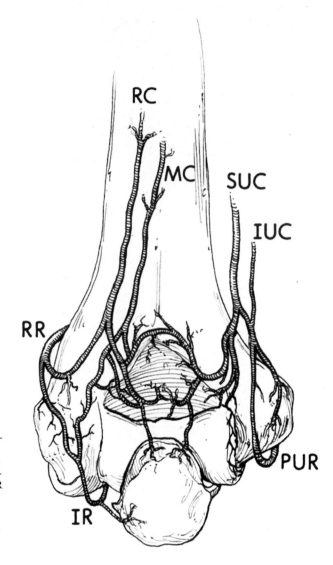

FIGURE 2–36 • Illustration of the posterior collateral circulation of the elbow. There are perforating vessels on the posterior aspect of the lateral epicondyle, in the olecranon fossa, and on the medial aspect of the trochlea. The tip of the olecranon is supplied by perforators from the posterior arcade in the olecranon fossa. The superior ulnar collateral artery (SUC) is seen terminating in the posterior arcade. IUC = inferior ulnar collateral artery; PUR = posterior ulnar recurrent artery; IR = interosseous recurrent artery; RR = radial recurrent artery; RC = radial collateral artery; and MC = middle collateral artery. (From Yamaguchi, K., Sweet, F. A., Bindra, R., Morrey, B. F., Gelberman, R. H.: The extraosseous and intraosseous arterial anatomy of the adult elbow. J. Bone Joint Surg. **79A**:1655, 1997.)

originate just distal to the origin of the ulnar artery. The anterior ulnar recurrent artery ascends deep to the humeral head of the pronator teres and deep to the medial aspect of the brachialis muscle to anastomose with the descending superior and inferior ulnar collateral arteries. The posterior ulnar recurrent artery originates with or just distal to the smaller anterior ulnar recurrent artery. The vessel then passes proximally and posteriorly between the superficial and deep flexors posterior to the medial epicondyle. This artery continues proximally with the ulnar nerve under the flexor carpi ulnaris to anastomose with the superior ulnar collateral artery. Additional extensive communication with the inferior ulnar and middle collateral branches constitutes the rete articulare cubiti (see Fig. 2–35).

The common interosseous artery is a large vessel originating 2.5 cm distal to the origin of the ulnar artery. It passes posteriorly and distally between the flexor pollicis longus and the flexor digitorum profundus just distal to the oblique cord, dividing into anterior and posterior interosseous branches. The interosseous recurrent artery originates from the posterior interosseous branch. This artery runs proximally through the supinator muscle to anastomose with the vascular network of the olecranon (see Fig. 2–36).

NERVES

Specific clinical and pertinent anatomic aspects of the nerves in the region of the elbow are discussed in subsequent chapters as appropriate. A general survey of the common anatomic patterns is given here (see Fig. 2–33).

Musculocutaneous Nerve

The musculocutaneous nerve originates from C5–8 nerve roots and is a continuation of the lateral cord. The musculocutaneous nerve innervates the major elbow flexors and the biceps and brachialis and continues through the brachial fascia lateral to the biceps tendon, terminating as the lateral antebrachial cutaneous nerve (Fig. 2–37). The motor branch enters the biceps approximately 15 cm distal to the acromion; it enters the brachialis approximately 20 cm below the tip of the acromion.[46]

Median Nerve

The median nerve arises from the C5–8 and T1 nerve roots. The nerve enters the anterior aspect of the brachium,

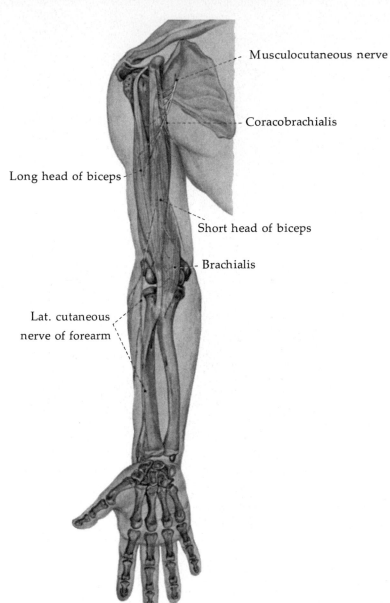

Musculocutaneous nerve

Coracobrachialis

Long head of biceps

Short head of biceps

Brachialis

Lat. cutaneous
nerve of forearm

FIGURE 2–37 • The musculocutaneous nerve innervates the flexors of the elbow and continues distal to the joint as the lateral cutaneous nerve of the forearm. (From Langman, J., and Woerdeman, M. W.: Atlas of Medical Anatomy. Philadelphia, W. B. Saunders Co., 1976.)

crossing in front of the brachial artery as it passes across the intermuscular septum. It follows a straight course into the medial aspect of the antecubital fossa, medial to the biceps tendon and the brachial artery. It then passes under the bicipital aponeurosis. The first motor branch is given to the pronator teres, through which it passes.[2, 38] It enters the forearm and continues distally under the flexor digitorum superficialis within the fascial sheath of this muscle.

There are no branches of the median nerve in the arm (Fig. 2–38). In the cubital fossa, a few small articular branches are given off before the motor branches to the pronator teres, the flexor carpi radialis, the palmaris longus, and the flexor digitorum superficialis. All of these arise medially, thus allowing safe medial retraction of the nerve during exposure of the anterior aspect of the elbow.

The anterior interosseous nerve arises from the median nerve near the inferior border of the pronator teres and travels along the anterior aspect of the interosseous membrane in the company of the anterior interosseous artery.

This branch innervates the flexor pollicis longus and the lateral portion of the flexor digitorum profundus.

Radial Nerve

The radial nerve is a continuation of the posterior cord and originates from the C6, C7, and C8 nerve roots with variable contributions of the C5 and T1 roots. In the midportion of the arm, the nerve courses laterally just distal to the deltoid insertion to occupy the groove in the humerus that bears its name. It then emerges in a spiral path inferiorly and laterally to penetrate the lateral intermuscular septum. Before entering the anterior aspect of the arm, it gives off motor branches to the medial and lateral head of the triceps, accompanied by the deep branch of the brachial artery. After penetrating the lateral intermuscular septum in the distal third of the arm, it descends anterior to the lateral epicondyle behind the brachioradialis. It innervates the brachioradialis with a single branch to this muscle. In the antecubital space, the nerve divides into the superficial and

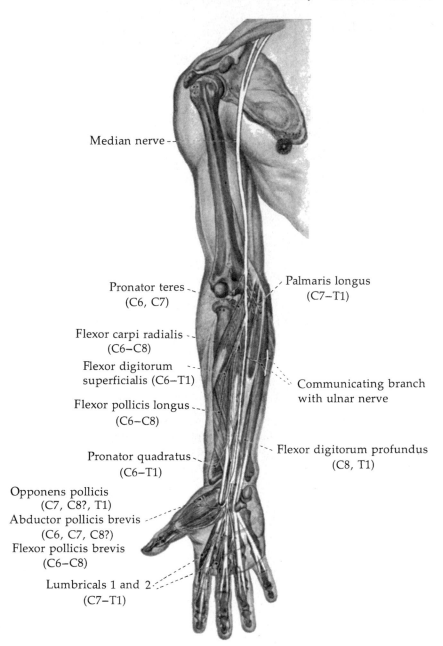

Median nerve

Pronator teres
(C6, C7)

Flexor carpi radialis
(C6–C8)

Flexor digitorum
superficialis (C6–T1)

Flexor pollicis longus
(C6–C8)

Pronator quadratus
(C6–T1)

Opponens pollicis
(C7, C8?, T1)
Abductor pollicis brevis
(C6, C7, C8?)
Flexor pollicis brevis
(C6–C8)

Lumbricals 1 and 2
(C7–T1)

Palmaris longus
(C7–T1)

Communicating branch
with ulnar nerve

Flexor digitorum profundus
(C8, T1)

FIGURE 2–38 • The median nerve innervates the flexor pronator group of muscles about the elbow, but there are no branches above the joint. (From Langman, J., and Woerdeman, M. W.: Atlas of Medical Anatomy. Philadelphia, W. B. Saunders Co., 1976.)

deep branches. The superficial branch is a continuation of the radial nerve and extends into the forearm to innervate the mid-dorsal cutaneous aspect of the forearm (Fig. 2–39).

The motor branches of the radial nerve are given off to the triceps above the spiral groove except for the branch to the medial head of the triceps, which originates at the entry to the spiral groove. This branch continues distally through the medial head to terminate as a muscular branch to the anconeus. Hence, surgical approaches that reflect the anconeus[11, 42, 67] can be performed while preserving the innervation of the muscle.

In the antecubital space, the recurrent radial nerve curves around the posterolateral aspect of the radius, passing deep to the supinator muscle, which it innervates. During its course through the supinator muscle, the nerve lies over a "bare area," which is distal to and opposite to the radial tuberosity.[20] The nerve is believed to be at risk at this site

with fractures of the proximal radius.[79] It emerges from the muscle as the posterior interosseous nerve, and the recurrent branch innervates the extensor digitorum minimi, the extensor carpi ulnaris, and, occasionally, the anconeus. The posterior interosseous nerve is accompanied by the posterior interosseous artery and sends further muscle branches distally to supply the abductor pollicis longus, the extensor pollicis longus, the extensor pollicis brevis, and the extensor indicis on the dorsum of the forearm. The nerve is subject to compression as it passes through the supinator muscle or from synovial proliferation.[14, 22, 25] Compression and entrapment problems are described in detail in Chapter 71.

Ulnar Nerve

The ulnar nerve is derived from the medial cord of the brachial plexus from roots C8 and T1. In the midarm, it

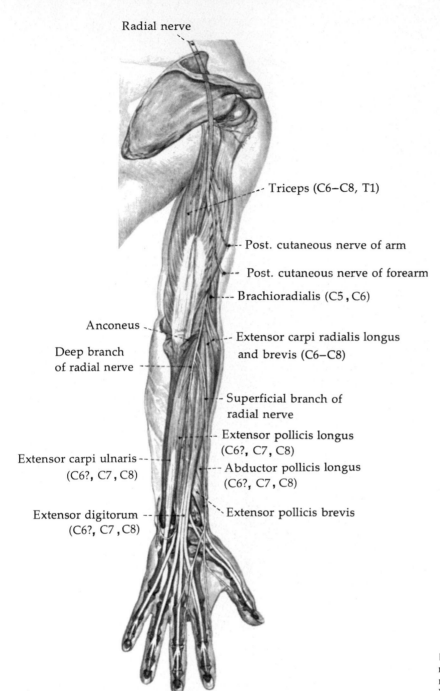

Radial nerve

Triceps (C6–C8, T1)

Post. cutaneous nerve of arm

Post. cutaneous nerve of forearm

Brachioradialis (C5, C6)

Anconeus

Extensor carpi radialis longus
and brevis (C6–C8)

Deep branch
of radial nerve

Superficial branch of
radial nerve

Extensor pollicis longus
(C6?, C7, C8)

Extensor carpi ulnaris
(C6?, C7, C8)

Abductor pollicis longus
(C6?, C7, C8)

Extensor digitorum
(C6?, C7, C8)

Extensor pollicis brevis

FIGURE 2–39 • The muscles innervated by the right radial nerve. (From Langman, J., and Woerdeman, M. W.: Atlas of Medical Anatomy. Philadelphia, W. B. Saunders Co., 1976.)

passes posteriorly through the medial intermuscular septum and continues distally along the medial margin of the triceps in the company of the superior ulnar collateral branch of the brachial artery and the ulnar collateral branch of the radial artery. There are no branches of this nerve in the brachium (Fig. 2–40). The ulnar nerve passes into the cubital tunnel under the medial epicondyle and rests against the posterior portion of the medial collateral ligament, where a groove in the ligament accommodates this structure.

The ulnar nerve may undergo compression as it passes behind the medial epicondyle (ME), emerging into the forearm through the cubital tunnel.[52] The roof of the cubital tunnel has been defined by a structure termed the cubital tunnel retinaculum (CTR).[63] Its absence accounts for congenital subluxation of the ulnar nerve. Furthermore, this tunnel is found to flatten with elbow flexion, thus decreasing the capacity of the cubital tunnel (Fig. 2–41).[63] This is particularly noticed as stimulating ulnar nerve symptoms when osteophytes are present on the ulnar or medial epicondyle.[70] During extension, the cubital tunnel retinaculum relaxes, allowing greater accommodation of the nerve (Fig. 2–42). This accounts for the clinical observation of ulnar nerve paresthesia and compression, which occurs when the elbow is fully flexed for a period of time. Similarly, elbow instability can compromise the integrity of the nerve.[49] A

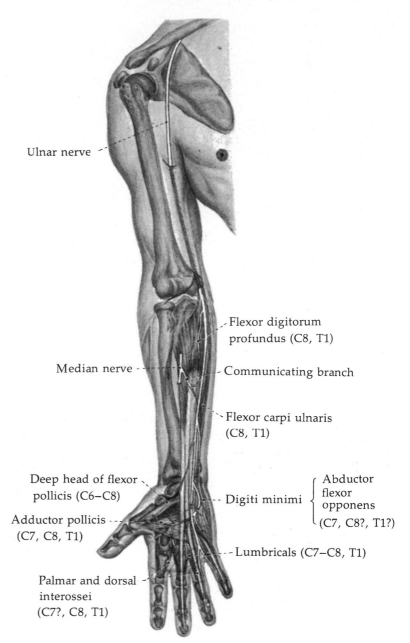

Ulnar nerve

Flexor digitorum
profundus (C8, T1)

Median nerve

Communicating branch

Flexor carpi ulnaris
(C8, T1)

Deep head of flexor
pollicis (C6–C8)

Digiti minimi

{ Abductor
flexor
opponens
(C7, C8?, T1?)

Adductor pollicis
(C7, C8, T1)

Lumbricals (C7–C8, T1)

Palmar and dorsal
interossei
(C7?, C8, T1)

FIGURE 2–40 • Muscles innervated by the right ulnar nerve. There are no muscular branches of this nerve above the elbow joint. (From Langman, J., and Woerdeman, M. W.: Atlas of Medical Anatomy. Philadelphia, W. B. Saunders Co., 1976.)

few small twigs are given to the elbow joint in this region and are the most obvious source of innervation of the capsule.[8] The first motor branch is a single nerve to the ulnar origin of the pronator and another one to the epicondylar head of the flexor carpi ulnaris. Distally, the nerve sends a motor branch to the ulnar half of the flexor digitorum profundus. Two cutaneous nerves arise from the ulnar nerve in the distal half of the forearm and innervate the skin of the wrist and the hand.

MUSCLES

Relevant features of the origin, insertion, and function of the muscles of the elbow region are covered in other chapters dealing with surgical exposure, functional examination, and biomechanics. This information is also dis-

cussed in various chapters when dealing with specific pathology. The following description will serve as a simple overview. The origin and insertion of these muscle groups are illustrated in Figure 2–43 through Figure 2–46, and the superficial musculature is shown in Figure 2–47 through Figure 2–50.[37]

Elbow Flexors

BICEPS

The biceps covers the brachialis muscle in the distal arm and passes into the cubital fossa as the biceps tendon, which attaches to the posterior aspect of the radial tuberosity (Fig. 2–47). The constant bicipitoradial bursa separates the tendon from the anterior aspect of the tuberosity, and an interosseous cubital bursa has been described as separating the tendon from the ulna and the muscles covering the

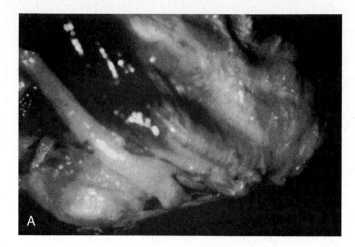

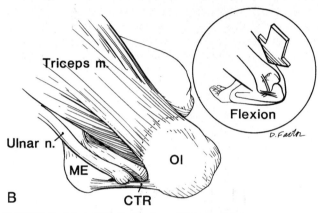

FIGURE 2–41 • With flexion the cubital tunnel flattens, compressing the ulnar nerve (A and B). Ol = olecranon. (From O'Driscoll, S. W., Horii, E., Carmichael, S. W., and Morrey, B. F.: The cubital tunnel and ulnar neuropathy. J. Bone Joint Surg. **73B**:613, 1991.)

radius (see Fig. 2–9). The bicipital aponeurosis, or lacertus fibrosus, is a broad, thin band of tissue that is a continuation of the anterior medial and distal muscle fasciae. It runs obliquely to cover the median nerve and brachial artery and inserts into the deep fasciae of the forearm and possibly into the ulna as well.[17]

The biceps is a major flexor of the elbow that has a large cross-sectional area but an intermediate mechanical advantage because it passes relatively close to the axis of rotation. In the pronated position, the biceps is a strong supinator.[6] The distal insertion may undergo spontaneous rupture,[57, 78] and this condition is discussed in detail later (see Chapter 35).

BRACHIALIS

This muscle has the largest cross-sectional area of any of the elbow flexors but suffers from a poor mechanical advantage because it crosses so close to the axis of rotation. The origin consists of the entire anterior distal half of the humerus, and it extends medially and laterally to the respective intermuscular septa (see Fig. 2–43). The muscle crosses the anterior capsule with some fibers inserting into the capsule that are said to help retract the capsule during

elbow flexion. More than 95 percent of the cross-sectional area is muscle tissue at the elbow joint,[48] a relationship that may account for the high incidence of trauma to this muscle and the development of myositis ossificans with elbow dislocation.[84] The insertion of the brachialis is along the base of the coronoid and into the tuberosity of the ulna.

The muscle is innervated by the musculocutaneous nerve, and the lateral portion covers the radial nerve as it spirals around the distal humerus. The median nerve and brachial artery are superficial to the brachialis and lie behind the biceps in the distal humerus.

BRACHIORADIALIS

The brachioradialis has a lengthy origin along the lateral supracondylar bony column that extends proximally to the level of the junction of the middle and distal humerus (see Fig. 2–43). The origin separates the lateral head of the triceps and the brachialis muscle. The lateral border of the cubital fossa is formed by this muscle, which crosses the

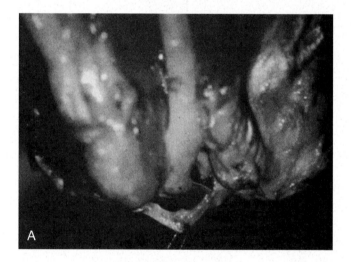

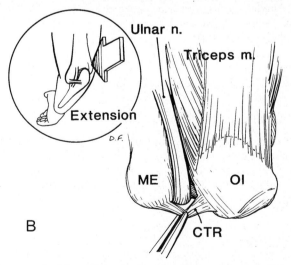

FIGURE 2–42 • With extension the cubital tunnel retinaculum (CTR) relaxes, allowing greater accommodation of the nerve (A and B). ME = medial epicondyle; Ol = olecranon. (From O'Driscoll, S. W., Horii, E., Carmichael, S. W., and Morrey, B. F.: The cubital tunnel and ulnar neuropathy. J. Bone Joint Surg. **73B**:613, 1991.)

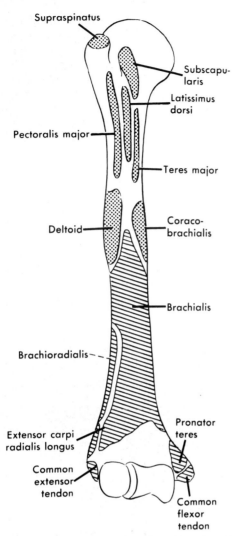

FIGURE 2–43 • Anterior humeral origin and insertion of muscles that control flexion of the elbow joint.

with that of the extensor carpi radialis brevis have been implicated in the pathologic anatomy of tennis elbow by Nirschl (see Chapter 40).

EXTENSOR CARPI RADIALIS BREVIS

The extensor carpi radialis brevis originates from the lateral superior aspect of the lateral epicondyle (see Fig. 2–43). Its origin is the most lateral of the extensor group and is covered by the extensor carpi radialis longus. This relationship is important as the most commonly implicated site of lateral epicondylitis. The extensor digitorum communis originates from the common extensor tendon and is just medial or ulnar to the extensor carpi radialis brevis. In the proximal forearm, the muscle fibers of the extensor carpi radialis longus and the extensor digitorum are almost indistinguishable from those of the extensor carpi radialis brevis (see Fig. 2–48). The latter muscle shares the same extensor compartment as the longus as it crosses the wrist under the extensor retinaculum and inserts into the dorsal base of the third metacarpal. The function of the extensor carpi radialis brevis is pure wrist extension, with little or no radial

elbow joint with the greatest mechanical advantage of any elbow flexor. It progresses distally to insert into the base of the radial styloid (Fig. 2–48; see Fig. 2–46). The muscle protects and is innervated by the radial nerve (C5, C6) as it emerges from the spiral groove. Its major function is elbow flexion. Rarely, the muscle may be ruptured.[33]

EXTENSOR CARPI RADIALIS LONGUS

The extensor carpi radialis longus originates from the supracondylar bony column joint just below the origin of the brachioradialis (see Fig. 2–48). The origin of this muscle is identified as the first fleshy fibers observed proximal to the common extensor tendon. As it continues into the midportion of the dorsum of the forearm, it becomes largely tendinous and inserts into the dorsal base of the second metacarpal. Innervated by the radial nerve (C6, C7), the motor branches arise just distal to those of the brachioradialis muscle.

In addition to wrist extension, its orientation suggests that this muscle might function as an elbow flexor.

Clinically, the origin of this muscle and its relationship

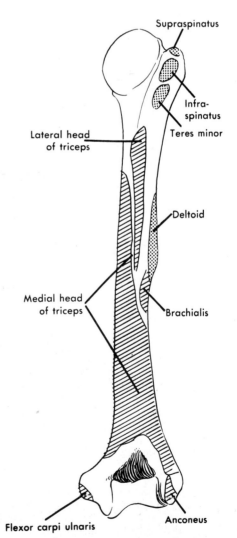

FIGURE 2–44 • Posterior view of the humerus demonstrating the broad surface over which the origin of the triceps lies.

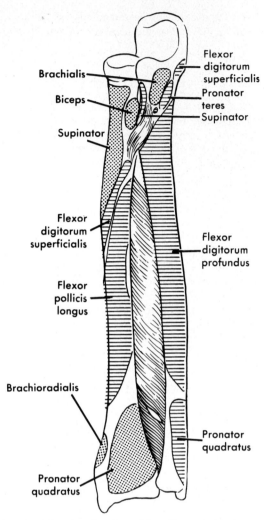

FIGURE 2–45 • Anterior view of the radius and ulna demonstrating the insertion of the major motors of the elbow joint.

or ulnar deviation.[1] The extensor carpi radialis brevis is innervated by fibers of the sixth and seventh cervical nerves. The motor branch arises from the radial nerve in the region of its division into deep and superficial branches.

EXTENSOR DIGITORUM COMMUNIS

Originating from the anterior distal aspect of the lateral epicondyle, the extensor digitorum communis accounts for most of the contour of the extensor surface of the forearm (see Fig. 2–48). The muscle extends and abducts the fingers. According to Wright, the muscle can assist in elbow flexion when the forearm is pronated. This observation is not, however, confirmed by our cross-sectional studies.[1] The innervation is from the deep branch of the radial nerve, with contributions from the sixth through eighth cervical nerves.

EXTENSOR CARPI ULNARIS

The extensor carpi ulnaris originates from two heads, one above and the other below the elbow joint. The humeral origin is the most medial of the common extensor group

(Fig. 2–49; see Fig. 2–43). The ulnar attachment is along the aponeurosis of the anconeus and at the superior border of this muscle. The insertion is on the dorsal base of the fifth metacarpal after crossing the wrist in its own compartment under the extensor retinaculum. The extensor carpi ulnaris is a wrist extensor and ulnar deviator. Fibers of the sixth through eighth cervical nerve routes innervate the muscle from branches of the deep radial nerve.

SUPINATOR

This flat muscle is characterized by the virtual absence of tendinous tissue and a complex origin and insertion. It originates from three sites above and below the elbow joint: (1) the lateral anterior aspect of the lateral epicondyle; (2) the lateral collateral ligament; and (3) the proximal anterior crest of the ulna along the crista supinatoris, which is just anterior to the depression for the insertion of the anconeus. The form of the muscle is approximately that of a rhomboid, as it runs obliquely, distally, and radially to wrap around and insert diffusely on the proximal radius, beginning lateral and proximal to the radial tuberosity and continuing distal to the insertion of the pronator teres at the

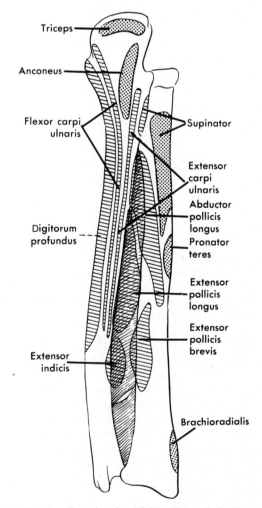

FIGURE 2–46 • Posterior view of the radius and ulna demonstrating the insertion of the extensors of the elbow as well as the origin of the forearm musculature.

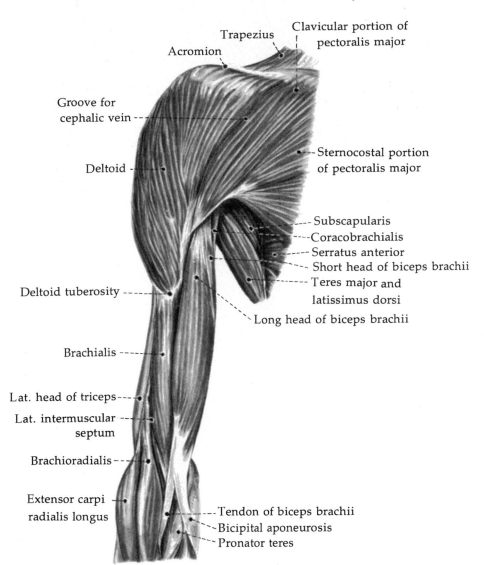

Trapezius

Acromion

Clavicular portion of
pectoralis major

Groove for
cephalic vein

Deltoid

Sternocostal portion
of pectoralis major

Subscapularis
Coracobrachialis
Serratus anterior
Short head of biceps brachii
Teres major and
latissimus dorsi

Deltoid tuberosity

Long head of biceps brachii

Brachialis

Lat. head of triceps

Lat. intermuscular
septum

Brachioradialis

Extensor carpi
radialis longus

Tendon of biceps brachii
Bicipital aponeurosis
Pronator teres

FIGURE 2–47 • Anterior aspect of
the arm and elbow region demonstrating the major flexors of the joint, the
brachialis, and the biceps muscles.
(From Langman, J., and Woerdeman,
M. W.: Atlas of Medical Anatomy. Philadelphia, W. B. Saunders Co., 1976.)

junction of the proximal and middle third of the radius (see Fig. 2–49). It is important to note that the radial nerve passes through the supinator to gain access to the extensor surface of the forearm. This anatomic feature is clinically significant with regard to exposure of the lateral aspect of the elbow joint and the proximal radius and in certain entrapment syndromes.[76]

The muscle obviously supinates the forearm but is a weaker supinator than the biceps.[36] Unlike the biceps, how-ever, the effectiveness of the supinator is not altered by the position of elbow flexion. The innervation is derived from the muscular branch given off by the radial nerve just prior to and during its course through the muscle with nerve fibers derived primarily from the sixth cervical root.

Elbow Extensors

TRICEPS BRACHII

The entire posterior musculature of the arm is composed of the triceps brachii (see Fig. 2–39). Two of its three heads originate from the posterior aspect of the humerus (see Fig. 2–44). The long head has a discrete origin from

the infraglenoid tuberosity of the scapula. The lateral head originates in a linear fashion from the proximal lateral intramuscular septum on the posterior surface of the hu-merus. The medial head originates from the entire distal half of the posteromedial surface of the humerus bounded laterally by the radial groove and medially by the intramus-cular septum. Thus, each head originates distal to the other, with progressively larger areas of origin. The long and lateral heads are superficial to the deep medial head, blend-ing in the midline of the humerus to form a common muscle that then tapers into the triceps tendon and attaches to the tip of the olecranon with Sharpey's fibers.[13] The tendon usually is separated from the olecranon by the subtendinous olecranon bursa. The distal 40 percent of the triceps mechanism consists of a layer of fascia that blends with the triceps distally.

Innervated by the radial nerve, the long and lateral heads are supplied by branches that arise proximal to the entrance of the radial nerve into the groove. The medial head is innervated distal to the groove with a branch that enters proximally and passes through the entire medial head to terminate by innervating the anconeus, an anatomic feature

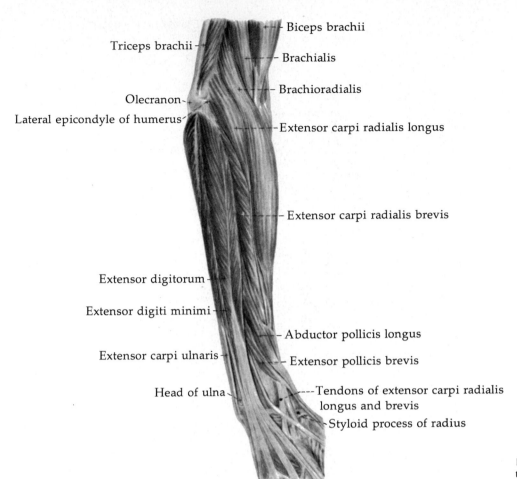

Triceps brachii

Biceps brachii

Brachialis

Brachioradialis

Olecranon

Lateral epicondyle of humerus

Extensor carpi radialis longus

Extensor carpi radialis brevis

Extensor digitorum

Extensor digiti minimi

Abductor pollicis longus

Extensor carpi ulnaris

Extensor pollicis brevis

Head of ulna

Tendons of extensor carpi radialis longus and brevis

Styloid process of radius

FIGURE 2–48 • The musculature of the posterolateral aspect of the right forearm. (From Langman, J., and Woerdeman, M. W.: Atlas of Medical Anatomy. Philadelphia, W. B. Saunders Co., 1976.)

of considerable importance when considering some approaches (e.g., Kocher, Bryan-Morrey, Boyd, and Pankovitch) to the joint.

The function of the triceps is to extend the elbow. Lesions of the nerve in the midportion of the humerus usually do not prevent triceps function that is provided by the more proximally innervated lateral and long heads.

ANCONEUS

This muscle has little tendinous tissue because it originates from a rather broad site on the posterior aspect of the lateral epicondyle and from the lateral triceps fascia and inserts into the lateral dorsal surface of the proximal ulna (see Fig. 2–49). It is innervated by the terminal branch of the nerve to the medial head of the triceps. Curiously, the function of this muscle has been the subject of considerable speculation.[5, 87] Possibly the most accurate description of the anconeus function is that proposed by Basmajian and Griffin and by DaHora, who suggest that its primary role is that of a joint stabilizer.[19] The muscle covers the lateral portion of the annular ligament and the radial head. For the surgeon, the major significance of this muscle is its position as a key landmark in various lateral and posterolat-

eral exposures and is used for some reconstructive procedures.

Flexor Pronator Muscle Group

PRONATOR TERES

This is the most proximal of the flexor pronator group. There are usually two heads of origin: The largest arises from the anterosuperior aspect of the medial epicondyle and the second from the coronoid process of the ulna, which is absent in about 10 percent of individuals (see Fig. 2–37).[38] The two origins of the pronator muscle provide an arch through which the median nerve typically passes to gain access to the forearm. This anatomic characteristic is a significant feature in the etiology of the median nerve entrapment syndrome and is discussed in detail in Chapter 71. The common muscle belly proceeds radially and distally under the brachioradialis, inserting at the junction of the proximal and middle portions of the radius by a discrete broad tendinous insertion into a tuberosity on the lateral aspect of the bone. Obviously, a strong pronator of the forearm, it also is considered a weak flexor of the elbow joint.[1, 7, 82] The muscle usually is innervated by two motor

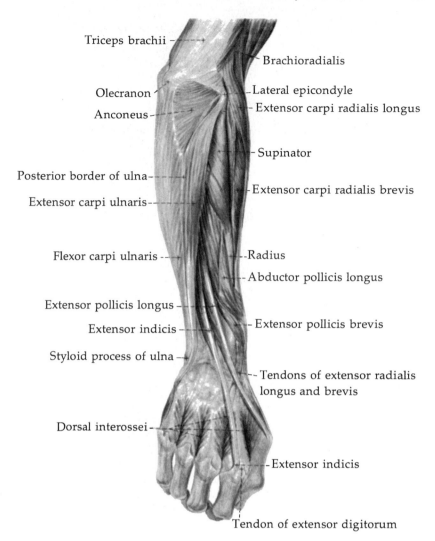

Triceps brachii

Olecranon

Anconeus

Posterior border of ulna

Extensor carpi ulnaris

Flexor carpi ulnaris

Extensor pollicis longus

Extensor indicis

Styloid process of ulna

Dorsal interossei

Brachioradialis

Lateral epicondyle

Extensor carpi radialis longus

Supinator

Extensor carpi radialis brevis

Radius

Abductor pollicis longus

Extensor pollicis brevis

Tendons of extensor radialis longus and brevis

Extensor indicis

Tendon of extensor digitorum

FIGURE 2–49 • The extensor aspect of the forearm demonstrating the deep muscle layer after the extensor digitorum and extensor digiti minimi have been removed. (From Langman, J., and Woerdeman, M. W.: Atlas of Medical Anatomy. Philadelphia, W. B. Saunders Co., 1976.)

branches from the median nerve before the nerve leaves the cubital fossa.

FLEXOR CARPI RADIALIS

The flexor carpi radialis originates just inferior to the origin of the pronator teres and the common flexor tendon at the anteroinferior aspect of the medial epicondyle (see Fig. 2–43). It continues distally and radially to the wrist, where it can be easily palpated before it inserts into the base of the second and sometimes the third metacarpal. Proximally, the muscle belly partially covers the pronator teres and palmaris longus muscles and shares a common origin from the intermuscular septum, which it shares with these muscles. The innervation is from one or two twigs of the median nerve (C6, C7), and its chief function is as a wrist flexor. At the elbow, no significant flexion moment is present.[1, 21]

PALMARIS LONGUS

The palmaris longus muscle, when present, arises from the medial epicondyle, and from the septa it shares with the flexor carpi radialis and flexor carpi ulnaris (see Fig. 2–43).

It becomes tendinous in the proximal portion of the forearm and inserts into and becomes continuous with the palmar aponeurosis. It is absent in approximately 10 percent of extremities.[69] Its major function is as a donor tendon for reconstructive surgery, and it is innervated by a branch of the median nerve.

FLEXOR CARPI ULNARIS

The flexor carpi ulnaris is the most posterior of the common flexor tendons originating from the medial epicondyle (see Figs. 2–38 and 2–43). A second and larger source of origin is from the medial border of the coronoid and the proximal medial aspect of the ulna. The ulnar nerve enters and innervates (T7–8 and T1) the muscle between these two sites of origin with two or three motor branches given off just after the nerve has entered the muscle. These are the first motor branches of the ulnar nerve, and the function of the flexor carpi ulnaris is therefore useful in localizing the level of an ulnar nerve lesion. The muscle continues distally to insert into the pisiform, where the tendon is easily palpable, because it serves as a wrist flexor and ulnar deviator. With an origin posterior to the axis of rotation, weak elbow extension may also be provided by the flexor carpi ulnaris.[1]

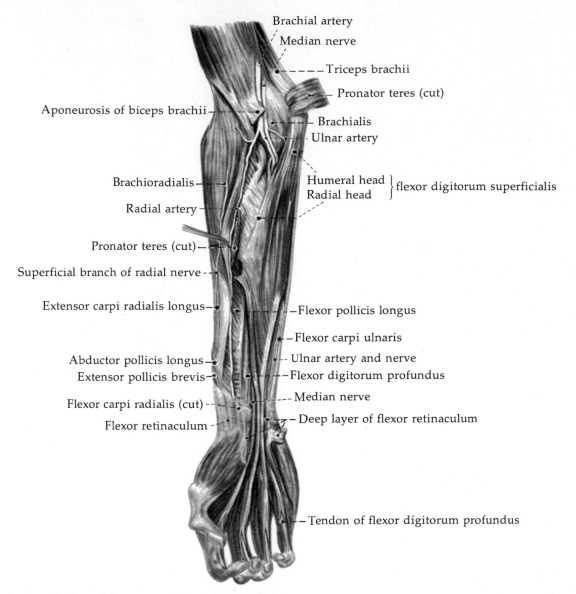

Brachial artery
Median nerve
Triceps brachii
Pronator teres (cut)
Aponeurosis of biceps brachii
Brachialis
Ulnar artery
Humeral head
Radial head } flexor digitorum superficialis
Brachioradialis
Radial artery
Pronator teres (cut)
Superficial branch of radial nerve
Extensor carpi radialis longus
Flexor pollicis longus
Flexor carpi ulnaris
Abductor pollicis longus
Ulnar artery and nerve
Extensor pollicis brevis
Flexor digitorum profundus
Median nerve
Flexor carpi radialis (cut)
Deep layer of flexor retinaculum
Flexor retinaculum
Tendon of flexor digitorum profundus

FIGURE 2–50 • The flexor digitorum superficialis is demonstrated after the palmaris longus and flexor carpi radialis has been removed. The pronator teres has been transected and reflected. The important relationships of the nerves and arteries should be noted. (From Langman, J., and Woerdeman, M. W.: Atlas of Medical Anatomy. Philadelphia, W. B. Saunders Co., 1976.)

FLEXOR DIGITORUM SUPERFICIALIS

The flexor digitorum superficialis muscle is deep to those originating from the common flexor tendon but superficial to the flexor digitorum profundus; thus, it is considered the intermediate muscle layer. This broad muscle has a complex origin (Fig. 2–50). Medially, it arises from the medial epicondyle by way of the common flexor tendon and possibly from the ulnar collateral ligament and the medial aspect of the coronoid.[36] The lateral head is smaller and thinner and arises from the proximal two thirds of the radius. The unique origin of the muscle forms a fibrous margin under which the median nerve and the ulnar artery emerge as they exit from the cubital fossa. The muscle is innervated by the median nerve (C7, C8, T1) with branches that originate before the median nerve enters the pronator teres. The action of the flexor digitorum superficialis is flexion of the proximal interphalangeal joints.

FLEXOR DIGITORUM PROFUNDUS

The flexor digitorum profundus originates from the proximal ulna distal to the elbow joint and is discussed only as appropriate for the given topic in subsequent chapters.

REFERENCES.

1. An, K. N., Hui, F. C., Morrey, B. F., Linscheid, R. L., and Chao, E. Y.: Muscles across the elbow joint: a biomechanical analysis. J. Biomechan. **14(10):**659, 1981.
2. Anson, B. J., and McVay, C. B.: Surgical Anatomy. Vol. 2., 5th ed. Philadelphia, W. B. Saunders Co., 1971.
3. Atkinson, W. B., and Elftman, H.: The carrying angle of the human arm as a secondary sex character. Anat. Rec. **91:**49, 1945.
4. Barnard, L. B., and McCoy, S. M.: The supracondyloid process of the humerus. J. Bone Joint Surg. **28(4):**845, 1946.
5. Basmajian, J. V., and Griffin, W. R.: Function of anconeus muscle. J. Bone Joint Surg. **54A:**1712, 1972.
6. Basmajian, J. V., and Latif, A.: Integrated actions and functions of

the two flexors of the elbow: a detailed myographic analysis. J. Bone Joint Surg. **39A:**1106, 1957.

7. Basmajian, J. V., and Travell, A.: Electromyography of the pronator muscles in the forearm. Anat. Rec. **139:**45, 1961.

8. Bateman, J. E.: Denervation of the elbow joint for the relief of pain: a preliminary report. J. Bone Joint Surg. **30B:**635, 1948.

9. Beals, R. K.: The normal carrying angle of the elbow. Clin. Orthop. Rel. Res. **119:**194, 1976.

10. Bert, J. M., Linscheid, R. L., and McElfresh, E. C.: Rotatory contracture of the forearm. J. Bone Joint Surg. **62A:**1163, 1980.

11. Boyd, H. B.: Surgical exposure of the ulna and proximal third of the radius through one incision. Surg. Gynecol. Obstet. **71:**86, 1940.

12. Boyd, H. D., and Anderson, L. D.: A method for reinsertion of the biceps tendon brachii tendon. J. Bone Joint Surg. **43A:**1141, 1961.

13. Bryan, R. S., and Morrey, B. F.: Extensive posterior exposure of the elbow: a triceps-sparing approach. Clin. Orthop. **166:**188, 1982.

14. Capener, N.: The vulnerability of the posterior interosseous nerve of the forearm: a case report and anatomic study. J. Bone Joint Surg. **48B:**770, 1966.

15. Carp, L.: Tennis elbow (epicondylitis) caused by radiohumeral bursitis. Arch. Surg. **24:**905, 1932.

16. Chen, J., Alk, D., Eventov, I., and Weintroub, S.: Development of the olecranon bursa: an anatomic cadaver study. Acta Orthop. Scand. **58:**408, 1987.

17. Congdon, E. D., and Fish, H. S.: The chief insertion of the biceps after neurosis in the ulna: a study of collagenous bundle patterns of antebrachial fascia and bicipital aponeurosis. Anat. Rec. **116:**395, 1953.

18. Cunningham, D. J.: Textbook of Anatomy, 12th ed. Edited by Romanes, G. J. New York, Oxford University Press, 1981.

19. DaHora, B.: Musculus Anconeus. Thesis, University of Recife, Recife, Brazil, 1959. Cited by Basmajian, J. V., and Griffin, W. R.: J. Bone Joint Surg. **54A:**1712, 1972.

20. Davies, F., and Laird, M.: The supinator muscle and the deep radial (posterior interosseous nerve). Anat. Rec. **101:**243, 1948.

21. Duchenne, G. B.: Physiology of Motion. Translated and edited by Kaplan, E. B. Philadelphia, J. B. Lippincott Co., 1949.

22. El-Hadidi, S., and Burke, F. D.: Posterior interosseous nerve syndrome caused by a bursa in the vicinity of the elbow. J. Hand Surg. **12B(1):**23, 1987.

23. Evans, E. M.: Rotational deformity in the treatment of fractures of both bones of the forearm. J. Bone Joint Surg. **27:**373, 1945.

24. Eycleshymer, A. C., and Schoemaker, D. M.: A Cross-Section Anatomy. New York, D. Appleton, 1930.

25. Field, J. H.: Posterior interosseous nerve palsy secondary to synovial chondromatosis of the elbow joint. J. Hand Surg. **6(4):**336, 1981.

26. Fuss, F. K.: The ulnar collateral ligament of the human elbow joint. Anatomy, function and biomechanics. J. Anat. **175:**203, 1991.

27. Gardner, E.: The innervation of the elbow joint. Anat. Rec. **102:**161, 1948.

28. Grant, J. C. B.: Atlas of Anatomy, 6th ed. Baltimore, Williams & Wilkins, 1972.

29. Gray, H.: Anatomy, Descriptive and Applied, 35th ed. Edited by Warwick, R., and Williams, P. L. Philadelphia, W. B. Saunders Co., 1980, pp. 429.

30. Gruber, W.: Monographie der Bursae mucosae cubitales. Mem. Acad. Sc. Petersburg **VII(7):**10, 1866.

31. Gruber, W.: Monographie les canalis supracondyloideus humeri. Mem. Acad. Sc. Petersburg. Cited by Morris, H.: Human Anatomy, 3rd ed. Philadelphia, Blakiston, 1953.

32. Guttierez, L. F.: A contribution to the study of the limiting factors of elbow fixation. Acta Anat. **56:**146, 1964.

33. Hamilton, A. T., and Raleigh, N. C.: Subcutaneous rupture of the brachioradialis muscle. Surgery **23:**806, 1948.

34. Henle, J.: Handbuch der Systematischen Anatomie des Menschen Muskellehre. Berlin, Braunschweig, 1866, p. 224.

35. Henry, A. K.: Extensile Exposure, 2nd ed. Baltimore, Williams & Wilkins, 1966.

36. Hollinshead, W. H.: The Back and Limbs. *In* Anatomy for Surgeons. Vol. 3, New York, Harper & Row, 1969, p. 379.

37. Hollinshead, W. H., and Markee, J. E.: The multiple innervation of limb muscles in man. J. Bone Joint Surg. **28:**721, 1946.

38. Jamieson, R. W., and Anson, B. J.: The relation of the median nerve to the heads of origin of the pronator teres muscle: a study of 300 specimens. Q. Bull Northwestern Univ. Med. School **26:**34, 1952.

39. Johansson, O.: Capsular and ligament injuries of the elbow joint. Acta Chir. Scand. (Suppl.) 287, 1962.

40. Kapandji, I. A.: The Physiology of Joints. Vol. I: Upper Limb, 2nd ed. Baltimore, Williams & Wilkins, 1970.

41. Keats, T. E., Teeslink, R., Diamond, A. E., and Williams, J. H.: Normal axial relationships of the major joints. Radiology **87:**904, 1966.

42. Kocher, T.: Textbook of Operative Surgery, 3rd ed. Translated by Stiles, H. J., and Paul, C. B. London, A. & C. Black, 1911.

43. Kolb, L. W., and Moore, R. D.: Fractures of the supracondylar process of the humerus. J. Bone Joint Surg. **49A(3):**532, 1967.

44. Langman, J., and Woerdeman, M. W.: Atlas of Medical Anatomy. Philadelphia, W. B. Saunders Co., 1976.

45. Lanz, T., and Wachsmuth, W.: Praktische Anatomie. ARM, Berlin, Springer, 1959.

46. Linell, E. A.: The distribution of nerves in the upper limb, with reference to variables and their clinical significance. J. Anat. **55:**79, 1921.

47. Lipmann, K., and Rang, M.: Supracondylar spur of the humerus. J. Bone Joint Surg. **48B(4):**765, 1966.

48. Loomis, L. K.: Reduction and after-treatment of posterior dislocation of the elbow: with special attention to the brachialis muscle and myositis ossificans. Am. J. Surg. **63:**56, 1944.

49. Malkawi, H.: Recurent dislocation of the elbow accompanied by ulnar neuropathy: a case report and review of the literature. Clin. Orthop. **161:**170, 1981.

50. Martin, B. F.: The annular ligament of the superior radial ulnar joint. J. Anat. **52:**473, 1958(a).

51. Martin, B. F.: The oblique cord of the forearm. J. Anat. **52:**609, 1958(b).

52. Masear, V. R., Hill, J. J., Jr., and Cohen, S. M.: Ulnar compression neuropathy secondary to the anconeus epitrochlearis muscle. J. Hand Surg. **13A(5):**720, 1988.

53. McCormick, L. J., Cauldwell, E. W., and Anson, B. J.: Brachial and antebrachial artery patterns: a study of 750 extremities. Surg. Gynecol. Obstet. **96:**43, 1953.

54. Monro, A.: A Description of All the Bursae Mucosae of the Human Body. London, 1788.

55. Morrey, B. F., and Chao, E. Y.: Passive motion of the elbow joint. A biomechanical analysis. J. Bone Joint Surg. **58A:**501, 1976.

56. Morrey, B. F., and An, K. N.: Functional anatomy of the elbow ligaments. Clin. Orthop. **201:**84, 1985.

57. Morrey, B. F., Askew, L., An, K. N., and Dobyns, J.: Rupture of the distal tendon of the biceps brachii. J. Bone Joint Surg. **67A:**418, 1985.

58. Morrey, B. F., Tanaka, S., and An, K. N.: Valgus stability of the elbow. A definition of primary and secondary constraints. Clin. Orthop. **265:**187, 1991.

59. Morris, H.: Human Anatomy, 11th ed. Edited by Schaeffer, J. P. Philadelphia, Blakiston, 1953.

60. O'Driscoll, S. W., Morrey, B. F., and An, K. N.: Intraarticular pressure and capacity of the elbow. Arthroscopy **6(2):**100, 1990.

61. O'Driscoll, S. W., Horii, E., and Morrey, B. F.: Anatomy of the attachment of the medial ulnar collateral ligament. J. Hand Surg. **17:**164, 1992.

62. O'Driscoll, S. W., Horii, E., Morrey, B. F., and Carmichael, S. W.: Anatomy of the ulnar part of the lateral collateral ligament of the elbow. Clin. Anat. **5:**296–303, 1992.

63. O'Driscoll, S. W., Horii, E., Carmichael, S. W., and Morrey, B. F.: The cubital tunnel and ulnar neuropathy. J. Bone Joint Surg. **73B(4):**613, 1991.

64. O'Driscoll, S. W., Bell, D. F., and Morrey, B. F.: Posterolateral rotatory instability of the elbow. J. Bone Joint Surg. **73A(3):**440, 1991.

65. Ogilvie, W. H.: Discussion on minor injuries of the elbow joint. Proc. R. Soc. Med. **23:**306, 1930.

66. Osgood, R. B.: Radiohumeral bursitis, epicondylitis, epicondylalgia (tennis elbow). Arch Surg. **4:**420, 1922.

67. Pankovich, A. M.: Anconeus approach to the elbow joint and the proximal part of the radius and ulna. J. Bone Joint Surg. **59A:**124, 1977.

68. Polonskaja, R.: Zur Frage der Arterienanastomosen im Gebiete der Ellenbogenbeuge des Menschen. Anat. Anz. **74:**303, 1932.

69. Reimann, A. F., Daseler, E. H., Anson, B. J., and Beaton, L. E.: The palmaris longus muscle and tendon: a study of 1600 extremities. Anat. Rec. **89:**495, 1944.

70. St. John, J. N., and Palmaz, J. C.: The cubital tunnel in ulnar entrapment neuropathy. Musculoskeletal Rad. **158:**119, 1986.
71. Schwab, G. H., Bennett, J. B., Woods, G. W., and Tullos, H. S.: The biomechanics of elbow stability: the role of the medial collateral ligament. Clin. Orthop. Rel. Res. **146:**42, 1980.
72. Shiba, R., Siu, D., and Sorbie, C.: Geometric analysis of the elbow joint. J. Ortho. Research **6:**897, 1988.
73. Simon, W. H., Friedenberg, S., and Richardson, S.: Joint congruence. J. Bone Joint Surg. **55A:**1614, 1973.
74. Sorbie, C., Shiba, R., Siu, D., Saunders, G., and Wevers, H.: The development of a surface arthroplasty for the elbow. Clin. Orthop. **208:**100, 1986.
75. Spalteholz, V.: Hand Atlas of Human Anatomy, 2nd ed. Edited and translated by Baker, L. F. Philadelphia, J. B. Lippincott Co., 1861.
76. Spinner, M., and Kaplan, E. B.: The quadrate ligament of the elbow: its relationship to the stability of the proximal radio-ulnar joint. Acta Orthop. Scand. **41:**632, 1970.
77. Steindler, A.: Kinesiology of the Human Body, 5th ed. Springfield, IL, Charles C Thomas, 1977.
78. Stimson, H.: Traumatic rupture of the biceps brachii. Am. J. Surg. **29:**472, 1935.
79. Strachan, J. H., and Ellis, B. W.: Vulnerability of the posterior interosseous nerve during radial head resection. J. Bone Joint Surg. **53B:**320, 1971.
80. Tanaka, S., An, K. N., and Morrey, B. F.: Kinematics of ulnohumeral joint under varus-valgus stress. J. Musculoskel. Res. **2:**45, 1998.
81. Terry, R. J.: New data on the incidence of the supracondylar variation. Am. J. Phys. Anthropol. **9:**265, 1926.
82. Thepaut-Mathieu, C., and Maton, B.: The flexor function of the m. pronator teres in man: a quantitative electromyographic study. Eur. J. Appl. Physiol. **54:**116, 1985.
83. Thomas, T. T.: A contribution to the mechanism of fractures and dislocations in the elbow region. Ann. Surg. **89:**108, 1929.
84. Thompson, H. C., III, and Garcia, A.: Myositis ossificans: aftermath of elbow injuries. Clin. Orthop. **50:**129, 1967.
85. Tillman, B.: A Contribution to the Function Morphology of Articular Surfaces. Translated by Konorza, G. Stuttgart, Georg Thieme, P. S. G. Publishing, 1978.
86. Travell, A., and Basmajian, J. V.: Electromyography of the supinators of the forearm. Anat. Rec. **139:**557, 1961.
87. Travell, A. A.: Electromyographic study of the extensor apparatus of the forearm. Anat. Rec. **144:**373, 1962.
88. Trotter, M.: Septal apertures in the humerus of American whites and negroes. Am. J. Phys. Anthropol. **19:**213, 1934.
89. Weiss, A-P., Hastings, H. II: The anatomy of the proximal radioulnar joint. J. Shoulder Elbow Surg. **1(4):**193–199, 1992.
90. Wright, W. B.: Muscle Function. New York, Hoeber, 1928; Hafner, 1962.
91. Yamaguchi, K., Sweet, F. A., Bindra, R., Morrey, B. F., Gelberman, R. H.: The extraosseous and intraosseous arterial anatomy of the adult elbow. J Bone Joint Surg. **79A:**1653–1662, 1997.

CHAPTER 3

Biomechanics of the Elbow

• KAI-NAN AN and BERNARD F. MORREY

INTRODUCTION

Upper extremity use depends largely on a functional elbow joint. A complex joint, the elbow serves as a link in the lever arm system that positions the hand, as a fulcrum of the forearm lever, and as a load-carrying joint. Mobility and stability of the elbow joint are necessary for daily, recreational, and professional activities. Loss of function in the elbow, possibly more than that in any other joint, can jeopardize individual independence.

In our practice, a working knowledge of biomechanics has been extremely important and rewarding. Clinical relevance includes elbow joint design and technique, the rationale and execution of trauma management, and ligament reconstruction. In short, a clear understanding of biomechanics provides a scientific basis for clinical practice.[10]

From the clinician's perspective, we have found the topic of elbow mechanics best discussed according to motion (kinematics), stability (constants), and strength (force transmission).

KINEMATICS

The elbow is described as a trochoginglymoid joint. That is, it possesses 2 degrees of freedom (motion): flexion-extension and supination-pronation. The articular components include the trochlea and capitellum on the medial and lateral aspects of the bifurcated distal humerus, and distally the upper end of the ulna and the head of the radius. The joint is thus composed of three articulations: the radiohumeral, the ulnohumeral, and the radioulnar.

Flexion-Extension

Because of the congruity at the ulnohumeral articulation and surrounding soft tissue constraint, elbow joint motion is considered primarily a hinge type. Yet, two separate three-dimensional studies of passive motion at the elbow revealed that the elbow does not function as a simple hinge joint.[49, 62] The position of the axis of elbow flexion, as measured from the intersection of the instantaneous axis with the sagittal plane, follows an irregular course. A type of helical motion of the flexion axis has been demonstrated.[62] This pattern was previously suggested[25, 48, 60] and was attributed to the obliquity of the trochlear groove along which the ulna moves.[50] An electromagnetic tracking device that allows a three-dimensional measurement of simulated active elbow joint motion reveals the amount of

potential varus-valgus and axial laxity that occurs during elbow flexion to average about 3 to 4 degrees. This has been confirmed with more advanced electromagnetic tracking technology.[97]

Center of Rotation

The axis of motion in flexion and extension has been the subject of many investigations.[59] Fischer (1909), using Reuleaux's technique, found the so-called locus of the instant center of rotation to be an area 2 to 3 mm in diameter at the center of the trochlea (Fig. 3–1). Subsequent experiments with the same technique described a much larger locus.[31] In a three-dimensional study of passive motion of the elbow joint, the observations of Fischer were confirmed by using the biplanar x-ray technique.[62] Based on direct experimental study as well as analytic investigation, Youm and associates[102] concluded that the axis does not change during flexion-extension. In our study, however, variations of up to 8 degrees in the position of the screw axis from individual to individual have been shown. As seen from below, the axis of rotation is internally rotated 3 to 8 degrees relative to the plane of the epicondyles. In the coronal plane, a line perpendicular to the axis of rotation forms a proximally and laterally opening angle of 4 to 8 degrees with the long axis of the humerus.[52] These data, coupled with the clinical information regarding implant loosening, have inspired the development of semiconstrained elbow joint replacement designs. It recently has been demonstrated that these designs do function as semiconstrained implants and allow for the normal out-of-plane rotations noted earlier (see Chapter 49).[77]

From a practical point of view, despite the different findings of various investigators, the deviation of the center

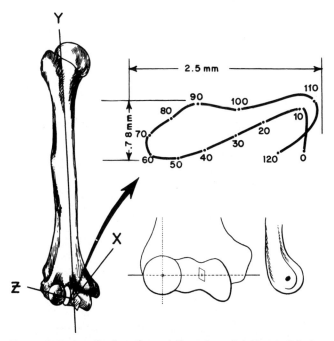

FIGURE 3–1 • Configuration and dimensions of the locus of the instant center of rotation of the elbow. This axis runs through the center of the articular surface, as viewed on both the anteroposterior (AP) and the lateral planes.

of joint rotation is minimal and the reported variation is probably due to limitations in the experimental design. Thus, the ulnohumeral joint could be assumed to move as a uniaxial articulation except at the extremes of flexion and extension. The axis of rotation passes through the center of the arcs formed by the trochlear sulcus and capitellum.[55]

The center of rotation can be identified from external landmarks. In the sagittal plane, the axis lies anterior to the midline of the humerus[88] and lies on a line that is colinear with the anterior cortex of the distal humerus.[62] The coronal orientation is defined by the plane of the posterior cortex of the distal humerus.[18] This axis emerges from the center of the projected center of the capitellum and from the anteroinferior aspect of the medial epicondyle (see Fig. 3–1).

Forearm Rotation

The radiohumeral joint, which forms the lateral half of the elbow joint, has a common transverse axis with the elbow joint, which coincides with the ulnohumeral axis during flexion-extension motion. In addition, the radius rotates around the ulna, allowing for forearm rotation or supination-pronation. In general, the longitudinal axis of the forearm is considered to pass through the convex head of the radius in the proximal radioulnar joint and through the convex articular surface of the ulna at the distal radioulnar joint.[33, 93] The axis therefore is oblique to the longitudinal axes of both the radius and the ulna (Fig. 3–2), and rotation is independent of elbow position.[43]

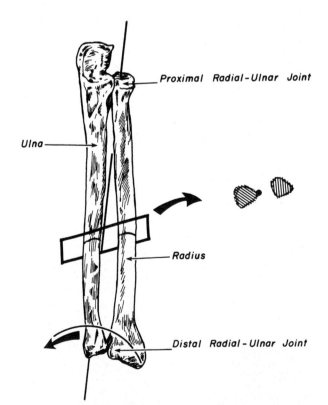

Proximal Radial-Ulnar Joint

Ulna

Radius

Distal Radial-Ulnar Joint

FIGURE 3–2 • The longitudinal axis of pronation-supination runs proximally from the distal end of the ulna to the center of the radial head. The axis is at the ulnar cortex in the distal one third of the forearm.

Mori has characterized the axis of forearm rotation as passing through the attachment of the interosseous membrane at the ulna in the distal fourth of the forearm (see Fig. 3–2).[61] This may have particular applications with regard to the sensitivity of forearm rotation to angular deformity in this particular portion of the bone. Clinically and experimentally, less than 10 percent angulation of either the radius or the ulna causes no functionally significant loss of forearm rotation.[87]

In the past, ulnar rotation was described as being coupled with forearm rotation.[100] This observation could not be reproduced in a subsequent study by Youm and associates.[102]

By using a metal rod introduced transversely into the ulna, extension, lateral rotation, and then flexion of the ulna was described with rotation from pronation to supination. The axial rotational movements of the ulna were also observed by others.[13, 21, 29, 42, 62, 85, 102]

Ray and associates[85] also suggested that varus-valgus movement of the ulna occurs if the forearm rotates on an axis extending from the head of the radius to the index finger. O'Driscoll and associates[74] have demonstrated external axial rotation of the ulna with forearm supination. Internal rotation or closure of the lateral ulnohumeral joint occurs with pronation.

Finally, the radius has been shown to migrate proximally with pronation.[66] This observation had not been reported previously but has been confirmed by observations at the wrist.[81]

Carrying Angle

The carrying angle is defined as that formed by the long axis of the humerus and the long axis of the ulna. It averages 10 to 15 degrees in men and is about 5 degrees greater in women.[1, 17, 51, 93]

However, uncertainty has arisen over the use of the term *carrying angle* in the dynamic setting. Dempster[27] described an oscillatory pattern during elbow flexion, while Morrey and Chao[62] reported a linear change with the valgus angle being the greatest at full extension and diminishing during flexion. The confusion arises because three descriptions based on different reference systems have been adopted for the measurement of carrying angle changes.

Definition 1. The carrying angle is the acute angle formed by the long axis of the humerus as the long axis of the ulna projects on the plane containing the humerus (Fig. 3–3A).

Definition 2. The carrying angle is described as the acute angle formed by the long axis of the ulna and the projection of the long axis of the humerus onto the plane of the ulna (see Fig. 3–3B).

Definition 3. The carrying angle is defined analytically as the abduction-adduction angle of the ulna with respect to the humerus when eulerian angles are being used to describe arm motion.

From an anatomic point of view, it is not difficult to conclude that the existence of the carrying angle is due to the existence of obliquities, or cubital angles, between the proximal humeral shaft, the trochlea, and the distal ulnar shaft. By assuming that the ulnohumeral joint is a pure hinge joint and that the axis of rotation coincides with the

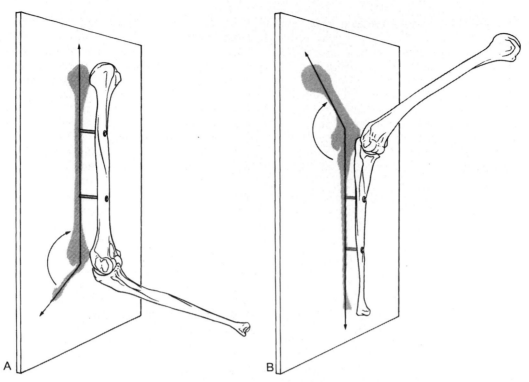

FIGURE 3–3 • A, Carrying angle between the humerus and the ulna as measured by viewing from the direction perpendicular to the plane containing the humeral and the flexion axes. Conventionally, the acute angle instead of the obtuse angle shown is used as the carrying angle measurement. B, Carrying angle between humerus and ulna as measured by viewing from the direction perpendicular to the plane containing the ulnar and flexion axes. Conventionally, the acute angle instead of the obtuse angle shown is based as the carrying angle measurement. (From An, K. N., Morrey, B. F., and Chao E. Y. S.: Carrying angle of the humeral elbow joint. J. Orthop. Res. 1:371, 1984.)

axis of the trochlea, the change in the carrying angle during flexion can be defined as a function of anatomic variations of the obliquity of the articulations according to simple trigonometric calculations.[7] If the first or second definition is accepted, the carrying angle changes minimally during flexion.

Restriction of Motion

In normal circumstances, elbow flexion ranges from 0 degree or slightly hyperextended to about 150 degrees in flexion. Forearm rotation averages from about 75 degrees (pronation) to 85 degrees (supination) (see Chapter 2). The cartilage of the trochlea forms an arc of about 320 degrees, while the sigmoid notch creates an arc of about 180 degrees. Generally, the arc of the radial head depression is about 40 degrees,[93] which articulates with the capitellum, presenting an angle of 180 degrees.

The significance of the 30-degree anterior angulation of the trochlea with the 30-degree posterior orientation of the greater sigmoid notch to flexion and extension and stability of the elbow joint is discussed in detail in Chapter 1 (Fig. 3–4). Kapandji[50] suggests that the factors limiting joint extension are the impact of the olecranon process on the olecranon fossa and the tension of the anterior ligament and the flexor muscles. Others have described tautness of the anterior bundle of the medial collateral ligament as serving as a check to extension.[39] The anterior muscle bulk of the arm and forearm, along with contraction of the triceps, is also reported to prevent active flexion beyond

145 degrees.[50] However, the factors limiting passive flexion include the impact of the head of the radius against the radial fossa, the impact of the coronoid process against the coronoid fossa, and tension from the capsule and triceps.

For pronation and supination, Braune and Flugel[19] found that passive resistance of the stretched antagonist muscle restricts the excursion range more than that of the ligamentous structures.[19] Spinner and Kaplan, however, have shown that the quadrate ligament does provide some static constraint to forearm rotation.[92] Impingement of tissue restrains pronation, especially by the flexor pollicis longus, which is forced against the deep finger flexors. The entire range of

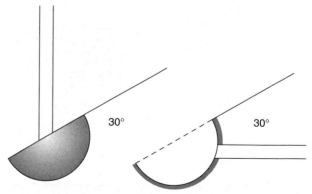

FIGURE 3–4 • The distal humeral forward flexion is complemented by a 30-degree posterior rotation of the opening of the greater sigmoid notch. (With permission, Mayo Foundation.)

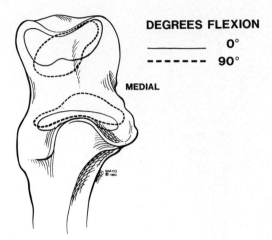

DEGREES FLEXION

——————— 0°

- - - - - - - 90°

MEDIAL

FIGURE 3–5 • Contact in the sigmoid fossa moves toward the center of the fossa during elbow flexion. (Redrawn from Walker, P. S.: Human Joints and Their Artificial Replacements. Springfield, IL, Charles C Thomas, 1977.)

active excursion in an intact arm is about 150 degrees, whereas when the muscles are removed from a cadaver specimen the range increases to 185 to 190 degrees. With cutting the ligaments, the range increased up to 205 to 210 degrees.

Capacity and Contact Area of the Elbow Joint

The capacity of the elbow joint recently has been shown to average about 25 ml. The maximum capacity is observed to occur with the elbow at about 80 degrees of flexion.[76] This explains the clinical observation that stiff elbows tend to have fixed deformities at about 80 to 90 degrees of flexion.[68]

Accurate measurement of the contact points of the elbow is extremely difficult, and several techniques have been applied to this highly congruous joint.[95] Silicone casting,

Fuji Prescale film, and reversible cartilage staining are most commonly used. Each has advantages and disadvantages. The contact area of the articular surface during elbow joint motion has been investigated by Goodfellow and Bullough, using a staining technique.[38] They found that the central depression of the radial head articulates with the dome of the capitellum and that the medial triangular facet was always in contact with the ulna. The upper rim of the radial head made no contact at all. At the humeroulnar joint, the articular surfaces were always in contact during some phases of movement. At a particular angle, there were two narrow bands of contact across the trochlear surface in young specimens, but a more diffuse contact area was present in older specimens. Others have verified these observations.[101] The contact areas on the ulna occurred anteriorly and posteriorly and tended to move together and slightly inward from each side from 0 to 90 degrees of flexion and with increasing load.[30, 73] Using wax as a casting material, the shape and size of the contact were shown to change areas in different elbow positions.[36] In full extension, the contact was observed to be on the lower medial aspect of the ulna, while in other postures the pressure areas described a strip extending from posterolateral to anteromedial. The radiocapitellar joint also revealed contact during flexion under no externally applied load. Investigations in our laboratory show that the contact areas of the elbow occur at four "facets"—two at the coronoid and two at the olecranon (Fig. 3–5). Similar patterns were present when both casting and staining techniques were used, and only a slight increase in total surface area occurred with elbow flexion and with a sevenfold increase in load.[95] An analysis[30] showed, with 10N load, about 9 percent contact of the articular surfaces, and with 1280 N, the area increased to about 73 percent.

When varus and valgus loads are applied to the forearm, the contact changes medially and laterally. This implies a pivot point about which the radioulnar articulation rotates on the humerus in the anteroposterior (AP) plane in extension with varus and valgus stress. In vivo experiments have demonstrated the varus-valgus pivot point of the elbow to

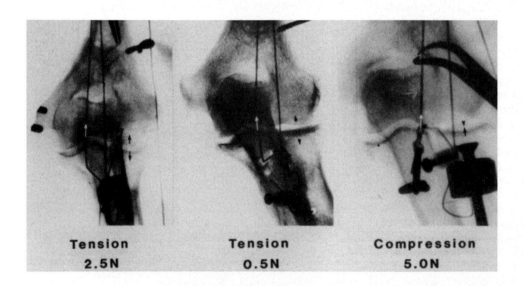

Tension 2.5N   **Tension 0.5N**   **Compression 5.0N**

FIGURE 3–6 • The line of action in the muscles produces a compression force at the radial head when situated just lateral to the middle of the lateral face of the trochlea, and a tension force on the radial head is situated just medial to this point. This indicates that the varus-valgus pivot point in the elbow lies at that point on the AP plane. (From Morrey, B. F., An, K. N., and Stormont, T. J.: Force transmission through the radial head. J. Bone Joint Surg. **70A**:254, 1988.)

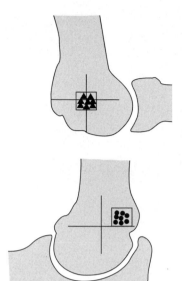

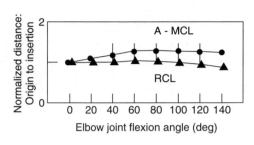

FIGURE 3–7 • The anterior medial collateral ligament remains more taut during elbow flexion than does the posterior segment of the ligament. The radial collateral ligament originates at the axis of rotation for elbow flexion; hence, the ligament has little length variation during flexion and extension. (With permission, Mayo Foundation.)

reside in the midpoint of the lateral face of the trochlea (Fig. 3–6).

ELBOW STABILITY

The elbow is one of the most congruous joints of the musculoskeletal system and, as such, is one of the most stable. This feature is the result of an almost equal contribution from the soft tissue constraints and the articular surfaces.

The static soft tissue stabilizers include the collateral ligament complexes and the anterior capsule. The descriptions of the anatomy of the lateral collateral ligament provided by Morrey and associates[65] and elaborated on by O'Driscoll and associates[75] and others[35, 78, 91] have been discussed previously (see Chapter 2). The lateral collateral ligament originates from the lateral condyle at a point through which the axis of rotation passes. Conversely, the medial collateral ligament has two discrete components, neither of which originates at a site that lies on the axis of rotation.[64, 89] The anterior bundle has been further subdivided according to function. The anterior portion of the anterior bundle is taut in extension; the converse is true for the posterior fibers of the anterior bundle. Because elbow joint motion occurs about a nearly perfect hinge axis through the center of the capitellum and trochlea, different parts of the medial collateral ligament complex will be taut at different positions of elbow flexion (Fig. 3–7). The lateral collateral ligament lying on the axis of rotation, however, will assume a rather uniform tension, regardless of elbow position. The description of the anatomy of the lateral ulnar collateral ligament has been expanded.[22, 64, 75, 79] This ligament inserts on the ulna and, as such, helps to stabilize the lateral ulnohumeral joint (Fig. 3–8). In experiments performed in our laboratory, O'Driscoll and associates have demonstrated that the lateral ulnar collateral ligament is essential to control the pivot shift maneuver (see Chapter 4). Further evidence of the contribution of the lateral ligament complex to elbow stability is offered by

Søjbjerg and associates.[90] These investigators attributed a major role in varus and valgus stability to the annular ligament. Although our work suggests that the major component in the varus and rotatory stability is the structure termed the *lateral ulnar collateral ligament*, the parallel findings of these investigators suggest that the lateral complex is, in fact, a major stabilizer of the elbow joint and functions with or without the radial head. This lateral complex is also an important stabilizer in forced varus and external rotation.[80]

Articular and Ligamentous Interaction

The influence of the ligamentous and articular components on joint stability are usually studied with the use of the materials testing machine by imparting a given and controlled displacement to the elbow.[45, 63, 84] The relative contribution of each stabilizing structure can be demonstrated by sequentially eliminating each element and observing the load recorded by the load cell for the constant displacement imparted, usually 2 to 5 degrees[91] (Fig. 3–9).

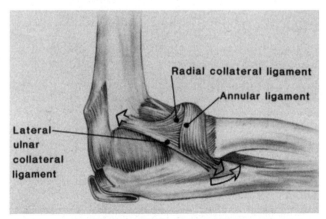

FIGURE 3–8 • The orientation and attachment of the lateral collateral ligament stabilizes the ulna to resist varus and rotatory stresses just as the medial ligament resists valgus stress.

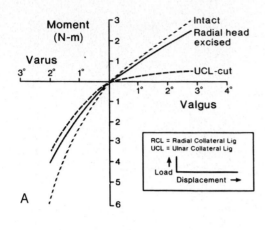

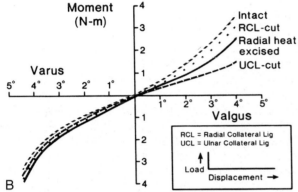

FIGURE 3–9 • Force displacement curves demonstrate relative contribution of elements to elbow stability in extension *(A)* and flexion *(B)*. (From Morrey, B.F., and An, K.N.: Articular and ligamentous contributions to the stability of the elbow joint. Am. J. Sports Med. **11**:315, 1983.)

• TABLE 3–1 • **Percent Contribution of Restraining Varus-Valgus Displacement**			
Position	Component	Varus	Valgus
Extension	MCL*	—	30
	LCL†	15	—
	Capsule	30	40
	Articulation	55	30
Flexion	MCL*	—	55
	LCL†	10	—
	Articulation	75	35

*MCL = medial collateral ligament complex.
†LCL = lateral collateral ligament complex.

A simplified summary of the observations from such an experiment is shown in Table 3–1. In extension, the anterior capsule provides about 70 percent of the soft tissue restraint to distraction, whereas the medial collateral ligament assumes this function at 90 degrees of flexion. Varus stress is checked in extension equally by the joint articulation (55 percent) and the soft tissue, lateral collateral ligament, and capsule. In flexion, the articulation provides 75 percent of the varus stability. Valgus stress in extension is equally divided between the medial collateral ligament, the capsule, and the joint surface. With flexion, the capsular contribution is assumed by the medial collateral ligament, which is the primary stabilizer (54 percent) to valgus stress at this position. Furthermore, for all practical purposes, the anterior portion of the medial collateral ligament provides virtually all of the structure's functional contribution.

Limitations of this experimental model have resulted in an overestimation of the role of the radial head in resisting valgus load.[45, 63, 86] This has prompted the development of an experimental technique that allows simultaneous and accurate measurement of three-dimensional angular and translational changes under given loading conditions (Fig. 3–10). Using the electromagnetic tracking device, an accurate technique for measuring the function of the articular and capsuloligamentous structures was developed.[67] More accurate and relevant data were generated.[67] Valgus stability is resisted primarily by the medial collateral ligament. With an intact medial collateral ligament, the radial head does not offer any significant additional valgus constraint (Fig. 3–11). With a released or compromised medial collateral ligament, the radial head does resist valgus stress (Fig. 3–12). This important experiment documents that the radial head is a secondary stabilizer for resisting valgus stress, whereas the medial collateral ligament is the primary stabilizer against valgus force (Fig. 3–13). In a laboratory investigation, the hyperextension trauma produces lesions of the anterior capsule, the avulsion of proximal insertions of both medial and lateral collateral ligaments.[99] The degree of extension increased by 17 degrees and induced signifi-

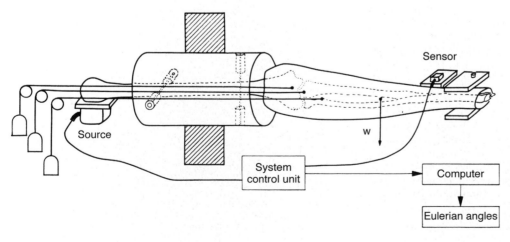

FIGURE 3–10 • The arrangement of the electromagnetic tracking device allows varus-valgus stresses applied to the elbow during simulated motion with the flexor and extensor muscles. Real-time simultaneous three-dimensional motion of the forearm may be monitored with reference to the humerus.

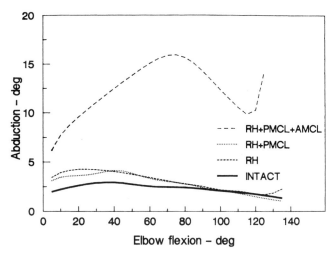

FIGURE 3–11 • With removal of the radial head, little increased valgus stress is noted. With subsequent release of the medial collateral ligament, the elbow subluxes. (With permission from Morrey, B. F., Tanaka, S., and An, K. N.: Valgus stability of the elbow. Clin. Orthop. Rel. Res. **265**:187, 1991.)

cant joint laxity in forced valgus internal-external rotation, but not varus.[99]

The contribution of the articular geometry to elbow stability was further evaluated by serial removal of portions of the proximal ulna, as shown in Figure 3–14.[8] Valgus stress, both in extension and at 90 degrees of flexion, was primarily (75 to 85 percent) resisted by the proximal half of the sigmoid notch, whereas varus stress was resisted primarily by the distal half, or the coronoid portion of the articulation, both in extension (67 percent) and in flexion (60 percent).

As demonstrated in subsequent chapters, for instability the critical role of the coronoid is emerging. As serial portions of the coronoid are removed the elbow becomes progressively more unstable (Fig. 3–15). This is especially

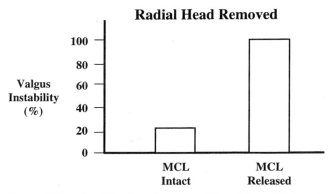

FIGURE 3–13 • The schematic representation of the stabilizing role of the radial head to valgus stress. The fact that the radial head is important only when the medial collateral ligament is released defines the radial head as the secondary stabilizer against valgus stress.

true if the radial head has been resected (Fig. 3–16). In this instance, as little as 25 percent resection causes elbow subluxation at about 70 degrees of flexion. Clinically, we have observed the useful observation that a line from the tip of the olecranon parallel with the ulna shaft passes through the middle of the trochlea.[69] This allows the clinician to estimate the critical 50 percent coronoid loss (Fig. 3–17).

FORCE ACROSS ELBOW JOINT

Study of the force across the elbow joint is not an easy task. The analysis can be performed at various degrees of sophistication. It can be either two-dimensional or three-dimensional, static or dynamic, with or without the hand activities. The clinical implications of these forces are obvious, but the magnitudes are not common knowledge. Consequently, in this section, the factors that affect the

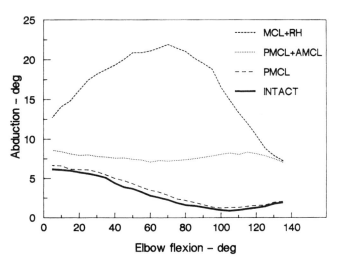

FIGURE 3–12 • When the medial collateral ligament is first released, a valgus stress produces some increased laxity of about 5 to 10 degrees. When the radial head is then removed, the elbow subluxes. (From Morrey, B. F., Tanaka, S., and An, K. N.: Valgus stability of the elbow. Clin. Orthop. Rel. Res. **265**:187, 1991.)

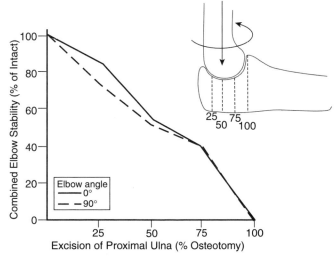

FIGURE 3–14 • Removal of successive portions of the proximal ulna was studied for its effect on various modes of joint stability. A linear decrease of combined stability is observed, with removal of the olecranon. Note a similar effect for both the extended and the 90-degree flexed positions.

Tricep Strength Tension Relationship

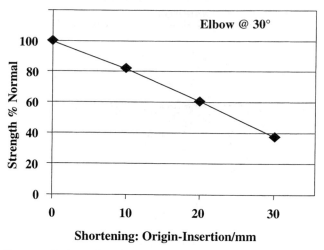

FIGURE 3-24 • Length-tension relationship for the triceps with the elbow at 30 degrees of flexion.

contraction and to show the phasic distribution of muscular activities for a given task.

FLEXORS

Surface electrodes along the belly of the biceps were first used[96] to record electrical activity during dynamic flexion and extension, with and without load. This early study showed a decrease in biceps activity in pronation compared with supination, and that the biceps acted in extension to "brake" the forearm.

Subsequent studies have presented inconsistent data, but in almost all investigations the biceps demonstrates no[15] or decreased activity when flexion occurs in pronation.[34, 58, 94] As expected, little influence is reflected in the brachialis muscle with forearm rotation.[34, 94] The brachioradialis demonstrates electrical activity with flexion, especially with the forearm rotated to the neutral position[16, 28] or in pronation.[34, 53, 94]

These data are summarized for the 90-degree flexion position, because this is the position of maximum strength[14, 53] and of greatest electrical activity of the elbow flexors.[34]

EXTENSORS

Electromyographic investigations of the elbow extensor muscles were first completed by Travill in 1962.[98] The medial head of the triceps and anconeus muscles were found to be active during extension; the lateral and long head of the triceps acted as auxiliaries. The anconeus also was active during resisted pronation and supination. In fact, the anconeus has been demonstrated to be active during flexion and abduction-adduction resisted motions.[34, 82] Thus, the anconeus may be considered a stabilizer of the elbow joint, being active with almost all motions.

In 1972, Currier studied the same muscles at 60, 90, and 120 degrees of elbow flexion. The greatest electrical activity occurred at the 90-degree and 120-degree positions, consistent with the position of greatest strength.[23] Others[54] found there was no difference between position and muscular electrical activity.

Electromyographic data of the elbow muscles have thus provided the following information: (1) the biceps is generally less active in full pronation of the forearm, probably owing to its secondary role as a supinator; (2) the brachialis is active in most ranges of function and is believed to be the "workhorse" of flexion; (3) there is an increase of electrical activity of the triceps with increased elbow flexion, probably secondary to an increased stretch reflex; (4) the anconeus shows activity in all positions and, hence, is considered a dynamic joint stabilizer; and (5) generally speaking, the different heads of the triceps and biceps are active in the same manner through most motion.

FOREARM MUSCLES

Some of the forearm muscles originating at the medial and lateral aspects of the distal humerus had been considered in stabilizing the elbow joint. Flexor carpi ulnaris and flexor digitorum superficialis muscles, because of their positions and proximities over the medial collateral ligaments, were potentially the muscles best suited to provide medial elbow support.[24] However, in the electromyographic investigations, no significant activities of these muscles were noted when valgus and varus stresses were applied.[34] In a recent study of baseball pitchers with medial collateral ligament insufficiency, the data did not demonstrate increased electrical activity of these muscles.[41] These findings suggested that the muscles on the medial side of the elbow do not supplement the role of medial collateral ligaments.[41]

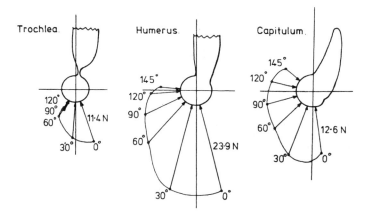

FIGURE 3-25 • Orientation and magnitude of forces at the humeral articular surface during flexion, per unit of force at the hand. (From Amis, A. A., Dowson, D., and Wright, V.: Elbow joint force predictions for some strenuous isometric actions. J. Biomech. 13:765, 1980.)

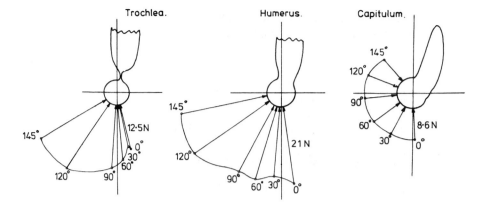

FIGURE 3–26 • Orientation and magnitude of forces at the humeral articulating surface during extension, per unit of force at the hand. (From Amis, A. A., Dowson, D., and Wright V.: Elbow joint force predictions for some strenuous isometric actions. J. Biomech. **13**:765, 1980.)

DISTRIBUTIVE FORCES ON THE ARTICULAR SURFACES

Joint compressive forces on various facets of the elbow joint have been reported in the literature.[3, 72] During the activities of resisting flexion and extension moments at various elbow joint positions, the components of force along the mediolateral direction, causing varus-valgus stress, are small compared with those acting in the sagittal plane directed anteriorly or posteriorly. The resultant joint forces on the trochlea and capitellum have been described in the sagittal plane for flexion (Fig. 3–25) and extension (Fig. 3–26) isometric loads. With the elbow extended and axially loaded, the distribution of stress across the joint has been calculated to be approximately 40 percent across the ulnohumeral joint and 60 percent across the radiohumeral articulation (Fig. 3–27).[40, 101] More recently, based on a cadaveric study,[44, 57] it has been noted that with the elbow in valgus realignment, only 12 percent of the axial load is transmitted through the proximal end of the ulna, but with

the elbow in varus alignment, 93 percent of the axial force is transmitted to proximal ulna. Because of the poor mechanical advantage with the elbow in extension, the largest isometric flexion forces occur in this position (see Fig. 3–26).[3, 46] Isometric extension produces a posterosuperior compressive stress across the distal humerus. These analytic calculations have undergone experimental confirmation. Using a force transducer at the proximal radius, the greatest force was transmitted across the radiohumeral joint in full extension, a position in which the muscles have poor mechanical advantage.[66]

When the elbow is flexed, inward rotation of the forearm against resistance imposes large torque to the joint. The magnitudes have been calculated as approaching twice body weight tension in the medial collateral ligament and three times body weight at the radiohumeral joint.[4] Experimental data from the force transducer study suggest that the analytic estimate is probably too high. The greatest force on the radial head from the transducer data occurs with the forearm in pronation (Fig. 3–28). Even in this position, however, the maximum possible force transmission at the radiohumeral joint was measured as approximately 0.9 times the body weight.[66]

Considerably less knowledge is available regarding the

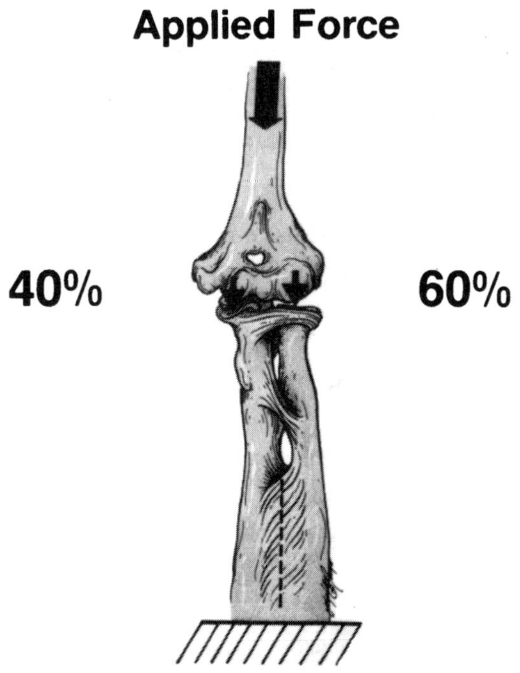

Applied Force

40%   **60%**

FIGURE 3–27 • Static compression of the extended elbow places more force on the radiohumeral than the ulnohumeral joint.

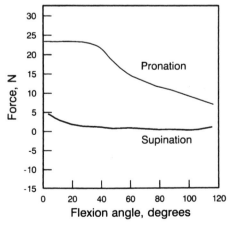

FIGURE 3–28 • Consistently greater force transmission occurs with the forearm in pronation than in supination. This indicates that a screwhole mechanism exists with the proximal radial migration occurring during this maneuver. (From Morrey, B. F., An, K. N., and Stormont, T. J.: Force transmission through the radial head. J. Bone Joint Surg. **70A**:250, 1988.)

dimensional quantitative motion analysis of the elbow joint. J. Jpn. Orthop. Assoc. **53**:989, 1979.

50. Kapandji, I. A.: The Physiology of the Joint: The Elbow: Flexion and Extension, 2nd ed. Vol. 1. London, Livingstone, 1970.
51. Keats, T. E., Tuslink, R., Diamond, A. E., and Williams, J. H.: Normal axial relationship of the major joints. Radiology **87**:904, 1966.
52. Von Lanz, T., and Wachsmuth, W.: Praktische Anatomie. Berlin, Springer-Verlag, 1959.
53. Larson, R. F.: Forearm positioning on maximal elbow-flexor force. Phys. Ther. **49**:748, 1969.
54. LeBozec, S., Maton, B., and Cnockaert, J. C.: The synergy of elbow extensor muscles during static work in man. Eur. J. Appl. Physiol. **43**:57, 1980.
55. London, J. T.: Kinematics of the elbow. J. Bone Joint Surg. **63A**:529, 1981.
56. McGarvey, S. R., Morrey, B. F., Askew, L. J., and An, K. N.: Reliability of isometric strength testing—temporal factors and strength variation. Clin. Orthop. **185**:301, 1984.
57. Markolf, K. L., Lamey, D., Yang, S., Meals, R., and Hotchkiss, R.: Radioulnar load-sharing in the forearm: A study in cadavera. J. Bone Joint Surg. **80A**:879, 1998.
58. Maton, B., and Bouisset, S.: The distribution of activity among the muscles of a single group during isometric contraction. Eur. J. Appl. Physiol. **37**:101, 1977.
59. Meissner, G.: Lokomotion des Ellbogengelenkes Ber ubd. Fortschr. d. Anat. u Physiol., 1856.
60. Messier, R. H., Duffy, J., Litchman, H. M., Pasley, P. R., Soechting, J., and Stewart, P. A.: The electromyogram as a measure of tension in the human biceps and triceps muscles. Int. J. Mech. Sci. **13**:585, 1971.
61. Mori, K.: Experimental study on rotation of the forearm. J. Jpn. Orthop. Assoc. **59**:611, 1985.
62. Morrey, B. F., and Chao, E. Y. S.: Passive motion of the elbow joint. J. Bone Joint Surg. **58A**:501, 1976.
63. Morrey, B. F., and An, K. N.: Articular and ligamentous contributions to the stability of the elbow joint. Am. J. Sports Med. **11**:315, 1983.
64. Morrey, B. F., and An, K. N.: Functional anatomy of the ligaments of the elbow. Clin. Orthop. **201**:84, 1985.
65. Morrey, B. F., Askew, L. J., and An, K. N.: Strength function after elbow arthroplasty. Clin. Orthop. **234**:43, 1988.
66. Morrey, B. F., An, K. N., and Stormont, T. J.: Force transmission through the radial head. J. Bone Joint Surg. **70A**:250, 1988.
67. Morrey, B. F., Tanaka, S., and An, K. N.: Valgus stability of the elbow. Clin. Orthop. **265**:187, 1991.
68. Morrey, B. F.: Post-traumatic contracture of the elbow: Operative treatment including distraction arthroplasty. J. Bone Joint Surg. **72A**:601, 1990.
69. Morrey, B. F.: Complex instability of the elbow. J. Bone Joint Surg. **79A**:460, 1997.
70. Motzkin, N. E., Cahalan, T. D., Morrey, B. F., An, K. N., and Chao, E. Y. S.: Isometric and isokinetic endurance testing of the forearm complex. Am. J. Sports Med. **19**:107, 1991.
71. Nemoto, K., Itoh, Y., Horiuchi, Y., and Sasaki, T.: Advancement of the insertion of the biceps brachii muscle: A technique for increasing elbow flexion force. J. Shoulder Elbow Surg. **5**:433, 1996.
72. Nicol, A. C., Berme, N., and Paul, J. P.: A biomechanical analysis of elbow joint function. *In* Joint Replacement in the Upper Limb. London, Institute of Mechanical Engineers, 1977, p. 45.
73. Nobuta, S.: Pressure distribution on the elbow joint and its change according to positions. J. Jpn. Soc. Clin. Biomech. Res. **13**:17, 1991.
74. O'Driscoll, S. W., Bell, D. F., and Morrey, B. F.: Posterolateral rotatory instability of the elbow. J. Bone Joint Surg. **73A**:440, 1991.
75. O'Driscoll, S. W., Horii, E., Morrey, B. F., and Carmichael, S.: Anatomy of the ulnar part of the lateral collateral ligament of the elbow. Clin. Anat. **5**:296, 1992.
76. O'Driscoll, S. W., Morrey, B. F., and An, K. N.: Intraarticular pressure and capacity of the elbow. Arthroscopy **6**:100, 1990.
77. O'Driscoll, S. W., Tanaka, S., An, K. N., and Morrey, B. F.: The kinematics of the semiconstrained total elbow prosthesis. J. Bone Joint Surg. **74B**:297, 1992.

78. Olsen, B. S., Henriksen, M. G., Søjbjerg, J. O., Helmig, P., and Sneppen, O.: Elbow joint instability: A kinematic model. J. Shoulder Elbow Surg. **3**:143, 1994.
79. Olsen, B. S., Vaesel, M. T., Søjbjerg, J. O., Helmig, P., and Sneppen, O.: Lateral collateral ligament of the elbow joint: Anatomy and kinematics. J. Shoulder Elbow Surg. **5 (2 Pt 1)**:103, 1996.
80. Olsen, B. S., Søjbjerg, J. O., Dalstra, M., and Sneppen, O.: Kinematics of the lateral ligamentous constraints of the elbow joint. J. Shoulder Elbow Surg. **5**:333, 1996.
81. Palmer, A. K., Glisson, R. R., and Werner, F. W.: Ulnar variance determination. J. Hand Surg. **7**:376, 1982.
82. Pauly, J. E., Rushing, J. L., and Schieving, L. E.: An electromyographic study of some muscles crossing the elbow joint. Anat. Rec. **159**:47, 1967.
83. Pauwels, F.: Biomechanics of Locomotor Apparatus. Translated by P. Maquet and R. Furlong. Berlin, Springer-Verlag, 1980.
84. Pryble, C. R., Kester, M. A., Cook, S. D., Edmund, J. O., and Brunet, M. E.: The effect of the radial head and prosthetic radial head replacement on resisting valgus stress at the elbow. Orthopedics **9**:723, 1986.
85. Ray, R. D., Johnson, R. J., and Jameson, R. M.: Rotation of the forearm: An experimental study of pronation supination. J. Bone Joint Surg. **33A**:993, 1951.
86. Regan, W. D., Korinek, S. L., Morrey, B. F., and An, K. N.: Biomechanical study of ligaments around the elbow joint. Clin. Orthop. **271**:170, 1991.
87. Sarmiento, A., Ebramzadeh, E., Brys, D., and Tarr, R.: Angular deformities and forearm function. J. Orthop. Res. **10**:121, 1992.
88. Schlein, A. P.: Semiconstrained total elbow arthroplasty. Clin. Orthop. **121**:222, 1976.
89. Schwab, G. H., Bennett, J. B., Woods, G. W., and Tullos, H.: Biomechanics of elbow instability: The role of the medial collateral ligament. Clin. Orthop. **146**:42, 1980.
90. Søjbjerg, J. O., Ovesen, J., and Gundorf, C. E.: The stability of the elbow following excision of the radial head and transection of the annular ligament. Arch. Orthop. Trauma Surg. **106**:248, 1987.
91. Søjbjerg, J. O., Ovesen, J., and Nielsen, S.: Experimental elbow stability after transection of the medial collateral ligament. Clin. Orthop. **218**:186, 1987.
92. Spinner, M., and Kaplan, E. B.: The quadrate ligament of the elbow: Its relationship to the stability of the proximal radio-ulnar joint. Acta Orthop. Scand. **41**:632, 1970.
93. Steindler, A.: Kinesiology of the Human Body Under Normal and Pathological Conditions. Springfield, IL, Charles C Thomas, 1955, p. 493.
94. Stevens, A., Stijns, H., Reybrouck, T., et al.: A polyelectromyographical study of the arm muscles at gradual isometric loading. Electromyogr. Clin. Neurophysiol. **13**:465, 1973.
95. Stormont, T. J., An, K. N., Morrey, B. F., and Chao, E. Y.: Elbow joint contact study: Comparison of techniques. J. Biomech. **18**:329, 1985.
96. Sullivan, W. E., Mortensen, O. A., Miles, M., and Greene, L. S.: Electromyographic studies of m. biceps brachii during normal voluntary movement at the elbow. Anat. Rec. **107**:243, 1950.
97. Tanaka, S., An, K.-N., and Morrey, B. F.: Kinematics and laxity of ulnohumeral joint under valgus-varus stress. J. Musculoskel. Res. **2**:45, 1998.
98. Travill, A. A.: Electromyographic study of the extensor apparatus of the forearm. Anat. Rec. **144**:373, 1962.
99. Tyrdal, S.: Combined hyperextension and supination of the elbow joint induces lateral ligament lesions: An experimental study of the pathoanatomy and kinematics in elbow ligament injuries. Knee Surg. **6**:36, 1998.
100. Von Meyer, H. Cited in Steindler, A.: Kinesiology of the Human Body Under Normal and Pathological Conditions. Springfield, IL, Charles C Thomas, 1955, p. 490.
101. Walker, P. S.: Human Joints and Their Artificial Replacements. Springfield, IL, Charles C Thomas, 1977, p. 182.
102. Youm, Y., Dryer, R. F., Thambyrajah, K., Flatt, A. E., and Sprague, B. L.: Biomechanical analysis of forearm pronation-supination and elbow flexion-extension. J. Biomech. **12**:245, 1979.

Diagnostic Considerations

• CHAPTER 4 •

PHYSICAL EXAMINATION OF THE ELBOW

• WILLIAM D. REGAN and BERNARD F. MORREY

GENERAL CONSIDERATIONS

Observations regarding the systematic elbow examination has been discussed elsewhere.[5, 9, 11, 15] This chapter focuses on the pathologic expectations of the examination.

HISTORY

A precise history is essential to accurately identify the singular nature of a problem. Pain is the most common complaint. The severity of the pain and whether it is intermittent or constant, the quantity and type of analgesia used, and the association of night pain are all important characteristics. The functional compromise experienced, whether it be recreational activity or activities of daily living, should be discussed. Frequently, the patient who has lived with chronic pain, such as that accompanying rheumatoid arthritis, has learned certain accommodative activities that have assisted in lessening or eliminating pain from a conscious level.

Functionally, the elbow is the most important joint of the upper extremity, because it places the hand in space away from or toward the body. It provides the linkage, allowing the hand to be brought to the torso, head, or mouth. Because the elbow is one of three important joints of the upper extremity that permit the hand to be placed in an infinite variety of positions, the examiner must be aware of the interplay of shoulder and wrist function as they complement the usefulness of the elbow. However, a considerable limitation of elevation and abduction function can exist at the shoulder complex without producing an appreciable compromise in most activities of daily living. This is true because only a relatively small amount of shoulder flexion and rotation is necessary to place the hand about the head or posteriorly about the waist or hip, and scapulothoracic motion can compensate for glenohumeral motion loss. Full pronation and supination can be achieved only when both the proximal and distal radioulnar joints are normal in their relationships for the full length of the radius. Thus, a loss of forearm rotation may suggest not only a problem with the elbow but also residual shortening or, more importantly, malrotation of the radius secondary to fracture.[24] There also may exist distal radioulnar joint incongruence, congenital or idiopathic abnormality of either radius or ulna.[6]

Conditions involving the lateral compartment of the elbow—that is, the radiocapitellar articulation—generally provoke pain that extends over the lateral aspect of the elbow with radiation proximally to midhumerus or distally over the forearm. The pain may be superficial directly over the lateral epicondyle or radial head, for example, or deep, localized poorly in the area of the proximal common extensor muscle mass supplied by the posterior interosseous nerve.

Conditions such as rheumatoid arthritis cause pain in a periarticular distribution. This contrasts markedly with pain arising from a neuropathy. Pain from a median neuropathy is localized anteromedially and may be reproduced with resisted forearm pronation and wrist flexion. An ulnar neuropathy arising in the cubital tunnel usually is described as lancinating pain, producing paresthesia into the ulnar two rays of the hand. Less commonly, nonspecific symptoms poorly localized to the medial aspect of the elbow can represent ulnar nerve pathology, medial epicondylitis, or arthrosis.

Symptoms arising from cervical radiculopathy can be distinguished usually by neck or shoulder pain in addition to elbow discomfort plus a specific radicular distribution of pain and associated neurologic abnormality of the upper extremity. Pain brought on by changes in the posture of the cervical spine, attempts at elevation of the upper extremity above the horizon, or lifting activities is characteristic.

PHYSICAL EXAMINATION

Inspection

The trained examiner can gain considerable information from visual inspection of the elbow joint. Because much

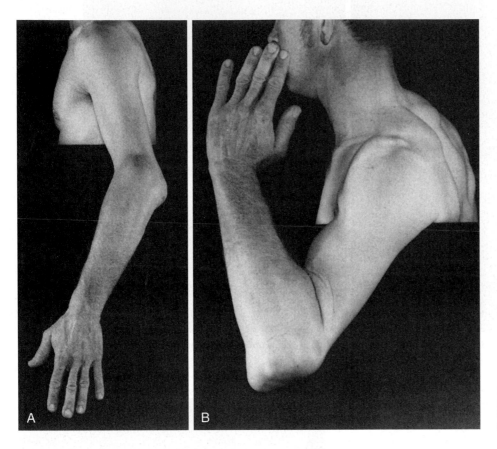

A

B

FIGURE 4–4 • Gross deformity of the elbow from a malunion of a condylar fracture. The excellent function is typical of condylar but not T-Y type malunions.

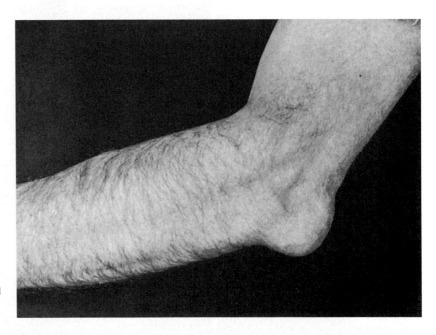

FIGURE 4–5 • An inflamed or enlarged olecranon bursa is one of the more dramatic diagnoses made by observation in the region of the elbow. (From Polley, H. G., Hunder, G. G.: Rheumatologic Interviewing and Physical Examination of the Joints, 2nd ed. Philadelphia, W.B. Saunders Co., 1978.)

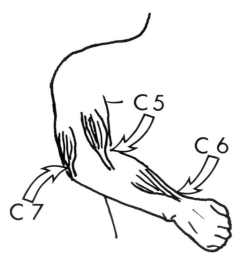

FIGURE 4–6 • The biceps, brachioradialis, and triceps reflexes allow evaluation of the C5, C6, and C7 nerve roots, respectively.

Associated Joints

No examination of the elbow is complete without a review of the cervical spine and all other components of the upper extremity. If the elbow pain has a radicular pattern, it is important to review the patient's cervical spine alignment and range of motion and perform neurologic testing of the entire upper extremity. The main nerve roots involved with elbow function include C5–7 (Fig. 4–6). The biceps, being a combination of C5–C6 roots, is a flexor of the elbow and forearm supinator. The reflex is primarily C5 but has C6 components.

The C6 muscle group of most interest is the mobile wad of three, consisting of the extensor carpi radialis longus and brevis and the brachioradialis muscles. These also are known as the radial wrist extensors and should be assessed for strength and reflex testing. The reflex is primarily C6 function, with some C5 component.

The primary muscle about the elbow innervated by C7 is the triceps, which should always be assessed for strength and reflex. Wrist flexion and finger extension also are primarily supplied by C7, with some C8 innervation (see Fig. 4–6).

There is considerable overlap in the sensory dermatomes of the upper extremity. The general distribution of sensory levels includes C5, the lateral arm; C6, the lateral forearm; C7, the middle finger; and C8 and T1, the medial forearm and arm dermatomes, respectively.

Elbow pain may be referred from the shoulder; therefore, a visual inspection of the shoulder for muscle wasting and alignment should be undertaken, followed by an appropriate functional assessment. Specific attention should be directed toward the spectrum of impingement tendinitis and associated rotator cuff pathology, which often is manifested by pain in the brachium.

Examination of the wrist, especially the distal radioulnar joint, is also important. For normal forearm rotation, there must be a normal anatomic relationship between the proximal and distal radioulnar joint. A loss of forearm rotation will result from inflammatory changes involving either the elbow or the wrist or both. A disruption of the normal relationship of the distal radioulnar joint will be character-

ized by a dorsally displaced prominence of the distal ulna. Dorsal displacement of the distal ulna is exaggerated by pronation and is lessened by supination. Because pronation is the common resting position of the hand, dorsal subluxation of the ulna at the wrist is often readily identifiable by inspection.

PALPATION

Bony Landmarks

Inspection and palpation of the medial and lateral epicondyles and the tip of the olecranon form an equilateral triangle when the elbow is flexed (Fig. 4–7). Fracture, malunion, unreduced dislocation, or growth disturbances involving the distal end of the humerus can be assessed clinically in this fashion.

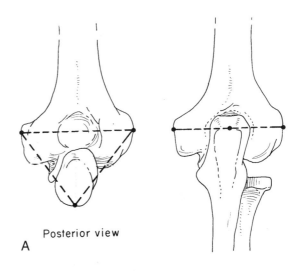

Posterior view

A

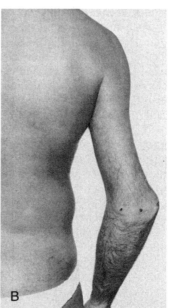

B

FIGURE 4–7 • With the elbow flexed to 90 degrees, the medial and lateral epicondyles and tip of the olecranon form an equilateral triangle when viewed from posterior. When the elbow is extended, this relationship is changed to a straight line connecting these three bony landmarks (A). The relationship is altered with displaced, intra-articular distal humeral fractures (B).

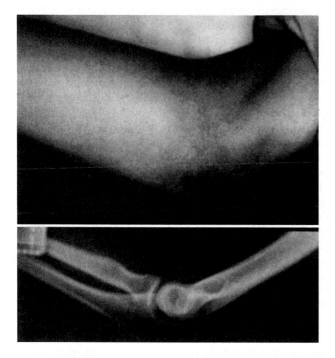

FIGURE 4–20 • With partial flexion or sometimes simple pronation of the forearm, the elbow is reduced and the dimple is obliterated. (From O'Driscoll, S. W.: Posterolateral rotatory instability of the elbow. J. Bone Joint Surg. **73A**:440, 1991.)

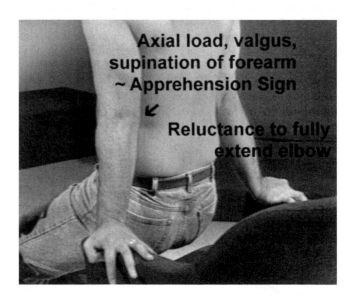

FIGURE 4–21 • Using the arms to rise from a chair can replicate the instability pattern of posterolateral rotatory instability (PLRI).

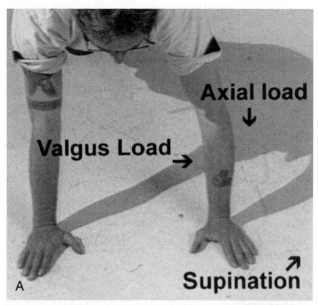

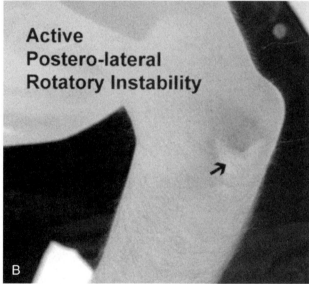

FIGURE 4–22 • *A,* The patient has done a push-up with hands in neutral and his arms wider than shoulder (valgus) and is at a terminal extension (axial load) of his unaffected elbow. He has apprehension in his affected left elbow (axial load + valgus). *B,* A close-up of the postero-lateral dislocation.

REFERENCES

1. American Academy of Orthopedic Surgeons: Joint Motion: Method of measuring and recording. Chicago, American Academy of Orthopedic Surgeons, 1965.
2. Askew, L. J., An, K. N., Morrey, B. F., and Chao EY: Functional evaluation of the elbow: normal motion requirements and strength determination. Orthop. Trans. **5**:304, 1981.
3. Atkinson, W. B., and Elftman, H.: The carrying angle of the human arm as a secondary symptom character. Anat. Rec. **91**:49, 1945.
4. Beals, R. K.: The normal carrying angle of the elbow. Clin. Orthop. **119**:194, 1976.
5. Beetham, W. P., Jr., Polley, H. F., Slocumb, C. H., and Weaver, W. F.: Physical examination of the joints. Philadelphia, W. B. Saunders Co., 1965.
6. Bert, J. M., Linscheid, R. L., and McElfresh, E. C.: Rotatory contracture of the forearm. J. Bone Joint Surg. **62A**:1163, 1980.
7. Boone, D. C., and Azen, S. P.: Normal range of motion of joints in male subjects. J. Bone Joint Surg. **61A**:756, 1979.
8. Childress, H. M.: Recurrent ulnar nerve dislocation at the elbow. Clin. Orthop. **108**:168, 1975.
9. Daniels, L., Williams, M., Worthingham, C.: Muscle Testing: Techniques of Manual Examination, 2nd ed. Philadelphia, W. B. Saunders Co., 1946.
10. Elkins, E. C., Ursula, M. L., and Khalil, G. W.: Objective recording of the strength of normal muscles. Arch. Phys. Med. Rehabil. **33**:639, 1951.
11. Hoppenfeld, S.: Physical Examination of the Spine and Extremities. New York, Appleton-Century-Crofts, 1976.
12. Johansson, O.: Capsular and ligament injuries of the elbow joint. Acta Chir. Scand. Suppl. **287**:1, 1962.
13. Keats, T. E., Teeslink, R., Diamond, A. E., and Williams, J. H.: Normal axial relationships of the major joints. Radiology **87**:904, 1966.
14. Lanz, T., Wachsmuth, W.: Praktische Anatomie. Berlin, ARM, Springer-Verlag, 1959.
15. McRae, R.: Clinical orthopedic examination. London, Churchill Livingstone, 1976.
16. Morrey, B. F., and Chao, E. Y.: Passive motion of the elbow joint. A biomechanical study. J. Bone Joint Surg. **61A**:63, 1979.
17. Morrey, B. F., Askew, L. J., An, K. N., and Chao, E. Y.: A biomechanical study of normal functional elbow motion. J. Bone Joint Surg. **63A**:872, 1981.
18. O'Driscoll, S. W., Morrey, B. F., and An, K. N.: Intra-articular pressuring capacity of the elbow. Arthroscopy **6**:100, 1990.
19. O'Driscoll, S. W., Morrey, B. F., and An, K. N.: Intra-articular pressuring capacity of the elbow. J. Bone Joint Surg. **73A**:440, 1991.
20. O'Neill, O. R., Morrey, B. F., Tanaka, S., and An, K. N.: Compensatory motion in the upper extremity after elbow arthrodesis. Clin. Orthop. Aug. (281):89, 1992.
21. Provins, K. A., and Salter N.: Maximum torque exerted about the elbow joint. J. Appl. Physiol. **7**:393, 1955.
22. Rasch, P. J.: Effect of position of forearm on strength of elbow flexion. Res. Q. **27**:333, 1955.
23. Regan, W. D., Korinek, S. L., Morrey, B. F., and An, K. N.: Biomechanical study of ligaments about the elbow joint. Clin. Orthop. **271**:170, 1991.
24. Schemitsch, E. H., Richards, R. R., and Kellam, J. F.: Plate fixation of fractures of both bones of the forearm. J. Bone Joint Surg. **71B**:2:345, 1989.
25. Wagner, C.: Determination of the rotary flexibility of the elbow joint. Eur. J. Appl. Physiol. **37**:47, 1977.
26. Williams, M., Stutzman, L.: Strength variation through the range of motion. Phys. Ther. Rev. **39**:145, 1959.
27. Youm, Y., Dryer, R. F., Thambyrajahk, K., Flatt, A. E., and Sprague, B. L.: Biomechanical analysis of forearm pronation-supination and elbow flexion-extension. J. Biomechan. **12**:245, 1979.

CHAPTER 5

Functional Evaluation of the Elbow

• BERNARD F. MORREY and KAI-NAN AN

Involvement of the upper limb accounts for about 10 percent of all compensation paid in the United States for disabling work-related injuries.[39, 55] In addition, dysfunction of the upper extremity cost about 5.5 million lost work days in 1977.[54] Elbow function may be summarized in three activities: (1) to allow the hand to be positioned in space, (2) to provide the power to perform lifting activities, and (3) to stabilize the upper extremity linkage for power and fine work activities. One may consider essential components of joint junction as motion, strength, and stability. However, the final determinant of function is ultimately determined by pain and the ability to perform activities of daily living.

ELBOW MOTION

Normal Motion

Normal flexion and forearm rotation at the elbow are estimated clinically with the handheld goniometer. Such measurement devices were described centuries ago[61] and are adequate for measurements required at the elbow. Forearm rotation is measured with the elbow at 90 degrees of flexion, often with the subject holding a linear object, such as a pencil, to make the measurement more objective.[69] In spite of obvious limitations, investigators have concluded that a standard handheld goniometric examination by a skilled observer allows measurement of elbow flexion-extension and pronation-supination with a margin of error of less than 5 percent.[29, 83] In fact, flexion-extension is reliably measured by the same observer with different goniometric designs with a reliability correlation coefficient of 0.99.[67] Different trained observers also provide measurements that are statistically equivalent.[26, 67]

Normal passive elbow flexion has been reported to range between 0 and 140 to 150 degrees.[1, 7, 37, 69] Greater variation of normal forearm rotation has been described but averages about 75 degrees pronation and 85 degrees supination.[1, 7, 37, 80] What is of particular importance, however, is the amount of motion used for daily activity.

Simultaneous Measurement of Active Motion

To measure the three-dimensional joint motion in daily activities, any one of several rather sophisticated experimental techniques can be used.[1, 83] For the elbow joint, the triaxial electrogoniometer[2, 12, 50] can be easily adapted to the subject for examination of a wide spectrum of daily activities and can simultaneously measure more than one joint system (Fig. 5–1).[59] In addition to flexion and rotation, a change in carrying angle can also be recorded by this device. Repeated testing of individual subjects at different times demonstrates the high reproducibility and reliability of this instrument.[46] Video telemetry and computer-simulated motion have also been developed in recent years and are of primary value at this time as investigative tools.[68] More recently, the application of the electromagnetic sensors for three-dimensional kinematic measurement has been found to be very feasible.[2, 59, 77]

Functional Motion

For most activities, the full potential of elbow motion is not needed or used. Loss of terminal flexion is more disabling than is the same degree of loss of terminal extension.[10, 58] Using the electrogoniometer just described, study of 15 activities of daily living established that most functions can be performed using an arc of 100 degrees of flexion between 30 and 130 degrees (Fig. 5–2) and 100 degrees of forearm rotation equally divided between pronation and supination (Fig. 5–3).

The motion requirements of the elbow joint needed for daily activities are really a measurement of the reaching ability of the hand. The extent to which this function is impaired by loss of elbow flexion or extension can also be estimated analytically (Fig. 5–4). If an individual has limited motion from 30 to 130 degrees, the potential area reached by the hand is reduced by about 20 percent. Thus, the range of elbow flexion between 30 and 130 degrees corresponds with about 80 percent of the normal reach capacity of the forearm and hand in a selected plane of shoulder motion. The functional impact of further loss of the flexion arc is also not equally distributed between flexion and extension. Our clinical experience indicates that flexion is of more value than extension in a ratio of about 2:1. Hence, a 10-degree further loss of flexion (120 degrees) is roughly equivalent to 20 degrees further loss of extension (Fig. 5–5).

The optimal position of elbow fusion to accomplish activities of daily living has been accepted as 90 degrees.[76] To further assess this issue, O'Neill and colleagues from our laboratory[59] assumed that the optimal position would be associated with a minimal amount of compensatory shoulder motion. It was surprising to observe that for discrete and fixed positions of the elbow, increasing the amount of shoulder motion did not provide greater use or increased function. It was also noted that for greater degrees of fixed elbow flexion, efforts to perform daily functions were accompanied by a tendency of the humerus to assume a less elevated and more lateral circumduction position (Fig. 5–6). This is consistent with the mechanical functions of these two joints; a ball and socket joint providing rotatory motion does NOT provide compensatory motion for hinge type motion that occurs only in a single plane. Furthermore, this laboratory investigation confirmed the clinical impression that the elbow joint fused in 90 degrees is the optimum for most activities.

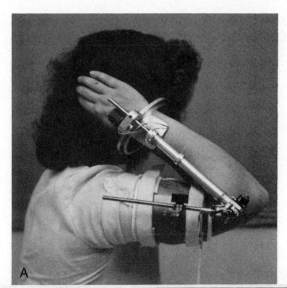

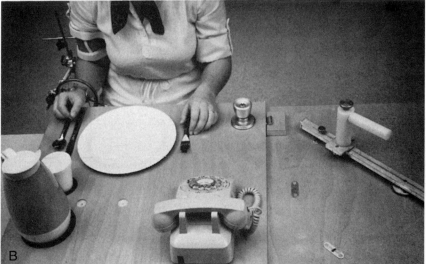

FIGURE 5–1 • The elbow electrogoniometer may be used to measure activities of daily living. *A,* Elbow flexion and forearm rotation to reach the back of the head. *B,* The subject is sitting at the activities table. (From Morrey, B. F., Askew, L. J., and Chao, E. Y.: A biomechanical study of normal functional elbow motion. J. Bone Joint Surg. **63A:**872, 1981.)

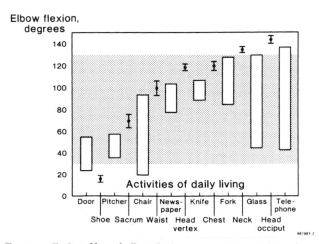

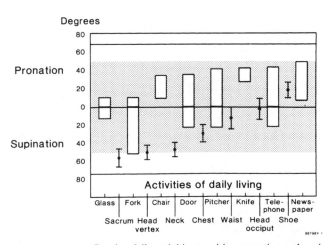

FIGURE 5–2 • Normal elbow flexion positions for activities of hygiene and those requiring arcs of motion are demonstrated. Most functions can be performed between 30 and 130 degrees of elbow flexion.

FIGURE 5–3 • Routine daily activities requiring pronation and supination or arcs of motion are performed between 50 degrees pronation and 50 degrees supination.

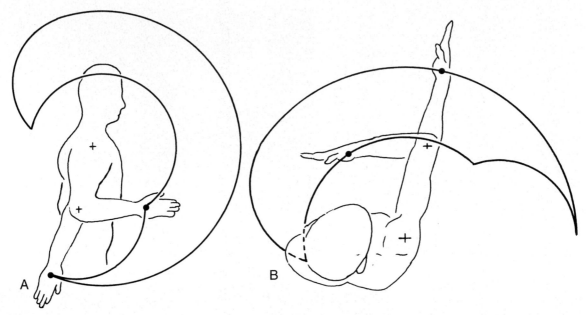

FIGURE 5–4 • The reaching area of the hand in the sagittal *(A)* and transverse *(B)* planes, with simultaneous movement of the elbow and shoulder. If the elbow is held at approximately 90 degrees of flexion, marked reduction of reach potential occurs. Note also that the circumduction motion of the shoulder does not compensate for the hinged type motion of the elbow joint.

STRENGTH

To understand the value and limitations of clinical strength assessment, it will be helpful to briefly review the types of muscle contraction, the major factors affecting strength, different measurement techniques, and the results of previous investigations.[11]

Types of Muscle Contraction

There are several types of muscle contraction classified according to changes in length, force, and velocity of contraction (Fig. 5–7).[4, 27, 48]

If there is no change in muscle length during a contraction, it is called isometric. When the external force exceeds the internal force of a shortened muscle and the muscle lengthens while maintaining tension, the contraction is called an *eccentric* or lengthening contraction. In contrast, if the muscle shortens while maintaining tension, a *concentric* contraction occurs. For elbow flexion, eccentric force exceeds isometric force by about 20 percent, and isometric force exceeds concentric force by about 20 percent (Fig. 5–8).[19, 75] However, it is known that eccentric exercise is associated with muscle fiber damage. This may lead to alterations in muscle receptors that can alter joint position sense.[9]

Force Considerations

If the muscle produces a constant internal force that exceeds the external force of the resistance, the muscle short-

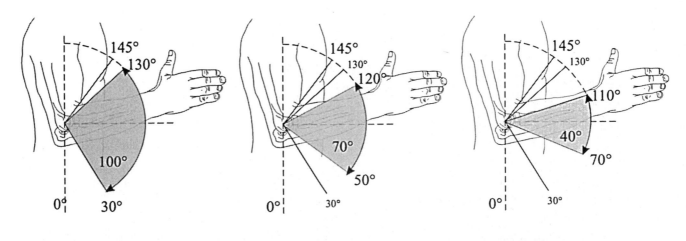

Functional Arc   **Optimum 70° Arc**   **Optimum 40° Arc**

FIGURE 5–5 • The further loss of motion from the ideal 30 to 130 degree arc is better tolerated as extension loss than as flexion loss.

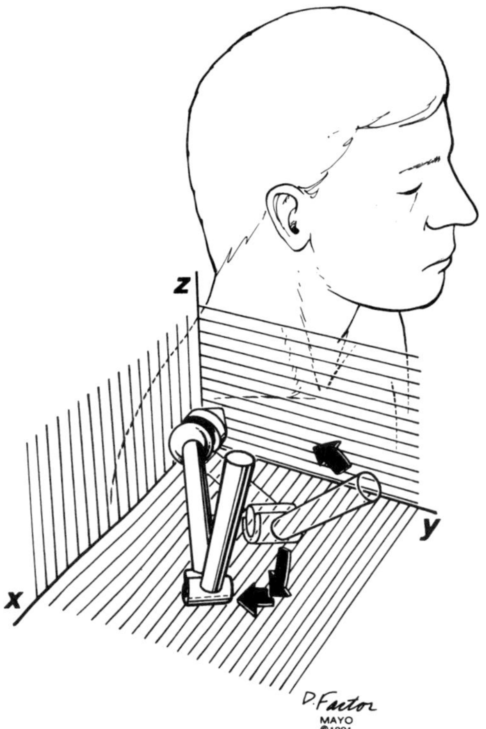

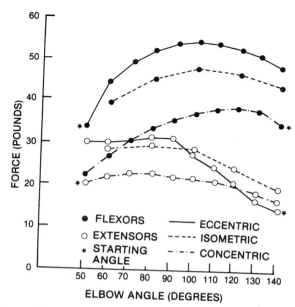

FIGURE 5–8 • Comparison of isometric, concentric, and eccentric flexion and extension contraction strength for different positions of elbow flexion. Note that approximately 20 percent greater strength may be generated with an eccentric than with an isometric contraction; the isometric contraction, on the other hand, is approximately 20 percent greater than the concentric type of contraction. (Modified from Singh, M.: Isotonic and isometric forces of forearm flexors and extensors. J. Appl. Physiol. **21:**1436, 1966.)

FIGURE 5–6 • As the fixed position of elbow fusion increases toward 90 degrees, activities of daily living are accomplished with the humerus less elevated and more laterally circumducted.

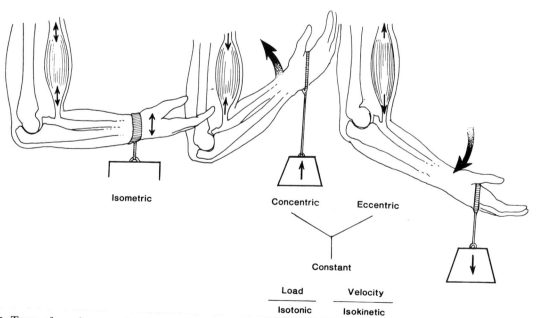

FIGURE 5–7 • Types of muscle contractions classified according to change in muscle length with a constant load and velocity. An isometric contraction results in no change of muscle length with a constant load and velocity. The concentric contraction is defined as a shortening of the muscle, whereas the eccentric contraction occurs with lengthening of the muscle. These latter two contractions may be subclassified according to whether a constant load (isotonic) or a constant velocity (isokinetic) condition is met.

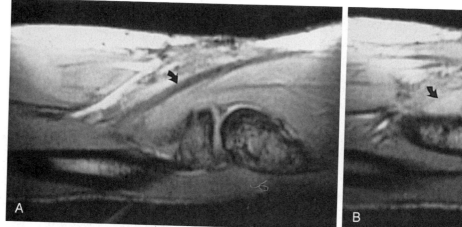
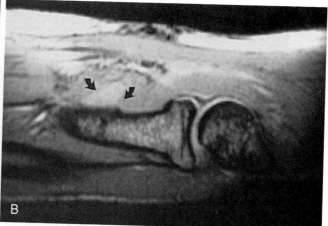

FIGURE 6–23 • Sagittal gradient echo images in different degrees of supination. *A*, The biceps tendon (*arrow*) is in the image plane. *B*, The tendon is snapping over the ganglion (*small arrows*).

provide advantages over CT and other imaging techniques.[6, 7, 23] Intra-articular contrast injection using gadolinium affords advantages provided with conventional arthrography and additional information regarding subtle synovial and cartilage abnormalities.

Surface coils generally are used to improve image quality. For patient comfort, the arm should be placed at the side when possible. When the arm is raised above the head, there is often motion artifact resulting in image degradation.[6, 7]

Magnetic resonance pulse sequences are designed to demonstrate contrast differences between normal and abnormal tissues. Multiple pulse sequences and image planes are required to identify and stage pathology. Often, the axial plane is combined with sagittal (Fig. 6–22) or coronal images for initial screening.[6, 7] In certain situations, fast scan techniques are used to allow motion (pronation-supination or flexion-extension) studies to be performed. Pronation-supination maneuvers (Fig. 6–23) are most easily performed, because magnetic resonance gantry size limits ranges of flexion and extension.

Significant progress has been made since the introduction of clinical MR imaging.[6–8, 23] It is the technique of choice for identification and staging of neoplasms. Evaluation of subtle soft tissue pathology (muscle, ligament, tendon, and neurovascular) is most easily assessed with MR imaging (Fig. 6–24; see Fig. 6–23).[6, 7, 26] New faster pulse sequences provide more flexibility for motion studies and positioning and improve patient throughput. In many cases, MR imaging has replaced arthrography, CT, and other techniques as the second examination following screening radiographs.[7, 23]

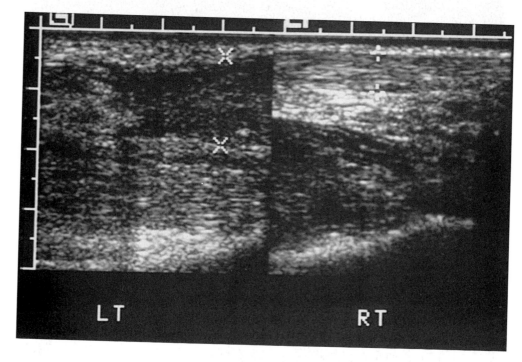

FIGURE 6–24 • Longitudinal ultrasonographic image of a normal (*right*) and ruptured (*left*) tendon.

ULTRASONOGRAPHY

Ultrasonographic applications for musculoskeletal imaging have expanded dramatically from the late 1970s. Improved technology and image quality permit more accurate depiction of normal anatomy and pathologic lesions. Ultrasonography is also more readily available and less expensive than MR imaging.[8, 23, 28]

Ultrasonography uses mechanical vibrations whose frequencies are beyond audible human perception (about 20,000 Hz or cycles per second). Ultrasonographic imaging uses frequency in the 2 to 10,000 MHz range. Doppler ultrasonography for peripheral vascular studies is performed in the 8 MHz range. New Doppler scanners provide color flow data that allow different flow rates (venous, arterial) to be easily demonstrated.[8, 23]

The central component of ultrasonographic instruments is the transducer, which contains a piezoelectric crystal. The transducer serves as a transmitter and receiver of sound waves. By applying the vibrating transducer to the skin surface (through an acoustic coupling medium such as mineral oil or gel), the mechanical energy is transmitted into the underlying tissues as a brief pulse of high energy sound waves. Sound waves reach different tissue interfaces (acoustic impedances), resulting in reflection or refraction. The reflected sound waves return to the transducer where they are converted into electrical energy used to produce the image.[8, 23, 28]

Ultrasonography, once limited to evaluating solid and cystic soft tissue lesions, is now commonly employed to evaluate articular and periarticular abnormalities. In the elbow, ultrasonography is well suited to evaluating tendon pathology. Tendon tears are demonstrated as gaps or areas of abnormal echo texture compared to the normal tendon (see Fig. 6–24). Avulsed bone fragments or calcification are hyperechoic with posterior acoustic shadowing.[23] The cost and flexibility of this technique will, no doubt, result in increased orthopedic use.[8]

REFERENCES

1. Arger, P. H., Oberkircher, P. E., and Miller, W. T.: Lipohemarthrosis. Am. J. Roentgenol. **121:**97, 1974.
2. Ballinger, P. W.: Merrill's Atlas of Radiographic Positions and Radiologic Procedures. 8th ed. St. Louis, C.V. Mosby Co., 1995.
3. Bassett, L. W., Mirra, J. M., Forrester, D. M., Gold, R. H., Bernstein, M. L., and Rollins, J. S.: Post-traumatic osteochondral "loose body" of the olecranon fossa. Radiology **141:**635, 1981.
4. Beals, R. K.: The normal carrying angle of the elbow: a radiographic study of 422 patients. Clin. Orthop. **119:**194, 1976.
5. Bernau, A., and Berquist, T. H.: Positioning Techniques in Orthopedic Radiology. Orthopedic Positioning in Diagnostic Radiology. Baltimore, Urban and Schwartzenberg, 1983.
6. Berquist, T. H.: MR imaging of the elbow and wrist. Magn. Reson. Imaging **1:**15, 1989.
7. Berquist, T. H.: MRI of the Musculoskeletal System, 3rd ed. New York, Lippincott-Raven Press, 1996.
8. Berquist, T. H.: Imaging of Orthopedic Trauma, 2nd ed. New York, Raven Press, 1992.
9. Berquist, T. H.: Diagnostic/therapeutic injections as an aid to musculoskeletal diagnosis. Semin. Intervent. Radiol. **10:**326, 1993.
10. Bledsoe, R. C., and Izenstark, J. L.: Displacement of fat pads in disease and injury of the elbow. A new radiographic sign. Radiology **73:**717, 1959.
11. Bohrer, S. P.: The fat pad sign following elbow trauma. Clin. Radiol. **21:**90, 1970.
12. Brown, R., Blazina, M. E., Kerlan, R. K., Carter, V. S., Jobe, F. W., and Carlson, G. J.: Osteochondritis of the capitellum. J. Sports Med. **2:**27, 1974.
13. Carlson, D. H.: CT evaluation of intra-articular fractures. South. Med. J. **73:**820, 1980.
14. Corbett, R. H.: Displaced fat pads in trauma to the elbow. Injury **9:**297, 1978.
15. Eto, R. T., Anderson, P. W., and Harley, J. D.: Elbow arthrography with the application of tomography. Radiology **115:**283, 1975.
16. Freiberger, R. H., and Kaye, J. J.: Arthrography. New York, Appleton Century Crofts, 1979.
17. Godefray, G., Pallardy, G., Chevrot, A., and Zenny, J. C.: Arthrography of the elbow: anatomical and radiological considerations and technical considerations. Radiology **62:**441, 1981.
18. Greenspan, A., and Norman, A.: The radial head, capitellar view. Useful technique in elbow trauma. Am. J. Roentgenol. **138:**1186, 1982.
19. Greenspan, A., and Norman, A.: The radial head, capitellar view. Another example of its usefulness. Am. J. Roentgenol. **139:**193, 1982.
20. Hall, F. H.: Morbidity from shoulder arthrography. Am. J. Roentgenol. **136:**59, 1981.
21. Hasselbacker, P.: Synovial fluid eosinophilia following arthrography. J. Rheumatol. **5:**173, 1978.
22. Hudson, T. M.: Elbow arthrography. Radiol. Clin. North Am. **19:**227, 1981.
23. Jacobson, J. A., and van Holsbeeck, M. I.: Musculoskeletal ultrasonography. Orthop. Clin. North Am. **29:**135, 1998.
24. Kohn, A. M.: Soft tissue alterations in elbow trauma. Am. J. Roentgenol. **82:**867, 1959.
25. London, J. T.: Kinematics of the elbow. J. Bone Joint Surg. **63A:**329, 1981.
26. Martin, C. E., and Schweitzer, M. E.: MR imaging of epicondylitis. Skel. Radiol. **27:**133, 1998.
27. McCullough, C., and Coulam, C. M.: Physical and dosimetric aspects of diagnostic geometrical and computer assisted tomography. Radiol. Clin. North Am. **14:**3, 1976.
28. Merritt, C. R. B.: Doppler color flow imaging. J. Clin. Ultra. **15:**591, 1987.
29. Mink, J. H., Eckardt, J. J., and Grant, T. T.: Arthrography in recurrent dislocation of the elbow. Am. J. Roentgenol. **136:**1242, 1981.
30. Murry, R. C.: Transitory eosinophilia localized to the knee joint. J. Bone Joint Surg. **32:**74, 1950.
31. Murry, W. A., and Siegel, M. J.: Elbow fat pads with new signs and extended differential diagnosis. Radiology **124:**659, 1977.
32. Norell, H. G.: Roentgenologic visualization of the extracapsular fat. Its importance in the diagnosis of traumatic injuries to the elbow. Acta Radiol. **42:**205, 1954.
33. Obermann, W. R., and Loose, H. W. C.: The os supratrochlear dorsale: a normal variant that may cause symptoms. Am. J. Roentgenol. **141:**123, 1983.
34. Pavlov, H., Ghelman, B., and Warren, R. F.: Double contrast arthrography of the elbow. Radiology **130:**87, 1979.
35. Resnick, D.: Diagnosis of Bone and Joint Diseases. Philadelphia, W. B. Saunders Co., 1995.
36. Roback, D. L.: Elbow arthrography: brief technical considerations. Clin. Radiol. **30:**311, 1979.
37. Rogers, S. L., and MacEwan, D. W.: Changes due to trauma in the fat plane overlying the supinator muscle: a radiographic sign. Radiology **92:**954, 1969.
38. Schwartz, J. L., and Crooks, L. E.: NMR imaging produces no observable mutations or cytotoxicity in mammalian cells. Am. J. Roentgenol. **139:**583, 1982.
39. Singson, R. D., Feldman, F., and Rosenberg, Z. S.: The elbow joint: assessment with double contrast CT arthrography. Radiology **160:**167, 1986.
40. Smith, D. N., and Lee, J. R.: The radiological diagnosis of post-traumatic effusion of the elbow joint and its clinical significance: the displaced fat pad sign. Injury **10:**115, 1978.
41. Weston, W. J., and Dalinka, M. K.: Arthrography. New York, Springer Verlag, 1980.
42. Yousefzadeh, D. K., and Jackson, J. H.: Lipohemarthrosis of the elbow joint. Radiology **128:**643, 1978.

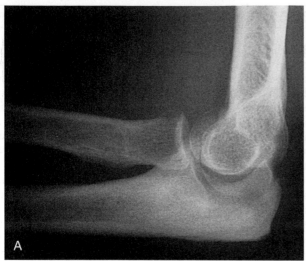

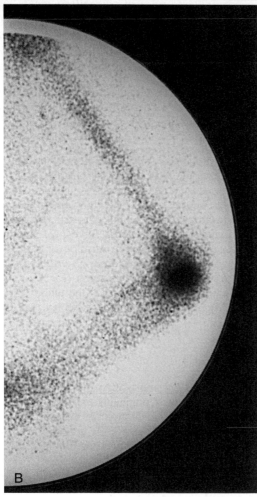

FIGURE 7–1 • Plain film reveals generalized sclerosis in the olecranon of 24-year-old man with pain of spontaneous onset of 2 years' duration (A). The bone scan was markedly abnormal (B). The patient was cured by excision of an osteoid osteoma of the olecranon.

inflammation. The sequence of studies listed earlier is also helpful. The intra-articular injection is not specific but is helpful. The early phase of the technetium Tc-99m bone scan may help to identify a soft tissue lesion, and the arthroscopic examination with biopsy may be definitive.

Ligaments

Typically, ligament disorders are the result of a single insult, but in throwers, such as baseball pitchers, they can result from chronic overuse.[5] A lesion of the anterior bundle of the medial collateral ligament can be distinguished by a valgus force. Occasionally, a subtle hint of instability is observed with this maneuver; however, a tear in continuity shows no instability, only pain after hard throwing. Arthrography may or may not show a bulge in the capsule medially; however, at arthroscopy a loose joint does allow easier passage of the scope at the ulnohumeral joint, suggesting this particular diagnosis (Fig. 7–3). Fluoroscopy centering on the olecranon fossa during the varus and valgus movements is usually diagnostic.

Muscle

The first step is to isolate the muscle by palpating and with active contraction against resistance. A careful history that elicits the exact onset and discrete palpation to determine the precise anatomic location of the pain is most rewarding. Next, injection of a limited amount of lidocaine in the most tender area determines whether the pain can be defined and controlled. A possible distal biceps tendon rupture can present with pain and crepitus at the biceps insertion,[4] although radial bicipital bursitis can also occur at this exact site, and distinguishing between the two is most difficult. Local injection in the area followed by objective strength tests reveals weakness on supination if there is a partial disruption and a return to normal if the problem is bursitis.

• TABLE 7–2 • Diagnostic Categories by Tissue Type

Articular Lesions
Inflammatory
  Infectious
    Bacterial
    Nonbacterial
  Postinfectious
    Reiter's disease
  Noninfectious
    Connective tissue
      Rheumatoid arthritis
      Ankylosing spondylitis
      Systemic lupus erythematosus
      Others
    Crystalline deposition disease
      Gout
      Pseudogout
      Hydroxyapatite crystals
    Neoplastic osteoid osteoma
Noninflammatory
  Traumatic
    Chondromalacia
    Osteochondritis
  Primary degenerative joint disease
Extra-articular Lesions
Capsular
Muscular/tendinous
  Epicondylitis
  Distal biceps insertion tendonitis
Bursitis
Neural
  Entrapment
  Reflex dystrophy

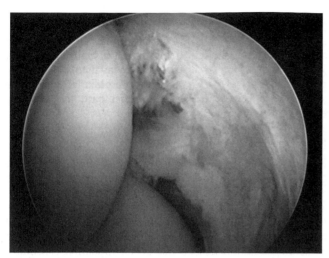

FIGURE 7–2 • After 2 years of refractory symptoms diagnosed as tennis elbow, arthroscopy revealed an intra-articular component to the process.

Magnetic resonance imaging (MRI) is usually performed but its utility varies.

Nerve

There are two common problems of neural origin and one rare one that can be great masqueraders at the elbow. Most consider the cubital tunnel syndrome to be associated with classic radicular symptoms felt in the fourth and fifth digits. We have, however, observed that ulnar neuritis may be associated with vague medial joint pain without radicular features. Tinel's sign is usually positive in this type of patient, but not always. This may be a very difficult diagnosis. Cubital tunnel syndrome is usually observed in patients who have osteoarthritis or mild and subtle medial collateral ligament insufficiency that allows valgus laxity and nerve

irritation. A second problem of neural origin at the elbow is posterior interosseous entrapment at the arcade of Frohse. The significance of this relates to differentiating the lesion from lateral epicondylitis, and the reader is again reminded that 5 percent of patients with legitimate lateral epicondylitis have associated posterior interosseous nerve entrapment (see Chapter 40).[12] In our judgment, a localized injection at the arcade of Frohse that eliminates the symptoms is diagnostic of this condition. We do not rely on electromyography (EMG) to make the diagnosis, because the patient can have significant involvement and symptoms and normal EMG findings. Finally, Bassett has clearly documented entrapment of the sensory portions of the musculocutaneous nerve just proximal to the lateral joint as a source of vague elbow pain.[2]

Blood Vessels

We have not appreciated any significant vascular problem that presents at the elbow. We have seen a prominent venous vascular network compressing the posterior interosseous nerve at the arcade of Frohse, and distended vessels may accompany the ulnar nerve that is demonstrating symptoms of ulnar neuritis. Typically, these are uncommon presentations for such conditions. We and others have also identified pain at the lateral elbow joint apparently due to a compartment syndrome of the anconeus os relieved by release of the anconeus fascia.[1] Others have also replicated a chronic compartment syndrome as causing vague proximal forearm pain.[6]

INVESTIGATIONS

Laboratory Studies
ANALYSIS OF BLOOD AND SYNOVIAL FLUID

A central question is whether the elbow is the only site of pain or whether other joints are involved. This helps to distinguish between localized and generalized processes.

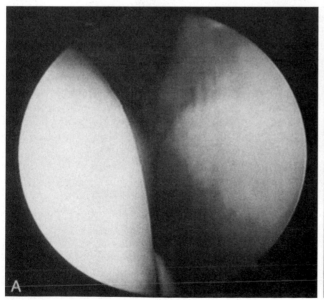
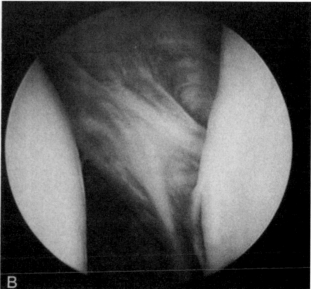

FIGURE 7–3 • Post-traumatic elbow pain with subtle instability escaped diagnosis by the usual means. Arthroscopy revealed a radiohumeral joint (A) that separated with varus stress (B).

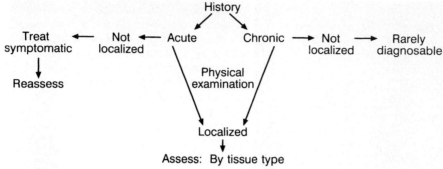

Cartilage: Intra-articular inject., ^{99m}Tc, arthroscopy
Bone: ^{99m}Tc, tomogram
Ligament: Fluoro stress, pivot shift, arthrogram, arthroscopy
Muscle: Objective strength measure, extra-art. inject., MRI (rare)
Nerve: PE, inject., EMG

CG135866B-1

FIGURE 7–6 • A flow chart for evaluation of the painful elbow. Workup should
proceed from left to right and from top to
bottom in individual categories.

features of the history, considering tissue type and diagnostic modality, is presented in Figure 7–6. Simple exploration
of the elbow with little or no idea of the underlying
pathology must be avoided.

REFERENCES

1. Abrahamsson, S. O., Sollerman, C., Soderberg, T., Lundborg, G., Rydholm, U., and Pettersson, H.: Lateral elbow pain caused by anconeus compartment syndrome. A case report. Acta Orthop. Scand. **58**:589–591, 1987.
2. Bassett, F., and Nunley, J.A.: Compression of the musculocutaneous nerve at the elbow. J Bone Joint Surg. **64A**:1050–1052, 1982.
3. Bateman, J.E.: The Shoulder and Neck. Philadelphia, W.B. Saunders Co., 1972, p. 99.
4. Bourne, M.H., and Morrey, B.F.: Partial rupture of the distal biceps tendon. Clin. Orthop. **291**:143, 1981.
5. Jobe, F.W., Stark, H., and Lombardo, S.J.: Reconstruction of the ulnar collateral ligament in athletes. J. Bone Joint Surg. **68A**:1158, 1986.
6. Kutz, J.E., Singer, R., and Lindsay, M.: Chronic exertional compartment syndrome of the forearm: a case report. J. Hand Surg. **10A**:302–304, 1985.
7. Morrey, B.F.: Reoperation for failed tennis elbow surgery. J. Shoulder Elbow Surg. **1**:47, 1992.
8. O'Driscoll, S.W., and Morrey, B.F.: Arthroscopy of the elbow: diagnostic and therapeutic benefits and hazards. J. Bone Joint Surg. **74A**:84, 1992.
9. Rettig, A., and Goris, J.E.: Osteoid osteoma of the olecranon. Orthopedics **19**:977–979, 1966.
10. Singson, R.D., Feldman, F., and Rosenberg, Z.S.: Elbow joint: assessment with double-contrast CT arthrography. Radiology **160**:167, 1986.
11. Tompkins, D.G.: Exercise myopathy of the extensor carpi ulnaris muscle. Report of a case. J. Bone Joint Surg. **59A**:407–408, 1977.
12. Werner, C.O.: Lateral elbow pain and posterior interosseous nerve entrapment. Acta Orthop. Scand. Suppl. **174**:1–62, 1979.

Surgery and Rehabilitation

• CHAPTER 8 •

Surgical Exposures of the Elbow

• BERNARD F. MORREY

Few joints require familiarity with as many surgical exposures as does the elbow. Depending on the lesion and the surgical goal, the joint and the surrounding region may be approached from the lateral, posterior, medial, or anterior direction.

Exposures from the medial and lateral aspects that once allowed the removal of loose bodies and the treatment of certain localized fractures are rarely used today. Instead, some form of an extensile posterior exposure is used for most complex fractures and joint reconstructive procedures, and this is considered the universal approach to the joint.

It is not the purpose of this chapter to discuss all of the approaches to the joint but rather to provide a comprehensive collection and critique of those exposures that may prove helpful to the practicing orthopedic surgeon.

It should be noted that those approaches used primarily for loose body removal are virtually obsolete, having been replaced by arthroscopy (see Chapter 39).[30]

GENERAL PRINCIPLES

As others have noted,[7, 8, 31] rigorous adherence to the principles of good surgical technique is of no greater importance in any anatomic part than at the elbow. The most appropriate surgical approach depends on the specific goal of the surgical intervention and on the lesion. As for any orthopedic procedure, the choice of the surgical approach should be based on the following criteria:

1. Potential to be extended to meet unforeseen circumstances.
2. Capability for providing adequate visualization to define and completely correct the problem.

3. Safety: avoidance of vital structures or visualization of these structures to avoid injury during the procedure.
4. Preservation of the normal anatomy as much as possible during the exposure, the procedure, and at closure.
5. Dissection along natural tissue planes rather than across muscle, tendon, or ligamentous structures.
6. Provision of careful hemostasis and adequate drainage after extensile exposures and dissections.
7. Satisfactory soft tissue closure that reliably heals and ensures rapid and predictable rehabilitation.

A thorough understanding of the anatomy of the elbow region is important to selecting the exposure that best satisfies these requirements. The cross-sectional anatomy is depicted in Figure 8–1.

LATERAL APPROACHES

The lateral exposure, probably the most commonly used approach to the elbow joint, offers many variations. It is used for radial head excision, removal of loose bodies, and repair of lateral ligaments to fix condylar and Monteggia fractures and release the joint capsule and remove osteophytes. Access to the radiohumeral articulation has been described by several authors.[6, 16, 19, 22, 33] The techniques differ according to the muscle interval entered and the means of reflecting the muscle mass from the proximal ulna. With any of the lateral exposures to the joint or to the proximal radius, the surgeon must be constantly aware of the possibility of injury to the posterior interosseous or recurrent branch of the radial nerve.

Kaplan has described an approach through the interval between the extensor digitorum communis and the extensor carpi radialis longus and brevis muscles. Because of the proximity of the radial nerve, pronation of the forearm during exposure has been recommended to assist in carrying the radial nerve out of the surgical field. The effect of this maneuver has been quantified by Strachan and Ellis, who found that approximately 1 cm of mediolateral radial nerve translation can occur with forearm pronation (Fig. 8–2).[38] Even with this maneuver, however, the radial nerve is precariously close to the surgical field, so this approach is used less often than that described by Kocher. Knowledge of Kaplan's interval[22] is useful to expose the posterior interosseous nerve when decompression is performed in conjunction with tennis elbow release (see Chapter 40).

We describe in detail only Kocher's exposure, as it is the most frequently used approach to the lateral aspect of the joint. Furthermore, it has the advantage of being exten-

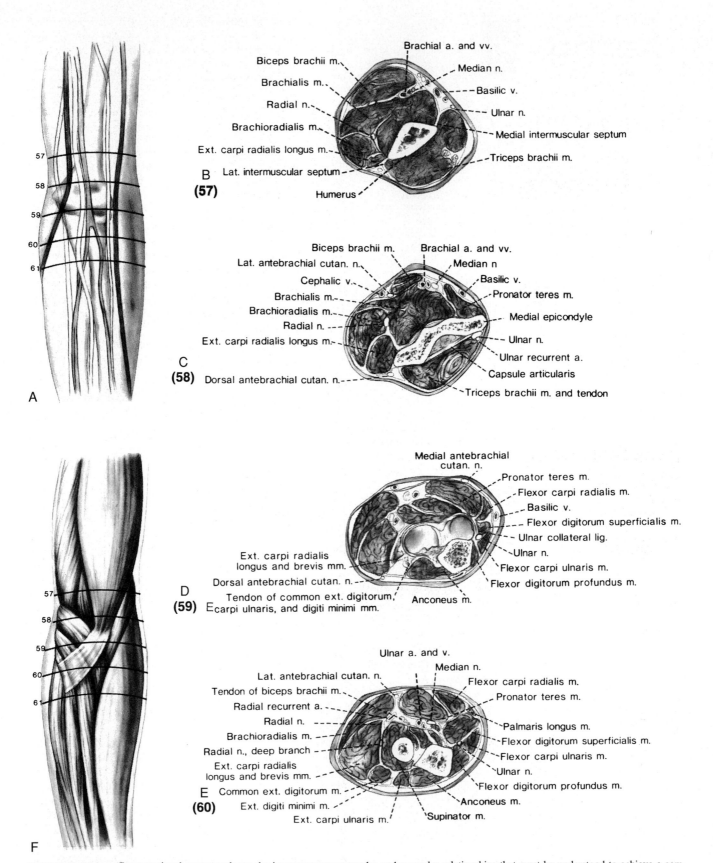

FIGURE 8–1 • Cross-sectional anatomy shows the important neurovascular and muscular relationships that must be understood to achieve a complication-free exposure of the elbow. (Modified from Eycleshymer, A. C., and Schoemaker, D. M.: A Cross Section Anatomy. New York, D. Appleton and Co., 1930. *In* Darrach, W.: Surgical approaches for surgery of the extremities. Am. J. Surg. **67**:93, 1945.)

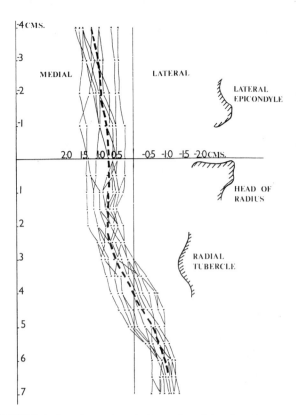

FIGURE 8–2 • Approximately 1 cm of medial to lateral translation of the posterior interosseous nerve occurs as the forearm is rotated from supination to pronation. (From Strachan, J. H., and Ellis, B. W.: Vulnerability of the posterior interosseous nerve during radial head resection. J. Bone Joint Surg. **53B**:320, 1971.)

sile, affording a full complement of surgical options as the exposure is extended.

Kocher's Approach

This approach enters the joint through the interval of the anconeus and extensor carpi ulnaris, thus providing protection to the deep radial nerve. The interval is also anterior to the lateral ulnar collateral ligament, which reduces the likelihood of severing it at arthrotomy. In addition to providing a limited exposure for radial head excision and loose body removal, the particular value of this technique is that it may be converted to an extensile posterolateral approach to the entire distal humerus (see below).

Description of Technique. The skin incision begins just proximal to the lateral epicondyle of the humerus in the avascular interval. It is extended distally and posteriorly approximately 6 cm in an oblique manner over the fascia of the anconeus and extensor carpi ulnaris muscles (Fig. 8–3). This interval is identified either visually or by palpation and is best seen after the forearm fascia has been entered. The dissection is then carried down to the joint capsule. The nerve is a safe distance from the dissection and is protected by the extensor carpi ulnaris and extensor digitorum communis muscle mass. The origin of the anconeus is released subperiosteally from the humerus and retracted posteriorly to permit adequate exposure of the capsule. A longitudinal incision is made through the capsule to expose the radiocapitellar joint.

Approach. Modified distal Kocher's.

Indications. Reconstruction of the lateral ulnar collateral ligament.[29]

Comment. A simple maneuver to reflect the anconeus allows adequate exposure to reconstruct the lateral ulnar collateral ligament and is a minor modification of the distal Kocher "J" approach.

Description of Technique. The development of Kocher's interval reveals the lateral joint capsule. The anconeus is then reflected posteriorly, exposing the crista supinatoris (Fig. 8–4A). The anconeus is reflected proximally and posteriorly along with the lateral aspect of the triceps tendon, while the extensor carpi ulnaris and the common extensor tendon are released from the lateral epicondyle and are reflected anteriorly, exposing the lateral capsular complex (see Fig. 8–4B). The periosteal elevator separates the anterior musculature, allowing identification of the anterior aspect of the joint, and provides sufficient exposure for lateral ligamentous reconstruction.

Approach. Transepicondylar lateral approach.[11]

Indications. Uncommon fractures of the lateral condyle; resurfacing elbow replacement.

Comment. Excellent exposure of the radiohumeral articulation may be achieved by performing an osteotomy of the lateral epicondyle. The clinical applications for this exposure are limited, however, because other techniques provide similarly adequate visualization of the joint without requiring union of the osteotomy and the common extensor origin.

Description of Technique. The incision is begun approximately 5 cm proximal to the lateral epicondyle of the humerus and extends distally over the avascular interval and across the epicondyle, ending about 3 to 4 cm distal to the joint along the posterolateral surface of the olecranon. The lateral border of the humerus is exposed by subperiosteal dissection of the triceps posteriorly and of the origin of the extensor carpi radialis longus and the brachioradialis anteriorly. The radial nerve is avoided, because it lies close to the proximal angle of the wound. Using a small osteotome, the lateral epicondyle, which is the common origin of the extensor muscle mass and the radial collateral ligament, is removed, and the complex is retracted distally, exposing the radiohumeral joint. The deep branch of the radial nerve is protected as it enters the supinator muscle. The brachioradialis and the extensor carpi radialis longus muscles are elevated where they originate on the anterior aspect of the distal humerus, and the capsule is incised to expose the lateral aspect of the elbow joint.

Comment. The value of this approach is limited, because alternative exposures are available that do not require release of the ligament.

POSTEROLATERAL EXPOSURES

When exposure of the olecranon and of the radiohumeral joint is required, several variations of a posterolateral approach described by Boyd may be used. Depending on the need to expose the proximal ulna or the distal humerus, these approaches can be extended and thus provide significant versatility.[37]

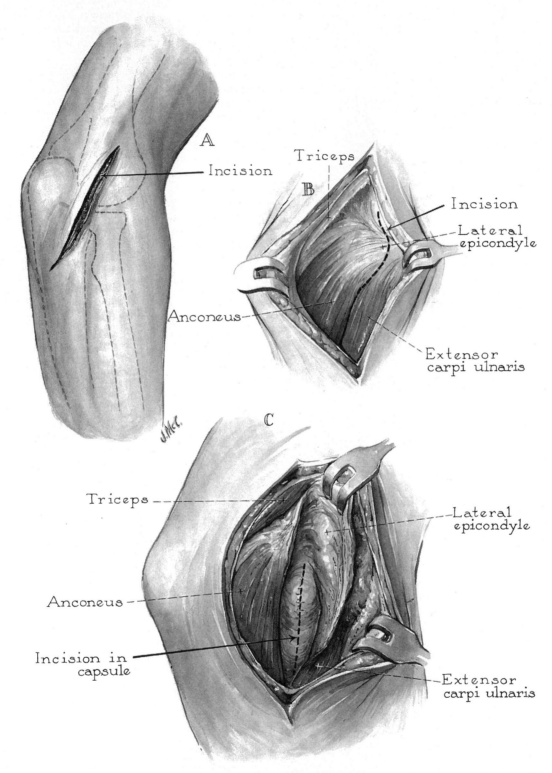

FIGURE 8–3 • The distal Kocher approach. *A*, The incision begins approximately 2 to 3 cm above the lateral epicondyle over the supracondylar bony ridge and extends distally and posteriorly for approximately 4 cm. *B*, The interval between the anconeus and the extensor carpi ulnaris is identified. *C*, Development of this interval reveals the capsule.

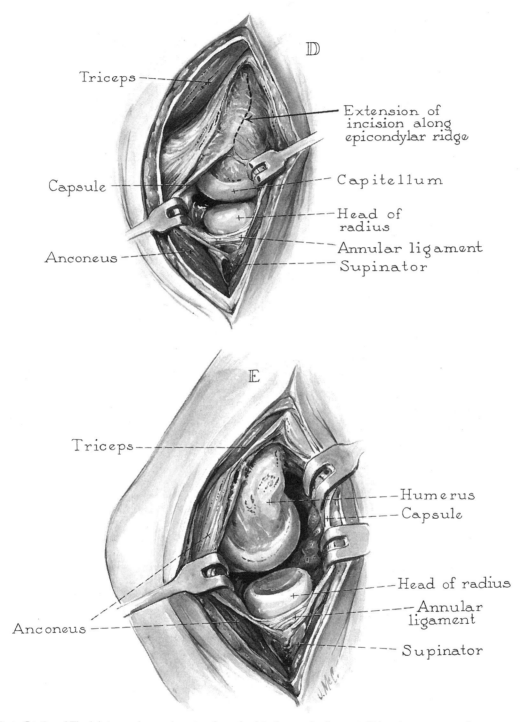

FIGURE 8–3 • *Continued* The joint capsule may be entered proximal to the annular ligament *(D)*, and a more extensive exposure may be obtained by extending the capsular incision proximally *(E)*, thus providing adequate exposure of the radiohumeral articulation. (From Banks, S. W., and Laufman, H.: An Atlas of Surgical Exposures of the Extremities. Philadelphia, W. B. Saunders, 1953.)

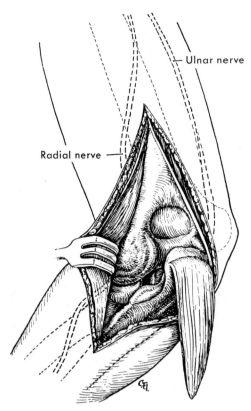

FIGURE 8–9 • The Campbell (Van Gorder) approach. The triceps aponeurosis is identified and reflected distally. The remaining fibers of the triceps are then split in the midline and reflected from the humerus, and the anconeus is reflected subperiosteally from the ulna to expose the joint. (From Crenshaw, A. H.: Surgical approaches. *In* Edmonson, A. S., and Crenshaw, A. H. [eds.]: Campbell's Operative Orthopaedics, 6th ed. St. Louis, C. V. Mosby, 1980.)

8–10*D*). Routine closure in layers is performed, but the radiocollateral ligament should be reattached to the bone through holes placed in the lateral epicondyle.

MAYO MODIFIED EXTENSILE KOCHER'S EXPOSURE

Indications. Release of ankylosed joint; interposition, replacement arthroplasty.

Description of Technique. A modification and extension of Kocher's extensile approach (Fig. 8–11) consists of reflecting the anconeus and triceps expansion from the tip of the olecranon by sharp dissection, as in the Mayo approach (Fig. 8–12). In this way, the entire extensor mechanism may be reflected medially, allowing the elbow to be opened with varus stress more readily than when the joint is tightly contracted. The triceps is reattached in a fashion identical to that described for the Mayo approach (see Fig. 8–12).

Comment. This step can easily be added to the initial Kocher extensile approach when circumstances require greater exposure posteriorly or anteriorly.

BRYAN-MORREY POSTEROMEDIAL, EXTENSILE TRICEPS-SPARING EXPOSURE[9]

Indications. Joint arthroplasty, elbow dislocation, supracondylar T and Y fractures, synovial disease, infection, and ulnar nerve or medial collateral ligament lesions.

Comment. This exposure is selected when exposure of the ulnar collateral ligament or ulnar nerve and extensive joint exposure is needed.

Description of Technique. The patient is placed supine with a sandbag under the scapula. A pneumatic tourniquet is applied high on the arm, which is brought across the chest after draping (see Fig. 8–12). A straight posterior incision is made medial to the midline, approximately 9 cm proximal and 8 cm distal to the tip of the olecranon. The ulnar nerve is identified proximally in the epineural fat at the margin of the medial head of the triceps and, depending on the procedure, is either protected or carefully dissected free of the cubital tunnel to its first motor branch.

The medial aspect of the triceps is elevated to the posterior capsule. The superficial fascia of the forearm is then incised distally for about 6 cm, to the periosteum of the medial aspect of the proximal ulna. The periosteum and fascia complex is carefully reflected laterally. The medial part of the complex is the weakest portion of the reflected tissue; therefore, care must be taken to maintain continuity of the triceps mechanism at this point. The remaining portion of the triceps mechanism then is reflected. If exposure of the radial head is desired, the anconeus is removed subperiosteally from the proximal ulna and reflected laterally with the triceps mechanism, widely exposing the entire joint.

The tip of the olecranon may be removed for clear visualization of the trochlea. The ligaments may be released either medially or laterally from the humerus. Depending on the nature of the procedure, if stability is important these ligaments should be repaired back to the humerus. For semiconstrained joint replacement repair is not considered necessary. The triceps is returned to its anatomic position and sutured directly to the bone or the proximal end of the ulna. The periosteum then is sutured to the superficial forearm fascia as far as the margin of the flexor carpi ulnaris. The tourniquet is deflated, hemostasis is secured, and the wound is drained and closed in layers.

Osteocutaneous Flap[43]

Indications. An extensile triceps-reflecting procedure similar in concept to the Mayo approach and most often used for joint replacement arthroplasty, it also may be used for distal humeral fractures.

Description of Technique. The patient is placed supine with the arm draped free across the chest. A straight posterior incision is made over the lateral subcutaneous border of the ulna and proximally in the midline of the brachium just lateral to the tip of the olecranon (Fig. 8–13). The ulnar nerve is identified and protected but not translocated. An incision is made along the subcutaneous border of the ulna and the medial aspect of the triceps (see Fig. 8–13*A*). The triceps attachment is released from the ulna by osteotomizing the attachment with a thin wafer of bone. This is the essential difference from the Mayo approach. The medial aspect of the triceps is elevated proximally, and the triceps attachment, with the wafer of bone, is elevated from the lateral aspect of the ulna in continuity with the anconeus muscle and the fascia (see Fig. 8–13*B*). The lateral collateral ligament is exposed and, for joint replacement, released from the humerus while the medial collateral liga-

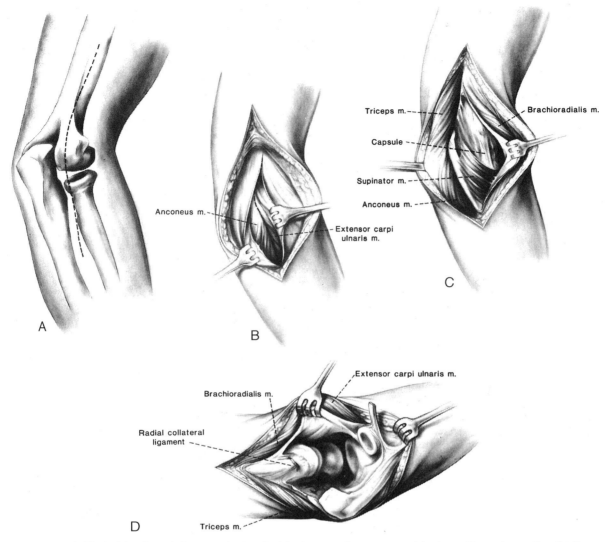

FIGURE 8–10 • *A*, The incision is made 8 cm proximal to the joint just posterior to supracondylar bony ridge and extending distally over the anconeus for approximately 6 cm. *B*, The interval between the anconeus and the extensor carpi ulnaris is identified and entered. *C*, The anconeus is reflected subperiosteally from the proximal ulna along with its fascial attachment to the triceps, which is likewise reflected medially, exposing the supinator muscle. The insertion of the triceps on the tip of the olecranon is released by sharp dissection, and the supinator muscle is released from the proximal portion of the ulna and the humerus as necessary to expose the capsule, which is entered via a longitudinal incision. *D*, The release of the radiocollateral ligament at its humeral origin allows joint subluxation to expose the entire distal humerus.

ment is elevated from its ulnar attachment. Rotation of the forearm and angular stress open the joint.

After the surgical procedure, the olecranon osteotomy is secured to its bed by 20 nonabsorbable sutures placed through bone holes. Interrupted sutures are used to repair the remaining distal portion of the extensor mechanism (see Fig. 8–13*C*).

Comment. The authors have noted excellent extension and reliable healing of the osseous attachment to the olecranon.[43] This exposure is similar in many ways to that described by Bryan and Morrey, except that, instead of the triceps' being reflected from the tip of the olecranon, the extensor mechanism is released with a wafer of bone. Furthermore, this approach exposes only the ulnar nerve, whereas the Mayo approach translocates the nerve.

TRICEPS-PRESERVING TECHNIQUE

Medial and lateral stabilization of the triceps exposes the proximal humerus adequately for distal humeral shaft frac-

tures.[3] We recently found that the triceps can be left intact when the distal humerus is to be or has been resected.

Surgical Approach. Posterior triceps-sparing.[27]

Indications. Tumor resection, joint reconstruction for resection of humeral nonunion, or revision joint replacement.[27]

Description of Technique. The technique is usually used for failed reconstructive procedures, so the previous skin incision is followed when possible. Otherwise, a posterior incision is made either medial or lateral to the tip of the olecranon. Medial and lateral skin flaps are elevated with as much subcutaneous tissue and fascia as possible. The medial and lateral aspects of the triceps are identified, and the ulnar nerve is isolated unless it was previously translocated anteriorly (Fig. 8–14). The tumor is resected, or the distal humeral nonunion is sharply mobilized through the pseudarthrosis. The lateral collateral attachment to the humerus is severed along with the common extensor tendon (see Fig. 8–14). The common flexor tendon and muscle

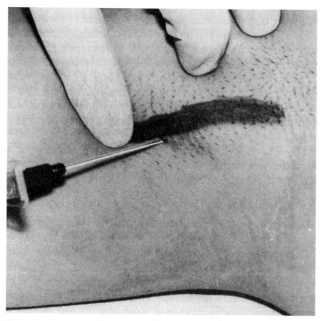

FIGURE 9–1 • The axillary artery is palpated and marked. The insertion of the needle occurs just distal and posterior to the palpated artery.

mally in the axillary sheath, parallel to the artery. The stimulator is set at a frequency of 1 Hz and is turned on to a low amperage immediately after the needle is inserted through the skin. This is done to stimulate the median nerve in its superficial course in the axillary sheath. A high amperage may result in a vigorous motor response that could dislodge the needle and decrease patient compliance with the procedure. The amperage may be increased to 2 mA as the needle is passed gently through the tissues.

Evoked Motor Response. Evoked motor responses to the stimulus will result in identification of the axillary (arm abduction, shoulder elevation); musculocutaneous (forearm flexion, supination); radial (hand, wrist, elbow extension); median (forearm pronation, internal thumb rotation, wrist flexion); and ulnar (flexion of the wrist and fourth and fifth fingers, thumb adduction) nerves.[5] The amperage may be decreased until only a minimal motor response is elicited. The needle is manipulated to elicit the maximal motor response while using the least amperage, usually 0.5 mA. An evoked motor response at 0.5 mA indicates close proximity between the tip of the needle and the nerve.[5] The plastic cannula is advanced over the needle once the desired motor evoked response is identified. The insulated needle then is withdrawn, leaving the plastic cannula in place.

Catheter Placement. The axillary catheter is passed through the cannula into the axillary sheath. The catheter is clearly marked in 1-cm increments up to 15 cm and comes with a threading assist guide. It is passed approximately 12 cm from the skin insertion site in the direction of the cords[6, 7] (Fig. 9–2). Passing the catheter more than 12 cm does not appear to add any clinical benefit and usually results in coiling or kinking of the catheter within the nerve sheath.[7] The cannula is withdrawn after catheter placement. An adapter is attached to the distal end of the catheter to facilitate anesthetic fluid infusion.

Testing the Catheter. Aspiration of the catheter at the adapter is performed with an empty 3- or 5-ml syringe. It is a negative aspiration if no blood or other fluid is drawn back through the catheter. Intermittent test boluses of local anesthetic may be given at this time. A test bolus of 3 ml of 0.5 percent bupivacaine with 1:200,000 epinephrine may be administered. An immediate tachycardic response, tinnitus, or circumoral numbness indicates that the catheter is intravascular or that rapid absorption is occurring. The catheter should be withdrawn and replaced if this happens.

Catheter Fixation. The catheter is sutured in place at the skin insertion site, the site is covered with povidone-iodine (Betadine) ointment, and a sterile transparent dressing is applied. Excess length of the catheter is gently looped and securely taped to the patient (Fig. 9–3).

Evaluating Results. Placement of a continuous axillary brachial plexus catheter is usually successful on the first attempt. The catheter is replaced if upper extremity anesthesia and analgesia are not adequate. Placement of the catheter into the median, ulnar, or radial neurovascular sheaths does not appear to provide a significant advantage in time of onset or intensity of brachial plexus blockade. No adverse reactions were found among any of the patients studied, confirming the safety of this technique.[4]

Anesthetic Agents

Administration. An anesthetizing dose of local anesthetic, usually 40 ml of 0.5 percent bupivacaine with 1:200,000 epinephrine, is administered prior to connecting and initiating a continuous infusion of a selected anesthetic agent. To avoid plasma anesthetic levels in the toxic range, the continuous infusion is not started until a satisfactory anesthetic neuromuscular block has been achieved and at least 45 to 60 minutes have elapsed since the initial bolus dose. The low-dose local anesthetic infusion can be supplemented with a patient-controlled or activated bolus dose for additional analgesia. On-demand bolus dosage is more responsive to rapidly changing pain levels, such as pain resulting from increased range of motion exercises or vigorous physical therapy. The initial bolus dose may result in peak plasma bupivacaine levels near 2 μ/ml.[11] Continuous infusions of bupivacaine have resulted in peak plasma levels between 0.5 and 1.8 μg/ml, depending on the dosage.[2, 11, 16] Plasma bupivacaine levels above 4 μg/ml would be expected to produce objective toxic reactions.[11]

Several different anesthetic agents have been used successfully for continuous axillary brachial plexus blockade. Lidocaine or mepivacaine, 1 to 1.5 percent in 20- to 40-ml bolus amounts, is often used initially for more rapid onset. These may be repeated safely in bolus fashion every 1 to 2 hours. The current regimen of choice is bupivacaine 0.25 percent at a rate of 8 to 10 ml/h; 0.125 percent at a rate of 10 to 14 ml/h may also be effective.[1, 17]

Anesthetic Toxicity. The rate of drug absorption into the circulation, redistribution to inactive tissue sites, and metabolic clearance determines the plasma concentrations of local anesthetics. Excess plasma concentrations of these drugs lead to signs of systemic toxicity. The rate of systemic absorption is dependent on the dosage, injection site, vascularity, presence of vasoconstrictive agents, and properties of the drug.

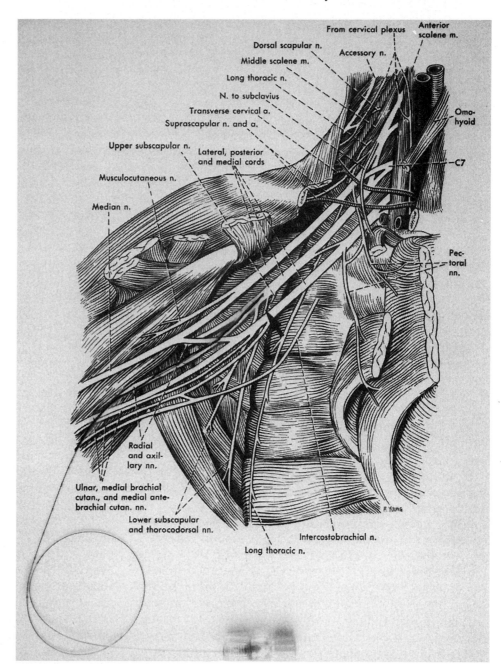

FIGURE 9–2 • The axillary catheter has been inserted percutaneously and passed about 12 cm from the skin insertion site to lie in proximity to the axillary musculocutaneous and ulnar nerves.

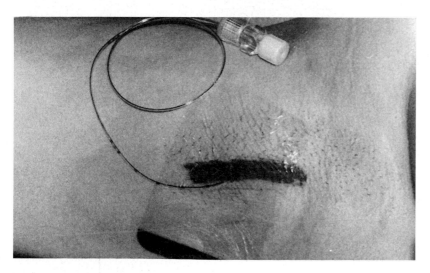

FIGURE 9–3 • Fixation of the axillary catheter by the combination of suturing and transparent dressing in a patient in the recovery room.

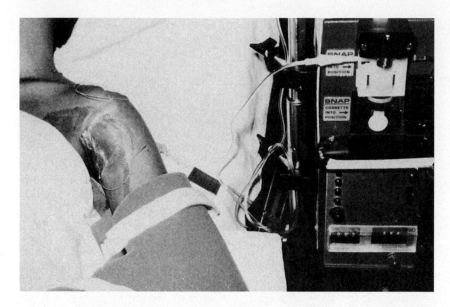

FIGURE 9–4 • Continuous infusion of the anesthetic agent.

Toxicity either is immediate, through intravascular injection, or is delayed, through systemic absorption. The threshold for toxicity may vary significantly among patients. The cardiovascular toxic effects of anesthetic agents may be accentuated during pregnancy.[14]

Signs and Symptoms. Initial signs of toxicity may include numbness of the tongue and circumoral tissues. The patient may exhibit restlessness and complain of tinnitus, vertigo, and difficulty with visual focusing. As concentrations in the central nervous system increase, slurred speech, drowsiness, and twitching of skeletal muscles may occur. The twitching is observed first in the face and extremities and is usually a premonition of the onset of tonic-clonic seizures. Seizures, apnea, cardiac dysrhythmias, and profound cardiovascular depression with hypotension are end-stage results.

Treatment. Immediate treatment of local anesthetic–induced seizures includes ventilation with 100 percent oxygen, correction of the resultant metabolic and respiratory acidosis, and intravenous administration of benzodiazepines. Vasopressors are used to treat hypotension (bretylium in anesthetized dogs is the preferred drug for anesthetic-induced ventricular dysrhythmias).[10]

Continuous Passive Motion. The arm may be placed in a continuous passive motion machine as soon as satisfactory analgesia is achieved. The continuous infusion of choice is usually 0.25 percent bupivacaine at a rate of 8 to 10 ml/h (Fig. 9–4). Both the rate and the concentration can be modified, depending on individual patient response to daily increases in the range of motion setting on the continuous passive motion machine. Breakthrough discomfort may require an increase in the flow rate of the anesthetic agent or, ideally, the instillation of small boluses of 0.5 percent bupivacaine through the catheter, as needed. Alternatively, the continuous infusion with on-demand bolus dosage methods provides flexibility with improved response to changing analgesic requirements. If sympatholysis for treatment or prevention of vasospasm or sympathetic pain is the primary therapeutic goal, 0.125 percent bupivacaine at 8 to 12 ml/h may be used. Upper extremity complex regional pain syndrome (reflex sympathetic dystrophy) responds to continuous infusion with patient-controlled anesthesia via a small portable infusion device (CADD APII Infusion Pump; Baxter Health Care Corp).[3]

KEY POINTS AND PITFALLS

Certain details promote rapid, precise catheter placement. The radial nerve axillary sheath for catheter positioning is preferred because of its direct course, allowing for farthest proximal placement. The catheter tip location comes closest to the brachial cords, with the greatest nerve cross-sectional density providing superior results (see Fig. 9–2). Proximal placement with distribution of an anesthetic agent will involve the musculocutaneous and often the axillary nerves (Fig. 9–5). Another benefit is that this placement rarely

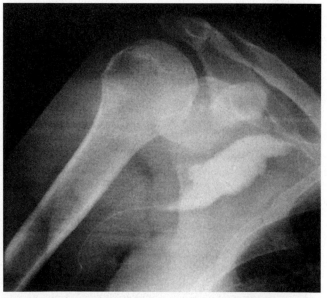

FIGURE 9–5 • Contrast material demonstrating spread of agent injected through an axillary catheter.

results in any back leakage of the agent through the skin insertion site. The median nerve sheath allows advancement only as far as the origin of the terminal nerve, which is formed by parts of the lateral and medial cord. The ulnar nerve curves around the axillary artery, interfering with catheter placement[6] (Fig. 9–6). This may result in subcutaneous or intrafascial coiling of the catheter as advancement is attempted (Fig. 9–7). It is also important to advance the plastic cannula only 3 to 5 mm off the insulated needle once an axillary nerve sheath is identified and selected for catheter placement. Any vigorous attempts at further advancement usually result in kinking or collapse of the cannula.[6]

An alternative technique to electric nerve stimulation is to elicit nerve paresthesias with a "finder needle." Dilation of the neurovascular sheath with 30 ml of 0.9 percent NaCl is performed on identification. This may help dilate the potential space, rupture fascial septa, and ease subsequent passage of the catheter.[6]

COMPLICATIONS: POTENTIAL AND REPORTED SIDE EFFECTS

There are several reported or potential complications and side effects of continuous axillary brachial plexus blockade. Bacterial colonization of the catheter, without evidence of local or systemic infection, has been noted to occur 6 to 10 days after insertion. The catheter is usually removed by 4 days after insertion because of decreased analgesic requirements, and culture samples taken from catheters at 4

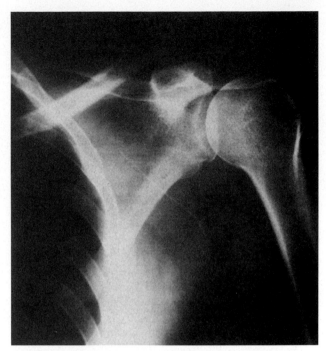

FIGURE 9–7 • In some cases, while threading the catheter, resistance may be noted, which indicates catheter curling. Curled catheter can still result in a complete nerve block and adequate postoperative pain relief.

days after insertion have shown no bacterial colonization.[6] Potential complications include intra-arterial injection and rapid venous absorption with local anesthetic toxicity. Incorrect placement has resulted in incomplete or absent anesthesia rates as high as 20 percent, nerve injury, hematoma formation, and catheter migration.[8, 9, 13, 16, 18] Subcutaneous or intrafascial kinking or coiling of the catheter has not interfered with anesthetic infusion or subsequent removal of the catheter[7] (see Fig. 9–7). Back-leakage of anesthetic solution through the skin insertion site has been a problem with catheters advanced 5 cm or less, thus complicating infusion rates and site hygiene. This has not been a problem with catheters inserted to 12 cm.[7] Horner's syndrome secondary to a continuous axillary catheter is a reported side effect.[12] To allay any apprehension, the patient should be informed that this troubling but clinically benign syndrome may occur.

Continuous auxillary brachial plexus blockade has been used extensively at the Mayo Clinic. Adherence to proper placement method coupled with clinical vigilance has resulted in minimal risk.[4] This system requires a dedicated, skilled, and responsive team of health care providers to overcome technical obstacles and maximize patient satisfaction. The procedure has been found to be safe and reliable, and its use to facilitate early postoperative mobilization, sympathectomy, and pain management is recommended.

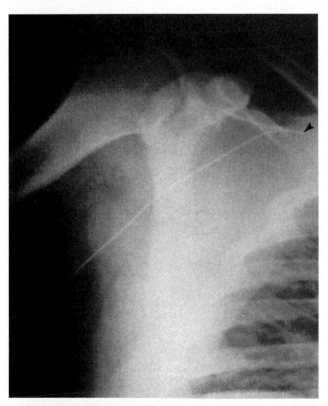

FIGURE 9–6 • Placement of the catheter in the radial axillary sheath allows for the most proximal advancement and superior clinical effect.

REFERENCES

1. Buttner, J., Kemmer, A., Argo, A., Klose, R., and Forst, R.: Axillare blockade des plexus brachialis. Reg. Anaesth. **11**:7, 1988.
2. Buttner, V. J., Klose, R., and Hammer, H.: Die kontinuierliche axillare

Katheter-plexusanasthesia: eine Methode zur postoperativen Analgesie und Sympathikolyse nach handchirugischen Eingriffen. Handchir. Mikrochir. Plast. Chir. **21**:29, 1989.

3. CADD APII Infusion Pump product brochure, Baxter, Health Care Corp., Deerfield, Il., 60015.
4. Davis, W. J., and Lennon, R. L.: Brachial plexus anesthesia for outpatient surgical procedures on an upper extremity. Mayo Clin. Proc. **66**:470, 1991.
5. Galindo, A.: Regional Anesthesia. Atlanta, Ga., R. M. Scientific Publications, 1982.
6. Gaumann, D. M., Lennon, R. L., and Wedel, D. J.: Continuous axillary block for postoperative pain management. Reg. Anaesth. **13**:77, 1988.
7. Hall, J. A., Wedel, D. J., and Lennon, R. L.: Axillary catheter technique for brachial plexus blockade in upper extremity surgery. Reg. Anaesth. **15**:546, 1990.
8. Haynsworth, R. F., Heavner, J. E., and Racz, G. B.: Continuous brachial plexus blockade using an axillary catheter for treatment of accidental intra-arterial injections. Reg. Anaesth. **10**:187, 1985.
9. Hobelmann, C. F., and Dellon, A. L.: Use of prolonged sympathetic blockade as an adjunct to surgery in the patient with sympathetic maintained pain. Microsurgery **10**:151, 1989.
10. Kasten, G. W., and Martin, S. T.: Bupivacaine cardiovascular toxicity: comparison of treatment with bretylium and lidocaine. Anesth. Analg. **64**:911, 1985.
11. Kirkpatrick, A. F., Bednarczyk, L. R., Hime, G. W., Szeinfeld, M., and Pallares, V. S.: Bupivacaine blood levels during continuous interscalene block. Anesthesia **62**:65, 1985.
12. Lennon, R. L., and Gammel, S. A.: Horner's syndrome associated with brachial plexus anesthesia using an axillary catheter. Letter to the editor. Anesth. Analg. **74**:311, 1992.
13. Merrill, D. G., Brodsky, J. B., and Hentz, R. V.: Vascular insufficiency following axillary block of the brachial plexus. Anesth. Analg. **60**:162, 1982.
14. Morishima, H. O., Pedersen, H., Finster, M., et al.: Bupivacaine toxicity in pregnant ewes. Anesthesia **63**:134, 1985.
15. Morrey, B. F.: Post-traumatic contracture of the elbow, operative treatment, including distraction arthroplasty. J. Bone Joint Surg. **4**:601, 1990.
16. Randalls, B.: Continuous brachial plexus blockade. Anaesthesia **45**:143, 1990.
17. Sada, T., Kobayashi, T., and Murakami, S.: Continuous axillary brachial plexus block. Can. Anaesth. Soc. J. **30**:201, 1983.
18. Selander, D.: Catheter technique in axillary plexus block. Acta Anaesthesiol. Scand. **21**:324, 1977.
19. Selander, D., Dhuner, K.-G., and Lundborg, G.: Peripheral nerve injury due to injection needles used for regional anesthesia. Acta Anaesth. Scand. **21**:182, 1977.

CHAPTER 10

Rehabilitation

• ROBERT P. NIRSCHL and
BERNARD F. MORREY

Elbow rehabilitation has received relatively little attention except as it relates to the athlete (see Chapters 40 and 43). In this edition, the concepts of continuous motion and splinting are described in Chapters 11 and 12. Hence this chapter deals with basic principles, and the concepts discussed are mainly the result of our experience over the last decade. Although the specific applications may vary, the principles have been expanded to encompass the broad scope of elbow pathology. It is our intention to present an organized and systematic basis for the rehabilitative process.

ANATOMIC CONSIDERATIONS

The anatomy of the elbow region was discussed in detail in Chapter 2. Some aspects that influence the rehabilitation plan or philosophy should be emphasized. The unique three-bone, four-joint articulation has a high degree of congruence. Further, the capsular reaction to trauma accounts for much of the difficulty experienced in obtaining normal function after injury or surgery.

Articulations

Ulnohumeral Joint. The high degree of congruence of the ulnohumeral joint originates in part from the presence of the posterior articular facets of the olecranon. The need to accommodate the olecranon in extension makes the elbow vulnerable to a mechanical block in the olecranon fossa. The high degree of congruity results in both anterior and posterior capsular scarring having an effect on both flexion and extension.

Radiohumeral Joint. This articulation is involved in flexion-extension movement as well as in forearm rotation. Any mechanical distortion of the lateral compartment will directly affect either motion and occasionally may be a severely compromising factor in the rehabilitative process.

Proximal and Distal Radioulnar Joints. The elbow is unique in that it provides pronation and supination motions. The two articulations that allow this function are intimately related, and the distal joint can affect forearm rotation as well as can the proximal rotation.

Ligaments and Capsule

The anterior capsule of the elbow joint is usually a relatively thin, pliable structure. The capsule is, however, very sensitive to injury, and major alterations in its anatomy are a common clinical factor compromising normal elbow flexion and extension (Fig. 10–1). The medial ligamentous structures originate primarily from the medial epicondyle to insert at the proximal ulna. The medial ligament is subject to rupture, contracture, and, occasionally, calcification,[10] the effects of which can contribute to loss of elbow extension and flexion.[9] Post-traumatic thickening of the lateral ligamentous structures can also cause motion limitation. Deficiency can cause subtle subluxation instability[10] (see Chapter 44). The annular ligament also may give rise to pain or restrictive motion when the radial head is deformed or misshapen.

Musculotendinous Factors

With the exception of the pronator teres, the muscles of the common flexor origin, comprising the flexor carpi radialis and ulnaris and the palmaris longus, traverse both the elbow and the wrist joints. Major alterations of these muscle-tendon units may severely compromise elbow function, which may in turn be aggravated by wrist dysfunction or pathology.

Muscles originating from the lateral epicondyle area, the common origin of the extensor tendons, the extensor carpi radialis brevis and longus, and the brachioradialis may affect normal elbow excursion and strength. These muscle-tendon units, except the brachioradialis, cross both the elbow and the wrist joints. In addition, the extensor brevis originates just anterior and distal to the lateral epicondyle. During elbow flexion and extension, this muscle origin glides over the outer lateral capsule and over the bony aspects of the lateral condyle. Alterations in the shape of the lateral condyle or scar tissue at the under-surface of the extensor brevis can alter normal elbow extension.

The anterior anatomy of the elbow is unique because the brachialis muscle inserts into the capsule and crosses the anterior aspect as a muscle, not as tendinous tissue.[13] Hemorrhage into the brachialis at this level, therefore, has a high potential for significant scar formation and joint contracture or even ectopic bone formation (e.g., myositis ossificans) (see Chapter 32).

Neurovascular Considerations

In a chronic flexion contracture, rehabilitative attempts to attain full extension may cause mechanical compression of either the brachial artery or the median nerve, or both. Because the ulnar nerve has little tolerance as it passes through the cubital tunnel, it is vulnerable to compression or inflammation during rehabilitative efforts. This is particularly true if the ulna is scarred in its position and increased elbow motion is attained without releasing the tethers to the nerve. Splints sometimes can cause neural irritation, usually of the ulnar nerve at the elbow and the superficial radial nerve at the wrist.

SPECIFIC REHABILITATIVE CONSIDERATIONS

As with other joints, rehabilitation of the elbow will vary according to the specific pathology involved: overuse, sin-

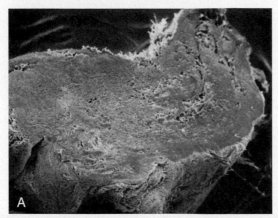

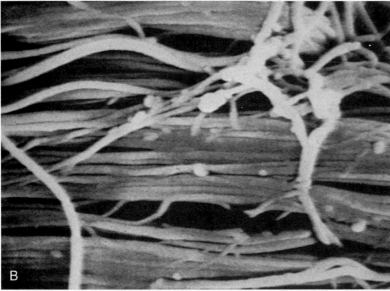

FIGURE 10–1 • The normal anterior capsule of the elbow is thin and translucent. When injured, this structure becomes thickened to 3 to 4 mm (*A*), which accounts for the typical flexion contracture seen after elbow injury. Note fibril thickening and cross-linking (*B*).

gle event trauma, surgical trauma, systemic inflammatory process, and the like. The stages of rehabilitation include control of the inflammatory response, allowance of healing, and restoration of function (Table 10–1). It does little good to know the appropriate concepts but to apply them with poor timing or improper implementation.[19] A more detailed discussion of these elements is appropriate.

Control of Inflammation and Pain

It should be kept in mind that rehabilitation essentially starts at the time of injury. If the inflammatory phase of healing including pain can be minimized, more complete and rapid rehabilitation will be attained. The time-tested scheme represented by the mnemonic PRICEMM (protection, rest, ice, compression, elevation, medication, and mo-

dalities) is highly appropriate in the early stages of healing of any tissue, whether bone, articular, ligamentous, or muscular.[19, 21, 23] These methods are enhanced by medications and other modalities (Table 10–2). Inability to control pain and inflammation frustrates all rehabilitative efforts (see Chapter 12).

Protection. Protection does not necessarily imply immobilization or lack of use of the injured parts. The technique of protection with various types of immobilization devices is discussed subsequently.

Rest. Rest implies restriction of the functional use or aggravation of the injured area, not total inactivity. Although not always possible, every effort should be made to encourage activity of the uninjured adjacent joints.

• TABLE 10–1 • **Stages of Rehabilitation**

Control inflammation and pain
Allow and encourage healing
Restore function
Strength
Flexibility (motion)
Endurance

• TABLE 10–2 • **Mnemonic for Remembering the Elements Used to Control Inflammation and Pain**

P—Protection
R—Rest
I—Ice
C—Compression
E—Elevation

M—Medication
M—Modalities

Ice. Cryotherapy is a time-honored modality used to minimize edema and hemorrhage and to control inflammatory exudation.[12, 15] It is used on a regular basis in the early postoperative period and in the early phase of inflammation and intermittently after exercise in the later stages of rehabilitation.[1]

Compression. Compression is useful in the early stages of injury or after surgery. Both static and intermittent air-compression devices may also be used. Although the ability to objectively demonstrate efficacy is difficult, we have recently documented the statistical advantage of compression cryotherapy after total elbow arthroplasty (Aircast) (Fig. 10–2). In a prospective study of 60 patients undergoing elbow replacement, a statistically significant reduction in swelling was recorded in 30 patients, as compared with 30 control subjects ($P<.05$).[1] All other parameters, pain, blistering, and motion also favored the cryo-compression–treated group.

Elevation. The elbow is relatively easy to elevate, at least to a moderate extent, above the level of the heart. Prolonged periods of elevation may be difficult if the shoulder is also involved with disease, as in rheumatoid arthritis.

Medications and Modalities. The inflammatory process

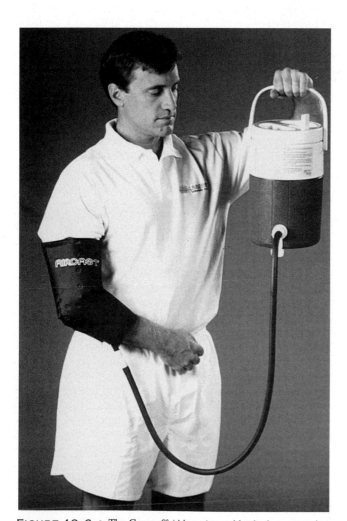

FIGURE 10–2 • The Cryocuff (Aircast) provides both compression and cold to the involved joint.

also can be controlled by pharmacologic methods. Aspirin is ill advised, however, in acute stages of trauma, as there is a potential for local hemorrhage. In some instances, high-voltage galvanic stimulation also has proved helpful in controlling the inflammatory process by initiating involuntary muscle contractions that relieve edema and provide muscle re-education. If immobilization is necessary, a device may be designed that allows the application of this additional modality. We rarely use plaster immobilization for elbow soft tissue problems. But selective use of an elbow immobilizer can be helpful.

Promotion of Healing

The healing process involves an inflammatory phase, but relief of pain by injection or oral medication must not be misinterpreted as assisting the healing process. If a patient is allowed to return to full activity without an appropriate period of rehabilitation, the underlying problem may well recur or become worse once the effects of the anti-inflammatory agent have ceased. It is therefore extremely important to distinguish the aspects of a rehabilitative program that provide pain relief from those that assist the true healing process.[21] Comfort therefore is not specifically reflective of biologic cure.

The following rehabilitative elements have, in our opinion, the potential to promote healing:

1. Early rehabilitation and fitness exercise of noninjured areas
2. Early protected rehabilitation exercises for injured areas
3. High-voltage galvanic stimulation
4. Continuous passive motion in selective presentations
5. Active motion

The relationship of the specific elements of strength and flexibility exercises and ultimate return to full function are illustrated in Figure 10–3. This illustrates the interdependence and sequence of motor and flexibility components of the rehabilitation process.

Early Exercise of Noninjured Areas. Basic research at the cellular level is incomplete, but there is little question about the beneficial effects of early function as a basic rehabilitative modality.[2, 3, 23] Observed clinical events include apparent enhancement of local circulation, maintenance of strength and tissue compliance, reduction of edema or fluid extravasation, and resolution of the hematoma.[5, 20] Even passive motion decreases the development of atrophy in the experimental animal.[24] The exercise programs, of course, must be designed in such a manner that the injured part is not violated. This concept is dealt with in detail in Chapter 11.

Early Protective Exercise for Injured Areas. Observations of bone and cartilage healing have demonstrated the effectiveness of protective exercise for promoting this process. The same principles apply to soft tissue injury. To prevent further injury, the program must have an appropriate timing sequence and must be supervised closely to achieve the rehabilitative objectives. Semirigid immobilization or functional counterforce bracing is appropriate at this stage. Motion is allowed to occur in a safe, prescribed arc that can be attained actively or passively without exces-

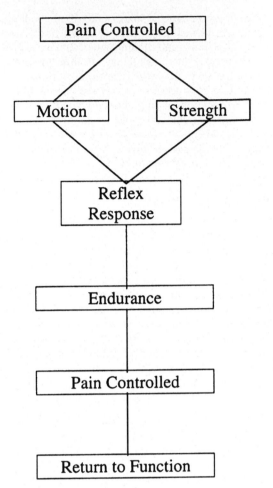

FIGURE 10–3 • After pain is controlled, strength and motion recovery lead to enhanced endurance and ultimately return of full function.

sive pain or stress to the healing tissue. Extremes of position that may injure bone, ligament, or muscle should be avoided. Protection, therefore, during the healing and rehabilitative phases can and should be modified according to the specific need of the individual. If the injury has caused instability due to fracture or ligament damage, rigid immobilization is appropriate. In most instances, however, because the joint is so congruent, early motion often is allowed with a ligament injury if proper protective splinting is provided.

Electrical Stimulation. High-voltage electrical stimulation is believed to play a role in the enhancement of bone healing and may have a role in soft tissue healing as well. In my opinion (RN), the benefits of high-voltage electrical stimulation may be summarized as follows:

1. Lessens local accumulation.
2. May enhance involuntary muscle contracture.
3. Enhances local blood flow.
4. Has a local analgesic effect.
5. Dissipates edema.

Continuous Passive Motion. Continuous passive motion is prescribed in that arc of known stability and one that will not injure tissue (discussed in detail in Chapter 11); decreased wound edema, lessened joint effusion, and increased range of motion have been observed in both postsurgical[5] and post-traumatic[11] joints. This modality should be avoided in patients with poor tissue or circulatory impairment; immobilization rather than motion is prescribed for such patients.

Restoration of Function

Once the pain or inflammatory process is controlled and an appropriate stage of healing has been attained, restoration of function to the injured area can be addressed.[19, 21, 23] There are significant differences in the goals and potential recovery of function in post-traumatic, rheumatoid, and athletic patients. For example, a several-fold difference in the oxygen consumption of skeletal muscle has been documented in sedentary and highly trained individuals.[14] In many athletic patients with soft tissue injury, an overuse syndrome is present. Thus, full flexibility generally is best introduced after there has been some reasonable progress in the program to increase strength. Endurance should be sought near the end of the process. This strategy may be entirely different from the goals and rehabilitation sequence sought in persons suffering from a generalized arthritic process or in those who have sustained an injury that has damaged multiple tissues around the joint. The general guidelines of the rehabilitation program are described later. Programs for specific conditions are discussed in those chapters.

MOTION

Because of the tight congruity of the elbow joint, the closely applied and vulnerable soft tissues, and the proximity of the muscles, stiffness is both common and extremely difficult to overcome. Immobilization adversely influences the orientation and mechanical properties of periarticular soft tissue.[2] Joint stiffness is believed to be due not only to scarred static structures (see Fig. 10–1) but also, in part, to the actin-myosin in cross-bridges[14] that cause muscle stiffness. This aspect of muscle stiffness must be addressed. Furthermore, excessive passive stretch of the joint is to be strictly avoided.

Early Motion. The scientific basis of the benefits of early motion is emerging as the harmful influence of increased synthesis of collagen cross-linking during immobilization has been shown.[3] Passive joint motion not only provides nourishment to the articular cartilage but also has the beneficial effect of clearing hematoma formation from the joint.[20] Further, early active motion must also be initiated as soon as the inflammatory process has been controlled and to the extent that the healing phase will allow. The initial arc of motion should be limited to one that does not aggravate inflammation or retard healing. If joint stiffness has occurred or if stiffness is anticipated, dynamic bracing also may be used.[17] A slow continuous force that stretches the damaged contracted tissue must be distinguished from the sudden, quick maneuver (manipulation) that tears tissue and may evoke a response that results in further contracture[8, 18] (see Chapter 12).

Manipulation. Although manipulation generally is not advocated and is even discouraged as an adjunct to rehabilitation of the elbow, one experience with 11 individuals with post-traumatic stiffness revealed that 55 percent did have improved motion with manipulation under anesthesia.[6] The value of manipulation has also been demonstrated in the patient with a closed-head injury.[7] One of us (BFM) regularly examines the postsurgical or post-trauma elbow under anesthesia. This examination sometimes increases the arc of motion that is present when the patient is awake; however, great care is taken to avoid quick moves or to deliver a force that will cause significant tearing and damage to the soft tissue.

BRACING

Five types of braces or splints are used in the postoperative or post-injury management of the elbow. These include (1) static resting splints, (2) a hinged splint with or without motion stops, (3) dynamic splints, (4) static adjustable splints, and (5) functional counterforce bracing. Each has a specific role in the management of various pathologies and they are discussed in detail in Chapter 12.

STRENGTH

A description of the physiology of muscle contraction is presented in Chapter 5, and the specifics of strength training are described in Chapter 41. In the less motivated patient or in one suffering from a generalized arthritic process, limited benefits should be anticipated. Isometric exercises to improve flexion and extension, pronation, supination, and grip strength are readily performed at home. The isometric contraction is held for 3 to 5 seconds and is followed by 3 to 5 seconds of relaxation. It is usually recommended that the elbow be held at 90 degrees for flexion and extension exercises and that the forearm be placed in the neutral position for pronation and supination isometric exercises. A series of 15 to 20 efforts performed two to three times a day is the usual recommendation. Complete relaxation is needed during the exercise period, and total muscle relaxation between contractures is important.[20] In those with radiohumeral problems, all flexion exercise should be done with the forearm in supination, as pronation increases radiohumeral stress.[16]

Probably the most common method of rehabilitation of elbow flexion and extension strength is the use of weights. The elbow is ideally suited to exert flexion and extension motions against the resistance of a hand-held weight. Such exercises result in both eccentric and concentric contracture of the muscles, and because the weight (force) is constant, the effect is further classified as an isotonic exercise. (The mechanical leverage advantage of the muscles changes with joint position, as the resistance decreases with successive flexion motions and increases with extension. By using an elastic tension cord classified as isoflex exercise, a progressive increase in tension occurs with increasing elbow flexion, thus accommodating the mechanical disadvantage of free weight isotonic resistance.)

Although such exercises may be extremely difficult or impossible to perform in a patient with rheumatoid arthritis, isotonic and "isoflex" concentric and eccentric contracture done in combination with proper sequence is an important feature in the rehabilitation program.[19, 21, 23] A series of 15 to 20 efforts performed two to three times per day is

the usual program, starting with approximately 1 kg. The exercise is performed in the sitting position, with the elbow flexed from extension through an arc of 130 to 140 degrees in 1 to 3 seconds. It should be noted that the more rapid rates of movement result in less force across the joint. Extension exercises are conducted with the patient either lying supine, with the elbow flexed and the arm elevated at a right angle to the torso, or standing, with the arm raised overhead. In this way, the effect of gravity is negated, and the extensor musculature may be adequately exercised. Starting with approximately 1 kg, additional weight is added in 1-kg increments to attain the maximal force that has been determined according to the patient's needs and goals and the status of the joint. For more specific details about strength testing, see Chapter 5. With a limited arc of motion, strength exercises should not be delayed until a full range of motion is obtained but should be begun simultaneously with flexibility exercises.

The concepts discussed are applicable not only to elbow but also to wrist motion. It should be noted that the exercises for tennis elbow are in large part focused at the wrist and include wrist flexion, extension, radial and ulnar deviation, and forearm pronation and supination (see Chapter 40). It should also be appreciated that the shoulder, upper back, and neck muscles are often weak in association with elbow dysfunction. As the shoulder is the platform of the elbow, these deficiencies, when present, must also be addressed.

Other Considerations

Personal motivation and pending litigation also are important variables and cannot be ignored when attempting to return the elbow to normal function.[4, 22] Realistic expectations also must be clearly set forth prior to initiating the rehabilitation effort. The condition of the person with severe rheumatoid arthritis and adjacent joint involvement is markedly improved with a total elbow replacement, offering 100 degrees of painless motion. In this patient, occupational therapy may be the most effective means not only of restoring motion but also of encouraging the use of other joints on a regular basis. For the competitive athlete, on the other hand, anything short of normal function with the potential of obtaining above-average strength and endurance is inadequate. Implicit in this discussion, therefore, is the recommendation that the physician devote adequate time to clearly explaining the goals of the treatment offered and carefully supervising the rehabilitation process.

REFERENCES

1. Adams, R., and Morrey, B. F.: The effect of cryo-compression on the elbow: a prospective randomized study. AAOS Annual meeting, Anaheim, CA, Feb., 1999.
2. Akeson, W. H., Amiel, D., and Woo, S. L. Y.: Immobility effects on synovial joints. The pathomechanics of joint contracture. Biorheology 17:95, 1980.
3. Amiel, D., Akeson, W. H., Harwood, F. L., and Frank, C. B.: Stress deprivation effect on metabolic turnover of the medial collateral ligament collagen—a comparison between 9 and 12 week immobilization. Clin. Orthop. 172:265, 1983.
4. Burton, K., Polatin, P. B., and Gatchel, R. J.: Psychosocial factors and the rehabilitation of patients with chronic work-related upper extremity disorders. J. Occup. Rehab. 7:139–153, 1997.

5. Coutts, R. D., Toth, C., and Kaita, J.: The role of continuous passive motion in the rehabilitation of the total knee patient. *In* Hungerford, D. (ed.): Total Knee Arthroplasty—A Comprehensive Approach. Baltimore, Williams & Williams, 1992.
6. Duke, J. B., Tessler, R. H., and Due, P. C.: Manipulation of the stiff elbow with the patient under anesthesia. J. Hand Surg. 16A:19, 1991.
7. Garland, D. E., Rozza, B. E., and Waters, R. L.: Forceful joint manipulation in hand-injured adults with heterotopic ossification. Clin. Orthop. 169:133, 1982.
8. Green, D. P., and McCoy, H.: Turnbuckle orthotic correction of elbow-flexion contractures. J. Bone Joint Surg. 61A:1092, 1979.
9. Guttierez, L. P.: A contribution to the study of the limiting factors of elbow flexion. Acta Anat 56:146, 1964.
10. Jobe, F. W., Stark, H., and Lombardo, S. J.: Reconstruction of the ulnar collateral ligament in athletes. J. Bone Joint Surg. 68A:1158, 1986.
11. Korcok, M.: Motion, not immobility, advocated for healing synovial joints. J.A.M.A. 246:2005, 1981.
12. Lehman, J.: Therapeutic Heat and Cold. Baltimore, Williams & Wilkins, 1982, pp. 404, 563.
13. Loomis, L. K.: Reduction and after-treatment of posterior dislocation of the elbow with special attention to the brachialis muscle and myositis ossificans. Am. J. Surg. 63:56, 1944.
14. Margar, D. L.: Separation of active and passive components of short-range stiffness of muscle. Am. J. Physiol. 232:45, 1977.
15. McMaster, W. C., and Liddle, S.: Cryotherapy influence on post-traumatic limb edema. Clin. Orthop. 150:282, 1980.
16. Morrey, B. F., An, K. N., and Stormont, T. J.: Force transmission through the radial head. J. Bone Joint Surg. 70A:250, 1988.
17. Morrey, B. F.: Post-traumatic contracture of the elbow: operative treatment, including distraction arthroplasty. J. Bone Joint. Surg. 72A:601, 1990.
18. Morrey, B. F.: The use of splints for the stiff elbow. Perspect. Orthop. Surg. 1:141, 1990.
19. O'Connor, F., Sobel, J., and Nirschl, R.: Five step treatment for overuse injury. Phys. Sports Med. 20:128, 1992.
20. O'Driscoll, S. W., Kumar, A., and Salter, R. B.: The effect of continuous passive motion on the clearance of a hemarthrosis from a synovial joint: an experimental investigation in the rabbit. Clin. Orthop. Rel. Res. 176:305, 1983.
21. Nirschl, R., and Sobel, J.: Arm Care. Arlington, VA. Medical Sports Publishing, 1996.
22. Sainbury, P., and Gebson, T. G.: Symptoms in anxiety and tension and the accompanying physiological changes in the muscular system. J. Neurol. Neurosurg. Pyschiatr. 17:216, 1954.
23. Sobel, J., and Nirschl, R.: Conservative treatment of tennis elbow. Phys. Sports Med. 9:42, 1981.
24. Wouter, J. A. D., O'Driscoll, S. W., van Royen, B. J., and Salter, R. B.: Effects of immobilization and continuous passive motion on post-operative muscle atrophy in mature rabbits. Can. J. Surg. 31:185, 1988.

• CHAPTER 11 •

Continuous Passive Motion

• SHAWN W. O'DRISCOLL

BIOLOGIC CONCEPT OF CONTINUOUS PASSIVE MOTION (CPM)

In 1960, Salter and Field[10] showed that immobilization of a rabbit knee joint under continuous compression, provided by either a compression device or forced position, resulted in pressure necrosis of cartilage. In 1965, Salter and colleagues[11] reported the deleterious effects of immobilization on the articular cartilage of rabbit knee joints and the resultant lesion that they termed "obliterative degeneration of articular cartilage. Salter[9] believed that, "The relative place of rest and of motion is considerably less controversial on the basis of experimental investigation than on the basis of clinical empiricism." He reasoned that since immobilization is obviously unhealthy for joints, and if intermittent movement is healthier for both normal and injured joints, then perhaps continuous motion would be even better. Because of the fatiguability of skeletal muscle, and because a patient could not be expected to move his or her own joint constantly, he concluded that for motion to be continuous it would also have to be passive. Thus, he invented the concept of *continuous passive motion*, which has come be known as simply CPM. Salter also believed that CPM would have an added advantage; namely, that if the movement was reasonably slow, it should be possible to apply it immediately after injury or operation without causing the patient undue pain.

FOUR STAGES OF ELBOW STIFFNESS

Because the elbow is so prone to post-traumatic and post-surgical stiffness, CPM should be especially useful in maintaining motion and preventing such stiffness. The rationale for this is much clearer if one understands the stages of stiffness, of which there are four.

The first stage, occuring within minutes to hours following surgery or trauma, is caused by bleeding. The second stage, which occurs during the next few hours and days is very similar but progresses more slowly. It is due to *edema*. Both bleeding and edema result in swelling of the periarticular tissues, thereby diminishing their compliance. The immediate effect is to limit joint motion and make it more painful and therefore less acceptable to the patient. Thus, stiffness in these first two stages is avoided by preventing swelling. This can be accomplished by ensuring that the joint is moved through its entire range of motion right from the start, rather than only a portion of its range. CPM is required for this purpose.

The third stage results from the formation of *granulation tissue* during the first few days and weeks. The stiffness is still soft but may require the use of splints to regain motion. The fourth stage results from *fibrosis* and is amenable only to splinting or surgical treatment.

PRINCIPLES OF USE

Based on an understanding of how stiffness develops, the principles of use of CPM are readily understandable. Motion should commence as soon as possible following surgery, ideally in the recovery room (which is not always practical). Until motion is started, it is preferable to elevate the limb with the elbow in full extension and wrapped in a compressive Jones dressing to minimize swelling. A drain is usually useful to prevent intra-articular accumulation of blood. Prior to starting CPM, all circumferential wrapping (e.g., Jones, cling) should be removed and replaced with a single elastic sleeve.

Once CPM is started, it is necessary that the full range of motion be utilized (Fig. 11–1A and B). Essentially the tissues are being squeezed alternately in flexion and extension. CPM causes a sinusoidal oscillation in intra-articular pressure.[1, 5] This not only rids them of excess blood and fluid but prevents further edema from accumulating.[4] In the first 24 hours, swelling can develop in minutes (due to bleeding), so CPM should be continuous. Only bathroom privileges are allowed. As the number of days following surgery increases, the amount of time required for swelling to develop increases also, so that longer periods out of the machine are permitted.

Continuous passive motion requires close supervision by someone skilled with its use, so it is mandatory that the patient and family are involved and educated from the beginning regarding the principles of use and how to monitor the limb. Frequent checking and slight adjustments of position prevent pressure-related problems. The arm tends to slip out of the machine, so it must frequently be pulled back into it. Nurses do not always have sufficient time, or sometimes the experience, to look after these needs. The patients and their families develop a keen sense of responsibility very quickly and become an invaluable asset.

The CPM should be used long enough to get the patient through the period during which he or she will be unable to accomplish the full range of motion by himself or herself. This can be several days to a month.

PAIN CONTROL

Such use of CPM immediately raises questions and concerns regarding uncontrollable pain. Pain control in these patients requires that we depart from traditional teaching. Rather than adjusting the motion according to the level of pain, the analgesia is adjusted instead. This is no different from the principles of anesthesia for surgery. Some patients have more pain than others, and appropriate modifications need to be made for them.

We favor the use of an indwelling catheter for continuous brachial plexus block anesthesia (Fig. 11–1C).[7–11] This permits a range from analgesia to anesthesia by varying the

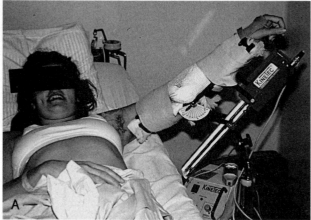

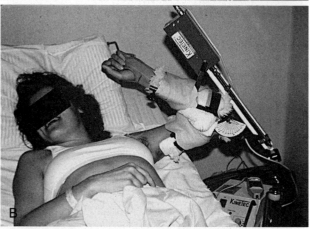

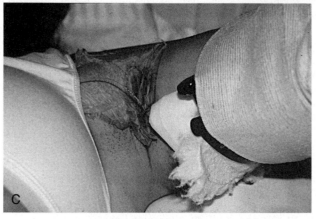

FIGURE 11–1 • *A* to *C*, The range of motion on continous passive motion should be full. This permits the tissues to be squeezed alternately in flexion and extension. Analgesia is accomplished with an indwelling catheter for continuous brachial plexus block anesthesia using bupivacaine, a long-acting local anesthetic.

dose of bupivacaine, a long-acting local anesthetic. In many cases, the dose employed initially is sufficient to cause a complete or near-complete motor and sensory block. Motor blockade requires splinting of the wrist to protect it. Moderate or complete anesthesia, as opposed to analgesia with minimal anesthesia, requires careful attention to the status of the limb overall, as the patient's protective pain response is no longer present.

The catheter is left in place for 3 days in hospital, then removed. At that time the patient is usually able to maintain

the same range of motion with either no or only oral analgesics. The goal is to have the patient leave the hospital capable of moving the elbow from about 10 to 130 degrees of motion actively. Of course, more is better.

A patient-controlled analgesia pump with morphine has also been used effectively if a brachial plexus block is contraindicated, unsuccessful, or not available.

ADVANTAGES

There are a number of advantages to the use of CPM. Most surgeons are aware from the total knee experience that analgesic consumption is diminished because the patients are more comfortable (though not always during the first day or two). Swelling is diminished.

My personal experience using CPM in strict accordance with the principles just outlined has convinced me that the final range of motion obtained is greater than that obtained without the use of CPM, despite the studies that failed to show such a benefit in the knee (Fig. 11–2*A* and *B*).[4, 12, 13] This can be explained on the basis of how CPM has been routinely used. Typical protocols involve starting with a small range of motion tolerated by the patient, for example 30 degrees, and gradually increasing the range each day. This pattern of use is not in compliance with the essential principles of CPM.

COMPLICATIONS

In using CPM for the elbow, I have not experienced any serious permanent complications; however, complications can occur. Bleeding is increased but rarely sufficiently to require a transfusion, although some patients have been taken back to the operating room for evacuation of a hematoma under such circumstances. On several occasions, the posterior skin flap turned dark and its viability looked questionable. Those elbows were treated by being placed back into a well-padded Jones dressing with an anterior plaster slab holding the elbow in extension, then elevating the arm for 2 to 4 days. No patients lost a flap, although a few have had small areas of necrosis that healed by secondary intention without further treatment. One patient almost fell out of bed from lying so close to the edge while using the machine.

A word of caution is required. No circumferential wrapping (e.g., cling) should be left on the elbow once the CPM is started. A single fish-net or elastic tube grip sleeve is best.

I do not generally use CPM in the presence of ligament injuries or potential joint instability because it is not possible to keep the elbow perfectly aligned with the axis of rotation of the machine. Malalignment would stress the ligaments and bony stabilizers of the joint.

INDICATIONS AND CONTRAINDICATIONS

Continuous passive motion is indicated to prevent stiffness and to maintain motion obtained at the time of surgery,

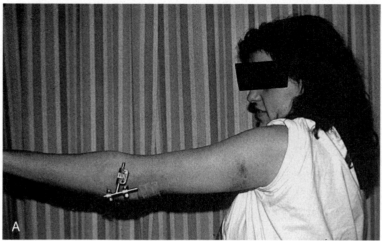
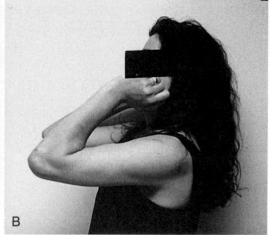

FIGURE 11-2 • Typical range of motion seen 3 weeks postoperatively *(A)* and 1 year postoperatively *(B)* following a distraction interposition arthroplasty treated postoperatively using continuous passive motion.

particularly following contracture release, synovectomy, and excision of heterotopic ossification. The same is true following the replacement of arthritic joints that were stiff preoperatively. If is relatively contraindicated if the soft tissue constraints (ligaments) are insufficient, if fixation of fractures has not been rigid, or if the elbow is unstable.

HOME USE

The home rental market for CPM machines is being served by at least two domestic companies at the time of this writing, so home use of CPM is practical. The typical requirement is in the range of 4 weeks for an elbow that has been stiff before surgery, and 1 to 2 weeks for elbows requiring assistance to prevent stiffness from developing.

REFERENCES

1. Breen, T. F., Gelberman R. H., Ackerman, G. N.: Elbow flexion contractures: Treatment by anterior release and continuous passive motion. J. Hand Surg. **13-B**:286, 1988.
2. Brown, A. R., Weiss, R., Greenberg, C., Flatow, E. L., Bigliani, L. U.: Interscalene block for shoulder arthroscopy: comparison with general anesthesia. Arthroscopy. **9**:295, 1993.
3. Gaumann, D. M., Lennon, R. L., Wedel, D. J.: Continuous axillary block for postoperative pain management. Reg. Anesth. **13**:77, 1988.
4. O'Driscoll, S. W., Kumar, A., Salter, R. B.: The effect of continuous passive motion on the clearance of a hemarthrosis from a synovial joint: an experimental investigation in the rabbit. Clin. Orthop. **176**:305, 1983.
5. O'Driscoll, S. W., Kumar, A., Salter, R. B.: The effect of the volume of effusion, joint position and continuous passive motion on intra-articular pressure in the rabbit knee. J. Rheumatol. **10**:360, 1983.
6. Pope, R. O., Corcoran, S., McCaul, K., Howie, D. W.: Continuous passive motion after primary total knee arthroplasty. J. Bone Joint Surg. Br. **79**:914, 1997.
7. Rice, A. S. C.: Prevention of nerve damage in brachial plexus block. XVI Annual European Society of Regional Anaesthesia Congress. London, 1997.
8. Romness, D. W., Rand, J. A.: The role of continuous passive motion following total knee arthroplasty. Clin. Orthop. **226**:34, 1988.
9. Salter, R. B.: Motion vs. rest. Why immobilize joints? J. Bone Joint Surg. **64-B**:251, 1982.
10. Salter, R. B., Field, P.: The effects of continuous compression on living articular cartilage. An experimental investigation. J. Bone Joint Surg. **42-A**:31, 1960.
11. Salter, R. B., McNeill, O. R., Carbin, R.: The pathological changes in articular cartilage associated with persistent joint deformity. An experimental investigation. Studies of the rheumatoid diseases. Third Canadian Conference on Research in Rheumatic Diseases. Toronto, 1965, pp. 33–47.
12. Schroeder, L. E., Horlocker, T. T., Schroeder, D. R.: The efficacy of axillary block for surgical procedures about the elbow. Anesth. Analg. **83**:747, 1996.
13. Stinson, L. J., Lennon, R., Adams, R., Morrey, B.: The technique and efficacy of axillary catheter analgesia as an adjunct to distraction elbow arthroplasty: a prospective study. J. Shoulder Elbow Surg. **2**:182, 1993.

CHAPTER 12

Splints and Bracing at the Elbow

• BERNARD F. MORREY

The elbow joint is frequently managed with the use of static or adjustable braces. By far the most complex and important of these two categories is the adjustable brace for the stiff elbow. Specifically, the four types of braces or splints used in the postoperative and postinjury management of the elbow include resting and hinged splints, and dynamic and static adjustable splints.[6]

STATIC AND PROTECTIVE SPLINTS

Static splinting for the elbow is commonly used for short periods as a protective measure after injury or surgery. As a long-term modality, this type of splinting is uncommonly indicated (Fig. 12–1).

If the issue is instability, a hinged splint is used (Fig. 12–2). By initially locking the hinge, the same device can be used as a resting static splint; then it can be converted to a movable stabilizing device by unlocking it. Hinged splints allow active motion and are employed primarily for ligament healing. Occasionally, they are prescribed for the resected elbow, but compliance is quite variable.

ELBOW STIFFNESS

The most common complication of elbow injury, and even in some arthritic conditions, is stiffness. The most im-

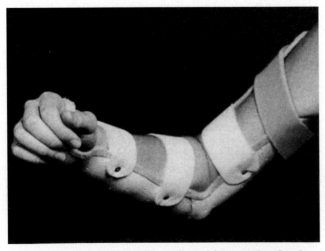

FIGURE 12–1 • Resting splint rarely used for more than 2 to 3 weeks.

portant means of avoiding this after a fracture is rigid fixation. Early motion has been shown to be effective in decreasing this sequela after fractures and injury at the elbow (see Chapter 23). After fracture dislocation, it has been demonstrated that immobilization lasting for more than 4 weeks resulted in a less than satisfactory outcome in every instance.[2] But despite the recognized need for and value of early motion and because of limitations imposed by the injury or by limitations in executing the treatment, and owing to the inherent biology and response to injury, stiffness of the elbow is a common problem in the orthopedic practice. Unfortunately, in the author's experience the use of aggressive physical therapy to address post-traumatic stiffness is not always successful and, in fact, as often as not, makes the contracture worse. To understand the rationale of splinting for this condition, therefore, it is necessary to understand the pathology of the process.

PATHOLOGY OF ELBOW CONTRACTURE

The exact reason that the elbow is so prone to joint contracture is not known with complete certainty. What is recognized is that the elbow is one of the most congruous joints in the body (see Chapter 2). It has also been observed that the typically translucent anterior capsule of the elbow undergoes a marked hypertrophy, with extensive cross-linking of the fibrils, as demonstrated on scanning electron microscopy (Fig. 12–3). This process is seen after direct injury, such as elbow dislocation, but it is also seen after minimal trauma. In some instances, a severe elbow contracture has been observed after surgery for lateral epicondylitis and after elbow trauma that appears to result only in hemarthrosis without any articular or extensive soft tissue damage. Under these circumstances, the elbow may contract rapidly, often within 2 to 3 weeks. An explanation of the rapid development of elbow contracture may be provided by the basic investigations on wound contracture. Experimental data demonstrate that dermal wounds undergo approximately 80 percent of the contracture within the first 3 weeks[1] (Fig. 12–4). Continuous motion, if properly used, has been shown to be an important adjunct to successful treatment.

This effect is designed at maintaining collagen length, thus maintaining the length of the capsule and ligaments. The use of continuous passive motion is discussed in detail in Chapter 11. This modality is used with confidence, particularly if rigid fixation has been afforded to the fracture and if pain and inflammation can be controlled. After 3 to 8 weeks of treatment and if the fracture has been rigidly fixed and it is thought that force could be applied, the use of splints may be introduced in order to gain further motion. In general, the author's philosophy is that the continuous motion machine maintains motion but does not gain motion. The use of static adjustable splints gains motion both in flexion and in extension. The question then arises as to the best method of providing a force to stretch the periarticular soft tissues. There are three possibilities: physical therapy, dynamic splinting, and static adjustable splinting.

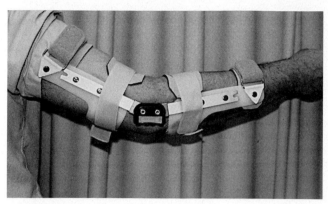

FIGURE 12–2 • Hinged splint allows static support when the mechanism is locked, and active motion thereafter as desired.

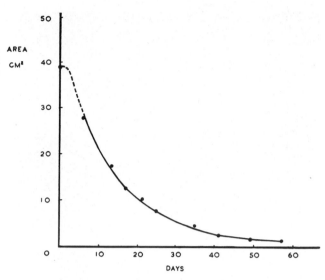

FIGURE 12–4 • Experimental data showing that the majority of tissue contracture occurs in the first 3 weeks. (With permission from Billingham, R. E., and Russell, P. S.: Studies on wound healing, with special reference to the phenomenon of contracture in experimental wounds in rabbits' skin. Ann. Surg. [144]: 961–981, 1956, p. 964.)

MANAGEMENT OF ELBOW STIFFNESS

Physical Therapy

Physical therapy must be executed with extreme caution in the post-traumatic or inflamed elbow. The reason for this is that passive stretch, in and of itself, can introduce the very inflammation that one is trying to treat in the course of the therapy. Inflammation results in contracture and thus is an obstacle to the treatment goal. If referral to a well-trained physical therapist who understands this principle is possible, then the cautious use of physical therapy may be of value. Such access is not possible in the author's practice; therefore, I have never prescribed physical therapy for a patient of mine with elbow stiffness.

Dynamic Splinting

Dynamic splinting is probably the most popular means of treating impending or developing stiffness. The concept

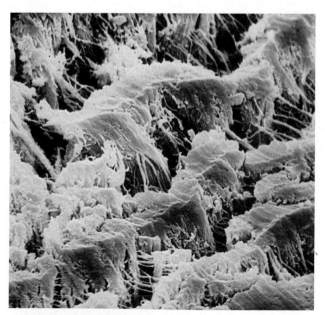

FIGURE 12–3 • Scanning electron microscopy (×30) showing dense hypertrophy of collagen fibrils with extensive cross-linkage sites.

has been used in hemophiliacs by employing a system of reverse dynamic slings both at the knee and at the elbow.[3] This is also an attractive concept at the elbow, as force may be delivered by readily available commercial devices (Fig. 12–5). To comprehend the rationale of dynamic or static adjustable splinting, some understanding of the soft tissue about the elbow as viscoelastic tissue is necessary. If the soft tissue at the elbow can be considered viscoelastic tissue, its response to a constant versus a variable force is different.[8] The theoretical response to a constant force is shown in Figure 12–6. This load results in soft tissue deformation, which is called creep.[5] However, what is not demonstrated in this illustration is the biologic response to this constant load, inflammation. Inflammation can, therefore, alter this idealized curve, and, in the author's opinion, inflammation is a common byproduct of dynamic splinting. Nonetheless, this remains an attractive option for many.[7]

Static Adjustable Splinting

The last philosophical approach to the stiff elbow is the use of static adjustable splints. In this modality, a constant force is applied to the elbow that results in stress and strain being imparted to the tissue. However, the force is not continuously applied, allowing a stress relaxation to occur over a period of time. This type of treatment has been employed extensively at the knee by serial casting and has also been effectively used at the elbow.[9] It is felt that the stress-free relaxation eliminates or lessens the likelihood of inflammation, and thus the elbow in our practice and opinion is more amenable to this type of load application (Fig. 12–7). The constant force is applied so as to exceed the elastic limits of the tissue or result in a stretch. But if this load is maintained at a constant and is not further increased, tissue relaxation should occur over time. Finally, to further avoid the likelihood of inflammation, the patient controls the amount and duration of tension being applied.

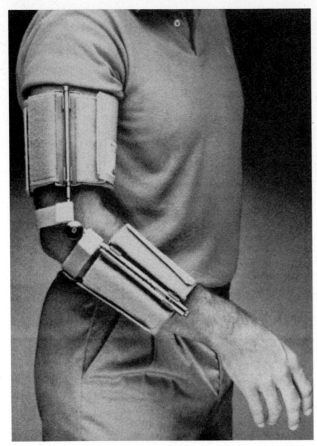

FIGURE 12–5 • Commercially available dynamic splint. The tension and excursion may be adjusted by the patient.

This is done within a very discrete set of recommendations and a very defined program (see later).

STATIC ADJUSTABLE SPLINTS

The classic static adjustable splint is a turnbuckle type. Its effectiveness has been reintroduced by Green and associates.[4] In this instance, approximately an 80 percent success

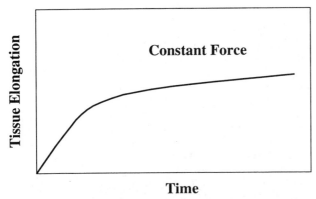

FIGURE 12–6 • Viscoelastic tissue response to a constant force resulting in gradual stretching of the tissue. The potential for inflammation, however, is not demonstrated by this curve but is possible if the force is constantly present, which is the case in dynamic loading.

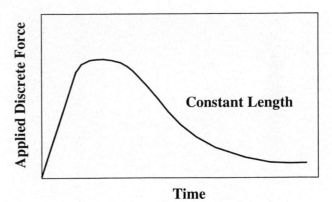

FIGURE 12–7 • The tissue response to the application of a single discrete force results in stress relaxation of the viscoelastic tissue.

rate in treating elbow contractures from various etiologies and at various stages of development was reported. These patients were primarily those developing flexion contracture, and the turnbuckle was used to gain extension. However, there are two problems associated with the use of these splints.

The first is the ability to attain full extension. As the contracture decreases to less than 30 degrees, the effectiveness of a turnbuckle in extension decreases. Second, when the elbow is at 90 degrees, a turnbuckle applied to the elbow imparts approximately 70 percent of the effective force in extending the elbow and 30 percent in separating the ulna from the humerus. Both are desirable characteristics; however, at 30 degrees of extension the mechanics change. Applying an extension load with a turnbuckle when the elbow is at 30 degrees results in the majority of the force going to separate the hinges and less then 25 percent of the force actually extending the elbow (Fig.

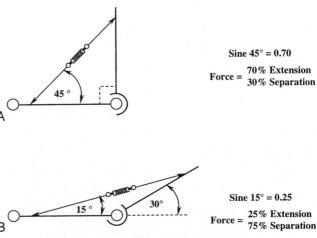

FIGURE 12–8 • A, With the elbow at 90 degrees, the anteriorly placed turnbuckle provides an effective force, approximately 70 percent of which is directed at extending the elbow and 30 percent in separating the joint itself. B, When the elbow is at 30 degrees, the turnbuckle is working through an angle of 15 degrees. The sine function of 15 degrees is .25. This means that 75 percent of the force is going to separate the hinge and distract the two components of the brace, and only 25 percent of the force is actually extending the elbow. These types of braces become inefficient as the elbow gets closer toward full extension.

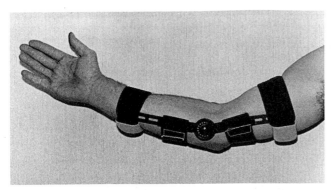

FIGURE 12–9 • A static adjustable splint currently used by the author in which the force is directly applied to the axis of rotation.

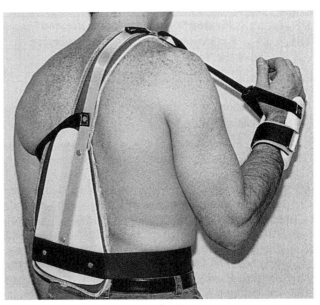

FIGURE 12–11 • To avoid the soft tissue impingement associated with straps supporting braces about the elbow, a hyperflexion splint that frees the elbow of any encumbrance is based at the shoulder, with flexion across the elbow by way of the wrist.

12–8). Hence, a means of delivering an extension moment without excessive axial distraction to the splint is necessary.

After several attempts, a means has been developed to apply the force through a gear mechanism at or about the flexion arc; the entire force is then directed toward extension, with no tendency to separate the splint hinge (Fig. 12–9). Furthermore, many patients have both flexion and extension loss. In patients with severe loss of motion, the splint that is currently used may be reversed and the same splint may be used to obtain flexion. This splint is, therefore, called the universal splint and is particularly effective is providing extension all the way to 0 and in improving flexion past 100 degrees (Fig. 12–10). If, however, more than 100 degrees of motion is needed, which is the case in the vast majority of instances, this brace and all others that are forearm- and brachium-based with straps are of limited value. The soft tissue tends to "bunch up" in flexion, and this tendency limits further flexion. For this reason, the ability to apply a flexion force was developed that had no cumbersome straps or any bracing around the elbow itself. This brace, called the hyperflexion brace, is stabilized on the thorax and the elbow is flexed through a mechanism applied to the wrist and an adjustable strap. The patient once again becomes responsible for the use of the brace, following the program described later. The splint is used after 100 degrees of flexion is obtained with the universal brace, noted earlier (Fig. 12–11). This brace is termed the *hyperflexion device*.

MAYO EXPERIENCE

Over the period 1984 through 1997, we have prescribed approximately 360 braces for patients with various expressions of stiff elbow. It is this experience that has resulted in the program that is currently employed. These splints are now commercially available.* A great deal of time is spent with the patient in the explanation of the rationale of brace management and specific discussion of the program, based on the specific goals of treatment (Fig. 12–12). Information given to the patient is shown in Appendix 1.

GENERAL INSTRUCTIONS FOR THE USE OF STATIC ADJUSTABLE SPLINTS

Appendix 1. The following general guidelines for the use of the turnbuckle splints may be modified, or instructions may be given to you, depending on your individual needs and progress.

I. General Goals
  A. To attain improved motion of your elbow, inflammation must be avoided. This is done with the use of the anti-inflammatory agents, heat and ice, and education of the patient to the signs of inflammation.
II. Cardinal Signs of Inflammation
  A. Increased soreness, increased discomfort, swelling,

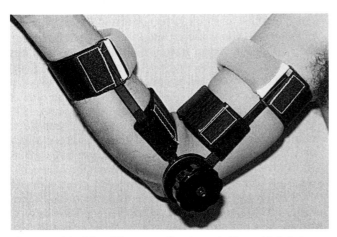

FIGURE 12–10 • The same splint shown in Figure 12–9, but reversed and being used in the flexion mode; hence, the splint is called the universal splint in our practice.

*Prosthetic Laboratories of Rochester, Inc., 201 1st Ave. S.W., Rochester, MN 55902.

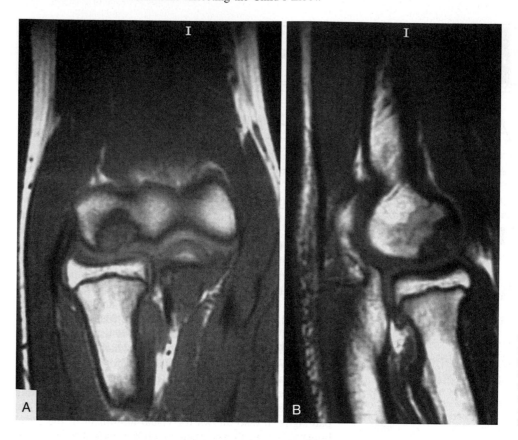

FIGURE 13-1 • Magnetic resonance imaging of a 13-year-old male with elbow pain, coronal (A) and sagittal (B) views. T1-weighted images show a defect in the capitellum. No loose body is seen. Clinical diagnosis was Panner's disease, and symptoms resolved in a few months without specific therapy.

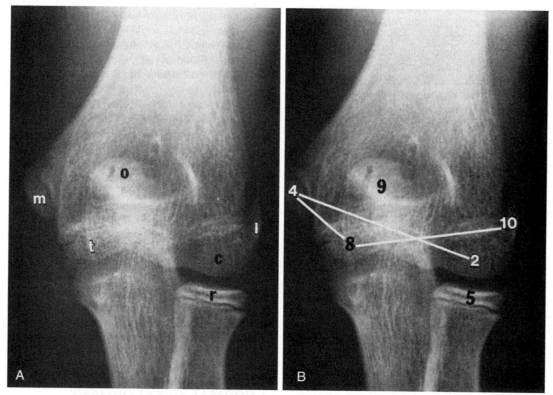

FIGURE 13-2 • A, Normal left elbow showing the secondary centers: capitellum (c); medial epicondyle (m); radial head (r); trochlea (t); olecranon (o); and lateral epicondyle (l). B, The approximate age at time of appearance of these centers is indicated in years. The cross connecting the secondary centers of the distal humerus serves as a reminder of the order of ossification of these centers (Modified from Brodeur, A. E., Silberstein, M. J., Graviss, E. R., and Luisiri, A.: The basic tenets for appropriate evaluation of the elbow in pediatrics. Curr. Probl. Diag. Radiol. 12:1, 1983.)

of the normal sequence and timing of the appearance of ossification centers and maturation patterns is important for an understanding of the radiographic appearances of the elbow in children (Fig. 13–2). Several mnemonics have been suggested to help remember the time of appearance of the ossification of these centers. We find that the cross (see Fig. 13–2B) connecting ossification centers is particularly helpful in remembering at least the order of ossification of these centers. An atlas, *Radiology of the Pediatric Elbow,*[4] shows standards for elbow maturation in children. To consistently evaluate the developing elbow, one must analyze each of the secondary centers of ossification, accounting for its appearance, configuration during development, and associated changes as it matures and eventually fuses with the humeral shaft. The descriptions that follow are brief, but they outline the major points of development and maturation of the centers.

Capitellum

The capitellum, the first of the elbow's six centers to ossify, generally becomes radiographically visible during the first and second years of life. Initially spherical, it flattens posteriorly to conform to the adjacent distal end of the humerus. The physis is broader posteriorly than anteriorly, giving the capitellum the appearance of a downward tilt; however, this appearance gradually disappears during the first decade (Fig. 13–3). During maturation, the capitellum fuses with the trochlea and the lateral epicondyle before it unites with the humeral shaft (Fig. 13–4).

The orientation of the capitellum with the humerus can be evaluated with a true lateral projection. The anterior surface of the humerus is gently bowed posteriorly, from the insertion of the deltoid muscle to the superior aspect of the coronoid fossa. A line drawn along the anterior surface

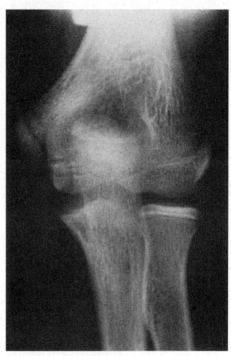

FIGURE 13–4 • A 13-year-old girl in whom the capitellum has joined with the lateral epicondyle and trochlea prior to fusion with the humeral shaft. Note the normal sclerotic radial epiphysis that is wider than the radial neck.

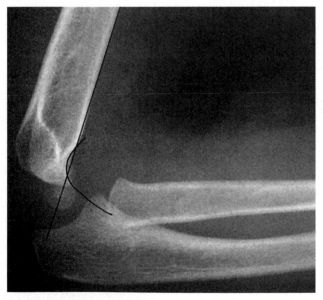

FIGURE 13–3 • Lateral elbow radiograph of a 2.5-year-old. A line along the anterior humeral shaft normally intersects the posterior half of the middle third of the capitellum. The continuation of the curved coronoid line just touches the anterior edge of the ossified capitellum. The angle formed by the coronoid line and humeral shaft line should contain the majority of the ossified capitellum.

of the humerus, from the deltoid insertion to the top of the coronoid fossa, should pass through the middle third of the capitellum. For practical reasons, most lateral examinations of the elbow do not include the deltoid insertion; therefore, one must use the most proximal portion of the humerus included on the radiograph. These two points determine the anterohumeral line, which passes precisely through the posterior half of the middle third of the capitellum. The capitellum is oriented anteriorly to the distal humerus. One also may draw a curvilinear line along the coronoid fossa. The extension of that line inferiorly should touch the anterior portion of the capitellum.

These two lines permit the detection of subtle supracondylar fractures, particularly Salter-Harris type I supracondylar fractures, with minimal posterior displacement of the distal humeral epiphysis with the capitellar ossification center.

Radiocapitellar Line

The radiocapitellar line is a line drawn through the long axis of the proximal radial shaft that should, in the absence of dislocation, pass through the middle of the capitellum ossification center. This is generally true in anteroposterior, lateral, or any oblique projection. In early development, however, the radial metaphysis is wedged so that on the anteroposterior projection a normal radial shaft line may appear to extend laterally to the capitellum. However, on the lateral projection, the normal radiocapitellar line can be appreciated (Fig. 13–5). In older patients, although it may appear that the radiocapitellar line is normal in one projection in a patient with a radial head dislocation, it

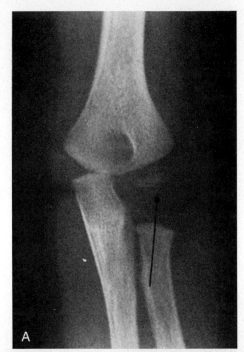

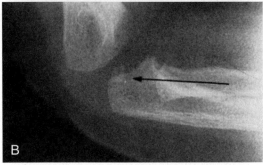

FIGURE 13–5 • *A,* Normal 7-month-old girl with apparent abnormal radiocapitellar line on the anteroposterior radiograph because of wedging of the metaphysis. *B,* The relationship between the radial shaft and capitellum is normal on the lateral radiograph.

invariably will be abnormal in the projection taken at right angles, generally the lateral projection.[15]

Medial Epicondyle

The medial epicondyle is the second elbow ossification center to appear in the normal sequence, usually at about 4 years. Lying posteromedially, it is often best appreciated on the lateral projection (Fig. 13–6). Frequently, it develops from more than one ossific nucleus. Although it is the second humeral ossification center to appear, its development is slow, and it is usually the last center to unite with the humeral shaft in the normal child, sometimes as late as 15 or 16 years of age.[14] This center may fuse with the trochlea before uniting with the humeral shaft. Injuries involving the nonunited medial epicondyle are relatively common and are among the most difficult to evaluate. Consequently, to avoid errors, Rodgers suggests making a habit of identifying the presence and the position of the medial epicondyle ossification center in each case.[12] A classic example of the importance of appreciating the se-

quence of humeral ossification center appearance is avulsion and displacement of the medial epicondyle ossification center. This frequently results in the displacement of the medial epicondyle into the normal position of the trochlear ossification center. In a child between 4 and 8 years of age—the time of appearance of the medial epicondyle and the trochlear ossification centers—a radiograph suggesting a trochlear ossification center, without visualization of a medial epicondyle center, should suggest that fracture and dislocation of the medial epicondyle have in fact occurred.[9]

Radial Head Epiphysis

The initial ossification of this epiphysis is fairly predictable and usually occurs in the fifth year (see Fig. 13–2B). Although usually beginning as a sphere, the radial head epiphysis often matures as one or more flat sclerotic centers. This pattern may be mistakenly interpreted as a fracture. With maturation, the physis on the anteroposterior radiograph is wider laterally than medially, and this appearance, combined with the medial angulation of the radius at the junction of its shaft and neck, may suggest dislocation on anteroposterior views. Lateral projection of the elbow will not confirm a suspected dislocation. With further maturation of ossification of the proximal radial ossification center, the normal relationship of the radius and capitellum can be seen on anteroposterior radiographs. Notches or clefts of the metaphysis of the proximal radius often are seen as normal variations of ossification during maturation.[7, 8]

Because fractures of the radial neck are extracapsular, they will not be associated with hemarthrosis and abnormalities of the humeral fat pads.[16]

Trochlear Epiphysis

Ossification of the trochlea appears at about 8 years and often is initially multicentric (Fig. 13–7; Fig. 13–8B). The trochlea frequently maintains an irregular contour during its development and should not be confused with abnormal processes such as trauma or avascular necrosis (Fig. 13–9). The trochlea will fuse with the capitellum prior to fusion with the distal humeral shaft. It is seldom fractured, except when associated with the vertical component of a supracondylar fracture or when its lateral edge is involved with a lateral condylar fracture.

Olecranon

The ossification center of the olecranon usually develops at 9 years of age, shortly after the trochlea and just before the lateral epicondylar epiphysis. The proximal end of the ulna flattens and becomes sclerotic just before the olecranon physis ossifies. Two ossification centers most often develop, and there is great variability in the configuration of the epiphysis. This results in an occasional misdiagnosis of acute fracture. The posterior ossification center is usually bigger than the anterior ossification center (Fig. 13–10), and these separate centers generally will unite prior to fusion with the proximal humerus. This process usually begins at about 14 years of age.

The pattern of closure of the olecranon physis is distinct,

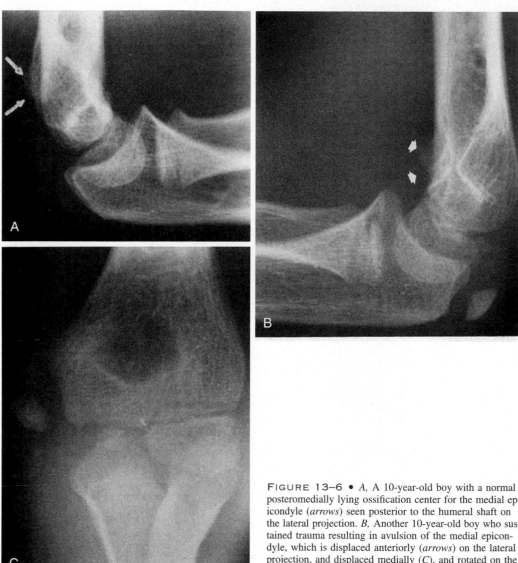

FIGURE 13–6 • A, A 10-year-old boy with a normal posteromedially lying ossification center for the medial epicondyle (arrows) seen posterior to the humeral shaft on the lateral projection. B, Another 10-year-old boy who sustained trauma resulting in avulsion of the medial epicondyle, which is displaced anteriorly (arrows) on the lateral projection, and displaced medially (C), and rotated on the anteroposterior projection.

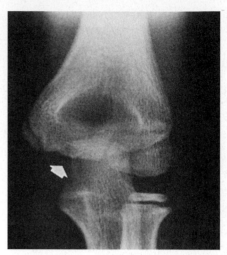

FIGURE 13–7 • Multiple ossification nuclei of developing trochlea (*arrow*) in a 9-year-old boy.

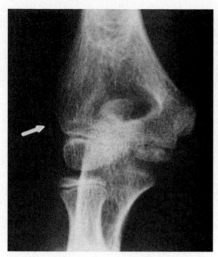

FIGURE 13–9 • A 9-year-old boy with beginning ossification of the lateral epicondyle (*arrow*) from a thin sliver widely separated from the metaphysis. Note the irregular outline of the developing ossification center of the trochlea.

with fusion occurring first along the joint line and then extending posteriorly. Frequently, fractures are wedged in the opposite direction.[13]

The olecranon physis has prominent sclerotic margins just prior to closure. Fusion proceeds posteriorly from the joint side or the anterior surface (Fig. 13–11). During its development, the physeal line remains relatively perpendicular to the ulnar shaft. As a result of differential growth, often with maturation, the olecranon growth plate, which initially is proximal to the elbow joint, comes to lie at a midelbow joint level by the time of fusion. This "wander-

ing physeal line of the olecranon" does not occur in all individuals.[4]

Although the majority of olecranon fractures are intracapsular and are associated with alterations of fat pads, some are not. The tip of the olecranon is not within the capsule in some individuals. The only other common site of fracture related to the elbow that lies outside the joint capsule is the radial neck (see Chapter 17).[4]

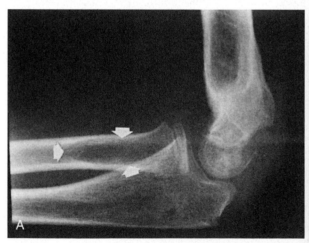

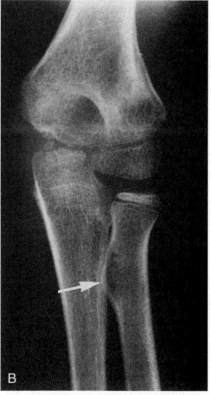

FIGURE 13–8 • *A*, Lateral radiograph with lucent region in the proximal radial shaft (*arrows*). *B*, Anteroposterior view shows prominent but normal radial tuberosity (*arrow*). Residual changes from previous transcondylar fracture of the humerus are seen.

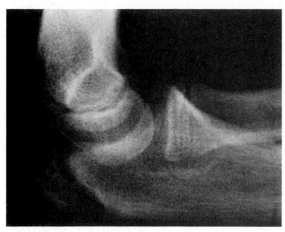

FIGURE 13–10 • A 13-year-old boy with double ossification center of the olecranon. The anterior nucleus is smaller.

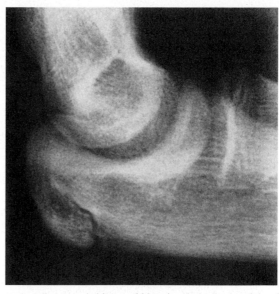

FIGURE 13–11 • A 14-year-old boy in whom closure of the olecranon growth plate has begun anteriorly. Note the sclerotic margin of that portion of the growth plate that remains unfused.

Lateral Epicondyle

The ossification center of the lateral epicondyle is the last of the elbow centers to appear. Usually, this center is first seen at 10 or 11 years of age, and it fuses to the humeral shaft at about 14 years of age. Unlike the other ossification centers of the elbow, the lateral epicondyle appears first as a thin sliver rather than as a round or spherical ossific nucleus (see Fig. 13–9).

Ossification commences at the lateral portion of the cartilaginous mold so that the physis appears particularly wide. The inferior aspect of the ossification begins at the junction between the distal humerus and the capitellum.[3]

Because of the relatively short time between the appearance and fusion of this center, it is not always certain in individual cases whether ossification is delayed or fusion to the humerus already has occurred. To avoid confusion about this point, it must be realized that prior to ossification, the humerus has a sharp, straight, sloping metaphyseal line that changes to a sloping, curving margin at the capitellum. The fused lateral epicondyle, on the other hand, has a smooth, curved margin that is continuous with the capitellum (Fig. 13–12).

NORMAL VARIANTS

In addition to the confusing appearances caused by the normally developing elbow, there are a few variations from normal or unusual appearances that should be noted.

The radial tuberosity lies medially at the junction of the medial shaft and the neck. On lateral views, it may appear as an undermineralized focus and may be misinterpreted as a destructive lesion of the bone (see Fig. 13–8). On the anteroposterior view of the elbow, the thin humeral olecranon fossa occasionally appears to be entirely lucent, the so-called perforated olecranon fossa (Fig. 13–13). In some instances, there is a bridge of bone crossing or a separate ossicle within a perforated olecranon fossa.

A rare anatomic anomaly is a bony projection from the anterior medial distal humerus known as the supracondylar process (Fig. 13–14), which is discussed in Chapter 2.

FIGURE 13–12 • A, A 9-year-old boy in whom ossification of the lateral epicondyle is about to begin. The metaphysis has a sharp, straight, sloping margin. B, The fusing lateral epicondyle in this 14-year-old boy, in contrast, has a smoother, rounded margin.

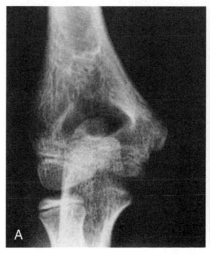
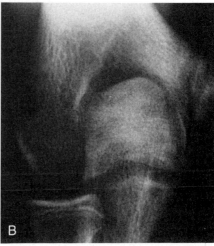

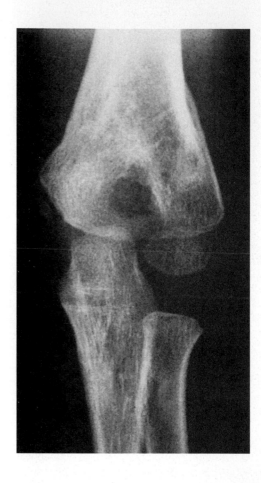

FIGURE 13–13 • A 6-year-old boy with perforated olecranon fossa. There has been a previous supracondylar fracture.

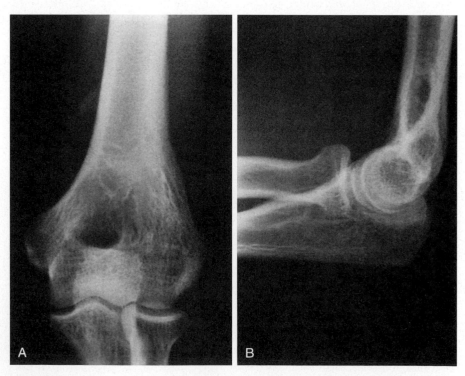

FIGURE 13–14 • Supracondylar process in a mature elbow. Anteroposterior (A) and lateral (B) radiographs.

REFERENCES

1. Barr, L. L.: Elbow. Clin. Diag. Ultrasound. **30**:135, 1995.
2. Beltran, J., Rosenberg, Z. S., Kawelblum, M., Montes, L., Bergman, A. G., and Strongwater, A.: Pediatric elbow fractures: MRI evaluation. Skel. Radiol. **23**:277, 1994.
3. Brodeur, A. E., Silberstein, M. J., Graviss, E. R., and Luisiri, A.: The basic tenets for appropriate evaluation of the elbow in pediatrics. Curr. Probl. Diag. Radiol. **12**:1, 1983.
4. Brodeur, A. E., Silberstein, M. J., and Graviss, E. R.: Radiology of the Pediatric Elbow. Boston, G. K. Hall, 1981.
5. Davidson R. S., Markowitz R. I., Dormans J., and Drummond D. S.: Ultrasonographic evaluation of the elbow in infants and young children after suspected trauma. J. Bone Joint Surg. **76A**:1804, 1994.
6. Gordon, A. C., Friedman, L., and White, P. G.: Pictorial review: magnetic resonance imaging of the paediatric elbow. Clin. Radiol. **52**:582, 1997.
7. Keats, T. E.: An Atlas of Normal Roentgen Variants That May Simulate Disease, 5th ed. St. Louis, Mosby Year Book, 1992, pp. 395–420.
8. Schmidt, H., and Freyschmidt, J.: Köhler/Zimmer Borderlands of Normal and Early Pathologic Findings in Skeletal Radiology, 4th ed. New York, Thieme Medical Publishers, 1993.
9. Markowitz R., Davidson R. S., Harty M. P., Bellah R. D., Hubbard A. M., and Kotlus Rosenberg H.: Sonography of the elbow in infants and children. Am. J. Roentgenol. **159**:829, 1992.
10. McCauley, R. G. K., Schwartz, A. M., Leonidas, J. C., Darling, D. B., Bankoff, M. S., and Swan, C. S., II: Comparison views in extremity injury in children: an efficacy study. Radiology **131**:95, 1979.
11. Merten, D. F.: Comparison radiographs in extremity injuries of childhood: current application in radiological practice. Radiology **126**:209, 1978.
12. Rodgers, L. F.: Radiology of Skeletal Trauma. New York, Churchill Livingstone, 1982, p. 435.
13. Silberstein, M. J., Brodeur, A. E., Graviss, E. R., and Luisiri, A.: Some vagaries of the olecranon. J. Bone Joint Surg. **63A**:722, 1981.
14. Silberstein, M. J., Brodeur, A. E., Graviss, E. R., and Luisiri, A.: Some vagaries of the medial epicondyle. J. Bone Joint Surg. **63A**:524, 1981.
15. Silberstein, M. J., Brodeur, A. E., and Graviss, E. R.: Some vagaries of the capitellum. J. Bone Joint Surg. **61A**:244, 1979.
16. Silberstein, M. J., Brodeur, A. E., and Graviss, E. R.: Some vagaries of the radial head and neck. J. Bone Joint Surg. **64A**:1153, 1982.

• CHAPTER 14 •

Congenital Abnormalities of the Elbow

• PETER C. AMADIO and
JAMES H. DOBYNS

Elbow function and configuration are affected by conditions both proximal and distal to the elbow as well as by abnormalities at the elbow itself. With this proviso, this chapter discusses congenital anomalies of the region between the shaft-metaphyseal junction of the humerus proximally and the bicipital tuberosity distally, and reviews the current state of knowledge for evaluation and treatment in that region.

CAUSES OF CONGENITAL ANOMALIES

The causes of congenital elbow anomalies follow the same patterns of genetic or somatic damage to the embryo that are seen in other congenital anomalies. The most common problem, radial head subluxation or dislocation, may be congenital, developmental, or post-traumatic. If not present at birth, it may be induced by a relatively trivial injury or merely by a short ulna from any cause. Because so much of the elbow area is cartilaginous at birth, it is difficult to rule out trauma as a possible agent in some dislocations and deformities. In addition, infections, tumors (congenital or infantile), and diseases (e.g., hemophilia) occasionally involve the elbow and may simulate congenital anomaly. Conditions that commonly involve the elbow are constitutional diseases of bone, metabolic abnormalities, and syndromes featuring limb formation and differentiation failure.[31, 36, 42, 66, 73] Some of the syndromes can be grouped under broad categories such as osteochondrodysplasia,[3, 26, 29, 73] dysostoses,[16] primary growth disturbances, primary metabolic abnormalities, and congenital myopathies (Table 14–1). Most, however, are chromosomal syndromes from the common dislocation of the radial head[54] through fairly well known syndromes such as trisomy 18, fibrodysplasia ossificans progressiva and the Antley-Bixler syndrome,[7] to such rarities as the Bruck syndrome (osteogenesis imperfecta with congenital joint contractures) and a congenital mirror hand syndrome. The most difficult problem when a congenital elbow condition is suspected is to decide whether the presenting deformity is entirely congenital or perhaps developmental or possibly even traumatic and whether one or more of these etiologies are interacting.

CLASSIFICATION

A multitissue defect classification can be based on the most obvious and most inhibiting tissue defect known to be present. Some degree of defect in other tissues is also commonly noted. The classification consists of three major categories: (1) bone and joint anomalies, (2) soft tissue anomalies, and (3) anomalies involving all tissues. Bone and joint abnormalities at the elbow may include major absences, but more commonly the skeletal structures are present but malformed. The common bone and joint problems are synostosis (Fig. 14–1), ankylosis (Figs. 14–2 to 14–4), and instability (Fig. 14–5). Soft tissue anomalies include malformations with contractures, control deficiencies, isolated tissue anomalies (Fig. 14–6), and congenital tumors (Fig. 14–7). Complete absence or disorganization of the whole limb, including elbow structures, may occur, as in phocomelia (Fig. 14–8); usually, recognizable though dysplastic structures are present (Fig. 14–9). Similar involvement, although more isolated to the elbow area, occurs in the pterygium syndromes.

With reference to the bone and joint deformities only it has been useful to many authors to classify them as follows:

I. Congenital
II. Developmental
III. Post-traumatic

There is much confusion and interplay between these diagnoses, particularly with reference to radial head subluxation or dislocation. In this classification, *congenital* refers to a primary genetic dysplasia of the skeleto-articular structure of the elbow, resulting in an observed deformity. Other congenital anomalies or a familial history of similar anomalies helps confirm this as an etiology. *Developmental* refers to elbow skeletal structures that are relatively normal at birth but are then secondarily deformed by abnormal stresses (perhaps from a congenital shortening of the ulna); by paralysis or other limited motion (arthrogryposis); neural, metabolic, endocrine, or dyscrasia disturbances (e.g., hemophilia, loss of pain recognition, hemochromatosis); tumor or hamartomatous involvement (e.g., fibromatosis, osteochondromata), and disease (e.g., sicklemia, Gorham's disease, infections). The post-traumatic etiologic grouping is only included in this chapter because of the continuing confusion over early radial head dislocations, which are often post-traumatic either as a variant of Monteggia fracture dislocation or as a pure dislocation of the soft cartilaginous radial head pulling through the annular ligament (see Chapter 21) and its residua. Both early and late, dislocation of the radial head is often diagnosed as a congenital subluxation or dislocation, but it often is not. A radial head subluxation or dislocation in an elbow with normal neural, muscular, and skeletal structures in both elbow and forearm is post-traumatic until proven otherwise; the condition of an elbow with abnormal skeletal forearm structures is probably caused by developmental stresses, but additional trauma may play a part. The condition of an elbow with a synostosis from birth or other skeletal deformity and no evidence of peribirth trauma is caused by congenital causes, but again trauma may be an additional factor.

Text continued on page 171

• TABLE 14–1 • Elbow Deformities in Congenital Syndromes

Syndrome	Syndrome Characteristics	Catalog Numbers*	Inheritance	Number of Patients†
Achondroplasia	O-1	10080	ASD	>100
Mesomelic dwarfism	O-1	15623, 24970	ASD, ASR	>100
Nievergelt	O-1	16340	ASD	<50
Werner	O-1	27770	ASR	>100
Ellis-Van Creveld	O-1	22550	ASR	<50
Acrodysostosis	O-1	10180	ASD	<50
Acromesomelic dwarfism	O-1	20125	ASR	<50
Ulna, fibula hypoplasia	O-1	19140	ASD	>25
Type 1 acrocephalopolysyndactyly	O-1	10110, 20100, 10112, 20102, 16420, 10120, 10130, 10140, 10160	ASD	>100
Multiple cartilaginous exostoses	O-2	13370	ASD, ASR	>100
Metaphyseal chondrodysplasia	O-3	26040, 25401, 20090, 25022, 25023, 25025, 15640, 25030, 15650, 24270, 15640, 15650, 21505, 25022, 25023, 25025, 25030, 25040, 25041	ASD	<100
Cranial dysostosis	D-1	12350, 12290, 21835, 30411	ASD	<100
Familial radioulnar synostosis	D-3	17930	ASD	<100
Pterygium	D-3	26500, 31215, 19100, 11950, 19360, 17820	ASD, ASR	>50
Radial aplasia	D-3	21860	ASD, S	>100
Idiopathic osteolysis		26580, 26570, 27795, 25960, 16630	ASD, ASR	<50
Mucopolysaccharidoses	PMA	25270, 23000, 22380, 25280, 30990, 25290, 25292, 25293, 25294, 25300, 25301, 25320, 25322, 25323	ASR	>100
Mucolipidoses	PMA	25240, 25250, 25260, 25265	ASR	>100
Lipidoses	PMA	21280, 30150, 24680, 23050, 23060, 23065, 21208, 25010, 25720	ASR	<50
VATER complex		19235, 10748	ASD	<50
Craniocarpotarsal dystrophy		19370, 27772	ASD	>50
Craniosynostosis		2310, 27235, 20100, 10120, 10160, 10140, 20155, 31410, 21850, 21853, 21855, 21860, 25922, 12315	ASD	>100
De Lange dwarfism		12247	ASD	>100
Diastrophic dysplasia		22260	ASR	<50
Nail-patella	D-2	16120	ASD	<50
Otopalatodigital		31130	X	<100
Rubenstein-Taybi		26860	ASR	>100
Silver-Russell		27005	ASR	>50
Klinefelter		27330	ASR	>50
Thalidomide embryopathy		27360	T, ASR	
Holt-Oram		14290	ASD	>100
Acrofacial dyostosis (Nager)		15440	S, ASD	>50
LADD		14973	ASD, S	<50
Fanconi anemia		22765, 22766	ASR	>100
TAR		27400	ASR	>100
Auriculo-osteodysplasia		10900	ASD	<25
Ehlers-Danlos		13000, 13001, 13002, 13005, 22535, 30520, 22540, 13006, 22541, 13008, 30415, 22531, 14790	ASD, ASR	>100
Phocomelia		26900	ASR	<50
Larsen's		15025, 24560	ASD, ASR	>50
Oculomelic complexes		16420, 25790, 25792, 16430, 25795, 16431	ASD, ASR	
Otopalatodigital		31130	X	<50
Amelia of arm		10440	S, ASD	<25
Peromelia of humerus		10030, 10330	ASD	<25
Humeroradial synostosis		14305, 23640	ASD, ASR	>50
Femoral-fibula-ulna complex		22820	ASR	>100
Focal dermal hypoplasia (Goltz)		30560	X	>50
Split hand		18360	ASD	>100
Ulnar mammary		19145	ASD	<25
Ulnar deficiency		13575, 19140, 20070, 24960, 10790, 31436, 27170, 20060, 20061	ASD, ASR	>100

O-1, defects of growth of tubular bones; O-2, disorganized development of cartilage and fibrous skeletal elements; O-3, abnormalities of diaphyseal cortical density or metaphyseal modeling; D-1, dysostosis with cranial and facial involvement; D-2, dysostosis with predominant axial involvement; D-3, dysostosis with predominant extremity involvement; PMA, Primary metabolic abnormalities; PGD, Primary growth disturbances; ASD, autosomal dominant; ASR, autosomal recessive; S, sporadic; X, linked to sex chromosome; T, Teratogenic.

*Catalog numbers are those used in McKusick, V. A.: Mendelian Inheritance in Man, 6th ed. Baltimore, Johns Hopkins University Press, 1983.

†Approximate number so far reported.

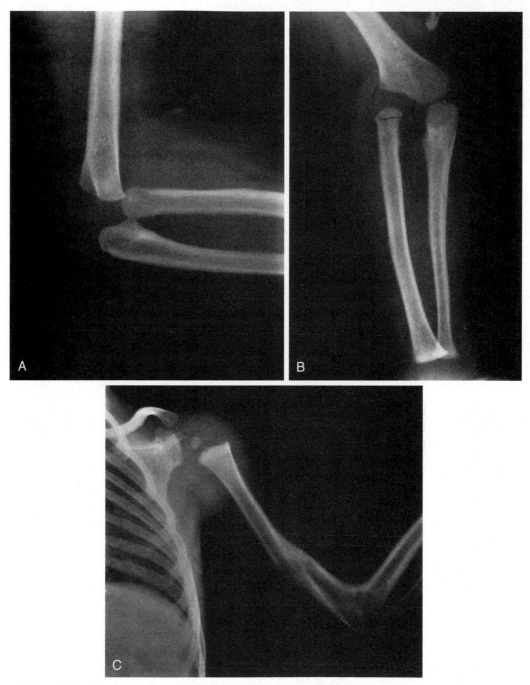

FIGURE 14–1 • Lateral (A) and anteroposterior (B) radiographic views of a hypoplastic distal humerus and an apparent radial head subluxation certainly reveal a deformity but probably not a subluxation. Clinically, there was no evidence of a dislocated radial head. The opposite elbow (C) showed a radiohumeral synostosis and also a recent fracture just proximal to the synostosis. This case demonstrates the difficulties of differentiation between subluxation, dislocation, and synostosis about the elbow, but the etiology is clearly congenital.

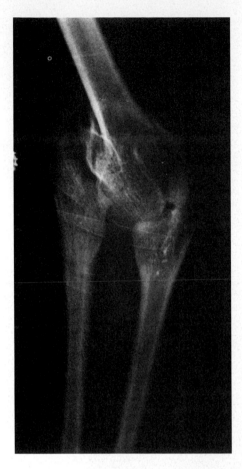

FIGURE 14–2 • This anteroposterior view of an elbow in congenital ulnar dimelia shows no radiohumeral joint but two ulnohumeral joints. The appearance is unusual, as expected, but no dislocation is noted. Both elbow and forearm motion are limited more than 50 percent.

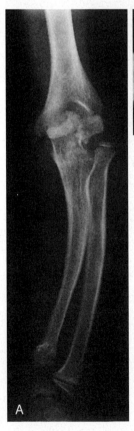

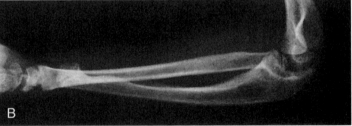

FIGURE 14–3 • A, Elbow and forearm function are, to date, nearly normal in this teenaged boy in whom the anteroposterior radiographic view shows ulnar hypoplasia and bowing, distortion of the distal ulnar physis-metaphysis, and subluxation of the radial head. B, The lateral radiographic view shows a similar epiphysis-physis-metaphysis distortion of the proximal ulna with associated joint surface irregularity and shaft bowing. No diagnosis has been confirmed, but this is probably an osteochondrodysplasia. The elbow abnormalities are developmental.

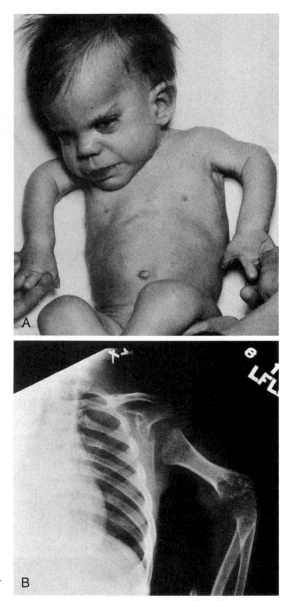

FIGURE 14–4 • This 18-month-old infant with chondrodysplasia punctata has developmental contractures of many joints including the elbows (A), where broad metaphyses and irregular, calcified epiphyses (B) are seen.

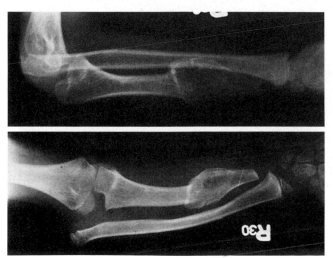

FIGURE 14–5 • This case further demonstrates the overlap between congenital and developmental abnormalities of the elbow. Gradual radial head subluxation due to unequal length of forearm bones is well known in multiple exostosis. These anteroposterior and lateral radiographs demonstrate a severe dislocation of the radial head that was present at birth and was associated with a severe osteochondroma deformity of the distal ulna with inhibition of ulnar growth.

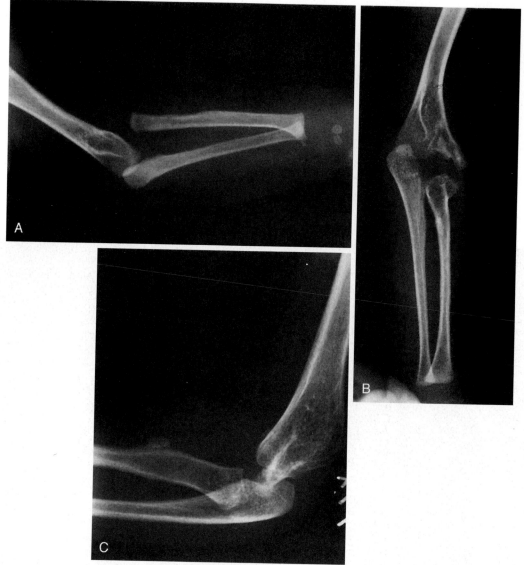

FIGURE 14–11 • *A*, Anteroposterior radiographic view of an *apparent* radiohumeral dislocation similar to that shown in Figure 14–2 is seen preoperatively. *B*, A postoperative anteroposterior radiographic view 4 years later shows repositioning of what was determined to be a congenital displaced radiohumeral joint without a dislocation of the radial head. *C*, A lateral postoperative view of the same elbow. Repositioning was obtained when the radius was shortened by removing a segment of the radial shaft. This segment of excised radius was then used to block the repositioned lateral condyle in its new position. This surgical procedure improved the radiographic position of the elbow but did not change function, which demonstrated, both preoperatively and postoperatively, mild loss of extension-flexion and moderate loss of supination-pronation.

resulting deformity is milder than that seen in definite congenital hypoplasia at the elbow. This may be so, but the so-called criteria for classifying a radial head dislocation as congenital (see later) may be seen after any early radial head dislocation regardless of cause (Fig. 14–12). By contrast, when traumatic dislocation is unreduced in the older child, the development of the radial head and the capitellum remains fairly normal, displaying only minimally those radiographic features said to be characteristic of congenital radial head dislocation. These features are: (1) dislocated or subluxed radial head, (2) underdeveloped radial head, (3) flat or dome-shaped radial head, (4) a more slender radius than normal, (5) a longer radius than normal, (6) underdeveloped capitellum humeri, and (7) lack of anterior angulation of the distal humerus.[4, 18, 44, 50, 71] Bilaterality, especially symmetric bilateral dislocation, is usually also

considered evidence for a congenital etiology, but this is not an absolute requirement.[39] However, many if not all of the features of congenital dislocation can also be seen with developmental dislocation, due to mild degrees of ulnar or capitellar hypoplasia. In such cases the radial head may slowly dislocate with growth, as the paired forearm bones continue to grow at dissimilar rates.[4]

There may be only one absolute criterion of congenital elbow dislocation: dislocation with severe hypoplasia of all the osseous elements of the elbow. Absence of the capitellum is probably an example of congenital aplasia, but hypoplasia of the capitellum may occur after dislocation from any cause, as may a deformity of the radial head (see Chapter 21).

When radial head dislocation is familial, bilateral, or seen at birth, or when it occurs with other musculoskeletal

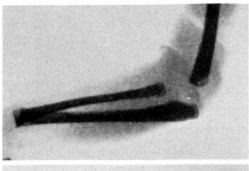

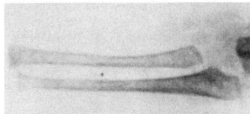

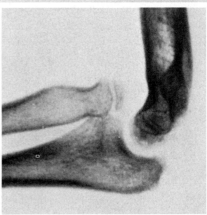

FIGURE 14–12 • Anterior dislocation of the radial head is demonstrated at initial diagnosis (age 2 weeks), at age 4 months, and at age 11 years. In addition to the dislocation, there is a reversal of the ulnar curve and some convexity of the radial head. The etiology is probably post-traumatic.

anomalies, particularly anomalies in the same upper limb, the evidence is strong that the radial head dislocation is congenital. Cases diagnosed later in life may be associated with a discrepancy in length of the paired forearm bones and therefore may fall within the "developmental" category. It is well known that inadequate length of the ulna from any cause will result in increased compressive stresses along the radius, gradually leading to a subluxation and perhaps a dislocation of the radial head.[33, 38, 63] Such subluxations, therefore, also may be a secondary phenomenon.[39]

Roughly half of all patients with isolated congenital radial head dislocation will have a problem bilaterally.[2, 39, 44] Bell and associates[4] have classified isolated congenital dislocations of the radial head as type I, subluxation; type II, posterior dislocation with minimal displacement; and type III, posterior dislocation with significant proximal migration of the radius. Type I is the least common dislocation but the one most likely to be associated with pain. Types II and III appear to be roughly equally prevalent. Type III is associated with the most loss of motion, usually supination. Deformity of the radial head without subluxation has also been reported.[20] Finally, Wiley and colleagues[69] have reported congenital anterior and lateral dislocations.

OTHER BONY PROBLEMS

Hypoplasia of the distal humerus may occur; the resulting deformity may cause ulnar neuropathy, either immediately, from synovial cysts, or chronically, due to abnormal elbow growth and nerve traction.[58] Congenital pseudarthrosis of the olecranon has been reported but is exceedingly rare.[52]

Soft Tissue Anomalies

Soft tissue anomalies or absences may interfere with elbow function as much as bone or joint deformities. These anomalies have been subdivided into syndromes with contractures (pterygium syndromes, congenital muscular atrophy, and myopathy syndromes), control deficiencies, isolated tissue anomalies (triceps absence or contracture), and congenital soft tissue tumors.

CONTRACTURES

The classic malformation with contracture is pterygium cubitale, in which almost every soft tissue is abnormal and a severe flexion contracture exists.[21, 22] The condition has also been called cutaneous webs and webbed elbow; it is but one manifestation of a congenital syndrome that may affect the neck, axilla, elbow, knee, or digits. A survey of 240 cases of cutaneous webs reported in the literature included 29 in the region of the elbow.[21] The web may be unilateral or bilateral, symmetric or asymmetric. The condition has been reported to result from both an autosomal dominant and a recessive gene. Associated abnormalities involving almost every body system have been reported.[31, 66] Other conditions resulting in formidable contractures about the elbow include fibrodysplasia ossificans progressiva and arthrogryposis.

CONTROL DEFICIENCIES

Arthrogryposis and its related syndromes are also included in this group. Both flaccid and spastic palsies affect elbow control and range of motion. Simple absences or deficiencies of tissue also affect elbow control. Hypoplasia of the elbow includes deficient growth not only of osseous structures but also of the related soft tissue control elements and cover structures.[12, 46, 65] Most characteristic is probably the extension contracture of arthrogryposis.[70]

ISOLATED TISSUE ANOMALIES

The skin may be deficient or missing, with absence, hypoplasia, or scarring of the underlying tissues. Nerve, vascular, and lymphatic anomalies in the region of the elbow are common.[31] The anconeus epitrochlearis occasionally is present as an anomalous muscle and may cover the ulnar nerve in the cubital tunnel area, contributing to the possibility of entrapment. Other anomalous muscles that may cause nerve entrapment problems are (1) Gantzer's muscle, an anomalous head of the flexor pollicis longus or flexor profundus that usually originates from the medial epicondyle or the coronoid process of the ulna and occasionally is a factor in anterior interosseous nerve compression; (2) a solitary head of the supinator and other anomalies of this muscle; (3) accessory muscles of the anterolateral aspect of the elbow, including the accessory brachialis or accessory brachioradialis; (4) variations in the head, origin, or insertion of the pronator teres; (5) variations of a similar nature in the flexor carpi radialis, the flexor carpi ulnaris, and the palmaris longus[67]; and (6) an aberrant medial head of the triceps, which may snap over the medial epicondyle and irritate the ulnar nerve.[15]

CONGENITAL SOFT TISSUE TUMORS

Tumors of the soft tissue are rare but include a wide variety of abnormalities, ranging from overgrowth to neoplasms and from multitissue hamartomas to single tissue entities. Probably the two most common tumors in the infant are the fibromatoses and vascular tumors. If the elbow area is involved, there is usually some limitation of motion.

Combined Bone and Soft Tissue Anomalies

Soft tissue anomalies may coexist with mild osseous anomalies, such as those related to the supracondyloid process.[12, 64, 67] The supracondyloid process is an anomalous bony prominence extending from the anteromedial aspect of the distal third of the humerus. Struthers[65] in 1848 described the ligament associated with this process, and, since then, various anomalies have been reported in connection with it. These include a more proximal branching of the ulnar artery off the brachial artery above the bony spur, a more proximal insertion of the pronator teres on the bony process, and various relationships of the neurovascular structures with bone and ligament. The symptoms—pain, tingling, numbness, and so on—usually are neuralgic, but they may be vascular.

Many of the congenital anomalies already discussed are manifest in both osseous and soft tissues. These abnormalities may be equivalent, as in the supracondyloid process syndrome just discussed, or predominantly in one tissue, as in fibromatosis. More severe changes are seen with severe pterygium cubitale and severe forms of ulnar hypoplasia and phocomelia. In pterygium cubitale, or congenital webbed elbow, a skin web extends from the upper arm across the volar elbow to the forearm. Flexion is usually possible, but extension, pronation, and supination are severely limited. The muscles and neurovascular structures are incompletely developed. The bones are hypoplastic and deformed, and the elbow joint often is dislocated or severely hypoplastic. Fibrous strands represent missing muscles or tendons. Muscle hypoplasia is present posteriorly as well as anteriorly.

Severe ulnar hypoplasia is marked by radial head dislocation, diminishing segments (ranging from small to nonexistent) of the proximal ulna, variable but seldom normal motion and stability, and muscle and neurovascular abnormalities. Conditions are more normal proximal to the elbow, but distally, more abnormalities are apparent; the ulnar forearm and hand structures are particularly dysplastic. Phocomelia may present with similar findings, or the elbow may be even more dysplastic or absent altogether (hand, wrist, or forearm may be attached directly to the shoulder or trunk).

TREATMENT OF BONE AND JOINT DYSPLASIAS

Treatment of Synostosis

The treatment of synostosis of the elbow joint, whether radiohumeral[47] or ulnohumeral, is dictated by the position of the forearm-wrist-hand unit and the function of the wrist-hand unit. If the hand is absent or nonfunctional, repositioning of a synostotic elbow is clearly less important. If the hand is functional and the elbow is in a "functional" position (i.e., somewhere near midflexion), especially if the contralateral limb is normal, no treatment is likely to be necessary. For bilateral synostoses, some consideration probably should be given to positioning one arm in relative flexion and the other in relative extension. Frequently, only one forearm bone is well represented, and this may be bowed or deformed in some manner as well as short. In addition, there may be a rotational deformity. The forearm-wrist-hand unit may point directly posterior when the upper limb is in its usual dependent position beside the torso. Although simple rotational deformities can be corrected by osteotomy at any level, multiplane deformities should be corrected at the site of maximum deformity—that is, the humeral-forearm junction—perhaps extending the correction distally in the forearm (Fig. 14–13). One such method involves a posterior approach and a multiple-segment corrective osteotomy, making one or more of the segments trapezoidal in shape and rotating it 180 degrees, if necessary, to realign the unit as desired. If only one limb is involved, this desired position is usually at maximum length, with the forearm, wrist, and hand in the midposition. Derotation should be accomplished in the direction that causes the least torsion of the neurovascular structures, commonly from an internally rotated position through a clockwise rotation to a forearm midposition. Hyperextension, if present, is corrected simply to neutral or slight flexion, and the osteotomy segments are adjusted to make the best contact in the desired position; a segment may be excised if this is needed for contouring. If both limbs are involved, enough elbow flexion angle should be included on one side to allow one of the limbs to reach the face and the head. Arthroplasty has been attempted,[27, 28, 34, 45] but with indifferent results; the usual result is recurrence.

Proximal forearm synostosis may occur with elbow synostosis, in which case the elbow is derotated as described previously. If, however, proximal radioulnar synostosis occurs in the presence of a functioning elbow joint, derotation of the forearm alone may be required. The indications for this procedure seem limited. Most patients have little functional deficit.[11] Compensatory rotation at the wrist appears to be an important factor in minimizing symptoms.[49] Although many authors have attempted and a few have claimed success for passive and even active mobilization of the forearm,[8, 14, 17, 24, 32, 43] there is no body of literature that substantiates these results in a significant number of patients who have been followed for an adequate period of

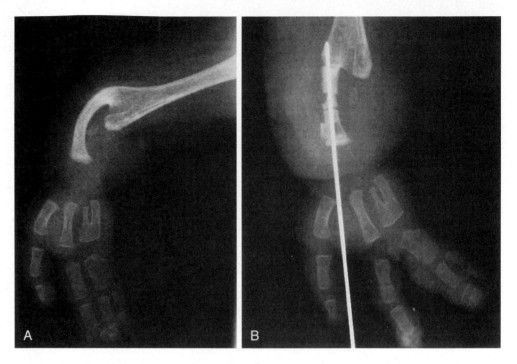

FIGURE 14–13 • *A*, Typical congenital radiohumeral synostosis with marked curving of the radial segment. The elbow synostosis resulted in a posterior pointing forearm, wrist, and hand. *B*, A "shish kabob" corrective osteotomy was carried out with temporary internal fixation. Excellent correction resulted and there were no complications.

time. When attempted, these procedures usually involve excision of the proximal radius, including the synostotic mass; division of the entire length of the interosseous membrane; interposition of some material between the contact areas of the radius and the ulna; and tendon transfers, such as rerouting the extensor carpi radialis longus to the volar wrist for supination and the flexor carpi radialis to the dorsal wrist for pronation. A similar procedure involving the interposition of a metallic swivel has been described by Kelikian and Doumanian,[32] but few long-term results have been reported.

A more reliable procedure is that of derotation osteotomy.[24, 60] This procedure is best outlined by Green and Mital,[22, 43] who perform the rotational osteotomy through the synostosis itself. It is indicated primarily when the forearm is fused in the extreme of either pronation or supination; forearms synostotic in neutral or close to neutral function well and, because of this, often are diagnosed only later in infancy or childhood. The synostosis is approached through a dorsal incision and is transversely osteotomized. A radioulnar (in the coronal plane) K-wire or Steinmann pin is then placed distal to the osteotomy site and is left protruding externally on both sides. A longitudinal (in the sagittal plane) pin is then placed from the olecranon across the osteotomy site, and corrective rotation is carried out as desired. Because the indication is an extreme pronated or supinated position, in most cases, 70 to 90 degrees of rotation from pronation toward supination is required. If circulatory deficits appear during or after this derotation, less rotation is accepted, although an additional amount may be carried out 10 to 15 days later. The radioulnar pin may be fixed by either a plaster cast or an external fixation apparatus. Internal fixation should not be used because alteration of forearm rotation may be necessary to diminish circulatory difficulties. Goldner and Lipton[19] claim that these circulatory problems may be minimized by the use of derotation in the distal forearm (radius only

in younger patients, radius and ulna in older patients). Their results have yet to appear in the literature except in abstract form, but the rationale seems reasonable and the technique appropriate. They recommend cross-pin fixation in children and plate fixation in adolescents and adults.

Treatment of Ankylosis

Ankylosis that does not involve synostosis, subluxation, or dislocation of the elbow may occur. Paralyses, muscle disease, and other soft tissue abnormalities commonly restrict motion; treatment of these abnormalities is discussed elsewhere (see Chapters 62 and 63). Abnormalities of joint shape and joint cartilage occur but are usually treated only by physical therapy. Rotation ankylosis due to soft tissue abnormalities occurs but has minimal effect on the elbow; its treatment requires release not only of the proximal radioulnar area but also in the forearm and wrist.[5]

Treatment of Instability

Treatment of infantile dislocations of the radial head, whether congenital, developmental, or traumatic, depends on the degree of hypoplasia present in the forearm and elbow area. If the clinician is in doubt about the configuration of the various components of the elbow joint, an arthrogram should be performed.[48] This may show that there is no dislocation at all but merely a deformed elbow joint with the radiocapitellar joint displaced from the usual position (see Fig. 14–11). Attempts at open reduction have been made, but the result is often recurrence unless both annular ligaments and ulnar length and configuration are restored (Fig. 14–14). Most authors do not advise the procedure,[4, 44, 69] although recently Sachar and Mih[56] reported good short-term results (maintenance of reduction and improved forearm rotation) in 10 of 12 children with congenital radial head dislocation who underwent surgery

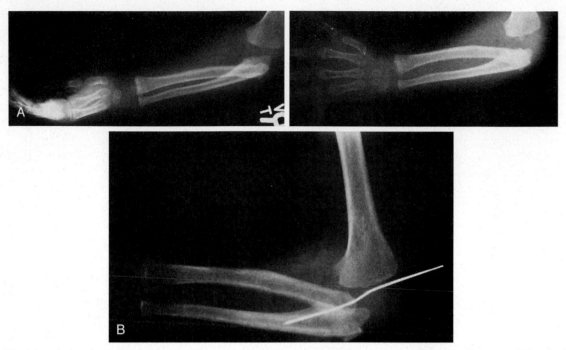

FIGURE 14-14 • *A*, Anteroposterior and lateral radiographic views of a radial head dislocation in a limb with other congenital anomalies but with a fairly normal skeleton at the elbow. Although this fulfills the requirements usually listed for congenital dislocation, the dislocation may simply be developmental, related to the unequal length of the two forearm bones. *B*, Postoperative lateral radiographs after open reduction of the dislocated radial head and internal fixation. A second operation was carried out a year later, at which time the radius was shortened and the annular ligaments were reconstructed; repeat reduction of the radial head was also performed.

between the ages of 7 months and 6 years. They reported that the most common finding was an interposition of the annular ligament, which they divided and then repaired in its anatomic position. Follow-up was short, however, averaging less than 2 years, with the longest being only 41 months.

The alternative to attempted reduction of congenital or infantile radial head dislocation is to accept the imposed disability (some limitation of forearm rotation, ranging from a few degrees to more than 90 degrees; occasional limitation of elbow motion; and infrequent pain) and proceed with radial head excision, if needed, at maturity.[17, 18, 20, 31, 39, 63] As noted in a long-term follow-up study,[4] painful arthritis is typical only of the least common type I deformity. Relief of pain and cosmesis are more likely to benefit from surgical excision; motion is seldom improved.[4]

TREATMENT OF SOFT TISSUE DYSPLASIAS

Treatment of most soft tissue problems at the elbow level is discussed in other chapters. Arthrogryposis, as well as other flaccid palsies, is covered in Chapter 62. Spastic neurogenic problems are discussed in Chapter 63, and nerve entrapment around the elbow is discussed in Chapter 71. Successful treatment for other soft tissue dysplasias at the elbow is rare. Aplasia cutis congenita has occurred in the elbow area. In the author's experience, it was associated with scarring and hypoplasia of the regional forearm muscles plus reactive deformity of the underlying bones. Resurfacing with a skin and subcutaneous flap was eventually

necessary, followed by tendon transfers, which in this case were required to provide extensor function of the wrist and hand. Muscle anomalies may result in either mechanical problems (snapping or catching)[15] or neurovascular entrapment, as discussed in Chapter 71.

TREATMENT FOR COMBINED BONE AND SOFT TISSUE DYSPLASIAS

Pterygium cubitale remains an unsolved challenge. Attempts at treatment have included Z-plasty, skin grafts, and release of other tight structures. Improvement has been limited, and risks are high.[21, 22] Because there is no substantial report in the literature describing a reliable and useful method of treatment, no recommendations for surgical treatment are offered. Techniques of bone shortening to permit a greater safe excursion of the neurovascular structures or techniques of vascular and nerve grafting have been attempted, but adequate reporting is not yet available. The lengthening-stretching techniques of Ilizarov have been tried by a few investigators, so far with limited success. The hands in pterygium cubitale are often deficient also, but because limited excursion of the elbow is available in flexion, at least they are usually able to reach the upper trunk, the face, and the head.

In severe forms of ulnar dysplasia, the elbow often displays adequate range and stability. Occasionally, the displaced radial head is sufficiently limiting or symptom-provoking that treatment is offered. Although excision of the radial head and a sufficient portion of the shaft to resolve the mechanical block might suffice, the desire to stabilize and lengthen the forearm plus the fear of recurrent encroachment by the radial shaft usually lead to a recommendation for a one-bone forearm procedure (Fig. 14–15).[9] This is carried out as follows:

1. Use a long lateral incision that covers the distal half of the arm, the elbow, and the proximal half of the forearm.

2. Mobilize the anterior flap, identify and protect the radial nerve, and identify and mobilize the anteriorly and radially dislocated radius.

3. Mobilize the posterior flap, identify the short ulnar fragment, and uncover the interosseous space.

4. With both bones visualized through both anterior and posterior intervals (obviously, the procedure can be performed through an anterior approach only or through both a proximal anterior and a distal posterior approach, but we have found that access and safety are preferable this way), the maximum forearm length that the soft tissue will accept is judged by manual displacement.

5. The radius then is osteotomized at the length just determined, and the proximal fragment is removed.

6. The distal fragment is aligned with the short ulnar fragment, and contact is maintained by an intramedullary pin drilled through the olecranon, along the ulnar medullary cavity, across the osteotomy site, and along the radial intramedullary space until it penetrates the radial cortex at some point. (The forearm position—usually the midportion—should be set before this distal penetration occurs.)

7. The usual support dressings (long arm splint-dressing combination initially, perhaps changed to a long arm cast later for the older child) are used until healing occurs (4 to 6 weeks). The supports are then discontinued, and the pin is removed.

In phocomelia, the elbow is seldom the site of the infrequent surgical attention given to this condition, but there may be an occasional indication for a one-bone forearm procedure or for simultaneous lengthening and stabilization at an unstable elbow segment.[61]

COMPLICATIONS

Overtreatment. In many cases, the severe upper limb anomaly, particularly if of the sporadic variety, is associated with a completely normal contralateral upper limb. In such cases, surgical treatment may have little effect on the long-term functional level of the patient.[6] Therefore, it also is important to consider the likely practical gains from therapy before proposing an intervention. As has been noted, many synostotic forearms function well, even if in a poor position owing to compensatory hyper-rotation at the wrist. Such factors need to be considered carefully before embarking on a surgical adventure.

Unwarranted Treatment Due to Misdiagnosis. This problem, present in any medical management situation, is a particular hazard with congenital anomalies. In the infant,

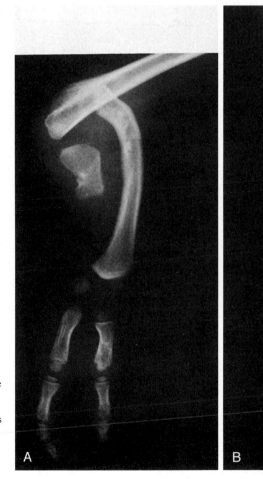

FIGURE 14–15 • *A*, A lateral view of an elbow in ulnar agenesis shows an apparent dislocation proximally and anteriorly of the radial head. Although the ulnar agenesis is congenital, the dislocation is probably developmental. Clinical findings suggested that this was a true dislocation. *B*, There is occasional need for excision of the dislocated radial head and combination of the proximal ulna and distal radius to form a one-bone forearm as seen here. This changes both the appearance and the function of the elbow as well as of the forearm (the range of motion of the elbow is usually improved; the forearm position becomes fixed).

testing of the neurovascular supply, dynamic and static control elements, and structural and support elements is difficult and uncertain. Interpretation of radiographs, when so much of the skeletal tissue is still cartilaginous, is deceptive. Nevertheless, the best review possible is needed if surgery is contemplated. This may require examination under sedation or special radiographic techniques such as arthrography, computed tomography or magnetic resonance imaging studies, cineradiographic motion and stress studies, and others. It should be recalled that "hands-on" examination is particularly valuable in the child because much cartilage is not yet bone and much muscle and tendon can be palpated better than tested.

Infection. This is a serious problem after any surgical procedure, and the usual wound management preventive measures are employed. The ability to apply a splint-dressing that will maintain the desired position and stay in place is important in infants but must not override the need for wound inspection if infection is suspected.

Vascular Compromise. Vascular damage due to direct insults, compartment pressure increase, or indirect damage from stretch or torsion does occur. The stretch-torsion injury is a particular risk in the corrective osteotomies used to treat synostosis. For this reason, circulation should be checked during the osteotomy procedure. For osteotomies in the proximal forearm or elbow, fixation that can be removed or adjusted to decrease vascular stress is necessary. The circulatory pattern in congenitally abnormal arms is almost always abnormal; if further, extensive alteration in anatomy is anticipated, preliminary angiography may be helpful. Doppler assessment before and during surgery is invaluable.

Nerve Damage. Nerve injury caused by dissection or compression at anatomic entrapment points during postoperative reaction, stretch, or torque stress may also occur. Torque stress usually can be monitored by assessing the effect of the stress on the vascular supply. The other possibilities are best controlled by adequate exposure and careful dissection. Regardless, close and skilled postoperative monitoring is essential.

Physis Damage. Partial or total destruction of the physis may result from bone cutting, pin or other fixation, or damage to the local physis circulation. Care should be taken to avoid physeal damage, particularly because most such limbs are hypoplastic and short already. A pin passing near the center of and at right angles to the physis seems to run the least risk of serious damage.

Joint Damage. Incongruous, malformed, and abnormally surfaced joints are common with congenital problems, and the investing soft tissue, motor units, and even skin also may limit normal joint function. Careful preservation of the available joint structures is therefore important; this includes avoiding pin breakage in the elbow joint. Many surgeons, for instance, fix the ulna and radius rather than the humerus and radius to minimize the chances of intraarticular pin breakage after radial head reduction. Recurring elbow or forearm stiffness after operations for congenital elbow area anomalies is the most depressingly common complication of all. Pharmacologic suppression of scar formation and early continuous passive motion for these tiny arms may help, and both treatments should be available in the future.

SUMMARY

Congenital elbow dysplasia is a more common problem than is generally realized. If mild, elbow function is minimally affected; if severe, problems of the entire limb or the wrist and hand often take precedence. In the few instances, when the elbow abnormality is isolated and relatively severe, surgical assistance is available but is less than satisfying. The most common and provocative problem is that of radial head subluxation-dislocation, in which the abnormality may be due to one or more of three differing etiologies: congenital, traumatic, or developmental (resulting from congenital, traumatic, infectious, tumor, or other causes). Effective management protocols have been developed, but unsolved problems still abound.

REFERENCES

1. Abbott, F. C.: Congenital dislocation of radius. Lancet 1:800, 1892.
2. Almquist, E. E., Gordon, L. H., and Blue, A. L.: Congenital dislocation of the head of the radius. J. Bone Joint Surg. 51A:1118, 1969.
3. Bailey, J. A.: Elbow and other upper limb deformities in achondroplasia. Clin. Orthop. 80:75, 1971.
4. Bell, S. N., Morrey, B. F., and Bianco, A. J.: Chronic posterior subluxation and dislocation of the radial head. J. Bone Joint Surg. 73A:392, 1991.
5. Bert, J. M., McElfresh, E. C., and Linscheid, R. L.: Rotary contracture of the forearm. J. Bone Joint Surg. 62A:1163, 1980.
6. Blair, S. J., Swanson, A. B., and Swanson, G. D.: Evaluation of impairment of hand and upper extremity function. Instr. Course Lect. 38:73, 1989.
7. Bottero, L., Cinalli, G., Labrune, P., Lajeunie, E., and Renier, D.: Antley-Bixler syndrome. Description of two new cases and a review of the literature. Childs Nervous System 13:275–280, 1997.
8. Brady, L. P., and Jewett, E. L.: A new treatment of radioulnar synostosis. South. Med. J. 53:507, 1960.
9. Broudy, A. S., and Smith, R. J.: Deformities of the hand and wrist with ulnar deficiency. J. Hand Surg. 4:304, 1979.
10. Caravias, D. E.: Some observations on congenital dislocations of the head of the radius. J. Bone Joint Surg. 39B:86, 1957.
11. Cleary, J. E., and Omer, G. E.: Congenital proximal radioulnar synostosis. J. Bone Joint Surg. 67A:539, 1985.
12. Crotti, F. M., Mangiagalli, E. P., and Rampini, P.: Supracondyloid process and anomalous insertion of pronator teres as sources of median nerve neuralgia. J. Neurolog. Sci. 25:41–44, 1981.
13. Danielsson, L. G., and Theander, G.: Traumatic dislocation of the radial head at birth. Acta Radiol. 22:379, 1981.
14. Dawson, H. G. W.: A congenital deformity of the forearm and its operative treatment. B. M. J. 2:833, 1912.
15. Dreyfuss, U., and Kessler, I.: Snapping elbow due to dislocation of the medial head of the triceps. J. Bone Joint Surg. 60B:56, 1978.
16. Falvo, K. A., and Freidenberg, Z. B.: Osteo-onychodysplasia. Clin. Orthop. 81:130, 1971.
17. Ferguson, A. B. Jr: Orthopedic surgery in infancy and childhood, 2nd ed. Baltimore: Williams & Wilkins., 1963.
18. Fox, K. W., and Griffen, L. L.: Congenital dislocation of the radial head. Clin. Orthop. 18:234, 1960.
19. Goldner, J. L., and Lipton, M. A.: Congenital radioulnar synostosis: diagnosis and treatment based on anatomic and functional assessment. Orthop. Trans. 6:466, 1982.
20. Good, C. J., and Wicks, M. H.: Developmental posterior dislocation of the radial head. J. Bone Joint Surg. 65B:64, 1983.
21. Green, D. C.: Operative Hand Surgery. New York: Churchill-Livingstone, 1982, pp. 267–308.
22. Green, W. T., and Mital, M. A.: Congenital radioulnar synostosis: surgical treatment. J. Bone Joint Surg. 61A:738, 1979.
23. Gunn, D. R., and Pillay, V. K.: Congenital posterior dislocation of the head of the radius. Clin. Orthop. 34:108, 1964.
24. Hansen, O. H., and Anderson, N. O.: Congenital radioulnar synostosis: report of 37 cases. Acta. Orthop. Scand. 41:225, 1970.

25. Hoffer, M. M.: Joint motion limitation in newborns. Clin. Orthop. **148**:94, 1980.
26. Hollister, D. W., and Lachman, R. S.: Diastrophic dwarfism. Clin. Orthop. **114**:61, 1976.
27. Hunter, A. G. W., Cox, D. W., and Rudd, N. L.: The genetics of and associated clinical findings in humeroradial synostosis. Clin. Genet. **9**:470, 1976.
28. Jacobsen, S. T., and Crawford, A. H.: Humeroradial synostosis. J. Pediatr. Orthop. **3**:96, 1983.
29. Kaitila, I. I., Leistei, J. T., and Rimoin, D. L.: Mesomelic skeletal dysplasia. Clin. Orthop. **114**:94, 1976.
30. Kasser, J., and Upton, J.: The shoulder, elbow and forearm in Apert syndrome. Clin. Plast. Surg. **18**:381, 1991.
31. Kelikian, H.: Congenital Deformities of the Hand and Forearm. Philadelphia, W. B. Saunders Co., 1974, pp. 310, 714, 902.
32. Kelikian, H., and Doumanian, A.: Swivel for proximal radioulnar synostosis. J. Bone Joint Surg. **39A**:945, 1957.
33. Kelly, D. W.: Congenital dislocation of the radial head spectrum and natural history. J. Pediatr. Orthop. **1**:245, 1981.
34. K'Iery, L., and Wouters, H. W.: Congenital ankylosis of joints. Arch. Chir. Neerl. **2**:173, 1971.
35. Leisti, J., Lachman, R. S., and Rimoin, D. L.: Humeroradial ankylosis associated with other congenital defects (the boomerang arm sign). Birth Defects **11**:306, 1975.
36. Lenz, W.: Genetics and limb deficiencies. Clin. Orthop. **148**:9, 1980.
37. Lloyd-Roberts, G. C., and Bucknill, T. M.: Anterior dislocation of the radial head in children: aetiology, natural history and management. J. Bone Joint Surg. **59B**:402, 1977.
38. Mann, R. A., Johnston, J. O., and Ford, J.: Developmental posterior dislocation of the radial head: ten cases resulting from ulnar hypoplasia. 38th Annual Meeting of the Western Orthopedic Association, Honolulu, Hawaii, October 5–12, 1974.
39. Mardam-Bey, T., and Ger, E.: Congenital radial head dislocation. J. Hand Surg. **4**:316, 1979.
40. McCredie, J.: Congenital fusion of bones: radiology, embryology, and pathogenesis. Clin. Radiol. **26**:47, 1975.
41. McFarland, B.: Congenital dislocation of the head of the radius. Br. J. Surg. **24**:41, 1936.
42. McKusick, V. A.: Mendelian Inheritance in Man, 6th ed. Baltimore: Johns Hopkins Press, 1983.
43. Mital, M. A.: Congenital radioulnar synostosis and congenital dislocation of the radial head. Orthop. Clin. North Am. **7**:375, 1976.
44. Miura, T.: Congenital dislocation of the radial head. J. Hand Surg. **15B**:377, 1990.
45. Mnaymneh, W. A.: Congenital radiohumeral synostosis. A case report. Clin. Orthop. **131**:183, 1978.
46. Murakami, Y., and Komiyama, Y.: Hypoplasia of the trochlea and the medial epicondyle of the humerus associated with ulnar neuropathy. J. Bone Joint Surg. **60B**:225, 1978.
47. Murphy, H. S., and Hansen, C. G.: Congenital humeroradial synostosis. J. Bone Joint Surg. **27**:712, 1945.
48. Ogden, J. A.: Skeletal Injury in the Child. Philadelphia: Lea & Febiger, 1982, 319.
49. Ogino, T., and Hikino, K.: Congenital radioulnar synostosis: compensatory rotation around the wrist and rotation osteotomy. J. Hand Surg. **12B**:173, 1987.
50. Pfeiffer, R.: Die angeborene Verrenkung des Speichenkopfchens als Teilerscheinung anderer kongenitaler Ellenbogengelenkmissbildungen. Mensch Vererb Konstitutionslehre **21**:530, 1938.
51. Phillips, S.: Congenital dislocation of radii. B. M. J. **1**:773, 1883.
52. Pouliquen, J. C., Pauthier, F., Kassis, B., and Glorion, C.: Bilateral congenital pseudarthrosis of the olecranon. J. Pediatr. Orthop. **6B**:223-224, 1997.
53. Powers, C. A.: Congenital dislocations of the radius. JAMA **41**:165, 1903.
54. Reichenbach, H., Hormann, D., and Theile, H.: Hereditary congenital posterior dislocation of radial heads. Am. J. Med. Genetics **55**:101, 1995.
55. Ryan, J. R.: The relationship of the radial head to radial neck diameters in fetuses and adults with reference to radial head subluxation in children. J. Bone Joint Surg. **51A**:781, 1969.
56. Sachar, K., and Mih, A.D.: Congenital radial head dislocations. Hand Clinics **14**:39, 1998.
57. Salter, R., and Zaltz, C.: Anatomic investigations of the mechanism of injury and pathologic anatomy of "pulled elbow" in children. Clin. Orthop. **77**:134, 1971.
58. Sato, K., and Miura, T.: Hypoplasia of the humeral trochlea. J. Hand Surg. **15A**:1004 1990.
59. Schubert, J. J.: Dislocation of the radial head in the newborn infant. J. Bone Joint Surg. **47A**:1019, 1965.
60. Simmons, B. P., Southmayd, W. W., and Riseborough, E. J.: Congenital radioulnar synostosis. J. Hand Surg. **9**:829, 1983.
61. Smith, R. J., and Lipke, R. W.: Treatment of congenital deformities of the hand and forearm, Part II. N. Engl. J. Med. **300**:402, 1979.
62. Smith, R. W.: Congenital luxations of the radius. Dublin Q. J. Med. Sci. **13**:208, 1852.
63. Southmayd, W., and Ehrlich, M. G.: Idiopathic subluxation of the radial head. Clin. Orthop. **121**:271, 1976.
64. Stone, C. A.: Subluxation of the head of the radius: report of a case and anatomical experiments. J. A. M. A. **1**:28, 1916.
65. Struthers, J.: A peculiarity of the humerus and humeral artery. Monthly J. Med. Sci. **28**:264, 1848.
66. Temtamy, S. A., and McKusick, V. A.: Carpal/tarsal synostosis. Birth Defects **14**:502, 1978.
67. Tubiana, R.: The Hand, Philadelphia: W. B. Saunders Co, 1981.
68. Uthoff, K., and Bosch, U.: Die proximale radioulnare Synostose im Rahmen des fetalen Alkoholsyndrom. Unfallchiru **100**:678, 1997.
69. Wiley, J. J., Loehr, J., and McIntyre, W.: Isolated dislocation of the radial head. Orthop. Rev. **20**:973, 1991.
70. Williams, P. F.: The elbow in arthrogryposis. J. Bone Joint Surg. **55B**:834, 1973.
71. Windfeld, P.: On congenital and acquired luxation of the capitellum radii with discussion of some associated problems. Acta. Orthop. Scand. **16**:126, 1946.
72. Wood, V. E., Sauser, D. D., and O'Hara, R. C.: The shoulder and elbow in Apert syndrome. J. Pediatr. Orthop. **15**:648, 1995.
73. Wynne-Davies, R.: Heritable Disorders in Orthopaedic Practice. Oxford: Blackwell Scientific Publications, 1973.

CHAPTER 15

Supracondylar Fractures of the Elbow in Children

• ANTHONY A. STANS and
RUDOLPH A. KLASSEN

Supracondylar humerus fractures are the most common fracture about the elbow in children and have the highest complication rate for elbow fractures in this age group.[6, 13, 33] These compelling facts continue to pique the interest and hold the attention of orthopedists who treat pediatric patients.

INCIDENCE AND ETIOLOGY

Supracondylar humerus fractures almost exclusively affect the immature skeleton.[35, 40] Eliason reported that 84% of supracondylar fractures occurred in patients younger than 10 years.[23] The peak age for supracondylar humerus fracture has been reported to be between 6 and 7 years, and the left arm is injured more frequently than the right.* Previous reports have suggested that supracondylar fractures were common in boys, but more recent studies have documented an equal sex distribution.†

Traditional teaching has held that the peak incidence for extension-type supracondylar humerus fractures occurs at approximately age 7 because that is the age of maximum elbow flexibility and hyperextension. This mechanism has been confirmed by recent research suggesting that a fall on a hyperextended elbow produces a supracondylar humerus fracture whereas a fall on an outstretched arm without elbow hyperextension is more likely to cause a distal radius fracture.[49] Hyperextension converts what would be an axial loading force to the elbow into a bending moment. The tip of the olecranon acts as a fulcrum, causing the fracture to occur through the relatively thin bone of the olecranon fossa (Fig. 15–1). The distinctive shape of the humeral metaphysis with the medial and lateral condyles and columns, and the narrow midpoint of the olecranon fossa, add to the instability of the fracture, particularly when there is rotation and tilting of the distal fragment.[51, 52]

Knowledge of elbow anatomy is important to understanding the cause of the injury, and to understanding effective treatment principles (see Chapters 2 and 3). The stability of the elbow derives from bony and soft tissue structures.[29, 50, 54] Soft tissue stability on the lateral aspect of the elbow is provided by an expansion of the triceps, anconeus, brachioradialis, and extensor carpi radialis lon-

gus. The thickened periosteum of a young child, both medially and laterally, is an important additional stabilizer of the fracture fragment and provides a medial or lateral hinge during attempted reduction (Fig. 15–2). Recent research by Khare has confirmed the importance of the triceps tendon's acting as a tension band to achieve fracture stability in the flexed elbow.[38]

Because angular deformity is a common complication of these fractures, the normal variations in pediatric anatomy should be understood. The carrying angle of the elbow joint is the angle formed by the intersection of the longitudinal axis of the arm and the forearm (Fig. 15–3). The normal elbow is usually in slight valgus alignment, but this varies among children.[1, 15, 64] Smith noted that, of 150 children aged 3 to 11, the carrying angle in boys averaged 5.4 degrees and ranged from 0 to 11 degrees, whereas in girls, it averaged 6 degrees and ranged from 0 to 12 degrees.[64] Aebi observed that the measurements were not constant and changed as the child matured, tending to decrease in magnitude and in variation between children.[1]

Although not commonly associated with abuse in the past, a recent report found that 36% of patients younger than 15 months when they sustained a supracondylar humerus fracture had sustained it as a result of abuse.[66] The same author found the incidence of abuse to be only 1% in children older than 15 months. Clinicians must exclude "nonaccidental trauma" as a potential cause of injury whenever an infant presents with a supracondylar humerus fracture.

CLASSIFICATION

A classification system should guide treatment, provide information on prognosis, and facilitate research by ensuring that similar injuries are compared in the literature. Supracondylar humerus fractures are first classified as either flexion or extension injuries, a distinction based on the radiographic appearance and the mechanism of injury. The distinction is important for treatment because the reduction maneuvers are essentially opposite for the two fracture types and flexion-type fractures are significantly more difficult to reduce by closed means.

Flexion-Type Fractures

Flexion-type fractures are the result of a direct fall onto a flexed elbow in which a powerful flexion force is applied to the distal humerus, usually through the olecranon. The distal humeral fragment is displaced anteriorly, and the fracture line crosses the humerus from the distal posterior to the proximal anterior aspect (Fig. 15–4). Flexion-type fractures are frequently completely displaced and are difficult to reduce by closed means.

Extension-Type Fractures

Extension-type fractures typically occur as the result of a fall onto an outstretched arm with a hyperextended elbow. The fracture line traverses the distal humerus from the proximal posterior to the distal anterior aspect. Displacement varies from none to marked displacement with frac-

---

*See references 11, 18, 20, 34, 35, 40, 41, 42, 44, and 63.
†See references 32, 34, 45, 46, 50, 58, 62, and 69.

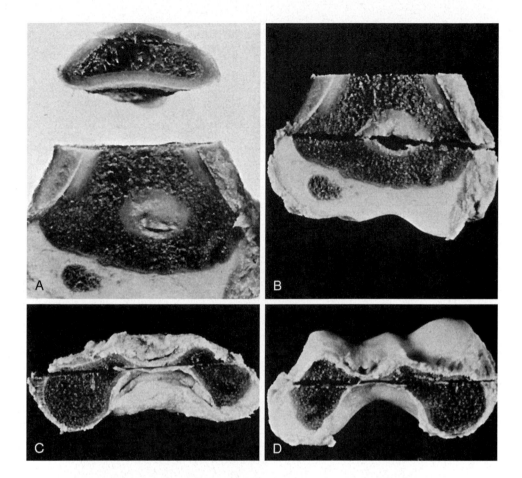

FIGURE 15–1 • *A*, Transverse and sagittal sections of the distal humerus. The shaft diameter is large above the supracondylar foramen. *B*, If, however, a cut is made through the supracondylar foramen, the "bicolumnar" nature of this region becomes evident, looking proximally (*C*) and distally (*D*). (From Ogden, J.: Skeletal Injury in the Child. Philadelphia, Lea & Febiger, 1983.)

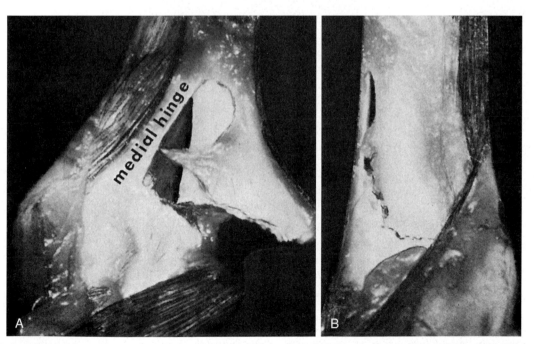

FIGURE 15–2 • An experimentally produced fracture shows the medial periosteal hinge and offers a glimpse of the posterior hinge. After reduction, the soft tissues hold the fragments in place. The better the reduction, the greater the security. (From Rang, M.: Children's Fractures, 2nd ed. Philadelphia, J. B. Lippincott, 1983.)

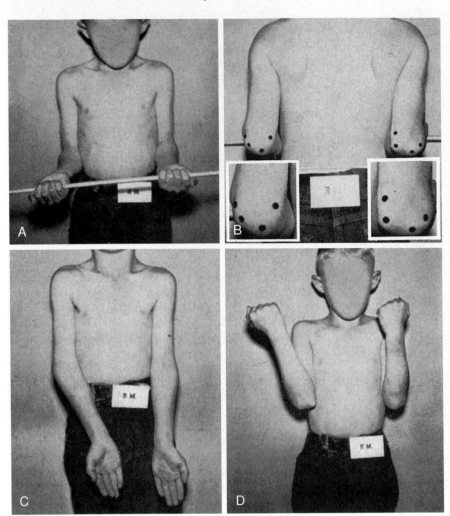

FIGURE 15–3 • *A*, Change in the carrying angle cannot be detected when the flexed elbows are examined from in front. *B*, Change in the carrying angle is apparent, however, when the flexed elbows are examined posteriorly. On the right, the bone prominences (*black dots*) can be seen to have tilted medially. *C*, With the arms extended, a 25-degree varus deformity of the right arm can be seen in a 9-year-old boy 2 years after a supracondylar fracture of the right arm. There is no limitation of motion. Note that the normal carrying angle of the left arm is 0 degrees. *D*, When the varus elbow is acutely flexed, the hand points laterally, away from the shoulder joint. This view also demonstrates the medial tilt of the bone prominences. (From Smith, L.: Deformity following supracondylar fractures. J. Bone Joint Surg. 42A:236, 1960.)

ture fragments separated by interposed soft tissue. Numerous classifications systems have been devised for extension-type supracondylar humerus fractures,[8, 22, 34, 35, 56] but the classification system attributed to Gartland is the most commonly accepted system in use today.[28] As described by Gartland, the classification system is simple, reproducible, helpful in guiding treatment, and provides information on prognosis and potential complications. Like much in our current English orthopedic literature, a very similar fracture classification system was published in the German literature of the early 20th century by Felsenreich.[24]

Type I

Type I fractures are nondisplaced (Fig. 15–5). In many patients the fracture line may not be visible on injury radiographs, but the posterior fat pad sign, palpable tenderness in the supracondylar region, and an appropriate mechanism of injury may allow the physician to establish the correct diagnosis. The diagnosis is often confirmed when periosteal callus is seen on radiographs taken 3 weeks after the injury. If recognized and treated appropriately, type I fractures should never be associated with neurovascular injury or malunion.

Type II

With type II fractures there is displacement or angulation at the fracture site, but a hinge of bone crossing the fracture site keeps the fragments in continuity. The distal fragment is most often displaced posteriorly, and apex anterior angulation at the fracture site results in a hyperextension deformity (Fig. 15–6). Variations of type II fractures have also been described that involve medial impaction or rotation, which can result in cubitus varus if it goes unrecognized (Fig. 15–7). While there are reports of neurovascular injury associated with type II fractures, such injuries are rare.[57]

Type III

Type III fractures are completely displaced fractures in which there is no continuity between fracture fragments (Fig. 15–8). The distal fragment is displaced posteriorly and may be displaced medially or laterally as well. There is a much higher incidence of neurovascular complications with type III fractures, and soft tissue is usually interposed between fracture fragments. The brachialis muscle is most often interposed, but the median nerve, radial nerve, or brachial artery may also be entrapped.

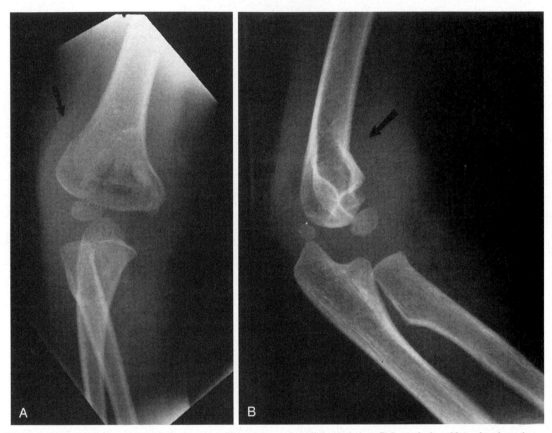

FIGURE 15–4 • *A*, Flexion-type supracondylar fracture with anterior and medial angulation. *B*, Lateral view. Note also that what appears to be an avulsion of the medial epicondyle is really due to the rotation of the distal humerus and the oblique orientation of the film.

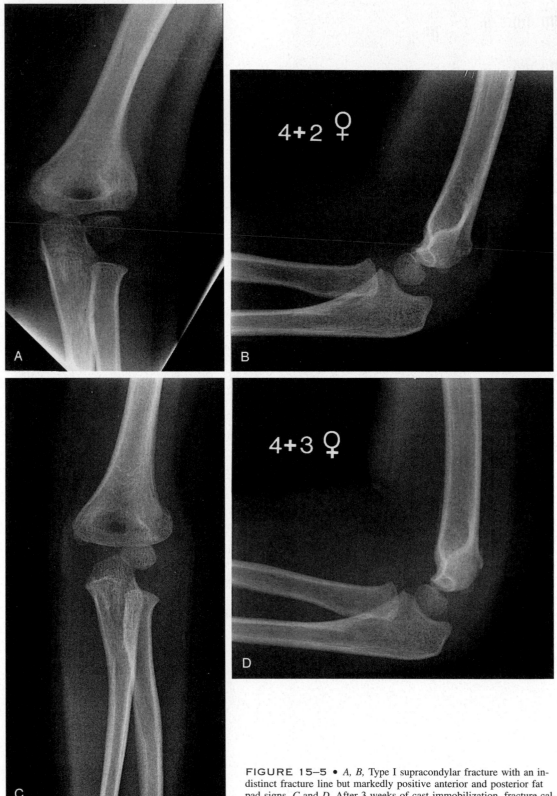

FIGURE 15–5 • *A, B,* Type I supracondylar fracture with an indistinct fracture line but markedly positive anterior and posterior fat pad signs. *C* and *D,* After 3 weeks of cast immobilization, fracture callus confirms the presence of a nondisplaced fracture.

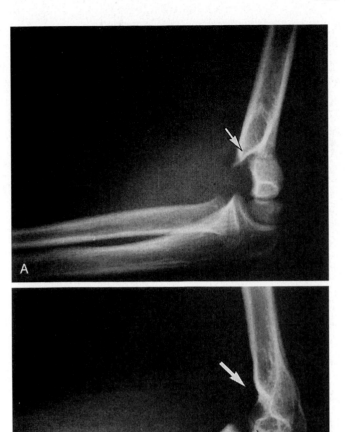

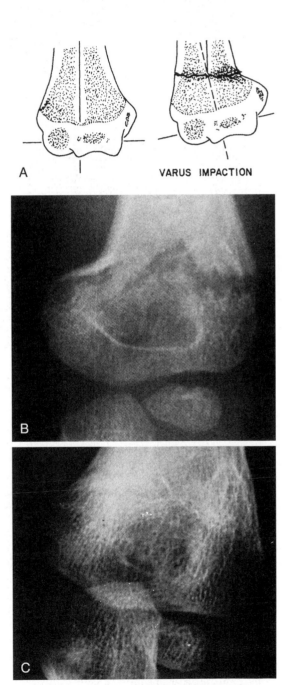

FIGURE 15–6 • *A*, Type II supracondylar fracture with anterior angulation. *B*, Treated with flexion of the elbow and casting, the injury shows excellent early alignment.

FIGURE 15–7 • *A*, Schematic view of greenstick type II fracture that is causing medial trabecular–cortical compression leading to cubitus varus. This condition must be corrected with manipulation. *B*, Acute cubitus varus in a 5-year-old child with a type II fracture that was not corrected. *C*, Mild cubitus varus can be seen 2 years later. (From Ogden, J. A.: Skeletal Injury in the Child. Philadelphia, Lea & Febiger, 1982.)

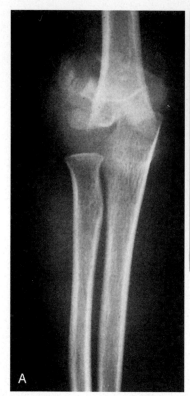
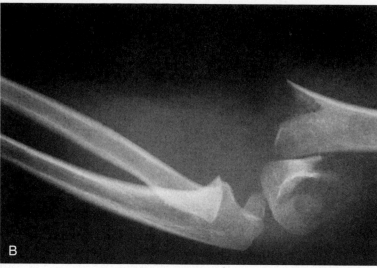

FIGURE 15–8 • *A* and *B*, Severe type III fracture with rotation and posterior and lateral displacement with associated neurovascular compromise.

DIAGNOSIS AND RADIOGRAPHIC EVALUATION

We define a supracondylar humerus fracture to be a transverse fracture traversing the entire width of the distal humeral metaphysis without involving the distal humeral physis. The primary challenge in establishing this diagnosis is to rule out other fractures of the distal humerus that do not meet these criteria. Fractures that can sometimes be confused with supracondylar humerus fractures include lateral condyle fractures, medial condyle fractures, and transphyseal fractures. Establishing the correct diagnosis is most difficult in patients younger than 4 years, whose ossific nuclei of the distal humerus are yet unossified.

Routine anteroposterior and lateral radiographs should be taken at 90 degrees to each other whenever a supracondylar humerus fracture is suspected. If the examiner is certain of the presence of a distal humerus fracture, because of focal point tenderness, mechanism of injury, and positive posterior fat pad sign, but is unable to identify the specific fracture pattern, 45-degree oblique radiographs often provide adequate visualization to establish the definitive diagnosis. On the other hand, if what may be a pathologic abnormality could possibly be a normal variant in a partially ossified distal humerus, comparison films of the opposite elbow allow identification of normal anatomy and determination of whether or not a fracture is present. Once a fracture is identified, the radiographic fracture classification system described earlier may be applied.

The anterior and posterior fat pad signs are often helpful in diagnosing intra-articular elbow fractures such as supracondylar humerus fractures (see Chapter 13). While very sensitive, the anterior fat pad sign is not very specific for intra-articular elbow fractures because the coronoid fossa of the humerus (occupied by the anterior fat pad) is much more shallow than the olecranon fossa (occupied by the posterior fat pad). Any insult that causes a joint effusion may cause the anterior fat pad to become visible on the lateral radiograph. A larger intra-articular fluid collection such as fracture hemarthrosis is necessary to displace the posterior fat pad enough for it to become visible on lateral radiographs; therefore, the posterior fat pad sign is much more reliable.

Additional radiographic measurements have been described to assess fracture alignment before and after reduction. The most commonly used measurement is Baumann's angle, the intersection of a line drawn along the longitudinal axis of the humerus and a line drawn along the physis between capitellum and distal lateral humeral metaphysis. The normal angle varies in magnitude but averages approximately 72 degrees, and it should always be compared to the uninjured contralateral elbow (Fig. 15–9).[72] A second useful radiographic reference line is the anterior humeral line (Fig. 15–10). If the capitellar ossific nucleus is displaced posterior to the anterior humeral line, fracture reduction should be considered. Fracture reduction should restore Baumann's angle to a measurement similar to that of the opposite elbow on the anteroposterior view, and on the lateral view should restore the capitellum to a position in which the central third is bisected by the anterior humeral line.

For all patients with supracondylar humerus fractures, the entire extremity should be examined and radiographs obtained of all areas where associated injuries might be present. Approximately 15% of patients with supracondylar fractures have associated injuries.[70]

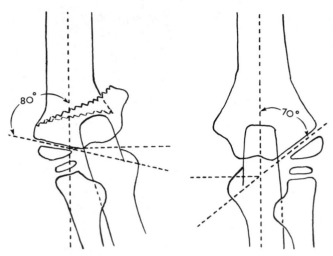

FIGURE 15–9 • Baumann's angle is the angle formed by a line perpendicular to the axis of the humerus and a line tangential to the straight epiphyseal border of the lateral part of the distal metaphysis. In the case illustrated, Baumann's angle is 80 degrees on the fractured left side and 70 degrees on the normal right side, indicating varus angulation of 10 degrees. The same holds true for lateral tilt and valgus angulation. (From Dodge, H. S.: Displaced supracondylar fractures of the humerus in children: treatment by dental extraction. J. Bone Joint Surg. 54A: 1411, 1972.)

TREATMENT

The goal of treatment is to obtain and safely maintain anatomic fracture alignment, measures that promote rapid healing and return to full and unlimited function with minimal risk of complications. Injury severity determines the ease with which this goal is attained and the most appropriate method of treatment. For extension-type supra-

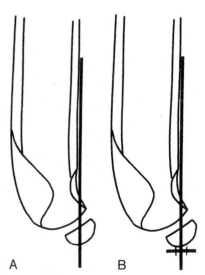

FIGURE 15–10 • The anterior humeral line (AHL). *A*, A line is drawn down the anterior humeral cortex. *B*, A second line is drawn perpendicular to the AHL from the anterior to the posterior extent of the capitellum and is divided into thirds. In normal cases, the AHL passes through the middle third of the capitellum. (From Rogers, L. F., et al.: Plastic bowing, torus and greenstick supracondylar fractures of the humerus: radiographic clues to obscure fractures of the elbow in children. Radiology 128:146, 1978.)

condylar fractures, Gartland's radiographic classification system is a helpful guide to injury severity and optimal treatment.

Type I Fractures

Because type I fractures are truly nondisplaced, there is minimal swelling and no significant risk of neurovascular injury. Immediate application of an above-elbow cast with the elbow at 90 degrees of flexion (and neutral angles of pronation and supination) is safe and is all that is necessary to prevent loss of reduction and to provide pain relief. If future swelling is a concern, the cast may be bivalved, splitting all fiberglass or plaster elements down to—but not through—the cast padding. The two halves of the cast are held together by the cast padding or with two or three circumferential bands of tape. Five to 10 days later, the cast is simply overwrapped with fiberglass. After 3 weeks of immobilization, the cast is removed and elbow range-of-motion exercises are begun. At 6 weeks, the fracture is essentially healed and the patient may resume full activity.

Type II Fractures

Despite an intact osseous hinge, type II fractures can vary significantly in displacement and injury severity, which determines treatment choice. In fractures in which the anterior humeral line does intersect the capitellum, reduction may not be necessary and immediate cast immobilization in 90 degrees of flexion is appropriate. Closed reduction warrants serious consideration for moderately displaced fractures when the anterior humeral line passes anterior to the capitellum. Given a cooperative patient and minimal swelling, gentle closed reduction may be performed under regional anesthesia or conscious sedation in the emergency department, and the fracture immobilized in an above-elbow cast that affords enough flexion to maintain the fracture reduction (see Fig. 15–6). If any swelling is present, close attention to the findings of the neurovascular examination is critical when immobilizing the elbow in more than 100 degrees of flexion. Fluoroscopic observation can be helpful in determining the minimum degree of flexion required to safely maintain fracture reduction.

Moderate, or severely displaced, or angulated type II fractures may be associated with neurovascular injury. Neurologic and vascular examinations, performed and documented meticulously, are essential. Significant swelling may also make it impossible to flex the elbow enough so that the fracture reduction can be sustained. In such situations, closed reduction and percutaneous pinning is indicated to maintain fracture reduction without compromising the neurovascular integrity of the limb. Moderately or severely displaced type II fractures may also be associated with medial column impaction, lateral column impaction, or rotation. If they go unrecognized, any of these three variations of a type II fracture can lead to malunion and angular deformity. Medial impaction, lateral impaction, and rotation all necessitate closed reduction, which is often most dependably maintained with percutaneous pinning.[17] After percutaneous pinning, a splint or bivalved cast is applied and, 5 to 10 days later, the bivalved cast may be overwrapped or the splint removed and an above-elbow cast applied.

Type III Fractures

Completely displaced supracondylar humerus fractures are intrinsically unstable, typically cause severe swelling, and are frequently associated with neurovascular injury (Fig. 15–11). These factors make management of type III fractures challenging and anxiety provoking.

Closed Reduction

Type III extension-type fractures have an intact posterior periosteal hinge which, in addition to the triceps tendon, provides some stability to the fracture when it is immobilized in flexion. Historically, immobilization in flexion has

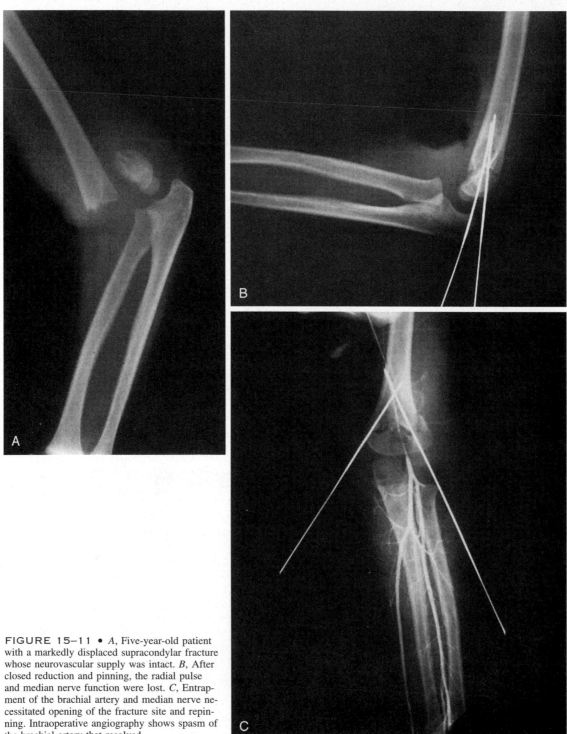

FIGURE 15–11 • *A*, Five-year-old patient with a markedly displaced supracondylar fracture whose neurovascular supply was intact. *B*, After closed reduction and pinning, the radial pulse and median nerve function were lost. *C*, Entrapment of the brachial artery and median nerve necessitated opening of the fracture site and repinning. Intraoperative angiography shows spasm of the brachial artery that resolved.

been common. Paradoxically, the completely displaced supracondylar fracture is just the fracture that requires elbow flexion greater than 100 degrees, to maintain adequate fracture reduction, but it is also the one least able to tolerate flexion beyond 100 degrees, at which point neurovascular compromise is a risk (Fig. 15–12).[43] Because of relatively high incidences of malunion and neurovascular compromise, immobilization in flexion has largely been replaced by other treatments.[39, 48, 53, 71, 73]

Percutaneous Pinning

In 1988, Pirone published a series of 230 displaced supracondylar humerus fractures and analyzed the results of (1) closed reduction and percutaneous pinning, (2) open reduction, (3) skeletal traction, and (4) closed reduction with casting.[53] Pirone reported significantly better results in the group treated with closed reduction and percutaneous pinning as compared with the other three groups. Subsequent studies have confirmed these results, and closed reduction with percutaneous pinning has become the most used and most accepted treatment nationwide.[10, 25, 30, 31, 71]

In the emergency department, a meticulous neurovascular examination should be performed and properly documented: median, radial, ulnar, and anterior interosseous nerve function among other findings. Because it has only a motor function, anterior interosseous nerve injury has been underdiagnosed in the past, but separate investigators have recently provided substantial evidence to suggest that the anterior interosseous nerve is the nerve most frequently injured in association with supracondylar fractures.[15, 19] Because of the severe nature of the injury, the amount of manipulation required for reduction, and the possible need to perform an open reduction, an attempt at closed reduction should *not* be made in the emergency department. A pulseless or dysvascular extremity requires immediate transport of the patient to surgery. While it is acceptable to splint and observe overnight a patient with a "neurovascularly intact" extremity, swelling quickly ensues that can make reduction and pinning significantly more difficult.

Therefore, we recommend bringing the patient to surgery as quickly as possible.

Closed reduction and percutaneous pinning can be performed successfully using a variety of techniques with the patient positioned supine, lateral, or prone. We prefer to perform the reduction with the patient positioned supine using the following series of steps. After general anesthesia has been administered, the patient is positioned toward the edge of the operating table with the affected extremity carefully supported over the side. C-arm fluoroscopy is brought in from the foot of the table, parallel to the table, so the patient's arm can rest on the C-arm.

Before prepping, with the arm less constrained by drapes, closed reduction is attempted. If the metaphyseal spike from the proximal fragment is tenting the skin and subcutaneous tissue, the brachialis is gently "milked" off of the fragment.[5] With the arm in a relaxed position at approximately 20 to 30 degrees of flexion, the medial-lateral displacement is corrected. When available, an assistant supports the forearm, and the operating surgeon places a thumb on the medial and lateral columns of the distal fragment. The final reduction maneuver involves the assistant's applying gentle longitudinal traction while the operating surgeon uses each thumb to manipulate the distal fragment distally and anteriorly. Simultaneously, the assistant flexes the elbow to maintain the reduction (Fig. 15–13).[47] If the initial displacement is posterior and medial, suggesting an intact medial periosteal hinge, the forearm is pronated. If the initial displacement is posterior and lateral, the forearm is supinated. When working alone, the operating surgeon can apply traction to the forearm and flexion to the elbow with one hand while applying distal and anterior pressure to the patient's olecranon with the other hand (Fig. 15–14).

The reduction is imaged with fluoroscopy on anteroposterior and lateral views. If the reduction is adequate or if it is clear that an adequate reduction is attainable with a second attempt, the elbow is extended to approximately 20 degrees of flexion, prepared, and draped. We prepare the hand into the field to allow neurovascular monitoring and

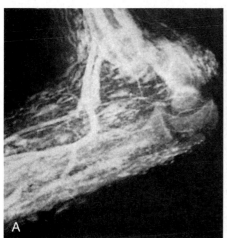 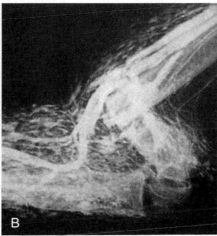 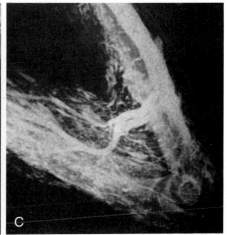

FIGURE 15-12 • Injection of a cadaver arm from an adolescent shows kinking of vessels. *A*, Vascular relationships at 90 degrees of flexion. *B*, In extension, the artery may be traumatized by the proximal fragment or kinked by soft tissue attachments. *C*, In hyperflexion, the vessels may be compressed in the edematous antecubital region. (From Ogden, J. A.: Skeletal Injury in the Child. Philadephia, Lea & Febiger, 1982.)

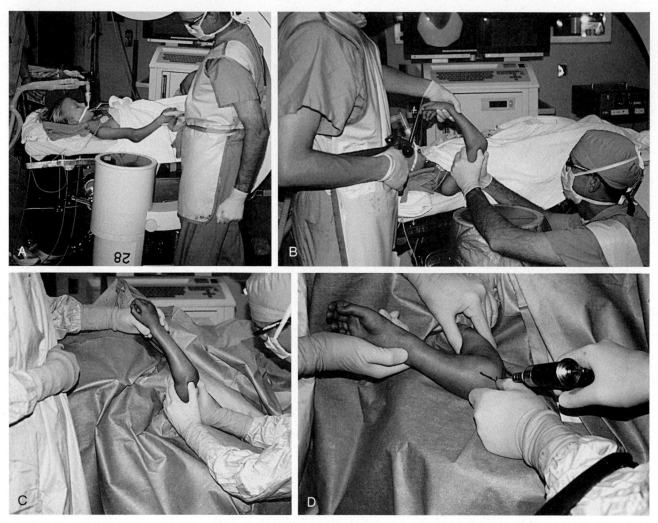

FIGURE 15–13 • Closed reduction of type III supracondylar humeral fracture. *A,* C-arm fluoroscopy is brought in from the foot of the operating table and used as the operating surface. *B,* Before surgical preparation and draping, and after medial-lateral displacement is corrected, the fracture is reduced. The operating surgeon places a thumb on the medial and lateral columns translating the fragment distally and anteriorly while the assistant flexes the elbow. *C,* After ensuring that a closed reduction can be obtained, the surgeon repeats the reduction maneuver after the arm has been prepared and draped. *D,* The operating surgeon retracts and protects the ulnar nerve with a thumb while placing the medial pin.

to the shoulder to allow for the use of a sterile tourniquet if necessary. The reduction maneuver is repeated, adequate alignment is confirmed fluoroscopically, and the elbow is temporarily held in a hyperflexed position to maintain the reduction.

Controversy persists about the optimal pin configuration that maintains adequate fracture reduction and minimizes potential complications. Crossed pins provide the greatest biomechanical stability but have the potential to cause ulnar nerve injury.[74] Recent reports suggest that the biomechanical stability sacrificed by using two or three lateral pins is not clinically significant and avoids iatrogenic ulnar nerve injury.[14, 68] If two lateral pins are used, great care must be taken to ensure that both pins cross through both fracture fragments with adequate spacing between the pins; otherwise, fracture reduction may be lost. If the crossed-pin technique is used, whether to pin the medial or lateral column first is a matter a little like religion: many surgeons have very strong opinions about the subject, but there is not much objective evidence to support one over the other. To pin the medial column first, the elbow is externally

rotated; to pin the lateral column internal rotation is used. Sometimes the fracture is more stable in internal or in external rotation, and this determines which column is pinned first. Because internal rotation of the elbow can result in posterior displacement of the medial distal fragment causing varus angulation, when possible we externally rotate the elbow and pin the medial column first.[52]

The operating surgeon palpates the medial epicondyle and uses a thumb to retract and protect the ulnar nerve posteriorly (see Fig. 15–13). A 0.062 Kirschner wire is then placed just anterior to the thumb on the medial epicondyle. The Kirschner wire is angled cephalad to travel within the medial column of bone and advanced until it just penetrates the opposite cortex. Using fluoroscopy, the position of the Kirschner wire is checked in anteroposterior and lateral planes. If placed in the correct site, this first pin often substantially improves fracture stability, allowing extension past 90 degrees to image the elbow and facilitate placement of the second pin. The second pin is placed within the lateral column of bone, crossing the first pin well above the fracture site (Fig. 15–15). The pins are left

protruding through
to ensure that they
postoperative dressi
pins has produced an
and loss of reductio

Occasionally, the
young to allow accu
In such instances the
may be made dire
tissues are spread v
condyle, and a smal
posterior to the pi
medial column pin
or three lateral pir
demonstrated that,
configuration was
fracture from the
aspect and a third
humeral shaft.[74]

Open Reductio

Inability to achiev
tissue interpositio
is interposed and
seal spike by cl
artery, median nei
between the frac
adequate closed
tures displaced
interposition of th
approached anter
posteromedially
radial nerve and
limited approach
ally be easily ex
reduction confirr
Past reluctance t
fractures for fea
to be unfounded
that open redu
increase the risl

While the ma
regain the pulse
is encountered
adequate reduc
Shaw and their
lar algorithms
reduction and
assessed. If the
sound and the
elbow is imm
tient is careful
not detectable
at the fracture
bers from both
radial pulse b
mediately. Al
transected, an
lished by free
ties) or by rep
ties). Using

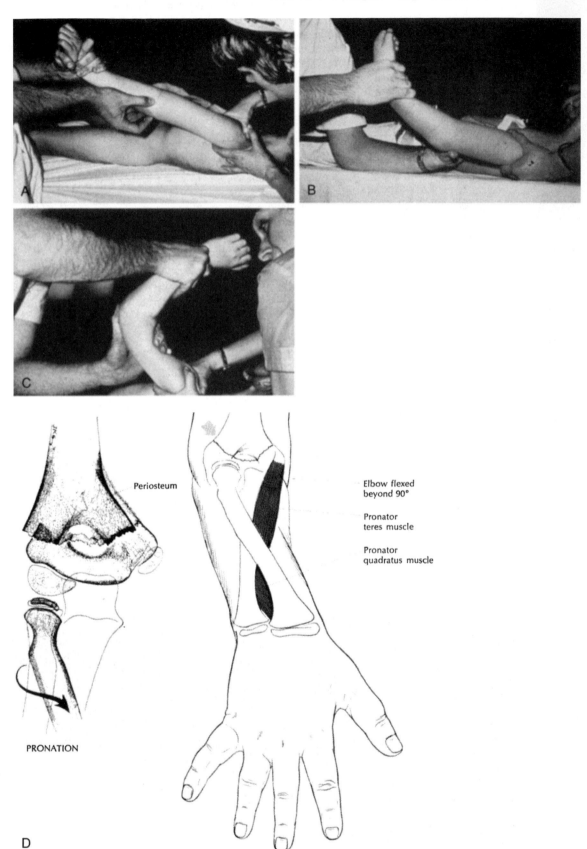

D

FIGURE 15–14 • *A*, Manipulative reduction is performed by exerting gentle traction in extension and supination. *B*, Direct pressure is exerted to realign the distal fragment. *C*, After realignment, the elbow is flexed to 120 degrees and appropriately pronated or supinated. *D*, Medial displacement of the distal fragment often requires pronation for stability, with the elbow flexed.

Illustration continued on following page

Brachioradialis
muscle

Supinator
muscle

SUPINAT

E

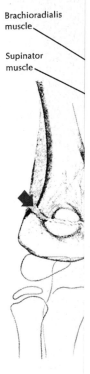

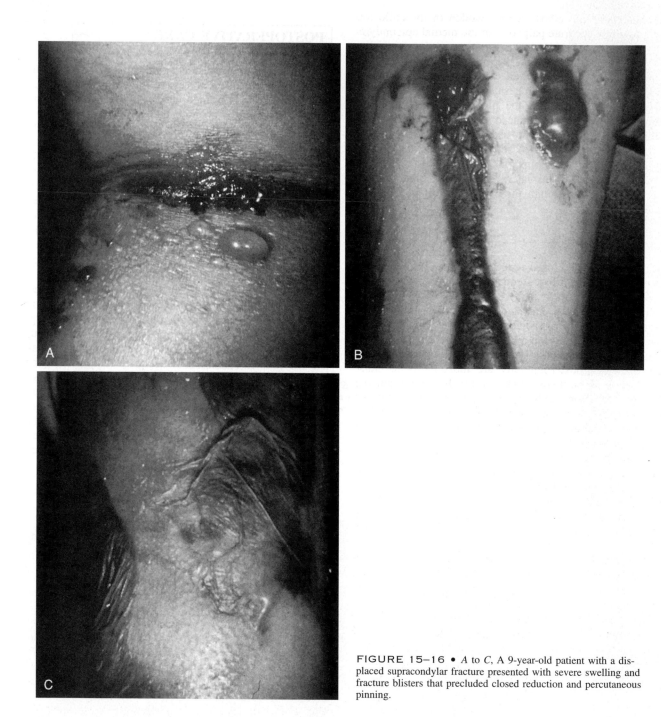

FIGURE 15–16 • *A* to *C*, A 9-year-old patient with a displaced supracondylar fracture presented with severe swelling and fracture blisters that precluded closed reduction and percutaneous pinning.

FIGURE 1
ture. *B*, Pins

com
and
on
the
witl
the
Fra
Wh
ear
cas

C

Co
tw
ate
an
oc
pr
tu

R

1

2

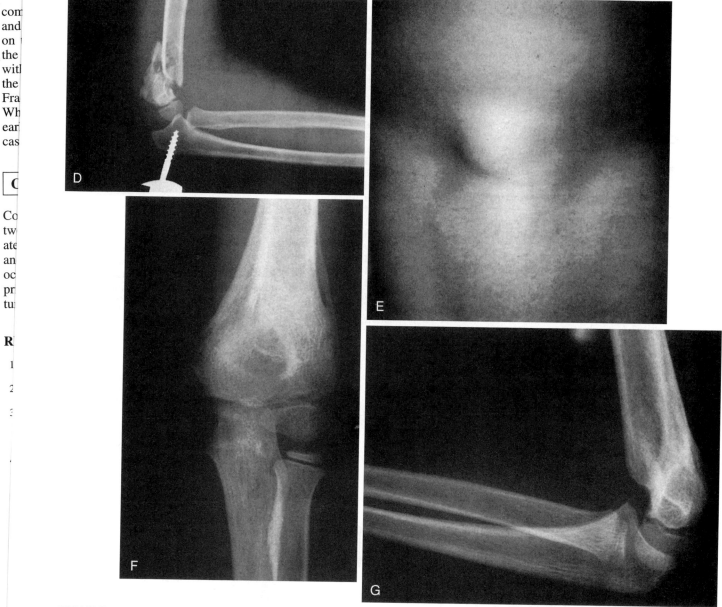

FIGURE 15–16 • *Continued D* and *E*, Overhead skeletal traction is used to safely obtain and maintain adequate fracture alignment. *F* and *G*, Six months after injury, the fracture is completely healed and the outcome excellent.

traction is applied in a lateral direction with the patient lying supine (Fig. 15–17). Pronation and supination of the forearm and varus or valgus tilt of the distal fragment are difficult to control and correct with this method of traction. The forearm tends to rotate into supination, resulting in a loss of stability that ordinarily is achieved when the forearm is maintained in the pronated position in most common fractures. This position also places the distal fracture fragment in some extension.

Because of these disadvantages, when traction is indicated we prefer to use skeletal traction with the arm held overhead. Under general or regional anesthesia, a Kirschner wire may be inserted through the proximal ulna at the palpable tip of the olecranon. An olecranon screw, which is inserted at the same level, is easier to insert and avoids risk to the ulnar nerve. Predrilling of the ulna and the use of image intensification are helpful for inserting the device.

Gross displacement is corrected at this time. The arm is suspended from an overhead frame with a sling under the forearm to control its position. Three to five pounds of traction is usually sufficient to reduce and stabilize the fracture. Too much weight elevates the shoulder and twists the thorax causing the child to shift position and losing control of the fracture fragment. Suspension of the forearm in this position permits rapid reduction of edema and good control of elbow flexion. Rotational deformity can be controlled by placing the arm in either a cephalad or a caudad position. If necessary, a lateral sling around the upper arm also may provide lateral traction to correct anterior displacement of the proximal fragment (Fig. 15–18). Smith used a traction bail attached to a Kirschner wire to provide more precise control of the tilt of the fracture, thus correcting varus and valgus positions, and he has documented the most successful use of traction with this method, noting no

45. Micheli, L. J., Santore, R., and Stanitski, C. L.: Epiphyseal fractures of the elbow in children. Am. Family Physician 22:107, 1980.

46. Micheli, L. J., Skolnick, D., and Hall, J. E.: Supracondylar fractures in the humerus in children. Am. Family Physician 19:100, 1979.

47. Minkowitz, B., and Busch, M. T.: Supracondylar humerus fractures. Current trends and controversies. Orthop. Clin. North Am. 25:581–594, 1994.

48. Mohammed, S., and Rymaszewski, L. A.: Supracondylar fractures of the distal humerus in children. Injury 26:487–489, 1995.

49. Nassar, A.: Correction of varus deformity following supracondylar fracture of the humerus. Poster Presentation, American Orthopedic Assoc., Annual Meeting, 1992.

50. Ogden, J.: Skeletal Injury in the Child. Philadelphia, Lea & Febiger, 1982, p. 240.

51. Ottolenghi, C. E.: Prophylactic due Syndrome de Volkmann dans des Humerus Supracondyliennes du Coude chez l'enfant. Rev. Chir. Orthop. 57:517, 1971.

52. Paradis, G., Lavallee, P., Gagnon, N., and Lemire, L.: Supracondylar fractures of the humerus in children. Technique and results of crossed percutaneous K-wire fixation. Clin. Orthop. 297:231–237, 1993.

53. Pirone, A. M., Graham, H. K., and Krajbich, J. I.: Management of displaced extension-type supracondylar fractures of the humerus in children. J. Bone Joint Surg. 70A:641, 1988.

54. Rang, M.: Children's Fractures, 2nd ed. Philadelphia, J. B. Lippincott, 1983.

55. Rodriguez Merchan, E. C.: Supracondylar fractures of the humerus in children: treatment by overhead skeletal traction. Orthop. Rev. 21:475–482, 1992.

56. Rogers, L. F., Malave, S. Jr., White, H., and Tachdjian, M. O.: Plastic bowing, torus and greenstick supracondylar fractures of the humerus: radiographic clues to obscure fractures of the elbow in children. Radiology 128:145, 1978.

57. Sairyo, K., Henmi, T., Kanematsu, Y., Nakano, S., and Kajikawa, T.: Radial nerve palsy associated with slightly angulated pediatric supracondylar humerus fracture. J. Orthop. Trauma 11:227–229, 1997.

58. Schickendanz, H., Schramm, H., Herrmann, K., and Jager, S.: Fractures and dislocations in the elbow in childhood. Am. Family Physician 13(2):1973.

59. Schoenecker, P. L., Delgado, E., Rotman, M., Sicard, G. A., and Capelli, A. M.: Pulseless arm in association with totally displaced supracondylar fracture. J. Orthop. Trauma 10:410–415, 1996.

60. Shaw, B. A., Kasser, J. R., Emans, J. B., and Rand, F. F.: Management of vascular injuries in displaced supracondylar humerus fractures without arteriography. J. Orthop. Trauma 4:25–29, 1990.

61. Sibly, T. F., Briggs, P. J., and Gibson, M. J.: Supracondylar fractures of the humerus in childhood: range of movement following the posterior approach to open reduction. Injury 22:456–458, 1991.

62. Smith, F. M.: Children's elbow injuries. Fractures and dislocations. Clin. Orthop. 50:7, 1967.

63. Siris, J. E.: Supracondylar fractures of the humerus analyzed: 330 cases. Surg. Gynecol. Obstet. 68:201, 1939.

64. Smith, L.: Deformity following supracondylar fractures. J. Bone Joint Surg. 42A:235, 1960.

65. Staples, O. S.: Complication of traction treatment of supracondylar fractures of the humerus in children. J. Bone Joint Surg. 41A:369, 1959.

66. Strait, R. T., Siegel, R. M., and Shapiro, R. A.: Humeral fractures without obvious etiologies in children less than 3 years of age: when is it abuse? Pediatrics 96 (4 pt 1):667–671, 1995.

67. Sutton, W. R., Green, W. B., Georgopoulos, G., and Dameron, T. B., Jr.: Displaced supracondylar humeral fractures in children. A comparison of results and costs in patients treated by skeletal traction versus percutaneous pinning. Clin. Orthop. 278:81–87, 1992.

68. Topping, R. E., Blanco, J. S., and Davis, T. J.: Clinical evaluation of crossed-pin versus lateral-pin fixation in displaced supracondylar humerus fractures. J. Pediatr. Orthop. 15:435–439, 1995.

69. Vahvanen, V., and Aalto, K.: Supracondylar fractures of the humerus in children. A long-term follow-up study of 107 cases. Acta Orthop. Scand. 49:225, 1978.

70. Wilkins, K. E.: Residuals of elbow trauma in children. Orthop. Clin. North Am. 21:291, 1990.

71. Wilkins, K. E.: Supracondylar fractures: what's new? J. Pediatr. Orthop. 6:110–116, 1997.

72. Williamson, D. M., Coates, C. J., Miller, R. K., and Cole, W. G.: Normal characteristics of the Baumann (humerocapitellar) angle: an aid in assessment of supracondylar fractures. J. Pediatr. Orthop. 12:636–639, 1992.

73. Williamson, D. M., and Cole, W. G.: Treatment of selected extension supracondylar fractures of the humerus by manipulation and strapping in flexion. Injury 24:249–252, 1993.

74. Zionts, L. E., McKellop, H. A., and Hathaway, R.: Torsional strength of pin configurations used to fix supracondylar fractures of the humerus in children. J. Bone Joint Surg. 76A:253–256, 1994.

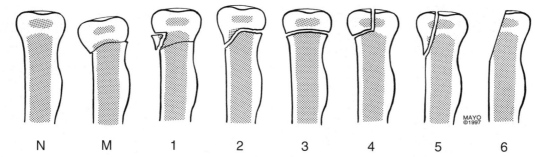

FIGURE 17–10 • Proximal radius. *N* = normal proximal radius; *M* = metaphyseal fracture; 1–6, Peterson-type physeal fractures.

elbow dislocation.[133] In most cases, there is relatively little displacement of the fragment. Immobilization of the elbow for 3 to 4 weeks usually is sufficient. Open reduction and internal fixation are usually unnecessary because these injuries tend to occur only in children approaching the age of skeletal maturity. The risk of associated growth arrest is minimal. Tardy ulnar nerve palsy has been reported.[77]

PROXIMAL RADIUS

The epiphysis of the radial head begins to ossify at about the age of 5 years. Although it may appear first as a sphere, ossification soon advances into one or two ovoid, flat, or wedge-shaped nuclei, which may be eccentrically located on the radial metaphysis[29] and misinterpreted as avulsion fractures of the epiphysis. Notches and clefts in the proximal radial metaphysis may closely resemble post-traumatic appearances.[3]

In children, fractures of the neck of the proximal radius (see Chapter 18) are more common than fractures involving the epiphyseal growth plate[141] (Fig. 17–10). These physeal fractures account for only 0.6 percent of all physeal injuries (see Table 17–1). The normal carrying angle of the elbow makes valgus injury more likely with a fall on the outstretched arm. The mechanism of injury of a fall on the outstretched hand drives the capitellum against the outer side of the head of the radius, tilting it and displacing it outward. The fracture may be, therefore, type 1, 2, 3, 4, or 5 (see Fig. 17–10), with type 1 being most common, and with decreasing frequency with each successive type. A

second mechanism is associated with posterior dislocation of the elbow with simultaneous compression of the capitellum on the anterior portion of the head of the radius.[138] This has the potential to produce the more serious type 4 and 5 fractures.

The joint capsule is attached to the radius in continuity with the annular ligament. Because the radial neck lies outside the joint capsule, fracture of the neck may not cause joint effusion or fat pad displacement. Fracture of the radial head, however, usually produces elbow effusion and a positive fat pad sign.[3]

Differentiating fractures that involve only the neck of the radius (metaphysis) from those that also involve the physis can be very difficult. Oblique radiographs and occasionally MRI can be helpful in making this differentiation. In a recent study,[136] fracture of the metaphysis (neck) was found to be the most common, followed in succession by types 1 and 2, which helps validate the Peterson classification[114] (Table 17–2).

The type 1 fracture is difficult to diagnose but is very common (Fig. 17–11). It is usually incorrectly called a neck fracture or type 2 fracture. It is distinguished by a transmetaphyseal fracture that extends to the physis. The transmetaphyseal fracture is often only a compression fracture that may not be visible on the initial radiographs. Transmetaphyseal sclerosis, however, is always present 3 to 6 weeks post fracture and verifies the compression component. The fracture line extending to the physis is also frequently difficult to visualize on routine anteroposterior and lateral views and is best seen on oblique views. This may be only a fracture line, but often there is a

		Extra-articular, *n* (%)		Intra-articular, *n* (%)		Total
Closed physis	Radial neck	16 (14)	Radial head	17 (15)		33 (28)
Open physis	Metaphyseal	42 (36)	P4	1 (1)		83 (72)
	P1	25 (22)	P5	4 (3)		
	P2	9 (8)	P6	1 (1)		
	P3	1 (1)				
TOTAL		93 (80)		23 (20)		116 (100)

• TABLE 17–2 • **Fractures of the Proximal Radius in Children***

*Ages 0 through 16 years.
P = Peterson type.
Data from Leung, A. G., and Peterson, H. A.: Fractures of the proximal radial head and neck, with emphasis on those that involve the articular cartilage. J. Pediatr. Orthop. (in press).

functional impairment and few, if any, cosmetic or clothes-fitting complaints. Even if complete closure of all physes about the elbow occurred in a young child, surgical lengthening of the involved humerus or forearm bones or surgical arrest of the contralateral elbow physes would rarely, if ever, be indicated.

Premature partial closure of the distal humerus is very rare and has not been reported in the proximal radius or ulna. Premature closure of the medial or lateral condyle theoretically may result in progressive cubitus varus or valgus, respectively. This could be determined only after many months of follow-up. In this rare occurrence, surgical closure of the remaining physis might be considered. Physeal bar excision for premature partial closure was performed at the Mayo Clinic in 173 cases between 1968 and 1997. None involved the elbow. Supracondylar osteotomy to correct angular growth is rarely necessary.

Premature closure of the central physis between the medial and lateral condyles occurs occasionally and has been called a fishtail deformity. The underlying cause of the arrest is multifactorial and may be due to a gap in reduction of an intracondylar fracture, avascular necrosis of the central or trochlear portion of the epiphysis, or central premature physeal arrest (bar formation) without a gap or avascular necrosis. This usually occurs in younger children and causes no pain and only minimal loss of motion. The deformity gradually produces functional disability in adults due to premature degenerative arthrosis. The intercondylar notch may predispose to subsequent intercondylar fracture. Thus, if the fishtail deformity is identified in a young child, surgical closure of the medial and lateral portions of the physis may prevent the deformity from progressing and result in only mild additional humeral length discrepancy.

An occasional concern is damage to the physeal cells between the medial metaphysis and the trochlea in young children. Because the trochlear ossification center is not radiographically visible at this early age, this damage cannot be diagnosed by routine radiographs, tomographs, arthrographs, CT scan, or scintigraphy. At the present time, MRI does not have the ability to evaluate such an injury early, and there has been no report of this use of MRI to date. It is best to observe these cases for months or years before making the diagnosis of premature partial physeal arrest.

REFERENCES

• ANATOMY

1. Silberstein, M. J., Brodeur, A. E., and Graviss, E. R.: Some vagaries of the capitellum. J. Bone Joint Surg. **61A:**244, 1979.
2. Silberstein, M. J., Brodeur, A. E., and Graviss, E. R.: Some vagaries of the lateral epicondyle. J. Bone Joint Surg. **64A:**444, 1982.
3. Silberstein, M. J., Brodeur, A. E., and Graviss, E. R.: Some vagaries of the radial head and neck. J. Bone Joint Surg. **64A:**1153, 1982.
4. Silberstein, M. J., Brodeur, A. E., Graviss, E. R., and Luisiri, A.: Some vagaries of the medial epicondyle. J. Bone Joint Surg. **63A:**524, 1981.
5. Silberstein, M. J., Brodeur, A. E., Graviss, E. R., and Luisiri, A.: Some vagaries of the olecranon. J. Bone Joint Surg. **63A:**722, 1981.

• EPIDEMIOLOGY

6. Havranek, P., and Hájkova, H.: Treatment of children's epiphyseal injuries in the elbow region. Acta Univ. Carol. **31:**243, 1985.

7. Mann, D. C., and Rajmaira, S.: Distribution of physeal and nonphyseal fractures in 2650 long-bone fractures in children aged 0–16 years. J. Pediatr. Orthop. **10:**713, 1990.
8. Mizuta, T., Benson, W. M., Foster, B. K., Paterson, D. C., and Morris, L. L.: Statistical analysis of the incidence of physeal injuries. J. Pediatr. Orthop. **7:**518, 1987.
9. Ogden, J. A.: Injury to the growth mechanisms of the immature skeleton. Skeletal Radiol. **6:**237, 1981.
10. Peterson, C. A., and Peterson, H. A.: Analysis of the incidence of injuries to the epiphyseal growth plate. J. Trauma **12:**275, 1972.
11. Peterson, H. A.: Physeal injuries of the distal humerus. Orthopedics **15:**799, 1992.
12. Peterson, H. A., Madhok, R., Benson, J. T., Ilstrup, D. M., and Melton, L. J. III: Physeal fractures: Part I. Epidemiology in Olmsted County, Minnesota, 1979–1988. J. Pediatr. Orthop. **14:**423, 1994.

• CLASSIFICATION

13. Peterson, H. A.: Physeal fractures: Part 2. Two previously unclassified types. J. Pediatr. Orthop. **14:**431, 1994.
14. Peterson, H. A.: Physeal fractures: Part 3. Classification. J. Pediatr. Orthop. **14:**439, 1994.
15. Peterson, H. A., and Burkhart, S. S.: Compression injury of the epiphyseal growth plate: Fact or fiction? J. Pediatr. Orthop. **1:**377, 1981.
16. Salter, R. B., and Harris, W. R.: Injuries involving the epiphyseal plate. J. Bone Joint Surg. **45A:**587, 1963.

• IMAGING AND DIAGNOSIS

17. Akbarnia, B. A., Silberstein, M. J., Rende, R. J., Graviss, E. R., and Luisiri, A.: Arthrography in the diagnosis of fractures of the distal end of the humerus in infants. J. Bone Joint Surg. **68A:**599, 1986.
18. Brodeur, A. E., Silberstein, M. J., and Graviss, E. R.: Radiology of the Pediatric Elbow. Boston, G. K. Hall Medical, 1981, p. 234.
19. Blane, C. E., Kling, T. F., Jr., Andrews, J. C., DePietro, M. A., and Hensinger, R. N.: Arthrography in the post-traumatic elbow in children. Am. J. Roentgenol. **143**(1):17, 1984.
20. Dias, J. J., Lamont, A. C., and Jones, J. M.: Ultrasonic diagnosis of neonatal separation of the distal humeral epiphysis. J. Bone Joint Surg. **70B:**825, 1988.
21. Grogan, D. P., and Ogden, J. A.: Pediatric elbow fracture need not be your nemesis. J. Musculoskeletal Med. May:64, 1986.
22. Hansen, P. E., Barnes, D. A., and Tullos, H. S.: Arthrographic diagnosis of an injury pattern in the distal humerus of an infant. J. Pediatr. Orthop. **2:**569, 1982.
23. Hoeffel, J. C., Blanquart, D., Galloy, M. A., Dinia, W., Mainard, L., Gerber, R., and Bretagne, M.C.: Fractures of the lateral condyle of the elbow in children. Radiological Aspects (in French). J. Radiol. **71:**407, 1990.
24. Holland, C. T.: A radiographic note of injuries to the distal epiphyses of the radius and ulna. Proc. R. Soc. Med. **22:**695, 1929.
25. Houben, J. J., van Elegem, P., Godart, S., and Blaimont, P.: Slipped epiphysis of the elbow in the young child. Diagnostic aspects. Acta Orthop. Belg. **49:**592, 1983.
26. Hudson, T. M.: Elbow arthrography. Radiol. Clin. North Am. **19:**227, 1981.
27. Marzo, J. M., d'Amato, C., Strong, M., and Gillespie, R.: Usefulness and accuracy of arthrography in management of lateral humeral condyle fractures in children. J. Pediatr. Orthop. **10:**317, 1990.
28. McCarthy, S. M., and Ogden, J. A.: Radiology of postnatal skeletal development. VI. Elbow joint, proximal radius, and ulna. Skeletal Radiol. **7:**239, 1982.
29. Nussbaum, A. J.: The off-profile proximal radial epiphysis: Another potential pitfall in the diagnosis of elbow trauma. J. Trauma **23:**40, 1983.
30. Resnik, C. S.: Diagnostic imaging of pediatric skeletal trauma. Radiol. Clin. North Am. **27:**1013, 1989.
31. Rogers, L. F.: Fractures and dislocations of the elbow. Semin. Roentgenol. **13:**97, 1978.
32. Yates, C., and Sullivan, J. A.: Arthrographic diagnosis of elbow injuries in children. J. Pediatr. Orthop. **7:**54, 1987.

• INJURY

Distal Humerus

Newborn to Age 2

33. Barrett, W. P., Almquist, E. A., and Staheli, L. T.: Fracture separation of the distal humeral physis in the newborn. Case report. J. Pediatr. Orthop. **4:**617, 1984.

34. Berman, J. M., and Weiner, D. S.: Neonatal fracture-separation of the distal humeral chondroepiphysis: a case report. Orthopedics **3:**875, 1980.

35. Blanquart, D., Hoeffel, J. C., Galloy, M. A., Mainard, L., and Bretagne, M. C.: Separation of the distal humeral epiphysis in young children. Radiologic features. Ann Pediatr. **37:**470, 1990.

36. Chand, K.: Epiphyseal separation of distal humeral epiphysis in an infant. A case report and review of the literature. J. Trauma **14:**521, 1974.

37. deJager, L. T., Hoffman, E. B.: Fracture-separation of the distal humeral epiphysis. J. Bone Joint Surg. **73B:**143, 1991.

38. DeLee, J. C., Wilkins, K. E., Rogers, L. F., and Rockwood, C. A.: Fracture-separation of the distal humeral epiphysis. J. Bone Joint Surg. **62A:**46, 1980.

39. Downs, D. M., and Wirth, C. R.: Fracture of the distal humeral chondroepiphysis in the neonate: a case report. Clin. Orthop. **169:**155, 1982.

40. Haliburton, R. A., Barber, J. R., and Fraser, R. L.: Pseudodislocation: an unusual birth injury. Can. J. Surg. **10:**455, 1967.

41. Holda, M. E., Manoli, A., II, and LaMont, R. L.: Epiphyseal separation of the distal end of the humerus with medial displacement. J. Bone Joint Surg. **62A:**52, 1980.

42. Kaplan, S. S., and Reckling, F. W.: Fracture separation of the lower humeral epiphysis with medial displacement. J. Bone Joint Surg. **53A:**1105, 1971.

43. Keon-Cohen, B. T.: Fractures of the elbow. J. Bone Joint Surg. **48A:**1623, 1966.

44. Marmor, L., and Bechtol, C. O.: Fracture separation of the lower humeral epiphysis. Report of a case. J. Bone Joint Surg. **24A:**333, 1960.

45. McIntyre, W. M., Wiley, J. J., and Charette, R. J.: Fracture-separation of the distal humeral epiphysis. Clin. Orthop. **188:**98, 1984.

46. Milton, L. P., and Port, R. B.: Separation of the distal humeral epiphysis in a neonate. Am. J. Dis. Child **139:**1203, 1985.

47. Omer, G. E., Jr., and Simmons, J. W.: Fractures of the distal humeral growth plate. South. Med. J. **61:**651, 1968.

48. Paige, M. L., and Port, R. B.: Separation of the distal humeral epiphysis in the neonate. Am. J. Dis. Child **139(2):**1203, 1985.

49. Perio, A., Mut, T., Aracil, J., and Martos, F.: Fracture-separation of the lower humeral epiphysis in young children. Acta Orthop. Scand. **52:**295, 1981.

50. Rogers, L. F., and Rockwood, C. A.: Separation of the entire distal humeral epiphysis. Radiology **106:**393, 1973.

51. Siffert, R. S.: Displacement of the distal humeral epiphysis in the newborn infant. J. Bone Joint Surg. **45A:**165, 1963.

52. Yngve, D. A.: Distal humeral epiphyseal separation. Orthopedics **8(1):**100, 1985.

Early Childhood (Ages 2–6)

53. Beghin, J. A., Bucholz, R. W., and Wenger, D. R.: Intracondylar fractures of the humerus in young children. A report of two cases. J. Bone Joint Surg. **64A:**1083, 1982.

54. Cothay, D. M.: Injury of the lower medial epiphysis of the humerus before development of the ossification centre. Report of a case. J. Bone Joint Surg. **49B:**766, 1967.

55. Mizuno, K., Hirohata, K., and Kashiwagi, D.: Fracture-separation of the distal humeral epiphysis in young children. J. Bone Joint Surg. **61A:**570, 1979.

56. Nwakama, A. C., Peterson, H. A., and Shaughnessy, W. J.: Fishtail deformity following fracture of the distal humerus in children: case presentations, discussion of etiology, and thoughts on treatment. Submitted for publication.

57. Smith, F. M.: Children's elbow injuries: fractures and dislocations. Clin. Orthop. **50:**7, 1967.

58. Sutherland, D. H., and Wrobel, L.: Displacement of the entire humeral epiphysis. Proceedings of the Western Orthopedic Association. J. Bone Joint Surg. **56A:**206, 1974.

59. Yoo, C. I., Suh, K. T., Kim, Y. J., Kim, H. T., and Kim, Y. H.: Avascular necrosis after fracture separation of the distal end of the humerus in children. Orthopedics **15:**959, 1992.

Ages 6–10

60. Amgwerd, M., and Sacher, P.: Treatment of fractures of the radial condyle of the humerus in children (in German). Z. Unfall. Versicherungsmed. **83:**49, 1990.

61. Attarian, D. E.: Lateral condyle fractures: Missed diagnoses in pediatric elbow injuries. Mil. Med. **155:**433, 1990.

62. Bede, W. B., Lefebvre, A. R., and Rosman, M. A.: Fractures of the medial humeral condyle in children. Can. J. Surg. **18:**137, 1975.

63. Chacha P. B.: Fracture of the medial condyle of the humerus with rotational displacement. Report of two cases. J. Bone Joint Surg. **52A:**1453, 1970.

64. Davids, J. R., Maguire, M. F., Mubarek, S. J., and Wenger, D. R.: Lateral condylar fracture of the humerus following posttraumatic cubitus varus. J. Pediatr. Orthop. **14:**466, 1994.

65. DeBoeck, H.: Surgery for nonunion of the lateral humeral condyle in children. Six cases followed for 1–9 years. Acta Orthop. Scand. **66(5):**401, 1995.

66. Dhillon, K. S., Sengupta, S., and Singh, B. J.: Delayed management of the lateral humeral condyle in children. Acta Orthop. Scand. **59:**419, 1988.

67. El Ghawabi, M. E.: Fractures of the medial condyle of the humerus. J. Bone Joint Surg. **57A:**677, 1975.

68. Fahey, J. J., and O'Brien, E. T.: Fracture-separation of the medial humeral condyle in a child confused with fracture of the medial epicondyle. J. Bone Joint Surg. **53A:**1102, 1971.

69. Finnbogason, T., Karlsson, G., Lindberg, L., and Mortensson, W.: Nondisplaced and minimally displaced fractures of the lateral humeral condyle in children: a prospective radiographic investigation of fracture stability. J. Pediatr. Orthop. **15:**422, 1995.

70. Flynn, J. C., and Richards, J. F.: Nonunion of minimally displaced fractures of the lateral condyle of the humerus in children. J. Bone Joint Surg. **53A:**1096, 1971.

71. Fowles, J. V., and Kassab, M. T.: Displaced fractures of the medial humeral condyle in children. J. Bone Joint Surg. **62A:**1159, 1980.

72. Gaur, S., Varma, A. N., and Swarup, A.: A new surgical technique for old ununited lateral condyle fractures of the humerus in children. J. Trauma **34:**68, 1993.

73. Gaur, S. C., Vishwakarma, D. P., and Varma, B.: An unusual injury of the lower humeral epiphysis in a child: a case report. Injury **16:**625, 1985.

74. Hardacre, J. A., Nahigian, S. H., Froimson, A. I., and Brown, J. E.: Fractures of the lateral condyle of the humerus in children. J. Bone Joint Surg. **53A:**1083, 1971.

75. Hennrikus, W. L., and Millis, M. B.: The dinner fork technique for treating displaced lateral condylar fractures of the humerus in children. Orthop. Rev. **22:**1278, 1993.

76. Holst-Nielsen, F., and Ottsen, P.: Fractures of the lateral condyle of the humerus in children. Acta Orthop. Scand. **45:**518, 1974.

77. Holmes, J. C., and Hall, J. E.: Tardy ulnar nerve palsy in children. Clin. Orthop. **135:**128, 1978.

78. Ingersol, R. E.: Fractures of the humeral condyles in children. Clin. Orthop. **41:**32, 1965.

79. Inoue, G., and Tamura, Y.: Osteosynthesis for long-standing nonunion of the lateral humeral condyle. Arch Orthop. Trauma Surg. **112:**236, 1993.

80. Jakob, R., Fowels, J. V., and Rang, M.: Observations concerning fractures of the lateral humeral condyle in children. J. Bone Joint Surg. **57B:**430, 1975.

81. Jeffrey, C. C.: Nonunion of the epiphysis of the lateral condyle of the humerus. J. Bone Joint Surg. **40B:**396, 1958.

82. Jones, K. G.: Percutaneous pin fixation of fractures of the lower end of the humerus. Clin. Orthop. **50:**53, 1967.

83. Kilfoyle, R. M.: Fractures of the medial condyle and epicondyle of the elbow in children. Clin. Orthop. **41:**43, 1963.

84. Kini, M. G.: Fractures of the lateral condyle of the lower end of the humerus with complications. J. Bone Joint Surg. **24:**270, 1924.

85. Kreusch-Brinker, R., Noack, W.: Injuries of the distal epiphysis of the humerus in the period of growth (in German). Unfallchirurgie **12:**60, 1986.

86. Kropfl, A., Genelin, F., Obrist, J., and Zirknitzer, J.: Malunion and growth disorders following fractures of the condylar radialis humeri in children (in German). Unfallchirurgie 15:113, 1989.
87. Makela, E. A., Bostman, O., Kekomaki, M., Sodergard, J., Vainio, J., Tormala, P., and Rokkanen, P.: Biodegradable fixation of distal humeral physeal fractures. Clin. Orthop. 283:237, 1943.
88. Masada, K., Kawai, H., Kawabata, H., Masatomi, T., Tsuyuguchi, Y., and Yamamoto, K.: Osteosynthesis of old, established nonunion of the lateral condylar of the humerus. J. Bone Joint Surg. 72A:32, 1990.
89. Micheli, L. J., Santori, R., and Stanitski, C. L.: Epiphyseal fractures of the elbow in children. Am. Fam. Physician 22:107, 1980.
90. Minami, A., and Sugawara, M.: Humeral trochlear hypoplasia secondary to epiphyseal injury as a cause of ulnar nerve palsy. Clin. Orthop. 228:227, 1988.
91. Mintzer, C. M., Waters, P. M., Brown, D. J., and Kasser, J. R.: Percutaneous pinning in the treatment of displaced lateral condyle fractures. J. Pediatr. Orthop. 14:462, 1994.
92. Mirsky, E. C., Karas, E. H., and Weiner, L. S.: Lateral condyle fractures in children: evaluation of classification and treatment. J. Orthop. Trauma 11:117, 1997.
93. Modrzcwski, K.: Late ulnar nerve paresis in adults after neglected treatment for fracture of the capitellum with part of the trochlea in children (in Polish). Chir. Narzadow Ruchn Orthop. Pol. 60:9, 1995.
94. Morrissy, R. T., and Wilkins, K. E.: Deformity following distal humeral fracture in childhood. J. Bone Joint Surg. 66A:557, 1984.
95. Perio, A., Mut, T., Aracil, J., and Martos, F.: Fracture-separation of the lower humeral epiphysis in young children. Acta Orthop. Scand. 52:295, 1981.
96. Roye, D. P., Jr., Bini, S. A., and Infosino, A.: Late surgical treatment of lateral condylar fractures in children. J. Pediatr. Orthop. 11:195, 1991.
97. Sharma, J. C., Arora, A., Mathur, N. C., Gupta, S. P., Biyani, A., and Mathur, R.: Lateral condylar fractures of the humerus in children: fixation with partially threaded 4.0 mm AO cancellous screws. J. Trauma 39:1129, 1995.
98. Shimada, K., Masada, K., Tada, K., and Yamamoto, T.: Osteosynthesis for the treatment of nonunion of the lateral condyle in children. J. Bone Joint Surg. 79A:234, 1997.
99. Stricker, S. J., Thomson, J. D., and Kelly, R. A.: Coronal-plane transcondylar fracture of the humerus in a child. Clin. Orthop. 294:308, 1993.
100. Smith, F. J., and Joyce, J. J., III.: Fractures of the lateral condyle of the humerus in children. Am. J. Surg. 87:324, 1954.
101. So, Y. C., Fang, D., Leong, J. C. Y., and Bong, S. C.: Varus deformity following lateral humeral condylar fractures in children. J. Pediatr. Orthop. 5:569, 1985.
102. Valdisseri, L., Venturi, B., and Busanelli, L.: External humeral condyle fracture in children. A long-term review of 30 cases reported. Chir. Organi. Mov. 78:105, 1993.
103. van Haaren, E. R., van Vugt, A. B., and Bode, P. J.: Posterolateral dislocation of the elbow with concomitant fracture of the lateral humeral condyle: case report. J. Trauma 36:288, 1994.
104. van Vugt, A. B., Severijnen, R. V. S. M., and Festen, C.: Fractures of the lateral humeral condyle in children: late results. Arch. Orthop. Trauma Surg. 107:206, 1988.
105. Vathana, P., and Prosartritha, T.: Repair of nonunion lateral humeral condyle: a case report. J. Med. Assoc. Thai. 81:146, 1998.
106. von Laer, L., Brunner, R., and Lampert, C.: Malunited supracondylar and condylar humeral fractures (in German). Orthopade 20:331, 1991.
107. Wadsworth, T. G.: Premature epiphyseal fusion after injury to the capitellum. J. Bone Joint Surg. 46B:46, 1964.
108. Wadsworth, T. G.: Injuries of the capitellar (lateral humeral condyle) epiphysis. Clin. Orthop. 85:127, 1972.
109. Wilkins, K. E.: Residuals of elbow trauma in children. Clin. Orthop. 21:291, 1990.

Ages 10 to Maturity

110. Ghawabi, M. H.: Fracture of the medial condyle of the humerus. J. Bone Joint Surg. 57A:677, 1975.
111. Godette, G. A., and Gruel, C. R.: Percutaneous screw fixation of intercondylar fracture of the distal humerus. Orthop. Rev. 22:466, 1993.
112. Kasser, J. R., Richards, K., and Millis, M.: The triceps-dividing approach to open reduction of complex distal humeral fractures in adolescents: a Cybex evaluation of triceps function and motion. J. Pediatr. Orthop. 10:93, 1990.
113. Papavasiliou, V. A., and Beslikas, T. A.: T-Condylar fractures of the distal humeral condyles during childhood: an analysis of six cases. J. Pediatr. Orthop. 6:302, 1986.
114. Peterson, H. A.: Triplane fracture of the distal humeral epiphysis. J. Pediatr. Orthop. 3:81, 1983.
115. Royle, S. G., and Burke, D.: Ulnar neuropathy after elbow injury in children. J. Pediatr. Orthop. 10:495, 1990.
116. Saraf, S. K., and Tuli, S. M.: Concomitant medial condyle fracture of the humerus in a childhood posterolateral dislocation of the elbow. J. Orthop. Trauma 3:352, 1989.

Medial Epicondyle

117. Carlioz, H., and Abols, Y.: Posterior dislocation of the elbow in children. J. Pediatr. Orthop. 4:8, 1981.
118. Case, S. L., and Hennrikus, W. L.: Surgical treatment of displaced medial epicondyle fracture in adolescent athletes. Am. J. Sports Med. 25:682, 1997.
119. Chessare, J. W., Rogers, L. F., White, H., and Tachdjian, M. O.: Injuries of the medial epicondylar ossification center of the humerus. Am. J. Roentgenol. 129:49, 1977.
120. Collins, R., and Lavine, S. A.: Fractures of the medial epicondyle of the humerus with ulnar nerve paralysis. Proc. Child. Hosp. D. C. 20:274, 1964.
121. Dunn, P. S., Ravn, P., Hansen, L. B., Burph, B.: Osteosynthesis of medial humeral epicondyle fractures in children. 8-Year follow-up of 33 cases. Acta Orthop. Scand. 65:439, 1994.
122. Fowles, J. V., Slimane, N., and Kassab, M. T.: Elbow dislocation with avulsion of the medial humeral epicondyle. J. Bone Joint Surg. 72B:102, 1990.
123. Hendel, D., Aghasi, M., and Halperin, N.: Unusual fracture dislocation of the elbow joint. Arch. Orthop. Trauma Surg. 104:187, 1985.
124. Josefsson, P. O., and Danielson, L. G.: Epicondylar elbow fracture in children. 35-Year follow-up of 56 unreduced cases. Acta Orthop. Scand. 57:313, 1986.
125. Low, B. Y., and Lim, J.: Fracture of humerus during arm wrestling: report of 5 cases. Singapore Med. J. 32:47, 1991.
126. Ogawa, K., and Ui, M.: Fracture-separation of the medial humeral epicondyle caused by arm wrestling. J. Trauma 41:494, 1996.
127. Partio, E. K., Hirvensalo, E., Bostman, O., and Rokkanen, P.: A prospective controlled trial of the fracture of the humeral medial epicondyle—how to treat? Ann. Chir. Gynaecol. 85:67, 1996.
128. Pritchett, J. W.: Entrapment of the medial nerve after dislocation of the elbow: case report. J. Pediatr. Orthop. 4:752, 1984.
129. Skak, S. V., Grossman, E., Wagn, P.: Deformity after internal fixation of fracture separation of the medial epicondyle of the humerus. J. Bone Joint Surg. 76B:272, 1994.
130. Sugita, H., Kotani, H., Ueo, T., Miki, T., Senzoku, F., Hara, T., Nakagawa, Y., Sakka, A., Nakagawa, T., and Seki, K.: Recurrent dislocation of the elbow (in Japanese). Nippon Geka Hokan. 63:181, 1994.
131. Szymanska, E.: Evaluation of AO kit screw fixation of medial condyle and epicondyle distal humeral epiphyseal fractures in children (in Polish). Ann Acad. Med. Stetin. 43:239, 1997.
132. Woods, G. W., and Tullos, H. S.: Elbow instability and medial epicondylar fractures. Am. J. Sports 5:23, 1977.

Lateral Epicondyle

133. Li, Y. H., and Leong, J. C.: Fractured lateral epicondyle associated with lateral elbow instability. Injury 26:267, 1995.

Proximal Radius

134. Gaston, S. R., Smith, F. M., and Baab, O. D.: Epiphyseal injuries of the radial head and neck. Am. J. Surg. 85:266, 1953.
135. Jeffery, C. C.: Fractures of the head of the radius in children. J. Bone Joint Surg. 32B:314, 1950.

136. Leung, A. G., and Peterson, H. A.: Fractures of the proximal radial head and neck, with emphasis on those that involve the articular cartilage. J. Pediatr. Orthop (in press).
137. McBride, E. E., and Monnet, J. C.: Epiphyseal fractures of the head of the radius in children. Clin. Orthop. **16:**264, 1960.
138. O'Brien, P. I.: Fractures involving the proximal radial epiphysis. Clin. Orthop. **41:**51, 1965.
139. Payne, J. F., and Earle, J. L.: Fracture dislocation of the proximal radial epiphysis. Minn. Med. **52:**479, 1969.
140. Reidy, J. A., and Van Gorder, G. W.: Treatment of displacement of proximal radial epiphysis. J. Bone Joint Surg. **45A:**1355, 1963.
141. Sessa, S., Lascombes, P., Prevot, J., and Gagneux, E.: Fractures of the radial head and associated elbow injuries in children. J. Pediatr. Orthop. **5:**200, 1996.

Proximal Ulna

142. Burrel, C. G., Strecker, W. B., and Schoenecker, P. L.: Surgical treatment of displaced olecranon fractures in children. J. Pediatr. Orthop. **17:**321, 1997.
143. Bracq, H.: Fracture of the coronoid apophysis. Rev. Chir. Orthop. **73:**472, 1987.
144. Parson, F. G.: Observations on traction epiphyses. J. Anat. Physiol. **38:**248, 1904.
145. Retrum, R. K., Wepfer, J. F., Olsen, D. W., and Laney, W. H.: Case report 355: delayed closure of the right olecranon epiphysis in a right-handed, tournament-class tennis player (post-traumatic). Skeletal Radiol. **15:**185, 1986.

CHAPTER 18

Fractures of the Neck of the Radius in Children

• ANTHONY A. STANS and JOHN H. WEDGE

Fractures of the neck and head of the radius in children are relatively rare, constituting 4 to 7 percent of elbow fractures and dislocations.[2, 6, 14, 16, 21, 23] A review of the early literature reveals considerable controversy on the significance, treatment, and late results of this injury.[12, 22, 23]

Sex frequency varies from series to series, but overall, there seems to be a slight female preponderance. The age range is 4 to 14 years, the mean age between 10 and 12 years. Some 30 to 50 percent of patients have associated injuries to the elbow region (Figs. 18–1 to 18–3).[10, 18, 30, 35]

The prognosis after this fracture seems to depend more on the severity of the injury, the associated injuries about the elbow, and the type of treatment than on the accuracy of the reduction.[10, 16, 22, 24] Although emphasis has been placed on the angulation of the radial head, it is actually the displacement of the fracture that is the more important component of the deformity.

The classic discussion on this subject is that of Jeffery,[10] whose observations in 1950 clarified the nature of the fracture, the mechanism of injury, the radiologic assessment, the method of reduction, and the prognosis. Complete remodeling of a fracture was demonstrated with perfect function after a residual angulation of 50 degrees.

Closed reduction seems to produce better results than open reduction, even taking into account that more severe injuries are more likely to require operation.[22, 24] Recently, significant technical advances have been made achieving percutaneous reduction of severely displaced or angulated fractures[1, 8, 20, 29, 32]; however, the functional result, regardless of the treatment, is generally good.[35]

MECHANISM OF THE FRACTURE

A fall on the outstretched arm produces a valgus thrust on the elbow that fractures the radial neck and often avulses structures on the medial side of the joint. The radial head tilts laterally because the forearm is usually supinated, but the exact direction of the tilt depends on the rotational position of the forearm at impact. This is the most common mechanism, but the fracture can also occur with posterior dislocation of the elbow, resulting in two types of displacement, depending on whether the radial head fractures during spontaneous reduction or in the course of "dislocating." The first type of fracture[10, 11] (reduction injury) leaves the separated proximal radial epiphysis tilted 90 degrees posteriorly beneath the capitellum of the humerus (Figs.

18–4 and 18–5). This mechanism of injury was recently confirmed in a report of an iatrogenic radial neck fracture that occurred during closed reduction of a posterior elbow dislocation.[33] With the second type of fracture[22] (dislocation injury), axial compression on the elbow results in anterior displacement of the radial head as the proximal radial epiphysis moving posteriorly is obstructed by the capitellum and fractures in the process (see Fig. 18–3). Less common injuries include anterior dislocation of the head of the radius with associated fracture of the radial neck; shear fracture through the neck of the radius with medial displacement of the shaft, which may become locked medial to the coronoid process of the ulna[17]; and osteochondral fracture of the epiphysis with an intra-articular loose body.

Associated injuries thus include fracture of the olecranon, avulsion of the medial epicondyle of the humerus, dislocation of the elbow, and avulsion of the medial collateral ligament from the distal humerus.[10] As many as 50 percent of these fractures have one of these injuries, which not only are important in themselves but also have implications for prognosis and treatment (see Figs. 18–1 to 18–3).[16, 35]

CLASSIFICATION

The fracture may be classified by the degree of angulation of the radial head,[23, 25] the mechanism of injury,[10] the type of epiphyseal plate disruption,[25, 27] the amount of fracture displacement, or combinations of these.[22] O'Brien[23] divided these fractures into three groups according to the degree of angulation:

Type I: less than 30 degrees
Type II: 30 to 60 degrees
Type III: More than 60 degrees

He also described an impaction fracture of the articular surface of the head, an injury that is more likely to be associated with lesser degrees of angulation.

It is important to recognize that the neck of the radius normally subtends an angle of 165 to 170 degrees with the shaft (see Chapter 3). The radius is not a straight bone, even in its proximal third.[16, 31] Thus, a measured angulation of 50 degrees may in reality represent only 35 to 40 degrees of true angulation. As in many pediatric injuries, comparison with the uninjured elbow is often helpful, or even essential, for accurate assessment of this feature.

The injury also may be classified according to the type of epiphyseal plate injury. Although some authors believe that the fracture may occur entirely through the metaphysis of the neck of the radius,[12, 34] this is unusual, both in the literature[22] and in our experience.[35]

The pattern of proximal radial physeal injuries, as traditionally classified by Salter and Harris, includes the following types:

Type I: Rare and usually associated with dislocation of the radial head or elbow
Type II: The most common pattern of fracture through the neck of the radius
Type III: Rare

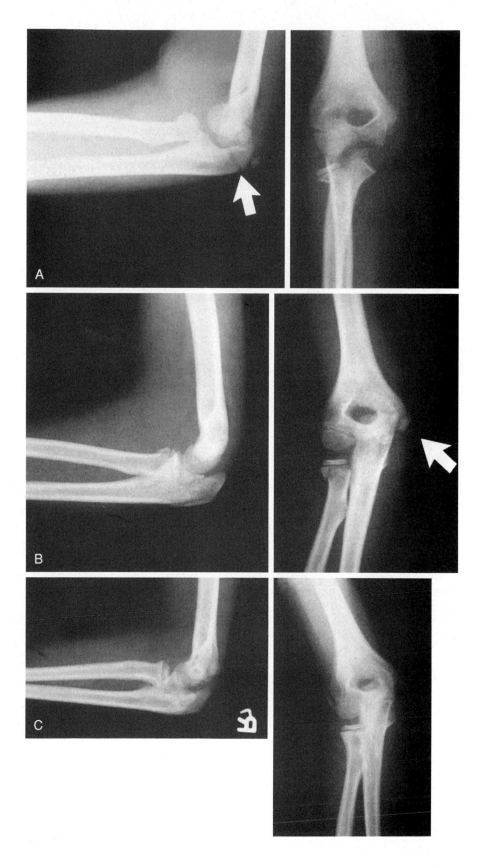

FIGURE 18–1 • *A*, A displaced and angulated fracture of the neck of the radius and fracture of the olecranon *(arrow)* in an 8-year-old girl. *B*, Three weeks after closed reduction and immobilization it is apparent that the capsular attachment has avulsed a portion of the medial epicondyle *(arrow)*. *C*, Three years later, the patient had perfect function and no pain.

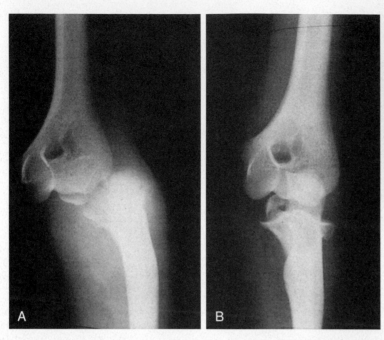

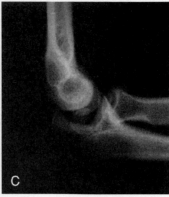

FIGURE 18–2 • *A* and *B*, A 12-year-old girl sustained a dislocation of the elbow, avulsion of the medial epicondyle, and fracture of the neck of the radius. *C*, After closed reduction, the medial epicondyle became trapped in the joint. This injury required open reduction.

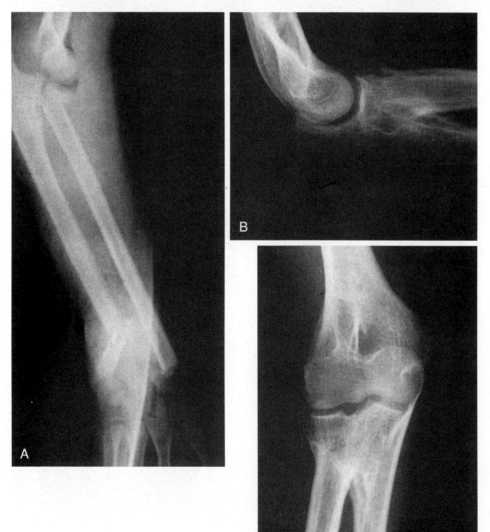

FIGURE 18–3 • *A*, An open dislocation of the elbow, fracture of the neck of the radius, and badly displaced fractures of the distal radius and ulna in a 10-year-old girl. Definitive treatment was not rendered until 8 days after the injury. Two years later (*B* and *C*), there was synostosis of the radius and ulna and enlargement and irregularity of the head of the radius.

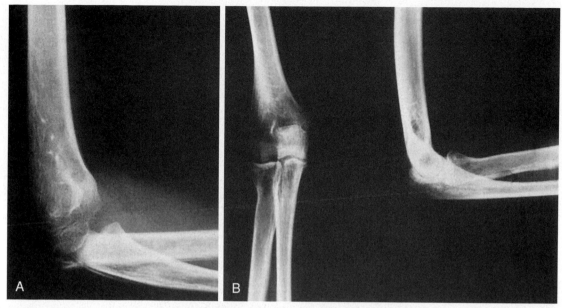

FIGURE 18–4 • *A*, Radiograph of the elbow of an 8-year-old girl who had fallen 6 weeks earlier. The radial head is tilted 90 degrees posteriorly and is not articulating with the joint surface of the capitellum. The presumed mechanism of this fracture pattern is a direct blow to a posteriorly dislocated elbow that reduces the dislocation but leaves the radial head displaced. *B*, In the same patient 22 years after open reduction, note the enlargement and irregularity of the radial head. She had a full range of motion and no pain. This is the only exception in our experience to the rule that stiffness usually follows late open reduction.

Type IV: Second in frequency (five in our series)[35] and associated with a poorer prognosis owing to marked displacement, irregularity of the radial head, and radioulnar synostosis (Figs. 18–6 and 18–7)

Type V: Seen in association with type II injuries. The crushing of the plate cannot be detected initially but is manifested by premature fusion of the physeal plate.

We prefer the classification of Wilkins,[26] which combines those of Jeffery[10] and Newman.[22] It is based primarily on the mechanism of injury, but it also describes the deformity to be corrected and suggests the severity of the injury and thus helps in formulating the prognosis.

I. Valgus fractures
  A. Type A: Salter-Harris type I and II injuries of the proximal physis
  B. Type B: Salter-Harris type III and IV injuries of the proximal radial physis
  C. Type C: Fractures involving only the proximal radial metaphysis
II. Fractures associated with dislocation of the elbow
  A. Type D: Reduction injuries
  B. Type E: Dislocation injuries

We have added Salter-Harris type III fractures to the type B classification. These may produce an intra-articular loose body consisting of articular cartilage and a portion of the epiphysis.

TREATMENT

Assessment of Injury

The entire extremity should be thoroughly examined for open wounds, other injuries, and neurovascular impair-ment. A fall on the outstretched hand can result in injury at multiple levels. As in adults, injury about the wrist must be specifically excluded, and fracture of the scaphoid has been reported (see Fig. 18–3).[10, 11]

Anteroposterior and lateral radiographs of both the elbow and the entire forearm should be examined for other injuries, particularly about the elbow. An estimate should also be made of the degree of angulation of the radial head and the amount of displacement.

The degree of angulation can be accurately determined only by an anteroposterior radiograph with the forearm in the position of rotation at the moment of impact. Jeffery[10] demonstrated that this is best achieved by taking radiographs in varying degrees of forearm rotation so that the radial head will cast shadows of different shapes. When the radial head forms as nearly perfect a rectangle as possible, the real degree of angulation can be determined. Oval shapes indicate that the radiographs have not been taken at a right angle to the plane of maximal angulation (Fig. 18–8). Comparison views of the uninjured forearm in the same degree of rotation are helpful in assessing the degree of angulation. Also, in children, normal variations in the radiographic appearance of the proximal radius must be considered when assessing injury.[28] Again, it is a basic principle of treating elbow fractures in children that radiographs of the injury must be compared with films of the opposite (uninjured) side.

Indications for Reduction

It is generally agreed that a fracture with angulation of more than 60 degrees or more than 3 mm of displacement will likely produce problems if it is not corrected.[2, 6, 22, 23, 35] It is also agreed (except in some of the older literature) that in fractured elbows, less than 30 degrees' angulation can safely be accepted.[10, 24, 31] There is also some support for

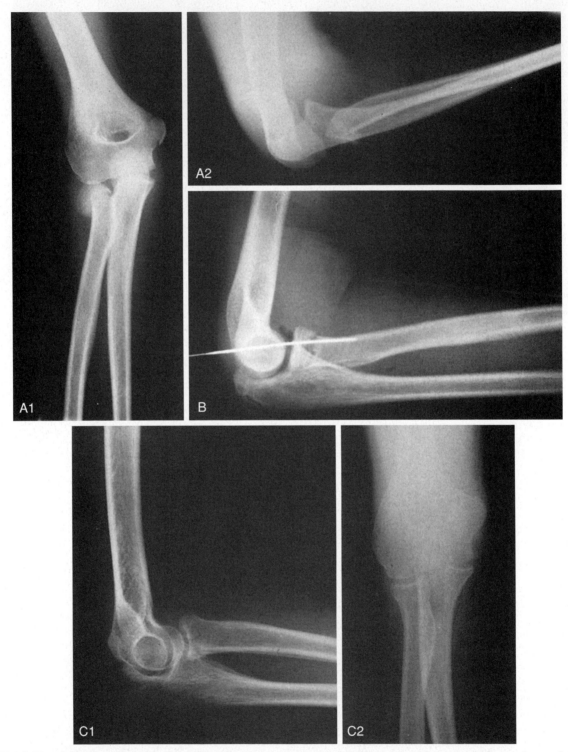

FIGURE 18–5 • *A,* Fracture of the neck of the radius in a 13-year-old girl with dislocation of the elbow and marked posterior angulation was treated *(B)* by open reduction and internal fixation with a wire passed through the capitellum into the radius. The high rate of complications associated with this method of fixation makes it an undesirable method of treatment. *C,* Three years later, there is deformity of the head of the radius, subluxation, and marked restriction of forearm rotation.

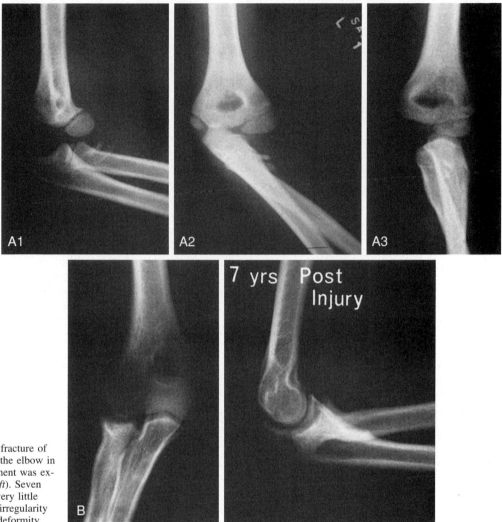

FIGURE 18–6 • *A*, A type IV fracture of the radial head and a dislocation of the elbow in an 8-year-old boy. *B*, The free fragment was excised, along with the radial head (*left*). Seven years later (*right*), that patient had very little forearm rotation, limited extension, irregularity of the articular surface, and valgus deformity.

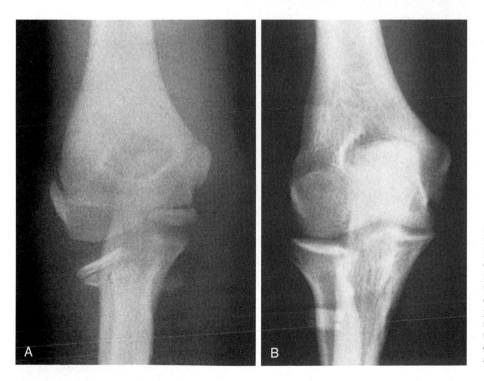

FIGURE 18–7 • *A*, A comminuted fracture of the head of the radius in a 13-year-old boy. Note the free fragment, which consisted of epiphysis, growth plate, and metaphysis, on the medial aspect of the ulna. The radial neck fracture was reduced open and the fragment was excised. *B*, Four years later the patient had full flexion, extension, and pronation, but no supination. Note the defect on the medial aspect of the head of the radius. The elbow was only occasionally painful.

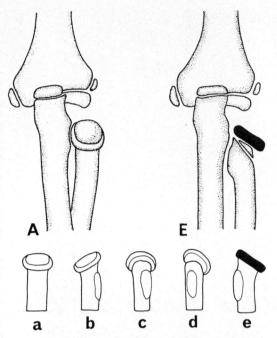

FIGURE 18–8 • Diagram of the radiographic appearance of the head of the radius in varying degrees of rotation, where A = a and E = e. When the film is taken at right angles to the plane of maximum angulation, the radial head is rectangular in shape as in Ee *(shaded epiphysis)*.

the position that fractures of no more than 45 degrees' angulation do not require open reduction.[2, 22, 23, 30, 35] The proper treatment approach is controversial when angulation is between 45 and 60 degrees. There is support both for and against open reduction of these fractures.[6, 18, 24, 25, 30, 35] Advocates of open reduction believe that, without it, significant loss of forearm rotation will ensue. Those who prefer closed reduction or acceptance of deformity believe that the complications of open reduction do not justify the risks, considering the minimal disability that is the legacy of fractures left with 50 to 55 degrees of angulation.

Recently, two other techniques have been reported to provide the benefits of better fracture reduction without the complications associated with open reduction. In several series, percutaneous reduction of radial neck fractures has been associated with fewer complications and less elbow stiffness as compared with open reduction (Fig 18–9).[1, 20, 29] Metaizeau has described a second method of reducing and stabilizing displaced or angulated radial neck fractures using an intramedullary K-wire.[20] Results of this closed technique are better than those from similar series of open reduction.[8, 20]

In our experience, angulation of less than 60 degrees may be accepted, as neither late pain nor significant loss of function is likely. Displacement, rather than angulation, leads to loss of forearm rotation. Angulation produces a defect at the joint surface and, therefore, does not obstruct rotation. Incomplete contact between articular surfaces is, theoretically, harmful, but enough remodeling usually occurs so that the incomplete contact appears to improve. Displacement, on the other hand, results in radial neck deformity and abutment on the edges of the radial notch (Fig. 18–10). This produces a cam effect during rotation,

an effect we have confirmed in cadaver studies: The radial neck was divided with a saw and fixed with Kirschner wires without angulation but with varying degrees of displacement. The observed effect on forearm rotation was that displacement greater than 3 mm resulted in loss of forearm rotation because of abutment of the radial head against the ulna.

Because closed or open reduction performed more than 5 to 7 days after injury leads to loss of forearm rotation and radioulnar synostosis,[18, 22, 30, 35] a fracture more than 1 week old is a relative contraindication to reduction. It is better to accept deformity.

Principles of Treatment

Review of the literature indicates that, regardless of the severity of the injury, closed treatment gives better results than open treatment. Fractures that require internal fixation also tend to have poorer results than do those treated by open reduction without internal fixation. Thus, as little internal fixation as possible is recommended.[2, 35] Transcapitellar fixation with a Kirschner wire passed through the capitellum of the humerus and across the joint into the head and medullary canal of the radius is associated with significant complications—among others, possible infection of the joint and breakage of the wire in the joint (leading to damage of the articular surface and making removal very difficult; see Fig. 18–6).[7, 19] Immobilization of the elbow for more than 3 to 4 weeks leads to stiffness, even in children.

Thus, the following principles apply to treating radial neck fractures:

1. Closed treatment generally gives better results than open reduction.
2. If open reduction is necessary, use as little internal fixation as possible.
3. Treat promptly.
4. Do not use transcapitellar wires.
5. Do not immobilize the fracture longer than 3 weeks.

RESULTS

When assessing the published results of fractures of the neck of the radius, it is apparent that any pain that might ensue from this injury is seldom disabling.[9, 21, 30, 35] Unsatisfactory results consistently are based on the degree of restriction of forearm motion.[6, 7, 10, 22, 25] It may be that permanent stiffness develops, not only because of a mechanical block to rotation but also, possibly, because of reflex inhibition to avoid a painful arc of motion. Even when irregularity of the joint surface results in stiffness, there is usually surprisingly little pain. On the other hand, a "successful" open reduction with a perfect anatomic result also may be associated with significant loss of forearm rotation. Our series of patients followed as long as 22 years confirms this impression: pain was not a prominent feature and was not the reason for poor results.[35]

Loss of 20 degrees of supination or as much as 40 degrees of pronation is not disabling, particularly when it occurs at a young age. "Fair" and "poor" results occur

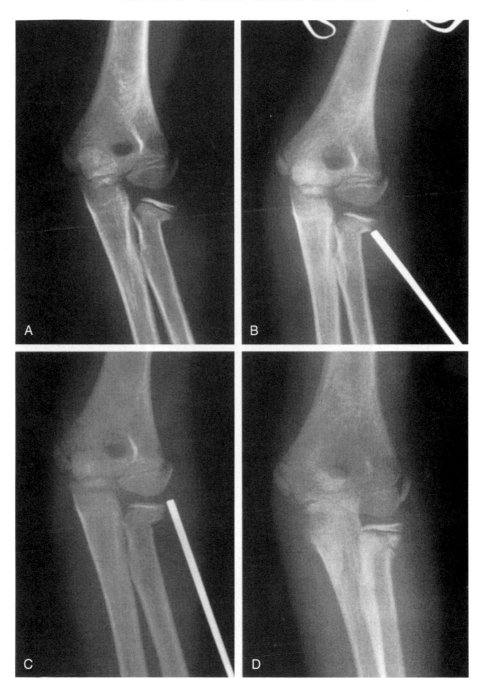

FIGURE 18–9 • *A*, Fracture of the radial neck angulated approximately 45 degrees. *B*, A Steinmann pin is inserted percutaneously. *C*, Using fluoroscopic guidance, the Steinmann pin is used to reduce the fracture. *D*, Normal anatomy is restored without open reduction, and the fracture is stable without internal fixation. (From Green N. E., Swiontkowski M. F.: Skeletal Trauma in Children, 2nd ed. Philadelphia, W. B. Saunders, 1998.)

when loss of forearm rotation is greater than 40 degrees. In contrast to the legacy of adults' radial neck fractures, loss of elbow flexion and extension is less common in children and not as disabling as loss of rotation. When a limitation develops, it is usually extension that is lost—and then seldom more than 30 to 35 degrees.

Avascular necrosis of the radial head, radioulnar synostosis,[1, 18, 22, 35] and removal of the radial head are associated with poor results.[1, 22, 35] The incidences of radioulnar synostosis and avascular necrosis of a substantial portion of the head of the radius are difficult to determine because of the small series of fractures of the neck of the radius in children. The problem is further complicated by the fact that these complications are associated with widely displaced fractures, those treated overenthusiastically, those treated

late, and those concomitant with dislocations of the elbow. These injuries, in turn, make up a smaller part of the total number of fractures. It is enough to say that, in almost every reported series, these complications are mentioned. In our experience, avascular necrosis and synostosis complicate 5 to 10 percent of fractures, are frequently intercurrent, and usually follow open reduction and fixation.

The unanticipated good result subsequent to acceptance of considerable deformity is related to remodeling of the deformity.[4, 9, 10, 18] This is surprising, because the plane of the fracture lies at right angles to the plane of motion of both the elbow and the radioulnar joints. This would seem to be an exception to the rule that remodeling in the child can be expected only if the fracture deformity is in the same plane of motion as the nearby joint. This remodeling

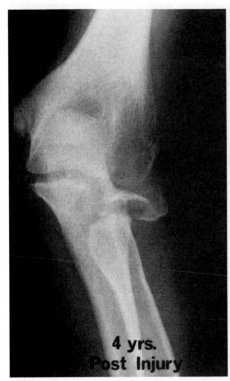
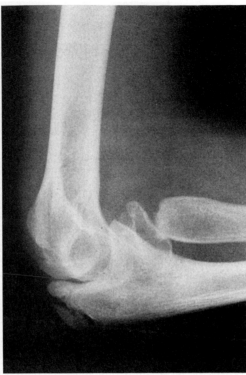

4 yrs.
Post Injury

FIGURE 18–14 • Nonunion of the neck of the radius 4 years after open reduction and fixation with a transcapitellar wire in a 12-year-old boy.

distal to the bicipital tuberosity of the radius. The elbow joint is entered anterior to the anconeus muscle. Do not interfere with the orbicular ligament even if torn, or stiffness may result. The radial head is "levered" into its proper position. It is usually sufficiently stable to make internal fixation unnecessary. If the radial head is unstable, the child's bone is often soft enough to allow use of a heavy absorbable suture on a stout cutting needle to hold it in place, introducing the needle at the articular margin of the radial head and passing it across the fracture into the neck of the radius and through the cortex. If this does not seem feasible, one or two fine, smooth Kirschner wires are inserted at the articular margin of the radial head, across the fracture, and just through the cortex of the radial neck. They should be cut off just deep to the skin to facilitate removal in 3 weeks.

A growing child's radial head must never be excised. Excision results in pain, increased carrying angle, radioulnar synostosis, or distal radioulnar dysfunction (see Figs. 18–7 and 18–13).[2, 3, 15] If stable reduction cannot be achieved, less than optimal reduction is acceptable and the radial head is excised later, at skeletal maturity. Delayed resection is not usually necessary.

The rare Salter-Harris type IV injury produces a dilemma. Often, the displaced fragment is too small to be fixed. In such cases, it may be excised. The result may not be very good, but the loss of motion after this fracture may be due to other factors, because the injury is usually produced by considerable forces (see Figs. 18–7 and 18–8).

Immobilization following open reduction is as described for closed treatment and should be continued for no more than 3 to 4 weeks. If Kirschner wires have been used, they should be removed at this time. Rehabilitation and follow-up are exactly as described for closed treatment.

SUMMARY

Fracture of the neck of the radius is a rare but serious injury, particularly when it is associated with marked angulation and displacement or with concomitant injuries to the elbow region. Every possible attempt should be made to treat this injury closed. Even though more serious fractures are treated by open reduction, clinical reports and personal experience suggest that surgical intervention has an adverse effect on the outcome. *Percutaneous* reduction techniques may permit reduction of more serious fractures without open surgical exposure. When open reduction is necessary, dissection and internal fixation should be kept to a minimum. Treatment 1 week after the injury leads to stiffness, as does external immobilization for longer than 4 weeks.

REFERENCES

1. Bernstein, S. M., McKeever, P., and Bernstein, L.: Percutaneous reduction of displaced radial neck fractures in children. J. Pediatr. Orthop. **13**:85–88, 1993.
2. Blount, W. P.: Fractures in Children. Baltimore, Williams & Wilkins, 1955, p. 56.
3. Bohrer, J. V.: Fractures of the head and neck of the radius. Ann. Surg. **97**:204, 1933.
4. Conn, J., and Wade, P. A.: Injuries of the elbow. A ten year review. J. Trauma **1**:248, 1961.
5. Dormans, J. P., and Rang, M.: Fractures of the olecranon and radial neck in children. Orthop. Clin. North Am. **21**:257, 1990.
6. Dougall, A. J.: Severe fracture of the neck of the radius in children. J. R. Coll. Surg. Edinb. **14**:220, 1969.
7. Fowles, J. V., and Kassab, M. T.: Observations concerning radial neck fractures in children. J. Pediatr. Orthop. **6**:51, 1986.
8. González-Herranz, P., Alvarez-Romera, A., Burgos, J., Rapariz, J. M., and Hevia, E.: Displaced radial neck fractures in children treated by closed intramedullary pinning (Metaizeau technique). J. Pediatr. Orthop. **17**:325–331, 1997.

9. Henriksen, B.: Isolated fractures of the proximal end of the radius in children. Epidemiology, treatment and prognosis. Acta Orthop. Scand. **40**:246, 1969.

10. Jeffery, C. C.: Fractures of the radius in children. J. Bone Joint Surg. **32B**:314, 1950.

11. Jeffery, C. C.: Fractures of the neck of the radius in children. Mechanism of causation. J. Bone Joint Surg. **54B**:717, 1972.

12. Jones, E. R. L., and Esch, M.: Displaced fractures of the neck of the radius in children. J. Bone Joint Surg. **53B**:429, 1971.

13. Kaufman, B., Rinott, M. G., and Tangman, M.: Closed reduction of fractures of the proximal radius in children. J. Bone Joint Surg. **71B**:66, 1989.

14. Landin, L. A., and Danielsson, L. G.: Elbow fractures in children. An epidemiological analysis of 589 cases. Acta Orthop. Scand. **57**:309–312, 1986.

15. Lewis, R. W., and Thibodeau, A. A.: Deformity of the wrist following resection of the radial head. Surg. Gynecol. Obstet. **64**:1079, 1937.

16. Lindham, S., and Hugosson, C.: The significance of associated lesions including dislocation in fractures of the neck of the radius in children. Acta Orthop. Scand. **50**:79, 1979.

17. Manoli, A.: Medial displacement of the shaft of the radius with a fracture of the radial neck. Report of a case. J. Bone Joint Surg. **61A**:788, 1979.

18. McBride, E. D., and Monnet, J. C.: Epiphyseal fractures of the head of the radius in children. Clin. Orthop. **16**:264, 1960.

19. Merchan, E. C. R.: Displaced fractures of the head and neck of the radius in children: open reduction and temporary transarticular internal fixation. Orthopedics **14**:697, 1991.

20. Metaizeau, J.-P., Lascombes, P., Lemelle, J.-L., Finlayson, D., and Prevot, J.: Reduction and fixation of displaced radial neck fractures by closed intramedullary pinning. J. Pediatr. Orthop. **13**:355–360, 1993.

21. Murray, R. C.: Fractures of the head and neck of the radius. Br. J. Surg. **9**:114, 1977.

22. Newman, J. H.: Displaced radial neck fractures in children. Injury **9**:114, 1977.

23. O'Brien, P. I.: Injuries involving the proximal radial epiphysis. Clin. Orthop. **41**:51, 1965.

24. Rang, M.: Children's Fractures. Philadelphia, J. B. Lippincott Co., 1974, p. 112.

25. Reidy, J. A., and Van Gorder, G. W.: Treatment of displacement of the proximal radial epiphysis. J. Bone Joint Surg. **45A**:1355, 1963.

26. Rockwood, C. A., Jr., Wilkins, K. E., and King, R. E. (eds.): Fractures in Children. Vol. 3. Philadelphia, J. B. Lippincott Co., 1984, p. 510.

27. Salter, R. B., and Harris, W. R.: Injuries involving the epiphyseal plate. J. Bone Joint Surg. **45A**:587, 1963.

28. Silberstein, M. J., Brodeur, A. E., and Graviss, E. R.: Some vagaries of the radial neck and head. J. Bone Joint Surg. **64A**:1153, 1982.

29. Steele, J. A., and Kerr Graham, H.: Angulated radial neck fractures in children. A prospective study of percutaneous reduction. J. Bone Joint Surg. **74B**:760–764, 1992.

30. Tibone, J. E., and Stoltz, M.: Fractures of the radial head and neck in children. J. Bone Joint Surg. **63A**:100, 1981.

31. Vahvanen, V., and Gripenberg, L.: Fracture of the radial neck in children. A long-term follow-up study of 43 cases. Acta Orthop. Scand. **49**:32, 1978.

32. van Rhijn, L. W., Schuppers, H. A., and van der Eijken, J. W.: Reposition of a radial neck fracture by a percutaneous Kirschner wire. A case report. Acta Orthop. Scand. **66**:177–179, 1995.

33. Ward, W. T., and Williams, J. J.: Radial neck fracture complicating closed reduction of a posterior elbow dislocation in a child: case report. J. Trauma **31**:1686–1688, 1991.

34. Weber, B. G., Brunner, C. H., and Freuler, F.: Treatment of fractures in children and adolescents. Berlin, Springer-Verlag, 1980, p. 172.

35. Wedge, J. H., and Robertson, D. E.: Displaced fractures of the neck of the radius in children. J. Bone Joint Surg. **64B**:256, 1982.

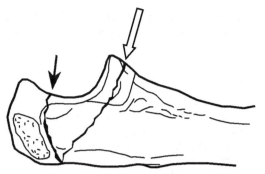

FIGURE 19–2 • Fracture of the apophysis may (*open arrow*) or may not (*closed arrow*) include the coronoid process.

to the precise degree of flexion of the elbow, possibly the rotation of the forearm, and the manner in which the muscles contracted at the time of impact. With fracture of the metaphysis, a varus or valgus force often occurs, causing additional fractures about the elbow. In four large series of proximal ulnar fractures, 20 percent had a documented associated fracture.[12] In some reports, as many as 50 to 70 percent had an additional injury, most commonly involving the radial head with a valgus stress at the time of impact (Fig. 19–3).[9, 11]

Classification

In 1981, Matthews[6] offered a classification based on radiographic appearance, degree of displacement, and associated

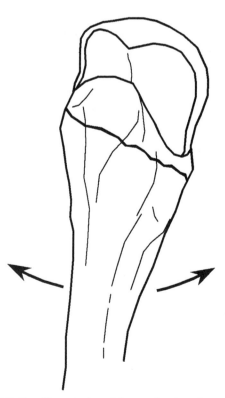

FIGURE 19–3 • The metaphyseal fracture involves the ossified proximal ulna. Varus or valgus angulation patterns assist in documenting the mechanism of injury.

injury (±4 mm being the limit). Wilkins[12] considered these by the mechanism of the fracture: (A) flexion; (B) extension; (1) valgus; (2) varus; and (C) shear injury. More recently, Graves and Canale[4] classified the fracture according to (1) displacement greater or less than 5 mm and (2) presence of compounding. This classification was subsequently modified by Gaddy and coworkers,[2] with a type I fracture being less than 3 mm and a type II greater than 3 mm. Thus, this fracture has the interesting characteristic of having almost as many classifications as episodes of occurrence.

Although metaphyseal fractures are extremely uncommon, as noted, they are more frequent than the physeal injury is, and they account for approximately 5 percent of all elbow injuries. Of these, only 10 to 20 percent require surgical management.

Diagnosis

Since the fracture involves ossified tissue, the metaphyseal fracture is relatively easily identified on the radiograph. Abrasion of the skin or compounding of the fracture gives some idea of the mechanism; that is, direct or indirect trauma, respectively. A further means of determining the extent of displacement and hence the need for open reduction and internal fixation is to observe whether the fracture separates with flexion and extension under fluoroscopy. If an excessive amount of motion is observed at the fracture site (3–5 mm), then open reduction and internal fixation are carried out.

Treatment

As implied from the above classification, the approach to treatment is a matter of displacement. Fortunately, most of these fractures are minimally displaced, leaving the need for open reduction and internal fixation in only 15 to 20 percent of individuals.

Reduction may be accomplished in most instances by reversing the mechanism, which provides some justification for Wilkins' mechanistic classification noted earlier.

For those fractures that are minimally displaced, simple immobilization for 1 to 3 weeks appears to be adequate and is the universal recommendation. For displacement of greater than 3 to 5 mm, depending on the classification, surgical treatment is necessary. It is rare to have greater than 4 mm displacement in patients under the age of 10; thus, open reduction and internal fixation are generally observed in the older age group. Several authors have noted that displacement found intraoperatively is often significantly greater than displacement appreciated on plain radiographs.[2, 4] Typically, the AO technique with smooth K-wire with circumferential tension band wire is adequate (Fig. 19–4). Internal fixation is typically removed 6 to 12 months postoperatively to ensure that premature closure of the proximal ulnar physis does not occur, and to relieve symptoms of proximal hardware. There have been no reported cases of premature proximal ulnar physeal closure using this internal fixation technique.

Results

In two series, a small but adequate number of patients have been reviewed. Graves and Canale[4] reported the results of

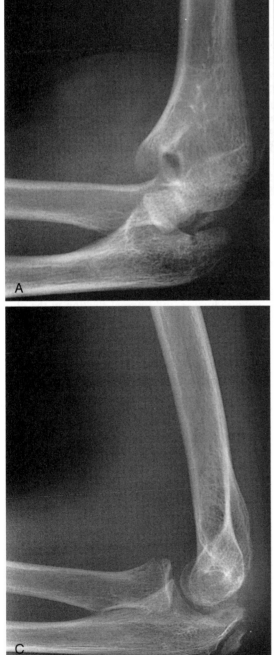

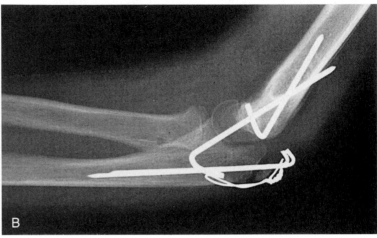

FIGURE 19–4 • A 10-year-old girl fell 3 feet from a desk directly onto her left elbow, sustaining a proximal ulnar fracture (A) and transcondylar humerus fracture associated with an intra-articular loose bone fragment. Four weeks after open reduction and internal fixation of the proximal ulna and distal humerus, anatomic alignment and periosteal healing is demonstrated (B). Two years following her fracture and 18 months following removal of the tension band wire, the fractures have completely healed, elbow motion is full and without limit, and the patient is entirely asymptomatic (C).

forces at the radiocapitellar joint, along with a tenuous blood supply to the region, may contribute to the development of this condition. Most affected persons are males, who initially note lateral elbow pain, loss of extension, and swelling. These symptoms are aggravated by activity and improve with 6 to 8 weeks of rest. Plain radiographs are usually sufficient to make the diagnosis, although tomography, CT, MRI, and arthroscopy may be necessary. It is important to distinguish osteochondritis dissecans from Panner's disease, a benign, self-limited condition that affects the capitellum in younger children.

Intact osteochondral lesions usually respond well to activity limitations. Many heal and patients are able to return to activities. Failed nonoperative treatment or a symptomatic loose body is an indication for surgery, which should aim to remove loose fragments. Curettage of the defect or drilling of the subchondral bone may be useful, but this remains to be proven. More aggressive surgical procedures have not been shown to be beneficial. The short-term prognosis is good, but a return to high-level competitive athletics involving throwing or gymnastic moves is not possible in all cases.

REFERENCES

1. Albright, J. A., Jokl, P., Shaw, R., and Albright, J. P.: Clinical study of baseball pitchers: correlation of injury to the throwing arm with method of delivery. Am. J. Sports Med. 6:15, 1978.
2. Andrews, J. R., and Carson, W. G.: Arthroscopy of the elbow. Arthroscopy 1:97, 1985.
3. Bauer, M., Jonsson, K., and Josefsson, P. O.: Osteochondritis dissecans of the elbow. A long-term follow-up study. Clin. Orthop. 284:156, 1992.
4. Brown, R., Blazina, M. E., Derlan, R. K., Carter, V. S., Jobe, F. W., and Carlson, G. J.: Osteochondritis of the capitellum. J. Sports Med. 2:27, 1974.
5. Clanton, T. O., and DeLee, J. E.: Osteochondritis dissecans. Clin. Orthop. 167:50, 1982.
6. Fritz, R. C., Steinbach, L. S., Tirman, P. F., and Martinez, S.: MR imaging of the elbow. An update. Radiol. Clin. North Am. 35:117, 1997.
7. Gardiner, J. B.: Osteochondritis dissecans in three members of one family. J. Bone Joint Surg. 37B:139, 1955.
8. Guhl, J. F.: Arthroscopy and arthroscopic surgery of the elbow. Orthopedics 8:1290, 1985.
9. Haraldsson, S.: On osteochondrosis deformans juvenitis, capituli humeri including investigation of intraosseous vasculature in distal humerus. Acta Orthop. Scand. Suppl. 38:1, 1959.
10. Janarv, P. M., Hesser, U., and Hirsch, G.: Osteochondral lesions in the radiocapitellar joint in the skeletally immature: radiographic, MRI, and arthroscopic findings in 13 consecutive cases. J. Pediatr. Orthop. 17:311, 1997.
11. Jackson, D. W., Silvino, N., and Reiman, P.: Osteochondritis in the female gymnast's elbow. Arthroscopy 5:129, 1989.
12. King, J. W., Brelsford, H. S., and Tullos, H. S.: Analysis of the pitching arm of the professional baseball pitcher. Clin. Orthop. 67:116, 1969.
13. Klekamp, J., Green, N. E., and Mencio, G. A.: Osteochondritis dissecans as a cause of developmental dislocation of the radial head. Clin. Orthop. 338:36, 1997.
14. Lindholm, T. S., Osterman, K., and Vankka, E.: Osteochondritis dissecans of elbow, ankle, and hip. Clin. Orthop. 148:245, 1980.
15. McManama, G. B., Michel, L. J., Berry, M. V., and Sohn, R. S.: The surgical treatment of osteochondritis of the capitellum. Am. J. Sports Med. 13:11, 1985.
16. Mitsunaga, M. M., Adishian, D. O., and Bianco, A. J. Jr.: Osteochondritis dissecans of the capitellum. J. Trauma 22:53, 1982.
17. Naguro, S.: The so-called osteochondritis dissecans of Konig. Clin. Orthop. 18:100, 1960.
18. Neilson, N. A.: Osteochondritis dissecans capituli humeri. Acta Orthop. Scand. 4:307, 1933.
19. Omer, G. E. J.: Primary articular osteochondroses. Clin. Orthop. 158:33, 1981.
20. Paes, R. A.: Familial osteochondritis dissecans. Clin. Radiol. 40:501, 1989.
21. Panner, H. J.: A peculiar affection of the capitellum humeri, resembling Calve-Perthes disease of the hip. Acta Radiol. 8:617, 1927.
22. Papilion, J. D., Neff, R. S., and Shall, L. M.: Compression neuropathy of the radial nerve as a complication of elbow arthroscopy: a case report and review of the literature. Arthroscopy 4:284, 1988.
23. Pappas, A. M.: Osteochondritis dissecans. Clin. Orthop. 158:59, 1981.
24. Roberts, N., and Hughes, R.: Osteochondritis dissecans of the elbow joint: a clinical study. J. Bone Joint Surg. 32B:348, 1950.
25. Rupp, S., and Tempelhof, S.: Arthroscopic surgery of the elbow. Therapeutic benefits and hazards. Clin. Orthop. 313:140, 1995.
26. Schenck, R. C., Athanasiou, K. A., Constantinides, G., and Gomez, E.: A biomechanical analysis of articular cartilage of the human elbow and a potential relationship to osteochondritis dissecans. Clin. Orthop. 299:305, 1994.
27. Singer, K. M., and Roy, S. P.: Osteochondrosis of the humeral capitellum. Am. J. Sports Med. 12:351, 1984.
28. Smillie, I. S.: Osteochondritis Dissecans: Loose Bodies in Joints; Etiology, Pathology, Treatment. Edinburgh, E. & S. Livingstone, 1960.
29. Tivnon, M. C., Anzel, S. H., and Waugh, T. R.: Surgical management of osteochondritis dissecans of the capitellum. Am. J. Sports Med. 4:121, 1976.
30. Torg, J. S.: Little League: the theft of a carefree youth. Physician Sports Med. 1:72, 1973.
31. Tullos, H. S., Erwin, W. D., Woods, G. W., Wukasch, D. C., Cooley, D. A., and King, J. W.: Unusual lesions of the pitching arm. Clin. Orthop. 88:169, 1972.
32. Woodward, A. H., and Bianco, A. J. Jr.: Osteochondritis dissecans of the elbow. Clin. Orthop. 110:35, 1975.

CHAPTER 21

Dislocations of the Child's Elbow

• R. MERV LETTS

Dislocations of the elbow in children, in contrast to dislocations of other joints in children, are common, constituting about 6 to 8 percent of elbow injuries.[66, 109] In general, however, because the attachments of ligaments and muscles are stronger than the adjacent growth plate, forces exerted about most joints tend to result in epiphyseal injury rather than dislocation of the adjacent joint. The elbow is unique in children because types I and II fractures through the distal humeral epiphysis are uncommon, and dislocations of the elbow are the most common type of dislocation encountered in the pediatric age group.

It is the purpose of this chapter to discuss the practical aspects of the cause, the recognition, and the management of dislocations about the elbow joint in children. Because the elbow is the most common joint injured in childhood, it is suggested that the reader be conversant with the various fractures that occur around this joint and that the chapters on fractures about the elbow joint (see Chapters 13, 15, 16, and 17) be prerequisite reading.

ANATOMIC FACTORS PREDISPOSING TO ELBOW DISLOCATION IN CHILDREN

Although the anatomy of the elbow joint was thoroughly discussed in Chapter 3, it is important to emphasize some of the anatomic differences that are unique to the pediatric elbow joint.

Growth Plates, Apophysis, and Secondary Centers of Ossification

To a casual observer, the radiograph of a child's elbow is an enigma—no two ever seem alike. The reason for this, of course, is that because the child is constantly growing, ossification centers are appearing and fusing, and cartilage is calcifying progressively until skeletal maturity is attained.

It is important to emphasize that there is usually a normal contralateral control that can be radiographed and compared with the radiograph of the injured elbow. This is not recommended as a routine practice, but sometimes it is necessary and useful, especially for those who treat elbow injuries in children only occasionally.

In general, the younger the child at the time of injury, the more difficult it is to assess the elbow, owing to the larger percentage of cartilage that is present about the elbow joint. For this reason, in the newborn or infant, it may be very difficult to diagnose an elbow injury or to determine whether it is a transcondylar fracture or a dislocation of the elbow (the former being much more common at this age). The ossific nuclei about the elbow joint are helpful in radiologic interpretation of elbow dislocation (see Chapter 13). The capitellum, whose center of ossification should be present by 6 months of age, facilitates the interpretation of radial head alignment, because a line drawn through the radial head should always intersect the capitellum no matter what view is taken (Fig. 21–1). This interpretation is improved even further with the appearance of the radial head secondary center of ossification, at around 5 years of age. The secondary center of ossification of the olecranon, which appears at about 9 years of age, allows a more accurate assessment of the position of the

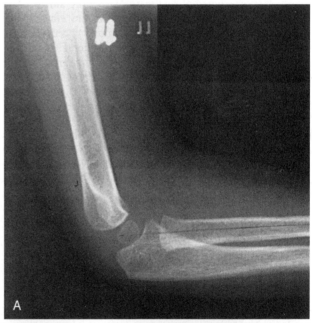
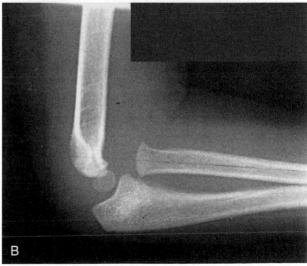

FIGURE 21–1 • *A*, A line drawn through the middle of the neck and head of the radius must always pass through the capitellum in every view. *B*, If it does not, dislocation of the radial head is present.

261

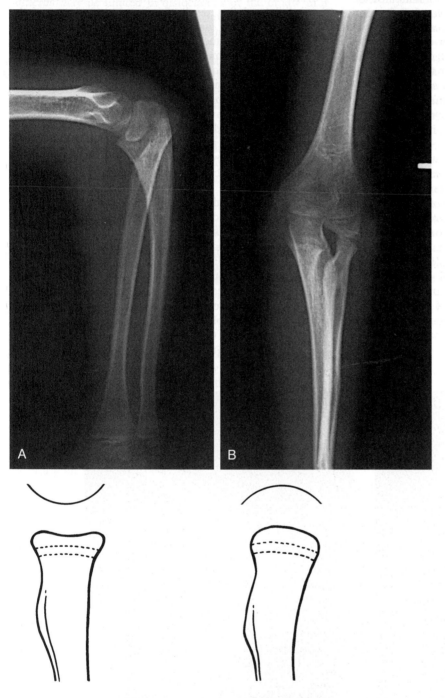

a. CONCAVE HEAD
   RECENT DISLOCATION

b. CONVEX HEAD
   CONGENITAL OR
   LONGTERM DISLOCATION

C

FIGURE 21–4 • Developmental or long-standing dislocation of the radial head. *A,* Note the rounded appearance of the head, convexity of the articular surface, and narrow neck typical of this deformity. *B,* Opposite normal elbow. *C,* Convexity of head develops if the radius is not in contact with the capitellum.

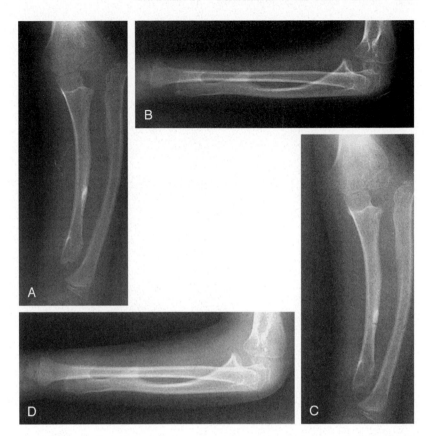

FIGURE 21–5 • *A–D*, Dislocation of the radial head posterolaterally in a patient with multiple exostoses.

or types, of posterior developmental radial head dislocation with characteristic radiographic appearance (Fig. 21–8). Types II and III are complete dislocations and are more obvious cosmetically but have relatively little functional loss except forearm rotation. Type I dislocations commonly are associated with late degenerative arthrosis and consist more of a subluxation than a frank dislocation.

Developmental dislocation of the radial head is seldom a functional disability. Clinically, the symptoms that occur with a gradual dislocation of the radial head seem to be much less severe than those occurring with acute dislocation of the radial head. There is probably little indication for operative treatment of developmental dislocation of the radial head unless it is recognized early. For example, a malunion of the radius and the ulna that is obviously directing the head of the radius laterally, posteriorly, or anteriorly should be corrected with an osteotomy to redirect the proximal radius or the deformed ulna.[15]

In cerebral palsy patients, if the bicipital tendon appears to be subluxating the radial head anteriorly, lengthening the biceps may prevent future dislocation. Once the dislocation is well established, attempts to relocate the radial head probably should not be made, and the dislocation should be accepted. Future resection of the radial head at skeletal maturity can be performed if the head is cosmetically or functionally a problem. The gradual nature of the dislocation and adjacent changes in the surrounding tissues and bone make this type of relocation of the radial head much more difficult than that in the acute traumatic dislocation.[22]

Relocation of the radial head by shortening the radius and reconstitution of the annular ligament are seldom indicated in the developmental dislocation.

RADIOGRAPHIC APPEARANCE

The radiographic appearance of a long-standing dislocated radial head is characterized by a rounded contour or convexity in contrast to the normal concave appearance (see Fig. 21–4). The posterior border of the ulna also may be concave rather than slightly convex in anterior dislocations of the radial head. Posterior dislocations result in a longer neck with a typical dome-shaped head. Even an isolated traumatic dislocation of the radial head, when it occurs in a very young child, may take on the appearance of a congenital or developmental dislocation with the passage of time. A relative increase in ulnar length in relation to the radius and the wrist is often noted in patients with developmental dislocation. With posterior dislocation, proximal ulnar bowing also is observed, and proximal radial migration of the radius may be present.[24] The capitellum may be hypoplastic or, occasionally, even absent.[34]

Other factors characteristic of congenital or developmental radial head dislocations have been reported to be bilaterality of involvement, association with other congenital anomalies, familial occurrence, absence of traumatic history, and the presence of the entity in a patient under 6 months of age[14–20] (see Chapter 14).

NATURAL HISTORY

Developmental dislocation of the radial head seldom causes any serious symptoms. Patients with developmental anterior dislocation of the radial head may complain of clicking

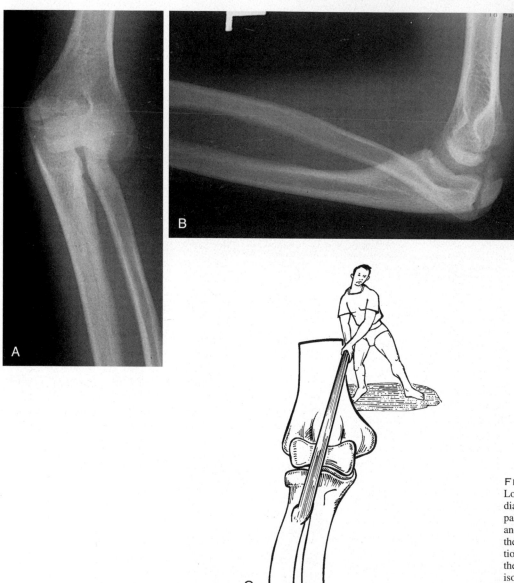

FIGURE 21–6 • *A* and *B*, Long-standing dislocation of the radial head in a child with cerebral palsy. The elongation of the neck and convexity of the head indicate the presence of a prolonged dislocation. *C*, Spasticity or contraction of the biceps tendon may contribute to isolated dislocation of the radial head in children.

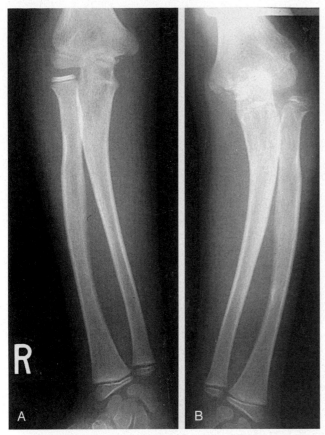

FIGURE 21–7 • *A* and *B*, A child sustained a fracture of the ulna and neck of the radius that healed in malunion. Four years later, the radial head is dislocating laterally owing to malposition of the proximal radial epiphyseal plate.

or impingement at the ulnohumeral joint with flexion of the elbow. This may be associated with some discomfort in teenagers and adults. Posterior dislocation of the radial head sometimes creates a cosmetic protuberance that also may be a source of pain with excessive elbow motion.[24] Aching in the region of the dislocation is common in the older child. A prominent ulna at the wrist and the resultant radioulnar subluxation at the distal end may result in some limitation of motion at the wrist and occasional discomfort. Most children with this abnormality do not have any complaints in childhood, although some may experience discomfort with excessive elbow motion in their teens and, later, as adults. There does not appear to be any progressive loss of motion with further growth, and the joint limitation, if present, remains static.[16, 24]

Traumatic Dislocation

Solitary dislocation of the radial head in children is uncommon but occurs much more frequently in younger children than in teenagers or adults. It is essential to differentiate this entity from a developmental dislocation of the radial head that has been noticed for the first time because of a radiograph that has been taken for a minor elbow injury.

The history may not be of much use in these cases because these children are often young, prone to frequent elbow injuries, and unable to make a reliable contribution

to the history. The radiograph, however, is usually diagnostic because it shows the rounded concave appearance of the radial head in the congenital or developmental dislocation (see Fig. 21–4).[1–13]

The use of arthrography to differentiate congenital from traumatic dislocation of the radial head has been recommended.[12, 34] The main differentiating feature has been the intra-articular nature of congenital dislocation as opposed to the extra-articular location of the radial head in traumatic dislocations.

CLINICAL FEATURES OF ISOLATED ANTERIOR DISLOCATION

Children who have sustained an anterior dislocation of the radial head usually have a history of trauma associated with inability or unwillingness to use the arm. Careful examination of the extremities and the radiograph may reveal some ulnar bowing. This is analogous to a Monteggia fracture-dislocation except that the ulna is simply bowed rather than fractured.

Radiographically, a line drawn through the shaft of the radius and the radial head will not intersect the capitellum when the radial head is dislocated (see Fig. 21–1). Children who have been subjected to child abuse may present with this particular injury, and again, the history will be difficult to elicit.

TREATMENT OF ACUTE ANTERIOR DISLOCATION

Closed Reduction

If the child is seen within 3 weeks of the dislocation, a closed reduction may be achieved. Direct pressure over the radial head with gradual flexion of the arm and immobilization in a flexed position of more than 100 degrees is usually successful.

If the radial head has been out of joint for some time or if the annular ligament has fallen back, preventing adequate reduction, an open reduction may have to be performed.

If the radial head can be reduced but is not stable, a Kirschner wire fixation to the ulna may be needed. Driving a pin across the elbow joint through the capitellum and into the radial head is *not* recommended because, in our experience, these Kirschner wires often break, making removal difficult. Breakage occurs because it is virtually impossible to immobilize the elbow completely in a child, and the constant minor motion, even in a cast, may result in a fatigue fracture of the wire. The elbow joint will then have to be opened unnecessarily to remove the fractured pin.

Open Reduction

TRICEPS FASCIAL RECONSTRUCTION

The technique of open reduction of an anterior dislocation of the radial head in children described by Lloyd-Roberts and Bucknill[16] is one I have used with success. This con-

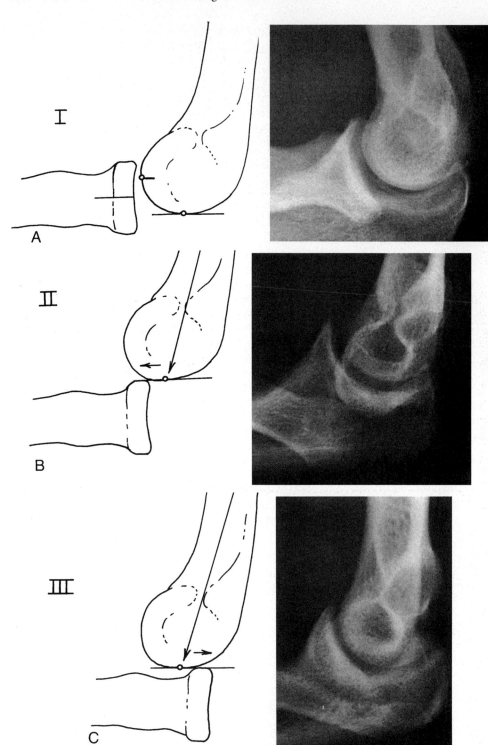

FIGURE 21-8 • The Mayo classification of posterior radial head instability. *A,* Type I is subluxation with characteristic radial head elongation and is associated with a poor functional result. *B,* Type II is complete dislocation but without subluxation. These patients typically have minimal pain but moderate loss of forearm rotation. Forearm prominence may be noticed *C,* Dislocation with posterior subluxation, type III, causes a marked cosmetic deformity but little functional impairment. Surgery is performed only for cosmetic reasons.

sists of using the lateral portion of the tendon of the triceps for reconstruction of the annular ligament (Fig. 21–9A).

A posterolateral incision is preferred rather than a posterior incision, which may disorient the surgeon to the position of the radial head. The triceps tendon is identified, and a long (10-cm) strip is removed from the lateral margin, ensuring attachment at the distal ulnar insertion. The tendon is increased in length by continuing the dissection through the periosteum of the ulna to a point opposite the neck of the radius, where it is then passed around the neck and sutured to itself and the ulnar periosteum with enough tension to hold the radial head in place. A Kirschner wire is then passed through the ulna into the radius to ensure solid fixation until the tendon has healed (see Fig. 21–9B). The extremity is kept immobilized in an above-elbow plaster cast for 6 weeks; gradual mobilization is begun at 6 weeks after the Kirschner wire has been removed. If there is any difficulty in reducing the radial head, careful inspec-

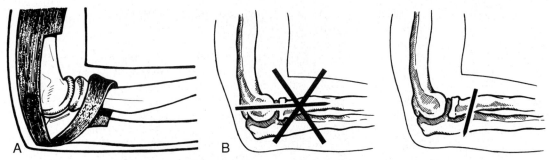

FIGURE 21–9 • *A,* Repair of radial head dislocation by reconstruction of annular ligament using triceps fascia (Lloyd Roberts-Bucknill technique). *B,* A Kirschner wire passed through the capitellum into the radial head *(left)* is not recommended owing to danger of pin fatigue and breakage. The radial head can be safely held in the reduced position by a pin across the radius and ulna *(right).*

tion of the joint capsule may reveal some infolding, which may have to be excised.

Care must be exercised when exposing the neck of the radius in a child because the normal guidelines that apply to adult anatomy do not apply to the young child. The radial nerve may be only a fingerbreadth below the head of the radius rather than the classic two fingerbreadths that is often used as a standard of measurement for locating the radial nerve in adults.

FASCIAL RECONSTRUCTION OF THE ANNULAR LIGAMENT

A method of reconstruction of the annular ligament has been described by Boyd[36] that is also a useful technique. A strip of fascia is dissected off the forearm muscles but is left attached to the proximal ulna. The length of this fascial strip should be about 5 inches by ½ inch. It is passed around the neck of the radius, proximal to the tuberosity and distal to the radial notch of the ulna, and is brought around and fastened to itself with nonabsorbable sutures (see Fig. 21–9). Care should be taken to ensure that the length of this fascial strip is adequate. Cross-radioulnar pin fixation for 4 weeks is recommended.

Untreated Anterior Dislocation of the Radial Head

A child with a long-standing anterior dislocation of the radial head actually may have good elbow function. The range of motion is usually functional, although the extremes of flexion and extension are usually limited by 20 or 30 degrees, and pain may develop at a later date. The cosmetic deformity is also a concern, and the elbow may appear somewhat grotesque, especially in a small, thin arm. Excision of the radial head at skeletal maturity will relieve most symptoms.

COMPLICATIONS

Relocation of an acute dislocation of the radial head in a child is usually successful, and few cases become recurrent. If the dislocation is not reduced, the child is left with limited motion in the elbow together with a cosmetic deformity. The dislocated radial head may also result in a rela-

tive shortening of the radius compared with the ulna, with subsequent subluxation at the radioulnar joint at the wrist. As a general rule, the radial head should not be excised in a child because this may further aggravate shortening of the radius by eliminating the proximal radial growth plate, which contributes about 30 percent of the final radial length. If there is pain or a grotesque appearance when the child is near skeletal maturity, the radial head then can be removed. In neglected patients, excision of the radial head may allow improved flexion and rotation and may alleviate complaints of pain and discomfort.

Attempts to reduce a long-standing dislocation of the radial head by shortening the radius and reconstructing the annular ligament are usually unsuccessful and, in most instances, are not indicated.

PEDIATRIC MONTEGGIA FRACTURE DISLOCATION

The Monteggia injury is uncommon in children but by no means rare. In the 5-year period from 1978 to 1982 at the Winnipeg Children's Hospital, 33 children were treated for a variety of Monteggia lesions. The true incidence of this fracture-dislocation is unknown, but it is more common than is generally appreciated. Olney and Menelaus[49] collected 102 cases of children with acute Monteggia lesions treated over a 25-year period.

Cause

The most common cause of dislocation of the radial head associated with an ulnar fracture in childhood is a hyperextension injury[40, 58]; a hyperpronation injury[41] of the elbow is less commonly the cause. In hyperpronation, Bado[35] pointed out that the bicipital tuberosity is the most posterior, thus predisposing the proximal radius to the greatest force during violent contraction of the bicipital tendon. In young children, the force generated by the biceps is less than that in the adult, and this mechanism probably is significant only in older children.

A direct blow over the posterior proximal ulna will produce a Monteggia lesion with anterior dislocation of the radial head, but this is an uncommon mechanism in children.

In our experience, this lesion is most frequently produced by a hyperextension injury. Further support for this theory is the observation that, in open type C injuries, the proximal ulnar fragment pierces the skin on the volar ulnar aspect of the forearm. This would not be possible if the arm were in full pronation because of imposition of the radius.

Because of the plasticity of the forearm bones, the radial head and neck may slip under the annular ligament and dislocate as the shaft of the radius bends. Indeed, many of the isolated traumatic dislocations of the radial head are undoubtedly variations of the Monteggia lesion[42-44] (Monteggia equivalent), in which the ulna has simply bent but not fractured. The radial shaft is bent to the extent that the head and neck are slipped from within the annular ligament, resulting in an apparent isolated dislocation of the radial head.[26, 39]

Classifications

Classifications of the Monteggia lesion are based largely on the injury in adults.[35] Because of differences in the configuration of the injury in childhood, the following classification has been devised to include dislocation of the radial head associated with the plasticity of the forearm bones in childhood (Fig. 21–10).

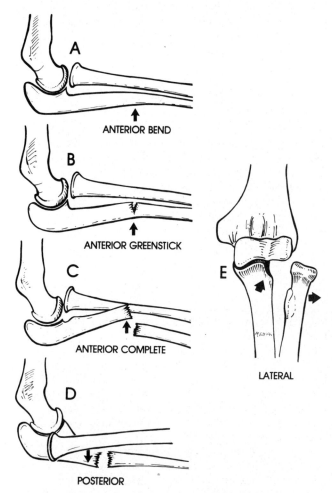

FIGURE 21-10 • Classification of the pediatric Monteggia fracture dislocation: types A through E.

Classification of Pediatric Monteggia Lesions

Type A: Anterior dislocation of the radial head with anterior bowing of the ulna (Fig. 21–11).
Type B: Anterior dislocation of the radial head with greenstick fracture of the ulna (Fig. 21–12).
Type C: Anterior dislocation of the radial head with transverse fracture of the ulna (Fig. 21–13).
Type D: Posterior dislocation of the radial head with bending or fracture of the ulna (Fig. 21–14).
Type E: Lateral dislocation of the radial head with fracture of the ulna (Fig. 21–15).

Types B and C are the most commonly encountered Monteggia lesions in children.[47]

Clinical Diagnosis

Like Monteggia himself, who explained this injury in a young woman in 1814, long before the advent of radiography, most physicians today should be able to identify the clinical configuration of this lesion in patients who are seen early, before the swelling clouds the clinical signs (see Fig. 21–15). The dislocation of the radial head is often evident on inspection of the lateral aspect of the elbow joint. Angulation of the ulna, whether fractured or not, necessitates careful appraisal of the position of the radial head. Dislocation of the radial head is frequently missed by those who treat pediatric elbow injuries only occasionally.[48-54] A mental line drawn through the shaft and the neck of the radius should intersect the capitellum in all views taken (see Fig. 21–1). If it does not, dislocation of the radial head is highly suspect.

In contrast to the lesion in adults, overlap of the ulnar fragments is not a prerequisite for dislocation of the radial head in a child. Disruption of the forearm parallelogram may occur as a result of ulnar bend when the radial head slips out of the annular ligament. A good rule of thumb is to obtain adequate films, such as anteroposterior and lateral views of the elbow joint in all fractures of the ulna. The apex of the ulnar bend or angulation is always in the direction of the radial head dislocation.[57-60]

The elbow must be carefully examined clinically and radiographically in any child who has an apparently intact radius associated with bowing, greenstick, or complete fracture of the ulna.

Treatment

In contrast to this lesion in adults, the Monteggia injury in children usually can be treated by closed methods.[27] Pressure directed over the dislocated radius usually will result in a stable ulnar reduction, provided that immobilization is imposed with the elbow flexed more than 90 degrees in types A, B, C, and E lesions. Supination assists in minimizing biceps pull. In the uncommon type D Monteggia lesion with posterior dislocation of the radial head, stability is obtained with extension, not flexion, of the elbow.

As long as the radial head is reduced and stable, angulation of the ulna of as much as 15 degrees can be accepted. Remodeling of this angulation will occur with further

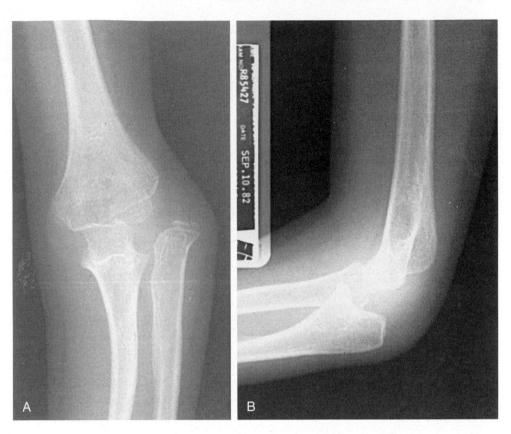

FIGURE 21–11 • *A* and *B,* Ulnar bend with lateral dislocation of the radial head, a type A Monteggia fracture dislocation.

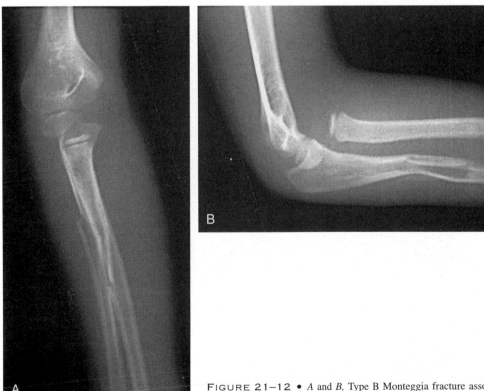

FIGURE 21–12 • *A* and *B,* Type B Monteggia fracture associated with a greenstick fracture of the ulna and anterior dislocation of the radial head.

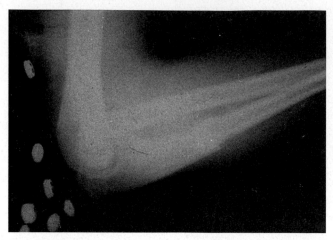

FIGURE 21–13 • Anterior dislocation of the radial head with transverse fracture of ulna.

growth. In children, stable reduction of the radial head is the first priority. A supination-pronation maneuver may facilitate repositioning of the annular ligament, which is seldom completely torn.

If it is impossible to obtain a stable reduction of the radial head, I approach the radial head through a Kocher incision and reapproximate the annular ligament around the neck. If stability is still precarious or if the annular ligament has had to be reconstituted, I recommend internal fixation of the radius to the ulna with a Kirschner wire (Fig. 21–16A). I would caution against maintenance of the reduction by a wire inserted through the capitellum and

into the radial head. No matter how rigid the postoperative immobilization may be, there is still a small degree of flexion and extension of the elbow joint that ultimately will result in fatigue breakage of the wire, necessitating re-exploration of the elbow joint (see Fig. 21–8B).

If the ulna is unstable in the older child, an open reduction with plate fixation may be necessary, but in my experience, this is seldom required in children under 10 years of age.[54]

Nerve Injury Associated with Monteggia Lesions

Anterior dislocation of the radial head may result in a traction injury to the posterior interosseous nerve as it passes dorsolaterally around the proximal radius to enter the substance of the supinator muscle mass between the superficial and deep layers (see Fig. 21–16B).[42, 56] Compression of the posterior interosseous nerve also may be aggravated by the fibrous arcade of Frohse, a firm fibrous band at the proximal edge of the supinator muscle.[55]

In children, nerve injury is less common than in adults, and recovery is the rule in closed injuries. In a large series of 102 Monteggia fractures, Olney and Menelaus[49] found a 10 percent incidence of nerve injuries, 6 percent involving the posterior interosseous nerve and 3 percent involving the radial nerve. All their nerve injuries healed completely within 6 months.

THE MISSED MONTEGGIA LESION

The missed dislocated radial head that is noticed after the ulna has healed is a common error made by less experi-

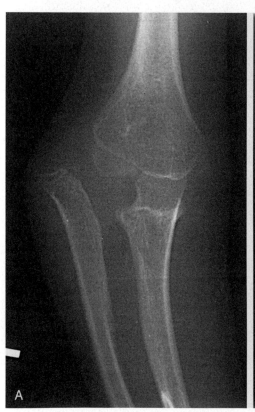

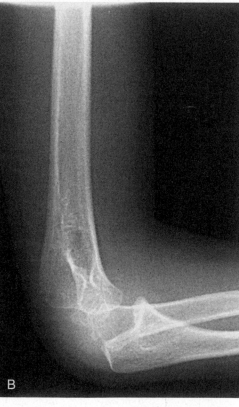

FIGURE 21–14 • A and B, Posterior lateral dislocation of the radial head with bending or fracture of the ulna.

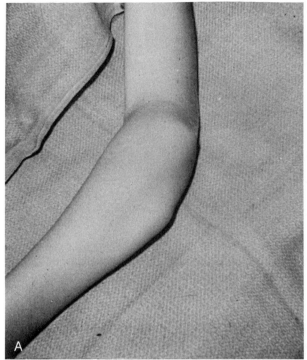

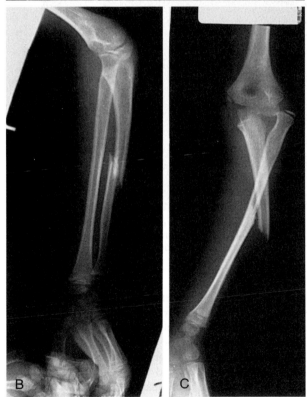

FIGURE 21–15 • Monteggia fracture with lateral dislocation of the radial head. *A*, Clinical appearance. *B* and *C*, Radiologic appearance.

diagnostic—the congenital lesion having a rounded convex head whereas the recently dislocated radius usually has a concave appearance. It can be appreciated that the younger the child, the more difficult it will be to make this interpretation, owing to the large cartilaginous component of the proximal radius.[36-40, 46]

Dislocation-Subluxation of the Radial Head Following Malunion of a Radial Neck Fracture

Fractures of the radial neck in children that have occurred after the age of 6 or 7 years may, if unreduced, result in a subluxation (see Fig. 21–7). When the angulation is more than 45 to 50 degrees, the growth plate becomes redirected laterally or posterolaterally. If there is not enough remodeling to allow the growth plate to reattain its normal transverse anatomy, increased prominence of the radial head results. As the child grows older, pain will be experienced, as well as irritation, cosmetic deformity, and, to a lesser extent, limitation of supination and pronation. This result can be avoided by ensuring that marked angulation of the radial neck is corrected by closed or open reduction to less than 40 to 45 degrees.

Dislocation of the radial head associated with malunion of the ulna may necessitate osteotomy of the ulna and an open reduction of the radial head. It is of course always prudent to attempt a closed reduction of the radial head if the injury has occurred recently (i.e., within 2 months) because the ulna may still be straightened. Usually, however, in the missed Monteggia lesion, an open reduction of the radial head will be necessary, and in this instance it will almost certainly be necessary to reconstitute the annular ligament—with the ligament itself, if possible, with fascia obtained from the triceps, or by using the Bell-Tawse procedure.[38, 40, 45] It also may require shortening of the radius to permit reduction. Internal fixation with Kirschner wires through the radius to the ulna is advisable. Relocation of the radial head should be attempted in children under 6 years of age. In older children in whom the lesion has been present for more than 1 year, it may be advisable to accept the dislocation because this is compatible with excellent function in most instances. Recent experience with a modified technique for reconstruction of the annular ligament has been reported by Peterson and Seel,[52] which appears to have good results in patients with long-standing radial head dislocations. If the radial head becomes cosmetically or functionally disabling, excision can be performed when skeletal maturity is attained. Removal of the radial head should not be considered until skeletal maturity is reached, because 30 percent of radial growth occurs at the proximal radial epiphysis.

PULLED ELBOW SYNDROME

Nursemaid's elbow, or pulled elbow syndrome, has been recognized since early in this century.[115] Some children seem to be particularly prone to this injury, and for them, even minor pulls on the arm result in the typical pain and failure of elbow motion that is always of concern to parents (Fig. 21–17A).[114, 115]

enced clinicians. In some instances, the dislocated radial head may not be identified for some time, even years later, after the initial injury has almost been forgotten (see Fig. 21–16C). Some confusion may occasionally arise in connection with the congenital dislocated radial head, but in general, the contour of the radial head should be

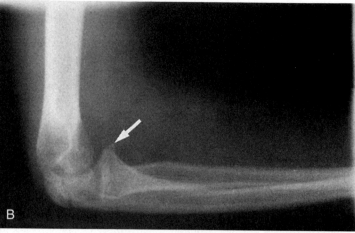

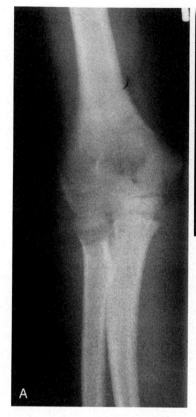

FIGURE 21–25 • *A* and *B,* Avulsion fracture of tip of coronoid process following dislocation of the elbow. The brachialis muscle often avulses a small portion of the coronoid process; when present, this is pathognomonic of a previous elbow dislocation.

neck, or the olecranon, this maneuver probably should not be attempted.

In our experience with children under age 12, it is best to proceed with a general anesthetic for complete relaxation, and this should be done within 6 hours of the trauma. It is not appropriate to allow the child to wait overnight because this encourages increased edema and resultant postreduction stiffness as well as being extremely uncomfortable for the child.

Once the child has been anesthetized, it is usually a simple matter to reduce the posterior dislocation of the elbow. Gentle traction on the forearm combined with some anterior pressure over the dislocated olecranon allows the joint to be reduced, usually with an audible and palpable clunk (Fig. 21–28).

Occasionally, in older children, the coronoid process becomes locked behind the humerus. In this instance, the arm should be put in extension, and with traction and good firm thumb pressure over the olecranon, the elbow usually can be reduced. Putting the elbow into hyperextension to lever the coronoid process under the humerus is a hazardous procedure, especially if vascular insufficiency is already present, because it places more stress on the brachial artery, which is often tented over the distal end of the humerus. Once the elbow is reduced, the integrity of the medial and lateral collateral ligaments should be tested, and the elbow should be moved through a full range of motion to ensure that no fragment, particularly the medial epicondyle, is caught within the joint. If the joint does not move freely or has a spongy feel to it, a mechanical problem with reduction exists. The reduction should always be checked radiographically, especially when a fracture is associated with the injury.[77, 85, 88]

Aspiration of the joint is recommended to assist in resolving the hematoma and improving joint motion after reduction.

Medial Epicondylar Entrapment

If it is known that the medial epicondyle is trapped within the joint, then during the reduction, a valgus strain placed on the elbow with flexion of the wrist may allow the attached flexor muscle mass to pull the trapped fragment out of the joint. Occasionally, this may yield an anatomic or nearly anatomic position. If the medial epicondyle is displaced more than 1 cm, it should be pinned back in place because it will add stability to the elbow subsequent to the dislocation and allow stable elbow motion to occur within 3 to 4 weeks. In children under the age of 5, when the medial epicondyle is not ossified, any springiness in the elbow joint subsequent to the reduction indicates an intra-articular position of the medial epicondyle. Ultrasonographic evaluation of the elbow might be helpful in confirming the presence of an intra-articular fragment.[68] If the medial epicondyle cannot be removed from the joint with manipulation, it must be removed surgically. The elbow is approached through a medial incision. The flexor muscle mass initially appears to be anatomically intact as it disappears into the joint; however, with valgus force and gentle pull on the muscle mass, the attached fragment can be removed from the joint, and the capsule can be repaired. The fragment then should be reattached to the distal medial humerus. Care should be taken not to injure the ulnar nerve. If there is any concern about this, the nerve should be identified and retracted with tapes until the repair has been completed.[61, 81, 86, 100]

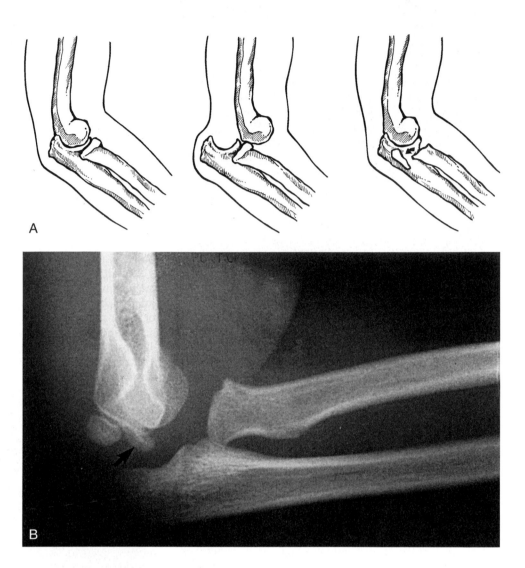

FIGURE 21–26 • *A,* Type I fracture of the proximal radial epiphysis with posterior displacement occasionally occurs in posterior dislocation of the elbow if reduction is forceful. *B,* Fracture of neck of radius secondary to dislocation of the elbow with forceful spontaneous reduction.

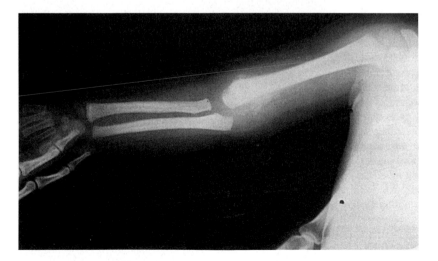

FIGURE 21–27 • Transcondylar fracture of the humerus in infancy may be misdiagnosed as a dislocation of the elbow. Arthrography or computed tomography scan is diagnostic.

the elbow systematically for evidence of skeletal injury coexisting with the dislocation. Particular care should be exercised to ensure that the radial head is in its proper relationship with the capitellum. Because most problems encountered in elbow dislocations in children are the result of missed diagnoses of associated injuries, the value of a thorough clinical and radiographic examination of the elbow cannot be overemphasized.

REFERENCES

• TRAUMATIC DISLOCATION OF THE RADIAL HEAD

1. Beddow, F. H., and Corckery, P. H.: Lateral dislocation of the radial humeral joint with greenstick fracture of the upper end of the ulna. J. Bone Joint Surg. **42B**:782, 1960.
2. De Lee, J. C.: Transverse divergent dislocation of the elbow in a child. J. Bone Joint Surg. **63A**:322, 1981.
3. Heidt, R. S., and Stern, P. J.: Isolated posterior dislocation of the radial head. Clin. Orthop. **168**:136, 1982.
4. Hudson, D. A., and DeBeer, De. V.: Isolated traumatic dislocation of the radial head in children. J. Bone Joint Surg. **68B**:378, 1986.
5. Lincoln, T. L., and Mubarek, S. J.: "Isolated" traumatic radial head dislocation. J. Pediatr. Orthop. **14**:454, 1994.
6. Schubert, J. J.: Dislocation of the radial head in the newborn infant. J. Bone Joint Surg. **47A**:1010, 1965.
7. Stelling, F. H., and Cote, R. H.: Traumatic dislocation of the head of the radius in children. J.A.M.A. **160**:732, 1956.
8. Storen, G.: Traumatic dislocation of the radial head as an isolated lesion in children. Acta Clin. Scand. **116**:144, 1958.
9. Vesely, D. G.: Isolated traumatic dislocation of the radial head in children. Clin. Orthop. **50**:31, 1967.
10. Wiley, J. J., Pegington, J., and Horwich, J. P.: Traumatic dislocation of the radius at the elbow. J. Bone Joint Surg. **56B**:501, 1974.
11. Wright, P. R.: Greenstick fractures of the upper end of the ulna with dislocation of the radial humeral joint or displacement of the superior radial epiphysis. J. Bone Joint Surg. **45B**:727, 1963.
12. Yates, C., and Sullivan, J. A.: Arthrographic diagnosis of elbow injuries in children. Pediatr. Orthop. **7**:54, 1987.
13. Zivkovic, T.: Traumatic dislocation of the radial head in a 5-year-old boy. J. Trauma **18**:289, 1978.

• DEVELOPMENTAL DISLOCATION OF THE RADIAL HEAD

14. Cummings, R. J., Jones, E. T., Reed, F. E., and Mazur, J. M.: Infantile dislocation of the elbow complicating obstetric palsy. J. Pediatr. Orthop. **16**:589, 1996.
15. Hirayama, T., Takemitsu, Y., Yagihara, K., and Mikita, A.: Operation for chronic dislocation of the radial head in children. Reduction by osteotomy of the ulna. J. Bone Joint Surg. **69**:639, 1987.
16. Lloyd-Roberts, G. C., and Bucknill, T. M.: Anterior dislocation of the radial head in children—etiology. Natural history and management. J. Bone Joint Surg. **59B**:402, 1977.
17. Pletcher, D., Hofer, M. M., and Koffman, D. M.: Non-traumatic dislocation of the radial head in cerebral palsy. J. Bone Joint Surg. **58A**:104, 1976.
18. Peeters, R. L. M.: Radiological manifestations of the Cornelia de Lange syndrome. Pediatr. Radiol. **3**:41, 1975.
19. Salama, R., Weintroub, S., and Weissman, S. L.: Recurrent dislocation of the radial head. Clin. Orthop. **125**:156, 1977.
20. Silberstein, M. J., Brodeur, A. E., and Graviss, E. R.: Some vagaries of the radial head and neck. J. Bone Joint Surg. **64A**:1153, 1982.
21. Southmayd, W., and Parks, J. C.: Isolated dislocation of the radial head without fracture of the ulna. Clin. Orthop. **97**:94, 1973.
22. Subbarao, J. V., and Kumar, V. N.: Spontaneous dislocation of the radial head in cerebral palsy. Orthop. Rev. **16**:457, 1987.

• CONGENITAL DISLOCATION OF THE RADIAL HEAD

23. Almquist, E. E., Gordon, L. H., and Blue, A. I.: Congenital dislocation of the head of the radius. J. Bone Joint Surg. **51A**:1118, 1969.
24. Bell, S. N., Morrey, B. F., and Bianco, A. J., Jr.: Chronic posterior subluxation and dislocation of the radial head. J. Bone Joint Surg. **73**:392, 1991.

25. Carevias, D. E.: Some observations on congenital dislocation of the head of the radius. J. Bone Joint Surg. **39B**:86, 1957.
26. Cockshott, W. P., and Omololu, A.: Familial posterior dislocation of both radial heads. J. Bone Joint Surg. **40B**:484, 1958.
27. Gattey, P. H., and Wedge, J. H.: Unilateral posterior dislocation of the radial head in identical twins. J. Pediatr. Orthop. **6**:220, 1989.
28. Gunn, D. R., and Pilley, V. K.: Congenital dislocation of the head of the radius. Clin. Orthop. **84**:108, 1964.
29. Kelikian, H. (ed): Dislocation of the radial head. *In* Congenital Deformities of the Hand and Forearm. Philadelphia, W. B. Saunders Co., 1974, p. 902.
30. Kelly, D. W.: Congenital dislocation of the radial head: spectrum and natural history. J. Pediatr. Orthop. **1**:295, 1981.
31. Mardam-Bey, T., and Ger, E.: Congenital radial head dislocation. J. Hand Surg. **4**:316, 1979.
32. Mital, M. A.: Congenital radial ulnar synostosis and congenital dislocation of the radial head. Orthop. Clin. North Am. **7**:375, 1976.
33. Miura, T.: Congenital dislocation of the radial head. J. Hand Surg. **15B**:477, 1990.
34. Mizuno, K., Usui, Y., Kohyama, K., and Hirohata, K.: Familial congenital unilateral anterior dislocation of the radial head: differentiation from traumatic dislocation by means of arthrography. J. Bone Joint Surg. **73A**:1086, 1991.

• MONTEGGIA FRACTURE-DISLOCATION OF THE ELBOW IN CHILDREN

35. Bado, J. L.: The Monteggia lesion. Clin. Orthop. **50**:71, 1967.
36. Boyd, H. B., and Boals, J. C.: The Monteggia lesion: a review of 159 cases. Clin Orthop **66**:94, 1969.
37. Bruce, H. E., Harvey, J. P. W., and Wilson, J. C., Jr.: Monteggia fractures. J. Bone Joint Surg. **56A**:1563, 1974.
38. Bell-Tawse, A. J. F.: The treatment of malunited anterior Monteggia fractures in children. J. Bone Joint Surg. **47B**:718, 1965.
39. Cappellino, A., Wolfe, S. W., and Marsh, J. S.: Use of a modified Bell Tawse procedure for chronic acquired dislocation of the radial head. J. Pediatr. Orthop. **18**:410, 1998.
40. Dormans, J. P., and Rang., M.: The problem of Monteggia fracture dislocations in children. Orthop. Clin. North Am. **21**:251, 1990.
41. Evans, E. M.: Pronation injuries of the forearm with special reference to the anterior Monteggia fracture. J. Bone Joint Surg. **31B**:578, 1949.
42. Fahmy, N. R. M.: Unusual Monteggia lesions in children. Injury **12**:399, 1981.
43. Freedman, L., Luk, K., and Leong, J. C.: Radial head reduction after a missed Monteggia fracture: brief report. J. Bone Joint Surg. **70**:846, 1988.
44. Hume, A. C.: Anterior dislocation of the head of the radius associated with undisplaced fracture of the olecranon in children. J. Bone Joint Surg. **39B**:508, 1957.
45. Hurst, L. C., and Dubrow, E. N.: Surgical treatment of symptomatic chronic radial head dislocation: a neglected Monteggia fracture. J. Pediatr. Orthop. **3**:227, 1983.
46. Kalamchi, A.: Monteggia fracture dislocation in children. Late treatment in two cases. J. Bone Joint Surg. **68**:615, 1986.
47. Letts, M., Locht, R., and Weins, J.: Monteggia fracture dislocations in children. J. Bone Joint Surg. **67**:724, 1985.
48. Mullick, S.: The lateral Monteggia fracture. J. Bone Joint Surg. **59A**:543, 1977.
49. Olney, B. W., and Menelaus, M. B.: Monteggia and equivalent lesions in childhood. J. Pediatr. Orthop. **9**:219, 1989.
50. Ovesen, O., Brok, K. E., Arreskov, J., and Bellstrom, T.: Monteggia lesions in children and adults: an analysis of etiology and long-term results of treatment. Orthopedics **13**:529, 1990.
51. Papavasiliou, V. A., and Nenopoulos, S. P.: Monteggia-type elbow fractures in children. Clin. Orthop. Rel. Res. **233**:230, 1988.
52. Peterson, H. A., and Seel, M. J.: Management of post-traumatic chronic radial head dislocation in children. Presented at the 1998 Annual Meeting of the Pediatric Orthopaedic Society of North America, Cleveland, Ohio, May 7, 1998.
53. Ravessoud, F. A.: Lateral condylar fracture and ipsilateral ulnar shaft fracture: Monteggia equivalent lesions. J. Pediatr. Orthop. **5**:364, 1985.
54. Ring, D., and Waters, P. M.: Operative fixation of Monteggia fractures in children. J. Bone Joint Surg. **78B**:734, 1996.
55. Spinner, M., Freundlich, B. D., and Teicher, J.: Posterior interosse-

ous nerve palsy as a complication of Monteggia fractures in children. Clin. Orthop. **58**:141, 1968.

56. Stein, F., Grabias, S. L., and Deffer, P. A.: Nerve injuries complicating Monteggia lesions. J. Bone Joint Surg. **53A**:1432, 1971.

57. Theodorou, S. D.: Dislocation of the head of the radius associated with fractures of the upper end of the ulna in children. J. Bone Joint Surg. **51B**:70, 1969.

58. Tompikins, D. G.: The anterior Monteggia fracture. Observations on etiology and treatment. J. Bone Joint Surg. **53A**:1009, 1971.

59. Wiley, J. J., and Galey, J. P.: Monteggia injuries in children. J. Bone Joint Surg. **69B**:728, 1985.

60. Wright, P. R.: Greenstick fracture of the upper end of the ulna with dislocation of the radiohumeral joint or displacement of the superior radial epiphysis. J. Bone Joint Surg. **45B**:727, 1963.

• ACUTE DISLOCATION OF THE ELBOW IN CHILDREN

61. Aitken, A. P., and Childress, H. M.: Inter-articular displacement of the internal epicondyle following dislocation. J. Bone Joint Surg. **20**:161, 1938.

62. Aufranc, O. E., Jones, W. M., Turner, R. H., and Thomas, W. H.: Dislocation of the elbow with fracture of the radial head and distal radius. J.A.M.A. **202**:131, 1967.

63. Beghin, J. L., Bucholz, R. W., and Wenger, D. R.: Intracondylar fractures of the humerus in young children. J. Bone Joint Surg. **64A**:1083, 1982.

64. Bilett, D. M.: Unreduced posterior dislocation of the elbow. J. Trauma **19**:186, 1979.

65. Blatz, D. J.: Anterior dislocation of the elbow in a case of Ehlers-Danlos syndrome. Orthop. Rev. **10**:129, 1981.

66. Caravias, D. E.: Forward dislocation of the elbow without fracture of the olecranon. J. Bone Joint Surg. **39B**:334, 1957.

67. D'Ambrosia, R., and Zink, W.: Fractures of the elbow in children. Pediatr. Ann. **11**:541, 1982.

68. Davidson, R. S., Markowitz, R. I., Dormans, J., and Drummond, D. S.: Ultrasonographic evaluation of the elbow in infants and young children after suspected trauma. J. Bone Joint Surg. **76A**:1804, 1994.

69. De Lee, J. C.: Transverse divergent dislocation of the elbow in a child. J. Bone Joint Surg. **63A**:322, 1981.

70. De Lee, J. C., Wilkens, K. E., Rogers, K. F., and Rockwood, C. A.: Fracture separation of the distal humeral epiphysis. J. Bone Joint Surg. **62A**:46, 1980.

71. Eppright, R. H., and Wilkins, K. E.: Fractures and dislocations of the elbow. *In* Rockwood, C. A., Jr., and Green, D. P. (eds.): Fractures, Vol. 1. Philadelphia, J. B. Lippincott Co., 1975, p. 487.

72. Fowles, J. V., Slimane, N., and Kassab, M. T.: Elbow dislocation with avulsion of the medial humeral epicondyle. J. Bone Joint Surg. **72**:102, 1990.

73. Grantham, S. A., and Tietjen, R.: Transcondylar fracture—dislocation of the elbow. J. Bone Joint Surg. **58A**:1030, 1976.

74. Heilbronner, D. M., Manili, A., and Little, R. E.: Elbow dislocation during overhead skeletal traction therapy. Clin. Orthop. **147**:185, 1981.

75. Holbrook, J. L., and Green, N. E.: Divergent pediatric elbow dislocation. A case report. Clin. Orthop. Rel. Res. **234**:72, 1988.

76. Kaplan, S. S., and Reckling, R. W.: Fracture separation of the lower humeral epiphysis with medial displacement. J. Bone Joint Surg. **53A**:1105, 1971.

77. Linscheid, R. L., and Wheeler, D. K.: Elbow dislocations. J.A.M.A. **194**:1171, 1965.

78. McAuliffe, T. B., and Williams, D.: Transverse divergent dislocation of the elbow. Injury **19**:279, 1988.

79. Meyn, M. A., Jr., and Quibley, T. B.: Reduction of posterior dislocation of the elbow by traction on the dangling arm. Clin. Orthop. **103**:106, 1974.

80. Oury, J. H., Roe, R. D., and Laning, R. C.: A case of bilateral anterior dislocations of the elbow. J. Bone Joint Surg. **12**:170, 1972.

81. Patrick, J.: Fracture of the medial epicondyle with displacement into the elbow joint. J. Bone Joint Surg. **28**:143, 1946.

82. Protzman, R. R.: Dislocation of the elbow joint. J. Bone Joint Surg. **60A**:539, 1978.

83. Rang, M.: Children's Fractures. Philadelphia, J. B. Lippincott Co., 1983.

84. Schwab, G. H., Bennett, J. B., Woods, G. W., and Tollos, H. S.: Biomechanics of the elbow instability—the medial collateral ligament. Clin. Orthop. **146**:42, 1980.

85. Smith, F. M.: Children's elbow injuries: fractures and dislocations. Clin. Orthop. **50**:7, 1967.

86. Smith, F. M.: Displacement of the medial epicondyle of the humerus into the elbow joint. Ann. Surg. **124**:410, 1946.

87. Sovio, O. M., and Tredwell, S. J.: Divergent dislocation of the elbow in a child. J. Pediatr. Orthop. **6**:96, 1986.

88. Tachdjian, M. O.: Pediatric Orthopaedics, Vol. 2. Philadelphia, W. B. Saunders Co., 1972, p. 1604.

• COMPLICATIONS OF DISLOCATION OF THE ELBOW IN CHILDREN

89. Boe, S., Holst-Neilson, F.: Intra-articular entrapment of the median nerve after dislocation of the elbow. J. Hand Surg. **12**:356, 1987.

90. Floyd, W. E., 3rd, Gebhardt, M. C., and Emans, J. B.: Intra-articular entrapment of the median nerve after elbow dislocation in children. J. Hand Surg. **12**:704, 1987.

91. Grimer, R. J., and Brooks, S.: Brachial artery damage accompanying closed posterior dislocation of the elbow. J. Bone Joint Surg. **67**:378, 1985.

92. Green, N. E.: Entrapment of the median nerve following elbow dislocation. J. Pediatr. Orthop. **3**:384, 1983.

93. Hallet, J.: Entrapment of the median nerve after dislocation of the elbow. J. Bone Joint Surg. **63B**:408, 1981.

94. Kerian, R.: Elbow dislocation and its association with vascular disruption. J. Bone Joint Surg. **51**:756, 1969.

95. Louis, D. S., Ricciardi, J., and Sprengler, D. M.: Arterial injuries: a complication of posterior elbow dislocation. J. Bone Joint Surg. **56A**:1631, 1974.

96. Matev, I.: A radiological sign of entrapment of the median nerve in the elbow joint after posterior dislocation. J. Bone Joint Surg. **58B**:353, 1976.

97. Noonan, K. J., and Blair, W. F.: Chronic median-nerve entrapment after posterior fracture-dislocation of the elbow. J. Bone Joint Surg. **77A**:1572, 1995.

98. Rubens, M. K., and Aulicino, P. L.: Open elbow dislocation with brachial artery disruption: a case report and review of the literature. Orthopaedics **9**:539, 1986.

99. Stiger, R. N., Larrick, R. D., and Meyer, T. F.: Median nerve entrapment following elbow dislocations in children. J. Bone Joint Surg. **51A**:381, 1969.

100. Tayob, A. A., and Shively, R. A.: A bilateral elbow dislocation with inter-articular displacement of medial epicondyle. J. Trauma **20**:332, 1980.

101. Thompson, H. C., and Garcia, A.: Myositis ossifans after massive elbow injuries. Clin. Orthop. **50**:129, 1967.

• RECURRENT DISLOCATION OF THE ELBOW IN CHILDREN

102. Beighton, P., and Horan, F.: Orthopaedic aspects of the Ehlers-Danlos syndrome. J. Bone Joint Surg. **51B**:444, 1969.

103. Hall, R. M.: Recurrent posterior dislocation of the elbow joint in a boy. J. Bone Joint Surg. **35B**:56, 1953.

104. Hassmann, G. C., Brunn, F., and Neer, C. S.: Recurrent dislocation of the elbow. J. Bone Joint Surg. **57A**:1080, 1975.

105. Hening, J. A., and Sullivan, J. A.: Recurrent dislocation of the elbow. J. Pediatr. Orthop. **9**:483, 1989.

106. Jacobs, R. L.: Recurrent dislocation of the elbow: a case report and review of the literature. Clin. Orthop. **74**:151, 1971.

107. Mantle, J.: Recurrent posterior dislocation of the elbow. J. Bone Joint Surg. **48B**:590, 1966.

108. Morrey, B. F.: Complex instability of the elbow. J. Bone Joint Surg. **79A**:460, 1997.

109. O'Driscoll, S. W., Bell, D. F., and Morrey, B. F.: Posterolateral rotatory instability of the elbow. J. Bone Joint Surg. **73A**:440, 1991.

110. Osborne, G., and Cotterill, P.: Recurrent dislocation of the elbow. J. Bone Joint Surg. **48B**:340, 1966.

111. Rames, R. D., and Strecker, W. B.: Recurrent elbow dislocations in a patient with Ehlers-Danlos syndrome. Orthopaedics **14**:707, 1991.

112. Trias, A., and Comeau, Y.: Recurrent dislocation of the elbow in children. Clin. Orthop. **100**:74, 1974.

• PULLED ELBOW

113. Amir, D., Frank, J., and Pogrund, H.: Pulled elbow and hypermobility of joints. Clin. Orthop. Rel. Res. **257**:94, 1990.

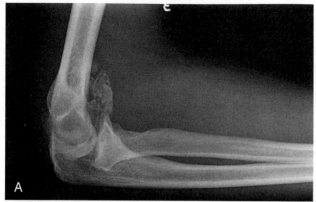

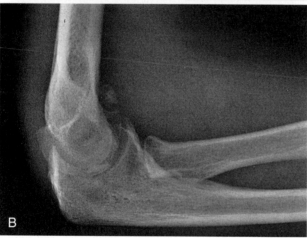

FIGURE 22–1 • *A*, A 16-year-and-10-month-old male sustained an injury to his right elbow while playing football, did not seek medical attention, and presented 2 years later with pain, locking, and elbow range of motion from −40 degrees extension to 130 degrees flexion. *B*, Six months following excision of ectopic bone, excision of loose bodies, anterior capsulotomy, radial head excision, and continuous passive motion with elbow range of motion from −30 degrees extension to 130 degrees flexion.

limitation, but it is reasonable to attempt to restore normal ROM through a trial of nonoperative treatment. We have found that the use of splints is helpful and better tolerated than physical therapy (see Chapter 12). Very seldom is surgical treatment indicated for patients with greater than −40 degrees of extension or greater than 125 degrees of flexion. Extension is the most common portion of the arc affected. Limitation of pronation and supination is observed almost exclusively after radial head and neck fractures and suggests involvement of the radiocapitellar joint or proximal radioulnar synostosis if no rotational motion is present.

STABILITY

Varus or valgus instability is classified by the method of Morrey.[13] The elbow is stable if there is no varus or valgus laxity. Mild instability exists if varus or valgus laxity is present but is less than 5 degrees in either direction. Elbows were considered moderately unstable if varus or valgus laxity was considered to be 5 to 10 degrees and associated with mild symptoms. Severely unstable elbows had greater than 10 degrees varus and valgus laxity and caused limitations in daily activities. Varus and valgus instability associ-

ated with elbow stiffness is uncommon in children unless bone has been resected.

Imaging Studies

PLAIN FILM RADIOGRAPHS

Anteroposterior and lateral radiographs are taken for all patients and provide helpful information regarding fracture union, fracture reduction, elbow alignment, loose bodies, and bone stock.

TOMOGRAMS

Although used less frequently than in the past, our experience suggests that standard plane tomograms provide the best means of imaging the osseous anatomy of the elbow. Lateral tomograms are obtained in elbows of patients sustaining intra-articular fractures to assess joint congruity. Anteroposterior tomograms are most helpful when assessing distal humeral anatomy.

Accurate imaging by tomography of loose bodies and other osseous pathology impeding elbow range of motion greatly facilitates preoperative planning and helps ensure that all pathologic conditions contributing to elbow stiffness are identified and addressed at surgery.

COMPUTED TOMOGRAPHY

Although computed tomography (CT) scanning provides the best axial images of the elbow, three-dimensional CT reconstructions in the coronal and sagittal planes are not as clear as standard tomographic reconstructions.

Because images in the coronal and sagittal planes are the most helpful views in assessing the etiology of elbow stiffness, we rarely use CT scans when imaging the elbow.

MAGNETIC RESONANCE IMAGING

Recent literature has recommended magnetic resonance imaging (MRI) of the stiff elbow.[1] However, MRI does not image osseous anatomy as well as standard radiographic techniques. For specific indications, MRI can provide helpful information. Evaluation for possible avascular necrosis, physeal injury, and soft tissue lesions is often facilitated by MRI. In general, as with CT, transverse images are not helpful in assessing elbow contracture.

TREATMENT: INDICATIONS AND CONTRAINDICATIONS

Nonoperative Treatment

The amount of time transpiring between the injury and the presence of an established contracture affects treatment. Early and aggressive passive ROM exercises have been demonstrated to cause heterotopic ossification in pediatric patients.[16]

During the first 2 months following injury, therefore, active ROM is used primarily. In the adult, the likelihood of improvement with nonoperative efforts such as therapy or even splinting is unlikely. The same is true of children in our experience (see Chapter 33).

PHYSICAL THERAPY

If decreased elbow ROM is present later than 2 months following injury, passive ROM exercises and stretching may be employed. Passive ROM and stretching should be limited by elbow swelling, pain, and inflammation. Any significant inflammation about the elbow caused by aggressive therapy may worsen elbow stiffness. The use of ice and a scheduled nonsteroidal anti-inflammatory drug (NSAID) often reduces inflammation and improves patient comfort, allowing greater progress to be made with therapy. Ideally, a physical therapist with an interest and competency in upper extremity rehabilitation instructs the patient on a home program of active and gentle passive stretching exercises that the patient performs daily and that are used in combination with ice and NSAIDs. In fact, because the likelihood of the therapist's being knowledgeable is limited, we prefer splinting to formal physical therapy.

SPLINTING

Previous authors have described the use of static and dynamic splinting to improve elbow range of motion. Green and McCoy[3] reported the use of a turnbuckle splint for elbow contracture, whereas others have advocated dynamic splinting.[5] Our current practice is to use a static splint primarily at night, with an adjustable hinge that can be fixed in any degree of flexion (see Chapter 12). Each night before retiring, the patient applies the brace to the affected elbow. Preferably this is immediately following a session of stretching. Patients with a primary limitation in extension place the elbow and splint in maximal extension to the point of tolerance and fix the hinge in this position. Conversely, patients with a primary limitation in flexion fix the splint in maximal flexion, again limited by pain. Patients with significant limitation in both planes alternate nights in flexion and extension. This nonoperative regimen of active and passive ROM exercises, NSAIDs, and splinting should be tried for a minimum of 1 and up to 3 months before its effectiveness can be determined.

Surgical Treatment

Patients whose injuries are more than 6 months old and who have failed an adequate trial of nonoperative treatment as described above, and who experience significant functional limitation due to elbow stiffness, may be considered for operative treatment. Successful surgical treatment addresses all extrinsic and intrinsic pathologic elements contributing to stiffness. In the pediatric patient, release of the extrinsic soft tissue contracture is typically performed in a manner similar to the technique described by Husband and Hastings[6] or Mansat and Morrey.[10] Anterior capsulectomy

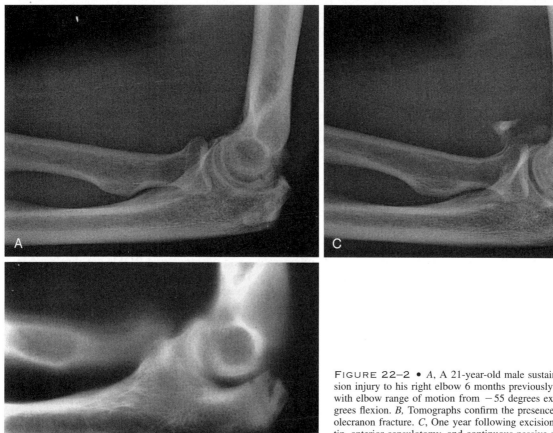

FIGURE 22–2 • A, A 21-year-old male sustained a hyperextension injury to his right elbow 6 months previously and presented with elbow range of motion from −55 degrees extension to 140 degrees flexion. B, Tomographs confirm the presence of a previous olecranon fracture. C, One year following excision of the olecranon tip, anterior capsulotomy, and continuous passive motion, radiographs demonstrate additional ectopic bone formation about the elbow. Range of motion measured −20 degrees extension and 140 degrees flexion.

three patients regained no motion or even lost motion after surgery.

COMPLICATIONS

The combination of previous surgery, extensive dissection, external fixation, and immediate ROM following surgery places surgical patients at risk for complications. In the Mayo series, there was one deep wound infection requiring surgical débridement, one transient radial nerve palsy, one postoperative hematoma that required surgical evacuation, and one patient with persistent contracture without improvement following surgery. Patients undergoing distraction arthroplasty or fascial interposition arthroplasty are at greater risk for complications than patients treated with surgical release without external fixation.[13]

AUTHORS' CURRENT PRACTICE

The assessment and surgical techniques for treating contracture in the child is similar to that of the adult. However, because of compliance issues as well as problems with less predictable response to surgery, we make every effort to avoid surgical release until the physes have closed. The use of splints before surgery is particularly helpful to improve the arc to the extent that surgery may be able to be avoided, it allows assessment of compliance, and splints can be used after surgery should this become necessary. As noted, a home splint therapy program is preferred to formal physical therapy and is most effective within 3 months of injury but is used up to 6 months after the onset of stiffness. Overall surgical treatment for elbow stiffness in the pediatric patient is to be avoided if possible, and the unpredictable result is carefully explained if surgery is undertaken.

REFERENCES

 1. Fortier, M. V., Forster, B. B., Pinney, S., and Regan, W.: MR assessment of post-traumatic flexion contracture of the elbow. J. Magnet. Res. Imag. 5:473–477, 1995.
 2. Gates, H. S., Sullivan, F. L., and Urbaniak, J. R.: Anterior capsulotomy and continuous passive motion in the treatment of post-traumatic flexion contracture of the elbow. J. Bone Joint Surg. 74A:1229–1234, 1992.
 3. Green, D. P., and McCoy, H.: Turnbuckle orthotic correction of elbow-flexion contractures after acute injuries. J. Bone Joint Surg. 61A:1092, 1979.
 4. Henrikson, B.: Supracondylar fracture of the humerus in children. Acta Chir. Scand. 369:1, 1966.
 5. Hepburn, G. R., and Crivelli, K. J.: Use of elbow Dynasplint for reduction of elbow flexion contracture. J. Sports Ther. 5:269, 1984.
 6. Husband, J. B., and Hastings, H.: The later approach for operative release of post-traumatic contracture of the elbow. J. Bone Joint Surg. 72A:1353, 1990.
 7. Jarvis, J. G., and D'Astous, J. L.: The pediatric T-supracondylar fracture. J. Pediatr. Orthoped. 4:697, 1984.
 8. Josefsson, O., Gentz, C., and Johnell, O.: Surgical versus nonsurgical treatment of ligamentous injuries following dislocations of the elbow joint. A prospective randomized study. J. Bone Joint Surg. 69A:605, 1987.
 9. Lal, H. M., and Bhan, S.: Delayed open reduction for supracondylar fractures of the humerus. Int. Orthoped. 15:189, 1991.
10. Mansat, P., and Morrey, B. F.: The column procedure: a limited lateral approach for extrinsic contracture of the elbow. J. Bone Joint Surg. 80A:1603, 1998.
11. Mih, A. D., and Wolf, F. G.: Surgical release of elbow-capsular contracture in pediatric patients. J. Pediatr. Orthop. 14:458, 1994.
12. Mital, M. A., Barber, J. E., and Stinson, J. T.: Ectopic bone formation in children and adolescent with head injuries: its management. J. Pediatr. Orthop. 7:83, 1987.
13. Morrey, B. F.: Post-traumatic contracture of the elbow. J. Bone Joint Surg. 72A:601, 1990.
14. Morrey, B. F., Askew, L. J., An, K. N., and Chao, E. Y.: A biomechanical study of normal functional elbow motion. J. Bone Joint Surg. 63A:872, 1981.
15. Papvasilious, V. A., and Beslikas, T. A.: T-condylar fractures of the distal humeral condyles during childhood: an analysis of six cases. J. Pediatr. Orthop. 6:302, 1986.
16. Pirone, A. M., Graham, H. K., and Krajbich, J. I.: Management of displaced extension-type supracondylar fractures of the humerus in children. J. Bone Joint Surg. 70A:641, 1988.
17. Thompson, H. G., and Garcia, A.: Myositis ossificans: aftermath of elbow injuries. Clin. Orthop. Rel. Res. 50:129, 1967.
18. Urbaniak, J. R., Hansen, P. E., Beissinger, S. F., and Aitken, M.: Correction of post-traumatic flexion contracture of the elbow by anterior capsulotomy. J Bone Joint Surg. 67A:1160, 1985.
19. Wedge, J. H., and Roberson, D. E.: Displaced fractures of the neck of the radius. J. Bone Joint Surg. 64B:256, 1982.

Adult Trauma

A. FRACTURES AND DISLOCATIONS

<table>
<tr><td>

• CHAPTER 23 •

Fractures of the Distal Humerus in Adults

• JESSE B. JUPITER and BERNARD F. MORREY

</td></tr>
</table>

Fractures involving the distal end of the humerus are among the most complex of fractures to manage effectively. Recommendations for treatment have ranged from essentially no treatment to operative reduction and extensive internal fixation.[1–13]

A number of reasons can be offered to explain why many clinicians have expressed pessimism about the outcome of these fractures. In the first place, the complex structural anatomy of the distal end of the humerus, with its unique orientation of articular surfaces supported by a meager amount of cancellous bone, presents a constant challenge to even the boldest and most experienced fracture surgeon. Figure 23–1 shows a section through the trochlear notch at 90 degrees to the coronal plane and demonstrates the precise articular relationships, which are often grossly disturbed and must be restored after a fracture. A similar view through the radial head and the capitellar articulation (Fig. 23–2) further illustrates the close tolerances.

Second, because these fractures tend to be uncommon, surgeons rarely can gain much experience in managing the variety of fracture patterns.

Finally, the sequelae of pain and loss of motion are well recognized after all forms of elbow trauma as are the more complex intra-articular fractures. The sensitivity of the surrounding joint capsule and soft tissue envelope to both trauma and surgical intervention can thwart even the most carefully planned and cautiously executed attempt at internal fixation.

INCIDENCE

Several large series suggest that fractures about the elbow account for approximately 7 percent of fractures treated.[14–17] Of these fractures, approximately a third involve the distal humerus, so distal humeral fractures account for approximately 2 percent of all fractures.

CLASSIFICATION

Many classifications of fractures of the distal end of the humerus have been based on the concept that the distal humerus terminates in two condyles (thus the terms *condylar*, *transcondylar*, and *bicondylar* fractures). Because classifications function best when they guide the treating physician's decision making, it may be better to view the distal end of the humerus as being composed of two diverging columns that support an intercalary articular surface. The

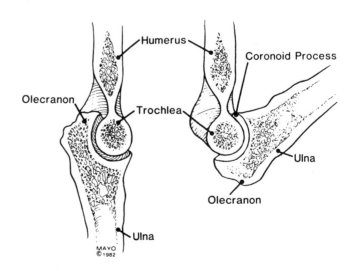

FIGURE 23–1 • A sagittal section through the trochlea demonstrates the precise relationship of the trochlea, the olecranon, and the fossae, which permit the extremes of flexion and extension.

293

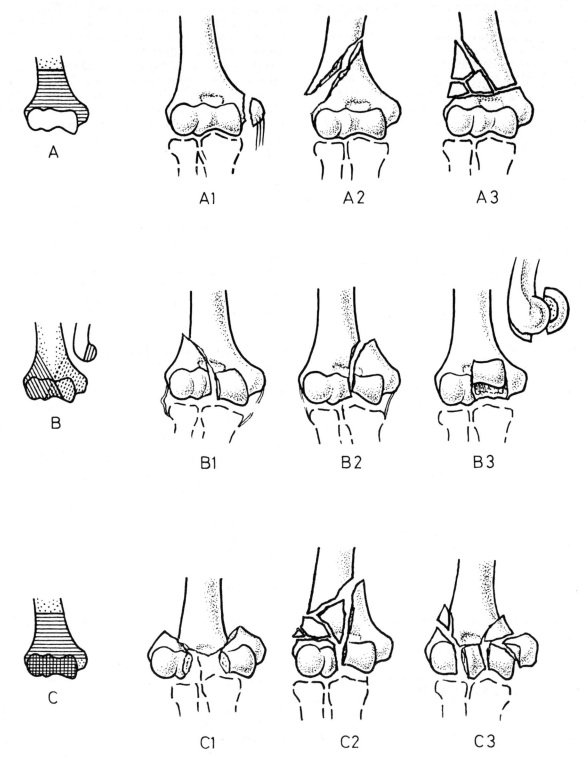

FIGURE 23–4 • The AO classification of fractures of the distal humerus. (From Müller, M. E., et al.: Comprehensive Classification of Fractures of Long Bones. New York, Springer-Verlag, 1990.)

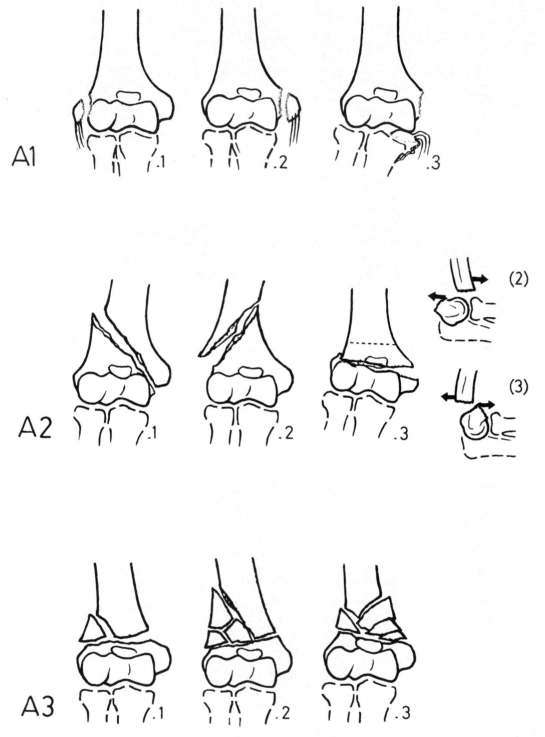

FIGURE 23–4 • *Continued*

posterior displacement of the distal fragment.

High Flexion. The fracture line is oblique, beginning anteroproximally and extending posterodistally, with anterior displacement of the distal fragment.

Low Extension. The fracture line is transverse or slightly oblique, with posterior displacement of the distal fragment (AO subgroup A2.3).

Low Flexion. The fracture line is transverse or slightly oblique, with anterior displacement of the distal fragment (AO subgroup A2.3).

Abduction. The fracture line is oblique, extending from lateral proximally to distal medially, with lateral displacement of the distal fragment (AO subgroup A2.1).

Adduction. The fracture line is oblique, extending from medial proximally to distal medially, with lateral displacement of the distal fragment (AO subgroup A2.2).

The AO group A3, with its three subdivisions, identifies fractures associated with metaphyseal comminution (see Fig. 23–4).

MECHANISM

Transcolumn fractures most often are the result of a fall on an outstretched hand with a posteriorly directed force on a flexed elbow. Although flexion injuries are much less common and are thought to be the result of an anteriorly directed force on the posterior aspect of the elbow,[42] in low-energy, low transcolumn fractures in elderly persons, anterior displacement of the distal fragment may be more common than was previously recognized (Fig. 23–9).[40] With secondary, more violent trauma, these fractures may

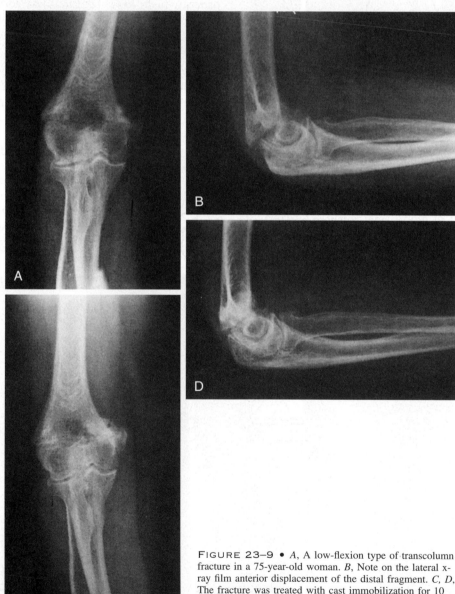

FIGURE 23–9 • *A*, A low-flexion type of transcolumn fracture in a 75-year-old woman. *B*, Note on the lateral x-ray film anterior displacement of the distal fragment. *C, D*, The fracture was treated with cast immobilization for 10 days in extension and then 5 days in flexion. (From Bryan, R. J.: Fractures about the elbow in adults. *In* The American Academy of Orthopaedic Surgeons: Instructional Course Lecture. Vol. 30. St. Louis, C. V. Mosby Co., 1981.)

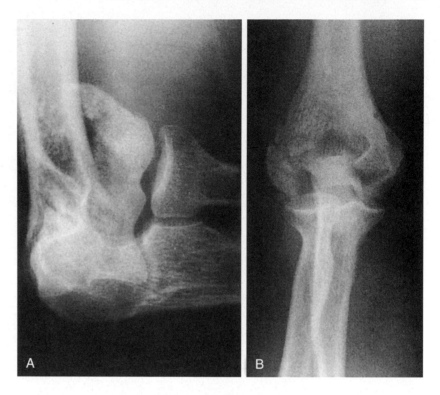

FIGURE 23-10 • A low transcolumn fracture in a 50-year-old woman. Anteroposterior radiograph *(A)* demonstrates the displaced fracture. An anteroposterior radiograph with traction applied to the forearm *(B)* proves a clearer picture of the fracture, suggesting some intra-articular involvement. (From Mehne, D. K., and Jupiter, J. B.: Fractures of the distal humerus. *In* Browner, B., Jupiter, J., Levine, A., and Trafton, P. [eds.]: Skeletal Trauma. Vol. II. Philadelphia, W. B. Saunders Co., 1991, p. 1171.)

be associated with significant soft tissue injury, including nerve and vascular disruption.[20]

DIAGNOSIS

Transcolumn fractures ordinarily present with visible deformity: The neurovascular status of the extremity must be carefully evaluated from the outset, because the brachial artery and all three major nerves can be injured with these fractures.[43] Routine anteroposterior and lateral radiographs generally are adequate to define the nature of the injuries. At times, however, it may not be possible to differentiate a low transcolumn fracture from a bicolumn injury, and an anteroposterior radiograph taken with traction applied to the elbow may allow better definition of the fracture (Fig. 23–10).

TREATMENT

It is difficult to appreciate the outcome of these fractures, because in studies they are often grouped with intra-articular fractures of the distal humerus[3, 7, 13] or injuries about the elbow.[24, 44, 45]

Closed Manipulation

Many authors have advocated closed reduction and plaster immobilization,[42, 45, 46] as they have for similar fractures in the pediatric age group. The techniques of closed reduction are the same as those for any displaced fracture. For extension injuries, longitudinal traction is used to overcome the pull of the triceps and the biceps. The surgeon uses a thumb to push the distal fragment distally and anteriorly

(Fig. 23–11). Reduction is confirmed fluoroscopically or with anteroposterior and lateral radiographs. A well-padded but properly molded splint should support the elbow in enough flexion to maintain the reduction, but considerable care must be exercised to preserve the circulation and avoid undue swelling. The forearm is kept in neutral rotation.

Reduction and immobilization of flexion fractures is more difficult. It must be kept in mind that they are more common in elders.[40] Sultanpur described a technique of cylindrical casting that may be effective for closed management of anteriorly displaced fractures.[42] It is designed to direct force posteriorly on the distal humeral fragment while holding the elbow in some flexion. Traction is applied in line with the axis of the humeral shaft, with the forearm in supination and the elbow flexed about 85 degrees. Circular plaster is applied to the brachium, which is then lifted forward as the elbow is flexed to 95 to 100 degrees. The cast is then extended below the elbow as pressure is applied along the line of the ulna. While the plaster is hardening, the surgeon places one hand posteriorly to support the cast and uses the other hand to push the patient's forearm posteriorly to maintain fracture reduction. The elbow is immobilized for a minimum of 2 weeks for impacted, stable fractures and for upward of 4 weeks for unstable, displaced fractures.

Skeletal Traction

Current indications for skeletal traction using an olecranon pin are similar to those for the pediatric age group. These include fractures associated with excessive soft tissue swelling and fractures in a polytrauma patient who needs temporary skeletal stabilization, maintaining alignment and soft tissue length until definitive treatment can be ren-

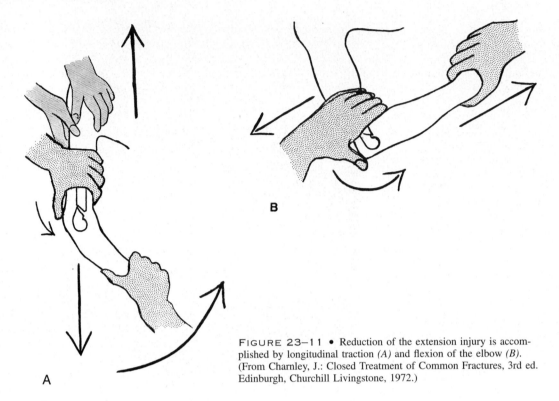

FIGURE 23–11 • Reduction of the extension injury is accomplished by longitudinal traction *(A)* and flexion of the elbow *(B)*. (From Charnley, J.: Closed Treatment of Common Fractures, 3rd ed. Edinburgh, Churchill Livingstone, 1972.)

dered.[47, 48] Avoidance of prolonged traction lessens the likelihood of internal fixation complicated by infection.

PERCUTANEOUS PIN FIXATION

In view of the fact that the prolonged bed rest required for skeletal traction may be poorly tolerated by adults and can lead to loss of reduction or pin tract infection, internal fixation has become increasingly accepted for management of these difficult fratures. The indications for percutaneous pin fixation are low transcolumn or supracondylar level fractures in (1) elderly persons, (2) those with advanced osteopenia, and (3) those whose clinical situation is believed to be inappropriate for open reduction and internal fixation (Fig. 23–12).

The technique was described as early as 1936 by Miller[49] and has been tremendously facilitated by the development of the image intensifier. With the elbow held in 90 degrees

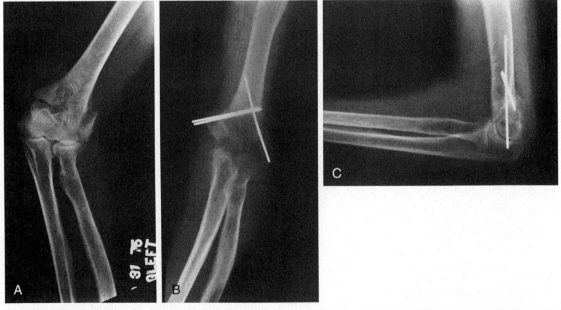

FIGURE 23–12 • Transcolumn fracture in a 65-year-old woman. *A*, Closed reduction could not be maintained, and, under a limited open procedure, the fracture was fixed with percutaneous Kirschner wires *(B, C)*. Final motion was 35 to 145 degrees (From Bryan, R. S.: Fractures about the elbow in adults. *In* The American Academy of Orthopaedic Surgeons: Instructional Course Lectures. Vol. 30. St. Louis, C. V. Mosby Co., 1981.)

of flexion, smooth (0.062-inch) pins are placed from each epicondyle across the fracture line into the opposite cortex. The pins should be directed at a 35- to 45-degree angle to the longitudinal axis of the humeral shaft. Permanent radiographs are recommended intraoperatively to accurately monitor pin placement and fracture reduction. The pins are cut off just below the skin and are covered with an antibiotic ointment and foam padding. A well-molded and well-padded posterior splint is applied with the elbow in 90 degrees of flexion and the forearm in neutral rotation. Percutaneous pins make it unnecessary to maintain the elbow in extreme flexion and even to use a circular cast in the face of soft tissue swelling.

Caution must be taken to minimize the possibility of injury to adjacent nerves, in particular the ulnar nerve. This can best be avoided by either exposing the nerve directly or using smooth pins placed into the anterosuperior aspect of the media epicondyle (thus avoiding the cubital tunnel).

Once postoperative swelling has diminished, the posterior splint is best converted to a circular, long-arm cast. The pins generally can be removed without anesthesia in the clinic between 4 and 6 weeks postoperatively. The timing of motion is begun, depending in part on the intrinsic stability of the reduction and radiographic evidence of union.

Open Reduction and Internal Fixation

Unstable intracapsular, extra-articular fractures are often difficult to reduce accurately by closed means. In addition, the limited bone stock may make percutaneous pin fixation unpredictable. Although gaining surgical access may be complex, the fracture fragments small, and a large portion

of the distal fragment covered with articular cartilage, well-planned and well-executed internal fixation is still considered the treatment of choice. The timing, techniques, and postoperative care are identical to those for intra-articular fractures (see section on Intra-articular Bicolumn Fractures).

Authors' Preferred Method of Treatment

Because many of these fractures occur in elderly persons with osteopenia, we would ordinarily attempt closed reduction and, if that were successful, percutaneous pin fixation. If this could not be satisfactorily accomplished, particularly in a more active person, our approach would likely be open reduction and internal fixation (Fig. 23–13).

Intra-articular Bicolumn Fractures (AO Group C3)

INCIDENCE

It is difficult to estimate the frequency of bicolumn intra-articular fractures, primarily because not all investigators have used a single classification system. Hitzrot reported that four of 34 distal humeral fractures in adults were of this type.[15] Lecestre and colleagues reported on 503 fractures of the distal humerus, of which 25 percent were simple fractures, and 37 percent comminuted bicolumn fractures.[50] Knight placed the incidence at about 5 percent of all distal humeral fractures in adults.[12]

MECHANISM OF INJURY

The common denominator of all split fractures of the trochlea and the distal humerus is believed to be the

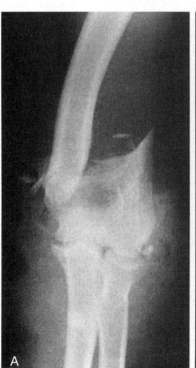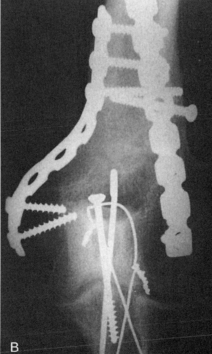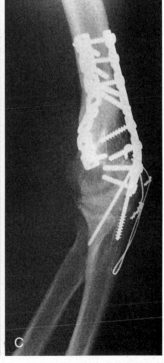

FIGURE 23–13 • A, An anteroposterior x-ray view of an open (grade I) transcolumn fracture in a 28-year-old man. Following thorough débridement and irrigation, stable internal fixation was accomplished with the plates extended distally to secure fixation to the distal fragment (B, C).

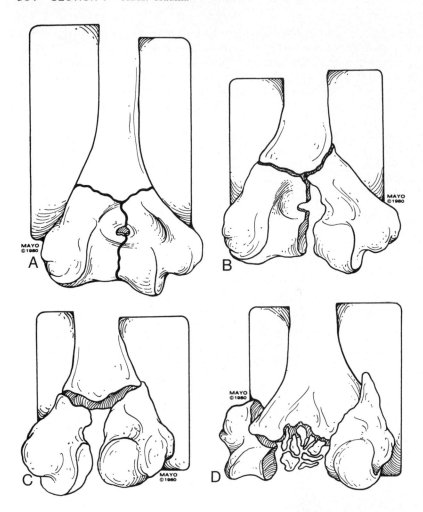

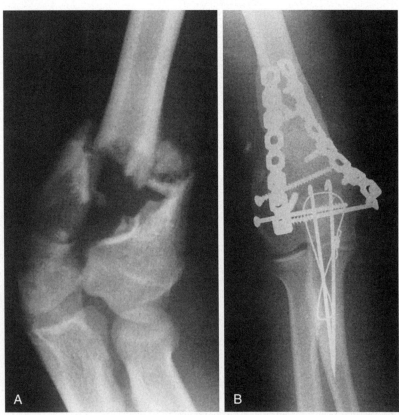

FIGURE 23–14 • *A*, Type I undisplaced T-condylar fracture of the elbow. *B*, Type II displaced but not rotated T-condylar fracture. *C*, Type III displaced and rotated T-condylar fracture. *D*, Type IV displaced, rotated, and comminuted T-condylar fracture. (From Bryan, R. J.: Fractures about the elbow in adults. *In* The American Academy of Orthopaedic Surgeons: Instructional Course Lectures. Vol 30. St. Louis, C. V. Mosby Co., 1981.)

FIGURE 23–15 • An example of a high T bicolumn, intra-articular distal humerus fracture *(A)* treated with stable internal fixation. Note the use of several interfragmentary screws *(B)*.

"wedge" effect of the longitudinal groove of the olecranon. The actual position of the elbow at the time of impact has been the subject of some debate. Smith[22] believed that the injury resulted from axial loading of the extended elbow, the coronoid process serving as the wedge. In 1936, Reich[51] observed that the cause of the fracture was usually a blow to the flexed elbow, the olecranon acting as the wedge, splitting the trochlea and distal humerus with or without associated comminution.[52, 53]

It is interesting that few mechanical studies have been directed at helping us understand the mechanism of intra-articular bicolumn fractures. In cadaver studies performed at the University of Southern California Biomechanics Laboratory, direct force applied to the olecranon with the elbow flexed at 90 degrees repeatedly produced transverse olecranon fractures. The same force directed to the olecranon with the elbow flexed beyond 90 degrees always produced a bicolumn fracture.[54] It seems clear that the contraction of the flexor and extensor muscle masses also contributes to the development of this fracture.

ASSOCIATED INJURIES

Bicolumn fractures are commonly associated with overlying soft tissue trauma. The incidence of open fractures has varied from 10 percent to as much as 50 percent in reported series.[7, 55–58] Associated vascular injury, however, is not common with these injuries in adults.[60, 61, 91] The prevalence of ulnar nerve dysfunction is becoming more widely recognized.[139, 140]

CLASSIFICATION

Although Desault[62] was the first to recognize the articular separation of these fractures in 1811, it was Reich, in 1936, who described them as T or Y fractures.[51] Riseborough and Radin, extended the classification in 1969, by subdividing these into four categories based on separation, rotation, and comminution of the distal articular surfaces (Fig. 23–14).[9]

The comprehensive AO classification of Müller and colleagues[19] further expanded these subdivisions (see Fig. 23–4). Type C, with its three major divisions and nine subdivisions based on the degree of complexity and articular and extra-articular fragmentation, has been particularly useful in evaluating treatment outcomes. The system is complex, however, and may not always be useful, in a practical sense, for preoperative planning for a particular fracture.

Another classification, proposed by Mehne and Matta,[41, 54] addresses specific characteristics of the anatomy of the injury to the skeletal columns. This approach is useful for preoperative planning of the type and placement of the internal fixation.

High T Fracture. A transverse line divides both columns proximal to or at the upper limits of the olecranon fossa. This fracture is the equivalent of AO subgroup C1.1 or C1.2 (Fig. 23–15).

Y Fracture. Oblique fracture lines cross each other, joining in the olecranon fossa to form a distal sagittal fracture line through the trochlea. The oblique fracture lines and large fragments produce broad fracture surfaces that facilitate stable internal fixation. This fracture is also the equivalent of AO subgroup C1.1 or C1.2 (Fig. 23–16).

Low T Fracture. This fracture is among the most common, especially in elderly persons, and is among the most difficult to treat. A transverse line crosses the olecranon fossa just proximal to the trochlea, resulting in relatively small distal fragments. This fracture is the equivalent of the AO subgroup C1.3 (Fig. 23–17).

H Fracture. The H pattern is that of a multifragmented fracture. Fracture lines cross each bony column, the medial column being fractured above and below the medial epicondyle. The lateral column is fractured in a T or Y configuration. The trochlea is rendered a free fragment and typically is comminuted. This fracture is the equivalent of the AO subgroup C3.3 (Fig. 23–18).

Medial Lambda Fracture. The most proximal fracture line exits medially and the lateral fracture line distal to the lateral epicondyle, leaving a small zone for internal fixation on the lateral side. This fracture is a variation of the AO group C2 (Fig. 23–19).

Lateral Lambda Fracture. In this pattern, the medial column remains essentially intact. The surgical exposure may vary from the medial fracture, but fixation tactics are similar to those applied to bicolumn fractures. The most proximal fracture line exits laterally, and the medial fracture line extends distal to the medial epicondyle and thus distal to the end of the medial skeletal column. This fracture also represents a variation of an AO group C2 pattern (Fig. 23–20).

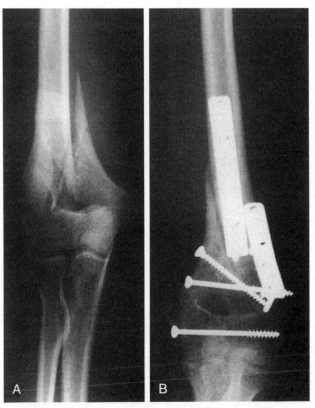

FIGURE 23–16 • *A*, An example of a Y-type bicolumn intra-articular fracture. The broad fracture lines made internal fixation relatively straightforward (*B*).

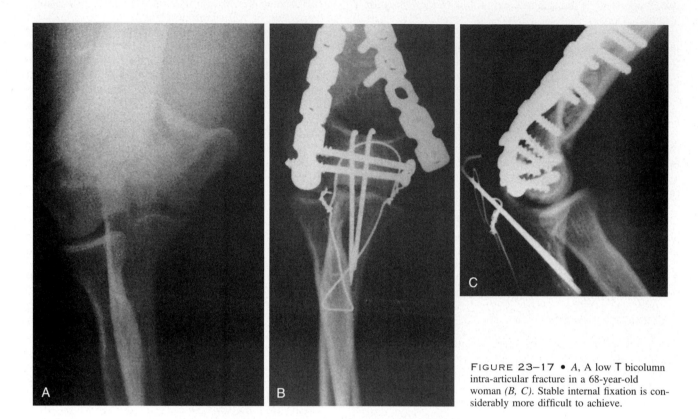

FIGURE 23-17 • *A*, A low T bicolumn intra-articular fracture in a 68-year-old woman *(B, C)*. Stable internal fixation is considerably more difficult to achieve.

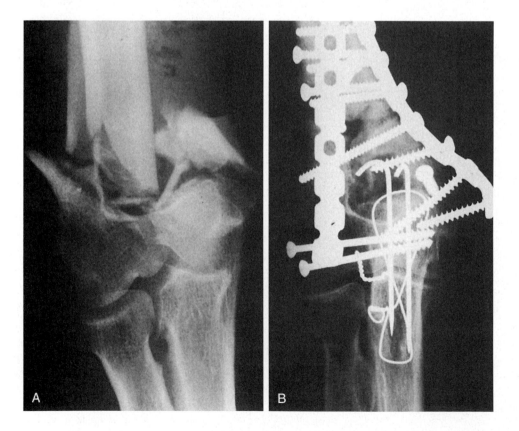

FIGURE 23-18 • *A*, An H-type intra-articular fracture represents an exceptionally difficult surgical procedure *(B)*.

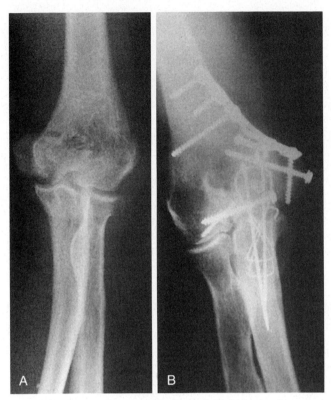

FIGURE 23–19 • An example of a medial lambda type fracture that has most of the lateral skeletal column intact *(A)*. Note the Hebert screws securing intra-articular fragments *(B)*.

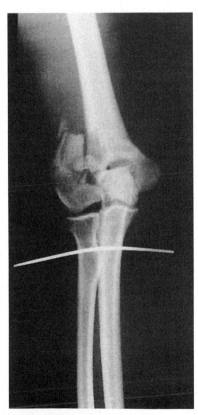

FIGURE 23–20 • An example of a lateral lambda type fracture, with the medial skeletal column intact.

The Mehne and Matta classification does not identify comminution in the fracture patterns (except for the H pattern) or the extent of displacement of the fragments. The surgeon must be wary of articular comminution, which may not be appreciated on the preoperative radiographs. In the operating room, an anteroposterior radiograph made while traction is applied to the forearm can further define the intra-articular anatomy, though not always completely (see Fig. 23–20).

As a further example of the unpredictability of preoperative assessment of the articular fracture patterns, a group of cases has been described that were characterized by disruption of the trochlea in both the sagittal and the coronal planes, in association with a more proximal fracture of the distal metaphysis. This fracture has been termed the *triplane distal humeral fracture* (Fig. 23–21).[63] In these cases, the coronal split of the articular surface could not be accurately assessed on preoperative radiographs.

TREATMENT

The goal of contemporary treatment of intra-articular bi-column fractures of the distal humerus is recovery of as much elbow motion as possible. Thus, surgical management has assumed greater acceptance and importance. By the same token, any surgeon who embarks on operative treatment of these complex injuries is well-advised to recognize the technical difficulties of obtaining secure fixation of the articular fragments.

It is for these reasons that it is always important to be mindful of the nonsurgical management options. Still, the published results of nonoperative treatment are difficult to interpret because rating systems, fracture classifications, data collection, and clinical interpretation vary much. To illustrate this, in one series, an excellent result could extend to include a residual 60-degree flexion contracture.[4]

Nonoperative Treatment
Until the past quarter century, nonoperative treatment was the standard management. The options ranged from closed reduction and casting, to skeletal traction through an olecranon pin, to early motion (the "bag-of-bones" treatment).[1]

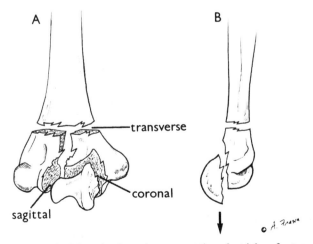

FIGURE 23–21 • A schematic representation of a triplane fracture of the distal humerus in which the trochlea is fractured in both the sagittal and the coronal planes.

Closed Reduction and Immobilization

Closed manipulative reduction generally is performed by applying longitudinal traction with the elbow flexed at 90 degrees and then molding the distal fragments together. Reich[51] recognized the rotational force of the flexor and extensor muscle groups and used ice tongs to press the condylar fragments together while applying traction to align the more proximal transverse fracture. Immobilization with the elbow at 90 degrees of flexion in a splint[15] or a cast for 4 to 6 weeks was standard practice in the past. Recognition of the deleterious effects of prolonged immobilization on elbow mobility has tempered enthusiasm for this approach.

Traction

Before better fixation devices and techniques of "small-fracture fixation" were developed, skeletal traction was the recommended treatment, particularly for multifragmented fractures.[9, 13, 47, 64, 65, 86] The most popular and effective method was overhead skeletal traction, with a pin or a wire placed through the olecranon (Fig. 23–22). Dunlop's traction, with the injured arm out to the side, also has been recommended. To minimize potential problems with pin tract infection,[14, 15] skin traction provided by a flat sling positioned across the proximal forearm with the elbow held at 90 degrees also has been advocated.[68]

Traction maintained for approximately 2 weeks is followed by an additional period of 2 to 3 weeks of immobilization in a splint or cast.[13, 65] Intermittent motion is permitted, depending on alignment, fracture stability, and patient compliance.

Miller[13] reported satisfactory results in seven of 11 patients treated with skeletal traction techniques, although the recorded average arc of motion was 47 degrees. Three other reviews reported combined results of four excellent, four good, and seven poor outcomes with traction (Fig. 23–23).[65, 69, 70] For this reason we prefer to fix even the "low" fractures, when possible.

Traction may be time consuming, and hospitalization may be prolonged, which can be a source of concern for both the patient and the health care administrator.

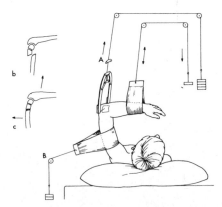

FIGURE 23–22 • Balanced overhead skeletal traction with a pin through the olecranon. This technique helps to achieve and maintain reduction of distal humeral fractures, and the elevation overhead helps to decrease edema. (From Smith, F. M.: Traction and suspension in the treatment of fractures. Surg. Clin. North Am., April, 1951.)

The Bag-of-Bones Approach

Eastwood,[5] in 1937, advocated fracture reduction with compressive manipulation of the distal articular fragments, followed by "collar and cuff," with the elbow flexed as far as possible within the limit imposed by swelling and the need to avoid circulatory embarrassment. Motion in the flexed position is begun at 2 weeks, and at 4 weeks, the elbow should achieve nearly 90 degrees of flexion. Hand and wrist mobilization is started at the outset of treatment, and shoulder mobility is allowed after the first 2 weeks.

Brown and Morgan[1] reported on 10 cases of intra-articular fractures treated with a collar and cuff. They discarded additional sling support by 6 weeks after treatment. Their patient group achieved an average range of motion of 95 degrees, but the authors noted that flexion must be gained by the first 3 weeks if it is to be gained at all. The older patients in their series achieved a greater ranges of motion than the younger ones. Evans observed that, although the older patients appeared to achieve greater arcs of motion than the younger patients with the bag-of-bones treatment, the outcome tended to be a weak and unstable elbow that was unsatisfactory to younger patients.[52]

This treatment is considered only occasionally and is reserved for infirm patients whose complex fractures are not amenable to surgical intervention.

Limited Exposure and Pinning

The rationale that has been given for this technique is that it restores the articular anatomy without further traumatizing surrounding soft tissues with extensive surgical exposure. The fracture is reduced and fixed first with Kirschner wires inserted to maintain the reduction and then with additional pins to secure the fixation. Introduced in 1936, this approach appears to have little application today.[49] Extreme care must be taken to avoid injuring the ulnar nerve. The surgeon should also be extremely careful that the pins do not block motion by intruding into the olecranon fossa (Fig. 23–24).

Open Reduction and Internal Fixation

Favorable results with open reduction and internal fixation have been reported by a number of authors.[3, 7, 10, 55–59, 61, 71, 82] However, careful preoperative planning, attention to detail in the surgical tactics, and a closely supervised postoperative program are essential to a successful outcome.

PREOPERATIVE PLANNING

Although good quality radiographs are essential to determine the particular fracture, the surgeon should plan to have a full set of instruments, which includes small and mini screws, routine and special contour plates, smooth and threaded Kirschner wires, and self-compressing Herbert screws. A sterile arm tourniquet, a fine-bladed oscillating saw, and thin osteotomes also are useful.

SURGICAL TIMING

The management of this fracture can require an exceptionally complex surgical procedure. It is advisable to proceed with the surgery when the equipment is complete, a trained operating team is available, and the surgeon is rested. This may not be possible if the fracture is open or is associated

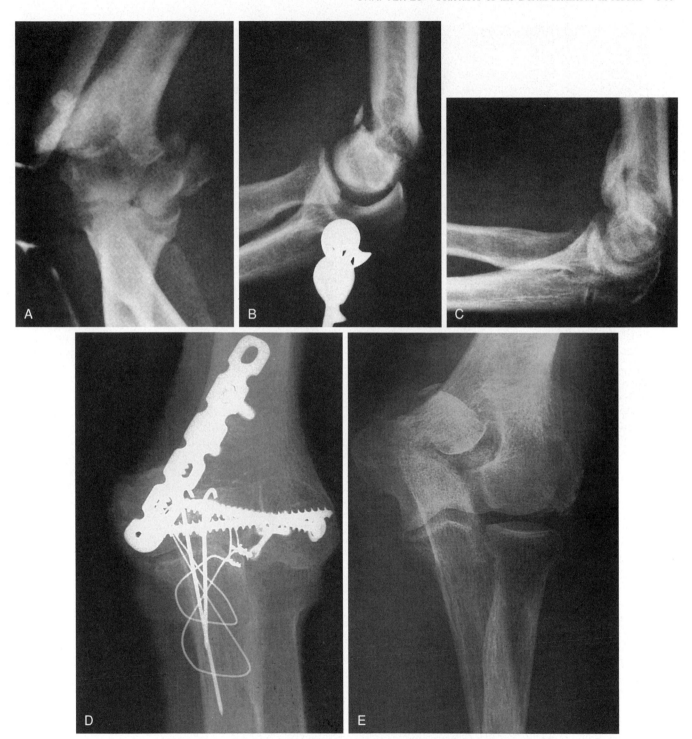

FIGURE 23–23 • *A,* This low T bicolumn fracture was displaced with limited bone stock for internal fixation. *B,* Alignment was obtained with a transolecranon pin. The fracture healed with a range of motion of 40 to 120 degrees at 6 months *(C).* Similar fracture *(D)* successfully treated with rigid fixation *(E).*

with nerve or blood vessel injury. In the presence of undue swelling, early surgery may decompress the fracture hematoma and reduce the pressure on the soft tissues.

In polytrauma patients this fracture must take second place to rapid stabilization of long bone fractures and attention to life-threatening visceral injuries. Although occasionally concern is expressed about the risk of myositis ossificans developing if surgery is delayed, there are few objective data that support such an association with closed intra-articular fractures in the absence of associated head or central nervous system trauma.

OPERATIVE APPROACH

General anesthesia ordinarily is preferred, and the patient is placed in the lateral decubitus position, which provides

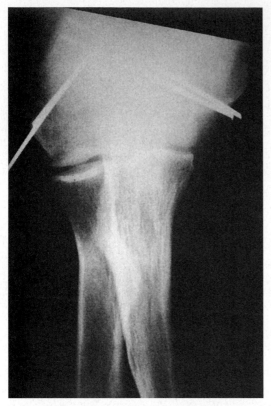

FIGURE 23–24 • A 50-year-old patient with rheumatoid arthritis had a closed reduction and percutaneous pinning for a transcolumn fracture.

ready access to the iliac crest should an autogenous bone graft be needed. Folded drapes or a bolster can be placed between the arm and the chest wall, which will suspend the arm and allow full mobility and ease of access.

The surgical approach must be extensile to offer full exposure to the complex intra-articular and extra-articular anatomy of the distal humerus. The posterior approach has been most widely used, although some (B.F.M.) have extended the lateral approach of Kocher, reflecting the triceps in continuity from the lateral to the medial aspect.[72, 77]

The transolecranon approach modified from that described initially by MacAusland tends to provide the best exposure of the articular fractures.[3] The ulnar nerve is first dissected free from surrounding soft tissue attachments for a distance of approximately 8 cm proximal and 5 cm distal to the cubital tunnel and is transposed into the adjacent soft tissue. The triceps insertion is identified, and the anconeus muscle is lifted up from its attachment to the proximal ulna on its lateral side, affording direct exposure of the articular surface of the olecranon. The midpoint of the olecranon is identified, and a chevron osteotomy is planned to extend across this region with its apex pointing distally (Fig. 23–25). The advantages of a chevron cut over a transverse osteotomy are the ease of repositioning the olecranon at the time of its fixation and a greater amount of cancellous bone in contact-enhancing union. Ideally, the first cut is made with a thin-bladed saw to the level of the subchondral bone of the olecranon's articular surface, and the osteotomy is completed with a thin, sharp osteotome.

This creates a slightly jagged cut of the cartilage, which also adds stability when reapproximated as the surgery is completed.

An oblique osteotomy across the proximal tip of the olecranon has been described, although this could put the attachment of the triceps at risk.[13] Van Gorder[53] popularized an approach first described by Campbell in 1932,[73] which reflects a tongue of triceps distally. Although this approach provides adequate visualization of the skeletal columns, it may offer less than optimal exposure of the intra-articular fracture fragments. Because of the time required for healing, this exposure also may be a limiting factor in regaining elbow motion in the early postoperative period. Reflection of the triceps from medial to lateral, as described by Bryan and Morrey,[74] or lateral to medial[77] also can provide excellent exposure without running the risk of failure of fixation of an olecranon osteotomy.

Alonso-Llames introduced a technique of medial and lateral release of the triceps from the humerus, leaving it attached distally to the olecranon and the ulna. This approach is more useful for extra-articular than for intra-articular fractures. These exposures are described in greater detail in Chapter 8.

FRACTURE STABILIZATION

After surgical exposure, for which in most cases we prefer a transolecranon approach, the proximal olecranon and attached triceps are carefully wrapped in moistened gauze and elevated proximally to expose the entire fracture. It is often only at this juncture that an accurate assessment can be made of the extent of articular involvement. The fracture

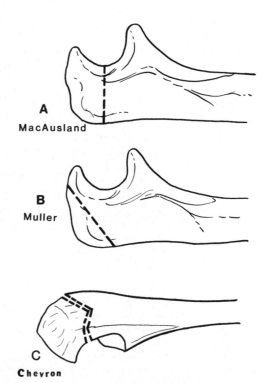

A MacAusland

B Muller

C Chevron

FIGURE 23–25 • Posterior exposure of the distal humerus can be obtained by osteotomizing the proximal ulna. A and B, The chevron cut enhances stability and union (C).

hematoma should be meticulously débrided using a fine dental pick or a pulsatile jet lavage.

The fundamental principle of the internal fixation is to restore the three arms of the anatomic triangular construction of the distal humerus. Although each internal fixation procedure must be tailored to meet the specific demands of the fracture pattern, a number of principles apply to all fractures:

1. Provisional fixation of the fracture fragments with smooth Kirschner wires.

2. Maintenance of normal width and alignment of the axis of the trochlea with the anterior cortex of the humerus.

3. Fixation of the articular fractures onto the bony columns with individually contoured plates.

4. Care to keep the hardware from violating the articular surfaces and the anatomic fossae, to avoid limiting mobility at extremes of the range.

5. Sufficient stability of fixation to permit postoperative mobilization.

In most instances, the surgeon begins by reassembling the fractured trochlea. The width of the trochlea must be preserved. If small fragments are present and cannot be replaced, consideration should be given to filling the defects with cancellous bone graft. When there is no comminution, the trochlear fragments are secured with one or two screws, placed between the fragments by overdrilling the near cortex. It may be preferable to direct the screw from the radial to the ulnar aspect,[50] because there would be less risk of injury to the ulnar nerve. If the radial articular fragment is small, it is preferable to pass the screw from ulnar to radial aspect. With comminution and bone loss, a fully threaded screw is placed across the trochlea without overdrilling the near cortex to avoid the possibility of compressing the fragments and thus reducing the width of the trochlea.

More complex is the situation when the surgeon is faced with a fracture of the trochlea in the coronal plane, where the fracture fragments are completely covered with articular cartilage (see Fig. 23–21). Fixation of these fragments is enhanced by using the double-threaded screw designed by Herbert,[75] which compresses the fragments and can be buried beneath the surface of the articular cartilage. Small, threaded wires can be used, as can bioabsorbable pins, although neither provides as firm a hold on the articular fragments as the Herbert screws (Fig. 23–26).

The reconstructed trochlea must now be reassembled onto the medial and lateral bony columns using individually contoured plates. The 3.5-mm reconstruction plate has become the most versatile implant for this purpose, because it can be bent in three dimensions to match the complex shape of the distal humerus.

Even in osteopenic patients, the marginal aspects of the skeletal columns often have sufficient cortical bone to accept screws.[83] The lateral plate should be applied posteriorly and as for distal as possible until it virtually abuts the posterior border of the capitellum. The most distal screw in this plate should be directed proximally and laterally to both avoid the capitellum and gain sound purchase in the lateral margin of the lateral skeletal column. Optimally, at least three screws should be placed into the lateral column proximal to the fracture line.

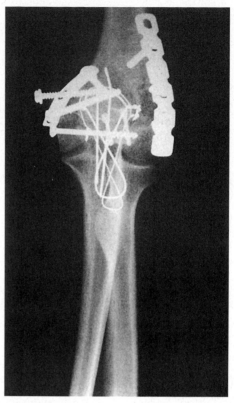

FIGURE 23–26 • A complex intra-articular fracture of the distal humerus in a 21-year-old woman in which the trochlea was fractured in both the sagittal and the coronal planes. The coronal fractures were fixed with Herbert self-compressing screws. Excellent function resulted, with 130 degrees of flexion and 20 degrees of full extension.

The medial plate can be applied in a number of ways. For high T or Y bicolumn fractures, the plate can be applied along the ridge of the medial column, ending at the level of the medial epicondyle. Applied along the ridge of the column, the plate sits at an angle of nearly 90 degrees to the lateral plate. Helfet and Hotchkiss, in a mechanical study, supported the concept that plates applied at right angles to each other provide greatest intrinsic stability.[76]

With the lower fractures, such as the low T type, the medial epicondyle can be "cradled" by placing a bend in the distal part of the plate to fit around the epicondyle. The two distal screws can then be positioned perpendicular to each other, providing a mechanical interlock. One alternative is to place a long screw through the plate from the cubital tunnel aimed proximally to gain purchase in the cortex of the lateral skeletal column proximal to the fracture (Fig. 23–27).

The sequence of steps in the internal fixation will vary with the the particular fracture pattern. On occasion, it may be advisable to fix the articular fragments directly to one of the columns (see Fig. 23–19).

Complex Intra-articular Bicolumn Fractures

One group of intra-articular distal humeral fractures are considerably more difficult to stabilize effectively with

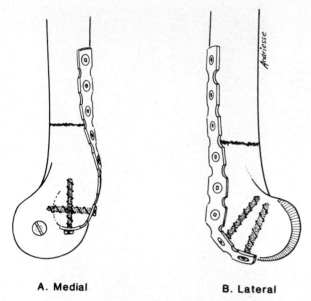

A. Medial   **B. Lateral**

FIGURE 23–27 • The medial epicondyle can be "cradled" with a contoured plate. The lateral column plate can extend just to the capitellum.

standard plate-and-screw applications. These include some fracture patterns seen in elderly or osteopenic patients that are characterized by the position of the transverse fracture lines—at or about the level of the olecranon sulcus. In addition, with fractures due to open injuries or high-energy trauma articular or bone structure may be lost.

The surgeon faced with such difficult fracture patterns in an elderly patient has several options. If the articular components can be reassembled and secured with one or two screws, the articular reconstruction can be reattached to the bony columns using either tension band wire constructs[84] or three strategically placed plates.[85, 86, 87] The tension band wire technique involves placing two parallel smooth Kirschner wires through each side of the distal fragments aimed proximally to gain fixation in the opposite column of bone. Smooth stainless wire can be looped around the bent tips of the wires and passed through drill holes in the ipsilateral bony column farther proximal.

Alternatively, by adding a third plate directly along the lateral column with the most distal screw securing purchase in the subchondral bone of the trochlea, this will create a construct with fixation points in multiple planes. Inadequate screw purchase can be enhanced with judicious use of methyl methacrylate to support the screws that fail to gain purchase.

Although several studies have reported encouraging results with operative fixation of these complex fractures in elderly, osteopenic patients,[83, 85] the complications of implant failure, nonunion, and loss of elbow mobility can be profound. In this content, the encouraging reports of primary total elbow arthroplasty[88] offer promise in the future as implant design and surgeon experience develop.

OLECRANON OSTEOTOMY FIXATION

The olecranon osteotomy can be secured with either a large 6.5-mm intramedullary cancellous bone screw incorporating a tension band wire or two obliquely placed Kirschner wires plus a tension band wire. The wires are directed anteriorly and penetrate the anterior cortex to avoid backing out (Fig. 23–28).

After secure fixation of the osteotomy, the elbow must be moved through a full range of motion, both to observe the stability of fixation and to make certain that the internal fixation has created no obstruction to full motion. The ulnar nerve also must be observed to make certain that it is neither tethered in the soft tissue nor in contact with the internal fixation. If there is any doubt, the nerve should be translated into the subcutaneous tissue.

The wound is closed in layers over a suction drain and a bulky soft tissue dressing is applied. The elbow is splinted overnight, preferably in extension, because, in the elbow, extension tends to be more difficult to maintain.

Optimally, motion should be initiated on the first postoperative day under the supervision of the surgeon with support from a trained therapist who is cognizant of the nature of the problem and the anticipated goals. Exercises begin, alternating between active extension and flexion motions, as the patient's contralateral hand supports the involved forearm. As radiographs demonstrate progression of bone healing, usually beginning between 4 and 6 weeks postoperatively, the patient is permitted to add a little resistance to these exercises. Passive exercises by a therapist should be avoided throughout the rehabilitation.

RESULTS

Meaningful comparison of the outcomes of the management of intra-articular distal humeral fractures has been made even more difficult by the fact that no standard evaluation criteria have been used in the literature. To gain insight into the outcomes of various treatment methods, Bryan and Morrey[77] used the outcome scale established by Bickel and Perry.[78] An excellent result is considered a stable, pain-free elbow with a "nearly normal" range of motion; a good-stable result is no deformity, 60 degrees of flexion and extension in a usable range, at least 50 percent of normal rotation, and no more than mild aching on heavy use; a fair-stable result is mild pain on normal use, significant loss of motion, and moderate deformity; and a poor result may include instability, pain, deformity, and greatly restricted range of motion.

Skeletal traction yielded satisfactory outcomes in approximately 50 to 60 percent of cases treated with traction alone[50, 69, 70, 92] or with open reduction and fixation followed

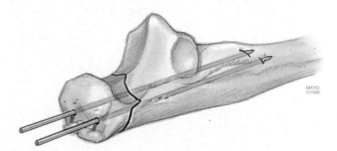

FIGURE 23–28 • Olecranon fixation is enhanced if Kirschner wires penetrate the cortex at the base of the coronoid.

by traction.[69, 70] With treatment by traction alone, for several investigators the mean arc of motion was 57 degrees, which, by contemporary standards, would be a less than satisfactory outcome.[13, 69, 79, 80]

The results of operative techniques, particularly those drawn from reports on the application of stable fixation with dual plates and early postoperative mobilization, are considerably better. Excellent or good results could be determined in more than 80 percent of 846 patients in the literature who were treated with stable internal fixation and postoperative mobilization for intra-articular distal humerus fractures.*

With fractures associated with high-energy trauma, gunshot wounds, or significant ipsilateral extremity injury, results will be less predictable.

COMPLICATIONS

Although the surgical management of distal humeral intra-articular bicolumn fractures has enhanced the possibility of improved functional outcome, the complications, particularly those associated with failed internal fixation, can be significant. These include delayed union or nonunion, elbow ankylosis, ulnar neuritis, and infection.[7, 87, 91, 93, 94, 95]

Nonunion, although rare, can be particularly disabling when it involves the dominant arm of an older patient. Treatment may be further complicated by disuse osteopenia or ankylosis of the elbow joint. Surgery for producing union has proved relatively successful, although the ultimate range of motion of the elbow was observed to be only satisfactory.[93] It has become apparent that, to improve the functional outcome, surgery to gain bony union should be performed in conjunction with elbow capsulotomy (see Chapter 24).

Nonunion of the olecranon osteotomy, also recognized in the literature,[7, 56] may be attributed to several causes. First, the surgically created smooth planes of an osteotomy do not interdigitate as an olecranon fracture does; thus, it would be intrinsically less stable. Second, problems may arise from use of an intramedullary screw because the olecranon and the proximal ulna are angled 7 degree from the longitudinal axis of the forearm and this can impede the screw's passage down the canal. In some younger patients, a narrow medullary canal could also be a factor in the screw's failure to apply satisfactory compression across the osteotomy.

A comprehensive assessment of complications and their management was presented by Lecestre and colleagues.[50] Among 388 fractures about the elbow, 110 of which were open injuries, there were 15 aseptic nonunions (4 percent), 21 deep infections (5.4 percent), 16 cases of postoperative paralysis (14 percent), and 31 loosened or broken implants (8 percent).

Total Elbow Arthroplasty for Distal Humeral Fracture

In older patients, fractures of the distal humerus often involve severe comminution and osteoporotic fragments. Under these circumstances the rigid fixation necessary for

early motion and a reliable functional result is often compromised. Under these circumstances, one of us (B.F.M.) has found immediate elbow replacement to be a reliable procedure that allows early motion and minimal physical therapy and has a low complication rate. Experience with 22 such procedures was reported by Cobb and associates.[143] The overall "satisfactory" rate was over 90%. The only measured complication was a fracture of one ulnar component, which occurred during a fall. While osteosynthesis remains the treatment of choice for this fracture, prosthetic replacement is a viable option in properly selected cases, specifically, badly comminuted fractures in persons older than 70 years (Fig. 23–29).

SINGLE-COLUMN (UNICONDYLAR) FRACTURES (AO GROUPS B1 or B2)

Single-column (condylar) fractures are uncommon and account for 3 to 5 percent[50, 96] of distal humeral fractures. The lateral column is fractured more often than its medial counterpart.[26, 29, 97, 98] These fractures can pose significant difficulties for the clinician unless the pathologic anatomy and precise nature of the fracture are appreciated. They traverse either the medial or the lateral skeletal column, extending distally through the intercolumnar portion of the distal humerus. The fracture fragment is the distal portion of the fractured skeletal column plus the adjacent part of the trochlea (Fig. 23–30). In fact, the size of the trochlear fragment that separates with the columnar fragment is directly related to the proximal extent of the columnar fracture and the intrinsic stability of the fracture. More proximal (high) fractures have more trochlea involved and are unstable because the ulna is displaced with the fracture fragment.

A clear distinction must be made between lateral-column fractures and the capitellar fractures (AO group B3). The lateral-column fracture occurs in the sagittal plane, involves the epicondyle, and contains some soft tissue attachments. Capitellar fractures, on the other hand, occur in the coronal plane and have no soft tissue attachments (Fig. 23–31).

MECHANISM

This fracture pattern has been extensively studied and discussed by Milch.[26, 46, 98] With lateral-column fractures, the medial margin of the radial head initiates the break as it strikes the sulcus between the capitellum and the trochlea in response to an axially directed load. The longitudinal groove of the sigmoid notch of the olecranon compresses the sulcus of the trochlea, causing a fracture of the trochlea. The energy is dissipated proximally, either laterally or medially. Although Milch suggested that these fractures might be the result of an abduction or an adduction force,[98] this has never been definitively proven.

CLASSIFICATION

Milch classified the single-column or unicondylar fractures into two types, based on whether the lateral wall of the trochlea remains attached to the humerus (type I) or to the fracture fragment (type II). Milch considered type II injuries to be fracture-dislocations, because the radius and the

---

*References 2, 7, 55–59, 61, 78, 81, 83, 87, 89, 90, 84, 96, 104.

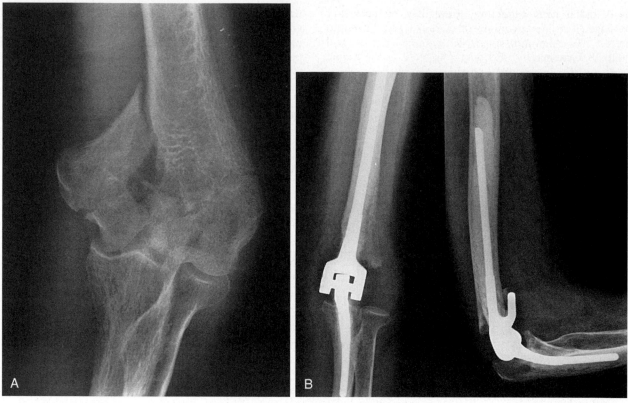

FIGURE 23-29 • *A*, Severely comminuted articulation in a low T condylar fracture in a 73-year-old woman. *B*, Patient has no pain and 20 to 135 degrees of motion after prosthetic replacement surgery with Coonrad-Morrey implant.

ulna are displaced along with the fracture fragment. On this basis, he suggested that type I injuries could be treated nonoperatively whereas type II injuries should be stabilized with internal fixation.[26] In addition, with lateral type II injuries, the medial collateral ligament often is disrupted, a condition that leads to wide displacement and the potential for traction injury to the ulnar nerve.[21] We have found it

convenient to remember this classification according to the number of contours ("lumps") involved: type I—one lump, lateral capitellar or medial face of trochlea; type II—two lumps, lateral capitellum and lateral or medial trochlea, both portions of the trochlea (see Fig. 23–30).

Considering the columnar concept of the surgical anatomy of the distal humerus, these fractures are classified on the basis of which column is fractured apart from the remaining intact humerus. High fractures include the majority of the trochlea, which is displaced with the radius and the ulna, and they are best managed by internal fixation, especially because there sufficient bone is available for the placement of internal fixation.

EXAMINATION

Standard anteroposterior and lateral radiographs of the elbow are often sufficient to diagnose a single-column frac-

FIGURE 23-30 • Single-column fractures of the distal humerus. A high fracture involves the majority of the trochlea (two contours, *arrows*) and is unstable as the ulna displaces with the fracture fragment. Low fractures (one contour, *arrow*) are inherently stable. (Modified from Mehne, D. K., and Jupiter, J. B.: Fractures of the distal humerus. *In* Browner, B., Jupiter, J., Levine, A., and Trafton, P. [eds.]: Skeletal Trauma. Vol. II. Philadelphia, W. B. Saunders Co., 1991, p. 1151.)

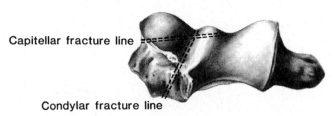

FIGURE 23-31 • Coronal view of the distal humerus demonstrates the fracture line of the single-column (unicondylar) fracture compared with the type I capitellar fracture.

ture. A radial head–capitellum view may be necessary to distinguish a lateral-column fracture from a capitellum fracture.[99] This view can also reveal an occult radial head fracture.[100] Tomography may also help to precisely define the extent of the skeletal and articular injury.

On examination, the elbow may be swollen and painful, and its motion restricted. High fractures are unstable and may exhibit varus or valgus deformity. The patient's neurovascular status should be evaluated and documented.

Management

NONOPERATIVE

Nondisplaced single-column fractures may be treated nonoperatively with splint or cast immobilization for 4 to 5 weeks, but considerable attention must be paid to monitoring the fracture radiographically, because loss of reduction can occur. Failure to detect displacement will likely lead to residual incongruity of the articular surface and post-traumatic arthrosis. In addition, managing intra-articular distal humerus fractures with cast treatment has certain drawbacks, in particular residual stiffness.

Displaced type I fractures may be successfully reduced by closed manipulation. For lateral-column fractures, the elbow is adducted, the forearm is supinated, and the wrist and digits are extended. An opposite maneuver is performed to reduce a displaced type I medial-column injury. If the maneuver is successful, the fracture is best stabilized by percutaneous wire or cannulated screws and immobilized in a cast for 4 to 5 weeks (Fig. 23–32). In actual fact, any column fracture in an adult is most reliably managed with open reduction and fixation.

OPERATIVE

Early open reduction and stable internal fixation is *recommended* for all condylar fractures but is *required* for displaced type I and all type II fractures.[97] Exposure to the lateral condylar injury is readily obtained by using Kocher's approach,[72] which can be extended proximally, if necessary (see Chapter 8). For medial condylar fractures, either the medial approach of Bryan and Morrey[77] or a transolecranon approach is recommended because complete visualization of the joint is required. In most cases, screws alone provide stable fixation, although a single plate may enhance stability in the presence of localized comminution[97] (Fig. 23–33).[97]

COMPLICATIONS

Nonunion and malunion of single-column fractures can lead to a mechanically unstable, deformed elbow.[103] Lateral-column fractures lead to ulnar neuritis and post-traumatic arthritis.[97] Malunion of type I fractures may in some cases be corrected with wedge osteotomy. Type II malunions are considerably more complex because the humeroulnar joint is not congruous and the joint is in subluxation. Angular correction and translation realignment of the distal fragment may be considered if the deformity is of relatively recent origin.[26] For late cases of nonunion or malunion, total elbow arthroplasty may be advisable (Fig. 23–34).[101] It is important to recognize that nonunion of this fracture is unique. Excellent function not only is possible but can be anticipated, in spite of gross deformity. Arthrosis develops only in the sixth or seventh decade of life.[102]

Fractures of the Capitellum

Isolated fractures of the capitellum are uncommon (estimated to account for 1 percent of all elbow fractures[39] and 6 percent of all fractures of the distal humerus).[12, 50] Hahn is credited with the first description of the fracture in 1853.[105] A palpable prominence in the anterolateral aspect of the elbow was confirmed at autopsy to be the capitellum, which though healed was displaced. The fracture may be more common in females and in adults.[106, 107] It may be associated with radial head fractures[100, 108, 109, 114–117] and posterior elbow dislocations.[113]

Classification

While there are some variations in fracture patterns, these injuries are essentially shear fractures in a coronal plane

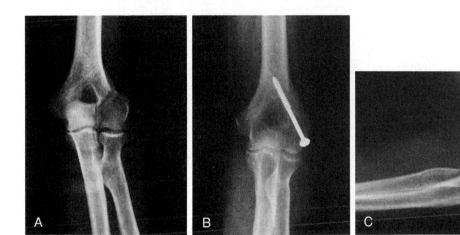

FIGURE 23–32 • *A*, Minimally displaced lateral single-column fracture in a 64-year-old woman. *B, C*, Reduction and internal fixation with a single malleolar screw. (From Bryan, R. J.: Fractures about the elbow in adults. *In* The American Academy of Orthopaedic Surgeons: Instructional Course Lecture. Vol. 30. St. Louis, C. V. Mosby Co., 1981.)

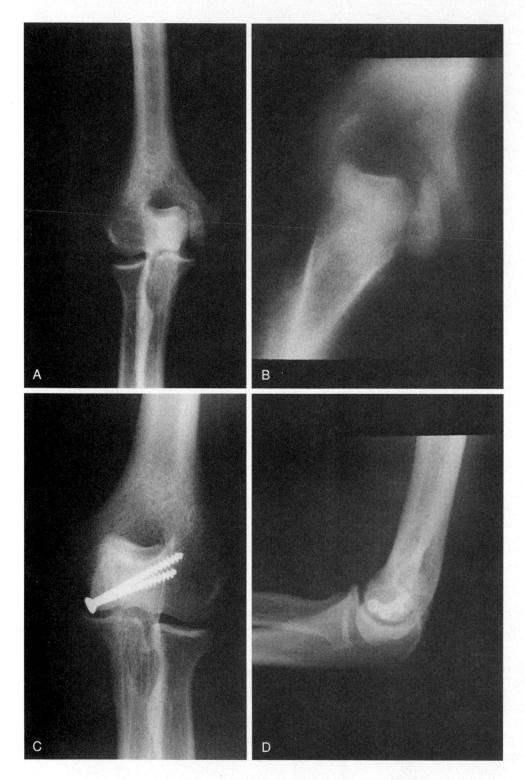

FIGURE 23–33 • A 28-year-old man with trauma from a high-speed motor vehicle. *A,* Anteroposterior radiograph reveals an unusual sagittal fracture of the trochlea. *B,* Tomogram reveals clearly the isolated fracture of the trochlea. *C, D,* Anteroposterior and lateral views show the stable internal fixation of the isolated trochlea fracture.

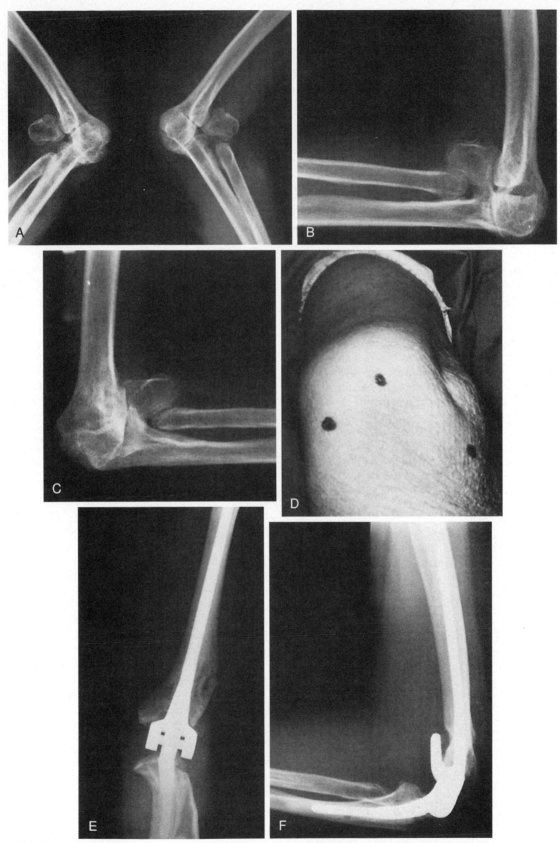

FIGURE 23–34 • *A,* Interesting case of bilateral type II lateral condylar fractures that occurred when the patient was 6 years old. At 62 years of age, the patient had painful limitation of motion and developed bilateral tardy ulnar nerve palsy. *B, C,* Lateral view demonstrates the almost identically altered anatomy. Bilateral injury nicely demonstrates a predictable and almost perfect mirror image deformity that results from the internal muscle forces and is common after lateral condylar type II injuries. *D,* Gross disruption of the posterior triangle is obvious. This patient was treated with total elbow arthroplasty *(E, F)* and is currently asymptomatic.

that displace the capitellum from the lateral column of the distal humerus. Historically, the complete shearing fracture was originally described by Hahn and then by Steinthal,[112] and it was called *the Hahn-Steinthal fracture* in subsequent publications.[113, 114] We call this a *type I injury.*

A second, less common, type II injury involves only the shell of the anterior cartilage of the capitellum and a thin layer of subchondral bone. This lesion has been called the *Kocher-Lorenz fracture.*[98, 102, 103, 107, 108]

Type III fractures are comminuted or compression fractures of the articular surface (Fig. 23–35).[6, 106, 110]

Mechanism of Injury

The most common fracture, type I, usually is associated with direct elbow trauma[107] or a fall on the outstretched hand. According to Lee,[105] the partially flexed, partially pronated elbow joint exposes the capitellum, making it vulnerable to fracture from a direct blow. Displacement almost always occurs anteriorly and superiorly. The less common type II slice fracture is usually the result of an indirect force transmitted across the joint. It can result from hammering, lifting, or a similar activity. The fragment is usually small and may not be displaced posteriorly. The type III fracture is caused by a fall on the outstretched hand, as exemplified in the report of Milch,[109] who observed an impaction of the capitellum into a fractured radial head.

Clinical Presentation

The clinical presentation of a capitellar fracture may be similar to that of a radial head fracture—swelling and tenderness localized along the lateral aspect of the elbow. Several characteristic features of the fracture have been described[118, 119]: pain independent of the position of the arm; maintenance of the normal anatomic landmarks; progressive loss of motion; palpable swelling in the antecubital fossa; and crepitus, especially with flexion and extension.

On examination, careful palpation over the posterolateral joint at about 45 degrees of flexion while rotating the forearm and flexing and extending the joint a few degrees often helps to localize the injury and detect an effusion. The contact of the capitellum with the radial head may cause painful crepitus, especially with valgus stress. Aspi-

ration of the joint may aid in diagnosis of the more subtle type II or type III injuries. If no blood is visible in the aspirate, a fracture is less likely.

Capitellar fractures are unique in the subtlety of the radiographic appearance. Although standard radiographs demonstrate the type I fracture in most cases, the anteroposterior view may look normal (Fig. 23–36). The type II lesion may be especially difficult to identify. The radiographic fat pad sign is important as a diagnostic clue.[120] The type II fracture may involve only a small fragment of bone. Because the mechanism of injury is often a force transmitted across the radial head, the radiograph must be carefully scrutinized to ensure that the fragments come from the capitellum and not from the radial head. As a rule, if the fracture fragment lies proximal to the radial head it is unlikely to have broken from the radius and a capitellar fracture should be suspected (Fig. 23–37). Tomography will be particularly important in revealing undisplaced fractures in patients with a positive fat pad sign.

Treatment

Because capitellar fractures are so uncommon, it would be unusual for any individual surgeon to have had a large clinical experience. The literature reflects a wide variety of recommendations—from closed treatment[106, 111, 121, 122] to open reduction and internal fixation[45, 107, 113] to excision of the fragment.[111, 118]

TYPE I

For large capitellar fractures without comminution, closed reduction can be considered, although is less successful than operative fixation. When this option is chosen, however, general or regional anesthesia is preferred because it affords complete muscle relaxation. With the patient in the supine position, an assistant applies traction to the supinated forearm with the elbow initially extended. Downward pressure is applied to the capitellar fragment in the antecubital fossa as the elbow is slowly flexed.[122] If successful anatomic reduction is achieved, the elbow should be immobilized in a well-molded posterior splint or a long-arm cast for 3 to 4 weeks. At that point, active assisted range-of-motion exercises can be initiated. Success with closed treatment is contingent on achieving an anatomic or nearly

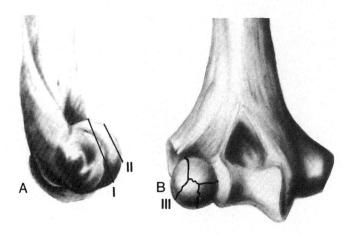

FIGURE 23–35 • The type I capitellar fracture involves a large portion of bone, often the entire structure. Type II is a shear fracture, often with minimal subchondral bone, and may displace posteriorly *(A)*. A type III fracture is a comminuted fracture with varying amounts of displacement of the fracture fragments *(B)*.

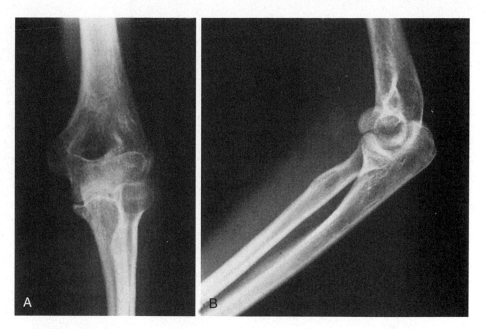

FIGURE 23–36 • Anteroposterior radiograph of the elbow does not show gross abnormality after a fall on the outstretched hand *(A)*. The lateral view *(B)* clearly demonstrates the type I fracture of the capitellum.

anatomic reduction. Mazel reported an instance of apparent anatomic reduction that was accompanied by restriction of flexion and forearm rotation. When the fracture fragment was removed, full range of motion returned.[119]

Open reduction and internal fixation is the recommended treatment. A lateral Kocher approach is recommended, with the incision beginning 2 cm proximal to the lateral epicondyle and extending 3 to 4 cm distal to the radial head. Additional exposure can be gained by cutting the lateral epicondyle with a sharp osteotome and reflecting the epicondyle with the origin of the common extensor muscle distally to expose the lateral elbow joint. The capitellar fragment is then reduced under direct vision and provisionally secured with Kirschner wires. Internal fixation then can be secured stably with small screws (2.7 or 4.0 mm) directed from posterior to anterior or with Herbert

screws, which can be placed from anterior to posterior and buried beneath the articular cartilage in the subchondral bone.[100, 114] Care is taken to avoid damaging the radial nerve lying between the brachioradialis and the brachialis muscles (Fig. 23–38).

Although the literature contains a wide range of outcomes for type I injuries, more stable techniques of internal fixation that permit early mobilization have improved the overall outcome. In a series of 22 single-column fractures treated at an AO center in Basel, Switzerland, five were type I capitellar injuries. All the patients were treated with early open reduction and stable internal fixation with postoperative mobilization. Three had normal function, and two noted some functional limitations. Four had nearly full elbow motion, but one had significant limitation. There was no medial or lateral instability. Follow-up radiographs showed no evidence of avascular necrosis.[97]

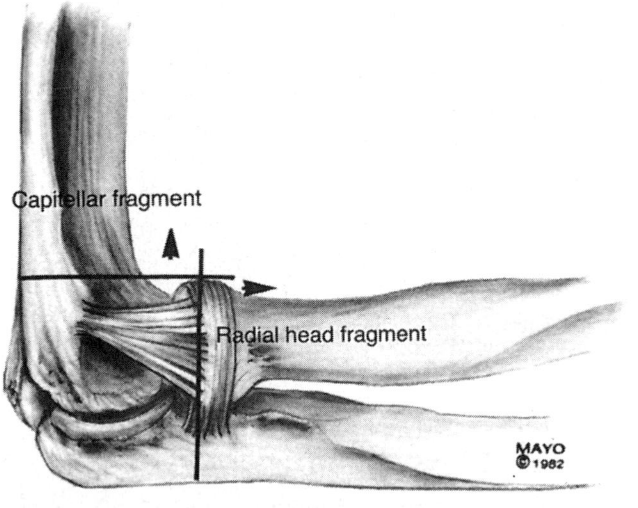

TYPES II AND III

Internal fixation of shearing or comminuted fractures is not an easy task. In most cases, excision of the fragments is advisable. The early results of excision can be expected to be favorable,[110, 111] but long-term results have been less predictable, as loss of motion or instability sometimes develops.[106, 107, 111]

COMBINED CAPITELLUM–RADIAL HEAD FRACTURE

There are few reports in the literature on combined fractures of the capitellum and the radial head[45, 100, 108, 109]—and only a few recommendations for treatment. McAusland and Wyman advocated open reduction and internal fixation of the capitellum along with excision of the radial head fracture fragments.[45] They advised against the reverse (that is, internal fixation of the radial head and excision of the capitellum) and also said that both should not be excised.

Hendel and Halperin reported good results in a case

FIGURE 23–37 • On the lateral view, fracture fragments after elbow dislocation may be identified as involving the capitellum if they are proximal to the anterior margin of the radial head. Fracture fragments distal to the capitellum typically originate from radial head.

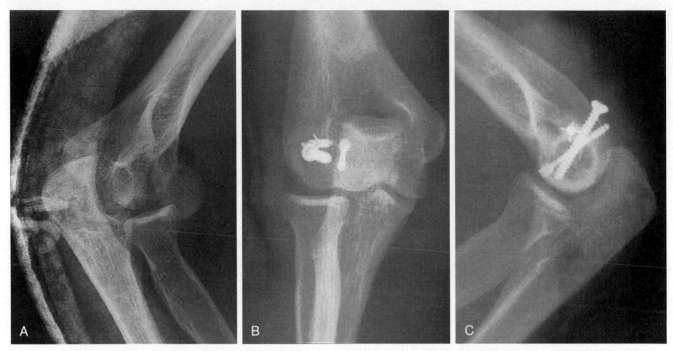

FIGURE 23–38 • *A*, A type I capitellar fracture. *B, C*, One year after injury, union is noted without any avascular necrosis and full function.

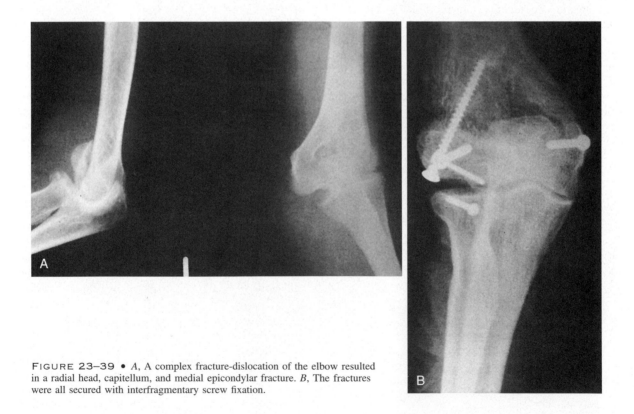

FIGURE 23–39 • *A*, A complex fracture-dislocation of the elbow resulted in a radial head, capitellum, and medial epicondylar fracture. *B*, The fractures were all secured with interfragmentary screw fixation.

associated with a medial collateral ligament tear in which the capitellum was treated by open reduction and internal fixation and the radial head was excised.[108] They cautioned that excising the capitellar fragment in the presence of a damaged medial ligament complex could result in a valgus deformity.

Ward and Nunley suggested that significant radial head fractures may be associated with capitellar fractures.[100] Seven of 13 (54 percent) capitellar fractures that were treated surgically at their center over 11 years had associated radial head fractures. They suggested that internal fixation of both fractures be attempted if the fragments are large enough to support stable internal fixation. This has been our approach as well (Fig. 23–39).

Complications

The principal complication of capitellar fractures is loss of elbow motion. Forearm rotation is not usually affected. Disruption of the medial collateral ligament can occur with fractures due to falls on the outstretched hand,[108] although this is uncommon.

Avascular necrosis has been reported but is also deemed uncommon.[110] In fact, it may be more common than generally is appreciated but may escape detection on radiographs because of rapid revascularization of the small fragments. Should avascular necrosis occur, however, fragment excision is recommended only if the patient becomes symptomatic.

Fractures of the Trochlea

Isolated fractures of the trochlea are extremely rare because this articulating unit has no capsule, muscle, or ligamentous attachment and is virtually cradled by the olecranon. Forces that are sufficient to fracture the trochlea usually disrupt the ulna, dislocate the elbow, or result in an intra-articular double-column distal humerus fracture. Very few authors have reported isolated trochlear fractures,[21, 66] but they are more likely to be associated with a coronal fracture of the capitellum.[118]

If a trochlear fracture is displaced, the joint must be explored to restore articular congruity. Although most surgeons support Smith,[21] who recommended excision of small trochlear fragments that cannot be replaced or anatomically secured, the availability of self-compressing Herbert screws and bioabsorbable pins has significantly enhanced the surgeon's ability to secure even small trochlear fragments (Fig. 23–40).

Small defects in the articular cartilage will fill with fibrous tissue and may be tolerated if motion is initiated within 3 to 5 days after injury. If motion is delayed, dense, adhesive bands likely will form between the trochlea and the ulna. We have successfully employed the distraction device to allow motion while unloading a tenuous fixation constraint of a trochlear fracture (Fig. 23–41).

MASSIVE TRAUMA TO THE ELBOW

Massive trauma to the elbow is characterized by involvement of all the major tissue systems—bone, joint, vessels, nerve, muscle, and skin. The most common causes are include gunshot wounds, auger injuries, and various combat injuries.

This type of massive injury was introduced into the orthopedic literature as the "sideswipe" or "car window" injury, which was common in the 1940s,[123, 124] before auto-

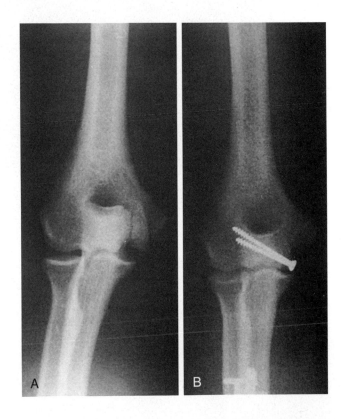

FIGURE 23–40 • *A,* An unusual sagittal fracture of the trochlea internally fixed with two lag screws *(B).*

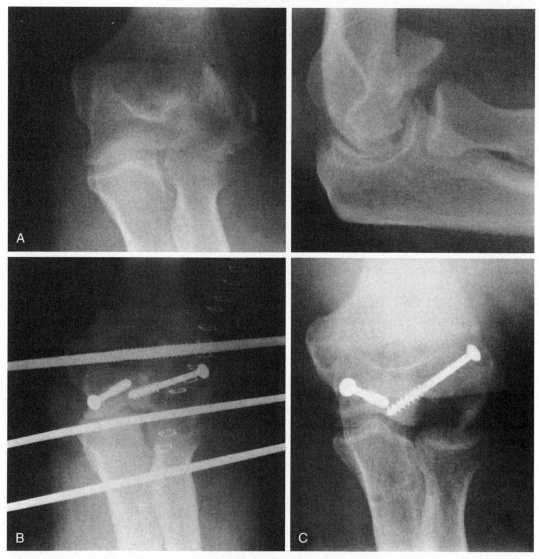

FIGURE 23–41 • Comminuted fracture of the trochlea (A) was fixed with internal fixation device supplemented by the distraction external fixator (B). The patient has a healed fracture, although there is a suggestion of an element of avascular necrosis (C).

mobiles were air conditioned. Typically, it involved the left elbow, which was struck by an oncoming car as it rested on the rolled-down window ledge. The pathologic findings usually consisted of a compound, comminuted fracture of the proximal ulna, a dislocation at the elbow, and a fracture of the distal humerus (Fig. 23–42). The devastating nature of the event was obvious by the associated 50 percent amputation rate.[125]

This lesion is mostly of historical interest, since the principles of management of massive limb injuries have been refined. Today, they include (1) judicious débridement of bone and soft tissue; (2) extensive lavage with a pulsatile jet stream; (3) reduction and internal fixation of the intra-articular fractures; (4) leaving the wound open but covering the joint expeditiously at the next surgical débridement; and (5) initiating motion as soon as possible.

The combination of ipsilateral fractures of the humerus and forearm creates an unstable intermediate articulation or a "floating elbow."[126, 128, 129, 130] In addition, associated neurovascular or soft tissue injury not only adds to the complexity of elbow management but also adversely affects the functional outcome. Pierce and Hodurski reviewed 21 cases of floating elbow injuries, noting residual neurologic dysfunction in more than half.[126] In fact, an overall good result, judged by both joint mobility and function, was reported in only 28 percent of their cases (Fig. 23–43).

Most authors have found that stable fixation of both the humeral and the forearm components provides the best chance for a functional outcome.[118, 120, 122] External skeletal fixation should be considered when the wounds are heavily contaminated,[126, 129, 131] when rapid skeletal stabilization is needed, or when the fractures are extremely comminuted, with or without segmental bone loss.[131–133] Because most external fixation is applied to the lateral surface of the humerus, considerable caution must be exercised in pin placement to avoid injury to the radial nerve. We have found excellent results with joint replacement in the devastating elbow injury in the absence of infection (Fig. 23–44).

Complications

Fractures of the distal humerus can have a number of serious complications. Because these problems can be exceedingly complex to understand and treat effectively, many are discussed in greater detail in separate chapters.

LOSS OF MOTION

Loss of motion is undoubtedly the most common complication of fractures about the elbow. Among the factors conditions that account for this are (1) soft tissue fibrosis and scarring, (2) articular malalignment (Fig. 23–45), (3) excessive callus formation, (4) myositis ossificans, and (5) internal fixation obstructing motion. Loss of motion is discussed in detail in Chapters 33 and 34.

NERVE INJURY

Injuries to all three major nerves can occur with fractures of the distal humerus, whether at the time of the original injury, with manipulation, or during surgery (Fig. 23–46). Postoperatively, ulnar nerve dysfunction is common.[50, 66,]

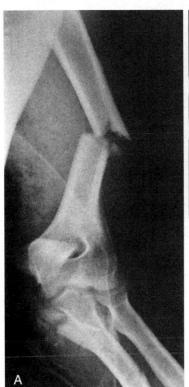
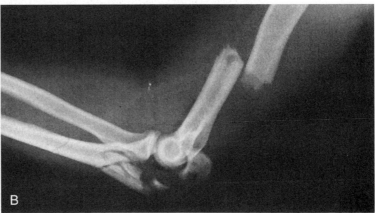

FIGURE 23–42 • Massive elbow trauma sustained in a snowmobile accident. An aggressive management program with rigid fixation of the humeral fracture and excision or fixation of the olecranon fracture is recommended, but such severe injuries portend a poor prognosis.

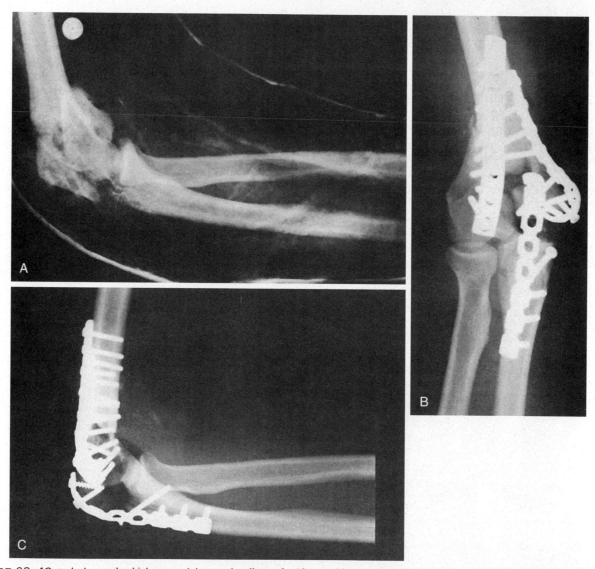

FIGURE 23–43 • *A*, A complex high-energy injury to the elbow of a 19-year-old man resulted in a multifragmented distal humerus and proximal ulna fracture. *B, C,* After extensive débridement and jet lavage, stable internal fixation was achieved. Note an area of bone loss in the olecranon, which was secondarily replaced with cancellous bone graft.

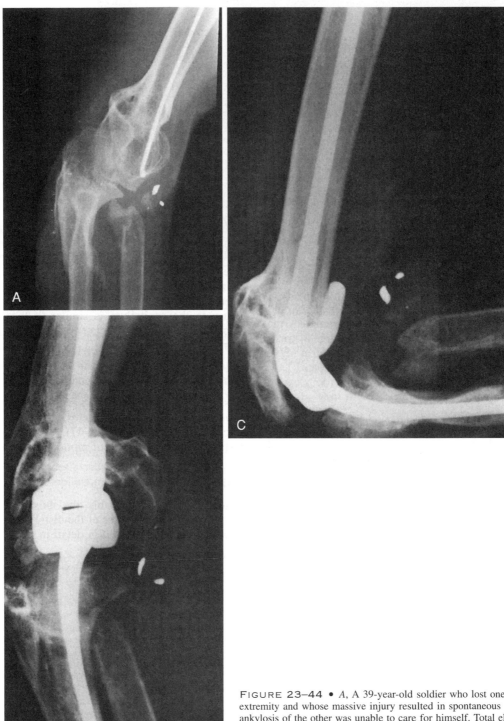

FIGURE 23–44 • *A*, A 39-year-old soldier who lost one extremity and whose massive injury resulted in spontaneous ankylosis of the other was unable to care for himself. Total elbow arthroplasty was successful in allowing him to perform activities of daily living *(B, C)*.

31. Marquis, J. W., Browner, A. J., and Keith, H. M.: Supracondylar process of the humerus. Proc. Staff Mayo Clin. **37**:691, 1957.
32. Genner, B. A.: Fracture of the supracondylar process. J. Bone Joint Surg. **18**:757, 1936.
33. Barnard, L. B., and McCoy, S. M.: The supracondylar process of the humerus. J. Bone Joint Surg. **28**:845, 1946.
34. Doane, C. P.: Fractures of the supracondylar process of the humerus. J. Bone Joint Surg. **18**:757, 1936.
35. Lund, H. J.: Fracture of the supracondylar process of the humerus. J. Bone Joint Surg. **12**:925, 1930.
36. Kolb, L. W., and Moore, R. D.: Fractures of the supracondylar process of the humerus. J. Bone Joint Surg. **49A**:532, 1967.
37. Hoyer, A.: Treatment of supracondylar fracture of the humerus by skeletal traction in an abduction splint. J. Bone Joint Surg. **34A**:623, 1952.
38. Wade, F. V., and Batdorf, J.: Supracondylar fractures of the humerus. A twelve-year review with follow-up. J. Trauma **1**:269, 1961.
39. Hotchkiss, R. N., and Green, D. P.: Fractures and dislocations of the elbow. *In* Rockwood, C. A. Jr., Green, D. P., and Bucholz, R. W. (eds.): Fractures in Adults, 3rd ed. Vol. I. Philadelphia, J. B. Lippincott Co., 1991, pp. 744–752.
40. Perry, C. R., Gibson, C. T., and Kowalski, M. F.: Transcondylar fractures of the distal humerus. J. Orthop. Trauma **3**:98, 1989.
41. Mehne, D. K., and Jupiter, J. B.: Fractures of the distal humerus. *In* Browner, B., Levine, A., and Trafton, P. (eds.): Skeletal Trauma. Philadelphia, W. B. Saunders Co., 1991.
42. Sultanpur, A.: Anterior supracondylar fracture of the humerus (flexion type): a simple technique for closed reduction and fixation in adults and the aged. J. Bone Joint Surg. **60B**:383, 1978.
43. Lipscomb, P. R., and Burleson, R. J.: Vascular and neural complications in supracondylar fractures of the humerus in children. J. Bone Joint Surg. **37A**:468, 1955.
44. Böhler, L.: The Treatment of Fractures, 5th ed. Vol. I. New York, Grune and Stratton, 1956.
45. MacAusland, W. R., and Wyman, E. T.: Fractures of the adult elbow. AAOS Instructional Course Lectures **24**:165, 1975.
46. Milch, H.: Fracture Surgery. A Textbook of Common Fractures. New York, Hoeber, 1959.
47. Erdman, P., and Lohr, G.: Supracondylar fractures of the humerus treated with olecranon traction. Acta Chir. Scand. **126**:505, 1963.
48. Smith, L.: Deformity following supracondylar fractures of the humerus. J. Bone Joint Surg. **42A**:235, 1960.
49. Miller, O. L.: Blind nailing of the T fracture of the lower end of the humerus which involves the joint. J. Bone Joint Surg. **21**:933–938, 1936.
50. Lecestre, R.: Round table on fractures of the lower end of the humerus. Société Française de Chirurgie Orthopédique et Traumatologie. Orthop. Trans. **4**:123, 1980.
51. Reich, R. S.: Treatment of intercondylar fractures of the elbow by means of traction. J. Bone Joint Surg. **18B**:997, 1936.
52. Evans, E. M.: Supracondylar Y fractures of the humerus. J. Bone Joint Surg. **35B**:381, 1953.
53. Van Gorder, G. W.: Surgical approach in supracondylar "T" fractures of the humerus requiring open reduction. J. Bone Joint Surg. **22**:278, 1940.
54. Mehne, D. K., and Matta, J.: Bicolumn fractures of the adult humerus. Presented at the 53rd Annual Meeting of the American Academy of Orthopaedic Surgeons, New Orleans, 1986.
55. Burri, C., Lob, G., and Feil, J.: Results of a study of 412 surgically treated patients with intra-articular fractures of the distal humerus. *In* Weller, S., Hierholzer, G., and Hermichen, H. G. (eds.): Late Results After Osteosynthesis. Tübingen, H. J. Köhler, 1984.
56. Gabel, G. T., Hanson, G., Bennett, J. B, Noble, P. C., and Tullos, H. S.: Intra-articular fractures of the distal humerus in the adult. Clin. Orthop. **216**:99, 1987.
57. Henley, M. B., Bone, L. B., and Parker, B.: Operative management of intra-articular fractures of the distal humerus. J. Orthop. Trauma **1**:24, 1987.
58. Letsch, R., Schmit-Neuerburg, K. P., Stürmer, K. M., and Walz, M.: Intra-articular fractures of the distal humerus. Clin. Orthop. **241**:238, 1989.
59. Wildburger, R., Mähring, M., and Hofer, H. P.: Supracondylar fractures of the distal humerus: results of internal fixation. J. Orthop. Trauma **5**:301, 1991.
60. Bryan, R. S., and Bickel, W. H.: "T" condylar fractures of the distal humerus. J. Trauma **11**:830, 1971.

61. Aitken, G. K., and Rorabeck, C. H.: Distal humeral fractures in the adult. Clin. Orthop. **207**:191, 1986.
62. Desault, P. J.: A Treatise on Fractures, Luxations, and Other Affections of the Bones, 2nd ed. Philadelphia, Kimber and Conrad, 1811.
63. Jupiter, J. B., Barnes, K. A., and Goodman, L. J.: The triplane intra-articular fracture of the distal humerus. J. Orthop. Trauma **7**:215, 1993.
64. Wickstrom, J., and Meyer, P. R.: Fractures of the distal humerus in adults. Clin. Orthop. **50**:43, 1967.
65. Suman, R. K., and Miller, J. H.: Intercondylar fractures of the distal humerus. J. R. Coll. Surg. Edinb. **27**:276, 1982.
66. Bryan, R. S.: Fractures about the elbow in adults. American Academy of Orthopaedic Surgeons: Instructional Course Lectures **30**:200. St. Louis, C. V. Mosby Co., 1981.
67. Smith, F. M.: Traction and suspension in the treatment of fractures. Surg. Clin. North Am. 1951.
68. Rogers, J., Bennett, B., and Tullos, H. S.: Management of concomitant ipsilateral fractures of the forearm and humerus. J. Bone Joint Surg. **66A**:552, 1984.
69. Lansinger, O., and Mare, K.: Intercondylar T fractures of the humerus in adults. Acta Orthop. Traumatol. Surg. **100**:37, 1982.
70. Horne, G.: Supracondylar fracture of the humerus in adults. J. Trauma **20**:71, 1980.
71. Helfet, D. L.: Bicondylar intra-articular fractures of the distal humerus in adults: their assessment, classification, and operative management. Adv. Orthop. Surg. **8**:223, 1985.
72. Kocher, T., Stiles, H., and Paul, C. (trans.): Textbook of Operative Surgery, 3rd ed. London, A & C Book Co., 1911.
73. Campbell, W. C.: Arthroplasty of the elbow. Ann. Surg. **76**:615, 1932.
74. Bryan, R. S., and Morrey, B. F.: Extensive exposure of the elbow—a triceps-sparing approach. Clin. Orthop. **166**:188, 1982.
75. Herbert, T. J., and Fischer, W. E.: Management of the fractured scaphoid using a new bone screw. J. Bone Joint Surg. **66B**:114, 1984.
76. Helfet, D. L., and Hotchkiss, R. N.: Internal fixation of the distal humerus: a biomechanical comparison of methods. J. Orthop. Trauma **4**:260, 1990.
77. Bryan, R. S., and Morrey, B. F.: Fractures of the distal humerus. *In* Morrey, B. F. (ed.): The Elbow and Its Disorders. Philadelphia, W. B. Saunders Co., 1985, p. 322.
78. Bickel, W. H., and Perry, R. E.: Comminuted fractures of the distal humerus. J.A.M.A. **184**:353, 1963.
79. Nieman, K.: Condylar fractures of the distal humerus in adults. South. Med. J. **70**:915, 1977.
80. Sotgiv, F., Melis, G. C., and Tolu, S.: Classification and treatment of intercondylar fracture of the humerus. Ital. J. Orthop. Traumatol. **2**:281, 1976.
81. Browne, A. O., O'Riordan, M., and Quinlan, W.: Supracondylar fractures of the humerus in adults. Injury **17**:184, 1986.
82. Johanssen, H., and Olerud, S.: Operative treatment of intercondylar fractures of the humerus. J. Trauma **11**:836, 1971.
83. John H., Rosso R., Neff, U., Boldosky A., Regazzoni, P., and Harder, E.: Operative treatment of distal humeral fractures in the elderly. J. Bone Joint Surg. **76B**:763–766, 1994.
84. Houber, P. F. J., Bongers, K. J., and von de Wildeberg, F. A. J. M.: Double tension band osteosythesis in supra- and transcondylar humeral fractures. Injury **25**:305–310, 1994.
85. Weirich, S., and Jupiter, J.: The management of trauma about the elbow in the aging population. *In* Koval, K., and Zuckerman, J. (eds): Fractures in the Elderly. New York, Raven Press, 1997, pp. 185–210.
86. Jupiter, J.: The surgical management of intraarticular fractures of the distal humerus. *In* Morrey, B. (ed): Master Techniques in Orthopaedic Surgery, The Elbow. New York: Raven Press, 1994, pp. 53–70.
87. Jupiter, J.: Complex fractures of the distal part of the humerus and associated complications. American Academy of Orthopaedic Surgeons Instructional Course Lectures. J. Bone Joint Surg. **76A**:1252–1264, 1994.
88. Cobb, T.K., and Morrey, B.F.: Total elbow arthroplasty as primary treatment for distal humeral fractures in elderly patients. J. Bone Joint Surg. **79A**:826–832, 1997.
89. Zagorski, J.B., and Jennings, J.J.: Comminuted intraarticular or

bicondylar fractures of the distal humerus. Orthop. Trans. **5**:403, 1981.

90. Jeshrani, M. K., and Bencivegna, A.: The management of intra-articular fractures at the lower end of the humerus. East Afr. Med. J. **55**:393, 1978.

91. Galbraith, K. A., and McCullough, C. J.: Acute nerve injury as a complication of closed fractures or dislocations of the elbow. Injury **11**:159, 1979.

92. Patterson, R. F.: A method of applying traction in T and Y fractures of the humerus. J. Bone Joint Surg. **17A**:476, 1935.

93. Ackermann, G., and Jupiter, J. B.: Nonunion of fractures of the distal end of the humerus. J. Bone Joint Surg. **70A**:75, 1988.

94. Jupiter, J., and Goodman, L. J.: The management of complex non-union of the distal humerus by triple plating, elbow capsulotomy, and ulnar nerve neurolysis. J. Shoulder Elbow Surg. **1**:37, 1992.

95. McKee, M., Jupiter, J., Toh, C. L., Wilson, L., Colton, C., and Karras, K. K.: Reconstruction after malunion and nonunions of intraarticular fractures of the distal humerus. J. Bone Joint Surg. **76B**:614–621, 1994.

96. Knight, R. A.: Fractures of the humeral condyle in adults. South. Med. J. **48**:1165, 1955.

97. Jupiter, J. B., Neff, U., Regazzoni, P., and Allgöwer, M.: Unicondylar fracture of the distal humerus. An operative approach. J. Orthop. Trauma **2**:102, 1988.

98. Milch, H.: Fracture of the external humeral condyle. J.A.M.A. **160**:641, 1956.

99. Greenspan, A., and Norman, A.: Radial head–capitellar view: an expanded imaging approach to elbow injuries. Am. J. Roentgenol. **8**:1186, 1982.

100. Ward, W. G., and Nunley, J. A.: Capitellum and radial head fractures. J. Orthop. Trauma **2**:110, 1988.

101. Morrey, B. F., and Adams, R. A.: Semiconstrained elbow replacement for distal humeral nonunion. J. Bone Joint Surg. **77B**:67–72, 1995.

102. Kolenak, A.: Ununited fracture of the lateral condyle of the humerus. A 50-year follow-up. Clin. Orthop. **124**:181, 1977.

103. Smith, F. M.: An 84-year follow-up on a patient with ununited fracture of the lateral condyle of the humerus. J. Bone Joint Surg. **55A**:378, 1973.

104. Holdsworth, B. J., and Mossad, M. M.: Fractures of the adult distal humerus. Elbow function after internal fixation. J. Bone Joint Surg. **72B**:362, 1990.

105. Lee, W. E., and Summey, T. J.: Fracture of the capitellum of the humerus. Ann. Surg. **99**:497, 1934.

106. Grantham, S. A., Norris, T. R., and Bush, D.C.: Isolated fracture of the humeral capitellum. Clin. Orthop. **161**:262, 1981.

107. Collert, S.: Surgical management of fractures of the capitulum humeri. Acta Orthop. Scand. **48**:603, 1977.

108. Hendel, D., and Halperin, N.: Fracture of the radial head and capitulum humeri with rupture of the medial collateral ligament of the elbow. Injury **14**:98, 1982.

109. Milch, H.: Unusual fracture of the capitulum humeri and capitulum radii. J. Bone Joint Surg. **13**:882, 1931.

110. Alvarez, E., Patel, M., and Nimberg, P., et al.: Fractures of the capitellum humeri. J. Bone Joint Surg. **57A**:1093, 1975.

111. Dusuttle, R., Coyle, M., Zawalsky, J., and Bloom, H.: Fractures of the capitellum. J. Trauma **25**:317, 1985.

112. Steinthal, D.: Die isolierte Fraktur der Eminentia Capetala in Ellenbogengelenk. Zentralbl. Chir. **15**:17, 1898.

113. Lansingen, O., and More, K.: Fractures of the capitellum humeri. Acta Orthop. Scand. **52**:39, 1981.

114. Simpson, L. A., and Richards, R. R.: Internal fixation of a capitellar fracture using Herbert screws. Clin. Orthop. **209**:166, 1986.

115. Wilson, P. O.: Fractures and dislocations in the region of the elbow. Surg. Gynecol. Obstet. **56**:335, 1933.

116. Palmer, I.: The validity of the rule of alternativity in traumatology. Acta Chir. Scand. **21**:481, 1961.

117. Rieth, P. C.: Fractures of the radial head associated with chip fracture in the capitellum in adults. Surgical considerations. South. Surgeon **14**:154, 1948.

118. Linden, M. C.: Fractures of the capitellum and trochlea. Ann. Surg. **76**:78, 1922.

119. Mazel, M. S.: Fracture of the capitellum. J. Bone Joint Surg. **17**:483, 1935.

120. Smith, D. N., and Lee, J. R.: The radiological diagnosis of post-traumatic effusion of the elbow joint and the clinical significance of the displaced fat pad sign. Injury **10**:115, 1978.

121. Rhodin, R.: Treatment of fractures of the capitellum. Acta Chir. Scand. **86**:475, 1942.

122. Christopher, F., and Bushnell, L.: Conservative treatment of fractures of the capitellum. J. Bone Joint Surg. **17**:489, 1935.

123. Highsmith, L. S., and Phalen, G. S.: Side swipe injuries. Arch. Surg. **52**:78, 1941.

124. Nicholson, J. T.: Compound comminuted fractures involving the elbow joint. J. Bone Joint Surg. **28**:565, 1946.

125. Wood, C. F.: Traffic elbow. Kentucky Med. J. **39**:78, 1941.

126. Pierce, R. D., and Hodurski, D.: Fractures of the humerus, radius, and ulna in the same extremity. J. Trauma **19**:182, 1979.

127. McKee, M.D., Jupiter, J., and Bamberger, H.B.: Coronal shear fractures of the distal end of the humerus. J. Bone Joint Surg. **79A**:49–54, 1996.

128. Lange, R. H., and Foster, R. J.: Skeletal management of humeral shaft fractures associated with forearm fractures. Clin. Orthop. **195**:173, 1985.

129. Staniski, C. L., and Micheli, L. J.: Simultaneous ipsilateral fractures of the arm and forearm in children. Clin. Orthop. **153**:218, 1980.

130. Viegas, S., Gogan, W., and Riley, S.: Floating dislocated elbow. Case report and review of the literature. J. Trauma **29**:886, 1989.

131. Smith, D., and Cooney, W.: External fixation of high energy upper extremity injuries. J. Orthop. Trauma **4**:7, 1990.

132. Levin, L. S., Goldner, R. D., Urbaniak, J.R., and Hardaker, W. T. Jr.: Management of severe musculoskeletal injuries of the upper extremity. J. Orthop. Trauma **4**:432, 1990.

133. Wild, J., Hausen, G., Bennett, J., and Tullos, H.: External fixation in the management of massive upper extremity trauma. Clin. Orthop. **164**:172, 1982.

134. Wang, K. C., Shin, H. N., Hsuk, Y., and Shih, C. H.: Intercondylar fracture of the distal humerus: routine subcutaneous transposition of the ulnar nerve in a posterior operative approach. J. Trauma **36**:770–773, 1994.

135. McKee, M. D., Jupiter, J. B., Bosse., G., and Goodman, L.: Outcome of ulnar, neurolysis during posttraumatic reconstruction of the elbow. J. Bone Joint Surg. **80B**:100–105, 1998.

136. Gay, J. R., and Love, J. G.: Diagnosis and treatment of tardy paralysis of the ulnar nerve. J. Bone Joint Surg. **29**:1087, 1947.

137. Johansson, O.: Capsular and ligament injuries of the elbow joint. Acta Chir. Scand. **287**(Suppl.):1, 1962.

138. Thompson, H. E. III, and Garcia, A.: Myositis ossificans. Clin. Orthop. **50**:129, 1967.

139. Mohan, K.: Myositis ossificans traumatica of the elbow. Int. Surg. **57**:475, 1972.

140. Jupiter, J. B.: Heterotopic ossification about the elbow. *In* The American Academy of Orthopaedic Surgeons: Instructional Course Lectures. Vol. 40. St. Louis, C. V. Mosby Co., 1991, p. 41.

141. Thompson, H. C. III, and Garcia, A.: Myositis ossificans: aftermath of elbow injuries. Clin. Orthop. **50**:129, 1967.

142. Cobb, T. K., and Linscheid, R. L.: Late correction of malunited intercondylar humeral fractures. J. Bone Joint Surg. **76B**:622–626, 1994.

143. Cobb, T. K. and Morrey B. F.: Total elbow arthroplasty as primary treatment for distal humeral fractures in elderly patients. J. Bone Joint Surg. **79A**:826–832, 1997.

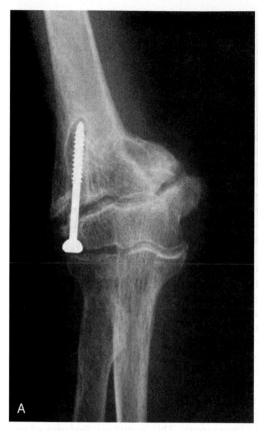

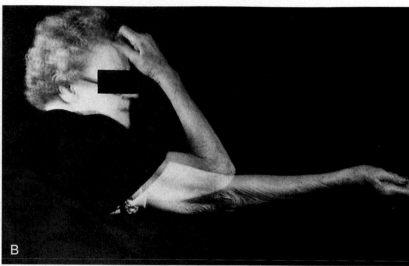

FIGURE 24–3 • A 75-year-old female sustained a nonunion after inadequate fixation of a low transcondylar fracture *(A)*. She has tolerated the nonunion without pain, requiring no additional surgery *(B)*.

nous iliac bone grafting. Biplanar plate fixation posteriorly and medially is recommended by Ackerman and Jupiter[1] for supracondylar fractures. Vascularized fibular grafting can also be considered in those with osseous deficiencies. In the past, an external fixator was necessary to obtain

rigid stabilization because of poor bone stock due to osteoporosis, but this is rarely necessary with current techniques.

In some patients with extensive joint damage and periarticular fibrosis, residual disability is certain, yet open reduction and fixation can restore the contour of the elbow

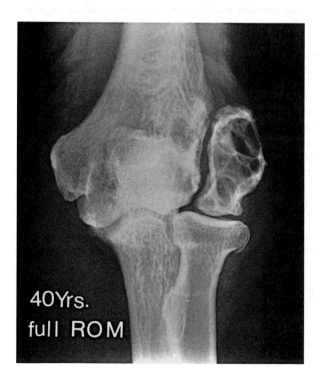

FIGURE 24–4 • A 40-year follow-up of a lateral Milch I nonunion. The patient is without significant symptoms and has motion from 15 to 140 degrees.

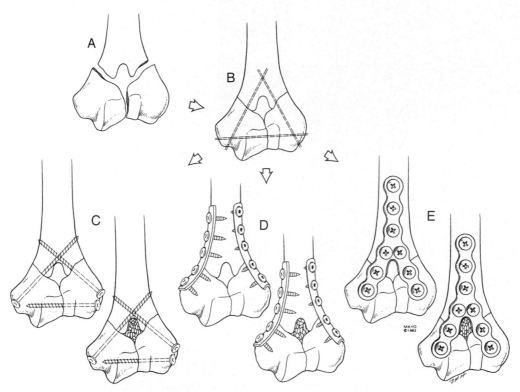

FIGURE 24–5 • Techniques of internal fixation of T-condylar fractures.

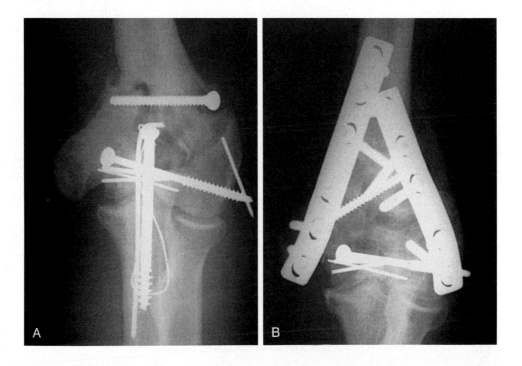

FIGURE 24–6 • Y-condylar nonunion *(A)* treated with mobilization, rigid fixation, and grafting *(B)*.

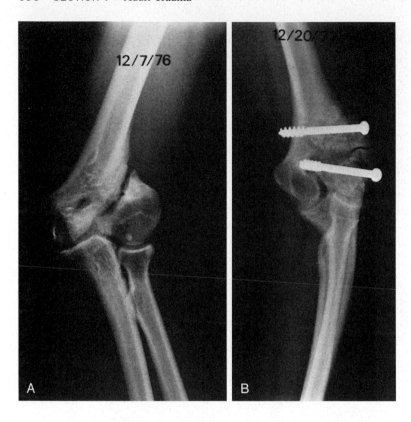

FIGURE 24–7 • *A*, A 24-year-old male with established nonunion of the lateral condyle. *B*, A solid union occurred 1 year following the use of a compression cancellous screw.

and preserve the bone stock and the collateral ligaments, allowing a more satisfactory resection, distraction,[12] or replacement at a later date (see Fig. 24–6).

Postoperative management of the elbow depends on the stability of fixation achieved at surgery. In supracondylar or isolated lateromedial condylar nonunion, solid fixation with compression plates and compression lag screws allows early active elbow motion within the first few days after surgery if there are no wound problems and if swelling is not extensive. In intra-articular T-condylar nonunion and when fixation is suboptimal because of osteoporosis and multiple previous surgical procedures, active elbow motion may be delayed, in which circumstances we employ continuous passive motion (see Chapter 11). When wound healing has occurred and when swelling and pain are diminished, active elbow motion may begin.

Results

Although much has been written about open or closed treatment of acute fractures, there is limited documentation of the relation between the initial treatment and a failed union.[5, 7, 8, 15, 16, 18, 27, 28] In the Mayo Clinic series of 32 nonunions, 19 fractures had been initially treated open and 13 had been treated closed. Of those fractures that were initially fixed operatively, material failure of the internal fixation occurred in 11.

Early experience with the management of these nonunions was not impressive. Mitsunaga and associates[22] reviewed the Mayo Clinic experience with 25 patients treated with open reduction and internal fixation. Of these, 22 achieved union after an average of 7.7 months (Fig. 24–7). However, 6 of the 22 patients required a second or third operation before union occurred, and in only about 30

patients were results considered satisfactory in terms of pain management and function. In the Boston experience, only 7 of 20 patients (34 percent) had satisfactory results despite a 95 percent union rate.[16] The improved union rate reflected the use of allograft reconstruction (10 percent) and a vascularized fibula in one patient.[1]

In a subsequent report, McKee and Jupiter[20] reported seven of eight successful results and emphasized the need to release the capsule and to free the ulnar nerve from such and protect it from harm. Results from a larger group of patients treated in several centers also revealed success in all 13 fractures treated.

Complications

The complication rate varies between 10 and 15 percent.[1, 9] Complications include transient or permanent nerve injury most often to the radial and then the ulnar nerve. Deep infection occurs in about 5 percent of patients. A persistent nonunion is uncommon today but occurs with a frequency of about 5 percent.

JOINT REPLACEMENT ARTHROPLASTY

Since Mitsunaga's initial study, significant improvements in the design of elbow joint replacement have allowed reliable replacement of the elbow with post-traumatic arthrosis (Fig. 24–8).[23] A particularly attractive feature of the Mayo-modified Coonrad device used at the Mayo Clinic is that distal humeral nonunion at the level of the roof of the olecranon fossa can be resected and the implant inserted without altering the original anatomic axis of rotation (Fig.

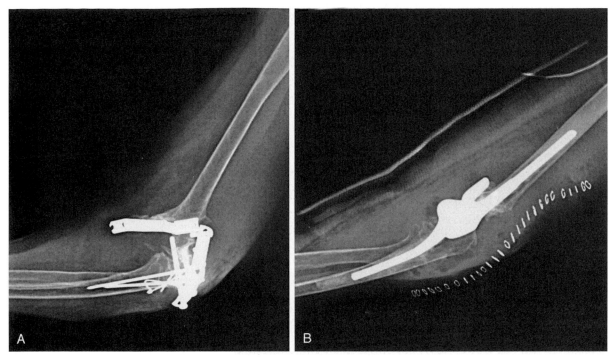

FIGURE 24–8 • *A,* A 71-year-old female with ununited comminuted T-condylar fracture at 5 months following surgery. *B,* Total elbow arthroplasty allowed 20 to 130 degrees of flexion and no pain.

24–9). This technique obviates the need for custom implants to treat most instances of distal humerus resection. In addition, the bone graft placed behind the anterior flange reliably incorporates and not only prevents the adverse posterior directed forces but also resists rotatory forces. This allows durable fixation in the tubular distal humerus after the condyles have been resected. The role of joint replacement for nonunions about the elbow is described in Chapter 53.

AUTHORS' PREFERENCE

For patients under the age of 55 years, osteosynthesis with the technique described earlier is the treatment of choice. If the ulnohumeral joint is severely ankylosed, the distraction device is used in conjunction with osteosynthesis or as a staged procedure. In patients over the age of 55 years or in whom the fracture involves only the articular elements or in whom the segments are markedly osteoporotic and not salvageable, joint replacement arthroplasty is the treatment of choice.

MALUNION

There is a paucity of information in the literature on the treatment of elbow malunion and most relates to the adoles-

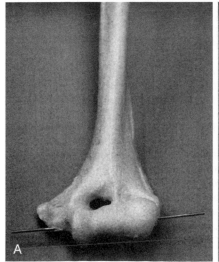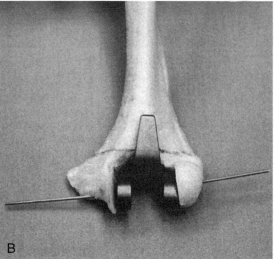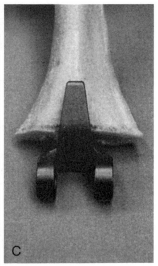

FIGURE 24–9 • Model of the distal humerus showing the normal axis of rotation *(A).* The axis of rotation is replicated by the Mayo-modified Coonrad implant with the condyles intact *(B).* If the condyles are removed, the axis is maintained at the anatomic location *(C).*

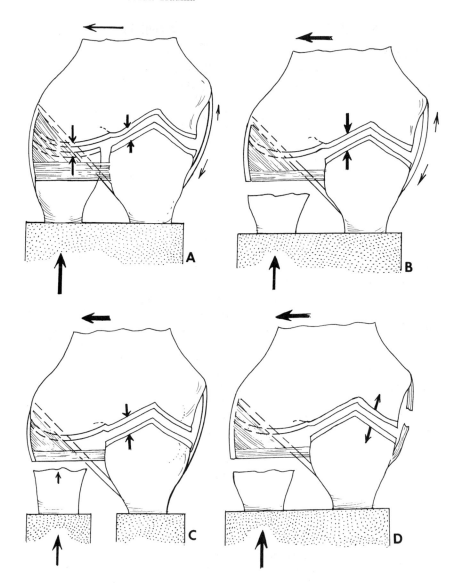

FIGURE 25–6 • *A*, Elbow stability requires articular and ligamentous integrity. *B*, Absence of the radial head does not cause instability if the ulnar collateral ligament and distal radioulnar joint are intact. *C*, Proximal migration can occur if distal ligaments are ruptured. *D*, Valgus laxity may be present if the ulnar ligament is violated.

able in the development of myositis ossificans.[81, 136] The significance and management of this complication are discussed later in this chapter and in Chapter 32.

FRACTURE MANAGEMENT

Most clinicians have personally experienced disappointment with the treatment of radial head fracture:

• • • In none of these cases should a too optimistic prognosis be given, for traumatic arthritis with painful restricted rotation may follow an apparently minor injury with or without displacement, regardless of treatment.[38] • • •

In general, the treatment of radial head fractures is based on the fracture type and the presence of any associated injury.

Uncomplicated Fractures

TYPE I

Treatment

There is little question that the type I fracture (Fig. 25–7), because of its favorable prognosis and lack of concurrent

soft tissue or other osseous injury, should be managed with early motion.[1, 5, 7, 23, 99, 101, 103, 144, 147] To facilitate immediate motion, a concept long advocated by Dehna and Torp,[33] aspiration of the joint, is recommended by some[108, 110] but does not appear to alter the final outcome.[62]

Results

Although cast immobilization is unheard of today, a study from India of 50 patients treated in a cast for relatively short periods reported an overall satisfactory result in 86 percent.[87] Early motion compared with prolonged immobilization does appear to offer advantages of early return of function. Mason and Schutkin, reporting a military experience, found a mean period of disability of 4 weeks in 18 patients treated with early motion, compared with 7 weeks in 7 individuals treated with 3 weeks of immobilization.[85] The major residuum is loss of extension rather than pain.[31] Adler and Shaftan[9] reported 23 excellent and 3 good results among 26 patients treated with early motion. No poor results were noted in 79 patients reported on by Gaston and colleagues[46] or in 55 patients reported on by Johnson[66] treated by early motion. Despite these optimistic accounts, this fracture may have been associated with an inexplicably poor outcome in 5[7, 103] to 13 percent of patients.[112] Mason[86] reported that about one third of his 62 patients with this fracture lost an average of 7 degrees of extension. Displacement following early motion was implicated as a factor in some of these treatment failures, and this may occur more often than is appreciated.

Complications

The most frequent complication of Type I fracture is displacement or nonunion (Fig. 25–8). If a nonunion of a fragment occurs, it is not always symptomatic, but, if necessary, delayed excision of the entire head may be considered.[25] Nonunion of the neck may sometimes be salvaged with osteosynthesis, but excision is the rule if there is no ligamentous injury. Increasingly, the nonunion is left intact if it involves the neck and if it is minimally symptomatic (Fig. 25–9).

TYPE II

Most of the controversy surrounding radial head fractures is focused on the proper management of type II fractures.

Nonoperative Treatment

Nonoperative treatment for type II fractures is similar to that described for type I fractures—that is, early motion as tolerated (Fig. 25–10). If displacement is considered possible, however, 2 to 3 weeks of immobilization is recommended. If nonoperative management is selected, some

information regarding the prognosis of delayed excision is necessary.

Delayed Excision of the Radial Head. As noted, recommendations for nonoperative treatment are predicated on the assumption that a delayed resection will salvage an unsatisfactory result from the nonoperative initial procedure. Yet there is little in the literature regarding delayed excision. Speed, in 1941,[125] stated that late excision is "of great help" but suggested that the results were not as good as those obtained by early surgery. If delayed more than 6 weeks, surgical excision is said to give poor results.[129]

Results. Gaston and associates[46] reported that in six patients with late excision 3 months to 16 years after fracture, flexion averaged 5 to 100 degrees, 63 degrees of pronation and 66 degrees of supination, a mean of 20 years after surgery.

Among 21 patients treated with delayed excision at the Mayo Clinic, Broberg and Morrey[11] reported 75 percent with decreased pain and 77 percent with improved motion. The time to delayed excision ranged from 1 month to 20 years (Fig. 25–11).

In summary, some considerable improvement in flexion and forearm rotation and moderate relief of pain can reasonably be expected.[11] If secondary arthrosis has intervened, the chances of a satisfactory result are compromised.

Complications. Complications that occur with nonoperatively managed type II or III fractures include residual pain and motion loss. The radiographic findings usually are those of a deformed radial head without subsequent arthrosis, lack of heterotopic bone, and a striking lack of correlation with the clinical results.[23]

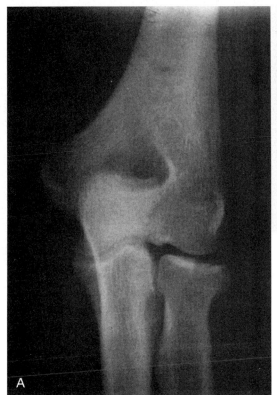
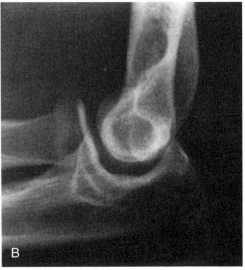

FIGURE 25–7 • *A,* Type I fracture involving approximately 50 percent of the head but with less than 2 mm of displacement. *B,* Minimally angulated neck fracture is also considered a type I fracture.

of longer than 16 years. Eighty-six percent had satisfactory results by all objective criteria. Ninety-four percent returned to their previous occupations. Only 22 percent had as much as 1 mm of shortening of the wrist. Despite these favorable results, these investigators recommend nonoperative treatment for type II fractures.

Mayo Experience and Comparative Studies

Mayo's study of cases of resection for type II fractures a mean of 20 years after surgery revealed over 80 percent satisfactory results.[92] A medial ulnohumeral osteophyte was commonly observed radiographically, but ulnohumeral symptoms were rare and mild. Proximal radial migration averaged 2 mm in the uncomplicated circumstance. Wrist symptoms were present in about 15 percent, but in no instance was this disabling to, or the major factor limiting, the patient's function.

A few studies have actually compared operative and nonoperative management of type II fractures. Adler and Shaftan[1] found roughly comparable good short-term results in 17 of 20 patients without surgery and in 13 of 18 with resection. Murray[97] compared 30 nonoperative cases with 16 surgically treated cases. Full motion was obtained in about 35 percent of both groups. The retrospective survey of Radin and Riseborough included 16 nonoperatively treated patients, six of whom were managed with early radial head excision.[112] The motion in these patients was "far greater" than that in the conservatively treated group. In Burton's experience, only two of nine nonoperatively treated patients had good results, compared with 22 of 25 patients after excision of the radial head.[16]

Open Reduction and Internal Fixation. Experience with open reduction and internal fixation is satisfactory in over 90 percent of cases.[39, 104, 118, 124]

Geel and coworkers[47] reported less than a 10-degree loss of extension and a 10-degree loss of pronation and supination in 19 patients who underwent open reduction and internal fixation. A similar outcome was observed by Sanders and French[116] in eight patients treated for difficult type III fractures. The Herbert screw has been reported to provide virtually normal function.[15] The traditional AO technique using the 2.0 or 2.7 screws has been reported as satisfactory in 100 percent of patients with Mason type II fractures but in only 33 percent of those with Mason type III fractures.[73] A small buttress plate can be used for radial neck fractures.[77] Overall, patients with associated injuries seem to benefit the most from such fracture management, particularly when considering the anticipated results of alternative procedures.[42, 105] Esser and colleagues[39] reported on 20 cases of osteosynthesis, 11 with type II and 9 with type III. All were graded as satisfactory after osteosynthesis. They emphasize the need to attain a special 45-degree anterior oblique radiograph to accurately ascertain the exact nature of the fracture.[104]

Comparative Data. One recent prospective study by Khalfayan and associates[72] compared the results of 16 patients treated by closed reduction and 20 by open reduction and internal fixation. The former had only 44 percent satisfactory results, compared with 90 percent in the group treated by open reduction and internal fixation.[72] Rochwerger and colleagues[115] compared the treatment of 22 type

II fractures. With mean surveillance of 5 years (2 to 23 years), osteosynthesis was found to be superior to resection, as the latter had satisfactory results in just over 50 percent of cases.

TYPE III (UNCOMPLICATED COMMINUTED)

Type III fracture is generally associated with a more severe injury and hence a worse prognosis than fractures of types I and II. Arthrography has demonstrated that up to 85 percent of these injuries have capsular or ligamentous disruption.[65] In addition, the degree of comminution is commonly more extensive than is suggested by the radiographic appearance (Fig. 25–18).[7, 104]

Treatment

There is relatively uniform agreement that comminuted radial head fractures are best treated by complete excision,[5, 21, 23, 31, 57, 61, 66, 70, 86, 97, 140, 149] which is preferred over simple removal of the more displaced fragments[97] and when osteosynthesis is not possible.

Early excision is more critical in this fracture than in type II injuries.[21, 23, 31, 65, 86, 118] The traditional wisdom of deferring radial head resection during growth has been questioned in a primate study, which showed virtually no alteration in growth or alignment as a result of radial head resection with open physes.[60] Although some investigators have reported satisfactory results with osteosynthesis, the extensive and badly comminuted fracture is not considered amenable to internal fixation.

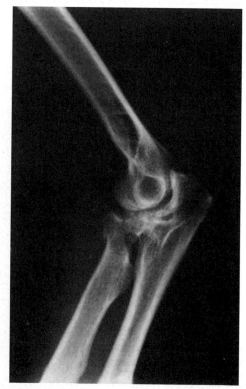

FIGURE 25–18 • Type III fracture demonstrating comminution.

Results

Because there is greater comminution in the type III fracture, less satisfactory results might be anticipated than after the type I or II injury. In Mason's series,[86] return to work was observed in 17 of 18 patients within 9.5 weeks. Yet Conn and Wade[28] reported good results in 28 of 33 patients with simple excision. Radin and Riseborough[112] observed satisfactory results in six of seven patients who underwent early excision, but outcome was poor with nonoperative treatment or late excision. The difference between objective and subjective results was noted by Carstam,[21] who reported satisfactory subjective results in 85 percent of patients but satisfactory objective results in only 55 percent.

There have been few attempts to compare different treatments. Cutler[31] reported that the early results of nonoperative treatment were better than those of operative treatment; at 1 year, however, the two groups were not comparable. Grossman[51] found operative and nonoperative treatment results comparable, whereas Arner and colleagues[5] demonstrated superior results with nonoperative treatment.

We and others[27] have reported long-term objective functional results in patients undergoing radial head excision for type III fractures an average of 21 years after surgery.[92] The mean range of motion in six patients was 5 to 137 degrees of flexion-extension, 63 degrees of pronation, and 66 degrees of supination. Losses of 12 percent of flexion strength, 8 percent of extension strength, 24 percent of pronation, 13 percent of supination, and 11 percent of grip strength were reported. The radiographic findings of these six patients revealed that five had minimal and one had moderate degenerative changes at the ulnohumeral articulation. These changes tend to be asymptomatic.[23, 92]

SEQUELAE OF SURGICAL EXCISION

Symptoms at the Wrist

Pain at the wrist from a concurrent disruption of the distal radioulnar joint was first reported in two patients by Brockman[13] in 1930 and later by Speed[125] and Curr and Coe.[30] In 1951, two additional cases were described by Essex-Lopresti,[40] and the injury has subsequently been associated with him. Given the frequency of radial head fracture and the relatively rare reports of concurrent wrist injury, this condition is uncommon, occurring in only about 1 to 2 percent of fractures.[78]

Concurrent wrist injury is not to be confused with the delayed process that occurs after radial head excision (Fig. 25-19).[41, 79, 89] Many investigators have noted an increase of 2 to 3 mm in proximal radial migration, with a frequency of 8,[21] 12,[7] 27,[78, 89] and even 54 percent.[134] Symptoms of the wrist are reported variously as insignificant[7, 21, 71] or as occurring with a frequency of 12[112] or even 87 percent.[134]

Arthrosis of the wrist is not a common finding and was not thought to be significant in 13 patients who had an average proximal radial migration of 1.9 mm and who were observed for an average of 20 years by Morrey and colleagues.[92]

Instability

Increased elbow valgus varies from 5 to 20 degrees and occurs in about 5 percent of patients.[7, 46, 97, 120] The largest and most carefully conducted study reported an average increase of 8 degrees valgus in 31 of 71 patients after total excision and 5.5 degrees if the fracture fragment alone had been removed.[21] Stress analysis of the elbow joint suggests that the elbow is stable to valgus stress[94] if the ulnar collateral ligament is intact, even if the radial head has been removed (see Fig. 25-6). Acute instability results from radial head excision with unrecognized medial collateral ligament injury (Fig. 25-20).

Instability in pronation and supination is uncommon,[46, 142] and its clinical relevance has not been generally recognized. We have experienced a significant number of patients with residual radioulnar impingement requiring a secondary debridement procedure. When performed for isolated symptoms, this is usually successful; when performed in conjunction with other pathologic conditions, the outcome is less predictable.

Loss of Strength

Loss of strength has rarely been quantitated after this injury or its treatment.[21] Measurements of 13 patients in our laboratory demonstrated an average loss of grip, pronation, and supination strength of about 18 percent. Flexion strength loss averaged 9 percent and extension weakness 6 percent.[92] No comparable data are available in a group treated nonoperatively; consequently, the specific functional loss due to the absent radial head compared with the direct effect of trauma is open to speculation.

Degenerative Arthritis

Arthritis at the ulnohumeral joint is observable radiographically after radial head excision, but no good studies are available for comparison with a similar, nonoperative group (Fig. 25-21). Radiographic arthritis was reported in 28 of 69 patients (41 percent) who were observed for an average of 9 years by Carstam.[21] Little significance has been attributed to these changes, but we correlated elbow pain with the more extensive radiographic changes seen in 13 patients who were observed for 10 to 30 years. The data suggest that mild but definite symptoms of arthrosis occur with longer surveillance.

Heterotopic Calcification

The presence of calcification after radial head excision has been variably reported (Fig. 25-22).[16, 18, 71] Rather significant calcification around the osteotomy site has been reported in 10[46] to 30 percent[142] of patients. However, there is relatively little clinical correlation with the presence and extent of such heterotopic bone.[86, 131] Proximal radioulnar synostosis due to extensive heterotopic bone is most frequently seen in children[71] or in fracture dislocation.[68]

Myositis Ossificans

Certainly the most dreaded complication of this type of fracture is myositis ossificans.[90] Thompson and Garcia found that the complication developed most commonly in radial head fractures with associated elbow dislocation.[136] Of the seven cases in which myositis ossificans was ob-

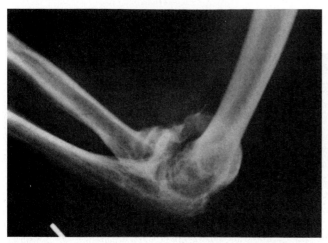

FIGURE 25–22 • Heterotopic ossification occurred in this elbow after radial head excision was performed about 5 days after a type IV injury occurred.

served in the 110 patients reported by Adler,[1] five had a type IV fracture. Excision has proved successful in about 75 percent in a recent review of our experience.

Neural Injury

An uncommon complication reported by Crawford[29] is late radial tunnel syndrome observed in two cases of radial head excision. We have also seen several instances of this particular problem. However, most commonly, radial nerve pathology occurs after injury, resection, or fixation and resolves over time.

Complicated Fractures

By definition, *complicated fracture* implies an associated fracture of the olecranon or coronoid, or injury of the ligamentous complex as well. This is considered a complex instability and is discussed in Chapter 30. The technique for open reduction and fixation is discussed earlier. It is reasonable to consider fracture dislocation and its treatment, including prosthetic replacement, in some detail.

FRACTURE-DISLOCATION (TYPE IV)

Elbow dislocation with radial head fracture is a rather common associated injury. A review of several series[1, 7, 21, 26, 46, 56, 97, 149] reveals 119 elbow dislocations complicating 1459 fractures, an incidence of about 8 percent.

The incidence of the inverse relation—that is, a radial head fracture with elbow dislocation—averages about 12 percent.[26, 80, 98, 149] Simply stated, approximately 10 percent of patients who sustain elbow dislocations have associated radial head fractures; similarly, about 10 percent of radial head fractures are complicated by elbow dislocation—that is, a type IV fracture. Most radial head fractures are displaced[57] type II or III fractures (Fig. 25–23).[12]

Treatment

Treatment consists of immediate reduction of the dislocation and treatment of the fractured radial head on its own

merit. Some clinicians do not alter the treatment plan because of the dislocation. McLaughlin[90] recommends immediate excision with a degree of urgency "to be measured in hours." Even Adler and Shaftan,[1] rather staunch advocates of nonoperative management of radial head fracture, emphasize that if surgery is necessary it should be done within the first 24 hours. After excision, immobilization of the elbow in the neutral position for 3 or 4 weeks has been recommended.[1, 28] This has been shown to be an excessively long period of immobilization, so we begin motion after about 1 week or sooner with a hinged splint.[12] In a detailed study of 22 patients with fracture dislocations of the elbow,[141] five different treatment options were used, a situation similar to that in a report from the Mayo Clinic.[12] Currently, we find the external fixator (DJD, Howmedica, Rutherford, NJ) of great assistance in these problems, as it can be applied percutaneously and allows for removal of the axis pin passing through the joint (see Chapter 34).

Results

More than half of all poor results associated with radial head fractures have been attributed to this type of fracture.[1] Flexion contracture of 15 to 30 degrees and 25 to 50 degrees of forearm rotation can be expected.[1, 56, 66] Early motion, beginning by the sixth day, has improved the outcome.[46] In our experience, no good outcome occurred if immobilization lasted for more than 4 weeks,[12] and early motion yielded results that were nearly as good as those achieved with uncomplicated fractures (Fig. 25–24).[12] In fact, using objective criteria, 75 percent of patients with this injury were observed to have satisfactory results.[12] One study reported a 90 percent satisfactory rate with emphasis on early motion.[141]

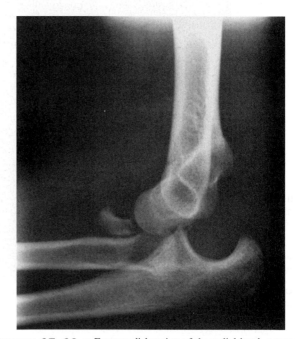

FIGURE 25–23 • Fracture-dislocation of the radial head, a type IV injury.

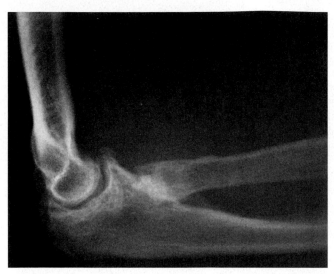

FIGURE 25–24 • This comminuted radial head fracture was excised in a patient with elbow dislocation. The patient had a good result 15 years after surgery but had radiographic evidence of arthritis.

PROSTHETIC REPLACEMENT

Background

The first English reference to prosthetic replacement of the radial head is that of Speed in 1941.[125] After extensive experimentation and several design modifications,[64] Vitallium ferrule caps were implanted in three patients. A decade later, Cherry[24] discussed a limited experience with an acrylic implant. The concept was later popularized by Swanson,[132] who used a silicone prosthesis.

Indications

Complicated radial head fracture is the indication for the use of the prosthesis. This occurs in six clinical settings[55]:

1. Dislocation of the elbow with radial head fracture (type IV fracture)
2. Concurrent medial collateral ligament disruption
3. Concurrent or residual lateral ulnar collateral ligament dysfunction.
4. Monteggia variant with olecranon and radial head fracture
5. Fracture of a major portion of the coronoid
6. Concurrent distal radioulnar joint injury (Essex-Lopresti)

If the elbow dislocates and if the radial head is excised, replacement with a radial head prosthesis might be considered if it enhances stability and allows early motion (Fig. 25–25). Increased valgus angulation, probably due to concurrent medial ligament injury,[6, 65, 119] can be addressed with use of the spacer.[83, 132] Instability of the proximal radius associated with severe fractures or excessive excision[83, 125, 134] can be lessened with the use of an implant. With large type II coronoid fractures, considerably enhanced stability is offered by the radial head, so the prosthesis may provide some element of stability in this clinical setting (Fig. 25–26). Finally, the implant stabilizes the

radius if the head is removed in the presence of interosseous membrane and distal radioulnar joint disruption.

Prosthetic Design

The early prostheses were made of Vitallium[125] or acrylic,[24] but the prosthesis made of Silastic and designed by Swanson is probably the most commonly used in the United States[88, 93, 133, 146] and abroad.[83, 84] However, the host of complications, coupled with the poor mechanical properties of Silastic in terms of withstanding axial load, has dramatically lessened the use of this material. Gupta and colleagues[52] recently assessed the mechanical properties of cobalt/chrome, titanium alloy, alumina ceramic, and ultra-high molecular weight polyethylene (UHMWPE). Although both metal and the UHMWPE showed acceptable resistance to axial load, the UHMWPE showed the best load transmission characteristics to the proximal ulna. What remains unclear is the tolerance of the cartilage to any of these materials.

The bipolar design of Judet represents, in our judgment, a real advance in design concept (Fig. 25–27).[67] Some concern regarding the extent of the exposure necessary to implant the device does exist, along with the length of the stem. Because of the increasing incidence of complex instability and because of the theoretical advantages of radial head replacement in this setting, renewed interest has been generated in prosthesis implant design. We conclude that newer designs must have several size options, flexibility at the articulation, and enhanced instrumentation to allow accurate and reproducible implantation.

Results

The successful use of the Silastic implant was reported in six patients with an average follow-up of 2.6 years by Swanson and colleagues.[133] Carn and associates[19] reviewed the experience in 10 patients treated with Silastic radial head implant replacement an average of more than 3 years after surgery; they found that only 50 percent had satisfactory results and over 50 percent had evidence of degenerative arthrosis. Similar disappointing results were reported by Trepman and Ewald,[137] and these two studies tend to reflect the current perception and accepted opinion that the Silastic radial head implant is not adequate to bear the stresses required of the radiohumeral joint and so should be avoided in most cases.

The Vitallium replacement provided satisfactory results in 12 cases of uncomplicated radial head fractures.[20] A careful and detailed description by Harrington and associates[55] of the use of 15 Vitallium and 2 Silastic replacements for unstable elbow joints documented 8 excellent, 6 good, 2 fair, and 1 poor result. These investigators wisely recommend use of the implant in complicated but not in uncomplicated radial head fractures. Experience with 18 Silastic implants for type II, III, and IV radial head fractures showed 7 excellent, 10 good, and 1 poor result after an average of 26 months of follow-up.[83] No increase in carrying angle was present in this group, but four patients had as much as 4 mm of distal subluxation, and one of these had pain and tenderness at the wrist.

Fourteen patients with simple radial head fractures

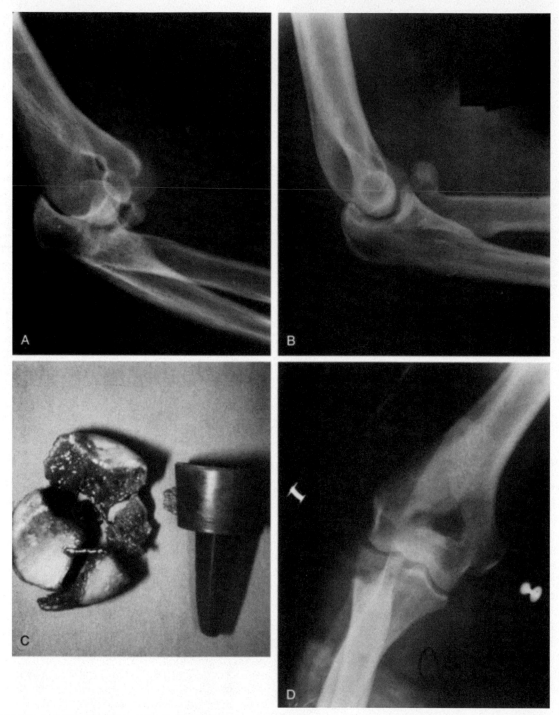

FIGURE 25–25 • *A,* Type IV injury of the dominant elbow in a 48-year-old man. *B,* A residual type III fracture was present after reduction. A Silastic implant *(C)* was used to replace the radial head *(D).*

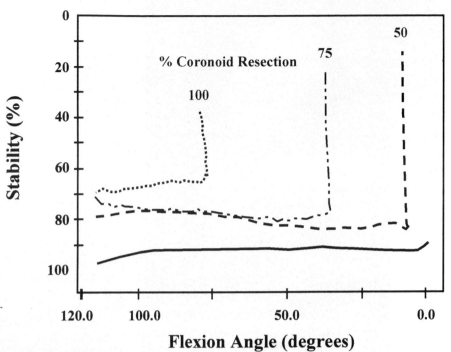

FIGURE 25–26 • Elbow stability after coronoid and radial head resection. Laboratory data reveal the value of the radial head when 50 percent or more of the coronoid has been removed.

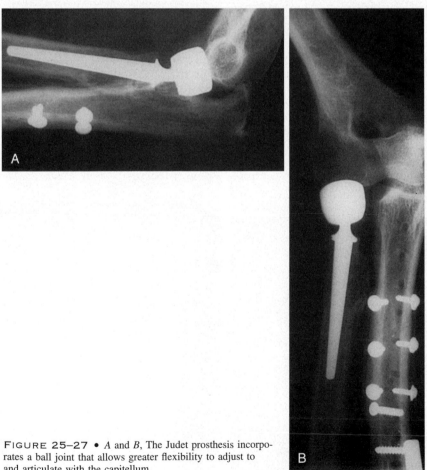

FIGURE 25–27 • A and B, The Judet prosthesis incorporates a ball joint that allows greater flexibility to adjust to and articulate with the capitellum.

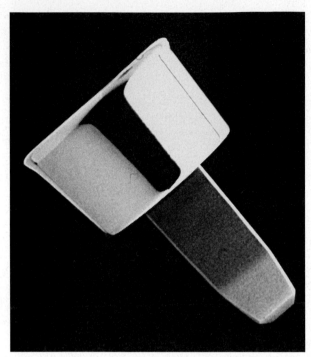

FIGURE 25–28 • A metallic device is used currently with greater confidence than that from the Silastic device. The optimum implant design has yet to appear.

treated by excision and metallic prosthetic replacement were compared with 11 patients with simple fractures treated by excision alone.[36] Satisfactory results were reported in 64 percent with excision and 76 percent with the device (Fig. 25–28).

The most recent information regarding the innovative implant of Judet is one of 12 patients followed at least 2 years. In all five elbows with implants inserted for acute fractures, results were satisfactory without complication.

In summary, the available data suggest that the prosthesis is useful in fractures associated with elbow or wrist insta-

bility. Expectations are of improved results with improved designs.

Complications

Numerous adverse effects have been associated with Silastic implants. Fatigue failure has occurred with both the acrylic[36] and the Silastic,[8, 88, 93] prostheses. In the report by Morrey and colleagues,[93] three of six Silastic implants showed fracture of the prosthesis (Fig. 25–29). Mayhall and associates[88] reported that 4 of 12 patients had symptomatic fractures of the device requiring revision of the prosthesis 9 to 36 months after surgery. Although poor technique may be responsible for some prosthetic failures, fatigue failure of the implant appears to account for most poor results. The inadequate material properties of the Silastic device for use at the radial head are generally accepted and have been confirmed by recent studies.[19, 137]

Finally, the synovitis reported to occur with Silastic hand implants can and does occur at the elbow.[22, 50, 150] Worsing and colleagues[150] observed clinical and experimental evidence of foreign-body giant cell reaction elicited by particulate Silastic debris. We have observed an articular reaction identical to that seen in the patient with rheumatoid arthritis.[139]

Thus, because of their inadequate material properties and demonstrable adverse biologic characteristics, Silastic replacements should rarely be used at the elbow. Even then, removal at 1 year is recommended.

Carr and Howard[20] reported no complications in 12 patients with the Vitallium cap. Harrington and Tountas[55] observed one dislocation among 15 patients with the metal prosthesis. The long-term effect of the metallic/capitellar articulation is also suspect.

ESSEX LOPRESTI INJURY

The Essex-Lopresti injury is a most troubling injury complex.[3] Several points have been made clear by Trousdale and associates[138] from Mayo and Edwards and Jupiter[37]

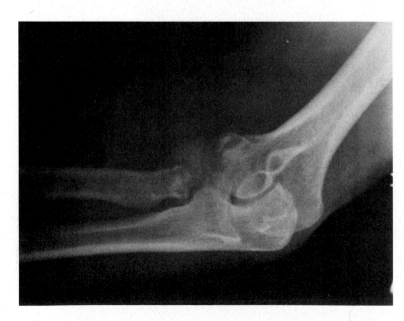

FIGURE 25–29 • Eight years after surgery, the prosthesis is deformed, with a fracture at the stem. The patient's condition, however, was rated as good with few symptoms. (From Morrey, B. F., Askew, L., and Chao, E. Y.: Silastic prosthetic replacement for the radial head. J. Bone Joint Surg. 63A:454, 1981.)

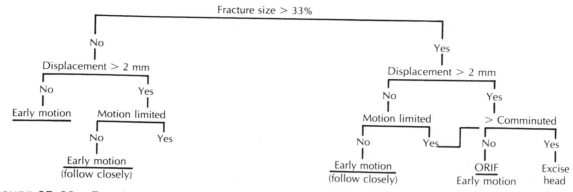

FIGURE 25-30 • Example of treatment logic that might be employed for the management of the uncomplicated radial head fracture.

from Massachusetts General Hospital. Early treatment from accurate immediate diagnosis can result in a successful outcome in about 80 percent of cases. However, if the diagnosis is delayed, reconstruction is successful in only about 33 percent. Hence, an accurate acute diagnosis seems to be more important than the actual mode of treatment.

The radial head is managed by leaving the type I, fixing the type II, and replacing the type III fragments, currently with a metallic device. The forearm is fully supinated after surgery. Further, the degree of axial radial instability is assessed at the time of surgery. If grossly unstable, then the radius is stabilized to the ulna for a period of 3 to 4 weeks with a cross pin inserted distally. The distal szabilizer may also be repaired.

AUTHOR'S PREFERRED TREATMENT

For all fracture types, treatment is initiated by a word of caution to the patient to expect some loss of motion. If

motion loss does not occur, so much the better. The overall thought process and treatment logic are summarized in Figure 25–30.

Type I Fractures

Type I fractures are treated by joint aspiration and lidocaine with epinephrine injection, a collar and cuff, and immediate motion as tolerated. If the fracture is stable, we see the patient in about 7 to 10 days; if it is unstable, re-evaluation is done at 3 to 5 days and at regular intervals for up to 3 months. We do not routinely use physical therapy in these patients.

Type II Fractures

Depending on the nature of the fracture and the presence or absence of associated injury, we tend to fix these fractures (Fig. 25–31).

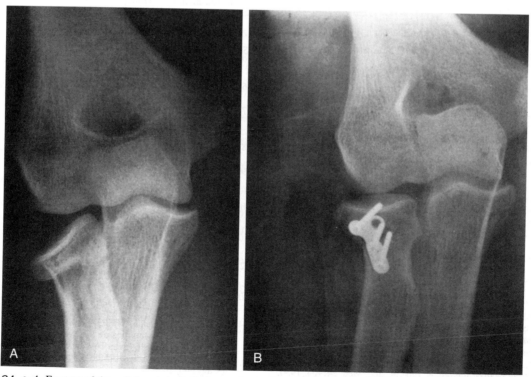

FIGURE 25–31 • A, Fracture of the radial neck typically is associated with deficiency of the medial collateral ligament. B, Open reduction and internal fixation is indicated in such patients, and a buttress plate using the minisystem has proved effective.

109. Pribyl, C. R., Kester, M. A., Cook, S. D., Edmunds, J. O., and Brunet, M. E.: The effect of the radial head and prosthetic radial head replacement on resisting valgus stress at the elbow. Orthopaedics 9:723, 1986.

110. Quigley, T. B.: Aspiration of the elbow joint in the treatment of fractures of the head of the radius. N. Engl. J. Med. 240:915, 1949.

111. Rabourdin, A. N.: Fractures of the head of the radius. Paris, Steinheill, 1910, p. 11.

112. Radin, E. L., and Riseborough, E. J.: Fractures of the radial head. J. Bone Joint Surg. 48A:1055, 1966.

113. Regan, W., and Morrey, B. F.: Fractures of the coronoid process of the ulna. J. Bone Joint Surg. 71A:1348, 1989.

114. Reith, P. L.: Fractures of the radial head associated with chip fracture of the capitellum in adults: surgical considerations. South. Surgeon 14:154, 1948.

115. Rochwerger, A., Bataille, J. F., Kelberine, F., Curvale, G., and Groulier, P.: Retrospective analysis of 78 surgically repaired fractures of the radial head. Acta Orthop. Belg. 62(suppl 1): 87, 1996.

116. Sanders, R. A., and French, H. G.: Open reduction and internal fixation of comminuted radial head fractures. Am. J. Sports Med. 14:130, 1986.

117. Scharplatz, D., and Allgower, M.: Fractures-dislocations of the elbow. Injury 7:143, 1976.

118. Shmueli, G., and Herold, H. Z.: Compression screwing of displaced fractures of the head of the radius. J. Bone Joint Surg. 63B:535, 1981.

119. Schwab, G. H., Bennett, J. B., Woods, G. W., and Tulloos, H. S.: The biomechanics of elbow stability: The role of the medical collateral ligament. Clin. Orthop. 146:42, 1980.

120. Schwartz, R., and Young, F.: Treatment of fractures of the head and neck of the radius and slipped radial epiphysis in children. Surg. Gynecol. Obstet. 57:528, 1933.

121. Sever, J.: Fractures of the head and neck of the radius: A study of end results. J.A.M.A. 84:1551, 1925.

122. Simpson, N. S., Goodman, L. A., and Jupiter, J. B.: Contoured LCDC plating of the proximal ulna. Injury 27:411, 1996.

123. Sojbjerg, J. O., Ovesen, J., and Gundorf, C. E.: The stability of the elbow following excision of the radial head and transection of the annular ligament: An experimental study. Arch. Orthop. Trauma Surg. 106:248, 1987.

124. Soler, R. R., Tarela, J. P., and Minores, J. M.: Internal fixation of fractures of the proximal end of the radius in adults. Injury 10:268, 1979.

125. Speed, K.: Ferrule caps for the head of the radius. Surg. Gynecol. Obstet. 73:845, 1941.

126. Speed, K.: Fracture of the head of the radius. Am. J. Surg. 38:157, 1924.

127. Spinner, M., and Kaplan, E. B.: The quadrate ligament of the elbow: Its relationship to the stability of the proximal radioulnar joint. Acta Orthop. Scand. 41:632, 1970.

128. Stankovic, P.: Über die operative Versorgung von Frakturen des proximalen Radiusendes. Chirurg. 49:377, 1978.

129. Stephen, I. B. M.: Excision of the radial head for closed fracture. Acta Orthop. Scand. 52:409, 1981.

130. Strachan, J. C. H., and Ellis, B. W.: Vulnerability of the posterior interosseous nerve during radial head resection. J. Bone Joint Surg. 53B:320, 1971.

131. Sutro, C. J.: Regrowth of bone at the proximal end of the radius following resection in this region. J. Bone Joint Surg. 17:867, 1935.

132. Swanson, A. B.: Flexible Implant Resection Arthroplasty in the Hand and Extremities. St. Louis, C. V. Mosby Co., 1973.

133. Swanson, A. B., Jaeger, S. H., and LaRochelle, D.: Comminuted fractures of the radial head: The role of silicone-implant replacement arthroplasty. J. Bone Joint Surg. 63A:1039, 1981.

134. Taylor, T. K. F., and O'Connor, B. T.: The effect upon the inferior radio-ulnar joint of excision of the head of the radius in adults. J. Bone Joint Surg. 46B:83, 1964.

135. Thomas, T. T.: Fractures of the head of the radius. Univ. Pa. Med. Bull. 18:184, 221, 1905.

136. Thompson, H. C., III, and Garcia, A.: Myositis ossificans: Aftermath of elbow injuries. Clin. Orthop. 50:129, 1967.

137. Trepman, E., and Ewald, F. C.: Early failure of silicone radial head implants in the rheumatoid elbow. J. Arthroplasty 6:59, 1991.

138. Trousdale, R. T., Amadio, P. C., Cooney, W. P., III, and Morrey, B. F.: Radio-ulnar dissociation spectrum of the Essex-Lopresti injury. J. Bone Joint Surg. 74A:1486, 1992.

139. VanderWilde, R. S., Morrey, B. F., Melberg, M. W., and Vinh, T. N.: Inflammatory arthrosis of the ulno-humeral joint after failed silicone radial head implant. J. Bone Joint Surg. 76B:78, 1994.

140. Vertonger, P.: Displaced fractures of the radial head. J. Bone Joint Surg. 43B:191, 1961.

141. Vichard, P. H., Tropet, Y., Dreyfuschmidt, G., Besancenot, J., Menez, D., and Pem, R.: Fractures of the proximal end of the radius associated with other traumatic lesions of the upper limb: A report of seventy-three cases. Ann. Chir. Main. 7:45, 1988.

142. Wagner, C.: Fractures of the head of the radius. Am. J. Surg. 89:911, 1955.

143. Ward, W. G., and Nunley, J. A.: Concomitant fractures of the capitellum and radial head. J. Orthop. Trauma. 2:110, 1988.

144. Watson-Jones, R.: Discussion of minor injuries of the elbow joint. Proc. R. Soc. Med. 23:323, 1930.

145. Watson-Jones, R.: Fractures and Other Bone and Joint Injuries, 2nd ed. Baltimore, Williams & Wilkins Co., 1941, p. 336.

146. Weingarden, T. L.: Prosthetic replacement in the treatment of fractures of the radial head. J. Am. Osteopath. Assoc. 77:804, 1978.

147. Weseley, M. S., Barenfeld, P. A., and Eisenstein, A. L.: Closed treatment of isolated radial head fractures. J. Trauma 23A:36, 1983.

148. Wexner, S. D., Goodwin, C., Parkes, J. C., II, Webber, B. R., and Patterson, A. H.: Treatment of fractures of the radial head by partial excision. Orthop. Rev. 14:83, 1985.

149. Wilson, P. D.: Fracture and dislocation in the region of the elbow. Surg. Gynecol. Obstet. 56:335, 1933.

150. Worsing, R. A., Engber, W. D., and Lange, T. A.: Reactive synovits from particulate Silastic. J. Bone Joint Surg. 64A:581, 1982.

CHAPTER 26

Fractures of the Olecranon

• MIGUEL E. CABANELA and
BERNARD F. MORREY

RELEVANT ANATOMIC OBSERVATIONS

Of the various anatomic fractures of the olecranon, the articular surface is particularly noteworthy. The layer of cartilage covering the sigmoid notch is usually interrupted by a transverse streak of uncovered bone situated between the olecranon and the coronoid process. Hence, anatomic reconstruction of a fracture through this area occurs from aligning the coronoid and olecranon, often based on the cortical fracture alignment. Posteriorly, the triceps tendon inserts into the olecranon, and its fascia has a medial and lateral expansion that helps prevent displacement of low-energy fractures. Because of its subcutaneous position, the olecranon is particularly vulnerable to direct trauma. Essentially all olecranon fractures are intra-articular and therefore tend to compromise the stability of the elbow joint. The ossification center for the olecranon appears at age 9 years and consistently fuses at the age of 14 to 14½ years. Persistent physeal lines, usually bilateral, have been reported and are easily differentiated from fractures.[50] They are often partial, are perpendicular to the ulnar shaft, and are not accompanied by soft tissue swelling. Patella cubiti,[35] an accessory ossicle in the triceps tendon adjacent to the olecranon, is also bilateral when present (see Chapter 74).

HISTORICAL ASPECTS

Early treatises on fractures of the proximal ulna recommended splinting in extension for a period of 4 to 6 weeks. The standard of plaster immobilization often resulted in a stiff elbow in a nonfunctional position, changed the position of immobilization to one of midflexion, and discouraged union by allowing separation of the fragments. Early motion appears to have been first mentioned by Elliot, who in 1934 advised no splint and active motion at 2½ weeks.[19] As long ago as 1884, surgical fixation was reported by Shelton,[58] and Lister utilized a wire loop to fix the fractured fragments[39]; this technique was also utilized by Berger[6] in 1902 and later adopted by Bohler[8] in 1929.

Daland in 1933 reported the first important series of olecranon fractures treated with a variety of materials: wire, nails, bone pegs, kangaroo tendon, and fascia lata.[17] Hey-Groves in 1939 advised open reduction and wiring of the fragments,[27] and Rush in the same year reported the use of an intramedullary rod for this fracture.[56] MacAusland in 1942 introduced the use of longitudinal screw or nail fixation.[40, 41] Since then, the array of internal fixation devices has continued to grow.

Excision of the fractured proximal fragment and repair of the triceps tendon was first reported by Fiolle[21] in 1918. Wainwright in 1942 reported 17 excellent results in 20 cases treated by excision of the olecranon fragment[66]; he believed that the advantages of this procedure were its technical ease, the rapid rehabilitation period, and the lack of arthritis on follow-up. Its disadvantages include limitation of elbow extension, loss of triceps power, loss of the point of the elbow, and the possibility of anteroposterior instability of the joint. This technique was reinforced by McKeever and Buck,[44] who in 1947 reported good strength and excellent range of motion in 10 patients treated with this method. They were the first to quantify that as much as 80 percent of the olecranon can be removed without fear of elbow joint instability. Our laboratory studies suggest the resection should be limited to about 30 percent.[4] Because some patients complained of frequent injury to the "crazy bone," they suggested anterior translocation of the ulnar nerve at the time of excision of the olecranon fragment.

MAYO CLASSIFICATION AND MECHANISMS OF INJURY

There have been several classification systems for these olecranon fractures. Colton[12] produced a scheme based on the anatomy of the fracture, its orientation, and the presence of an associated tear of the collateral ligament (Fig. 26–1). An increasingly discussed method has been advanced by Muller and the AO group in which fractures of the ulna are viewed in relation to (1) fractures of the proximal radius, (2) the level of the fracture, and (3) articular comminution. Variations within each group constitute a thorough but comprehensive description of the fracture (Fig. 26–2). Our experience with this fracture has been to simplify the consideration to the three factors that relate both to the selection of the optimal treatment and to prognosis: displacement, stability, and comminution (Table 26–1; Fig. 26–3).

Type I: Undisplaced Fracture

Type I fractures are typically noncomminuted, although occasionally minimal fragmentation is observed but less than 2 mm of displacement is present. This configuration accounts for 5 percent of olecranon fractures.

• TABLE 26–1 • Characteristics of Mayo Classification of Olecranon Fractures	
Type	**Fractures**
I	Undisplaced
	Displaced
II	Stable
A	Noncomminuted
B	Comminuted
III	Unstable
A	Noncomminuted
B	Comminuted

CLASSIFICATION OF OLECRANON FRACTURES (Morrey)

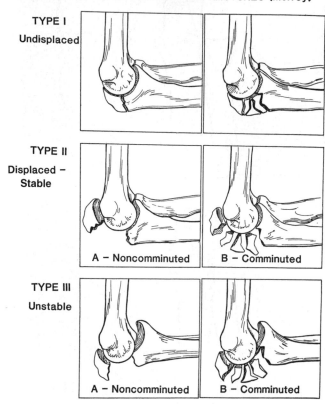

TYPE I
Undisplaced

TYPE II
Displaced –
Stable

A – Noncomminuted | B – Comminuted

TYPE III
Unstable

A – Noncomminuted | B – Comminuted

FIGURE 26–3 • The Mayo classification is based on three variables: displacement, stability, and comminution. Type I is an undisplaced fracture with minimal or no comminution. A type II fracture is displaced but stable, with subtypes comminuted or noncomminuted. The type III and least common fracture is one that is unstable. This is usually comminuted and with associated radial head fracture but occasionally presents as a noncomminuted fracture. Subtype A are noncomminuted, and subtype B comminuted fractures.

device also has been useful for this injury. This topic is discussed in detail later.

Prognosis. Prognosis is guarded.

BIOMECHANICS OF FIXATION

Several rather recent investigations have studied the static rigidity of the most popular modalities of internal fixation. These include the classic AO tension band technique of Weber and Vasey; that of an intramedullary screw, with or without a tension band wire; and plate fixation.[22, 28, 48] With the tension band, Murphy and colleagues[48] found a nonstatistical advantage in the use of a screw plus the wire, as compared with the AO tension band technique. Fyfe and associates,[22] on the other hand, found that the AO tension band with two tightening knots provided fixation superior to that afforded by the screw and wire. If the fracture line can be compressed, the screw and wire technique is preferable. However, it has been shown recently that the screw causes slight displacement in the clinical setting.[26] A modification of the wire placement into the anterior cortex may decrease the tendency to back out but is not more stable in the laboratory setting.[52] Similarly, the use of high tension cables offers no advantage to the standard 18-gauge wire.[37] Both Fyfe and coworkers[22] and Horner and colleagues,[28] however, agreed that the semitubular plate provided the most rigid fixation for comminuted fractures, and a further study showed no mechanical advantage of medial or lateral placement on the olecranon.[33]

TREATMENT METHODS

Rationale for Selecting a Treatment Plan

The goals of treatment in olecranon fractures are (1) restoration of articular congruity, (2) preservation of motor power, (3) restoration of stability, (4) restoration of normal (functional) motion, (5) avoidance or lessening of complications, and (6) rapid recovery. With this in mind, it is obvious that all these fractures, but especially displaced fractures, should be handled by surgery.

Undisplaced Fractures: Type I

Undisplaced fractures can easily be handled by immobilization for 1 to 3 weeks with a long arm cast or a simple posterior splint. The best position is one of mid-flexion and neutral forearm rotation. Full extension for more than a few days should be avoided.

A repeat radiograph is obtained at the initiation of motion. Generally, sufficient stability is present at 1 to 3 weeks to allow early motion; in the elderly patient, motion should be started even earlier. A dynamic extension splint is ideal to provide early motion with passive extension and active flexion (Fig. 26–4) (see Chapter 12). Flexion beyond 90 degrees should be avoided until the union is stable, usually at no earlier than 4, and typically 6, weeks.

Displaced Fractures: Type II

The two accepted methods of treatment are (1) open reduction and internal fixation, and (2) excision and reconstruction of the triceps mechanism.

INTERNAL FIXATION

Tension Band Wiring

Approximation of the fragments with a loop of various materials is obsolete.[2, 64, 66] However, cerclage wire has been superseded by tension band wiring introduced by Weber and Vasey of the AO group (see Fig. 26–4).[12, 47] The principle of this method (the tension band principle) is based on the transformation of distraction forces at the fracture site into compression forces across the fracture. After reduction, the fragments are temporarily fixed with two parallel intramedullary Kirschner wires or, more recently, anteriorly directed wires into the anterior cortex at the base of the coronoid (Fig. 26–5). Then, a figure-of-eight loop of stainless steel wire is advanced through a coronal drill hole in the distal fragment. The wire is then crossed over on the posterior surface of the olecranon, passed around the protruding end of the pins, which are then bent slightly inward, and tightened with a twist. When the wire is tightened, some gapping at the articular aspect of the fracture can be seen occasionally; however, active flexion corrects this force to one of compression to close

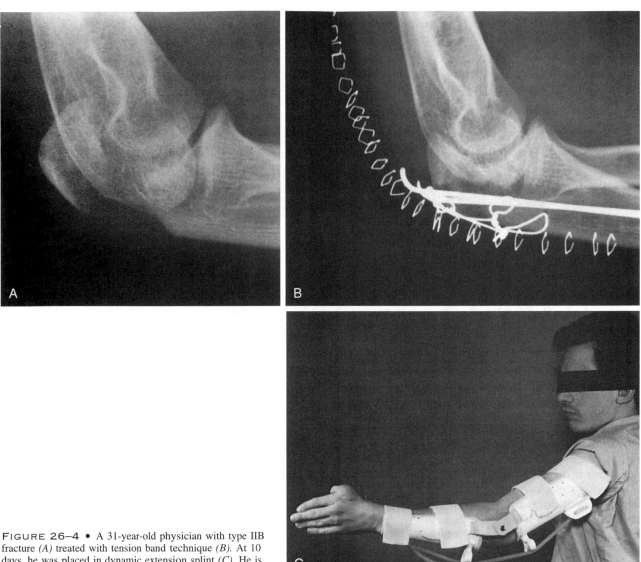

FIGURE 26–4 • A 31-year-old physician with type IIB fracture *(A)* treated with tension band technique *(B)*. At 10 days, he was placed in dynamic extension splint *(C)*. He is asymptomatic with normal motion 15 years later.

the gap. Weber has suggested that both sides of the figure-of-eight wire loop be twisted.[47] This improves the rigidity of the fixation and may equalize the compression forces on the medial and lateral aspects of the fracture. However, it also complicates the necessary removal of the Kirschner pins and the wire after fracture healing has occurred.

Tension band wiring can be difficult when there is a

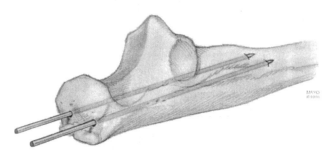

FIGURE 26–5 • Anteriorly directed K-wires penetrating the anterior cortex lessens the tendency for back-out requiring removal.

central cuneiform or comminuted fragment. Careful repositioning of the articular fragments is essential and may necessitate the use of a small cancellous graft to fill the void left after articular reconstruction. If central comminution is such that reconstruction is impossible but there is still a large intact proximal fragment, it may be possible to discard the comminuted fragments, produce smooth surfaces in the intact proximal and distal fragments by careful osteotomies, and fix them with the proximal fragment in a distally advanced position. Occasionally, the comminuted portion is ignored and the olecranon is fixed in some extension to bypass the deficiency created by the comminution. This requires accurate preservation of the trochlear curve to avoid articular incongruity.

The results of the application of the extension band treatment principle to more complicated fractures were recently reviewed by Wolfgang and associates.[72] This group treated 45 patients with displaced olecranon fractures. Twenty-one had radial head fractures or dislocations and were treated with supplemental internal fixation as necessary. Although, as expected, terminal extension was lost in

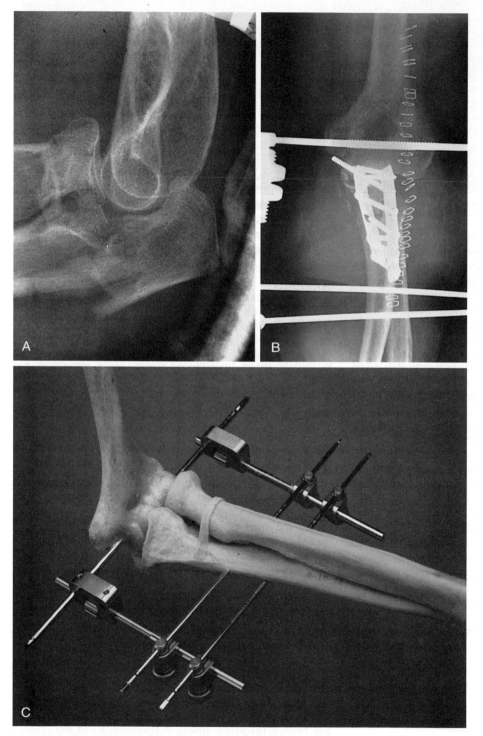

FIGURE 26–15 • Unstable type III fracture (A) treated by rigid plate fixation (B) and "neutralized" by Dynamic External Fixator (C).

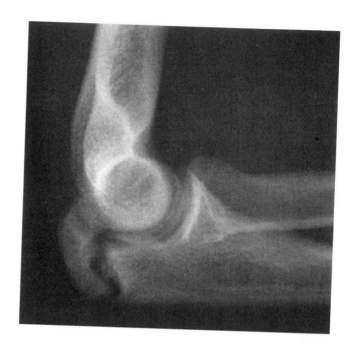

FIGURE 26–16 • Overuse fracture in 20-year-old male. Note sclerotic and rounded margins of the fragment.

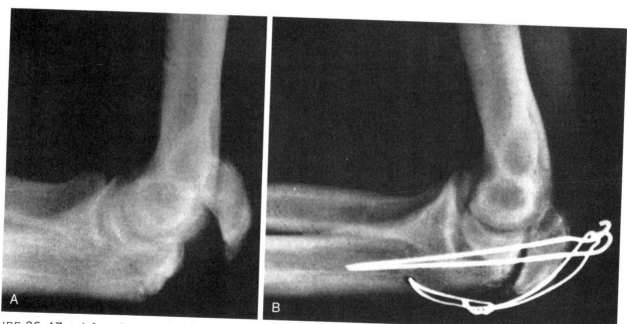

FIGURE 26–17 • A, Lateral radiograph of the left elbow, demonstrating fracture separation of the olecranon. The fracture surfaces are smooth and sclerotic. An anterior fat pad sign is present. B, Lateral radiograph of the left elbow 9 months later, demonstrating nonunion of the proximal olecranon secondary ossification center.

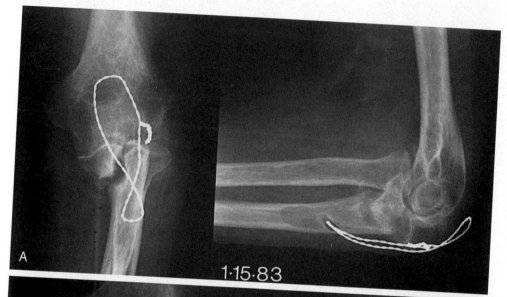

1·15·83

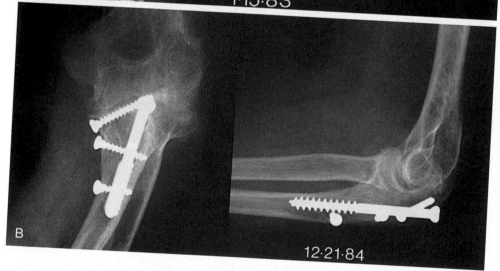

12·21·84

FIGURE 27–9 • Antero-posterior *(A)* and lateral radiographs of a 60-year-old woman who was right-hand dominant and presented with a painful nonunion 6 months after a fracture of the left olecranon treated initially with Kirschner wires in a tension band technique. Pins have been removed. Twenty-three months after open reduction and internal fixation of the nonunion with an intramedullary cancellous screw and a corticocancellous bone plate fixed with screws medially *(B)*. The patient had a good result with a stable painless elbow and a range of motion from 45 to 145 degrees of flexion and full pronation and supination. *(B,* With permission from Papagelopoulos, P. J., and Morrey, B. F.: Treatment of nonunion of olecranon fractures. J. Bone Joint Surg. Br. **76**:627, 1994.)

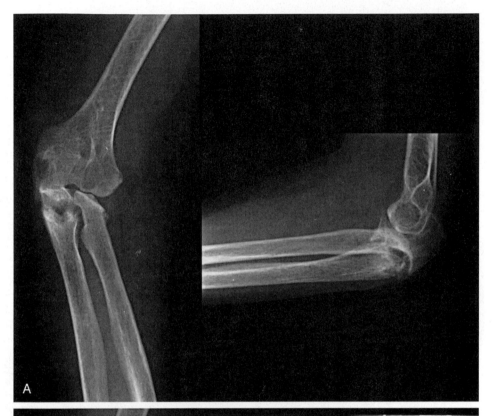

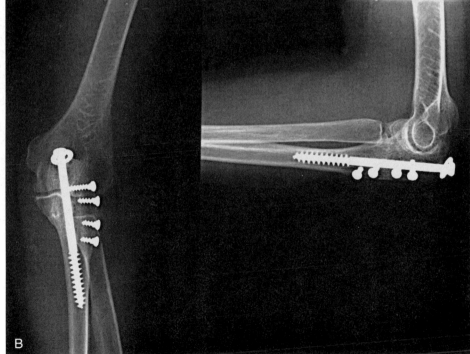

FIGURE 27–10 • *A,* Anteroposterior and lateral radiographs of a painful olecranon nonunion in a 58-year-old woman who was right-hand dominant. She presented 10 months after removal of tension band fixation. *B,* Three years after successful open reduction and internal fixation of olecranon nonunion with corticocancellous bone plate fixation combined with intramedullary screw fixation. The patient had a good result with a stable elbow, mild pain, flexion from 30 to 140 degrees, and full pronation and supination. (With permission from Papagelopoulos, P. J., and Morrey, B. F.: Treatment of nonunion of olecranon fractures. J. Bone Joint Surg. Br. **76**:627, 1994.)

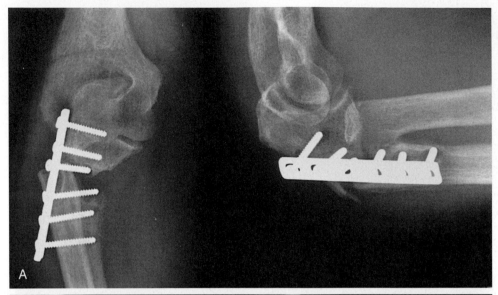

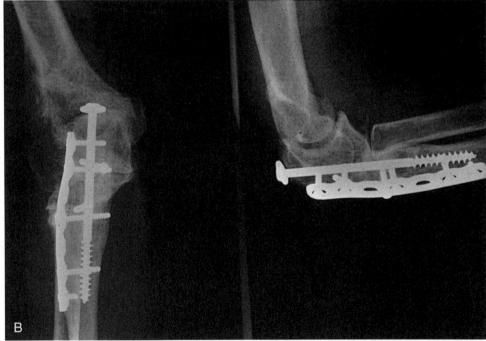

FIGURE 27–11 • *A*, Antero-posterior and lateral radiographs of a painful proximal ulna nonunion. The patient was treated initially elsewhere with plate and screw fixation for a fracture dislocation of the left elbow. *B*, Open reduction and internal fixation of olecranon nonunion with corticocancellous bone plate fixation combined with intramedullary screw and plate fixation.

If a large proximal fragment is present, either a spongiosa (cancellous) intramedullary screw (see Fig. 27–12) or a contoured DCP plate placed over the medial ulna cortex is used (Fig. 27–13). Great care is taken to avoid narrowing the coronoid and olecranon distance. Cancellous bone graft is packed around the nonunion site.

TREATMENT OF NONUNIONS OF THE OLECRANON WHEN ARTICULAR CARTILAGE HAS BEEN SEVERELY DAMAGED

This group of nonunions requires an entirely different approach from that used in the previous group. If the olecranon nonunion is an isolated problem and if the humeroulnar articular surface is destroyed beyond restoration from recent or old trauma, the factors of pain, malalignment, infection, age, and instability become important.[50] In a salvage situation and when articular surface destruction, the patient's pain, instability, and the overall assessment preclude lesser procedures, arthrodesis, total joint replacement, and allograft replacement are additional options.

Excision. If the nonunion is associated with articular distortion or loss of motion, excision of a proximal unstable fragment, if it constitutes less than 50 to 60 percent of the joint, may be the most reliable option. The postoperative period of rehabilitation is shortened as well.

Distraction Arthroplasty. In cases of nonunion of the olecranon with coexistent severe articular destruction, union initially must be achieved before the question of mobilization can be addressed. If tomograms show evidence of articular incongruity or loss and if attempts at mobilization with dynamic splinting and active exercise

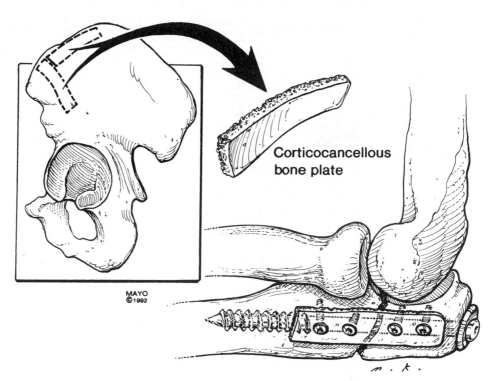

FIGURE 27–12 • Cortico-cancellous bone plate fixation of olecranon nonunion combined with intramedullary screw fixation. Bone plate of about 60 by 10 mm is harvested from the iliac crest. (By permission from Papagelopoulos, P. J., and Morrey, B. F.: Treatment of nonunion of olecranon fractures. J. Bone Joint Surg. Br. **76**:627, 1994.)

are unsuccessful, distraction arthroplasty may constitute a reasonable final treatment option (Fig. 27–14).

The concept of distraction arthroplasty has been used since the mid-1980s for treating the stiff elbow and has been adapted for the treatment of the olecranon nonunion. Thus, in those patients in whom there is contracture of soft tissue around the olecranon nonunion, the distraction device is an ideal adjunct because this may be combined with soft tissue release.[42]

When the distraction device is applied, the midportion of the lateral epicondyle, which is the projected center of the capitellum, is identified. The axis of rotation passes through the anteroinferior aspect of the medial epicondyle, and a threaded pin is placed across the distal humerus by using a specially designed targeting guide. The ulnar nerve must be identified and protected at the time of the placement of the threaded humeral pin. Two additional pins are placed across the ulna distal to the fixation provided for the nonunion. These pins are then coupled and appropriate tension adjusted so as to allow ulnohumeral motion while neutralizing or protecting the area of osteosynthesis.

In the Mayo series,[48] four patients were managed by distraction arthroplasty combined with internal fixation and bone grafting of the olecranon nonunion. In these patients, union was achieved and the arc of motion improved from a mean of 48 degrees to a mean of 95 degrees.

Arthrodesis. When stressful use of the elbow mandates a stable joint, such as in a manual laborer, arthrodesis is rarely a consideration for proximal ulna nonunions associated with significant articular distortion (see Chapter 61).

Joint Replacement. In a salvage situation, when pain and instability are paramount and only sedentary activity is acceptable, total joint replacement has been successful, using the semiconstrained types of prosthetic replacement. Joint replacement is effective in elderly patients with severe arthrosis, ankylosis, or osteoporosis (Fig. 27–15). In the Mayo Clinic series, all joint replacements were performed in older individuals who had fractures that precluded osteosynthesis.[48] One patient had severe rheumatoid arthritis, another had significant osteoporosis contraindicating internal fixation, and the last had severe post-traumatic arthritis. In the first patient, the olecranon fragment was excised. In two cases, the olecranon fracture was preserved and successfully fixed after joint replacement. All patients were treated successfully and the postoperative rehabilitation period averaged 3 months.

Allograft Composite Replacement. Similarly, composite frozen cadaver bone allograft replacement, either of the total elbow joint or of the olecranon, has been successful.[11] Late universal Charcot-like traumatic or degenerative arthritic changes can be anticipated. Infection is a major risk.

TREATMENT OF NONUNION WITH MONTEGGIA FRACTURE-DISLOCATION

Nonunion with anterior fracture dislocation is the most severe and most difficult injury of the proximal ulna because the coronoid is involved.[9, 17, 50] Cases are divided into two treatment groups: injuries with a restorable articular surface and those in which articular surface damage precludes restoration.

In the first group, accurate realignment and restoration of the articular surface is mandatory. After taking down and repositioning or shortening the fragments, rigid internal fixation must be achieved. The subluxed distal ulnar segment is reduced, and the anterior capsule is dissected from the coronoid process and tubercle to protect the vital anterior neurovascular structures. Exposure is generally achieved by the posterior approach described by Bryan and Morrey.[14] The medial collateral ligament is identified and repaired or reconstructed. Shortening of the ulna may be necessary to prevent pressure of the ulnar articular surface against the trochlea of the humerus. Internal fixation is best achieved with either a long lag screw or a six- to eight-hole tubular AO plate and screws. Early motion is initiated at 3 weeks.

When the sigmoid notch articular surface is destroyed and dislocation has existed so long that the articular surface of the lower humerus has been destroyed, the age and overall functional level of the patient is determined. If stressful use of the extremity is demanded, arthrodesis is still a consideration, and the technique is determined by the amount of bone stock present.

When chronic nonunion is associated with anterior dislocation and joint destruction, when pain or instability warrant reconstruction, and when sedentary use of the extremity is acceptable, total joint replacement with a semiconstrained prosthesis, with an adequate stem for the ulna, has been a satisfactory approach.

Complications of Treatment of Nonunions

The complications of treatment for nonunion of olecranon fractures include recurrent nonunion, heterotopic ossification, neurapraxia, diminished range of motion, traumatic arthritic changes, pain, reflex sympathetic dystrophy, and infection.[36, 48] When rigid internal fixation is achieved and early motion can be initiated at 5 to 7 days in the functional range of 30 to 130 degrees, less permanent contracture may be anticipated. Unless ossification occurs in the brachialis muscle or the anterior capsule, ectopic calcification is usually of little consequence.

In the Mayo series, there was only one patient with postoperative ulnar nerve paresthesias after operative treatment of olecranon nonunion.[48] Eriksson and associates[24] reported a higher rate of nerve complications (10 percent) with fresh olecranon fractures. Isolation and protection of the nerve are warranted for virtually all reconstructive surgeries for nonunion at the elbow. The use of a nerve

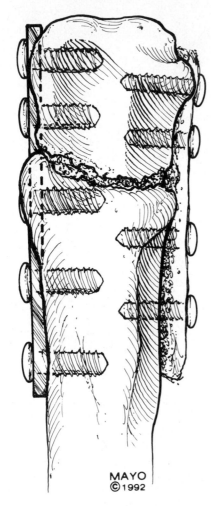

FIGURE 27–13 • Corticocancellous bone plate fixation of olecranon nonunion combined with DCP plate and screw fixation. The plate is contoured and placed laterally. Mini 2.5-mm screws are used medially for bone plate fixation. (With permission from Papagelopoulos, P. J., and Morrey, B. F.: Treatment of nonunion of olecranon fractures. J. Bone Joint Surg. Br. **76**:627, 1994.)

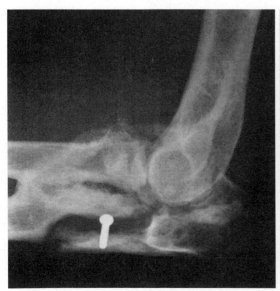
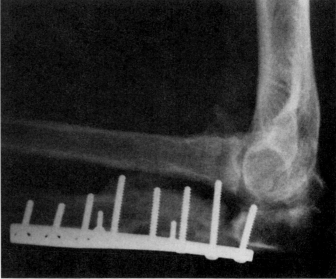

FIGURE 27–14 • Painful, stiff nonunion of proximal ulna in a 35-year-old man treated with plate and a bone graft screwed to the nonunion (the two smaller screws). The patient developed a union with residual stiffness that was treated secondarily with distraction arthroplasty.

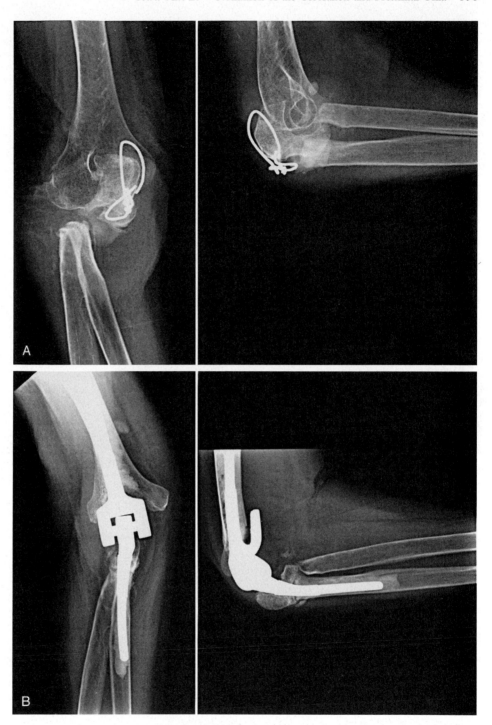

FIGURE 27–15 • *A,* Anteroposterior and lateral radiographs of a 75-year-old woman who was right-hand dominant at 1 year after right elbow olecranon fracture and failed osteosynthesis. *B,* Twenty-eight months postoperatively the patient had an excellent result with no pain. (With permission from Papagelopoulos, P. J., and Morrey, B. F.: Treatment of nonunion of olecranon fractures. J. Bone Joint Surg. Br. **76**:627, 1994.)

stimulator and high-power loops is helpful for dissection of scar tissue about the ulnar nerve.

Results

Papagelopoulos and Morrey[48] reported the Mayo Clinic experience in 24 consecutive patients treated from 1976 to 1991 for nonunion of olecranon fractures. The mean age of these patients was 42 years, and the mean interval from fracture to treatment for nonunion was 19 months. Management was by rehabilitation and activity as tolerated for 3 patients, continued immobilization for 1, and operative treatment for 20. Operations included excision of the olecranon fragment (1), osteosynthesis (16), and joint replacement (3). Four patients also had distraction arthroplasty. At a mean follow-up time of 18 months, no patient had severe residual elbow pain but 3 had moderate and 6 had mild symptoms. The mean arc of motion was 98 degrees, representing an average improvement of 11 degrees. Twelve patients had an excellent result, 4 good, 6 fair, and 2 poor. Union had been achieved in 15 of the 16 patients treated by osteosynthesis.

Danziger and Healy[21] reviewed five patients treated surgically for nonunion of the olecranon. Four of the five fractures leading to nonunion were comminuted or oblique. Three nonunions occurred after tension band wiring, one nonunion occurred after open reduction internal fixation with a semitubular plate, and one nonunion occurred after treatment with a cast. The median interval from fracture to treatment of nonunion was 8 months. All nonunions were treated surgically. Four patients were treated with a tension band plate technique. All nonunions united at a median of 3 months. The median follow-up period was 36 months (range, 12–48 months).

CONCLUSIONS

Olecranon nonunion is not a common complication and little has been written regarding its management. Treatment depends on patient age, characteristics of the fracture, bone quality, and joint and soft tissue status. No treatment is acceptable for painless "fibrous nonunion" with 90 degrees or more of flexion. Immobilization can be used in cases of stress nonunion of the olecranon epiphysis of adolescents. Osteosynthesis is the treatment of choice in young patients or in those without severe comminution. Bone grafting with a corticocancellous bone plate and a DCP plate or cancellous screw fixation is the treatment of choice. Soft tissue release with adjunctive use of the distraction fixator is helpful when marked loss of motion has occurred. Overall, an acceptable result is to be anticipated in about 70 percent of patients. Total elbow arthroplasty is a viable option for treatment in elderly patients with coexisting severe arthritis or osteoporosis.

REFERENCES

1. Adler, S., Fay, G. F., and McAusland, W. R., Jr.: Treatment of olecranon fractures. J. Trauma 2:597, 1962.
2. Bakalim, G., and Wilppula, E.: Fractures of the olecranon I, II, III. Ann. Chir. Gynaecol. Fenn. 60:95, 1971.
3. Barford, B.: Quoted in personal communication with drawing by Colton, C. L.: Fracture of the olecranon in adults: classification and management. Injury 5:121, 1973.
4. Bassett, C. A.: Contributions of endosteum, cortex and soft tissue to osteogenesis. Surg. Gynecol. Obstet. 112:145, 1961.
5. Bassett, C., and Andrew, L.: Pulsing electromagnetic fields: a new method to modify cell behavior in calcified and noncalcified tissues. Calcif Tiss Int 34:1–8, 1982.
6. Bassett, C., Andrew L., Valdes, M. G., and Hernandez, E.: Modification of fracture repair with selected pulsing electromagnetic fields. J. Bone Joint Surg. 64A:888, 1982.
7. Becker, R.: Bioelectric factors controlling bone structure. In Frost, H. M. (ed.): Bone Biodynamics. Boston, Little, Brown & Co., 1964.
8. Berger, P.: Le Traitement des Fractures de l'Olécrane et Particulièrement la Suture de l'Olécrane par un Procédé (Cedarg de l'Olécrane). Ga. 2 Hebd. de Med. 193, 1902.
9. Boyd, H. B., and Boles, J. C.: The Monteggia lesion. A review of 159 cases. Clin. Orthop. 66:94, 1969.
10. Boyd, H. B., Lipinski, S. W., and Wiley, J. H.: Observations on nonunions of the shafts of the long bones, with a statistical analysis of 842 patients. J. Bone Joint Surg. 43A:159, 1961.
11. Breen, T., Gelberman, R. H., Leffert, R., and Botte, M.: Massive allograft replacement of hemiarticular traumatic defects of the elbow. J. Hand Surg. 13A:6, 1988.
12. Brighton, C. T., Black, J., Friedenberg, Z. B., Esterhai, J. L., Day, L. J., and Connolly, J. F.: A multicenter study of the treatment of nonunion with constant direct current. J. Bone Joint Surg. 63:1, 1981.
13. Brooks, M.: The Blood Supply of Bone. New York, Appleton-Century-Crofts, 1971.
14. Bryan, R. S., and Morrey, B. F.: Extensive posterior exposure of the elbow. Clin. Orthop. 166:188, 1982.
15. Burge, P., and Benson, M.: Bilateral congenital pseudarthrosis of the olecranon. J. Bone Joint Surg. 69:460, 1987.
16. Colton, C. L.: Fractures of the olecranon in adults: classification and management. Injury 5:121, 1973.
17. Conn, J., and Wade, P. A.: Injuries of the elbow (a ten-year review). J. Trauma 1:248, 1961.
18. Coughlin, M. J., Slabaugh, P. B., and Smith, T. K.: Experience with the McAtee olecranon device in olecranon fractures. J. Bone Joint Surg. 61A:385, 1979.
19. Cozen, L.: Does diabetes delay fracture healing? Clin. Orthop. 82:134, 1972.
20. Crenshaw, A. H.: Delayed union and nonunion of fractures. In Edmonson A., and Crenshaw, A. H. (eds.): Campbell's Operative Orthopedics, 6th ed. St. Louis, C. V. Mosby Co., 1980.
21. Danziger, M. B., and Healy, W. L.: Operative treatment of olecranon nonunion. J Orthop Trauma 6:290–293, 1992.
22. Dell, P. C., and Sheppard, J. E.: Vascularized bone grafts in the treatment of infected forearm nonunions. J. Hand Surg. 9:653, 1984.
23. Dunn, N.: Operation for fracture of the olecranon. Br. Med. J. 1:214, 1939.
24. Eriksson, E., Sahlen, O., and Sandohl, U.: Late results of conservative and surgical treatment of fracture of the olecranon. Acta Chir. Scand. 113:153, 1957.
25. Foille, D. J.: Note sur les Fractures de l'Olecrane Par Projectiles de Guerre. Marseille Med 55:241, 1918.
26. Gainor, B. J., Moussa, F., and Schott, T.: Healing rate of transverse osteotomies of the olecranon used in reconstruction of distal humerus fractures. J South Orthop Assoc 4:263–268, 1995.
27. Gartsman, G. M., Sculco, T. P., and Otis, J. C.: Operative treatment of olecranon fractures. J. Bone Joint Surg. 63A:718, 1981.
28. Green, D. P., and Rockwood, C. A.: Fractures. Philadelphia, J. B. Lippincott Co., 1975.
29. Green, N.: Radiation induced delayed union of fractures. Radiology 93:635, 1969.
30. Heppenstall, R. B.: Fracture Treatment and Healing. Philadelphia, W. B. Saunders Co., 1980, p. 83.
31. Howard, J. L., and Urist, M. R.: Fracture dislocation of radius and ulna at the elbow joint. Clin. Orthop. 12:276, 1958.
32. Judet, J., and Jude, R.: L'Ostéogenèse et les Retards de Consolidation et les Pseudarthroses des Os Longs. Huitième Congres SICOT 1966, p. 315.
33. Kiviluoto, O., and Santauirta, S.: Fractures of the olecranon. Analysis of 37 consecutive cases. Acta Orthop. Scand. 49:28, 1978.
34. Kovach, J., Baker, B. E., and Mosher, J. F.: Fracture separation of the olecranon ossification center in adults. Am. J. Sports Med. 13:2, 1985.
35. Lehman, M. A.: Nonunion of an olecranon fracture following birth injury. Bull. Hosp. Joint Dis. 26:187, 1965.
36. Levy, R. N., and Sherry, H. S.: Complications of treatment of fractures and dislocations of the elbow. In Epps, C. H. (ed.): Complications in Orthopedic Surgery. Philadelphia, J. B. Lippincott Co., 1975, p. 237.
37. Mathews, J. G.: Fractures of the olecranon in children. Injury 12:207, 1980.
38. Mayer, P. J., and Evarts, C. M.: Nonunion, delayed union, malunion, and avascular necrosis. In Epps, C. H. (ed.): Complications in Orthopedic Surgery. Philadelphia, J. B. Lippincott, 1975, p. 159.
39. McKeever, F. M., and Buck, R. M.: Fracture of olecranon process of the ulna. J.A.M.A. 135:1, 1947.
40. Meals, R. A.: The use of a flexor carpi ulnaris muscle flap in the treatment of an infected nonunion of the proximal ulna. Clin. Orthop. 240:168, 1989.
41. Morrey, B. F., and An, K. N.: Functional anatomy of the ligaments of the elbow. Clin. Orthop. 201:84, 1985.
42. Morrey, B. F.: Distraction arthroplasty. Clinical applications. Clin Orthop 293:46–54, 1993.
43. Muller, M. E., Allgower, M., and Willenegger, H.: Manual of Internal Fixation. Berlin, Springer-Verlag, 1970.
44. Muller, M. E.: Treatment of nonunion by compression. Clin. Orthop. 43:83, 1965.
45. Murphy, D. F., Greene, W. B., Gilbert, J. A., and Dameron, T. B.: Displaced olecranon fracture in adults. Clin. Orthop. 2:224, 1987.
46. Newell, R. L. M.: Olecranon fractures in children. Injury 37:33, 1975.

47. Orava, S., and Hulkko, A.: Delayed unions and nonunions of stress fractures in athletes. Am. J. Sports Med. 16:517, 1988.
48. Papagelopoulos, P. J., and Morrey, B. F.: Treatment of nonunion of olecranon fractures. J. Bone Joint Surg. Br. 76:627, 1994.
49. Paterson, D. C., Lewis, G. N., and Cass, C. A.: Treatment of delayed union and nonunion with an implanted direct current stimulator. Clin. Orthop. 148:117, 1980.
50. Regan, W., and Morrey, B. F.: Fractures of the coronoid process of the ulna. J. Bone Joint Surg. 71A:1348, 1989.
51. Rettig, A. C., Waugh, T. R., and Evanski, P. M.: Fracture of the olecranon: a problem of management. J. Trauma 12:23, 1979.
52. Rothman, R.: The effect of iron deficiency anemia on fracture healing. Clin. Orthop. 77:276, 1971.
53. Sharrard, W. J. W., Sutcliffe, M. S., Robson, M. J., and Maceachern, A. G.: The treatment of fibrous nonunion of fractures by pulsing electromagnetic stimulation. J. Bone Joint Surg. 64B:189, 1982.
54. Silberstein, M. J., Bradeur, A. E., Graviss, E. R., and Luisiri, A.: Some vagaries of the olecranon. J. Bone Joint Surg. 63A:722, 1981.
55. Smith, F. M.: Surgery of the Elbow. Philadelphia, W. B. Saunders Co., 1972, p. 260.
56. Srivastava, K. P., Vyas, O. N., Varshney, A. K., and Singh, C. P.: Compression osteosynthesis in fractures of the olecranon. Int. Surg. 63:20, 1978.
57. Taylor, T. K. F., and Scham, S. M.: A posteromedial approach to the proximal end of the ulna for the internal fixation of olecranon fractures. J. Trauma 9:594, 1969.
58. Tonna, E. A.: The cellular complement on the skeletal system studied autoradiographically with tritiated thymidine (H$_3$DTR) during growth and aging. J. Biophys. Biochem. Cytol. 9:813, 1961.
59. Torg, J. S., and Moyer, R. A.: Nonunion of a stress fracture through the olecranon epiphyseal plate observed in an adolescent baseball pitcher. J. Bone Joint Surg. 59A:264, 1977.
60. Tullos, H. S., Schwab, G., Bennett, J. B., and Woods, W. G.: Factors influencing elbow instability. In American Academy of Orthopedic Surgeons: Instructional Course Lectures, Vol. 30. St. Louis, C. V. Mosby Co., 1981, p. 193.
61. Waddell, G., and Howat, T. W.: A technique of plating severe olecranon fractures. Injury 5:135, 1973.
62. Wadsworth, T. G.: Screw fixation of the olecranon after fracture of osteotomy. Clin. Orthop. 119:197, 1976.
63. Walker, L. G.: Painful olecranon physeal nonunion in an adult weight lifter. A case report. Clin. Orthop. 311:125, 1995.
64. Weber, B. G., and Cech, O.: Pseudarthrosis: Pathology, Biomechanics, Therapy, Results. Berne, Hans Huber Medical Pub., 1976.
65. Weber, B., and Vasey, H.: Osteosynthese bei Olecranon Fraktur. Z. Unfallmed. Berufskr. 2:90, 1963.
66. Weisband, I. D.: Tension band wiring technique for treatment of olecranon fractures. J. Am. Osteopath. Assoc. 77:390, 1978.
67. Weseley, M. S., Barnfield, P. A., and Einstein, A. I.: The use of the Zuelzer hook plate in fixation of olecranon fractures. J. Bone Joint Surg. 58A:859, 1976.
68. Wilkerson, R. D., and Johns, J. C.: Nonunion of an olecranon stress fracture in an adolescent gymnast. Am. J. Sports Med. 18:4, 1990.

CHAPTER 28

Coronoid Process and Monteggia Fractures

• WILLIAM D. REGAN
and BERNARD F. MORREY

THE CORONOID

As this fracture often occurs in conjunction with radial head fractures, and dislocation, it is discussed in some detail in Chapter 30.

Mechanism of Injury

Isolated coronoid fractures are uncommon and usually occur in association with elbow dislocation.[43] Theoretically, the coronoid is fractured with the elbow in 0 to 20 degrees of flexion during an axial load (Fig. 28–1).[1] This is a mechanism similar to that in elbow dislocation. With flexion past 30 degrees, radial head fractures occur. The combination of coronoid and radial head fracture has important implications for treatment, as discussed in Chapter 30. Of particular note is the fact that fractures involving more than 50 percent of the coronoid (Regan/Morrey type II) are associated with elbow instability if the radial head has been resected (Fig. 28–2).

Incidence

Fractures of the coronoid process are uncommon. The injury has been reported in 2 to 10 percent of patients with dislocation of the elbow (see Chapter 29). The fracture occurs in association with an olecranon fracture in about 5 percent of the olecranon fractures reported according to the Mayo IIIB fracture classification (Fig. 28–3). Other than a recent review of Mayo Clinic records that revealed 35 patients who had sustained fractures of the coronoid,[43] only a few case reports deal with this injury.[19, 50]

Classification

Review of Mayo records resulted in a simple classification of coronoid fractures as well as a rationale for treatment (Fig. 28–4). Type I is a fracture of the tip of the coronoid process caused by a shearing force as the coronoid process subluxates or dislocates over the trochlea. A type II injury involves a single or comminuted fragment constituting about half of the coronoid. A type III fracture involves more than half of the coronoid process. The type II or III fracture may be comminuted, and all three may be associated with dislocation of the elbow or with other injuries. Further, the comminution frequently occurs in the sagittal

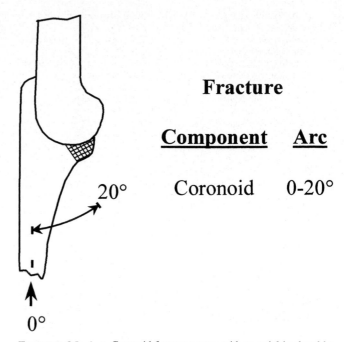

Fracture

Component	Arc
Coronoid	0-20°

20°

0°

FIGURE 28–1 • Coronoid fracture occurs with an axial load and between 0 and 20 degrees of flexion.

plane involving the medial portion of the coronoid and sometimes involving the medial collateral ligament (Fig. 28–5).

Association Injuries

Of the 14 patients identified with type I fractures, only 2 (28 percent) had clearly documented elbow dislocation. This compares with 6 of 16 (37 percent) with dislocations who had type II fractures and 4 of 5 (80 percent) with type

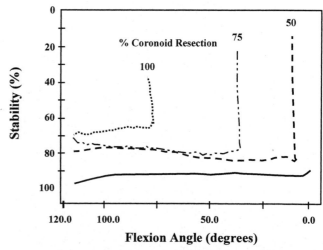

Elbow Stability After Coronoid and Radial Resection

% Coronoid Resection

100 75 50

FIGURE 28–2 • Experimental data depicting the stability of the ulnohumeral joint. With fractures involving 75 to 100 percent of the coronoid, the joint is grossly unstable. The type II, 50 percent fracture is stable except at nearly full extension, even with the radial head removed.

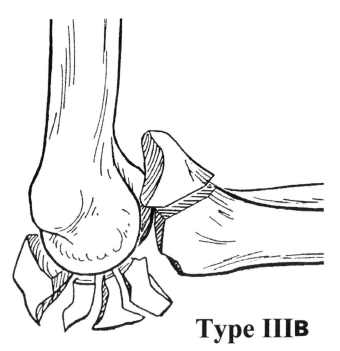

Type IIIB

FIGURE 28–3 • The Mayo IIIB olecranon fracture may also involve the coronoid.

III coronoid fractures who had elbow dislocations. In reality, today we consider virtually any coronoid fracture to have had an associated collateral ligament injury, even if only a strain. Fracture of the coronoid process is typically associated with other injuries. Thirty-five percent of the patients with type I, 56 percent of the patients with type II, and 80 percent of the patients with type III coronoid fractures had other identified injuries.[43]

Treatment

AUTHORS' PREFERENCE

Type I. The patient with type I fracture can be treated according to the concurrent pathology. The fracture itself generally indicates that the elbow has dislocated and might be managed on that basis. One recent report has implicated the fragment as a source of catching or impingement, both responding to arthroscopic excision.[26]

Type II. Type II fractures should be treated with early motion unless the elbow is unstable. In this circumstance, the fracture should be reduced if possible. If the process is comminuted and the elbow is unstable, a distraction device can be used to provide the initial stability while the soft tissue heals. Fixation of the smaller fragments alone may not stabilize the joint but should be considered if technically feasible. As a useful clinical tool, we have observed that determining the fracture type is assisted by a line from the tip of the olecranon through the residual coronoid. If this is parallel to the long axis of the ulna, a type II fracture has occurred (Fig. 28–6).

Type III. Type III fractures are virtually always associated with elbow instability. If the fracture is comminuted and is not amenable to fixation, the external fixation distraction device is mandatory. Failure to stabilize the elbow in type III fractures results in a painful subluxation of the

ulnohumeral joint, usually with marked limitation of motion (Fig. 28–7). The use of the distraction device has dramatically improved the potential to treat the chronic subluxation associated with type II and III unstable fractures (Fig. 28–8). However, open reduction and rigid fixation, with or without the distraction device, remains the treatment of choice (Fig. 28–9).

TECHNIQUE

If the radial head is fractured, and/or the elbow is grossly unstable, exposure and fixation of the coronoid is facilitated. The safest exposure is a straight posterior skin incision. Kocher's interval is used if the radial head is fractured. If the fracture is an isolated one, a medial approach is used (see Chapter 8). This is mandatory if a sagittal component is present and if the medial collateral ligament is involved.

With the use of the posterior incision, the ulnar nerve is exposed but not transferred. The flexor-pronator origin is released with a 1-cm cuff of tendon left on the medial epicondyle (Fig. 28–10). The brachialis muscle is elevated for the capsule, and the joint entered. Fixation is ideally accomplished with one or two compression screws. With comminuted fractures, a heavy No. 5 nonabsorbable suture is placed through the brachialis tendon, and then through the fracture, and is secured through drill holes in the ulna through the base of the fracture (Fig. 28–11).

Reconstruction. An absent coronoid may be reconstructed with a well-fashioned bone graft from the ilium. Moritomo and colleagues[31] have described reconstruction with the osteotomized portion of the olecranon. We have employed this technique and find it preferable to the iliac crest graft.

Results

The results of 35 patients with coronoid fractures are shown in Table 28–1. Using an elbow performance index, it is obvious that the chance of a satisfactory result directly correlates with the severity of the injury, as reflected by the coronoid fracture type. Pain is uncommon in type I and typical in type III injury. Our impression is that the results have improved over the last decade owing to: (1) a better understanding of the implications of associated injury; (2) more aggressive exposure; and (3) improved design of the external fixator.

STRESS FRACTURE

Although reported for the olecranon,[27, 54] stress fracture has not been reported for the coronoid. We have documented

Text continued on page 403

• TABLE 28–1 • **Results of Treatment According to Coronoid Fracture Type**			
	Type of Fracture		
	I	*II*	*III*
Pain, none (%)	50	67	20
Motion, mean lag (degrees)	4–136	12–127	39–100
Satisfactory (%)	92	74	20
Unsatisfactory (%)	8	26	80

been discontinued, active range-of-motion exercises are begun. Improvement occurs slowly, but passive stretching is not advisable.

The advent of rigid internal fixation methods has improved the prognosis for these potentially treacherous injuries.

REFERENCES

1. Amis, A. A., and Miller, J. H.: The mechanisms of elbow fractures: An investigation using impact tests in vitro. Injury 26:163, 1995.
2. Anderson, L. D.: Fractures of the shaft of the radius and ulna. In Rockwood, C. A., and Green, D. P. (eds.): Fractures. Philadelphia, J. B. Lippincott Co., 1975.
3. Austin, R.: Tardy palsy of radial nerve from a Monteggia fracture. Injury 7:202, 1976.
4. Bado, J. L.: The Monteggia lesion. Clin. Orthop. 50:71, 1967.
5. Beck, C., and Dabezies, E. J.: Monteggia fracture-dislocation. Orthopedics 7:329, 1984.
6. Bohler, L.: The Treatment of Fractures. Vienna, Wilhelm Mandrich, 1929.
7. Boyd, H. B.: Surgical exposure of the ulna and proximal third of the radius through one incision. Surg. Gynecol. Obstet. 71:86, 1940.
8. Boyd, H. B., and Boals, J. C.: The Monteggia lesion: A review of 159 cases. Clin. Orthop. 66:94, 1969.
9. Bruce, H. E., Harvey, J. P., and Wilson, J. C.: Monteggia fractures. J. Bone Joint Surg. 56A:1563, 1974.
10. Bryan, R. S.: Monteggia fracture of the forearm. J. Trauma 11:992, 1971.
11. Burghele, H., and Serban, N.: Fractures of the olecranon: Treatment by external fixation. Ital. J. Orthop. Traumatol. 8:159, 1982.
12. Chapman, M. W., Gordon, J. E., and Zissimos, A. G.: Compression-plate fixation of acute fractures of the diaphysis of the radius and ulna. J. Bone Joint Surg. 71A:159, 1989.
13. Cobb, T. K., and Morrey, B. F.: Use of distraction arthroplasty in unstable fracture dislocations of the elbow. Clin. Orthop. (312):201, 1995.
14. Conn, J., and Wade, P. A.: Injuries of the elbow: A ten-year review. J. Trauma 1:248, 1961.
15. DeLuca, P. A., Lindsey, R. W., and Ruwe, P. A.: Refracture of bones of the forearm after the removal of compression plates. J. Bone Joint Surg. 70A:1372, 1988.
16. Evans, E. M.: Pronation injuries of the forearm with special reference to the anterior Monteggia fracture. J. Bone Joint Surg. 31B:578, 1949.
17. Fiolle, D. J.: Note sur les fractures de l'olecrane par projectiles de guerre. Marseille Med. 55:241, 1918.
18. Givon, U., Pritsch, M., Levy, O., Yosepovich, A., Amit, Y., and Horoszowski, H.: Monteggia and equivalent lesions: A study of 41 cases. Clin. Orthop. (337):208, 1997.
19. Hanks, G. A., and Kottmeier, S. A.: Isolated fracture of the coronoid process of the ulna: A case report and review of the literature. J. Orthop. Trauma 4:193, 1990.
20. Hidaka, S., and Gustilo, R. B.: Refracture of bones of the forearm after plate removal. J. Bone Joint Surg. 66A:1241, 1984.
21. Inoue, G., and Shionoya, K.: Corrective ulnar osteotomy for malunited anterior Monteggia lesions in children: 12 patients followed for 1–12 years. Acta Orthop. Scand. 69:73, 1998.
22. Jessing, P.: Monteggia lesions and their complicating nerve damage. Acta Orthop. Scand. 46:601, 1975.
23. Joshi, R. P.: The Hastings experience of the Attenborough springs and Rush nail for fixation of olecranon fractures. Injury 29:455, 1997.
24. Kozin, S. H., Berglund, L. J., Cooney, W. P., Morrey, B. F., and An, K-N.: Biomechanical analysis of tension band fixation for olecranon fracture treatment. J. Shoulder Elbow Surg. 5:442, 1996.
25. Lichter, R. L., and Jacobsen, T.: Tardy palsy of the posterior interosseous nerve with a Monteggia fracture. J. Bone Joint Surg. 57A:124, 1975.
26. Liu, S. H., Henry, M., and Bowen, R.: Complications of type I coronoid fractures in competitive athletes: Report of two cases and review of the literature. J. Shoulder Elbow Surg. 5:223, 1996.
27. Maffulli, N., Chan, D., and Aldridge, M. J.: Overuse injuries of the olecranon in young gymnasts. J. Bone Joint Surg. 74B:305, 1992.
28. Mobley, J. E., and Janes, J. M.: Monteggia fractures. Proc. Staff Meet. Mayo Clin. 30:497, 1955.
29. Monteggia, G. B.: Instituzioni Chirurgiche, Vol. 5. Milan, Maspero, 1814.
30. Moore, T. M., Klein, J. P., Patzakis, M. J., and Harvey, J. B.: Results of compression plating of closed Galeazzi fractures. J. Bone Joint Surg. 67A:1015, 1985.
31. Moritomo, H., Tada, K., Yoshida, T., and Kawatsu, N.: Reconstruction of the coronoid for chronic dislocation of the elbow: Use of a graft from the olecranon in two cases. J. Bone Joint Surg. 80B:490, 1998.
32. Morrey, B. F.: Fractures and dislocations of the elbow. In Gustilo, R. B. (ed.): Fractures and Dislocations. Chicago, Year Book Medical Publishers, 1992.
33. Morrey, B. F.: Current concepts in the treatment of fractures of the radial head, the olecranon, and the coronoid. J. Bone Joint Surg. 77A:316, 1995.
34. Muller, M. E., Allgower, M., Schneider, R., and Willenegger, H.: Manual of Internal Fixation: Techniques Recommended by the AO Group, 2nd ed. New York, Springer-Verlag, 1979.
35. Murphy, D. F., Green, W. B., and Dameron, T. B.: Displaced olecranon fractures in adults: Clinical evaluation. Clin. Orthop. 224:215, 1987.
36. Murphy, D. F., Green, W. B., Gilbert, J. A., and Dameron, T. B.: Displaced olecranon fractures in adults: Biomechanical analysis of fixation methods. Clin. Orthop. 224:210, 1987.
37. O'Donoghue, D. H., and Sell, L. S.: Persistent olecranon epiphysis in adults. J. Bone Joint Surg. 24:677, 1942.
38. Pavel, A., Pitman, J. M., Lance, E. M., and Wade, P. A.: The posterior Monteggia fracture: A clinical study. J. Trauma 5:185, 1965.
39. Penrose, J. H.: The Monteggia fractures with posterior dislocation of the radial head. J. Bone Joint Surg. 33B:65, 1951.
40. Perruelo, N. N., and Platigorsky, H.: Fractura de olecranon-olecranectomia. Acta Ortoped.-Traumatol. Iberica 3:12, 1955.
41. Reckling, F. W.: Unstable fracture-dislocation of the forearm (Monteggia and Galeazzi lesions). J. Bone Joint Surg. 64A:857, 1982.
42. Reckling, F. W., and Cordell, L. B.: Unstable fracture-dislocations of the forearm: The Monteggia and Galeazzi lesions. Arch. Surg. 96:999, 1968.
43. Regan, W., and Morrey, B. F.: Fractures of the coronoid process of the ulna. J. Bone Joint Surg. 71A:1348, 1989.
44. Rettig, A. C., Waugh, T. R., and Evanski, P. M.: Fracture of the olecranon: A problem of management. J. Trauma 19:23, 1979.
45. Reynders, P., De Groote, W., Rondia, J., Govaerts, K., Stoffelen, D., and Broos, P. L.: Monteggia lesions in adults: A multicenter Bota study. Acta Orthop. Belgica 62 (Suppl 1):78, 1996.
46. Ring, D., Jupiter, J. B., Sanders, R. W., Mast, J., and Simpson, N. S.: Transolecranon fracture-dislocation of the elbow: J. Orthop. Trauma 11:545, 1997.
47. Ring, D., Jupiter, J. B., and Waters, P. M.: Monteggia fractures in children and adults. J. AAOS 6:215, 1998.
48. Rosson, J. W., and Shearer, J. R.: Refracture after the removal of plates from the forearm: An avoidable complication. J. Bone Joint Surg. 73B:415, 1991.
49. Scharplatz, D., and Allgower, M.: Fracture dislocation of the elbow. Injury 7:143, 1975.
50. Selesnick, F. H., Dolitsky, B., and Haskell, S. S.: Fracture of the coronoid process requiring open reduction with internal fixation. J. Bone Joint Surg. 66A:1304, 1984.
51. Speed, J. S., and Boyd, H. B.: Treatment of fractures of the ulna with dislocation of head of radius (Monteggia fracture). J.A.M.A. 115:1699, 1940.
52. Spinner, M., Freundlich, B. D., and Teicher, J.: Posterior interosseous nerve palsy as a complication of Monteggia fractures in children. Clin. Orthop. 58:141, 1968.
53. Tompkins, D. G.: The anterior Monteggia fracture: Observations on etiology and treatment. J. Bone Joint Surg. 53A:1109, 1971.
54. Wilkerson, R. D., and Johns, J. C.: Non-union of an olecranon stress fracture in an adolescent gymnast: A case report. Am. J. Sports Med. 18:432, 1990.
55. Yamamoto, K., Yanase, Y., and Tomihara, M.: Posterior interosseous nerve palsy as complication of Monteggia fractures. Arch. Jpn. Chir. 46:46, 1977.

CHAPTER 29

Elbow Dislocations

· SHAWN W. O'DRISCOLL

The elbow is the second most commonly dislocated joint, after the shoulder, in adults. In the pediatric age group, it is the joint most commonly dislocated. Despite the prevalence of this injury, there are few analyses of series of this dislocation in the literature.[6, 13, 15, 26, 32, 37, 43, 51, 64, 70, 88] Recently, our understanding of the basic biomechanics and mechanism of injury has improved, and along with this, so has our approach to treating patients with these injuries.

MECHANISM OF INJURY

The traditional teaching that the mechanism of dislocation is hyperextension cannot be completely substantiated by the data available. Some of the proponents of the accepted hypothesis have expressed uncertainty in this regard, noting that "the mechanism of posterolateral dislocation is poorly understood."[23]

Elbow dislocations or subluxations typically result from falls on the outstretched hand; motor vehicle accidents, direct trauma, and miscellaneous causes account for the rest. The elbow experiences an axial compressive force during flexion as the body approaches the ground. As the body rotates internally on the elbow (forearm rotates externally on the trunk), a supination moment occurs at the elbow. A valgus moment results from the fact that the mechanical axis is medial to the elbow (Fig. 29–1). This combination of valgus instability and supination with axial compression during flexion is precisely the mechanism that results in a posterolateral rotatory subluxation or dislocation of the elbow and can be reproduced clinically by the lateral pivot-shift test, which is described later.[56] We have documented this exact mechanism in two patients whose dislocations were caught on video camera during wrestling matches.

Osborne and Cotterill[61] first suggested a posterolateral rotational displacement as the mechanism of elbow dislocation. The radial collateral ligament and the lateral capsule are torn. They suggested a method of repair for recurrent dislocation based on this theory of mechanism, which involved imbrication of the lateral soft tissues. The method has been used with success.[26]

The forces acting on the joint, besides producing tensile forces that disrupt the ligamentous constraints, also produce substantial compressive and shear forces on the articular surfaces. Adjunctive fractures, such as those occurring in the radial head and neck or capitellum are therefore frequent.[2, 12] There is evidence from reports of dislocations treated by open means that chondral injuries to the capitellar and trochlear surfaces are probably much more common than was previously believed.[8, 21]

In the child, late nucleation and closure of the physes alter the response to dislocation forces and certainly increase the difficulty of radiographic interpretation. This is covered separately in Chapter 17.

Understanding the mechanism of injury is obviously important for appreciating a classification, interpreting the clinical and radiographic findings, instituting treatment, anticipating complications, and providing adequate follow-up care.

CLASSIFICATION

Acute elbow dislocations are classified as posterior, anterior, and divergent.

Posterior Dislocations

By far the most common dislocation occurs posteriorly (Fig. 29–2). Whether the forearm is medially or laterally displaced is irrelevant to the pathologic condition seen or the ultimate treatment.

Anterior Dislocations

Anterior dislocations are extremely rare and are usually seen in younger individuals (Fig. 29–3).[4] The forearm bones are displaced anterior to the distal humerus. The

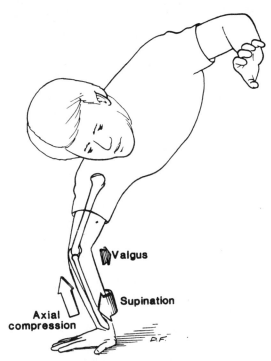

FIGURE 29–1 • Proposed mechanism of elbow dislocation. A fall on the outstretched hand with the shoulder abducted produces an axial force on the elbow as it flexes. As the body internally rotates on the hand and approaches the ground, external rotation and valgus moments are applied to the elbow. This is the same combination of forces and moments that are applied to the elbow during the lateral pivot-shift test for posterolateral rotatory instability. (From O'Driscoll, S. W., Morrey, B. F., Korinek, S., and An, K. N.: Elbow subluxation and dislocation: A spectrum of instability. Clin. Orthop. **280**:186, 1992.)

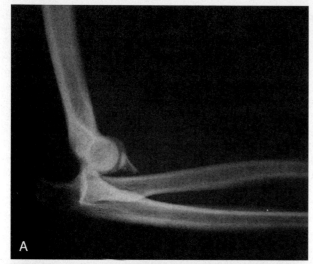

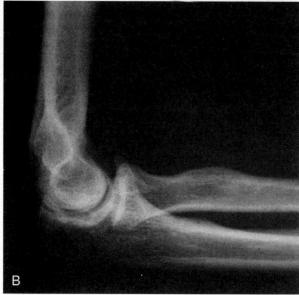

FIGURE 29–2 • A, Posterior dislocation of the elbow from a fall on the outstretched hand. Note the shear fracture of coronoid fragment, which is pathognomonic of an elbow subluxation or dislocation. Small "flake" fractures are not avulsion fractures because nothing attaches to the very tip of the coronoid. The brachialis inserts distally. B, Coronoid fragment has healed.

mechanism of injury may be similar to that described for posterior dislocations, but there is a forward rebounding response that allows the anterior projections after extensive hyperextension has allowed the olecranon to slide under the trochlea. In adults, the olecranon is usually fractured.

Divergent Dislocations

Displacement of the radius from the ulna with concomitant dislocation is a rare injury associated with energetic trauma.[7, 40] The interosseous membrane, annular ligament, and distal radioulnar joint capsule are necessarily torn.

PATHOMECHANICS OF ELBOW INSTABILITY

The pathoanatomy can be thought of as a circle of soft tissue disruption from lateral to medial in three stages (Figs. 29–4 and 29–5).

In stage 1, the ulnar part of the lateral collateral ligament is disrupted (the remainder of the lateral collateral ligament complex may be intact or disrupted). This results in posterolateral rotatory subluxation of the elbow, which reduces spontaneously.[56, 58]

With further disruption anteriorly and posteriorly, the elbow is capable of an incomplete posterolateral dislocation (stage 2). The concave medial edge of the ulna rests on the trochlea in such a way that a lateral radiograph gives one the impression that the coronoid is perched on the trochlea.[47]

Stage 3 has two parts. In stage 3A, all the soft tissues are disrupted around to and including the posterior part of the medial collateral ligament, leaving the important anterior band intact. This permits posterior dislocation by the previously described posterolateral rotatory mechanism. The elbow pivots around on the intact anterior band of the medial collateral ligament. In stage 3B, the entire medial collateral complex is disrupted. Gross varus and valgus as well as rotatory instability is present following reduction, owing to the fact that all ligaments and capsules are disrupted. Surgical exploration has established that the anterior medial collateral ligament usually is disrupted by a complete dislocation of the elbow.[6–8, 10] These pathoanatomic stages correlate with clinical degrees of elbow instability.

Dislocation is therefore the final of three sequential stages of elbow instability resulting from posterolateral

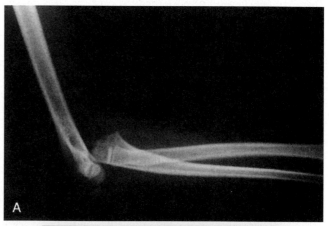

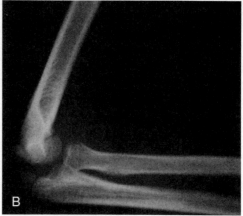

FIGURE 29–3 • A, Anterior dislocation, elbow. Avulsion olecranon fragment. B, Three weeks post-reduction.

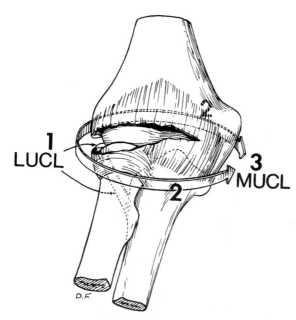

FIGURE 29–4 • Soft tissue injury progresses in a circle-like manner, from lateral to medial, in three stages. In stage 1, the lateral ulnar collateral ligament (LUCL) is disrupted. In stage 2, the other lateral ligamentous structures and the anterior and posterior capsule are disrupted. In stage 3, disruption of the medial ulnar collateral ligament (MUCL) can be partial with disruption of the posterior MUCL only (stage 3A), or complete (stage 3B). (From O'Driscoll, S. W., Morrey, B. F., Korinek, S., and An, K. N.: Elbow subluxation and dislocation: A spectrum of instability. Clin. Orthop. **280**:186, 1992.)

relevant. This hypothesis explains the spectrum of instability, from posterolateral rotatory instability to perched dislocation to posterior dislocation without or with disruption of the anterior medial collateral ligament, which occurs with further posterior displacement. Such a posterolateral rotatory mechanism of dislocation is compatible with those suggested by Osborne and Cotterill,[61] Roberts,[70] and others.[1, 5, 29, 60]

A posterolateral rotatory mechanism is also consistent with the observation that some patients experience recurrent dislocations requiring reduction and also have a positive lateral pivot-shift test.[56] Furthermore, such patients with recurrent dislocations typically do very well with surgical reconstruction of the lateral collateral ligament complex alone, without any attention paid to the medial side,[3, 4, 19, 21, 25, 50, 56] which suggests that the essential lesion of such an instability is on the lateral side. Finally, it has not been shown that the results of surgical repair of the anteromedial collateral ligament following acute dislocations are superior to those of nonoperative treatment.[9, 31] On the other hand, these observations do not preclude hyperextension as a cause of elbow dislocation in some instances. In fact, both the anterior band of the medial collateral ligament and the lateral ulnar collateral ligament may be considered analogous structures with similar functions.

ASSOCIATED INJURIES

Associated injuries with elbow dislocation are common.[30, 34, 59, 71, 74, 87, 89] Radial head and neck fractures occur in about 5 to 10 percent of cases secondary to compressive loading at the radiocapitellar joint. Avulsion of fragments from either the medial or the lateral epicondyles occurs in approximately 12 percent of cases, and fractures of the coronoid process occur in 10 percent of dislocations (see Fig. 29–2).

Displacement of the medial epicondyle in adolescents ranges from minimal to incarceration of the epicondyle within the joint (Fig. 29–6).[37, 65, 73, 81, 83, 90] The latter, if undetected, results in significant traumatic arthrosis (Fig. 29–7). Medial epicondylar fracture can predispose to late

ulnohumeral rotatory subluxation, with soft tissue disruption progressing from lateral to medial. In each stage, the pathoanatomy is correlated with the pattern and degree of instability. This has been confirmed in studies of cadaver elbows; 12 of 13 of the elbows could be dislocated posteriorly, with the anterior medial collateral ligament intact.[18] In all 13 elbows, the coronoid could be perched on the trochlea after release of the lateral collateral ligament complex and the lateral half of the anterior capsule. Following reduction, the elbows were clinically stable to valgus stress.

This mechanism of dislocation results in less soft tissue damage than would a hyperextension or a valgus mechanism; its kinematics are easily reproduced and clinically

FIGURE 29–5 • Clinical stages of elbow instability correlating with the pathoanatomic stages of capsuloligamentous disruption. Forces and moment responsible for displacements are illustrated. PLRI = posterolateral rotatory instability. See also Table 27–2. (From O'Driscoll, S. W., Morrey, B. F., Korinek, S., and An, K. N.: Elbow subluxation and dislocation: A spectrum of instability. Clin. Orthop. **280**:186, 1992.)

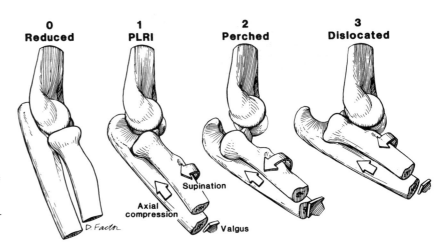

The relationship of the radial head to the ulnar part of the lateral collateral ligament has also been studied experimentally. O'Driscoll and associates[19, 20] demonstrated the clinical manifestation of an attenuated or torn lateral collateral ligament; posterolateral rotatory subluxation can occur in the presence or absence of the radial head. However, clinical experience suggests that elbows without a radial head do less well after reconstruction of the ulnar part of the lateral collateral ligament than do those in which the radial head is intact.[18] This suggests that the radial head provides some resistance to posterolateral rotatory instability but, once again, in a secondary capacity.

OLECRANON

The major determinant of stability of the elbow is clearly the ulnohumeral joint. Although the stabilizing influence of this joint has not been studied to any great extent, the relative contribution of the olecranon in resisting various loading configurations has been shown to be linearly correlated with the extent of resection of the proximal part of the ulna (Fig. 30–2).[1] The critical amount of articulation required for maintaining stability is about 50 percent. These data may be altered by dynamic forces, but this has not been studied.

CORONOID

The amount of the coronoid required for stability with or without ligamentous integrity and with and without the radial head is emerging. The experimental and clinical experience suggests that at least 50 percent of the coronoid must be present for the ulnohumeral joint to be functional (Fig. 30–3). Absence of the radial head further compromises the elbow with a coronoid deficiency. From a practi-

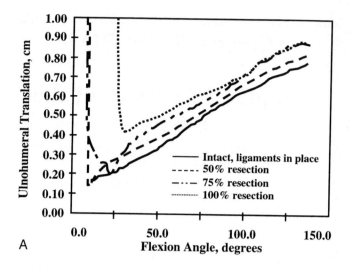

A

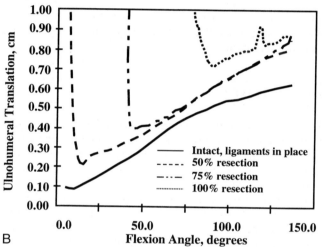

B

FIGURE 30–3 • Experimental study measuring ulnohumeral translation with resection of various portions of the coronoid demonstrates instability both with (A) and without (B) the radial head. However, when as much as 50 percent of the coronoid is present, the degree of instability is dramatically reduced and the ulnohumeral joint approaches normal. These data were obtained after releasing the ligaments, common flexor-extensor tendons, and capsule. The testing was performed with the elbow in the neutral (sagittal) plane and no unbalanced varus-valgus moments.

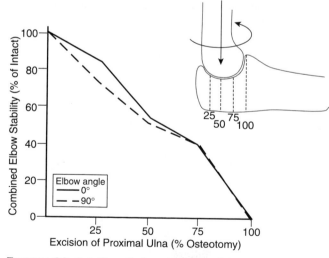

FIGURE 30–2 • The articular contribution of the proximal ulna in various loading modes and in various flexion positions demonstrates that the articulation contributes to stability to the extent that it is present. Thus, approximately 25 percent stability is lost when 25 percent is removed, 50 percent is lost when 50 percent is removed. However, the collateral ligaments are contained in the distal 25 percent; thus, at least 75 and ideally 50 percent of the olecranon should be present to provide ulnohumeral stability.

cal perspective, we have found it useful to observe that the typical 30-degree angle formed by a line from the intact olecranon and coronoid is reduced to 0 degrees when the critical 50 percent of the coronoid is present (Fig. 30–4A and B).

Ligamentous Contributions

The relative contributions of the medial and lateral collateral ligaments to varus-valgus stability with the elbow articulation intact and in flexion and extension have been studied experimentally.[16] Investigation has shown that the collateral ligaments provide approximately 50 percent of the varus-valgus stability of the joint, and the articular surfaces an additional 50 percent. The only exception is with the elbow in full extension: under this condition, the ulnohumeral joint and anterior capsule render the elbow stable to varus-valgus stress, even in the absence of collateral ligaments.

CLINICAL MANAGEMENT: PRINCIPLE

A basic principle underlying the treatment of complex instability of the elbow has been defined on the basis of careful evaluation of the experimental data and our clinical experience. This tenet is simply that it is essential that all treatment options take advantage of or restore a competent ulnohumeral joint. In this context, the management of complex instability is discussed according to the nature of the articular injury.

Fracture of the Radial Head with Attenuation or Tear of the Medial Collateral Ligament

The presentation of medial ligament injury can be extremely subtle. The prevalence is difficult to ascertain, but in my experience it has occurred in about 1 to 2 percent of patients who had a fracture of the radial head.[15] One should have a high level of suspicion that an injury to the ligament might be present when there is a compression fracture of the radial neck. However, some comminuted fractures may also be due to an axial load and severe valgus stress causing concurrent rupture of the medial collateral ligament. Ecchymosis on the medial side of the elbow should be an obvious clue.

TREATMENT

Treatment of this difficult problem is based on the realization that the radial head is an important secondary stabilizer when the medial collateral ligament has been disrupted. The primary goal of the treatment strategy is to restore ulnohumeral joint stability. However, a reconstructed medial collateral ligament has been observed to stretch in the absence of radial humeral integrity; hence if the radial head fracture is amenable to fixation, the stable arc is determined after fixation. If the arc is stable and within 40 degrees of

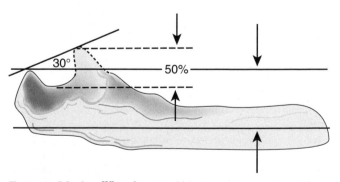

FIGURE 30–4 • When the coronoid is intact, the line between the tip of the olecranon and the coronoid makes approximately a 30-degree angle with the shaft of the humerus. However, when 50 percent of the coronoid is absent, a line through the remnant and the tip of the olecranon is approximately parallel to the shaft of the ulna. This information is useful to the clinician in assessing the amount of coronoid present, which has direct implications for treatment options and strategy.

extension, unrestricted passive motion is allowed after 7 to 10 days of protection. If dislocation occurs with extension of approximately 60 degrees, the elbow is immobilized for 2 weeks, after which motion in a hinged splint, with a 45-degree extension stop, is allowed for 2 weeks. In our practice, the collateral ligament is not repaired in selected cases in which it is already exposed or felt to enhance stability. Nonetheless, the popularity of suture anchors has prompted a more aggressive attitude toward ligament repair. Rodgers and colleagues[23] report 88 percent satisfactory results in 17 patients treated with suture anchors who had major elbow injuries.

If osteosynthesis is not possible, then restoration of the radiohumeral joint with the use of a prosthesis becomes a higher priority. Unfortunately, the Silastic implant does not reliably offer the material characteristics necessary for achieving stability. Therefore, the possibility of use of metal implants has been reintroduced,[5, 9, 11] although there is limited clinical evidence to document their efficacy. In some instances in which the medial collateral ligament has been disrupted, replacement of the radial head with an allograft has been performed as an alternative method of providing stabilization (Fig. 30–5A and B).

If the radiohumeral joint cannot be reconstructed, it is appropriate to address the injury of the medial collateral ligament directly and to repair it as soon as possible. The ligament may be avulsed from its origin or insertion, allowing direct reattachment. Midsubstance tears are more difficult to repair, and there is less likelihood of achieving immediate stabilization.

Finally, a hinged external fixator may be applied in any circumstances in which it is desirable to protect a fractured radial head, protect a ligament repair, or, on occasion, protect the ulnohumeral joint without either of the aforementioned adjunctive treatments (see Chapter 34).

If the fixator is not used, patients are fitted with a locked hinged brace for protection for about 2 weeks postoperatively; the brace is then unlocked, and motion is allowed in the stable arc. The hinged brace is worn for a total of at least 6 weeks or until the joint is stable.

There is insufficient clinical experience to provide clear expectations of the results of this combined injury to the metacarpophalangeal joint and radial head. However, treatment of the acute injury is accomplished much more reliably than is reconstruction for chronic or late instability (see Chapter 31).

Fractures of the Radial Head With Dislocation of the Elbow

This lesion is often referred to as a Mason type IV injury, an extension of the original Mason classification of fractures[7, 13] (see Chapter 25). There is little information in the literature to help to define the optimum treatment for fracture-dislocations.[2, 24] However, the simple principle defined earlier is followed. If it is clearly demonstrated that the coronoid is intact, the basic treatment principle is first to reduce the dislocation and then to determine the extent to which the ulnohumeral articulation provides stability. Additional treatment is determined according to the type of fracture.[13]

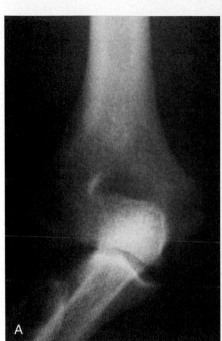

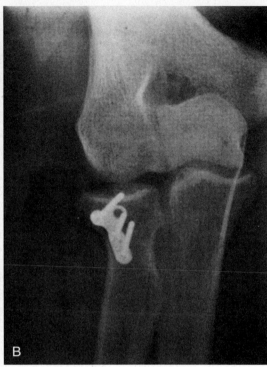

FIGURE 30–5 • *A*, Radiograph showing gross valgus instability in a patient who had resection of the radial head in the presence of an unrecognized disruption of the medial collateral ligament. *B*, Two years after reconstruction with an allograft, the patient had excellent function.

TYPE I FRACTURES

In type I injuries, if the elbow is stable to within 45 or 50 degrees of extension, nothing more need be done except to place the elbow in a splint with a 60-degree extension stop, which the patient wears for 1 to 2 weeks. Full extension is then allowed as tolerated while the elbow is protected with a hinged splint.

TYPE II FRACTURES

Type II fractures are treated by open reduction and internal fixation. These injuries are the most amenable to such treatment. King and associates[10] report a successful outcome in all eight patients so treated. It is essential that elbows with injuries of the collateral ligaments be treated with open reduction and internal fixation, as these injuries result in chronic instability if the radial head is resected.[4, 5, 9] Because these fractures are amenable to such treatment, repair of the collateral ligaments is not always necessary, but one of us (SOD) repairs the ligaments routinely. However, if the elbow remains unstable on examination through the arcs described earlier, enhanced stability may be obtained by repairing or stabilizing the collateral ligament. Josefsson and associates[8] reviewed their experience with 19 complex injuries of the elbow and recommended open reduction and internal fixation of the radial head fracture as well as repair of the ligament. However, treatment of 4 of 19 coronoid fractures had a poor result, suggesting that this component of the lesion must be specifically addressed.

In this setting, we would consider the use of the distraction external fixator.

TYPE III FRACTURES

These are the most difficult injuries to treat. Experience has suggested that the entire comminuted radial head should be excised acutely if it cannot be fixed.[2] Open reduction and internal fixation is technically difficult and was reported to be successful in only two of six instances by King and colleagues.[10] During operative excision, the elbow is tested according to the scheme described for type I fractures. If the elbow is unstable, then direct repair of the collateral ligaments might be considered. If sufficient stability cannot be achieved, a Silastic implant may be tried as a temporary spacer if it enhances stability sufficiently to permit motion.

Alternatively, a metal implant may be employed. Experience with a vitallium implant with a mean follow-up of 4.5 years has been reported by Knight and associates.[11] An overall success rate of 78 percent was observed. Dislocation of the elbow was an associated injury in 21 of these 31 patients. More recently, the so-called *floating radial head implant of Judet* was reported successful in all 12 cases at a mean of 43 months.[9] These authors particularly recommend the implant for the type III or type IV radial head fractures, that is, complex injuries. Alternatively, a cadaveric replacement may be an option; however, there has been little experience with the use of such a replacement in the acute setting. This has been reported as a successful treatment in five patients with wrist pain after an Essex-Lopresti injury.[25]

If stability remains a problem, a hinged external fixator that allows elbow motion is applied. The indication for use of the external fixator is a joint without a radial head or a healing radiohumeral joint with a torn medial collateral ligament that is inherently and grossly unstable (see Chapter 34). If use of an implant or open reduction and internal fixation of the radial head does not restore stability, the distraction device allows congruous alignment of the ulnohumeral joint, and motion lessens the likelihood of stiffness (Fig. 30–6*A* to *C*). The device is removed as early as the third to fourth week and as late as 12 weeks, after which adjustable splints are used to restore motion (see Chapter 12).

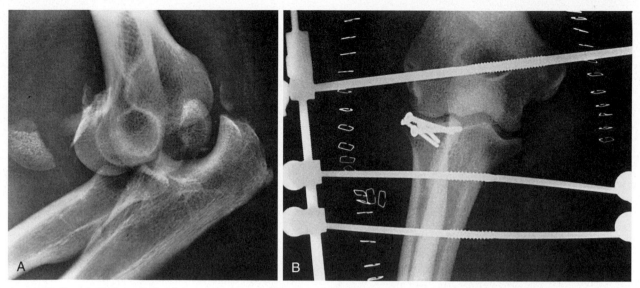

FIGURE 30–6 • *A*, Radiograph showing a severe fracture-dislocation of the elbow (a Mason type-III fracture of the radial head). The fracture of the radial head was treated with internal fixation. Because of gross instability, additional stabilization was achieved with use of the Dynamic Joint Distractor *(B)*.

Fracture of the Proximal Part of the Ulna

Fortunately, fractures of the proximal part of the ulna, the olecranon, or the coronoid that are associated with instability are the most uncommon of these injuries, as they pose the most difficult treatment problems.[15] Treatment consists of restoring the integrity of the ulnohumeral joint, as just described. Ideally, this is accomplished by reduction and stabilization of the fracture.

Fracture of the Olecranon

The Mayo classification scheme for fractures of the olecranon is based on displacement, comminution, and stability[15] (see Chapter 26). The injury discussed here is termed type III, meaning that the elbow is unstable because of injury both to a collateral ligament and from a displaced fracture of the olecranon (Fig. 30–7).

The type III fracture of the olecranon is accompanied by ligamentous disruption. The principle is again applied: stabilize the ulnohumeral joint (Fig. 30–8). If there is minimum comminution of the olecranon, rigid plate fixation restores the ulnohumeral joint. If the olecranon is rigidly fixed, then the unstable injury is converted to a stable one as the ulnohumeral joint is inherently stable. Hence, the technique for rigid fixation of the fracture is of paramount importance (Fig. 30–9A and B). A 3.5-mm dynamic compression (DC) or low-contour dynamic compression (LCDC) plate bent at an 80-degree angle and applied to the posterior surface of the ulna permits excellent fixation on the small proximal fragment.[19] Not uncommonly, one fragment may also involve the coronoid. If it does, this is the most important component of the reduction and fixation.

Fracture of the Coronoid

The coronoid is the most important portion of the ulnohumeral articulation. This is related to the posteriorly directed

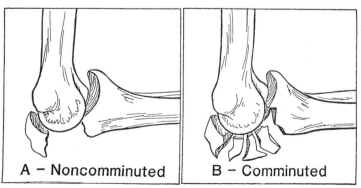

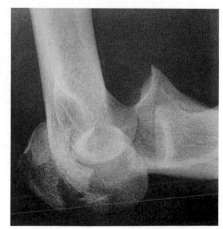

FIGURE 30–7 • *Left* and *Right Panels*, A Mayo type-III ulnar fracture may or may not be comminuted, but it is characterized by attenuation or disruption of the medial collateral ligament or the ulnar part of the lateral collateral ligament, or both. This is characterization by instability of the forearm.

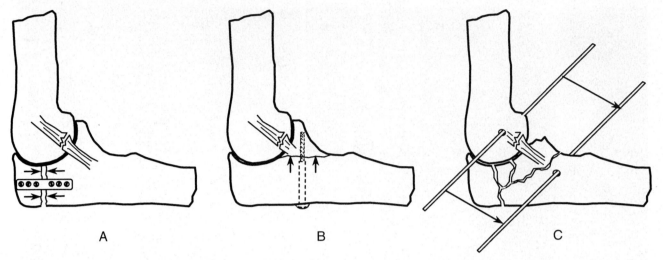

FIGURE 30–8 • When there has been disruption of the collateral ligament and alteration of the ulnohumeral joint, the ulnohumeral joint must be somehow stabilized. This may occur by rigid plate fixation if the fracture allows *(A)*, by rigid fixation of the coronoid if the fracture allows *(B)*, or by neutralization of the ulnohumeral relationship if the fractures do not allow rigid fixation *(C)*.

forces of both the biceps and the triceps that tend to "drive" the humerus into the coronoid fracture (Fig. 30–10). It also serves as a site of attachment for the collateral ligaments.

TYPE I FRACTURE

According to the classification of Regan and Morrey, type I fractures represent a small chip of the tip of the coronoid and serve mainly as an indicator that the elbow has dislocated or at least displaced sufficiently to have sustained an injury of the collateral ligaments.[21] The ulnohumeral joint is stable, and rehabilitation is similar to that recommended for type I fracture-dislocations of the radial head. Open reduction is not necessary if the elbow is stable.

TYPE II FRACTURE

In type II fractures, as much as 50 percent of the coronoid is involved and the elbow is usually unstable, especially if the radial head is also fractured. Careful examination with the patient under anesthesia reveals whether the joint is stable after reduction (see Fig. 30–10). The threshold for fixation varies with individual surgeons. If fixation is stable, motion within the stable arc, as described previously, may be allowed (Fig. 30–11). If posterior displacement occurs with less than 40 to 45 degrees of flexion, the articulation is considered inadequate, and the ulnohumeral joint must be stabilized. If the fracture fragment is large enough for fixation, osteosynthesis with a single screw is performed. If the fragment is too small for fixation, a heavy No. 5 suture is placed through the fragment (or fragments), which is brought to its anatomic location and tied through drill holes placed in the ulna. In the latter situation, or even if osteosynthesis has been carried out but there is concern about stability, the elbow may need to be neutralized by the application of a hinged external fixator—that is, the external fixator eliminates the dynamic forces that are ap-

plied to the fracture site by the muscles that flex and extend the elbow joint (see Fig. 30–11). The device allows motion of the ulnohumeral joint while a distal distraction force is placed on the ulna, thus protecting the articulation. The device is maintained for 3 to 6 weeks, depending on the nature of the injury.[3] Cobb and Morrey[3] reported on seven such injuries and documented a successful outcome in six. In that series, the coronoid fracture was treated as described earlier, and a distraction device was applied in each instance.

TYPE III FRACTURE

These injuries are the most difficult to treat, as, by definition, they render the ulnohumeral joint grossly unstable. If the coronoid is a large fragment and has not been comminuted (type IIIA), it may be fixed with a screw and the joint will be stable. However, because of the large forces transmitted through this relatively small surface area, as with the type II fractures, these injuries should be further neutralized with the distraction device.

The severely comminuted coronoid fracture (type IIIB) is a very uncommon injury. In this setting, I reduce the elbow and bring the fracture fragments into relative alignment with the use of a heavy suture. I avoid removing any bone fragments, as they may serve as a basis for substantive healing and formation of callus. The ulnohumeral relationship is maintained in a reduced position by the distraction device.

In every instance, the most important goal is to prevent posterior displacement of the ulna against the trochlea—thus, the concept of neutralization with an external fixator that permits flexion and extension while keeping the articulation aligned and eliminating the disruptive force from muscle contracture (Fig. 30–12). Once again, the principle of restoration of the ulnohumeral integrity has been followed.

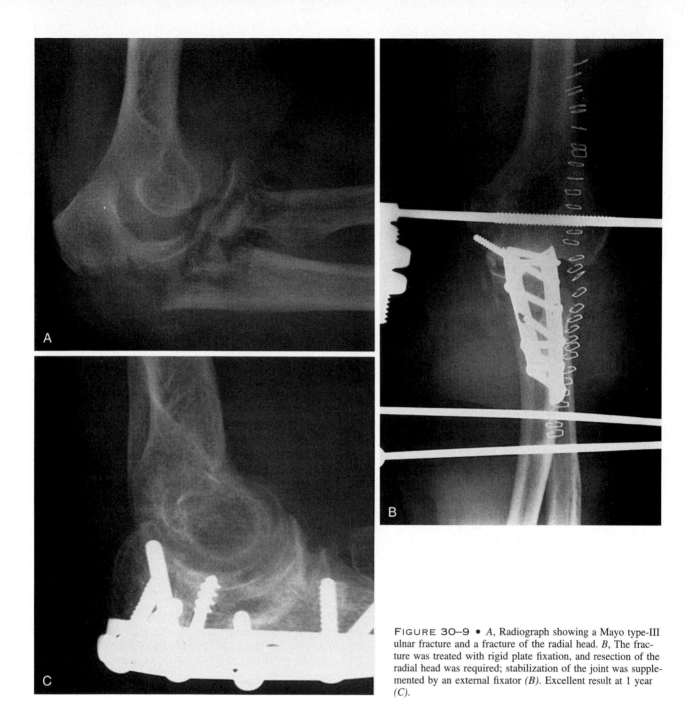

FIGURE 30–9 • *A*, Radiograph showing a Mayo type-III ulnar fracture and a fracture of the radial head. *B*, The fracture was treated with rigid plate fixation, and resection of the radial head was required; stabilization of the joint was supplemented by an external fixator *(B)*. Excellent result at 1 year *(C)*.

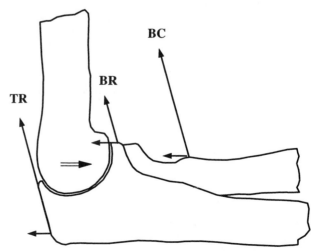

FIGURE 30–10 • The anterior displacement of the humerus into the coronoid is brought about by the posterior directed vector occurring with elbow flexion that is a component of triceps (TR), brachialis (BR), and/or biceps (BC) contraction. Thus, there is a tendency for posterior ulnar translation with both flexion and extension movements.

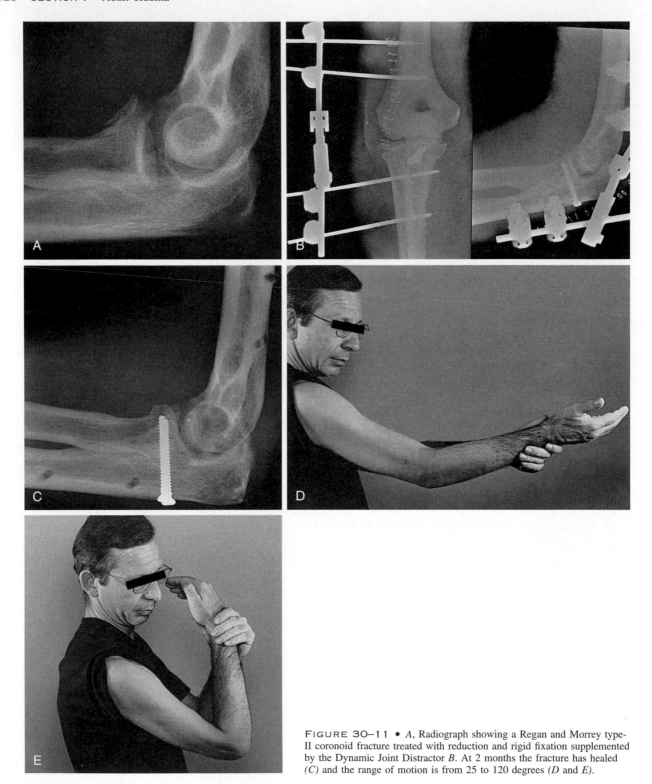

FIGURE 30–11 • *A*, Radiograph showing a Regan and Morrey type-II coronoid fracture treated with reduction and rigid fixation supplemented by the Dynamic Joint Distractor *B*. At 2 months the fracture has healed (*C*) and the range of motion is from 25 to 120 degrees (*D* and *E*).

FRACTURE OF THE RADIAL HEAD AND CORONOID WITH DISLOCATION

These injuries are the most difficult in this category to treat. The principle is the same as already discussed: the radial head must be fixed or replaced. The coronoid fracture is fixed, if possible, with use of a direct or retrograde screw. In either instance, the elbow may need to be protected by a hinged external fixator. This allows motion but eliminates force on the radial head and the coronoid.

OVERVIEW

The first principle for treating the complex injuries of the elbow is to restore the essential element, the ulnohumeral

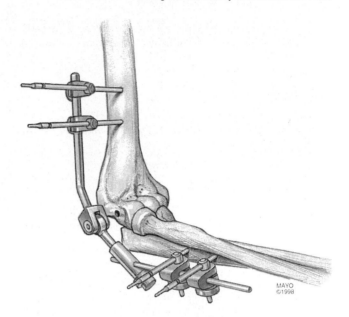

FIGURE 30–12 • When there has been internal fixation in the proximal ulna the dynamic joint distractor is applied in such a way as to result in a distal displacement force on the ulna that allows realignment of the ulnohumeral joint. Current design favors half pins and eliminates the axis pin, lessening the likelihood of infection.

joint (Fig. 30–13). This is done by reduction of the intact joint or, if the coronoid or the olecranon has fractured, by osteosynthesis. The second principle is that the radial head is an important secondary stabilizer, which must be fixed or replaced if the ulnohumeral joint cannot be restored to normal. Finally, the collateral ligaments should be repaired

if they have been injured. Efforts to restore the ulnohumeral articulation are enhanced by protection with a hinged external fixator that allows motion. The implications for rehabilitation and the exact degree of instability are best determined after the ulnohumeral joint has been reduced and the elbow has been moved through an arc of motion. If

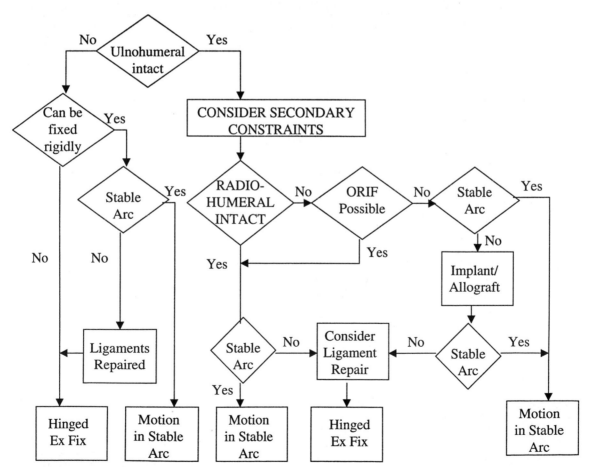

FIGURE 30–13 • Treatment logic for complex instability. Notice the pre-eminent status of the integrity of the ulnohumeral joint.

there is any tendency for the elbow to subluxate or dislocate within 45 degrees of extension, the primary or secondary constraints have not adequately been restored.

REFERENCES

1. An, K. N., Morrey, B. F., and Chao, E. Y. S.: The effect of partial removal of proximal ulna on elbow constraint. Clin. Orthop. **209:**270, 1986.
2. Broberg, M. A., and Morrey, B. F.: Results of treatment of fracture-dislocations of the elbow. Clin. Orthop. **216:**109, 1987.
3. Cobb, T. K., and Morrey B. F.: Use of distraction arthroplasty in unstable fracture dislocations of the elbow. Clin. Orthop. **312:**201, 1995.
4. Geel, C. W., Palmer, A. K., Ruedi, T., and Leutenegger, A. F.: Internal fixation of proximal radial head fractures. J. Orthop. Trauma **4:**270, 1990.
5. Harrington, I. J., and Tountas, A. A.: Replacement of the radial head in the treatment of unstable elbow fractures. Injury **12:**405, 1981.
6. Hotchkiss, R. N.: Displaced fractures of the radial head: Internal fixation or excision? J. AAOS **5:**1, 1997.
7. Johnston, G. W.: A follow-up of 100 cases of fracture of the head of the radius with a review of the literature. Ulster Med. J. **31:**51, 1962.
8. Josefsson, P. O., Gentz, C. F., Johnell, O., and Wendeberg, B.: Dislocations of the elbow and intraarticular fractures. Clin. Orthop. **246:**126, 1989.
9. Judet, T., de Loubresse, C. G., Piriou, P., and Charnley, G.: A floating prosthesis for radial-head fractures. J. Bone Joint Surg. **78B:**244, 1996.
10. King, G. J., Evans, D. C., and Kellam, J. F.: Open reduction and internal fixation of radial head fractures. J. Orthop. Trauma **5:**21, 1991.
11. Knight, D. J., Rymaszewski, L. A., Amis, A. A., and Miller, J. H.: Primary replacement of the fractured radial head with a metal prosthesis. J. Bone Joint Surg. **75-B:**572, 1993.
12. Moneim, M. S., and Garst, J. R.: Vascular injuries associated with elbow fractures and dislocations. Int. Angiol. **14:**307, 1995.
13. Morrey, B. F., and An, K.-N.: Articular and ligamentous contributions to the stability of the elbow joint. Am. J. Sports Med. **11:**315, 1983.
14. Morrey, B. F.: Complex instability of the elbow. J. Bone Joint Surg. **79A:**460, 1997.
15. Morrey, B. F.: Current concepts in the treatment of fractures of the radial head, the olecranon, and the coronoid: Instructional Course Lecture. J. Bone Joint Surg. **77-A:**316, 1995.
16. Morrey, B. F.: Fracture of the radial head. *In* Morrey, B. F. (ed.): The Elbow and Its Disorders, 2nd ed. Philadelphia, W. B. Saunders, 1993, pp. 383–404.
17. Morrey, B. F., Tanaka, S., and An, K.-N.: Valgus stability of the elbow: A definition of primary and secondary constraints. Clin. Orthop. **265:**187, 1991.
18. Nestor, B. J., O'Driscoll, S. W., and Morrey, B. F.: Ligamentous reconstruction for posterolateral rotatory instability of the elbow. J. Bone Joint Surg. **74A:**8:1235, 1992.
19. O'Driscoll, S. W., Morrey, B. F., Korinek, S., and An, K. N.: Elbow subluxation and dislocation. Clin. Orthop. **280:**186, 1992.
20. O'Driscoll, S. W.: Technique for unstable olecranon fracture-subluxations. Op Techniques Orthop. **4:**49, 1994.
21. Regan, W., and Morrey, B. F.: Fracture of the coronoid process of the ulna. J. Bone Joint Surg. **71-A:**1348, 1989.
22. Regel, G., Seekamp, A., Blauth, M., Klemme, R., Kuhn, K., and Tscherne, H.: Complex injury of the elbow joint. Unfallchirurg **99:**92, 1996.
23. Rodgers, W. B., Kharrazi, F. D., Waters, P. M., Kennedy, J. G., McKee, M. D., and Lhowe, D. W.: The use of osseous suture anchors in the treatment of severe, complicated elbow dislocations. Am. J. Orthop. **25:**794, 1996.
24. Scharplatz, D., and Allgower, M.: Fracture dislocation of the elbow. Injury **7:**143, 1975.
25. Szabo, R. M., Hotchkiss, R. N., and Slater, R. R., Jr.: The use of frozen-allograft radial head replacement for treatment of established symptomatic proximal translation of the radius: Preliminary experience in five cases. J. Hand Surg. **22:**269, 1997.

• CHAPTER 31 •

Chronic Unreduced Elbow Dislocation

• BERNARD F. MORREY

The spectrum of elbow instability is dealt with in various chapters, including those involving the pediatric patient (see Chapter 21) and simple and complex instability (see Chapters 29 and 30), and in the chapter on external fixation for the elbow (see Chapter 34). At Mayo we consider elbow instability according to three major variables: (1) temporal considerations, that is, duration to definitive treatment; (2) the extent of the dislocation; and (3) the direction of the dislocation (Table 31–1). Hence the instability pattern considered in this chapter is termed chronic unreduced complete dislocation. A chronic unreduced dislocation is very uncommon in this country and is principally seen in Third World nations. Thus, much of our understanding has come from contributions from South Africa, Thailand, and India.[8, 9, 11, 13]

CHRONIC UNREDUCED ELBOW JOINT

The two major types of chronic unreduced elbow joint depend on the extent. The most common is sometimes subtle and is a chronic unreduced subluxation. This chronic instability pattern is the most common in this country and is dealt with in the chapter on complex instability (see Chapter 30). The second is an unreduced complete dislocation that is quite rare except, as mentioned, in underdeveloped countries.

PRESENTATION

There are two chronic instabilities with different characteristics. Chronic unreduced complete dislocation has the following characteristics: (1) gross deformity; (2) motion is variable from complete ankylosis in approximately one third of cases to an arc of motion of greater than 40 degrees in one third, and motion between 0 to 40 degrees in the remaining one third[10]; (3) pain ranges from minimal to significant depending on the duration of the dislocation.

In the setting of chronic unreduced partial dislocation (subluxation), the characteristics are different. Gross deformity is rare. Motion is often functional and pain is variable but usually quite severe. Both cause marked dysfunction.

Occurrence and Clinical Presentation

The presentation of individuals with chronic unreduced elbow dislocation is such that two thirds have unacceptable function due to instability, pain, or both.[10] The frequency is highly dependent on the local medical customs dealing with the initial dislocation, experience, and expertise. The presence of traditional medical care (bone setters[3]) explains the reports from Africa documenting 81 cases over a 10-year period.[11] In Thailand, 135 patients were reported in a 15-year period from three hospitals.[9] The deformity may occur both in children and in adults. These patients often have sustained an associated fracture as well. Naidoo[11] noted that 13 of 23 patients undergoing treatment had an associated fracture. A similar rate of 45 percent (62 of 135) was reported from a large multicenter study by Mahaisavariya and associates.[9] About 50 percent simply have a posteriorly displaced, complete dislocation. The patients usually do not have neurologic deficit at the time of presentation, but if there is neural impairment, the ulnar nerve is most commonly symptomatic. It is extremely rare to have vascular compromise.

Treatment

The full spectrum of reconstructive options has been suggested as a treatment for the neglected dislocation. These options include reduction, reduction and interposition, resection, fusion, and replacement. Of these various treatment options, resection really is not a viable one. Today, in most practices and circumstances, fusion might be considered in some settings, but this is not usually considered in the United States. The techniques of interposition and replacement arthroplasty are discussed elsewhere (see Chapters 49 and 60). Several additional debated factors that in the past have surrounded the treatment of the condition include the age of the patient, the timing of the intervention, and the likelihood of successful reduction. In our opinion, these questions have been resolved in recent years, particularly with the excellent contribution of Naidoo. An attempt at closed reduction is recommended at all ages for dislocations of less than 3 weeks' duration. Although fusion and resection have both been considered for the chronic condition,[2, 4, 6] by far the most logical and accepted approach is open reduction (Fig. 31–1). Although this recommendation has been somewhat controversial in the past, open reduction outcomes are as good or better than other options even as late as 1 year after injury.[5]

• TABLE 31–1 • **Mayo Classification of Elbow Instability**			
Temporal	**Extent/Direction**		**Clinical Description**
Acute	Incomplete	Translation	Elbow subluxation
		Angulation	Ligament injury
	Complete	Translated	Elbow dislocation
Subacute	Incomplete	Translation	Subluxed joint
		Angulation	Ligament insufficiency
	Complete	Translation	
Recurrent	Incomplete	Translation	Recurrent subluxation
		Angulation	
		Rotation	Post lat ret subluxation
	Complete	Translocation	Recurrent dislocation
Chronic (unreduced)	Incomplete	Translocation	Chronic subluxation
	Complete	Translated	Chronic dislocation

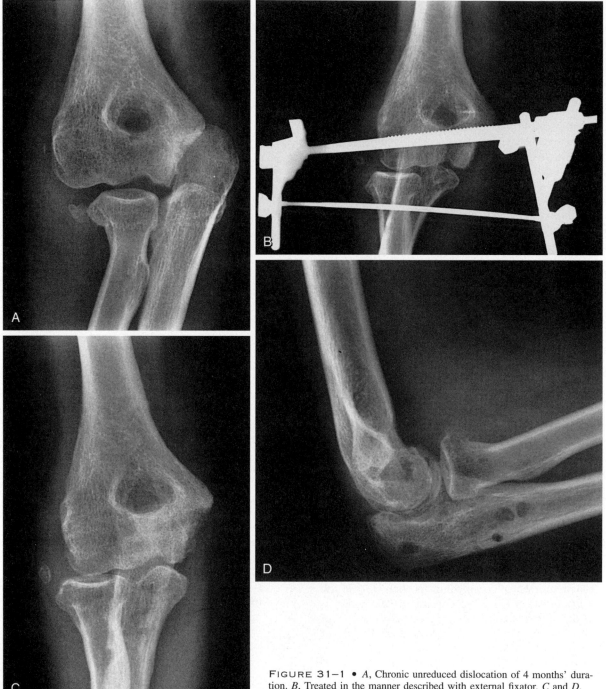

FIGURE 31–1 • *A*, Chronic unreduced dislocation of 4 months' duration. *B*, Treated in the manner described with external fixator. *C* and *D*, Well reduced and functional with a 105-degree arc of motion 1 year later.

Hence, we will review only the treatment strategy for open reduction. Joint replacement is recommended in patients over 60 years of age and is discussed in Chapter 53. The surgical approach is predicated on an understanding of the pathology and a flexible surgical treatment plan.

Pathology

The rationale and surgical strategy is predicated on recognizing and treating the pathology encountered. The pattern is rather consistent: (1) a contracted triceps tendon; (2) contracture of the medial and lateral collateral ligaments; (3) variable involvement of the ulnar nerve; (4) contracted anterior and posterior capsules; (5) fibrous membrane covering the articular surface; and (6) common (30 to 40 percent) associated fracture of the coronoid or a radial head.

TECHNIQUE

The surgical technique preferred by the author specifically addresses the pathology according to a defined sequence (Fig. 31–2).

1. A posterior skin incision is made. With gross deformity, the subcutaneous border of the ulna is identified as the distal landmark and the midportion of the humerus as the proximal landmark. An incision over these two landmarks is then joined to provide a straight incision after the deformity has been corrected (see Fig. 31–2A).

2. The dissection is carried medially to the ulnar nerve, which is identified and released to its first motor branch. A subcutaneous pocket is developed (see Fig. 31–2B).

3. The dissection is carried laterally. Kocher's interval is entered and the radial head exposed.

4. The lateral collateral ligament and extensor mass are elevated from the lateral epicondyle (see Fig. 31–2C). The dense adhesions that are almost always present are then released from the articular surface between the ulna and humerus and the radius and the humerus. The lateral contracted tissue is the limiting factor in preventing relocation, so this is aggressively released. The greater sigmoid notch is cleaned.

5. The posterior capsule is completely released (see Fig. 31–2D).

6. The anterior capsule is excised.

7. The medial collateral ligament is contracted and if

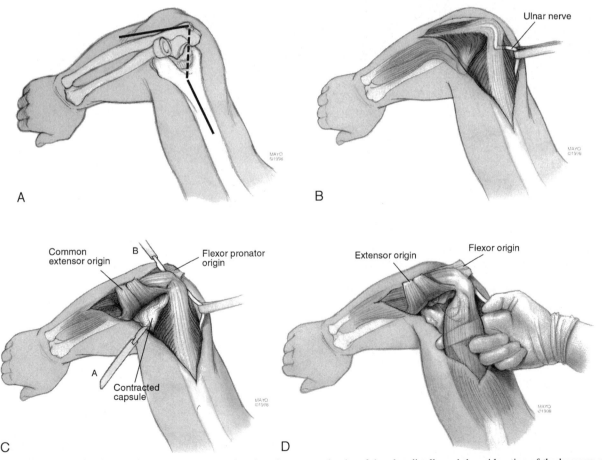

FIGURE 31–2 • *A*, Posterior incision is employed by using the subcutaneous border of the ulna distally and the midportion of the humerus proximally. The ends of each incision are joined to ensure proper orientation of the final incision for those with gross deformity. *B*, Medial and lateral flaps are elevated and the ulnar nerve is released. *C*, The lateral contracted ligament and extensor mechanism (A) is first released from the humerus followed by medial collateral ligament release (B) from the humerus if necessary. *D*, The joint is cleared of membrane and the posterior and anterior capsules are resected. The triceps is elevated from the humerus.

Illustration continued on following page

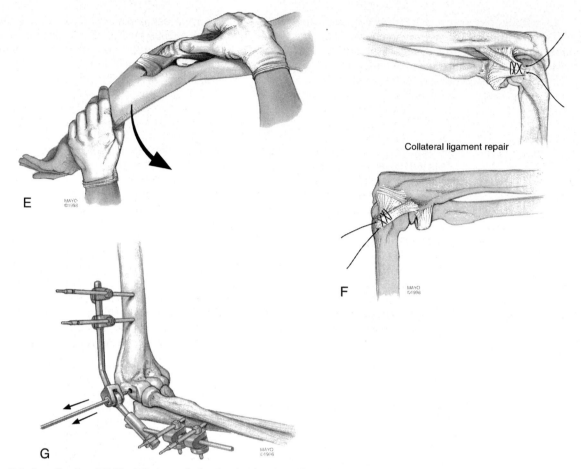

Collateral ligament repair

FIGURE 31–2 • *Continued E*, The joint is manipulated and reduced. *F*, The collateral ligaments are repaired. *G*, The construct is stabilized with dynamic external fixation, and the axis pin removed.

this prevents relocation it is then released from the medial epicondyle.

8. The elbow is gently manipulated in such a way as to reduce the radial humeral and ulnohumeral articulations (see Fig. 31–2E).

9. The lateral collateral ligament and, if necessary, the medial collateral ligaments are repaired with No. 5 Mersilene sutures placed through the ligament in a Bunnell fashion and attached to the anatomic origin through bone holes (see Fig. 31–2F).

10. Triceps repair. Management of the triceps is one of the most controversial issues of this treatment.[9] The elbow is flexed to assess the influence of the contracted triceps. If the elbow can be flexed to 110 degrees, no triceps reconstruction is performed, as it is felt that the musculotendinous complex will stretch out in time. If less than 100 degrees of flexion is possible, a tricepsplasty is performed. The anconeus is elevated from the bed. The anconeus and triceps are then repositioned over the tip of the olecranon, and, with the elbow in 90 degrees of flexion, it is reattached with nonabsorbable No. 5 suture.

11. An external fixator is applied and is essential to allow immediate motion and to preserve the collateral ligament reconstruction (see Chapter 34) (see Fig. 31–2G).

Postoperative Management

The arm is elevated for 2 days, after which a continuous passive motion (CPM) machine is used. The patient returns home in a portable CPM with as much motion as tolerated. The external fixator is maintained for 3 to 4 weeks. The patient then returns to the hospital, and, under a brief general anesthesia, the external fixator is removed (see Chapter 34). Flexion and extension splints are then used to regain the arc of functional motion (see Chapter 12).

RESULTS

Naidoo[11] described a satisfactory result in 23 of 25 patients treated in a manner similar to that just described but without a fixator. Arafiles[1] described a satisfactory outcome in 11 of 12 surgical procedures. Open reduction was reported as successful in 72 percent of 52 patients by Di Schino and associates.[5] Interestingly, these investigators also found complete resection of the elbow for the chronic cases to be successful in 80 percent of cases.[4] However, careful interpretation of these two reports suggests that these authors are referring to improvement of motion and admitted that the resected elbow was weak and had marked instability and hence they favor reduction over resection.

Motion

The improvement is marked but a functional status is not always attained. Of the 23 patients reported by Nadioo[11] with 13 with associated fractures, 8 patients remain with less than 60 degrees of motion (33 percent). Five had an arc of motion between 60 and 90 degrees (20 percent) and 10 (40 percent) had an arc of motion greater than 90 degrees. Naidoo also demonstrated that the overall outcome was not a function of age or duration of dislocation as had been previously thought. On the other hand, Arafiles[1] reports a mean of 105 degrees arc at 2 years in a group of 11 patients.

One major discussion in the literature relates to the management of the triceps. If operated on less than 3 months after injury, this generally need not be lengthened or addressed. However, as mentioned earlier, if the triceps is badly contracted and limits flexion, then some form of triceps augmentation and release is appropriate. Mahaisavariya and colleagues[9] demonstrated that leaving the triceps intact was associated with increased motion ($P < .05$) of 115 degrees in those in which the triceps was not altered, compared with 89 degrees in those with triceps release. In addition, they demonstrated that the flexion contracture was markedly greater (by 70 degrees) in those with a tricepsplasty, compared with 45 degrees in patients in whom tricepsplasty was not carried out. If the triceps is addressed, V-Y lengthening as described by VanGorder has been suggested by some; however, as noted, we prefer the anconeus slide technique.

Complications

This is difficult surgery, and, as might be expected, this type of injury and surgery are associated with significant complications. Transient nerve injury has been reported in 8 to 40 percent of cases.[7, 11] Infection occurs in approximately 5 percent.[1] Ectopic bone was reported in none of the 70 cases of Mahaisavariya and associates[9] and none of the 23 cases of Naidoo.[11] On the other hand, it was ob-

served in 8 percent of the patients reported by Fowles and colleagues[7] and one in four of the patients described by Billett.[3] The overall complication rate is approximately 20 to 25 percent. Complications that significantly affect the outcome occur at a rate of at least 10 percent.

AUTHOR'S EXPERIENCE

We have treated only four patients with complete, chronic dislocation with reduction and stabilization. Three of the four treatments have been successful, leaving patients with an arc of greater than 90 degrees and no or mild pain. One treatment was a failure.

Elbow Replacement

Because of the factors and prognosis noted previously, we prefer the reliable and functional outcome of elbow arthroplasty in patients over 60 years of age. Experience with joint replacement in patients with gross instability has been reported by Ramsey and associates.[12] A success rate of about 90 percent was documented a mean of 6 years after surgery (Fig. 31–3).

CONCLUSIONS

Ideally, of course, chronic unreduced elbow dislocation is best managed by prevention. In the absence of prevention, most patients with unreduced elbow dislocations should be managed according to the principles and technique described here. If this methodology is followed, it is expected that approximately 60 to 75 percent of the patients will have a satisfactory result, which includes minimal pain and an arc of motion of greater than 80 to 90 degrees. If the

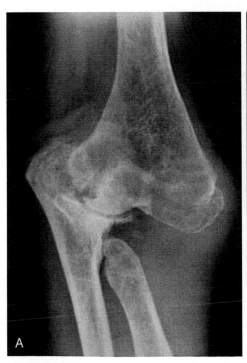

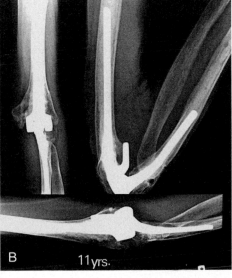

FIGURE 31–3 • *A*, Chronic instability of 3 years' duration and after two procedures. *B*, Excellent flexion and extension with no evidence of implant failures at 11 years.

surgeon reconstructs the collateral ligaments and employs an external fixation device, the well-recognized complication of elbow instability should be all but eliminated. The complication rate is significant and varies as a function of surgeon experience and expertise. Finally, joint replacement is the treatment of choice for patients over 60 years of age.

REFERENCES

1. Arafiles, R. P.: Neglected posterior dislocation of the elbow. A reconstruction operation. J. Bone Joint Surg. **69B**:199, 1987.
2. Ashby, M. E.: Old dislocations of the elbow. J. Nat. Med. Assoc. **66**:465, 1974.
3. Billett, D. M.: Unreduced posterior dislocation of the elbow. J. Trauma **19**:186, 1979.
4. Di Schino, M., Breda, Y., Grimaldi, F. M., Lorthioir, J. M., Merrien, Y.: Resection of the distal part of the humerus in neglected elbow dislocations. Apropos of 23 case reports. Med. Trop. **49**:415, 1989.
5. Di Schino, M., Breda, Y., Grimaldi, F. M., Lorthioir, J. M., and Merrien, Y.: Surgical treatment of neglected elbow dislocations. Report of 81 cases. Rev. Chir. Orthop. Repar. Appareil Moteur **76**:303, 1990.
6. Dryer, R. F., Buckwalter, J. A., and Sprague, B. L.: Treatment of chronic elbow instability. Clin. Orthop. **148**:254, 1980.
7. Fowles, J. V., Kassab, M. T., Douik, M.: Untreated posterior dislocation of the elbow in children. J. Bone Joint Surg. **66A**:921, 1984.
8. Krishnamoorthy, S., Bose, K., Wong, K. P.: Treatment of old unreduced dislocation of the elbow. Injury **8**:39, 1976.
9. Mahaisavariya, B., Laupattarakasem, W., Supachutikul, A., Taesiri, H., and Sujaritbudhungkoon, S.: Late reduction of dislocated elbow. Need triceps be lengthened? J. Bone Joint Surg. **75B**:426, 1993.
10. Martini, M., Benselama, R., and Daoud, A.: Neglected luxations of the elbow: 25 surgical reductions. Rev. Chir. Orthop. Repar. Appareil Moteur **70**:305, 1984.
11. Naidoo, K. S.: Unreduced posterior dislocations of the elbow. J. Bone Joint Surg. **64B**:603, 1982.
12. Ramsey, M., Adams, R. A., and Morrey, B. F.: Elbow displacement for gross instability. J. Bone Joint Surg. **81A**:38–47, 1999.
13. Silva JF: Old dislocations of the elbow. Ann. R. Coll. Surg. Engl. **22**:363, 1958.

• CHAPTER 32 •

Ectopic Ossification About the Elbow

• BERNARD F. MORREY

TERMINOLOGY

Three terms are used more or less interchangeably when referring to bone forming in an atypical location: ectopic bone, heterotopic bone, and myositis ossificans. The first two terms have a similar connotation, but myositis ossificans usually refers to bone formation in the muscle itself,[1] and for the purposes of this chapter, the term *ectopic bone* is used.

An additional distinction is also made between *calcification* and *ossification*. Calcific deposits do occur in tendons, articular cartilage, synovium, and articular capsule, and they typically consist of calcium pyrophosphates. These are usually globular deposits, are amorphous, and, most importantly, have no trabecular structure. This form of radiodensity is most commonly observed about the elbow in ligamentous tissue after injury.[9, 12, 45]

CLASSIFICATION

There are several discrete clinical circumstances in which ectopic bone develops around the elbow: (1) trauma, usually fracture; (2) closed head or spinal cord injury; (3) burn injury to the extremity; and (4) genetic conditions (Table 32–1). Recently, the process has also been reported to occur after adult respiratory distress syndrome[36] and after orthotopic liver transplant.[53]

The post-traumatic elbow can demonstrate several expressions of radiodensity.[9] Ectopic bone may develop within the zone of injury. Mineralization may occur within the three principal soft tissues that surround the elbow: muscle (myositis ossificans), capsule, and ligaments (Fig. 32–1).

Radiographically, ectopic bone is seldom seen before 3 weeks after injury or surgery, but it usually can be detected if one looks for it critically. The soft density on the radiograph can be visualized under a bright light. The extent of ectopic bone formation usually is evident by 12 weeks (Fig. 32–2). Bressler and colleagues[10] studied the maturation process of ectopic bone in 25 patients with computed tomographic scans. Persistent, unossified, low-density soft tissue areas were detected adjacent to mineralized areas up to 16 years after injury. In adults, after the maturation process is completed, the bone usually does not resorb. Resorption may occur in children younger than 16 years.

PATHOLOGY

The histology of ectopic bone reveals that it resembles normal bone. It is similarly mineralized, and the bone matrix–forming cells produce a highly organized bone containing secondary haversian systems as evidence of bone remodeling.

CLINICAL PRESENTATION

Pain and loss of range of motion are the common presenting complaints during the evolution of ectopic bone formation.[55] On physical examination, there may be swelling, erythema, and local warmth to the affected joint. Aggressive physical therapy with passive stretching beyond the pain-free arc of motion only exacerbates the formation of ectopic bone. The presentation can be confused with cellulitis, deep infection, thrombophlebitis, reflex sympathetic dystrophy, and other conditions that cause pain and swelling.

DIAGNOSTIC STUDIES

Several laboratory variables have been studied in an effort to identify high-risk patients. An increased incidence of the human leukocyte antigen (HLA) B18 in a group of patients with central nervous system injury and paraosteoarthropathy has been reported.[31, 39, 44, 50, 67]

Unfortunately, the predictive value of serum alkaline phosphatase determinations has not been consistent and the utility of the test in clinical practice is limited.[2, 28, 43, 51, 55] The test lacks specificity, and, in most cases, the ideal time to initiate prophylactic treatment may have passed.

The technetium bone scan is markedly positive during

• TABLE 32–1 • **Patients at Risk for Developing Ectopic Bone About the Elbow**

I. Trauma Patients
  A. Elbow Trauma
    1. Open elbow dislocations requiring extensive or multiple débridements
    2. Elbow dislocations associated with fractures requiring open reduction with internal fixation
    3. Radial head fractures treated with surgery more than 24 hours after injury
    4. Failed internal fixation about the elbow requiring revision fixation within 3 months
  B. Distal biceps tendon repair
  C. Repeated procedures with an improper exposure in the first 2 weeks
II. Patients with Central Nervous System Injury
  A. Traumatic brain injury
  B. Elbow trauma in patients with traumatic brain injury
III. Burn Patients
  A. Third-degree burns over 20% of total body area
  B. Third-degree burns over the elbow
  C. Long periods of bed confinement
IV. Patients with Genetic Conditions
  A. Fibrodysplasia ossificans progressiva
  B. History of ectopic bone formation

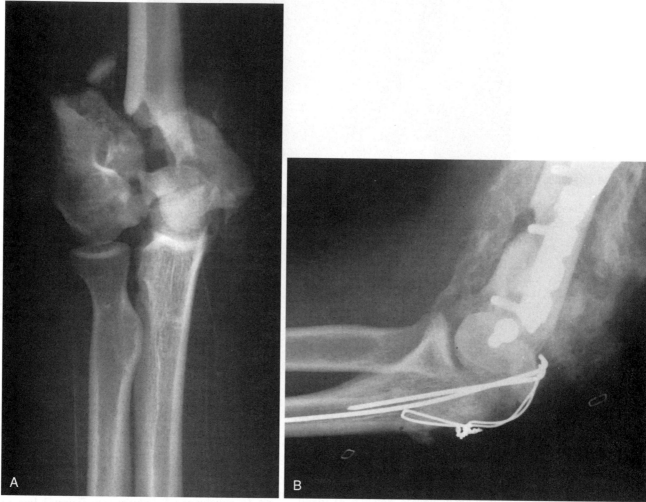

FIGURE 32–4 • Comminuted, compound fracture *(A)*. Three débridements and fixation occurred over a 10-day period. Extensive ectopic bone developed *(B)*.

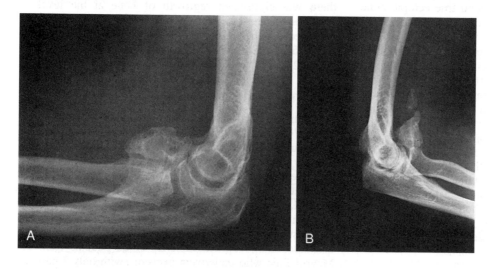

FIGURE 32–5 • *A* and *B*, Radial head fracture with dislocation develops a typical pattern of ectopic ossification after excision.

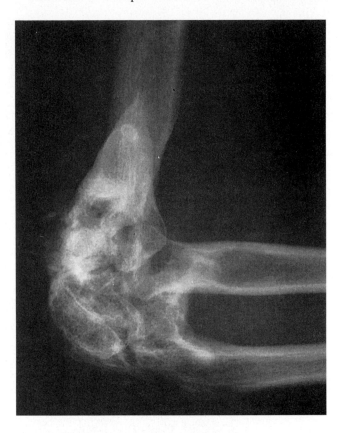

FIGURE 32–6 • Proximal radioulnar synostosis from radioulnar fracture.

be important, with no good or excellent results in patients operated on less than 12 months after injury or more than 3 years after injury. We use the radiographic appearance of discrete margins and mature trabeculation as the basis of when to resect the lesion. Bone scans and serum enzymes are of little value in deciding when to resect the lesion and hence I do not obtain these studies.

The less than ideal results of surgical treatment may be related to several factors,[22] including (1) size and anatomic features of the synostosis, (2) severity of the initial injury, (3) unsuccessful excision of the lesion intraoperatively, (4) postoperative complications requiring reoperation, and (5) the period of postoperative immobilization. Preoperative planning is necessary to choose the correct surgical approach to remove the entire lesion if this is deemed necessary. Computed tomographic scans or tomograms can be used to define the anatomy of the synostosis.

If possible, the entire lesion must be resected, and the radius and ulna in the area of the synostosis must be contoured to allow motion without impingement. The intimate proximity of neurovascular structures may limit this resection. Ideally, a free space of at least 5 mm should be created and maintained throughout the intraoperative arc of motion. We prefer not to interpose Silastic or other foreign material, but we do translocate fat into the defect. Patients can be expected to lose about 50 percent of the intraoperative motion achieved. Accordingly, the surgeon should attempt to achieve at least 120 degrees of combined supination and pronation intraoperatively.

In those cases in which the process is not amenable to excision, we have excised a 5- to 7-mm segment of radius

distal to the synostosis, creating an effective pseudoarthrosis and allowing surprisingly functional forearm rotation (Fig. 32–7).

Ectopic Bone Formation Following Central Nervous System Injury

First described during the First World War,[16] ectopic bone formation may occur after central nervous system (CNS) injury to the brain or spinal cord.[29, 61] Garland and others[29–35] extensively studied the orthopedic problems encountered by patients with both traumatic brain injury and spinal cord injury (see Chapter 63).

TRAUMATIC BRAIN INJURY WITHOUT ELBOW TRAUMA

In a review of 496 patients with traumatic brain injury, Garland and colleagues[32] found an incidence of periarticular bone formation in 100 joints in 57 patients (11 percent). Patients with spastic quadriparesis have the highest incidence of ectopic bone formation. The hip was the most common location, followed by the shoulder, elbow, and knee. Ectopic bone formation developed in 4 percent of the elbows. Anterior bone formation was deep to the biceps and brachialis muscles and anterior to the joint capsule, occasionally involving the entire brachialis muscle (Fig. 32–8). The posterior ectopic bone was beneath the triceps tendon in close association to the posterior capsule. In Garland's series, the ectopic bone was anterior in 6 and posterior in 17, and 8 of the elbows were completely

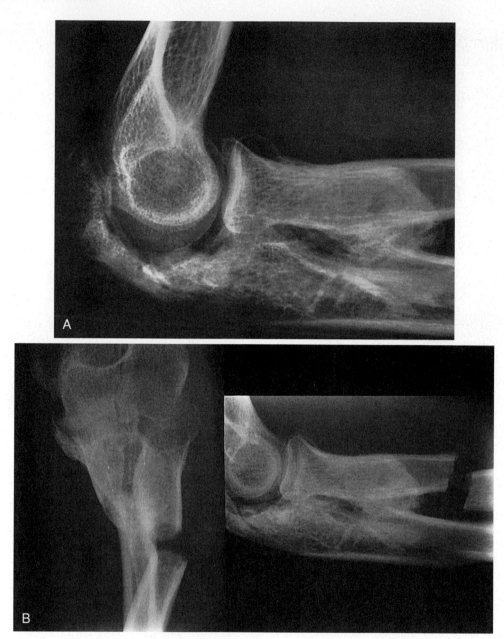

FIGURE 32–7 • Extensive proximal radioulnar synostosis (A) treated by excision of a segment of the radius distal to the synostosis (B).

ankylosed preoperatively. Posterolateral ectopic bone formation is the most common site of occurrence.[30]

A major determinant of potential successful surgical treatment is the residual neurologic deficit. Twenty-three patients underwent resection of ectopic bone about the elbow. In general, resection should be delayed until at least 18 months after CNS injury to allow maximum functional recovery. The results of excision correlate to the neurologic classification.[32] Complications include soft tissue infections and neurologic injury. Patients with severe neurologic deficits probably will not have significant functional improvement after surgery, but restoration of some elbow motion may aid in hygiene. In the severely compromised patient, the ectopic bone should be mature on radiographs and the alkaline phosphatase level should be near normal. Recurrence is closely associated with spasticity.[30]

Ectopic Bone Formation in Burn Patients

Significant ectopic bone formation in burn patients is a rare occurrence. Evans[20, 21] listed the following risk factors: (1) the percentage area, (2) the location of the burn, (3) the length of bed confinement, (4) osteoporosis, (5) superimposed trauma, and (6) genetic predisposition. The elbow, shoulder, and hip are the most commonly involved.[20, 21] In a study of more than 5000 cases at the U.S. Army Institute of Surgical Research, the incidence of ectopic bone formation was only 1.2 percent, with 82.5 percent of those cases involving the elbow. This is similar to the recent report of a 1.2 percent incidence after 1478 burns, of which 93 percent involved the elbow.[57] Although several studies have reported an incidence of ectopic bone formation varying from 2 to 35 percent,[20, 21, 54, 65, 71] the incidence of significant

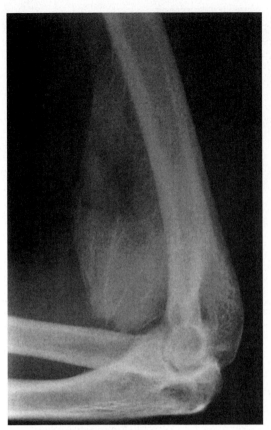

FIGURE 32–8 • The entire brachialis muscle has been replaced in this 30-year-old man after head injury without elbow trauma.

ectopic bone formation at the elbow that requires treatment is probably about 1 percent.[21]

The distribution of the ectopic bone about the elbow in the burn patient is posterior and medial along the medial border of the triceps and anterior in the plane of the brachialis from the anterior surface of the humerus to the coronoid (Fig. 32–9).[21]

Evans[21] and others[19] have noted that prevention of ectopic bone in the burn patient is best accomplished by reducing the period of bed confinement and the period of post-burn hypermetabolic state through the use of early wound excision and grafting. If ectopic bone formation does occur, passive stretching of the joint should be avoided. Active range of motion exercises of the joint within a pain-free arc may continue.[15]

Selection criteria for excision include (1) decreased range of motion sufficient to cause functional limitations, (2) maturation of new bone confirmed on the radiograph, (3) no evidence of acute inflammation, and (4) complete healing of the skin in the area of the ectopic bone. After excision, most patients have functional range of motion arcs and recurrence is uncommon.[15, 39] The most common complication is ulnar nerve irritation.[18]

Technical factors include anterior transposition of the ulnar nerve, excision of the ectopic bone and collateral ligaments if they are ossified, and excision of the radial head when forearm rotation is limited.[20] In my experience, however, radial humeral involvement very rarely occurs. If the anterior aspect of the elbow is significantly scarred by

third-degree burns, excision of the scarred areas with release of the contractures and excision of the ectopic bone is recommended.[17]

Fibrodysplasia Ossificans Progressiva

Genetic conditions may lead to ectopic ossification about the elbow. More than half of patients with this disorder experience ectopic bone formation about the elbow between the third and fourth decades of life. Connor and Evans[13] and others[63] have recommended against surgical treatment. Avoidable factors for the precipitation of ectopic bone in these patients include local trauma, careless venipuncture, intramuscular injections, biopsy of the lumps, and operations to excise heterotopic bone.

GENERAL PRINCIPLES OF TREATMENT

There are two components to treatment of ectopic bone: (1) prophylaxis at the time of initial injury and (2) resection of heterotopic bone with adjuvant measures to prevent its recurrence.

Not all ectopic bone formation about the elbow requires surgical treatment. The goal of surgery is to restore functional motion (see Chapter 5). One must perform a careful preoperative evaluation to ensure that the ectopic bone itself is blocking motion. Tomograms may be necessary to determine whether the joint surfaces are congruous. In traumatic circumstances, if the joint surfaces are not congruous, total elbow arthroplasty or distraction arthroplasty may be necessary. In general, we wait about 9 to 12 months after injury to allow maturation of the ectopic bone. The maturation is judged with plain radiographs. We do not employ laboratory tests or technetium bone scans, as they are of limited value for determining the timing of resection.

The surgical principles are simple and are a matter of routine in orthopedic practice. They include (1) atraumatic handling of the tissues; (2) careful hemostasis; (3) suction drainage of the wound; (4) postoperative compressive dressings; and (5) avoiding the creation and deposit of bone dust in the joint by the use of osteotomes rather than saws, meticulous lavage, and so forth. Careful preoperative planning is crucial to identify areas to be resected and the surgical approach.

Surgical Techniques

In all instances, the basic surgical strategy is to remove the ectopic bone at its narrowest portion, and with the least risk to the articulation. Avoid injury to cartilage by excision of enough bone to initiate some motion and define the joint line. Once some motion is initiated, additional bone is resected as necessary.

SURGICAL APPROACH

In most cases, a posterior skin incision is made. Subcutaneous dissection is performed laterally or medially depending on the location of the bridge.

For the posterolateral resection, the triceps mechanism

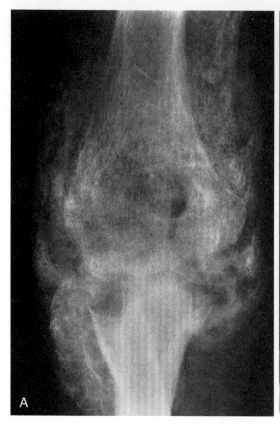
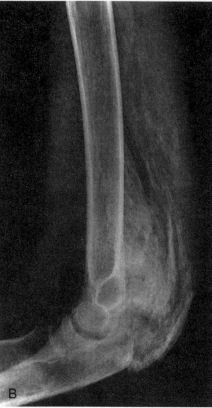

FIGURE 32–9 • A, Third-degree burn associated with extensive ectopic bone but a normal joint. B, Surgical excision reliably restores function.

is retracted medially without disturbing its insertion, and the ectopic bone is exposed subperiosteally. The central bridge of ectopic bone is resected initially. The elbow is then flexed, and attachments of the ectopic bone to the humerus and olecranon are removed. Anterior capsule release is not necessary. Varying amounts of the olecranon are excised to reduce olecranon impingement. The posterior bar is the easiest to resect and in our experience has an excellent prognosis.

Medial Excision. A medial exposure is employed when (1) posterior ectopic bone extends to the medial aspect of the elbow, (2) ulnar nerve transposition is necessary, and (3) the medial collateral ligament requires resection. The ulnar nerve is always identified first and in some cases is completely surrounded by bone. The triceps expansion is exposed and incised distally to the triceps insertion. The ectopic bone is subperiosteally exposed and resected. When the ectopic bone interferes with ulnar nerve function, the nerve is decompressed or transferred anteriorly if necessary.

Anterolateral Approach. If an anterior excision is necessary, the bone is exposed by elevating the origins of the brachioradialis and common extensor tendons. Occasionally an anterior approach is used. The interval between the brachioradialis and brachialis muscles is identified. The radial nerve is identified and retracted laterally. The brachialis muscle fibers are split at their most lateral border, and the muscle is elevated off the ectopic bone. The central bridge of bone is resected, allowing motion of the elbow, which further facilitates resection of the ectopic bone off the humerus and coronoid process.

POSTOPERATIVE MANAGEMENT

If the process involves muscle fibers, the surgical field is treated with 700 cGy radiation. Otherwise, 75 mg indomethacin is prescribed 3 weeks before and 8 weeks after surgery. The elbow is managed with continuous motion and splints as described in Chapters 11 and 12. When motion goals are not met, examination under anesthesia is performed 6 weeks after surgery.

Ulnar Neuropathy in Association With Ectopic Bone Formation

Late ulnar neuropathy may occur as a result of compression in the cubital tunnel from ectopic bone. Sometimes when completely encased in bone, it is further at risk if elbow motion increases while it remains tethered or compressed by the ectopic ossification. Although the brain-injured adult[32, 34, 41, 77] is the most common situation for ulnar neuropathy from ectopic bone, it occurs after burns[76] and trauma as well. In a 5-year period, 2.5 percent of the adult brain-injured population in one study developed late ulnar neuropathy.[41] Fourteen percent had a history of trauma, and 86 percent were found to have idiopathic heterotopic ossification associated with spasticity. Treatment consisted of ulnar nerve transposition anteriorly, with 85 percent of the patients having complete recovery. We completely free the nerve from the ectopic bone for a distance of 3 cm with preservation of function. Simple subcutaneous translocation of the nerve is adequate. If completely surrounded by bone, I usually release the nerve, remove the ectopic bone and replace it in its bed, or translocate the nerve if it is stretched by motion.

Adjuvant Treatment to Prevent Ectopic Bone Formation

There are three main adjuvants to reduce the likelihood of ectopic bone formation after excision: (1) oral nonsteroidal anti-inflammatory agents, (2) oral diphosphonates, and (3) low-dose external beam irradiation.

Several authors have shown that indomethacin is an effective agent[47, 60, 66] that significantly reduces the formation of ectopic bone about the hip. The recommended dosage is 75 mg daily for 6 weeks after surgery.[47, 60, 66] We typically begin the treatment 1 to 2 weeks before the surgery but have no scientific basis for this practice.

Oral diphosphonates have been used,[24, 72] and experimental data have shown this class of drug to delay the mineralization of osteoid.[58] Unfortunately, when these drugs are discontinued, the osteoid may mineralize.[68, 69]

Low-dose external beam irradiation has been shown to be an effective method of preventing ectopic bone formation about the hip after total hip arthroplasty[3, 4, 14, 43] and following acetabular fractures.[6] Recent studies noted effective control of ectopic bone with only 700 cGy in a single dose.[3, 4] External beam irradiation should be delivered to the high-risk patient within 24 hours and no later than 72 hours after surgery. Delay of radiation treatments beyond 72 hours significantly reduces its effectiveness. Potential or theoretical problems of low-dose irradiation include wound healing problems and nonunion. The risk of postirradiation sarcoma is extremely rare. In the past 10 years we have treated more than 100 patients with low-dose irradiation for control of ectopic bone formation about the elbow and hip, and we have never detected delayed wound healing that was attributable to the low-dose irradiation. When necessary, bone graft fracture sites may be shielded.[25] In our experience, there have been no nonunions directly attributable to the low-dose irradiation. There are more than 130 postirradiation sarcomas in the Mayo Clinic files, and none has been caused by the use of low-dose irradiation for the prevention of ectopic bone.[26] We have found no instance of sarcoma to have developed after doses of 3000 cGy or less.

REFERENCES

1. Ackerman, L. V.: Extraosseous localized nonneoplastic bone and cartilage formation (so-called myositis ossificans). J. Bone Joint Surg. 40A:279, 1958.
2. Andersen, P. K., Pedersen, P., Kristensen, S. S., Schmidt, S. A., and Pedersen, N. W.: Serum alkaline phosphatase as an indicator of heterotopic bone formation following total hip arthroplasty. Clin. Orthop. Rel. Res. 234:102, 1988.
3. Ayers, D. C., Evarts, C. M., and Parkinson, J. R.: The prevention of heterotopic ossification in high-risk patients by low-dose radiation after total hip arthroplasty. J. Bone Joint Surg. 68A:1423, 1986.
4. Ayers, D. C., Pellegrini, V. D., and Evarts, C. M.: Prevention of heterotopic ossification in high-risk patients by radiation therapy. Clin. Orthop. Rel. Res. 263:87, 1991.
5. Benjamin, A.: Injuries of the forearm. In Wilson, J. N. (ed.): Watson-Jones Fractures and Joint Injuries, 6th ed., vol. 2. New York, Churchill Livingstone, 1982, p. 650.
6. Bosse, M. J., Poka, A., Reinert, C. M., Ellwanger, F., Slawson, R., and McDevitt, E. R.: Heterotopic ossification as a complication of acetabular fracture. J. Bone Joint Surg. 70A:1231, 1988.
7. Botting, T. D. J.: Posttraumatic radioulnar cross union. J. Trauma 10:16, 1970.
8. Broberg, M. A., and Morrey, B. F.: Results of delayed excision of the radial head after fracture. J. Bone Joint Surg. 68A:669, 1986.
9. Broberg, M. A., and Morrey, B. F.: Results of treatment of fracture-dislocations of the elbow. Clin. Orthop. 216:109, 1987.
10. Bressler, E. L., Marn, C. S., Gore, R. M., and Hendrix, R. W.: Evaluation of ectopic bone by CT. Am. J. Roentgenol. 148:931, 1987.
11. Bunnell, S.: Surgery of the Hand, 2nd ed. Philadelphia, J. B. Lippincott, 1948, p. 591.
12. Buxton, J. D.: Ossification in the ligaments of the elbow joint. J. Bone Joint Surg. 20:709, 1938.
13. Connor, J. M., and Evans, D. A. P.: Fibrodysplasia ossificans progressiva: the clinical features and natural history of 34 patients. J. Bone Joint Surg. 64B:76, 1982.
14. Coventry, M. B., and Scanlon, P. W.: The use of radiation to discourage ectopic bone. J. Bone Joint Surg. 63A:201, 1981.
15. Crawford, C. M., Varghese, G., Mani, M., and Neff, J. R.: Heterotopic ossification: are range-of-motion exercises contraindicated? J. Burn Care Rehabil. 7:323, 1986.
16. Dejerine, A., and Ceiller, M. A.: Paraosteoarthropathies of paraplegic patients by spinal cord lesion. Clin. Orthop. Rel. Res. 263:3, 1991.
17. Dias, D. A.: Heterotopic para-articular ossification of the elbow with soft tissue contracture in burns. Burns 9:128, 1983.
18. Djurickovic, S., Meek, R. N., Snelling, C. F., Broekhuyse, H. M., Blachut, P. A., O'Brien, P. J., and Boyle, J. C.: Range of motion and complications after post burn heterotopic bone excision about the elbow. J. Trauma 41:825, 1996.
19. Elledge, E. S., Smith, A. A., McManus, W. F., and Pruitt, B. A.: Heterotopic bone formation in burned patients. J. Trauma 28:684, 1988.
20. Evans, E. B.: Orthopaedic measures in the treatment of severe burns. J. Bone Joint Surg. 48A:643, 1966.
21. Evans, E. B.: Heterotopic bone formation in thermal burns. Clin. Orthop. Rel. Res. 263:94, 1991.
22. Failla, J. M., Amadio, P. C., and Morrey, B. F.: Posttraumatic proximal radioulnar synostosis: Results of surgical treatment. J. Bone Joint Surg. 71A:1206, 1989.
23. Fielding, J. W.: Radioulnar crossed union following displacement of the proximal radial epiphysis: A case report. J. Bone Joint Surg. 46A:1277, 1964.
24. Finerman, G. A. M., Krengel, W. F., Lowell, J. D.: Role of diphosphonate (EHDP) in the prevention of heterotopic ossification after total hip arthroplasty: A preliminary report. In The Hip: Proceedings of the Fifth Open Scientific Meeting of the Hip Society. St. Louis, C. V. Mosby, 1977, p. 222.
25. Frassica, F. J., and Coventry, M. B.: Ectopic bone following total hip arthroplasty. In Morrey, B. (ed.): Joint Replacement Arthroplasty. New York, Churchill Livingstone, 1991, p. 867.
26. Frassica, F. J., Sim, F. H., Frassica, D. A., and Wold, L. E.: Survival and management considerations in postradiation osteosarcoma and Paget's osteosarcoma. Clin. Orthop. Rel. Res. 263:200, 1991.
27. Freed, J. H., Hahn, H., Meneter, R., and Dillon, T.: The use of the three phase bone scan in the early diagnosis of heterotopic ossification (HO) and in the evaluation of didronel therapy. Paraplegia 20:208, 1982.
28. Furman, R., Nicholas, J. J., and Jovoff, L.: Elevation of the serum alkaline phosphatase coincident with ectopic bone formation in paraplegic patients. J. Bone Joint Surg. 52A:1131, 1970.
29. Garland, D. E.: A clinical perspective on common forms of acquired heterotopic ossification. Clin. Orthop. Rel. Res. 263:13, 1991.
30. Garland, D. E.: Surgical approaches for resection of heterotopic ossification in traumatic brain-injured adults. Clin. Orthop. Rel. Res. 263:59, 1991.
31. Garland, D. E., Alday, B., and Venos, K. G.: Heterotopic ossification and HLA antigens. Arch. Phys. Med. Rehabil. 65:531, 1984.
32. Garland, D. E., Blum, C., and Waters, R. L.: Periarticular heterotopic ossification in head injured adults: Incidence and location. J. Bone Joint Surg. 62A:1143, 1980.
33. Garland, D. E., Hanscom, D. A., Keenan, M. A., Smith, C., and Moore, T.: Resection of heterotopic ossification in the adult with head trauma. J. Bone Joint Surg. 67A:1261, 1985.

34. Garland, D. E., and O'Halloren, R. M.: Fractures and dislocations about the elbow in the head injured adult. Clin. Orthop. Rel. Res. **168**:38, 1982.

35. Garland, D. E., and Orwin, J. F.: Resection of heterotopic ossification in patients with spinal cord injuries. Clin. Orthop. Rel. Res. **242**:169, 1989.

36. Goodman, T. A., Merkel, P. A., Perlmutter, G., Doyle, M. K., Krange, S. M., and Polisson, R. P.: Heterotopic ossification in the setting of neuromuscular blockade. Arthritis Rheum. **40**:1619, 1997.

37. Ilahi, O. A., Strausser, D. W., and Gabel, G. T.: Post-traumatic heterotopic ossification about the elbow. Orthopedics **21**:265, 1998.

38. Hoffer, M. M., Brody, G., and Ferlic, F.: Excision of heterotopic ossification about the elbows in patients with thermal injury. J. Trauma **18**:667, 1978.

39. Hunter, T., Dubo, H. I. C., Hildahl, C. R., Smith, N. J., and Schroeder, M. L.: Histocompatibility antigens in patients with spinal cord injury or cerebral damage complicated by heterotopic ossifications. Rheum. Rehabil. **19**:97, 1980.

40. Josefsson, P. O., Johnell, O., and Gentz, C. F.: Long-term sequelae of simple dislocation of the elbow. J. Bone Joint Surg. **66A**:927, 1984.

41. Keenan, M. A., Kauffman, D. L., Garland, D. E., and Smith, C.: Late ulnar neuropathy in the brain-injured adult. J. Hand Surg. **13A**:120, 1988.

42. King, B. B.: Resection of the radial head and neck: An end result of thirteen cases. J. Bone Joint Surg. **21**:839, 1939.

43. Klein, L., Van Den Noort, S., and Dejak, J. J.: Sequential studies of urinary hydroxyproline and serum alkaline phosphatase in acute paraplegia. Med. Serv. J. Can. **22**:524, 1966.

44. Larson, J. M., Michalski, J. P., Collacott, E. A., Eltorai, D., McCombs, C. C., and Madorsky, J. B.: Increased prevalence of HLAB27 in patients with ectopic ossification following traumatic spinal cord injury. Rheum. Rehabil. **20**:193, 1981.

45. Linscheid, R. L., and Wheeler, D. K.: Elbow dislocations. J.A.M.A. **194**:1171, 1965.

46. Mason, M. L.: Some observations on fractures of the head of the radius with a review of 100 cases. Br. J. Surg. **42**:123, 1954.

47. McLaren, A. C.: Prophylaxis with indomethacin for heterotopic bone after open reduction of fractures of the acetabulum. J. Bone Joint Surg. **72A**:245, 1990.

48. McLaughlin, H. L.: Some fractures with a time limit. Surg. Clin. North Am. **35**:553, 1955.

49. Mikic, Z. D., and Vukadinovic, S. M.: Late results in fractures of the radial head treated by excision. Clin. Orthop. Rel. Res. **181**:220, 1983.

50. Minaire, P., Betuel, H., Girard, R., and Pilonchery, G.: Neurologic injuries, paraosteoarthropathies, and human leukocyte antigens. Arch. Phys. Med. Rehabil. **61**:214, 1980.

51. Mollan, R. A. B.: Serum alkaline phosphatase in heterotopic para-articular ossification after total hip replacement. J. Bone Joint Surg. **61B**:423, 1979.

52. Morrey, B. F., Askew, L. J., An, K. N., and Dobyns, J. H.: Rupture of the distal tendon of the biceps brachii: A biomechanical study. J. Bone Joint Surg. **67A**:418, 1985.

53. Munin, M. C., Balu, G., and Sotereanos, D. G.: Elbow complications after organ transplantation. Case reports. Am. J. Phys. Med. Rehab. **74**:672, 1995.

54. Munster, A. M., Bruck, H. M., Johns, L. A., von Prince, K., Kikman, E. M., and Remig, R. L.: Heterotopic calcification following burns: A prospective study. J. Trauma **12**:1071, 1973.

55. Orzel, J. A., and Rudd, T. G.: Heterotopic bone formation: Clinical, laboratory, and imaging correlation. J. Nucl. Med. **26**:125, 1985.

56. Newman, J. H.: Displaced radial neck fractures in children. Injury **9**:114, 1977.

57. Peterson, S. L., Mani, M. M., Crawford, C. M., Neff, J. R., and Hiebert, J. M.: Post burn heterotopic ossification: insights for management decision making. J. Trauma **29**:365, 1989.

58. Plasmans, C. M. T., Kuypers, E. I. M., and Sloof, T. J. J. H.: The effect of ethane-1-hydroxy-1, l diphosphonic acid (EHDP) on matrix-induced ectopic bone formation. Clin. Orthop. Rel. Res. **132**:233, 1978.

59. Razemon, J. P., Decoulx, J., and Leclair, H. P.: Les synostoses radiocubitales posttraumatiques de l'adulte. Acta Orthop. Belgica **31**:5, 1965.

60. Ritter, M. A., and Sieber, J. M.: Prophylactic indomethacin for the prevention of heterotopic bone formation following total hip arthroplasty. Clin. Orthop. Rel. Res. **196**:217, 1985.

61. Roberts, P. H.: Heterotopic ossification complicating paralysis of intracranial origin. J. Bone Joint Surg. **50B**:70, 1968.

62. Roberts, P. H.: Dislocation of the elbow. Br. J. Surg. **56**:806, 1969.

63. Rogers, J. G., and Geho, W. B.: Fibrodysplasia ossificans progressiva: a survey of forty-two cases. J. Bone Joint Surg. **61A**:909, 1979.

64. Russell, T. A.: Malunited fractures. *In* Crenshaw, A. H. (ed.): Campbell's Operative Orthopaedics, 7th ed., vol. 3. St. Louis, C. V. Mosby, 1987, p. 2041.

65. Schiele, H. P., Hubbard, R. B., and Bruck, H. M.: Radiographic changes in burns of the upper extremity. Radiology **104**:13, 1972.

66. Schmidt, S. A., Kjaersgaard-Andersen, P., Pedersen, N. W., Kristensen, S. S., Pedersen, P., and Neilson, J. B.: The use of indomethacin to prevent the formation of heterotopic bone after total hip arthroplasty. J. Bone Joint Surg. **70A**:834, 1988.

67. Seignalet, J., Moulin, M., and Pelissier, J.: HLA and neurogenic paraosteoarthropathies. Tissue Antigens **21**:268, 1983.

68. Stover, S. L., Niemann, K. M., and Miller, J. M.: Disodium etidronate in the prevention of postoperative recurrence of heterotopic ossification in spinal cord injury patients. J. Bone Joint Surg. **58A**:683, 1976.

69. Stover, S. L., Niemann, K. M., and Tullos, J. R.: Experience with surgical resection of heterotopic bone in spinal cord injury patients. Clin. Orthop Rel. Res. **263**:71, 1991.

70. Sutro, C. J.: Regrowth of bone at the proximal end of the radius following resection in this region. J. Bone Joint Surg. **17**:867, 1935.

71. Tepperman, P. S., Hilbert, L., Peters, W. J., and Pritzker, K. P. H.: Heterotopic ossification in burns. J. Burn Care Rehabil. **5**:283, 1984.

72. Thomas, B. J., and Amstutz, H. C.: Results of the administration of diphosphonate for the prevention of heterotopic ossification after total hip arthroplasty. J. Bone Joint Surg. **67A**:400, 1985.

73. Thompson, H. C., and Garcia, A.: Myositis ossificans: Aftermath of elbow injuries. Clin. Orthop. Rel. Res. **50**:130, 1967.

74. Tooms, R. E.: Complications of treatment of injuries to the forearm. *In* Epps, C. H. (ed.): Complications in Orthopaedic Surgery, 2nd ed., vol. 1. Philadelphia, J. B. Lippincott, 1986, p. 325.

75. Vince, K. G., and Miller, J. E.: Cross-union complicating fracture of the forearm. Part 1. Adults. J. Bone Joint Surg. **69A**:640, 1987.

76. Vorenkamp, S. E., and Nelson, T. L.: Ulnar nerve entrapment due to heterotopic bone formation after a severe burn. J. Hand Surg. **12A**:378, 1987.

77. Wainapel, S. F., Rao, P. U., and Schepsis, A. A.: Ulnar nerve compression by heterotopic ossification in a head-injured patient. Arch. Phys. Med. Rehabil. **66**:512, 1985.

• CHAPTER 33 •

Extrinsic Contracture: "The Column Procedure," Lateral and Medial Capsular Releases

• PIERRE MANSAT, BERNARD F. MORREY, and ROBERT N. HOTCHKISS

Soft-Tissue Considerations

Of the numerous potential causes for elbow stiffness, the causes and pathophysiologic mechanisms dictate treatment and affect prognosis. Extrinsic contracture typically involves only the soft tissues around the elbow, sparing the joint space (Fig. 33–1).[36] Post-traumatic stiffness is one of the most frequent causes of this kind of contracture[7]; however, it can also occur in association with other causes, such as congenital or developmental disease, osteoarthritis or inflammatory arthritis, burns, and head injury. Intrinsic contracture is associated with joint articular involvement and is not discussed here (see Chapter 34).

Several treatment options have been proposed for treatment of elbow contracture. Conservative treatment sometimes gives good results if the contracture is of short duration[2, 3, 8, 11, 18, 31, 38]; however, its efficacy is unpredictable. With failure of nonoperative treatment, surgical release may be indicated. Some reports of this being done through an arthroscopic procedure recently appeared.[23, 28, 41, 43, 45, 49] Most employ an open procedure, and several have been described.*

ETIOLOGY AND INCIDENCE

An extrinsic contracture usually involves the periarticular soft tissue without involving the articulating surface. Contracture may involve the capsulo-ligamentous structures or muscle tissue. Ectopic ossification is also considered an extrinsic condition. Bone may form a bridge across the joint or form in the capsule or in the muscle crossing the joint. Trauma is the major cause of extrinsic stiffness, especially elbow dislocation, with or without fracture.[24, 33] The brachialis muscle that crosses the anterior capsule[29] tears with dislocation, developing scar tissue or ectopic bone when healing,[48] often associated with contracture of the capsule.[54] Pain, swelling, limited motion, and contracture after this type of elbow trauma then leads to the irreversible changes that constitute extra-articular ankylosis. Collateral injuries can contribute to elbow ankylosis from permanent contracture.[5, 19, 22] In trauma, length of immobilization has also been recognized as a major contributor to postinjury contracture. The precise incidence of elbow stiffness after trauma is difficult to identify and is as much a function of the severity of injury as of the initial treatment. In adults, nontraumatic elbow contractures are usually caused by a primary inflammatory process. With osteoarthritis, a mild inflammatory synovitis occurs with periarticular fibrosis and osteophytic new bone formation.[42] The articular surface of the joint is intact, but osteophytes are present at the tip of the olecranon and at the tip of the coronoid process. Hemophilia,[9] juvenile rheumatoid arthritis, acute or chronic septic arthritis, and periarticular new bone formation after head injury[14, 30, 34] all can produce ankylosis of the elbow, but often involve the joint space. Congenital stiffness is rare and is often associated with bone malformation or soft tissue dysplasia.[7, 10]

PRESENTATION AND CLASSIFICATION

Post-traumatic contracture of the elbow usually affects young, active patients around 40 years of age, who need the use of the elbow joint. Although such contractures are often related to intrinsic lesions, they can be associated with extrinsic stiffness. Osteoarthritis, on the other hand, involves patients in their mid-50s, predominantly men. At the beginning, the lesions are periarticular and can be considered an extrinsic condition.

Generally, the patient initially notices loss of full extension but no limitation of activity. The first complaint is pain in terminal extension. Concurrent with this is the recognition that midarc motion typically is not painful, a finding that confirms the extrinsic character of the stiffness. Occasionally, full flexion also produces pain. Flexion contracture develops progressively.

In addition to classifying elbow contracture according to extrinsic and intrinsic lesions, age of the patient, severity of the stiffness, and distribution of the contracture are also important for evaluating what might be expected from the surgery. Thus, the stiffness may be graded as very severe, severe, moderate, or minimal, depending on data on the amount of residual arc of flexion.[12, 40] The stiffness is considered *very severe* when the total arc is 30 degrees or

---

*See references 1, 4, 6, 12, 15, 17, 20, 21, 25–27, 32, 35, 44, 46, 47, 50–53, 55, 56.

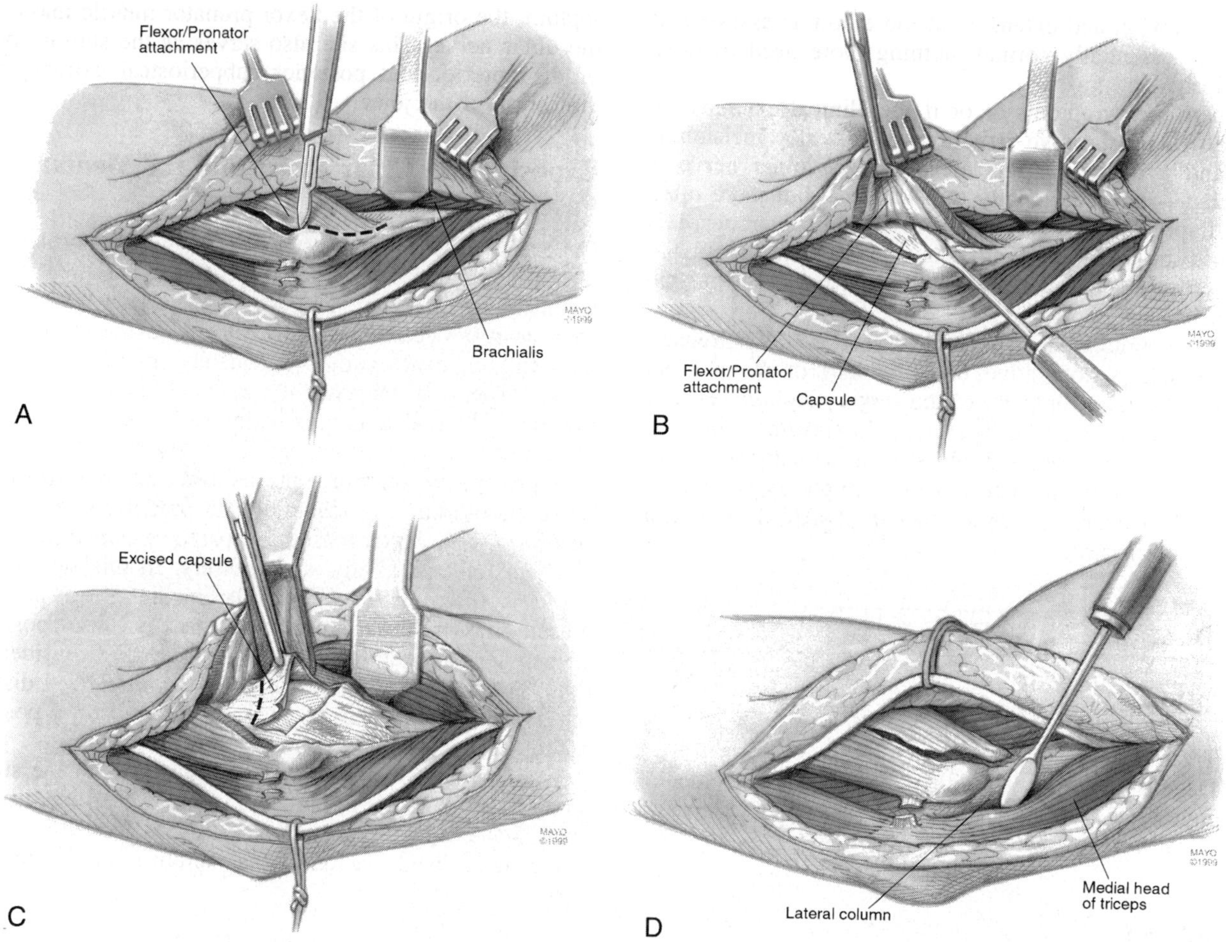

FIGURE 33–5 • *A*, After the ulnar nerve has been identified and protected and the septum excised, the flexor-pronator muscle mass is divided, leaving a cuff for reattachment. *B*, After the fibers of the brachialis are swept from the anterior capsule, a special elbow or Bennett retractor is placed across the joint and the interval between the capsule and muscle is developed further. Once the capsule has been adequately exposed, it is excised as far laterally as can be identified. *C*, The last fibers laterally may be incised if excision cannot be safely done. *D*, If contracture persists posteriorly, the medial aspect of the triceps is elevated, and the posterior capsule is identified and excised, along with any ectopic bone or spur formation.

muscle is encountered from the underside. This muscle should be kept anterior and elevated from the capsule and anterior surface of the distal humerus. Finding this plane requires careful attention. The dissection of the capsule from the brachialis muscle proceeds both laterally and distally.

At this point, it is helpful to feel for the coronoid process by gently flexing and extending the elbow. The first few times that this approach is used, the coronoid seems quite deep and far distal. A deep, narrow retractor is often helpful to allow the operator to see down to the level of the coronoid.

The extreme anteromedial corner of the exposure deserves special comment. In a contracture release, the anteromedial portion often requires release. To see this area, a small, narrow retractor can be inserted to retract the medial collateral ligament, pulling it medially and posteriorly. This affords visualization of the medial capsule and protection of the anterior medial collateral ligament.

The anterior capsule should be excised (see Fig. 33–5C) to the extent that that is practical and safe. When first performing this procedure, it is helpful first to incise the capsule from the medial to the lateral aspect along the

anterior surface of the joint. Once this edge of the capsule is incised, it can be lifted and excised as far distally as is safe. From this vantage, and after capsule excision, the radial head and capitellum can be visualized and freed of scar, as needed.

In cases of primary osteoarthritis of the elbow, removing the large spur from the coronoid is crucial. Using the Cobb elevator, the brachialis muscle can be elevated anteriorly for 2 cm from the coronoid process. With the elevator held in position, protecting the brachialis but anterior to the coronoid, the large osteophyte can be removed with an osteotome. The brachialis insertion is well distal to the tip of the coronoid.

Exposing and Excising the Posterior Capsule and Bone Spurs

The posterior capsule of the joint is exposed likewise to the anterior surface. The supracondylar ridge is again identified (see Fig. 33–5D). Using the Cobb elevator, the triceps is elevated from the posterior distal surface of the humerus. The exposure should extend far enough proximal to permit use of a Bennett retractor.

The posterior capsule can be separated from the triceps as the elevator sweeps from proximal to distal. The posterior medial joint line should also be identified, as it is often involved by osteophytes or heterotopic bone. In contracture release, the posterior capsule and posteromedial ligaments should be excised. The medial joint line up to the anterior medial ligament should also be exposed and the capsule excised. This area is the floor of the cubital tunnel.

In contracture release and in primary osteoarthritis, the tip of the olecranon usually must be excised to achieve full extension. The posteromedial joint line is easily visualized, but the posterolateral side must also be carefully palpated to ensure clearance.

Ulnar Nerve Transposition

After being reattached to the medial supracondylar region, the ulnar nerve should be transposed and secured with a capacious fascial sling to prevent posterior subluxation. The sling can be fashioned by elevating two overlapping rectangular flaps of fascia or by using a medially based flap attached to the underlying subcutaneous tissue. Once this maneuver is completed, the nerve must not be compressed or kinked. The joint should be flexed and extended to ensure that the nerve is free to move.

CLOSURE

Flexor-Pronator Muscle Origin

The flexor-pronator mass should be reattached to the supracondylar ridge with nonabsorbable braided 1-0 or 0 suture. If enough fibrous tissue was left behind, no holes need be drilled in bone. Otherwise, drill holes in the edge of the supracondylar ridge can be made to secure the flexor-pronator mass.

AFTERCARE

If the neurologic examination findings in the recovery room are normal, a brachial plexus block is established and maintained with a continuous pump through a percutaneous catheter.[16] The arm is elevated as much as possible, and mechanical continuous passive motion exercise is begun the day of surgery and adjusted to provide as much motion as pain or the machine itself allows (see Chapter 11). After 2 days the plexus block is discontinued, and, at day 3, the continuous passive motion machine is stopped.

Physical therapy is not used, but a detailed program of splint therapy is prescribed. Adjustable splints are prescribed,[38] depending on the motion before and after the procedure (see Chapter 12). The splints include a hyperextension or a hyperflexion brace, or both (Fig. 33–6). A detailed discussion regarding heat, ice, and anti-inflammatory medication, along with a visual schedule for bracing, is provided (Fig. 33–7). During the first 3 months, the patient sleeps with the splint adjusted to maximize flexion or extension, whichever is more needed, and yet not to be so uncomfortable as to prevent sleeping for at least 6 hours. On rising in the morning, the patient moves the elbow

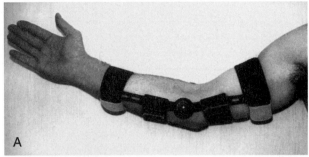

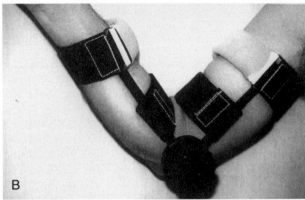

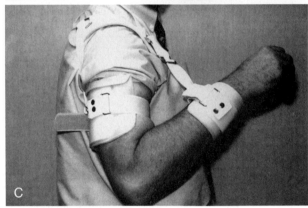

FIGURE 33–6 • *A* and *B*, A reversible flexion/extension splint is used to improve loss of extension and flexion less than 100 degrees. *C*, When flexion exceeds 100 degrees, a hyperflexion splint with a shoulder harness and adjustable Velcro strap is used.

actively in a tub of hot water for 15 minutes and then applies the other splint to hold the elbow at the opposite extreme of motion during the daytime. Between 8:00 in the morning and 12:00 noon, noon and 6:00 in the evening, and 6:00 in the evening and 12:00 midnight, the splint is removed for 1 hour and the patient is encouraged to move the elbow frequently through a full range of active motion. At bedtime, if the elbow is sore from the activity, ice is applied for 10 to 15 minutes. If the elbow is stiff but not sore, heat is applied for the same period. Because the principal objective is to gain motion but to avoid pain, swelling, and inflammation, routine use of an anti-inflammatory medication is prescribed. Therapy with splints is continued for about 3 months, during which time the patient is seen at 2- to 4- week intervals, if possible. Since often this is not feasible, the patient is asked to make tracings of the upper limb with the elbow in maximum

Flexion/Extension Splint Program

Rise	Flexion* Extension		Out#	Flexion* Extension	Out#	Flexion* Extension	Out#	Flexion* Extension	Rise
	8 AM	Noon	___ Hours	1 PM	___ Hours	6 PM	___ Hours	10 PM Sleep	

* Flexion/Extension sequence circled
\# Hours out of aid

FIGURE 33–7 • A printed prescription of the splint use program is provided to patients undergoing splint therapy.

flexion and maximum extension and to send them in for review. The angles so formed are measured with a goniometer to document the patient's progress. After 4 weeks, an arc of about 80 degrees of motion is obtained, and the amount of time that each splint is worn is gradually decreased. Splinting at night is continued for as long as 6 months if flexion contracture tends to recur when the splint is not used. Patients are advised that it may take a year to realize full correction.

RESULTS

Recent reports on the results of surgical arthrolysis reveal an absolute gain in the flexion-extension arc between 30 and 60 degrees.[1, 12, 20, 27, 35–37, 51] A functional arc of motion between 30 and 130 degrees is obtained in more than 50 percent of cases, and some improvement in motion in more than 90 percent of the cases has been reported in the literature.[1, 12, 20, 27, 35–37, 51] An anterior exposure popularized by Urbaniak produced good results for extrinsic stiffness, but patients with intrinsic stiffness did less well and were not considered ideal candidates for arthrolysis.[51] In Europe, a combined lateral and medial approach has been used for many years, and gains in flexion arc have averaged between 40 and 72 degrees (in approximately 400 procedures).[1, 12, 35] Results obtained with a lateral approach in seven patients with primarily extrinsic contractures were reported by Husband and Hastings.[20] Range of motion for extension contractures improved from 45 to 12 degrees and for flexion contractures from 116 to 129 degrees. The complication rate was low. A recent Scandinavian study reported that, after 5 years, range of motion was acceptable in 11 of the 13 cases.[53] Using the same approach, Kessler observed improvement in 13 of 14 elbows.[27] Schindler employed a lateral approach in 30 patients and obtained a mean improvement of flexion of 35 degrees, and 30 percent have a normal range of motion.[46]

The Mayo Clinic experience was recently reported by Mansat and coworkers. From 1989 through 1994, 38 elbows were operated on principally for extrinsic stiffness using this limited lateral approach called the column procedure.[32] Trauma was the cause of the contracture in 20 patients (53%). Primary osteoarthritis was responsible for the stiffness in seven patients, heterotopic ossification around the elbow secondary to head trauma or coma in five, a burn in three, congenital stiffness in two, and stiff-

ness due to excessive immobilization after distal biceps repair in one. The mean preoperative arc of total motion was 49 degrees (range 52 to 101 degrees). At an average of 42 months of follow-up, the mean arc of total motion was 92 degrees (range 28 to 120 degrees). The total gain in flexion and extension was 43 degrees, and 33 of 38 patients (87 percent) enjoyed greater range of motion (Fig. 33–8). Improvement was greater in those with severe or very severe stiffness and with combined flexion-extension contractures. Extrinsic stiffness had better results on improvement of motion.

Nerve Palsies

The ulnar nerve is particularly vulnerable. Care must be taken to mobilize and protect the nerve during contracture release and when hinged fixation is used. Even with these precautions, we have found that about 10 percent of patients have dysfunction of the nerve after release. Most of these problems resolve over a period of days or weeks. The radial nerve is also vulnerable, especially if excessive retraction is applied through the lateral approach. The other point of vulnerability is distal at the level of the posterior interosseous nerve.

COMPLICATIONS

In our study,[32] complications occurred in 4 of 38 elbows (10 percent): two cases of intra-articular bleeding, one

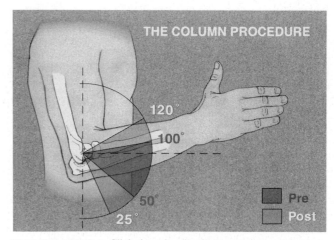

FIGURE 33–8 • Clinical results after 38 procedures performed at the Mayo Clinic.

of which impaired the final outcome; and two transient paresthesias of the ulnar nerve, both of which resolved spontaneously. The typical complication is loss of motion after surgery. Loss of the flexion arc after a period of improvement was seen in 10 patients (26 percent). Four patients ultimately lost the benefits of the procedure and, on average, had 25 degrees' less motion than before surgery.

REFERENCES

1. Allieu, Y.: Raideurs et arthrolyses du coude. Rev. Chir. Orthop. **75** (Suppl. I): 156–166, 1989.
2. Balay, B., Setiey, L., and Vidalain, J. P.: Les raideurs du coude. Traitement orthopédique et chirurgical. Acta Orthop. Belg. **41**:414–425, 1975.
3. Bonutti, P. M., Windau, J. E., Ables, B. A., and Miller, B. G.: Static progressive, stretch to reestablish elbow range of motion. Clin. Orthop. **303**:128–134, 1994.
4. Breen, T. F., Gelberman, R. H., and Ackerman, G. N.: Elbow flexion contractures: treatment by anterior release and continuous passive motion. J. Hand Surg. **13B**:286–287, 1988.
5. Buxton, J. D.: Ossification in the ligaments of the elbow. J. Bone Joint Surg. **20**:709, 1938.
6. Cauchoix, J., and Deburge, A.: L'Arthrolyse du coude dans les raideurs post traumatiques. Acta Orthop. Belg. **41**:385–392, 1975.
7. Cooney, W. P. III: Contractures of the elbow. In Morrey, B. F. (ed.): The Elbow and Its Disorders. 2nd ed. Philadelphia, W.B. Saunders, 1993, pp. 464–475.
8. Dickson, R. A.: Reversed dynamic slings. A new concept in the treatment of posttraumatic elbow flexion contractures. Injury **8**:35–38, 1976.
9. Dietrich, S. L.: Rehabilitation and nonsurgical management of musculoskeletal problems in the hemophilic patients. Ann. N.Y. Acad. Sci. **240**:328, 1975.
10. Dobyns, J. H., and Amadio, P. C.: Congenital abnormalities of the elbow. In Morrey, B. F. (ed.): The Elbow and Its Disorders, 2nd ed. Philadelphia, W.B. Saunders, 1993, pp. 189–205.
11. Duke, J. B., Tessler, R. H., and Dell, P. C.: Manipulation of the stiff elbow with patient under anesthesia. J. Hand Surg. **16A**:19–24, 1991.
12. Esteve, P., Valentin, P., Deburge, A., and Kerboull, M.: Raideurs et ankyloses post-traumatiques du coude. Rev. Chir. Orthop. **57** (Suppl. I): 25–86, 1971.
13. Figgie, M. P., Inglis, A. E., and Mow, C. S.: Total elbow arthroplasty for complete ankylosis of the elbow. J. Bone Joint Surg. **71A**:513–520, 1989.
14. Garland, D. E., and O'Hollarin, R. M.: Fractures and dislocations about the elbow in the head injury adult. Clin. Orthop. **168**:38, 1982.
15. Gates, H. S., Sullivan, R. N., and Urbaniak, J. R.: Anterior capsulotomy and continuous passive motion in the treatment of post-traumatic flexion contracture of the elbow. J. Bone Joint Surg. **74A**:1229–1234, 1992.
16. Gaumann, D. M., Lennon, R. L., and Wedel, D. J.: Continuous axillary block for postoperative pain management. Reg. Anesth. **13**:77–81, 1988.
17. Glynn, J. J., and Niebauer, J. J.: Flexion and extension contracture of the elbow. Surgical management. Clin. Orthop. **117**:289–291, 1976.
18. Green, D. P., and McCoy, H.: Turnbuckle orthotic correction of elbow-flexion contractures after acute injuries. J. Bone Joint Surg. **61A**:1092–1095, 1979.
19. Gutierrez, L. S.: A contribution to the study of the limiting factors of elbow extension. Acta Anat. **56**:146, 1964.
20. Husband, J. B., and Hastings, H.: The lateral approach for operative release of post-traumatic contracture of the elbow. J. Bone Joint Surg. **72A**:1353–1358, 1990.
21. Itoh, Y., Saegusa, K., Ishiguro, T., Horiuchi, Y., Sasaki, T., and Uchinishi, K.: Operation for the stiff elbow. Int. Orthop. **13**:263–268, 1989.
22. Johanson, O.: Capsular and ligament injuries of the elbow joint: clinical and arthrographic study. Acta Chir. Scand. Suppl. **287**:124, 1962.
23. Jones, G. S., and Savoie F. H. III: Arthroscopic capsular release of flexion contractures (arthrofibrosis) of the elbow. Arthroscopy **9**:277–283, 1993.
24. Josefsson, P. O., Johnell, O., and Gentz, C. F.: Long-term sequelae of simple dislocation of the elbow. J. Bone Joint Surg. **66A**:927, 1984.
25. Judet, J., and Judet, H.: Arthrolyse du coude. Acta Orthop. Belg. **41**:412–413, 1975.
26. Kerboull, M.: Le traitement des raideurs du coude de l'adulte. Acta Orthop. Belg. **41**:438–446, 1975.
27. Kessler, I.: Arthrolysis of the elbow. In Kashiwagi D (ed.): Elbow Joint, Proceedings of the International Seminar, Kobe, Japan. International Congress, Series 678. Amsterdam, Excerpta Medica, 1985, pp. 77–80.
28. Kim, S. J., Kim, H. K., and Lee, J. W.: Arthroscopy for limitation of motion of the elbow. Arthroscopy **11**:680–683, 1995.
29. Loomis, J. K.: Reduction and after-treatment of posterior dislocation of the elbow: with special attention to the brachialis muscle and myositis ossificans. Am. J. Surg. **63**:56, 1944.
30. Lusskin, R., Grynbaum, B. B., and Dhir, R. S.: Rehabilitation surgery in adult spastic hemiplegia. Clin. Orthop. **63**:132, 1969.
31. Mac kay-Lyons, M.: Low-load, prolonged stretch in treatment of elbow flexion contractures secondary to head trauma: a case report. Phys. Ther. **69**:292–296, 1989.
32. Mansat, P., and Morrey, B. F.: The "column procedure": a limited surgical approach for the treatment of stiff elbows. J. Bone Joint Surg. **80A**:1603–1615, 1998.
33. Mehlhoff, T. L., Noble, P. C., Bennett, J. B., and Tullos, H. S.: Simple dislocation of the elbow in the adult. J. Bone Joint Surg. **70A**:244, 1988.
34. Mendelson, L., Grosswassner, Z., Najenson, T., Sandbank, U., and Solzi, P.: Periarticular new bone formation in patients suffering from severe head injuries. Scand. J. Rehab. Med. **7**:141, 1975–1976.
35. Merle D'Aubigne, R., and Kerboul, M.: Les opérations mobilisatrices des raideurs et ankylose du coude. Rev. Chir. Orthop. **52**:427–448, 1966.
36. Morrey, B. F.: Post-traumatic contracture of the elbow. Operative treatment, including distraction arthroplasty. J. Bone Joint Surg. **72A**:601–618, 1990.
37. Morrey, B. F.: Surgical takedown of the ankylosed elbow. Orthop. Trans. **12**:734, 1988.
38. Morrey, B. F.: The use of splints for the stiff elbows. Perspect. Orthop. Surg. **1**:141–144, 1990.
39. Morrey, B. F., Adams, R. A., and Bryan, R. S.: Total replacement for post-traumatic arthritis of the elbow. J. Bone Joint Surg. **73B**:607–612, 1991.
40. Morrey, B. F., An, K. N., and Chao, E. Y. S.: Functional evaluation of the elbow. In Morrey, B. F. (ed.): The Elbow and Its Disorders, 2nd ed. Philadelphia, W. B. Saunders, 1993, pp. 86–97.
41. Nowicki, K. D., and Shall, L. M.: Arthroscopic release of a posttraumatic flexion contracture in the elbow: a case report and review of the literature. Arthroscopy **8**:544–547, 1992.
42. Oh, I., Smith, J. A., Spencer, G. E. Jr., Frankel, V. H., and Mack, R. P.: Fibrous contracture of muscles following intramuscular injections in adults. Clin. Orthop. **127**:214, 1977.
43. Phillips, B. B., and Strasburger, G.: Arthroscopic treatment of Arthrofibrosis of the elbow joint. Arthroscopy **14**:38–44, 1998.
44. Richards, R. R., Beaton, D., and Bechard, M.: Restoration of elbow motion by anterior capsular release of post-traumatic flexion contractures. J. Bone Joint Surg. **73B** (Suppl. II): 107, 1991.
45. Savoie, F. H III:, and Jones, G. S.: Arthroscopic management of arthrofibrosis of the elbow. In Operative Arthroscopy. McGinty, J. B., Caspari, R. B., Jackson, R. W., and Poehling, G. G.(eds.): Philadelphia, Lippincott Raven, 1996, pp. 887–896.
46. Schindler, A., Yaffe, B., Chetrit, A., Modan, M., and Engel, J.: Factors influencing elbow arthrolysis. Ann. Hand Surg. **10**:237–242, 1991.
48. Seth, M. K., and Khurana, J. K.: Bony ankylosis of the elbow after burns. J. Bone Joint Surg. **67B**:747–749, 1985.
47. Shahriaree, H., Sajadi, K., Silver, C. M., and Sheikholeslamzadeh, S.: Excisional athroplasty of the elbow. J. Bone Joint Surg. **61A**:922–927, 1979.
48. Thompson, HC III, and Garcia, A.: Myositis ossificans: aftermath of elbow injuries. Clin. Orthop. **50**:129, 1967.
49. Timmerman, L. A., and Andrews, J. R.: Arthroscopic treatment of posttraumatic elbow pain and stiffness. Am. J. Sports Med. **22**:230–235, 1994.
50. Tsuge, K., and Mizuseki, T.: Débridement arthroplasty for advanced primary osteoarthritis of the elbow. Results of a new technique used for 29 elbows. J. Bone Joint Surg. **76B**:641–646, 1994.

51. Urbaniak, J. R., Hansen, P. E., Beissinger, S. F., and Aitken, M. S.: Correction of post-traumatic flexion contracture of the elbow by anterior capsulotomy. J. Bone Joint Surg. 67A:1160–1164, 1985.
52. Weiss, A.P.C., and Sachar, K.: Soft tissue contractures about the elbow. Hand Clin. 10:439–451, 1994.
53. Weizenbluth, M., Eichenblat, M., Lipskeir, E., and Kesslser, I.: Arthrolysis of the elbow: 13 cases of post-traumatic stiffness. Acta Orthop. Scand. 60:642–645, 1989.
54. Wheeler, D. K., and Linscheid, R. L.: Fracture-dislocations of the elbow. Clin. Orthop. 50:95, 1967.
55. Willner, P.: Anterior capsulectomy for contractures of the elbow. J. Int. Coll. Surg. 11:359–362, 1948.
56. Wilson, P. D.: Capsulectomy for the relief of flexion contractures of the elbow following fracture. J. Bone Joint Surg. 26A:71–86, 1944.

CHAPTER 34

External Fixators of the Elbow

• BERNARD F. MORREY and
ROBERT N. HOTCHKISS

RATIONALE

The rationale of dynamic hinged external fixation is that a pin placed across the distal humerus, through the axis of rotation, can provide a stable element for construction of an external fixation system.[19] With a properly constructed device, the ulna may be separated or distracted from the humerus and still allow flexion and extension. The mechanics and anatomic landmarks to allow the design and application of such a device have been defined.[3, 9, 16, 18] The axis of rotation of the distal humerus passes through the tubercle of origin of the lateral collateral ligament and through the anteroinferior aspect of the medial epicondyle (Fig. 34–1).

INDICATIONS

There are several major indications for the use of an external fixation device that at once stabilizes the joint in varus and valgus but allows elbow flexion motion. In general, these include clinical circumstances in which flexion motion is allowed while translation and other rotational relationships are maintained (Fig. 34–2).[12] In trauma and reconstruction, the hinged fixator maintains an aligned and reduced ulnohumeral joint during motion, thereby protecting the healing repaired or reconstructed collateral ligaments. The requirement and usefulness of such an approach for managing the elbow is becoming more widely recognized. Although these goals may be attained with relatively simple designs, greater flexibility and broader utility have been introduced by Hotchkiss with a more complex design. Both the Mayo dynamic joint distractor (DJD)[13] and the Hotchkiss Compass Hinge[6] are discussed in this chapter.

Trauma

In many traumatic circumstances, the goal is to "neutralize" the forces across the joint while elbow motion is maintained. There are several acute and subacute clinical settings in which the attainment of these goals is required. The specific indications for dynamic external fixators of the elbow in acute trauma include the following:

1. Elbow dislocation in which gross instability due to extensive soft tissue injury exists even after reduction.[2]
2. Complex instability (fracture dislocation).[11] This in-cludes instability with fractures of the radial head,[10] some olecranon fractures (Mayo type III)[11] as well as Regan-Morrey type II and III coronoid fractures.[15] When a device is applied in these circumstances, its major role is one of neutralization or unloading of the stresses placed on the fracture fixation.

3. Residual subluxation after simple or complex fracture-dislocation. In this setting, a percutaneous application can assist in reducing a subluxated joint without having to revert to an open procedure. Maintenance of the device allows early motion without concern for frank redislocation or continued subluxation.

Reconstruction

The same basic goals obtain for the use of the fixator after reconstructive interventions.

Ankylosis. When arthrolysis for the post-traumatic joint stiffness is carried out, release of the collateral ligament is sometimes necessary.[5, 13] Application of the device protects the repaired collateral ligaments while allowing immediate motion after the arthrolysis. Furthermore, by dislocating the joint, the soft tissue envelope is stretched, allowing greater motion when the fixator is removed.

Interposition Arthroplasty. At least one collateral ligament must be released for exposure.[1] Hence, the goals in this setting are as follows:

1. To separate the joint surfaces, allowing the interposed tissue to heal to the humerus and/or the ulna
2. To provide motion during the healing phase
3. To allow the released or reconstructed ligament to heal without tension

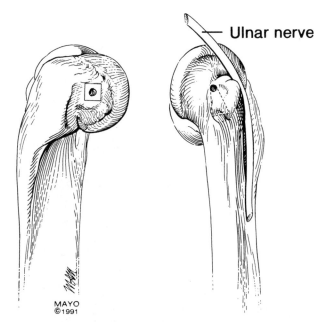

FIGURE 34–1 • On the medial side, placement of the axis pin is at the anteroinferior aspect of the medial epicondyle. On the lateral side, the center of rotation is at the tubercle of the lateral epicondyle, which is at the center of the projection of the curvature of the capitellum.

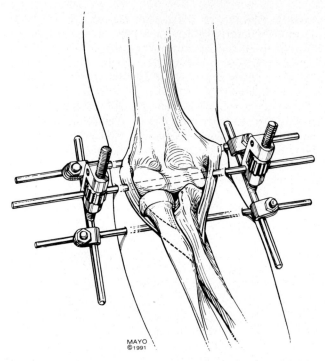

FIGURE 34–2 • An articulated external fixator (1) allows flexion motion, (2) protects the ligaments from varus and valgus stress, and (3) separates the joint.

CONTRAINDICATIONS

Contraindications for the use of this device are similar to those for other external fixators and include both absolute and relative contraindications.

Absolute

1. Local sepsis at the site of the pins. The external fixation pins should not be placed through infected bone or skin. The fixators can be used to stabilize a septic joint, which on occasion is helpful. However, care must be taken to ensure that the pins of the device are fixed to bone in sites free of infection.

2. When uncertainty exists regarding the anatomic location of the neurovascular structures due to post-traumatic disturbance of the anatomy. If a fixator is needed, a careful dissection with protection of the vulnerable nerves (usually the ulnar and radial) must be made.

Relative Contraindications

1. The presence of fracture fixation devices in the humerus or proximal ulna, making pin placement impossible. (There is some flexibility for pin placement. The presence of internal fixation does not absolutely preclude use.)

2. Inexperience with the use of external fixation devices, a relative contraindication.

TECHNIQUE

Mayo Dynamic Joint Distractor

PATIENT POSITIONING

The patient is placed in the position required for proper treatment of the primary pathologic condition. The distraction device itself may be applied with the patient in the prone, supine, or lateral decubitus position. In the practice of one of us (B.F.M.), the supine position is favored for most circumstances.

SURGICAL TECHNIQUE

The patient is supine with a sandbag under the scapula, and a nonsterile tourniquet is applied. The arm is draped free and brought across the chest.

In most cases of trauma or reconstruction, a posterior skin incision is used and the elbow joint is exposed either

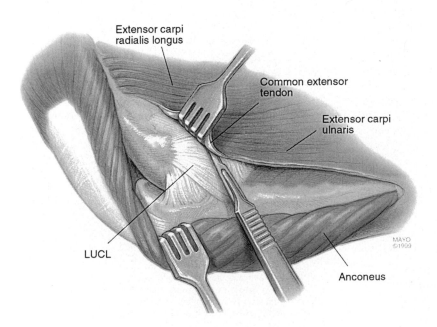

Extensor carpi radialis longus

Common extensor tendon

Extensor carpi ulnaris

LUCL

Anconeus

FIGURE 34–3 • A posterior skin incision is used while laterally the deep exposure is through Kocher's interval. LUCL = lateral ulnar collateral ligament.

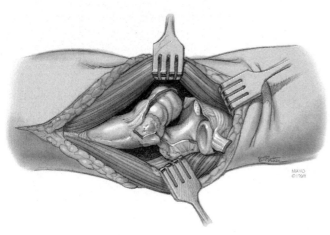

FIGURE 34-4 • The joint has been exposed and adequately released of scar tissue and intra-articular adhesions. The radial collateral ligament has been reflected, and the site of the anatomic axis of rotation at the projected center of rotation of the capitellum is identified.

medially or laterally according to the pathologic condition being addressed. In reconstructive procedures, the triceps is often reflected from the tip of the olecranon. If the elbow is stiff, a complete anterior and sometimes posterior capsular excision is required. The anterior capsule is exposed by elevating the common extensor tendon (Fig. 34-3). If the lesion is extrinsic to the joint and the articular cartilage is reasonably normal, the anterior capsule is excised but the lateral collateral ligament is preserved. In this case, the distraction device is usually not necessary.

If the joint is to be altered, or the joint is badly distorted, a more extensive exposure is required, and the lateral

collateral ligament is carefully elevated as a flap of tissue from its origin at the lateral condyle. This is tagged and reflected distally, providing full access to the joint (Fig. 34-4). The tip of the olecranon is always removed, and a complete anterior and posterior capsulectomy is performed. If the joint surface is destroyed, it must be refashioned, and some form of an interpositional arthroplasty is carried out. An autologous Achilles tendon is currently our tissue of choice becuase of its material properties and availability (see Chapter 60).

When the condition involves the joint surface that requires an extensive dissection, identification and protection of the ulnar nerve is necessary. This is accomplished through the same posterior incision. A subcutaneous dissection is carried out to the medial aspect of the triceps, and the ulnar nerve is identified but is usually not translocated anteriorly. Instead, it is simply protected, first during the capsular dissection and later at the time of joint axis pin placement. If ulnar nerve symptoms are present, then the nerve is decompressed with subcutaneous or submuscular translocation according to the nature of the pathologic condition and surgeon preference.

PLACING THE EXTERNAL FIXATOR

Once the elbow has been exposed and the pathologic condition addressed, the external fixator is applied. Several possible configurations are available and are used depending on the lesion and surgeon preference (Fig. 34-5). The essential landmarks of the flexion axis are identified. On the lateral aspect of the capitellum, a tubercle is present at the site of origin of the lateral collateral ligament (see Fig. 34-1). This tubercle also represents the geometric center

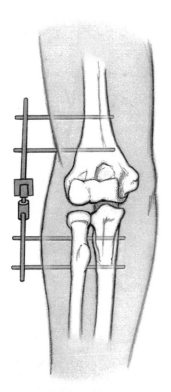
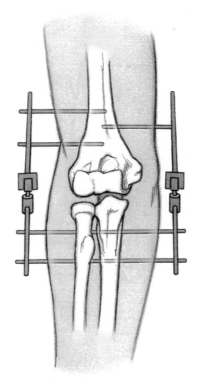
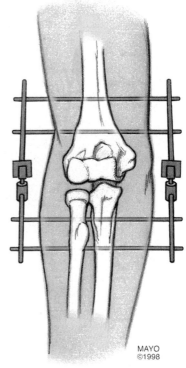

FIGURE 34-5 • Several configurations with half-pins and transfixing pins may be used with the current design of the dynamic joint distractor.

of curvature of the capitellum, which is also the lateral site of the flexion axis of the elbow and is the point through which the lateral pin must pass. If this anatomic feature has been altered by pathology, then the center of curvature of the ulnohumeral joint or reconstructed joint is identified as the axis of rotation.

On the medial aspect of the distal humerus, the axis of rotation lies just anterior and inferior to the medial epicondyle. This corresponds to the center of curvature of the medial contour of the trochlea. The axis pin is placed in this region, or slightly anterior and proximal to this location. This is a safe zone relative to the ulnar nerve, which is always identified and protected at the time of insertion of the medial humeral pin. Half-pins replicating the flexion axis are an attractive option when an interposition graft has been used. Recently, we have routinely used this method to apply the device, especially when the half-pin fixator is used.

An alignment guide is available and recommended when placing the transfixing pin and can also be used for insertion of the half-pins (Fig. 34–6). Because this pin is removed before closure, it may be placed directly through the epicondyles or percutaneously if desired.

If ligament reconstruction is necessary, 1- to 2-mm holes are made distal and proximal to the lateral axis pin for reattachment of the lateral collateral ligament. Two No. 5 nonabsorbable Bunnell sutures are placed through the radial (lateral) collateral ligament and through the holes drilled through the lateral column around the flexion pin (Fig. 34–7). These sutures are tied later, since it is more difficult to place the sutures when the axis pin is in place.

Once the axis pin or pins have been properly placed, stabilization of the distractor to the humerus is required. Under direct vision, transfixing pins or half-pins are inserted posterior to the radial nerve in the distal humerus and engage both cortices (Fig. 34–8). Medially, the ulnar nerve is visualized and avoided if a transfixing pin or half-pin is used. The center of the fixator is verified, and the device coupled to the humeral pins with the universal snap-on couplers. The elbow is flexed and extended to ensure proper alignment of the device. The ulnar transfixing or half-pins are then placed anterior and posterior to the axis center and secured to the distracting device (Fig. 34–9).

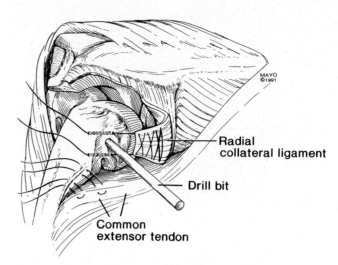

FIGURE 34–7 • To ensure stability after the external fixator is removed, the collateral ligaments are carefully reconstructed with care taken to avoid severing of the collateral suture by the permanent or temporary placement of the axis pin.

The ulnar transfixing or half-pins are then placed and secured to the distracting device. The axis pin or pins are removed after the humeral and ulnar coupling elements have been securely tightened.

If the triceps has been reflected, then it is reattached with a meticulous cruciate and transverse suturing technique. Crossed drill holes, as well as a transverse hole, are placed through the tip of the olecranon. A heavy (No. 5 nonabsorbable) suture is placed through the bone, across and into the triceps tendon in a criss-cross fashion and then back through the ulna. A second, transverse-type suture is placed through the ulna and through the triceps tendon. These sutures are then tied with the elbow at 90 degrees of flexion. The knots should be buried and placed to the side, avoiding the midline, and should not be palpable through the subcutaneous tissue.

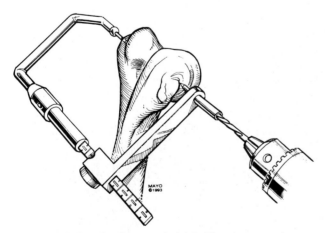

FIGURE 34–6 • An alignment device facilitates accurate placement of the axis pin(s).

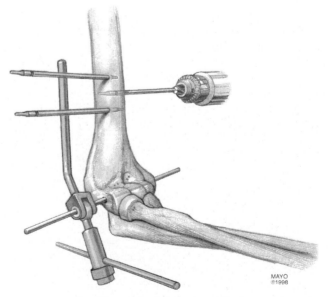

FIGURE 34–8 • The proximal fixator is stabilized to the distal shaft of the humerus by half-pins or transfixing pins.

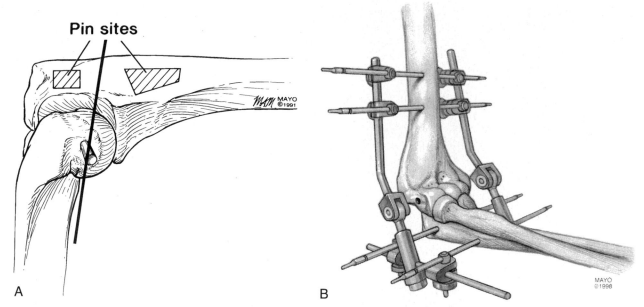

Pin sites

A   B

FIGURE 34–9 • Pins are placed across the ulna anteriorly and posteriorly to the axis of rotation *(A)* and the device secured with coupling devices *(B)*. Note that the axis pin has been removed.

The distraction of the ulna from the humeral joint surface is then accomplished after the axis pin has been removed by a counter-clockwise rotation of the mechanism using an Allen wrench. Typically, 2 to 3 mm of distraction of the joint surfaces is desired. Passive motion should be performed without crepitus or evidence of joint surface contact.

DISTAL ULNAR PIN PLACEMENT

The indication for distal ulnar pin placement is proximal ulnar fracture with instability. For some acute or subacute fractures in which the elbow is unstable due to coronoid deficiency, there is a tendency for the ulna to sublux posteriorly. In these cases, the dynamic joint distractor may sometimes be applied percutaneously under fluoroscopy to neutralize this tendency. The ulnar nerve is identified and the medial and lateral axis pins are placed under fluoroscopic control or under direct vision. The ulnar pins are placed distal to any internal fixation elements. This allows the distraction to occur down the axis of the ulna, thus affording the proper direction of force to reduce the ulno-humeral joint (Fig. 34–10). Full motion cannot be achieved by this slight asymmetrical distraction, but a flexion arc of 60 to 90 degrees of motion is usually attainable and this is considered adequate given the specific goals of this application.

The Compass Hinge

FRAME ASSEMBLY

The frame should be pre-built to confirm that proper ring size has been selected. In most adults, the 150-mm ring size is usually the best fit. It is important that the geared component is always medial, with the knob facing posterior.

When the frame has been assembled and appropriately

adjusted, it should slide along the axis pin without significant impingement or resistance (Fig. 34–11). If there is any, the components are probably out of alignment. The clinician should make sure to allow for swelling in the postoperative period, allowing at least 2 cm of clearance from the skin to the hinge block at the time of surgery.

PATIENT POSITIONING

For release of contracture and removal of heterotopic bone, the patient should be placed in the supine position with the

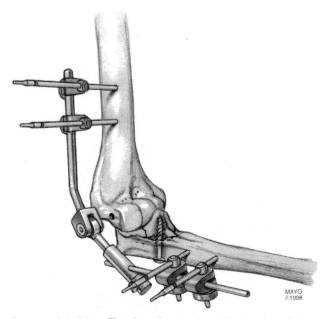

FIGURE 34–10 • The ulnar pins are placed distal to the articular fixation screws when treating complex instability or in instances in which proximal ulnar fixation is required, as with this coronoid fracture.

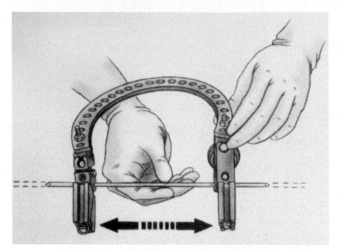

FIGURE 34–11 • Pre-assemble the frame so that the alignment of the axis elements freely slide on a 4-mm pin. (With permission, Smith & Nephew, Inc.)

arm on a radiolucent hand table. If the patient first requires a more extensive exposure of the distal humerus for fracture or reconstructive work, it may be useful to begin the operation with the arm over the chest when using one of the more standard posterior approaches to the elbow, either olecranon ostectomy or a triceps sparing exposure (Bryan-Morrey). In cases of gross instability, the prone position can be used, with the added benefit that gravity in this position tends to reduce the joint during hinge placement and operative ligament repair or reconstruction. However, exposure of the coronoid is quite difficult in the prone position.

EXPOSURE OF THE JOINT (STIFF, ANKYLOSED, OR POST-TRAUMATIC JOINT)

A modified "over the top" medial exposure of the elbow is most commonly used (see Chapter 8). Using the medial incision, the ulnar nerve can be mobilized and will allow exposure of both the anterior and posterior elbow joint (Fig. 34–12). The flexor pronator muscle mass is first elevated, followed by the brachialis and biceps being separated from the anterior capsule, thereby fully exposing the elbow joint. If there is extensive heterotopic bone or con-

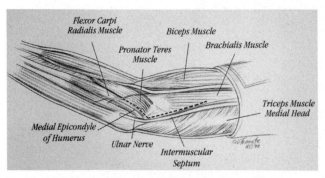

FIGURE 34–12 • For most applications involving stiff elbows or when the ulnar nerve is involved, a medial exposure is preferred (see Chapter 8). (With permission, Smith & Nephew, Inc.)

cern over contracture at the lateral side, it may be necessary to perform a lateral exposure through a supplementary incision along the supracondylar ridge of the distal humerus. This need only be as extensive as necessary to complete the capsular incision and removal of heterotopic bone. If necessary and similar to the anterior approach, a subperiosteal dissection and retraction of the triceps at the distal humerus is performed and the capsule of the posterior elbow joint can be exposed and excised.

AXIS PIN PLACEMENT

As with the dynamic joint distractor, a single temporary axis pin can be placed across the joint, or two half-pins can be inserted, one from the medial and the other from the lateral aspect of the joint. The alignment of the axis is crucial. It is important to take the time necessary to achieve perfect placement of this pin for alignment of the Compass Hinge at the elbow. Both an anteroposterior and lateral radiographs should be viewed to ensure adequate placement (Fig. 34–13). Once the two pins are coincident, entering at their respective centers of rotation, the frame should still be easy to slide from medial to lateral, back and forth, before securing the axis pin from the medial side (Fig. 34–14).

HUMERAL PIN PLACEMENT

The principle is to secure the humerus in two planes, without impaling any of the major muscle-tendon units or jeopardizing any neurovascular structures. It is helpful to

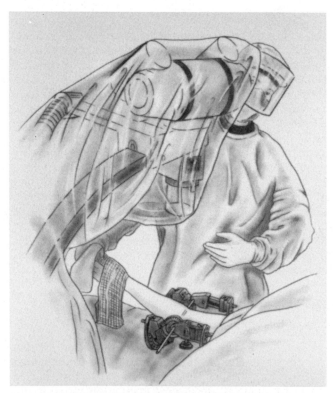

FIGURE 34–13 • Intraoperative fluoroscopy is helpful and in some instances is helpful to obtain proper orientation and alignment of the axis pin. (With permission, Smith & Nephew, Inc.)

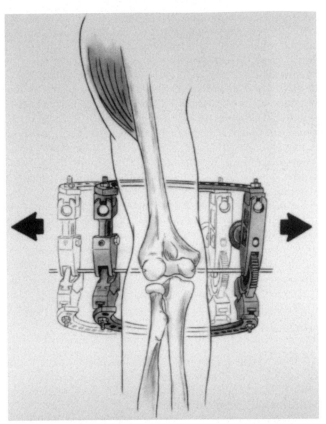

FIGURE 34–14 • Once the axis pin has been inserted, the preconstructed frame should slide freely medial to lateral on the axis pin. (With permission, Smith & Nephew, Inc.)

be familiar with the Rancho pin and cube system for half-pin placement. If there is internal fixation present, the pin placement can be adjusted to avoid the plates by customizing the frame. In general, two 5-mm half-pins, medial and lateral, are required. In larger elbows, or in cases in which internal fixation precludes use of the described sites, a third humeral pin may be used, usually placed laterally, superior to the spiral groove.

The medial pin is usually placed first through a two-hole Rancho cube on the undersurface of the upper ring. Both cortices should be engaged.

The lateral pin is usually placed using a two-hole post and a single-hole Rancho cube. The lateral flare of the humerus is used for placement. The drill guide rests on the lateral supracondylar ridge, directed anterior and distally. The radial nerve, at this level, is anterior to the pin (Fig. 34–15). Humeral fixation and alignment of the axis of the hinge must be achieved before fixation of the ulna.

PLACEMENT OF ULNAR FIXATION

One 5-mm and one or two 4-mm pins are used in the ulna. The more proximal pin (5-mm) provides optimal control of the joint and is placed from the dorsal surface through the coronoid. The smaller (4-mm) pins are used more distally in the ulna, again from the dorsal surface. If the elbow is grossly unstable, it is quite important to reduce the elbow by placing it in approximately 90 degrees of flexion when applying the ulnar fixation. Once the joint is

reduced and held in position, the first two proximal ulnar pins can be placed. Once the first two pins are in place, ranging through flexion and extension and ensuring reduction of the joint is important. If there is a tendency for the elbow to subluxate, then alignment has not been achieved and the bolts must be loosened and reduction achieved (see Fig. 34–15).

APPLICATION OF DISTRACTION

Once the joint has been reduced and all pins applied, distraction can then be applied to the system through the distraction mechanism. Distraction is achieved by turning the bolts located on the ulnar ring fixation blocks (Fig. 34–16). Both sides of the hinge should be distracted an equal amount. Use and extent of distraction should be done at the discretion of the surgeon.

AFTERCARE

The patient is assessed in the recovery room for neurovascular competence. A brachial plexus block is performed by an anesthesiologist, using a continuous infusion technique for 1 to 3 days. The extremity is placed in a continuous passive motion machine. The maximal amount of flexion and extension possible with the distraction device is at-

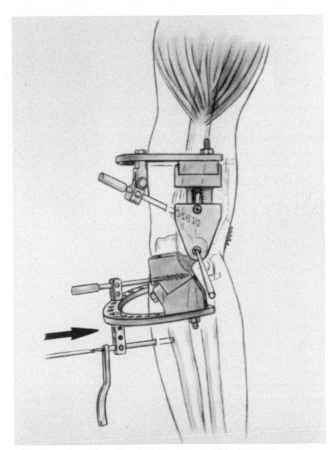

FIGURE 34–15 • The correct rotatory orientation of the ring referable to the humerus is perpendicular to the long axis of the humerus. The half-pins are inserted using the Rancho system through the alignment blocks, securing first the humerus followed by the ulnar components. (With permission, Smith & Nephew, Inc.)

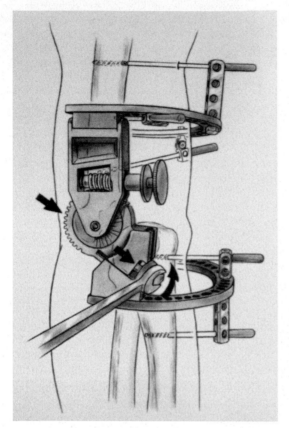

FIGURE 34–16 • Distraction is achieved by rotating the bolts under the ulnar ring. Both sides should be distracted an equal amount. (With permission, Smith & Nephew, Inc.)

tained immediately. A careful inspection of the elbow is made to check for swelling and to keep the skin from exerting pressure against the device. If there is no evidence of infection and there has been adequate progress, the patient is dismissed with a portable continuous passive motion unit about 3 to 4 days after surgery.

For aftercare of the Compass Hinge, passive mobilization is initiated using the gear mechanism. In the early postoperative period, the elbow is incrementally extended to the maximally tolerated position. As swelling subsides over the following days, incremental flexion is initiated. The patient then begins a schedule of maximizing the position of flexion or extension using the gear mechanism on alternating days. The device is usually left on the patient for 4 to 6 weeks.

After reconstructive procedures, the patient returns approximately 3 weeks after dismissal from the hospital, the distraction device is removed, and the elbow is examined under general anesthesia. Care is taken not to forcefully manipulate the elbow, but some sense of the firmness of the end points of motion is determined, since this is felt to have prognostic value.

After trauma, assessment is predicated on the severity of the injury, soft tissue integrity, and stability of the internal fixation. A common program is to see the patient at 1, 3, and 6 weeks. The device is removed between 3 and 6 weeks under a general anesthesia.

Splints (see Chapter 12). For patients treated for ar-

throlysis, static adjustable splints are employed when the device is removed, usually at about 3 weeks for stiffness and 4 to 6 weeks after fracture. The goal is to attain a degree of soft tissue stretch with a constant force allowing the soft tissue to "relax" under the constant pressure. For the first 3 weeks of application, the patient wears one or the other for approximately 20 to 21 hours a day. After 3 weeks, the program is individualized with the time in the splint decreasing to 10 to 16 hours, but the basic principles continue to be followed. For release of the stiff elbow, splint usage may be required at night and to maintain motion for up to 3 months or occasionally even up to 6 months.

Examination Under Anesthesia. If progress is not being achieved with the splints and there is no concern about fracture displacement, examination under anesthesia may be performed. If done, this is accomplished before 3 months. The most recent radiograph should be available to appreciate the articular pathologic lesion being addressed.

RESULTS

We have applied external fixators in approximately 200 cases. A general summary of the documented indications and results of the first 50 patients with the dynamic joint distractor are shown in Table 34–1.

For most surgeons, the value of this device will be in the management of trauma and its sequelae (Fig. 34–17).[7, 11] The results of the external fixators for arthrolysis have been reported as satisfactory in approximately 90 percent of patients.[13] As an adjunct in the management of complex instability, the technique has been described with an 80 percent success rate.[2] The results of such pathology do vary according to time of treatment from injury. The expectation when managing residual or neglected instability is only about 60 to 65 percent satisfactory outcomes[14] (Fig. 34–18). Interposition arthroplasty for pain from traumatic or inflammatory arthritis is successful in 67 percent of cases.[1]

For all indications, the outcome is not just to be attributed to the fixator; consideration of the prognosis of the condition being treated is equally relevant. This is particularly true for the management of the stiff joint. Satisfactory results without the external fixator can be expected in patients with extensive pathologic lesions.[4, 8, 17] We do, however, feel that this type device brings added value to interposition arthroplasty for management of intrinsic

• TABLE 34–1 • Experience with the Dynamic Distraction Device According to Indication (Mayo Experience)			
Indications	Experience (No. of Patients)	Satisfactory Result (%)	Reference
Ankylosis	26	90	Morrey[13]
Fracture	7	86	Cobb & Morrey[2]
Arthritis	13	70	Chen & Morrey[1]
Complex instability	16	75	McKee et al.[7]
Chronic instability	6	67	

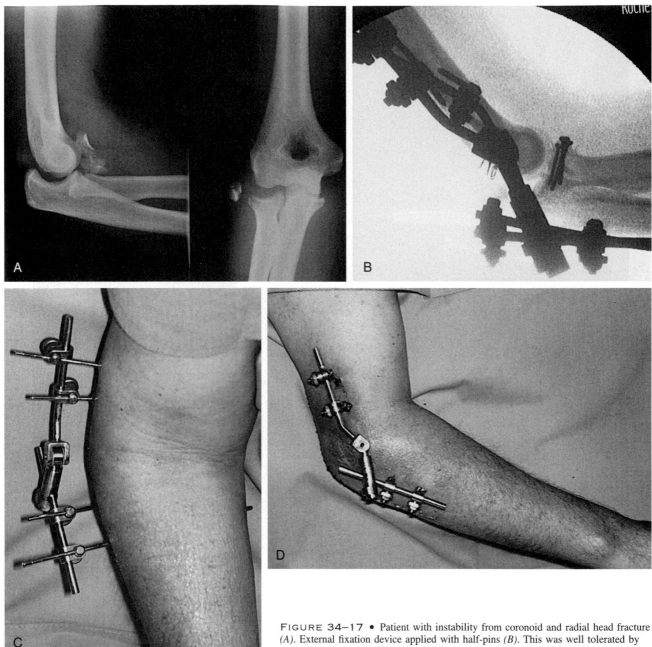

FIGURE 34–17 • Patient with instability from coronoid and radial head fracture *(A)*. External fixation device applied with half-pins *(B)*. This was well tolerated by the patient *(C and D)*. (With permission from R. N. Hotchkiss.)

pathologic conditions and is essential for the effective management of some complex instabilities.

COMPLICATIONS

The complications associated with these devices are listed in Table 34–2. Well-recognized complications associated with external fixators, infection, fracture, and nerve irritation are present with these devices as well.

Infection

Soft tissue pin site infection or irritation is a minor problem and is readily treated by pin removal. The transarticular pin used in the original design was a concern, as an infection at that site caused a deep infection of the joint, resulting in treatment failure. Although deep infection may occur, it should be noted that the patient population consists largely of those with post-traumatic conditions and a higher infection rate is recognized with surgical procedures in this group. Nonetheless, the current design of the dynamic joint distractor to eliminate a permanent articular pin, as was originally introduced with the Compass Hinge, is felt to be a major advantage in addressing this complication.

Neural Injuries

The incidence of neural injury relates to the underlying pathologic condition, to the surgical approach, and in a

CHAPTER 35

Injury of the Flexors of the Elbow: Biceps in Tendon Injury

• BERNARD F. MORREY

Except for epicondylitis, injury to the muscles or tendons about the elbow, as an isolated event, is rather uncommon.[3, 11, 14, 24, 55] Distal biceps tendon injury, usually avulsion from the radial tuberosity, although rare, is the most common tendinous injury in this region. Calcific tendinitis has been observed in the biceps tendon, but it is very uncommon.[45]

DISTAL BICEPS TENDON INJURY

The biceps muscle-tendon complex may be injured at the musculotendinous junction, by an in-continuity tear of the tendon, and by a complete or partial tear or avulsion from the radial tuberosity.

MUSCULOTENDINOUS JUNCTION

This is a quite uncommon injury and one rarely reported.[53] The mechanism is similar for all biceps injuries—an eccentric load against a contracting biceps muscle. It may have a predilection for persons with encephalopathy, a condition present in many who experience triceps rupture.

Treatment

Because of the delay in diagnosis, or owing to the frequency of underlying disease, our experience with surgical repair and reconstruction has not been favorable. I have used a Bunnell-type suture repair and augmentation with an LAD (commercial) graft. The elbow is protected in a splint for 3 weeks, with slow stretch and return to function over a 3-month period.

TEAR IN CONTINUITY

A tear of the tendon in continuity is very rare. This has been seen on occasion and I have used an LAD graft from the tuberosity to the muscle as a "stent" for the tendon insufficiency with success. Simple plication of the stretched tendon is not effective.

AVULSION

By far, the most common injury is tendon avulsion, and complete avulsion is much more common than a partial

injury. According to McReynolds, the first known diagnosis of a distal rupture was reported by Starks, in 1843.[42]

Incidence

Avulsion of the biceps tendon at its distal insertion was reported in three of 100 patients with biceps tendon rupture who were studied by Gilcreest.[17, 22, 23, 40, 57] The European literature suggests that distal avulsion injury accounts for some 3 to 10 percent of all biceps tendon ruptures.[27] The rarity of the condition is exemplified by the fact that only 24 cases were reported in a 43-year period after the original surgical descriptions by Johnson[31] in 1897 and Acquaviva[1] in 1898. Three hundred and fifty-five surgeons responded to a questionnaire Dobbie circulated in 1941 and added only 51 cases.[18] In addition, only three of this group had experience with as many as three cases. By 1956, the world literature contained 152 cases.[22] Currently, the injury is well-known—the incidence may be increasing or the lesion is recognized more often.[2, 5, 9, 26, 35, 37, 38, 54]

More reports in the literature notwithstanding, we have encountered only a single instance of involvement in a female in the English literature[42] and personally have no experience with a complete rupture in a female patient. In addition, more than 80 percent of the reported cases have involved the right dominant upper extremity, usually in a well-developed man[7, 50] whose average age is about 50 years[4, 18, 44] (range 21[51] to 70[18] years).

Mechanism of Injury

In virtually every reported case,[6, 18, 44] a single traumatic insult, often a force of 40 kg or more against resistance from an elbow in about 90 degrees of flexion, has been implicated. This mechanism, along with abuse of anabolic steroids, accounts for its surprisingly common occurrence in well-conditioned, healthy, but competitive weightlifters. Pre-existing degenerative changes in the tendon predispose

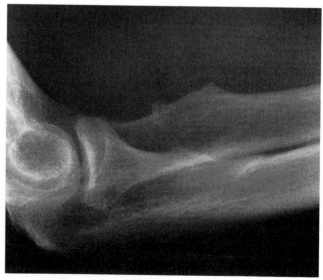

FIGURE 35–1 • Irregularity of the biceps tuberosity is frequently observed, suggesting that a degenerative process may be implicated, at least in part, in the causation of this condition.

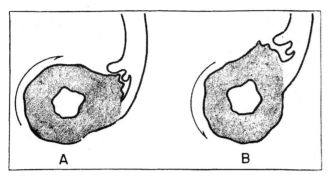

FIGURE 35–2 • Illustration of the pathophysiology of distal biceps rupture. Hypertrophic changes at the radial tuberosity cause irritation of the tendon, predisposing it to degenerative changes and rupture during pronation and supination. (From Davis, W. M., and Yassine, Z.: An etiologic factor in the tear of the distal tendon of the biceps brachii. J. Bone Joint Surg. 38A:1368, 1956.)

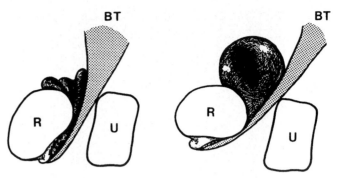

FIGURE 35–3 • Cubital bursitis may occur in association with degeneration of the distal biceps insertion. BT, biceps tendon. (From Karanjia, N. D., and Stiles, P. J.: Cubital bursitis. J. Bone Joint Surg. 70B:832, 1988.)

to rupture.[15, 16] Acute pain in the antecubital fossa is noted immediately. Rarely, a patient complains of a second episode of acute pain several days later. Such a history suggests the possibility of an initial partial rupture or of secondary failure of the lacertus fibrosus.[9, 12] Occasionally, forearm pain has been reported, but it is considered rather uncommon.

Etiology

The cause of the injury has been discussed by several authors and is considered in detail by Davis and Yassine.[15] The histologic pathology is that of degeneration of the biceps tendon, a finding that is consistent with the radiographic changes often observed on the volar aspect of the radial tuberosity (Fig. 35–1).[18, 29, 50] During pronation and supination, inflammation and subsequent attenuation of the biceps tendon is initiated by irritation from the irregularity of the radial tuberosity (Fig. 35–2) or from chronic cubital bursitis (Fig. 35–3).[32] Spurring of the radial tuberosity is common and is consistent with the degenerative nature of this injury.

Predisposition to this and other tendon injuries has been associated with hyperparathyroidism,[13, 51] chronic acidosis,[46] and systemic diseases such as lupus erythematosus.[56]

One interesting study has also implicated a hypovascular zone of tendon near its attachment as a cause or contributing factor to the injury.[52]

Presentation

SUBJECTIVE COMPLAINTS

The common symptom of distal biceps tendon rupture is a sudden, sharp, tearing-type pain followed by discomfort in the antecubital fossa or in the lower anterior aspect of the brachium. The intense pain usually subsides in several hours, but a dull ache persists for weeks. Immediately after the injury, activity is possible, but difficult. If surgical repair is not performed, chronic pain with activity is common.[30] Flexion weakness of about 15 percent inevitably develops but over time some flexion strength returns.[36] Loss of supination strength has been reported as the source of variable dysfunction but has been measured as averaging 40 percent,[44] and diminution of grip strength also has been recognized.[2, 36, 44]

OBJECTIVE COMPLAINTS

Ecchymosis is visible in the antecubital fossa,[18, 49] and occasionally over the proximal ulnar aspect of the elbow joint.[7] Extensive bleeding is uncommon but is seen occasionally (Fig. 35–4). With elbow flexion, the muscle con-

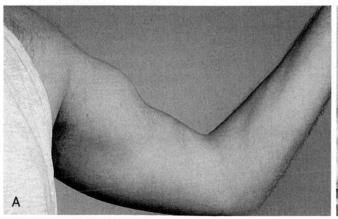

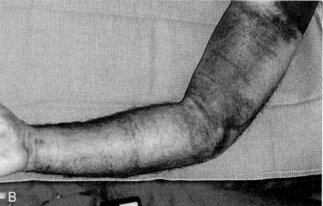

FIGURE 35–4 • A, The left forearm ecchymosis is vaguely seen in this patient, who presented 10 days after injury. B, Less commonly, extensive ecchymosis develops.

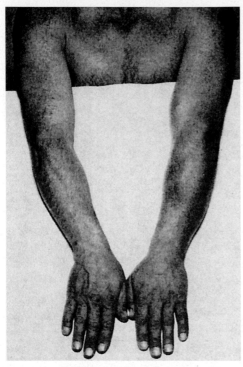

FIGURE 35–5 • Proximal retraction of the biceps muscle is the consistent and obvious finding and should allow the diagnosis to be readily made.

tracts proximally and a visible, palpable defect of the distal biceps muscle is obvious (Fig. 35–5). This contour, however, may be altered by a space-occupying lesion, such as a lipoma, or fibrosis of the biceps muscle.[21] Thus, assessment of strength alteration is essential to substantiate the diagnosis. Local tenderness is present in the antecubital fossa. The defect may be palpable; if it is not and if symptoms are otherwise consistent with the diagnosis, a partial rupture may have occurred. With partial rupture, crepitus or grinding is noted with forearm rotation.[9] Motion is not altered, except possibly as a result of pain at the extremes of flexion, extension, and supination. Flexion weakness usually is detectable by routine clinical examination. The loss of strength may be profound,[18] especially on supination immediately after injury. Loss of grip strength is variable in degree but is associated with most such injuries.

ROENTGENOGRAPHIC CHANGES

Some investigators recommended routine use of magnetic resonance imaging to make or to confirm the diagnosis.[37] Although ocasionally MRI is helpful (Fig. 35–6), we have not found it to be routinely necessary.

SURGICAL FINDINGS

If the biceps tendon is explored early, local hemorrhage is present in the antecubital space but usually is not extensive. The tendon may have recoiled into the muscle or may lie loosely curled in the antecubital fossa. Invariably, the separation is clean and from the radial tuberosity,[7, 18, 36, 40, 44, 49] a configuration that supports the hypothesis and

observations of Davis and of Chevallier that the underlying lesion is degeneration at the site of attachment.[12, 15] The lacertus fibrosus may be attenuated, but sometimes is not completely torn. After several months, typically the tendon has retracted into the substance of the biceps muscle and cannot be retrieved to be reattached. In such cases, the lacertus fibrosus is usually torn and retracted.

Treatment

ACUTE DISRUPTION

Reliance on the older literature is unwise. Nonoperative management has been reported to provide satisfactory results in about half of cases[29]; however, the functional superiority of surgical treatment is obvious when the results of cases treated with and without surgical intervention are reviewed.[44] The recent literature offers overwhelming documentation of the excellent results of early repair.[2, 5, 38, 48] With partial rupture, there is less functional loss or the tear may heal; thus, operative management may not be necessary acutely. Chronic pain may necessitate surgical repair.

SUTURE ANCHOR

Reattachment to the radius, by any one of several techniques,[4, 7, 20, 49, 54] is clearly the treatment of choice. The difficulty of performing the anterior exposure needed to avoid radial nerve injury has inspired the development of a second incision that is placed over the dorsal aspect of the forearm.[10] Curiously, this technique appears first to have been employed in 1937 by Plummer to reattach the

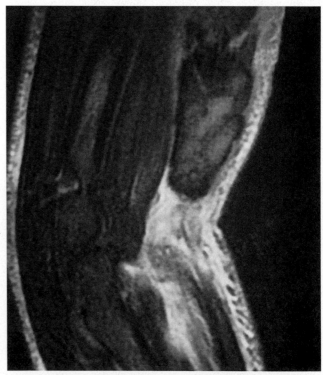

FIGURE 35–6 • MRI of the arm shown in Figure 35–1 4 days after the injury. This study was useful for demonstrating distal avulsion with retraction of the tendon and absence of tendon in the cubital fossa.

biceps tendon to the proximal ulna.[18] It is paramount to understand that the two-incision Boyd-Anderson technique originally described has been modified at the Mayo Clinic to reduce the likelihood of the development of ectopic bone between the radius and ulna. This point is explained later.

Because of concern over the development of ectopic bone associated with the two-incision technique, and with the advent of suture anchors, the anterior exposure using these anchors is gaining popularity. If the procedure is done promptly, the tract of the biceps tendon is still present and is easily identified. Later (more than 2 weeks after injury), the tract may be obliterated, making the exposure more difficult.[28]

Surgical Technique

TWO-INCISION TECHNIQUE (MAYO)

With the patient in the supine position, the extremity is prepared and draped in the usual fashion using an elbow table. A tourniquet is applied to the arm. A limited 3-cm transverse incision is made in the cubital crease (Fig. 35–7). The arm is grasped and milked distally to deliver the biceps tendon. In the majority of cases, the tendon is readily retrieved with this maneuver. The tendon is inspected and invariably is found to be cleanly avulsed from the radial tuberosity. The distal 5 to 7 mm of degenerative tendon is resected, and two No. 5 nonabsorbable Bunnell or whipstitch (Krackow) sutures are placed in the torn tendon (see Fig. 35–7). The tuberosity is palpated with the index fingers, and a blunt, curved hemostat is carefully inserted into the space previously occupied by the biceps tendon. The instrument slips past the tuberosity and is advanced below the radius and ulna so that its tip may be palpated on the dorsal aspect of the proximal forearm (see Fig. 35–7). A second incision is made over the instrument. The tuberosity is exposed by a muscle-splitting incision with the forearm maximally pronated. The ulna is *never* exposed.[20] A high-speed burr is used to evacuate a defect 1.5 cm wide and 1 cm deep in the radial tuberosity (see Fig. 35–7). Three holes are then placed 7 to 8 mm apart and at least 5 mm from the edge of the excavation. The tendon is delivered through the second incision, and the sutures are placed through the holes in the tuberosity. The tendon is carefully introduced into the excavation formed in the tuberosity, and, with the forearm in the neutral position, the sutures are pulled tight and secured. The wounds are closed in layers, and a suction drain is inserted in the depths of the wound, both anteriorly and posteriorly. The elbow is placed in 90 degrees of flexion with the forearm rotated between neutral position and supination. A compressive dressing is applied.

SUTURE ANCHOR TECHNIQUE

We have no personal experience with suture anchors for this problem. Which particular technique is chosen depends on three variables: exposure, type of anchor used, and method of reattachment. The exposure is usually a limited anterior approach. Usually, two or three suture anchors are used, most often they are placed directly into the unprepared tuberosity. The use of both the screw and the barb designs has been described (Fig. 35–8).

Results

Today, few surgeons attach the acutely ruptured tendon to the brachialis, but in the past this maneuver has been said to produce full function of the forearm,[11, 34] including adequate supination.[8, 50] Restoration of normal or nearly normal supination strength without anatomic reinsertion of the biceps tendon is incomprehensible. The result may be surprisingly good, but it is *not normal* and cannot restore supination strength. We have conducted isometric strength assessment tests on seven patients at least 15 months after the two-incision technique.[44] Restoration of strength approached normal in flexion and supination (Table 35–1). Nontreated distal biceps rupture results in loss of about 20 percent flexion and 40 percent supination strength.[44]

The objective measurements of restoration of normal strength have been reaffirmed by Agins and co-workers with the use of Cybex testing for not only strength but also endurance.[2] However, these investigators found restoration of normal strength only to the dominant extremity, and residual 20 to 30 percent weakness if the nondominant side was involved. Although this observation of different results by dominant extremity has also been made by others,[35] this certainly has not been our experience with isometric testing.

Complications

No individual report in the English literature specifically deals with the complications of surgical treatment for distal biceps tendon rupture. Transient radial nerve palsy with reattachment to the tuberosity has been,[18, 43] and continues to be, noted occasionally.[38, 48] The use of suture anchors is being considered to prevent injury to the nerve. Straugh reports three instances of successful treatment using a lim-

		Strength (%)*				
Treatment (No. of Patients)	Follow-Up per Month	Flexion	Extension	Pronation	Supination	Grip
None (2)	15	61	100	93	63	86
Early reattachment (2)	17	97	117	99	95	114
Late reattachment (1)	36	85	74	94	64	77
Insertion into brachialis (1)	20	87	105	113	43	100

• TABLE 35–1 • **Strength of Various Functions After Treatments for Distal Biceps Tendon Rupture**

*Percentage difference from opposite extremity, corrected for effect of the dominant side.

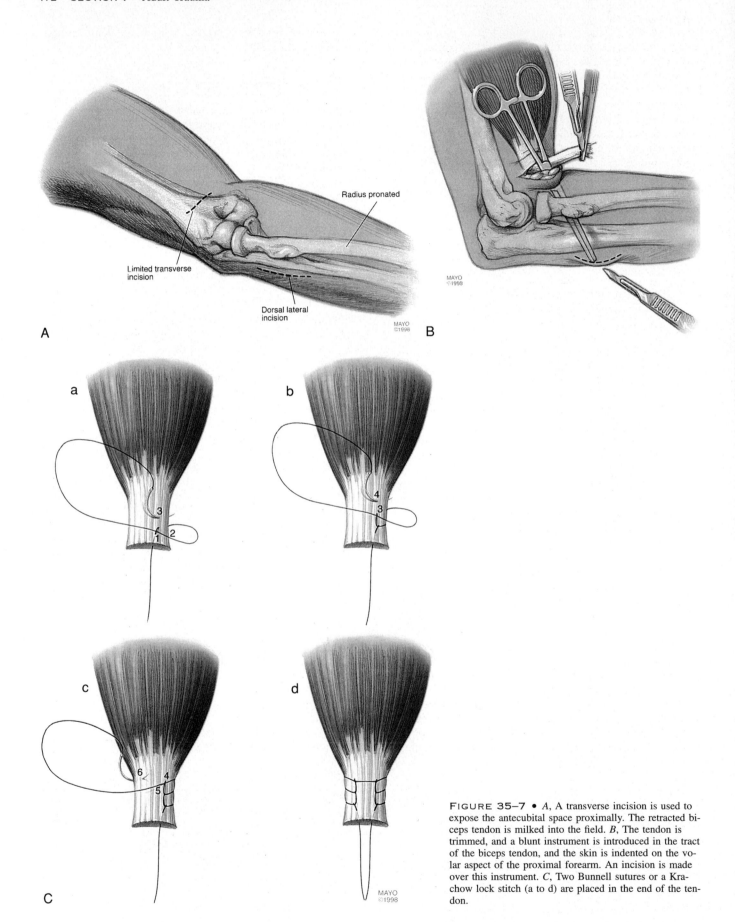

A

Radius pronated

Limited transverse
incision

Dorsal lateral
incision

MAYO
©1998

B

MAYO
©1998

a

3
1 2

b

4
3

c

6 4
5

d

C

MAYO
©1998

FIGURE 35–7 • *A*, A transverse incision is used to
expose the antecubital space proximally. The retracted biceps tendon is milked into the field. *B*, The tendon is
trimmed, and a blunt instrument is introduced in the tract
of the biceps tendon, and the skin is indented on the volar aspect of the proximal forearm. An incision is made
over this instrument. *C*, Two Bunnell sutures or a Kra-
chow lock stitch (a to d) are placed in the end of the tendon.

island flaps have been described in the past decade for use in orthograde or retrograde pedicle transposition or free tissue transfers. Island flaps are raised with a base consisting solely of a fully mobilized vascular pedicle, and they may include fascia, subcutaneous tissue, skin, and segments of vascularized muscle, bone, tendon, and cutaneous nerves, depending on the particular reconstructive needs. Some flaps used for elbow coverage are orthograde radial forearm, ulnar forearm, and posterior interosseous flaps and retrograde medial and lateral arm flaps.* Their arteriovenous pedicle and axial blood supply allow the widest possible arc of rotation and present relatively little risk of circulatory embarrassment. Coverage of small and moderate defects on all surfaces of the elbow is possible without microvascular anastomoses and upper extremity mobilization.[29] A parascapular flap may also be used to cover an above-elbow amputation stump.[46]

Antecubital Fasciocutaneous Transposition Flap

Described by Lamberty and Cormack,[49, 50] the antecubital fasciocutaneous flap is an axial-pattern, fasciocutaneous flap based on the inferior cubital artery. This vessel usually arises from the radial recurrent artery or from the radial artery proper and lies in the intermuscular septum between brachioradialis and pronator teres. It runs distally, paralleling the course of the cephalic vein in the superficial fascia from its origin 4 cm inferior to the midportion of the anterior interepicondylar line (Fig. 37–8). Venous drainage based on injection studies is provided principally by the cephalic vein.[50] A 4:1 length-width–ratio flap may safely be raised.

TECHNIQUE

The flap is incised through subcutaneous tissue and fascia initially medially and distally and then is raised, including the intermuscular septum between brachioradialis and the flexor-pronator muscles of the forearm. Proximally, the inferior cubital artery is identified as it passes through this septum and then is protected. Elevating the flap includes the cephalic vein, which is ligated and divided distally, and the lateral antebrachial cutaneous nerve. Its length and relatively narrow base allow it to be rotated to cover many elbow area defects.

Radial Forearm Island Flap

The cutaneous territory nourished by the radial artery includes the radial two thirds of the anterior forearm and its lateral aspect.[49] A fasciocutaneous flap based on an orthograde (proximal) pedicle provides excellent elbow coverage of moderate sized defects, including the posterior aspect of the region.[2, 17, 22, 28, 57] Some 9 to 17 cutaneous perforators from the radial artery supply the skin, including musculocutaneous vessels proximally and fasciocutaneous vessels distally by means of a deep prefascial plexus and a subdermal plexus.[95] Its chief advantages are its reliability, techni-

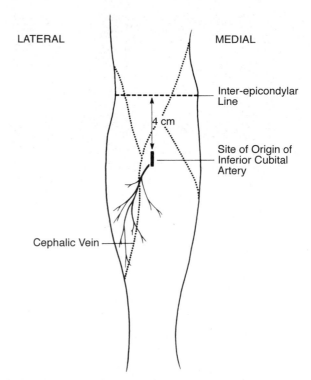

FIGURE 37–8 • The distribution of the inferior cubital artery. (From Lamberty, B. G. W., and Cormack, G. C.: Br. J. Plast. Surg. **35**:425, 1982.)

cal simplicity, and versatility, the results of its being a compound flap including fascia only, composite skin and fascia, vascularized brachioradialis, flexor carpi radialis, or palmaris longus tendon segment of the distal radius and its sensibility with lateral and medial antebrachial cutaneous nerves.[19, 29, 73] Its arc of rotation allows coverage of all aspects of the elbow joint but is limited proximally by its point of rotation at the radial artery origin 10 cm below the elbow joint.[95] The principal drawback of this method is the unsightly donor site, which requires split-thickness skin grafting unless a small area or fascia only is used.[40] Although the size of the radial cutaneous territory may be as large as 15 by 25 cm, flaps generally no larger than 16 by 8 cm (usually smaller) are considered for elbow defects that measure 6 to 8 by 14 to 6 cm.[17, 19, 49, 94] A complete deep palmar arch is necessary for adequate perfusion of the hand by the ulnar and (occasionally) median arteries. Because of donor site considerations, a fasciocutaneous flap is generally contraindicated for women.[73] One recent study demonstrated a 10 percent incidence of grip weakness and 50 percent incidence of paresthesias, and, inretrospect, 25 percent of patients expressed regret at having had the operation.[92]

TECHNIQUE

The course of the radial artery is marked with the help of a Doppler ultrasound probe and a timed Allen's test is performed to verify adequate distal circulation with the radial artery occluded. The donor area is outlined somewhat larger than the defect and is centered over the radial artery with a pedicle long enough to enable it to be trans-

*References 8, 13, 17, 19, 28, 29, 34, 40–43, 56, 61, 68, 73, 74, 79, 88–90, 94–96.

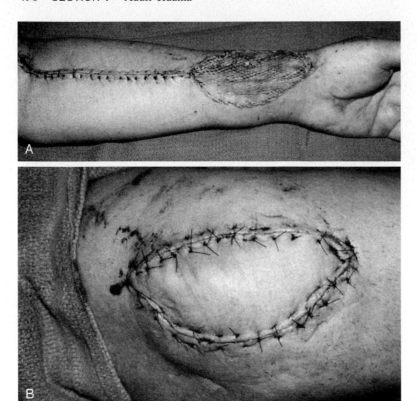

FIGURE 37–9 • Coverage of a posterior defect secondary to chronic olecranon bursitis with an orthograde radial forearm flap. Earlier, a brachioradialis flap had failed to cover the defect. *A*, The donor site with skin graft. *B*, The flap in place over the olecranon. (Courtesy of M. B. Wood, M.D.)

posed. The flap is then raised, protecting the superficial radial nerve but including the cephalic vein and lateral antebrachial cutaneous nerve. The margins are incised, including the antebrachial fascia. Distally, the radial artery is ligated and the flap, including the lateral intermuscular septum, radial vessels, and fasciocutaneous perforators, is raised as a proximally based island flap transposed to cover the elbow (see Fig. 37–8). Closure of the donor site requires split-thickness skin grafting (Fig. 37–9). Incomplete graft "take" is a common complication, but the risk may be minimized by preserving paratenon over distal tendons

and by immobilizing the wrist and digits for several days after surgery.[68, 96]

Retrograde Lateral Arm Flap

The lateral arm flaps described by Katsaros and colleagues have been widely used for upper limb reconstruction as a free flap transfer based on its fasciocutaneous supply by means of a terminal branch of the profunda brachii artery, the posterior radial circumflex artery.[43] This vessel contributes to the anastomotic blood supply of the elbow via the

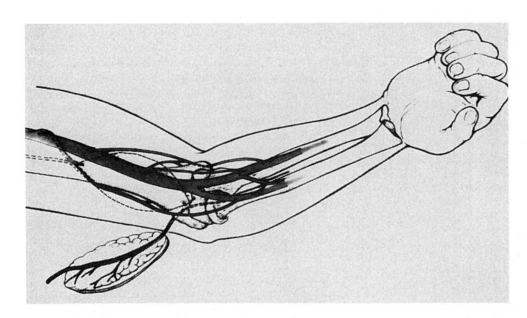

FIGURE 37–10 • Design of a reverse lateral arm flap for elbow coverage (From Culbertson, J. H., and Mutimer, K.: Ann. Plast. Surg. **18**:64, 1987.)

interosseous recurrent artery. Culbertson and Mutimer have described a retrograde island flap based on this distal circulation with reverse-flow venous drainage through venae comitantes in a fashion analagous to the reverse radial forearm flap (Fig. 37–10).[13, 56, 73] The flap may include fascia only, skin up to 8 to 10 cm as well as sensation by neurotization of the posterior brachial cutaneous nerve, triceps tendon, or even a segment of vascularized humerus.[43] Recently Kuek and Lanzetta and their respective colleagues revealed that local circulation supports greater distance to the forearm than had been previously described.[45, 51] This allows a broader indication than previously reported. As a retrograde flap, it covers all surfaces of the elbow and is indicated for burn cicatrix, olecranon area defects secondary to pressure sores, excision of rheumatoid nodules or bursitis, and local skin loss of other causes, provided that the anastomotic circulation is not disturbed. From measurements of the defects in flexion and extension a more accurate estimate of posterior coverage can be made.[99] It has the significant advantages of a minimal donor site problem (because usually the defect can be closed primarily) and no need to sacrifice a major vessel, two problems associated with the radial forearm flap. Yet, one recent study of almost 100 procedures reported concerns for appearance in 27 percent of patients and paresthesias in 59 percent, and the investigators recommended the procedures only for males.[27] A recent modification described by Hamdi and Coessens resulted in markedly greater patient satisfaction, so that recommendation may be revised.[30]

TECHNIQUE

The axis of the flap is a line from the deltoid insertion to the lateral humeral epicondyle. The course of the posterior radial circumflex artery is located with a Doppler ultrasound probe, and a flap of sufficient size and pedicle length to allow transposition to the elbow is outlined. The flap is elevated from the proximal to the distal aspect, including the biceps and triceps fascia and the lateral intermuscular septum. The vessels are identified and divided proximally and are included with the flap as a distally based pedicle. The flap is then rotated into the recipient site.

Other Fasciocutaneous Flaps

The medial arm, ulnar forearm, and posterior interosseous flaps also may be used for elbow coverage. The medial arm flap is not much used as a free flap because of its variable cutaneous blood supply through unnamed cutaneous arteries and biceps myocutaneous branches from the brachial artery. The anastomoses these vessels form with the superior ulnar collateral artery are various and not uniform.[43, 89] Its potential as a fasciocutaneous transposition flap for elbow coverage has been based on this anastomotic connection, but no clinical cases have been reported.[42]

The posterior interosseous flap described by Zancolli and Angrigiani in 1986, has been used primarily as a retrograde flap for hand coverage.[8, 79, 104] It also may be used as an orthograde fasciocutaneous flap based on some of the 7 to 14 fasciocutaneous perforators that arise from the posterior interosseous artery. These vessels run in the interval between the extensor carpi ulnaris and the extensor digiti minimi. The pivot of the flap is the point of emergence of the artery in the posterior forearm at the junction of the proximal and middle thirds of forearm, and the axis lies on a line drawn from the lateral humeral epicondyle to the ulnar head. A flap outlined in the distal third of the forearm will reach the antecubital fossa and olecranon (Fig. 37–11).[79]

An orthograde ulnar artery forearm flap also may cover the elbow, and it offers the potential for sensibility and composite tissue inclusion.[61] Its drawbacks are similar to those of the radial forearm flap, and it is seldom indicated.

MUSCLE PEDICLE FLAPS

Ger used muscle pedicle flaps to close complicated leg wounds in the lower extremity,[21] and extended to include overlying skin by recognition of musculocutaneous perforators.[8, 67, 98] For coverage about the elbow, a number of such flaps have been reported, including flexor digitorum superficialis, extensor carpi radialis longus, extensor carpi ulnaris, anconeus, brachioradialis, and latissimus dorsi.[6, 9, 23, 34, 47, 67, 76] Indications for muscle rotation to cover a cutaneous defect include infection, dead space that must be filled, and loss of motor function (restored by functional muscle transfer). Muscle flaps have been shown to diminish the bacteria count and to survive to a greater extent better than skin flaps.[11] They are probably preferred in cases of infection or significant risk thereof. Their bulk is useful to fill defects. Elbow flexion and extension and digit flexion have been restored by pedicled latissimus dorsi transfer.[4, 35, 83, 86, 91, 105] Because of significant functional loss with many of the aforementioned muscles or limited coverage secondary to small size and limited arc of rotation, only brachioradialis and latissimus dorsi transfers are used frequently about the elbow.[6, 34] The overall utility of and morbidity associated with pedicled forearm flaps was assessed from a survey of 267 patients from seven academic institutions in Germany and Switzerland. An overall satisfactory rate of 84 percent was reported.[36]

Brachioradialis

The brachioradialis is an expandable elbow flexor that arises from the upper two thirds of the lateral supracondylar

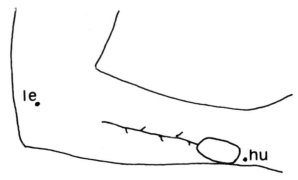

FIGURE 37–11 • An orthograde posterior interosseous flap for elbow coverage. (From Penteado, C. V., Masquelet, A. C., and Chevrel, J. P.: Surg. Radiol. Anat. **8**:214, 1986.)

coverage include thoracoepigastric flaps (based on internal mammary perforators), lateral thoracic flaps (thoracodorsal or lateral thoracic artery), external oblique fasciocutaneous flaps (myocutaneous perforators), pectoralis major flaps (muscle used as carrier for skin), and proximally based rectus abdominis pedicle flaps (Hartrampf's flap).* Several donor sites are illustrated in Figure 37–16. The interested reader is referred to the original salvage reference or to the second edition of this book for details.

FREE TISSUE TRANSFER

Free flaps are assuming an ever increasing role in reconstruction of upper extremity defects. The added operative time, need for microvascular anastomoses, and higher complication rate must be taken into consideration.[83] Nevertheless, in certain circumstances free tissue transfer is the procedure of choice, provided that the patient's health, age, and injuries allow surgery and that a skilled microvascular surgical team is available. In many instances, simpler methods are either inappropriate or less desirable.[15, 33, 103] For example, need for multiple tissue reconstruction may be possible in a single stage with a composite free flap. Distant pedicle flaps are contraindicated in a recipient site with marginal vascularity or when early limb mobilization is

---

*References 1, 3, 9, 16, 18, 23, 32, 62, 67, 84, and 102.

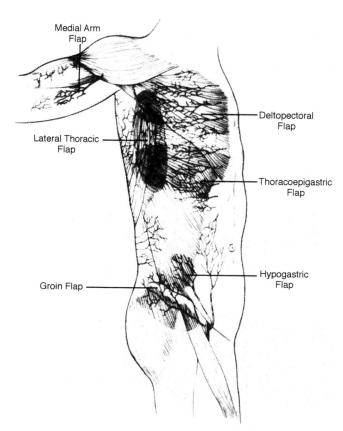

Medial Arm Flap

Deltopectoral Flap

Lateral Thoracic Flap

Thoracoepigastric Flap

Hypogastric Flap

Groin Flap

FIGURE 37–16 • Several potential temporary pedicle donor sites for upper extremity coverage. (From Gilbert, D. A.: Clin. Plast. Surg. 8:134, 1981.)

important. A local flap may be precluded by an external fixator, and free tissue transfer may be necessary. On the other hand, the free gastrocnemius muscle transfer to overcome the functional residua of Volkmann's contracture has been employed successfully for about 20 years.[60] The progressive advancement of the technique has broadened its indications. Thus, Minami and Ogino have progressed from using the latissimus dorsi muscle as a free pedicle to a free vascular flap.[71]

Choice of a flap is dictated by the size of the defect, the type of tissue required (skin, muscle, fascia, composite tissue), donor site morbidity, and the surgeon's preference. Skin (fasciocutaneous) flap choices for the elbow include the groin, scapular or parascapular, and lateral arm flaps.[5, 22, 31, 33, 37, 43, 72] Muscle is often preferable when dead space infection, or significant risk of infection is present, either with overlying skin or covered by a split-thickness graft. Manktelow and McKee pioneered free neurotized muscle transfers for functional reconstruction in the upper extremity.[65] The large variety of potential donor muscles includes latissimus dorsi, serratus anterior, rectus abdominis, gracilis, and triceps.[15, 26, 69, 77, 93] A recent addition is the triceps tendon and muscle.[26] A composite lateral arm free flap has been shown to take its blood supply from discrete vessels amenable to anastomosis rather than from the lateral arm fascia. Use of this flap causes no significant loss of extension strength.[26]

Vascularized bone is optimally provided with a composite groin flap based on the deep circumflex iliac vessels or a fibular graft including muscle, skin, or both, as needed. End-to-side arterial anastomosis to the brachial artery and end-to-end venorrhaphy to a vena comitante or cephalic vein is preferred for most elbow defects.[24]

REFERENCES

1. Abu Dalu, K., Muggia, M., and Schiller, M.: A bipedicled chest wall flap to cover an open elbow joint in a burned infant. Injury 13:292, 1982.
2. Akpuaka F. C.: The radial recurrent fasciocutaneous flap for coverage of posterior elbow defects. Injury 22:332, 1991.
3. Ariyan, S.: The pectoralis major myocutaneous flap. Plast. Reconstr. Surg. 63:73, 1979.
4. Axer, A., Segal, D., and Elkon, A.: Partial transposition of the latissimus dorsi: a new operative technique to restore elbow and finger flexion. J. Bone Joint Surg. 55A:1259, 1973.
5. Bartwick, W. J., Goodkind, D. J., and Serafin, D.: The free scapular flap. Plast. Reconstr. Surg. 69:779, 1982.
6. Bostwick, J., Nahai, F., Wallace, J. G., and Vasconez, L. D.: Sixty latissimus dorsi flaps. Plast. Reconstr. Surg. 63:31, 1979.
7. Brones, M. F., Wheeler, E. S., and Lesavoy, M. A.: Restoration of elbow flexion and arm contour with the latissimus dorsi myocutaneous flap. Plast. Reconstr. Surg. 69:329, 1982.
8. Büchler, U.: Retrograde posterior interosseous flap. J. Hand Surg. 16A:283, 1991.
9. Burstein, F. D., Salomon, J. C., and Stahl, R. S.: Elbow joint salvage with the transverse rectus island flap: a new application. Plast. Reconstr. Surg. 84:492, 1989.
10. Chang, L. D., and Goldberg, N. H.: Elbow defect coverage with a one-staged, tunneled latissimus dorsi transposition flap. Ann. Plast. Surg. 32:496, 1994.
11. Chang, N., and Mathes, S.: Comparison of the effect of bacterial inoculation in musculocutaneous and random pattern flaps. Plast. Reconstr. Surg. 70:1, 1982.
12. Cormack, G. C., and Lamberty, B. G. H.: A classification of fasciocutaneous flaps according to their patterns of vascularization. Br. J. Plast. Surg. 37:80, 1984.

13. Culbertson, J. H., and Mutimer, K.: The reverse lateral upper arm flap for elbow coverage. Ann. Plast. Surg. **18**:62, 1987.
14. Cuono, C. B.: Double Z-plasty repair of large and small rhombic defects: the double-Z rhomboid. Plast. Reconstr. Surg. **71**:658, 1983.
15. Daniel, R. K., and Weiland, A. J.: Free tissue transfers for upper extremity reconstruction. J. Hand Surg. **7**:66, 1982.
16. Davis, W. M., McCraw, J. B., and Carraway, J. H.: Use of a direct, transverse thoracoabdominal flap to close difficult wounds of the thorax and upper extremity. Plast. Reconstr. Surg. **60**:526, 1977.
17. Fatah, M. F., and Davies, D. M.: The radial forearm island flap in upper limb reconstruction. J. Hand Surg. **9B**:234, 1984.
18. Fisher, J.: External oblique fasciocutaneous flap for elbow coverage. Plast. Reconstr. Surg. **75**:51, 1985.
19. Foucher, G., Genechten, E., Merle, N., and Michon, J.: A compound radial artery forearm flap in hand surgery: an original modification of the Chinese forearm flap. Br. J. Plast. Surg. **37**:139, 1984.
20. Freshwater, M. F.: Ten signs for successful skin grafting. Plast. Reconstr. Surg. **72**:491, 1983.
21. Ger, R.: The operative treatment of the advanced stasis ulcer: a preliminary communication. Am. J. Surg. **3**:659, 1966.
22. Gilbert, A., and Teot, L.: The free scapular flap. Plast. Reconstr. Surg. **69**:601, 1982.
23. Gilbert, D. A.: An overview of flaps for hand and forearm reconstruction. Clin. Plast. Surg. **8**:129, 1981.
24. Godina, M.: Preferential use of end to side arterial anastomoses in free flap transfers. Plast. Reconstr. Surg. **64**:673, 1979.
25. Godina, M.: Early microsurgical reconstruction of complex trauma to the extremities. Plast. Reconstr. Surg. **78**:285, 1986.
26. Gosain, A. K., and Matloub, H. S.: The composite lateral arm free flap: vascular relationship to triceps tendon and muscle. Ann. Plast. Surg. **29**:496, 1992.
27. Graham, B., and Adkins, P.: Complications and morbidity of the donor and recipient sites in 123 lateral arm flaps. J. Hand Surg. **17B**:189, 1992.
28. Hallock, G. G.: Island forearm flap for coverage of the antecubital fossa. Br. J. Plast. Surg. **39**:533, 1986.
29. Hallock, G. G.: Soft tissue coverage of the upper extremity using the ipsilateral radial forearm flap. Contemp. Orthop. **15**:15, 1987.
30. Hamdi, M., and Coessens, B. C.: Distally planned lateral arm flap. Microsurgery **17**:375, 1996.
31. Hamilton, S. G. L., and Morrison, W. A.: The scapular free flap. Br. J. Plast. Surg. **35**:2, 1982.
32. Hartrampf, C. R., Scheflan, M., and Black, P. W.: Breast reconstruction with a transverse abdominal island flap. Plast. Reconstr. Surg. **69**:216, 1982.
33. Hing, D. N., Buncke, J. H., Alpert, B. S., and Gordon, L.: Free flap coverage of the hand. Hand Clin. **1**:741, 1985.
34. Hodgkinson, D. J., and Shepard, G. H.: Muscle musculocutaneous and fasciocutaneous flaps in forearm reconstruction. Ann. Plast. Surg. **10**:399, 1983.
35. Hovnanian, A. P.: Latissimus dorsi transplantation for loss of flexion or extension of the elbow. Ann. Surg. **143**:493, 1956.
36. Hulsbergen-Kruger, S., and Muller, K.: Donor site defect after removal of free and pedicled forearm flaps: functional and cosmetic results. Handchir. Mikrochir. Plast. Chir. **28**:70, 1996.
37. Ikuta, Y., Watari, S., Kuwamura, K.: Free flap transfers by end-to-side arterial anastomosis. Br. J. Plast. Surg. **28**:1, 1975.
38. James, J. H., and Watson, A. C. H.: The use of Opsite, a vapor permeable dressing on skin graft donor sites. Br. J. Plast. Surg. **28**:107, 1975.
39. Janevicius, R. V., and Greager, J. A.: The extensor carpi radialis longus muscle flap for anterior elbow coverage. J. Hand Surg. **17A**:102, 1992.
40. Jim, Y., Guam, W., Shi, T., Quian, Y., Xu, L., and Change, T.: Reversed island forearm fascial flap in hand surgery. Ann. Plast. Surg. **15**:340, 1985.
41. Jones, N. F., Hardesty, R. A., Goldstein, S. A., and Ward, W. T.: Upper limb salvage using a free radial forearm flap. Plast. Reconstr. Surg. **79**:468, 1987.
42. Kaplan, E. N., and Pearl, R. M.: An arterial medial arm flap: vascular anatomy and clinical applications. Ann. Plast. Surg. **4**:205, 1980.
43. Katsaros, J., Schusterman, M., Beppu, M., Banis, J. C., and Ackland, R. D.: The lateral upper arm flap: anatomy and clinical applications. Ann. Plast. Surg. **12**:489, 1984.
44. Krizek, T. J., Robson, M. C., and Kho, E.: Bacterial growth and skin graft survival. Plast. Surg. Forum **18**:518, 1967.
45. Kuek, L. B.: The extended lateral arm flap: a detailed anatomical study. Ann. Acad. Med. Singapore **21**:169, 1992.
46. Kumar, P., and Charndra, R.: Parascapular fasciocutaneous flap for covering an above-elbow amputation stump. Burns **17**:425, 1991.
47. Lai, M. F., Krishna, B. V., and Pelly, A. D.: The brachioradialis myocutaneous flap. Br. J. Plast. Surg. **34**:431, 1981.
48. Lalikos, J. F., and Fudem, G. M.: Brachioradialis musculocutaneous flap closure of the elbow utilizing a distal skin island: a case report. Ann. Plast. Surg. **39**:201, 1997.
49. Lamberty, B. G. H., and Cormack, G. C.: The forearm angiotomes. Br. J. Plast. Surg. **35**:420, 1982.
50. Lamberty, B. G. H., and Cormack, G. C.: The antecubital fasciocutaneous flap. Br. J. Plast. Surg. **36**:428, 1983.
51. Lanzetta, M., and Bernier, M.: The lateral forearm flap: an anatomic study. Plast. Reconstr. Surg. **99**:460, 1997.
52. Le Huec, J. C., and Liquois, F.: A study of the fasciocutaneous vascularization of the arm. Surgical applications. Surg. Radiol. Anat. **17**:121, 1995.
53. Lendrum, J.: Alternatives to amputation. Ann. R. Coll. Surg. Engl. **62**:95, 1980.
54. Levine, N. S., Lindberg, R. B., Mason, A. D., and Pruitt, B. A.: The quantitative swab culture and smear: a quick simple method for determining the number of viable aerobic bacteria in open wounds. J. Trauma **16**:89, 1976.
55. Lewis, V. L., and Cook, J. Q.: The nondelayed thoracoepigastric flap: coverage of an extensive electrical burn defect of the upper extremity. Plast. Reconstr. Surg. **65**:492, 1980.
56. Lin, S. D., Lai, C. S., and Chin, C. C.: Venous drainage in the reverse forearm flap. Br. J. Plast. Surg. **34**:431, 1981.
57. Lister, G.: The theory of the transposition flap and its practical application in the hand. Clin. Plast. Surg. **8**:115, 1981.
58. Lister, G. D., and Gibson, T.: Closure of rhomboid skin defects: the flaps of Limberg and Dufourmentel. Br. J. Plast. Surg. **25**:300, 1972.
59. Lister, G., and Schecker, L.: Emergency free flaps to the upper extremity. J. Hand Surg. **13A**:22, 1988.
60. Liu, X. Y., and Ge, B. F.: Free medial gastrocnemius myocutaneous flap transfer with neurovascular anastomosis to treat Volkmann's contracture of the forearm. Br. J. Plast. Surg. **45**:6, 1992.
61. Lovie, M. J., Duncan, G. M., and Glasson, D. W.: The ulnar artery forearm free flap. Br. J. Plast. Surg. **37**:486, 1984.
62. Luce, E. A., and Gottlieb, S. F.: The pectoralis major island flap for coverage in the upper extremity. J. Hand Surg. **7**:156, 1982.
63. Mackinnon, S. E., Weiland, A. J., and Godina, M.: Immediate forearm reconstruction with a functional latissimus dorsi island pedicle myocutaneous flap. Plast. Reconstr. Surg. **71**:700, 1983.
64. Manchot, C.: Die Hautarterien des Menschlichen Körpers. Leipzig, F. C. W. Vogel, 1889.
65. Manktelow, R. T., and McKee, N. H.: Free muscle transplantation to provide active finger flexion. J. Hand Surg. **3**:416, 1978.
66. Marty, F. M., Montandon, D., Gumener R., and Zbrodowski, A.: The use of subcutaneous tissue flaps in the repair of soft tissue defects of the forearm and hand: an experimental and clinical study of a new technique. Br. J. Plast. Surg. **37**:95, 1984.
67. McCraw, J. B., Dibbell, D. G., and Carraway, J. H.: Clinical definition of independent myocutaneous vascular territories. Plast. Reconstr. Surg. **60**:341, 1977.
68. McGregor, A.D.: The free radial forearm flap: the management of the secondary defect. Br. J. Plast. Surg. **40**:83, 1987.
69. Milloy, F. J., Anson, B. J., and McAfee, D. K.: The rectus abdominis muscle and the epigastric arteries. Surg. Gynecol. Obstet. **110**:293, 1960.
70. Milton, S. H.: Pedicled skin flaps: the fallacy of the length-width ratio. Br. J. Surg. **57**:502, 1970.
71. Minami, A., and Ogino, T.: The latissimus dorsi musculocutaneous flap for extremity reconstruction in orthopedic surgery. Clin. Orthop. **260**:201, 1990.
72. Moffett, T. R., and Madison, S. A.: An extended approach for the vascular pedicle of the lateral arm free flap. Plast. Reconst. Surg. **89**:259, 1992.
73. Mühlbauer, W., Herndl, E., and Stock, W.: The forearm flap. Plast. Reconstr. Surg. **70**:343, 1982.
74. Mühlbauer, W., Herndl, E., and Stock, W.: The forearm flap. Plast. Reconstr. Surg. **70**:336, 1982.
75. Nassif, T. M., Vidal, L., Bovet, J. L., and Baudet, J.: The parascapular flap: a new cutaneous microsurgical free flap. Plast. Reconstr. Surg. **4**:591, 1982.

76. Ohtsuka, H., and Imagawa, S.: Reconstruction of a posterior defect of the elbow joint using an extensor carpi radialis longus myocutaneous flap: case report. Br. J. Plast. Surg. 38:238, 1985.

77. Onishi, K., and Yu, M.: Cutaneous and fascial vasculature around the rectus abdominis muscle: anatomic basis of abdominal fasciocutaneous flaps. J. Reconstr. Microsurg. 2:247, 1986.

78. Orgill, D. P., and Pribaz, J. J.: Local fasciocutaneous flaps for olecranon coverage. Ann. Plast. Surg. 32:27, 1994.

79. Penteado, C. V., Masquelet, A. C., and Chevrel, J. P.: The anatomic basis of the fasciocutaneous flap of the posterior interosseous artery. Surg. Radiol. Anat. 8:209, 1986.

80. Pontéu, B.: The fasciocutaneous flap: its use in soft tissue defects of the lower leg. Br. J. Plast. Surg. 34:215, 1981.

81. Pruzansky, M., and Kelly, M.: Latissimus dorsi musculocutaneous flap for elbow extension. J. Surg. Oncol. 47:62, 1991.

82. Rohrich, R. J., Ingram, A. E. Jr: Brachioradialis muscle flap: clinical anatomy and use in soft tissue reconstruction of the elbow. Ann. Plast. Surg. 35:70, 1995.

83. Romm, S., and Massac, E.: A guide to skin grafting. Contemp. Orthop. 11:35, 1985.

84. Sbitany, U., and Wray, R. C. Jr.: Use of the rectus abdominis muscle flap to reconstruct an elbow defect. Plast. Reconstr. Surg. 77:988, 1985.

85. Schoofs, M., Bienfast, B., Calteux, N., Dachy, C., Vandermaeren, C., and de Coninck, A.: Le lambeau aponéurotique de l'avantbras. Ann. Chir. Main 2:197, 1983.

86. Schottstaedt, E. R., Larsen, L. J., and Bost, F. G.: Complete muscle transposition. J. Bone Joint Surg. 37A:897, 1955.

87. Solmon, M.: Artères de la Peau. Paris, Masson et Cie, 1936.

88. Song, R. S., Gao, Y., Song, Y., Yu, Y., and Song, Y.: The forearm flap. Clin. Plast. Surg. 9:21, 1982.

89. Song, R., Song, Y., Yu, Y., and Song, Y.: The upper arm free flap. Clin. Plast. Surg. 9:27, 1982.

90. Soutar, D. S., and Tanner, S. B.: The radial forearm flap in the management of soft tissue injuries of the hand. Br. J. Plast. Surg. 37:18, 1984.

91. Stern, P. J., Neale, H. W., Gregory, R. O., and Kreilein, J. G.: Latissimus dorsi musculocutaneous flap for elbow flexion. J. Hand Surg. 7:25, 1982.

92. Suominen, S., and Ahovuo, J.: Donor site morbidity of radial forearm flaps. A clinical and ultrasonographic evaluation. Scand. J. Plast. Reconst. Surg. Hand Surg. 30:57, 1996.

93. Takayanagi, S., and Tsukie, T.: Free serratus anterior muscle and myocutaneous flaps. Ann. Plast. Surg. 8:277, 1982.

94. Thornton, J. W., Stevenson, T. R., and Vander Kolk, C. A.: Osteoradionecrosis of the olecranon: treatment by radial forearm flap. Plast. Reconstr. Surg. 80:833, 1987.

95. Timmons, M. J.: The vascular basis of the radial forearm flap. Plast. Reconstr. Surg. 77:80, 1986.

96. Timmons, M. J., Missotten, F. E. M., Pode, M. D., and Davies, D. M.: Complications of radial forearm flap donor sites. Br. J. Plast. Surg. 39:176, 1986.

97. Tobin, G. R.: The compromised bed technique. Surg. Clin. North Am. 64:653, 1984.

98. Tolhurst, D. E., Haeseker, B., and Zeeman, R. J.: The development of the fasciocutaneous flap and its clinical applications. Plast. Reconstr. Surg. 71:597, 1983.

99. Tung, T. C. and Wang, K.C.: Reverse pedicled lateral arm flap for reconstruction of posterior soft-tissue defects of the elbow. Ann. Plast. Surg. 38:635, 1997.

100. Urbaniak, J. R., Koman, L. A., Goldner, R. D., Armstrong, N. B., and Nunley, J. A.: The vascularized cutaneous scapular flap. Plast. Reconstr. Surg. 69:772, 1982.

101. Webster, J. P.: Thoracoepigastric tubed pedicles. Surg. Clin. North Am. 17:145, 1937.

102. Winspur, I.: Distant flaps. Hand Clin. 1:729, 1985.

103. Wood, M. B., and Irons, G. B.: Upper extremity free skin flap transfer: results and utility as compared with conventional distant pedicle skin flaps. Ann. Plast. Surg. 11:523, 1983.

104. Zancolli, E. A., and Angrigiani, C.: Colgajo dorsal de antebrazo (en "isla" con pediculo de vasos interosseos posteriores). Rev. Assoc. Arg. Orthop. Traumatol. 51:161, 1986.

105. Zancolli, E., and Mitre, H.: Latissimus dorsi transfer to restore elbow flexion: an appraisal of eight cases. J. Bone Joint Surg. 55A:1265, 1973.

CHAPTER 38

Replantation About the Elbow

• MICHAEL B. WOOD

Since the first successful human limb reattachment in 1962,[1, 2] replantation of severed parts has become a relatively common surgical procedure. Nonetheless, limb replantation about the elbow is infrequent because there have been few appropriate candidates. Although the term *replantation* is restricted to reattachment of a completely severed part, there is probably a larger group of patients with physiologic rather than anatomic amputations about the elbow, to which much of the following discussion applies. Since the first editions of this book, the focus of this subject has shifted somewhat from techniques to functional expectations and a revisit of the indications and expectations.

CLASSIFICATION

The American Academy of Orthopaedic Surgeons Committee on the Upper Extremity[3] has defined 10 anatomic zones of amputation pertaining to replantation (Table 38–1). Three of these levels (6, 7, and 8) occur about the elbow and are discussed in this chapter.

Zone 8 is an amputation through the upper limb above the elbow (i.e., transhumeral at any level). In this group of patients, a plausible and worthwhile surgical goal may be the conversion of an above-elbow amputation to a functioning below-elbow level. Depending on other factors, additional function may result, including the use of the wrist and hand, which would augment the success of the procedure.

• TABLE 38–1 • **Classification of Upper Extremity Amputation Levels**

Zone	Level
1	Finger distal to insertion of superficialis tendon
2	Finger proximal to insertion of superficialis tendon
3	Through the metacarpal
4	Through the wrist
5	Through the forearm distal to the musculotendinous junction
6	Through the forearm proximal to the musculotendinous junction
7	Through the elbow joint
8	Through the arm above the elbow
9	Through the thumb (specify level)
10	Amputation of multiple digits

Zone 7 is an amputation level through the elbow joint. In this group of patients, it is implied that replantation requires sacrifice of the elbow joint. Hence, at this level, the goal of converting an above-elbow amputation to functioning at the below-elbow level is less likely. The possibility remains, however, of restoring function to the wrist and hand, and this should be considered along with the proper position of the fused or ankylosed joint or later implantation of an elbow endoprosthesis.

Zone 6 involves the forearm below the elbow but above the musculotendinous junction. In this group, it is generally implied that a functioning below-elbow amputation already exists, so the success of the procedure depends on recovery of function to the wrist and hand.

INCIDENCE

The true incidence of replantation about the elbow is difficult to determine. Most reports on this topic involve only a few cases or a large series without clear differentiation of the level of injury or whether the injury was a complete or incomplete amputation. My review of the literature yielded 257 reported apparent major limb replantations.[3–7] Of this number, 47 were above-elbow (zone 8), 12 were trans-elbow (zone 7), and 33 were proximal forearm amputations (zone 6). Thus, 36 percent of reported major limb replantations are about the elbow region (Fig. 38–1).

MECHANISM OF INJURY

There is, of course, great variation in the mechanism of all traumatic amputations at any level; however, certain trends are apparent with patients with amputations about the elbow. In general, above-elbow amputations (zone 8) are usually violent avulsions frequently associated with other major injuries. In our practice, they are most often agricultural injuries produced by a tractor power takeoff or an auger device.

Trans-elbow amputations (zone 7), by contrast, are most often sharp, guillotine-type injuries, perhaps with some local crushing. The literature and our own experience suggest that these are more commonly nonagricultural industrial injuries or the result of vehicular accidents.

The proximal forearm group (zone 6) does not appear to be associated with a clear pattern of injury. Sharp severance, frank avulsion, and crush amputations have been reported resulting from industrial and recreational activities.

GOALS OF TREATMENT

The goals of limb replantation about the elbow should be the restoration of limb function to excede that possible at the level of injury by available limb prostheses (see Chapter 64). It cannot be overemphasized that this goal must be commensurate with the patient's medical condition, age, economic resources, wishes, and realistic expectations.

In zone 8 (above-elbow level), the minimum expectation should be conversion of an above-elbow amputation to a

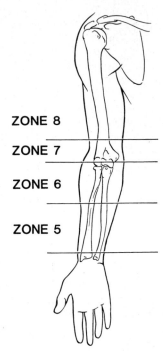

ZONE 8

ZONE 7

ZONE 6

ZONE 5

FIGURE 38–1 • Levels of amputation about the elbow.

functional below-elbow level. In zones 7 and 6, the minimal expectations should be a functioning hand unit that permits at least simple hook-grasp and prehension with protective sensibility.

INDICATIONS FOR REPLANTATION

The ideal situation for limb replantation about the elbow is a sharp, guillotine-type transsection that occurred as an isolated injury without direct damage to the elbow joint, with minimal contamination and minimal ischemic time in a young, emotionally stable patient. Unfortunately, the potential candidate most of us deal with strays from this description to a greater or lesser extent. Therefore, the indications for limb replantation about the elbow depend on a composite consideration of a number of factors, including the age and general medical condition of the patient, the presence of associated major injuries, the degree of damage within the amputated part, the duration of normothermic and hypothermic ischemia, the degree of wound contamination, and the mechanism of injury.[8]

Age. In general, age is a factor as it relates to the general medical state of the patient and to his or her economic situation in terms of a prolonged recovery and rehabilitation period. Limb replantation at this level is a major undertaking associated with prolonged anesthesia, considerable blood loss, possible metabolic acidosis, myoglobinemia and renal complications, and, frequently, multiple postreplantation surgical procedures. Maximal recovery is influenced primarily by the speed and adequacy of recovery of peripheral nerve function and may require a minimum of 2 or 3 years. Most authors agree that age 50 or 60 years, if the patient's general health is excellent, is the upper range for consideration of replantation at this level.[3]

Medical Condition of the Patient. For the reasons mentioned, a patient's medical condition may modify his or her candidacy for this procedure. Cardiopulmonary, peripheral vascular, renal, and metabolic factors require careful scrutiny. Not to be overlooked also is the psychiatric stability of the patient and his or her ability to deal with a prolonged rehabilitation program.

Associated Injuries. Associated injuries, particularly to the thorax and brachial plexus, are common. The appropriate management of open chest wounds should never be compromised by a zealous replantation effort and may be an absolute contraindication to the procedure. Brachial plexus avulsion should also be regarded as a contraindication[9] unless it is probably postganglionic and occurs in the very young patient. Head, abdominal, and other injuries require individual consideration and should be assigned appropriate priority.

Degree of Damage Within the Amputated Part. Injury distal to the site of amputation within the part is common. Although segmental vascular and nerve injuries can be successfully managed, they should be regarded as relative contraindications to replantation. Distal fractures should be evaluated and managed on their own merits and usually are not contraindications in themselves. Extreme distal crushing and shredding militates against consideration of replantation.

Ischemic Time. In any major limb amputation, the duration of normothermic and hypothermic ischemic time is critical.[9–15] Myonecrosis resulting in late irreversible loss of muscle function and immediate myoglobinemia and metabolic acidosis may become significant after 6 hours at room temperature and 12 hours with appropriate cooling. In general, revascularization of the part beyond these time limits is not advised.[3]

Degree of Wound Contamination. Because sepsis is one of the most common causes of failure with these patients,[16] the degree and type of wound contamination merits scrutiny. However, it is important to realize that radical débridement at the level of amputation with considerable skeletal shortening is both possible and advisable.[4] For this reason, a contaminated wound at the level of transsection frequently can be rendered tidy by appropriate débridement.

Mechanism of Injury. With any replantation procedure, sharp transsection is most ideal. Limited crush at the level of amputation is acceptable and can be managed by skeletal shortening. Massive crush is a definite contraindication to the procedure.[12, 17] Avulsion is a relative contraindication, depending on the extent of injury within the vascular structures. If limited, resection of the damaged structures and replacement by autogenous vein grafts may be possible.

MANAGEMENT

The initial management goal with these patients concerns successful general resuscitation. Control of bleeding at the level of amputation is typically not a major problem provided that the transsected vessels can retract. Bleeding is usually curtailed by direct pressure with a sterile compressive dressing. Direct clamping of the vessels in the proximal stump is to be avoided if at all possible because it may further damage the vessels more proximally.

The amputated part should be inspected to assess the level of injury, the presence of additional more distal injury in the limb, the degree of contamination, and, if possible, the mechanisms of injury. The transsected end should be thoroughly irrigated and a dressing moistened with saline or lactated Ringer's solution applied, and the amputated part should be placed in a clean or preferably sterile container. For amputations about the elbow, a sterile, surgical x-ray cassette polyethylene bag is convenient for this purpose. The wrapped limb should then be placed on ice in preparation for replantation.

The period after injury until re-establishment of circulation to the limb is critical for amputations about the elbow because of the large bulk of skeletal muscle within the severed part. These are true emergencies, and every effort should be made to minimize the period of ischemia and to cool the limb before reperfusion as efficiently as possible.[9, 10, 12, 18]

Surgical Technique

ORTHOTOPIC REPLANTATION

In the operating room, the initial goal of surgery is thorough and radical débridement of all obvious foreign material and contused or crushed skeletal muscle, both in the amputated part and proximally in the stump. Skeletal shortening is always carried out, at times for as much as 8 cm or more. Usually shortening is chiefly accomplished in the amputated segment unless this will compromise the integrity of the elbow joint or make internal skeletal fixation difficult. Although there is not uniform agreement, most authors believe that perfusion of the amputated part before replantation helps dilute accumulated toxic metabolites and lactic acid within the part.[1, 19] The author prefers to routinely perfuse the limb by gravity drip with 3 liters of lactated Ringer's solution containing one ampule of sodium bicarbonate per liter.

The process of reattachment begins with rigid osteosynthesis. The author prefers humeral or radial and ulnar osteosynthesis by compression plates. Trans-elbow injuries (zone 7) are not amenable to compression plate fixation and require Steinmann pins or Rush rods, often in conjunction with an exoskeletal fixation device. For amputations above the elbow (zone 8), bony fixation may be sufficiently stable to permit postoperative elevation of the limb by a skeletal traction pin in the olecranon (Fig. 38–2). This detail is extremely important for facilitating management of the wound and soft tissue defect, for minimizing postoperative lymphedema and fluid and protein losses, and for general nursing care.

After stabilization, repair of the remaining structures follows a sequential order from deep to superficial. We prefer large whipstitch coaptation of the muscle bellies, Bunnell crisscross, or Kessler side-locking sutures for cylindrical tendons (e.g., biceps), and multiple horizontal mattress sutures for flat tendons (e.g., triceps).

Nerve repairs should be executed carefully because they have a major influence on the ultimate functional result. The initial requirement in this regard is proper isolation

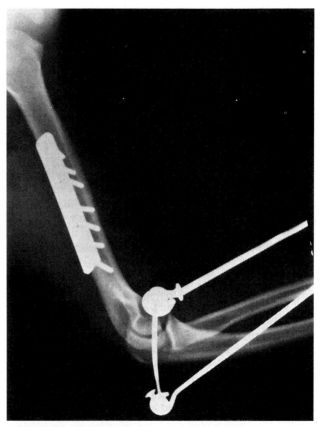

FIGURE 38–2 • Midhumeral replantation: immediate postoperative radiograph. Note the skeletal traction pin in the olecranon for elevation and the stable internal fixation plate.

and correct anatomic identification of the various nerves. No nerve length is débrided before the time of actual coaptation. At the time of neurorrhaphy, the nerve ends are resected, both proximally and distally, to a length that permits repair without tension. An epineural neurorrhaphy under magnification is then carried out. We prefer to accomplish this with multiple sutures of 8-0 nylon. There is no evidence to suggest that a group fascicular neurorrhaphy improves the quality of repair with this type of injury because it is impossible to be certain that the nerve ends are uninjured. Thus, extra surgical time expended on fascicular nerve repairs is not justified.

The vascular repairs are, of course, crucial to the immediate success of the procedure. In contrast to more distal replantations, in which the sequence of vascular repair is unimportant, for major limb reattachments, arterial repair should always precede the venous anastomoses. This is necessary because the reperfusion of the limb is urgent and the initial venous effluent containing high concentrations of lactic acid, myoglobin, and other myonecrotic products must be prevented from entering the central circulation. After arterial reperfusion of the limb is accomplished, multiple venous anastomoses should be carried out relatively swiftly to minimize blood loss and to curtail the massive swelling of the limb that characteristically occurs. In general, the more venous repairs accomplished, including both deep and superficial systems, the fewer are the problems related to swelling and fluid and protein losses

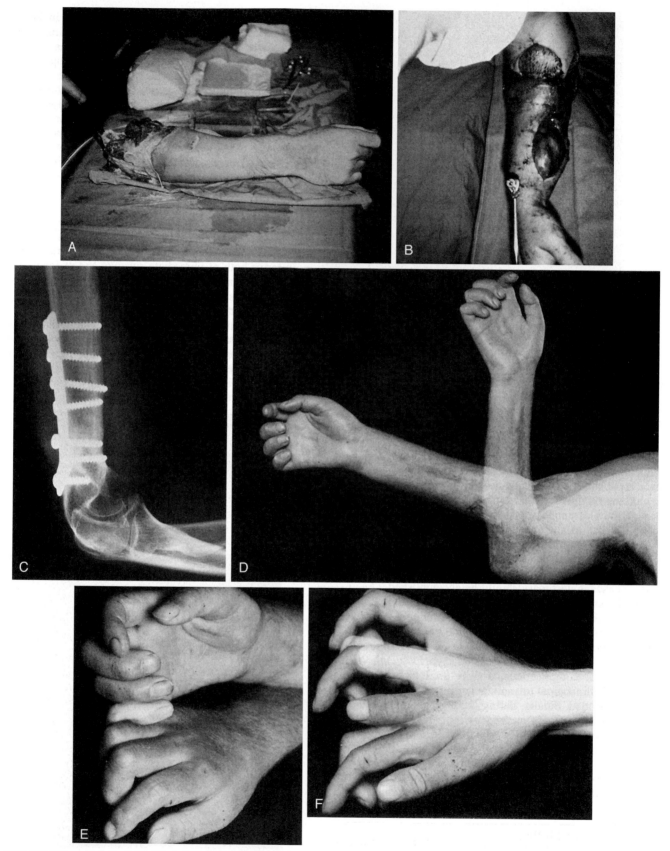

FIGURE 38–7 • *A*, Amputated limb, humeral supracondylar level. Note compression plate application and perfusion catheter in preparation for re-plantation. *B*, Immediate postoperative view. Note the open fasciotomy wounds and skeletal traction pin for elevation. *C*, Six months postoperatively. Note bone union at the replantation site. *D*, Range of active elbow flexion and extension. There was no interim surgery after replantation. *E*, Range of active forearm pronosupination. *F*, Range of active wrist extension and flexion.

larizations, with an overall limb survival rate of 73.4 percent.[3] Unfortunately, insufficient detail is usually given to allow assessment of the functional result at a given level.

At above-elbow levels (zone 8), we identified a limb survival rate of 50 percent among 36 cases.[1, 6, 7, 14, 22–32] Failure was due to sepsis in eight cases and to thrombosis in five, and death from intraoperative or postoperative complications occurred in four cases. Of the successful cases with a mean follow-up of 3.2 years, an average of 1.78 secondary procedures were necessary. Results in 9 of the 11 cases were rated good, and 2 were rated poor.

At the trans-elbow level (zone 7), only eight cases have been reported in detail,[22, 23, 25] with survival of the limb in seven. Of the five cases with sufficient follow-up, two were rated functionally good, one was fair, and two were poor.

At proximal forearm levels (zone 6) of 20 cases, with an overall limb survival rate of 65 percent,[23, 25, 26, 33–40] most failed because of vascular thrombosis. Of the eight survivors, one was rated functionally excellent, three were good, two were fair, and two were poor.

My experience with replantations about the elbow consists of 13 patients with follow-up of over 1 year. Overall, the limb survival rate is 69 percent. All the survivors have been rated functionally good to fair, although multiple secondary procedures are nearly always required for maximum function (mean, two procedures). Of the seven surviving patients with above-elbow replanted limbs, three achieved useful hand function in excess of that possible with a conventional prosthetic terminal device. The other four patients have regained good elbow control but do not have useful hand function.

COMPLICATIONS

Sepsis and vascular thrombosis are the chief complications leading to ultimate failure of the replantation effort. If the patient survives, poor recovery of neurologic function is the chief reason for an unsatisfactory functional outcome.

In addition, a spectrum of complications collectively called *replantation toxemia* may occur in this group,[10, 13–15, 41–43] particularly in above-elbow (zone 8) amputations. Included among these disturbances are metabolic acidosis from lactic acid accumulation in the limb,[41] hyperkalemia from excessive potassium losses from the limb,[44–46] and protein and fluid losses from edema of the replanted part.[10] Which of these factors, if any, are most important in terms of systemic effects is unclear. However, a number of deaths after major limb replantation have been attributed to toxemia.[5, 23, 26, 27] In addition, the renal complications occurring from myoglobinemia after replantation of a large amount of muscle undergoing rhabdomyolysis are perhaps of greater significance. Decreased limb ischemic time and effective cooling of the amputated part are thought to minimize the problems of toxemia as well as myoglobinemia.[10, 13, 14, 23, 41] In addition, preoperative perfusion of the amputated part, anastomosis of the arteries prior to veins, volume diuresis, alkalinization of the urine, and meticulous attention to serum electrolyte balance are helpful measures in preventing complications of this type.

AUTHOR'S PREFERRED TREATMENT METHOD

My preferred technique of limb replantation about the elbow was discussed earlier. I usually employ a prescribed protocol of monitoring and management. This includes serum electrolyte, lactate, arterial blood gases, and urine myoglobin levels and myoglobin determinations. Depending on the results of these studies, a high fluid diuresis is maintained by intravenous fluid and mannitol. Urine pH is monitored every 4 to 6 hours for the first 5 postoperative days, and sodium bicarbonate is used to maintain a urine pH above 6.0.

A broad-spectrum antibiotic, provided there is no allergic history to it, is given intravenously preoperatively and maintained postoperatively until wound culture results become available. Anticoagulation is usually limited to a combination of aspirin (10 grains) and dipyridamole (50 mg) three times a day postoperatively. In the absence of any bleeding difficulties, this regimen is continued for 2 to 4 weeks.

The principles of management can be synthesized, as applied in the following case report.

A 23-year-old farmer sustained an avulsion amputation of the right (dominant) upper limb at the supracondylar level of the humerus (Fig. 38–7A). After extensive débridement of the limb, perfusion with lactated Ringer's solution, and skeletal shortening, fixation was accomplished with an AO T-plate and seven screws (Fig. 38–7B). Triceps, biceps, and brachioradialis muscles or tendons, radial, ulnar, and median nerves; brachial artery; and four major veins were repaired in a 10-hour procedure. Revascularization was accomplished by 12.5 hours after injury with effective interim cooling. Volar forearm fasciotomy was done intraoperatively (Fig. 38–7C). The wounds were left open and the limb suspended in skeletal traction postoperatively. A high fluid output by intravenous fluid infusion and mannitol with alkalinization of the urine to maintain a urinary pH above 6.0 was carried out for the first 5 postoperative days. Serum myoglobin peaked at 25,000 ng/ml on the first postoperative day, but urinary myoglobin was negligible at 12 μg/ml. Serum myoglobin levels gradually decreased during the first postoperative week. Skin grafting was carried out 1, 3, and 4 weeks postoperatively, and the patient was released at 6 weeks. Bone union was confirmed at 6 months (Fig. 38–7D). At last evaluation, 22 months after the injury, the patient was an independent farmer, had good elbow and wrist control, was capable of light grasp activity, and had good protective tactile sensibility in the hand but poor pinch prehension (Figs. 38–7E–F). Functionally, the limb was used primarily in an assistive manner.

REFERENCES

1. Malt, R. A., and McKhann, C. F.: Replantation of the severed arm. J.A.M.A. **189**:114, 1964.
2. Malt, R. A., Remensynder, J. P., and Harris, W. H.: Longterm utility of replanted arms. Ann. Surg. **176**:334, 1972.
3. Results of microsurgery in orthopaedics. Committee on the Upper Extremity, American Academy of Orthopaedic Surgeons. Publication No. 6651981. June 4–5, 1981.
4. Balas, P.: The present status of replantation of amputated extremities. Vasc. Surg. **4**:190, 1970.

5. Engber, W. D., and Hardin, C. A.: Replantation of extremities. Surg. Gynecol. Obstet. **132**:901, 1971.
6. Nasseri, M., and Voss, H.: Late results of successful replantation of upper and lower extremities. Ann. Surg. **177**:121, 1973.
7. Shanghai Sixth People's Hospital: Extremity replantation. Chinese Med. J. **4**:5, 1978.
8. Bignardi, A., Barale, I., Leonardi, L., Rossi, F., Pisanu, R., Chiarpenello, R.: Reimplantation of the upper limb after tear lesion: long-term results. Chirg. Degli Organi di Movimento **82(4)**:409, 1997.
9. O'Brien, B. M., and Macleod, A. M.: *In* Daniller, A. I., and Strauch, B. (eds.): Symposium on Microsurgery. St. Louis, C. V. Mosby Co., 1976.
10. Eiken O., Nabseth, D. C., Mayer, R. F., and Deterling, R. A.: Limb replantation. Arch. Surg. **88**:70, 1964.
11. Fukunishi, H.: Studies on cause of shock following replantation of amputated extremity. J. Nara. Med. Assoc. **19**:127, 1968.
12. Herbsman, H., Lafer, D. J., and Shaftan, G. W.: Successful replantation of an amputated hand. Ann. Surg. **163**:137, 1966.
13. Kleinert, H. E., Jablon, M., and Tsai, T. M.: An overview of replantation and results of 347 replants in 245 patients. J. Trauma **20**:390, 1980.
14. McNeill, I. F., and Wilson, J. J. P.: The problems of limb replacement. Br. J. Surg. **57**:356, 1970.
15. Usui, M., Ishii, S., Muramatsu, J., and Takahata, N.: An experimental study on "replantation toxemia." J. Hand Surg. **3**:589, 1978.
16. Morrison, W. A., O'Brien, B. M., and Macleod, A. M.: Major limb replantation. Orthop. Clin. North Am. **8**:343, 1977.
17. O'Brien, B. M., Miller, G. D. H., Macleod, A. M., and Newing, R. K.: Saving the amputated digit and hand. Med. J. Aust. **1**:558, 1973.
18. O'Brien, B. M.: Replantation surgery in China. Med. J. Aust. **2**:255, 1974.
19. Shaftan, G. W., Herbsman, H., and Malt, R. A.: Replantation of limbs. Minn. Med. **48**:1645, 1965.
20. Carrel, A.: Results of transplantation of blood vessels, organs and limbs. J.A.M.A. **51**:1662, 1908.
21. Wood, M. B., and Cooney, W. P., III: Above-elbow limb replantation: Functional results. J. Hand Surg. **11A**:682, 1986.
22. Christeas, N., Balas, P., and Giannikas, A.: Replantation of amputated extremities. Am. J. Surg. **118**:68, 1969.
23. Ferriera, M. C., Marques, E. F., and Azze, R. J.: Limb replantation. Clin. Plast. Surg. **5**:211, 1978.
24. Halmagyi, A. F., Baker, C. B., Campbell, H. H., Evans, J. G., and Mahoney, L. J.: Reimplantation of a completely severed arm followed by reamputation because of failure of reinnervation. Can. J. Surg. **12**:222, 1969.
25. Ikuta, Y.: Method of bone fixation in reattachment of amputations in the upper extremities. Clin. Orthop. **133**:169, 1978.
26. O'Brien, B. M., Macleod, A. M., Hayhurst, J. W., Morrison, W. A., and Ishida, H.: Major replantation surgery in the upper limb. Hand **6**:217, 1974.
27. Peking Trauma Hospital: Replantation of severed limbs. Chinese Med. J. **1**:265, 1975.
28. Rosenkrantz, J. G., Sullivan, R. C., Welch, K., Miles, J. S., Salder, K. M., and Paton, B. C.: Replantation of an infant's arm. N. Engl. J. Med. **276**:609, 1967.
29. Shaftan, G. W., and McAlvanah, M. J.: *In* Daniller, A. I., and Strauch, B. (eds.): Symposium on Microsurgery. St. Louis, C. V. Mosby Co., 1976.
30. Ts'ui, C., Feng, Y., T'ang, C., et al.: Microvascular anastomosis and transplantation. Chinese Med. J. **85**:610, 1966.
31. Williams, G. R., Carter, D. R., Frank, G. R., and Price, W. E.: Replantation of amputated extremities. Ann. Surg. **163**:758, 1966.
32. Wright, P. E.: Convention Report, 67th Annual Meeting of the Clinical Orthopaedic Society **3**:1, 1979.
33. Ch'en, C. W., Ch'ien, Y. C., and Pao, Y. S.: Further experiences in the restoration of amputated limbs. Chinese Med. J. **82**:633, 1963.
34. Ch'en, C. W., Ch'ien, Y. C., and Pao, Y. S.: Further experiences in the restoration of amputated limbs. Chinese Med. J. **84**:225, 1965.
35. Ch'en, C. W., Qian, Y. Q., and Yu, Z. J.: Extremity replantation. World J. Surg. **2**:513, 1978.
36. Paletta, F. X., Willman, V., and Ship, A. G.: Prolonged tourniquet ischemia of extremities. J. Bone Joint Surg. **42A**:945, 1960.
37. Ramirez, M. Z., Duque, M., Hernandez, L., Londono, A., and Cadvid, G.: Reimplantation of limbs. Plast. Reconstr. Surg. **40**:315, 1967.
38. Shorey, W. D., Schneewind, J. H., and Paul, H. A.: Significant factors in the reimplantation of an amputated hand. Bull. Soc. Int. Chir. **24**:44, 1965.
39. Tamai, S., Hori, Y., Tatsumi, Y., et al.: Major limb, hand and digital replantation. World J. Surg. **3**:17, 1979.
40. Worman, L. W., Darin, J. C., and Kritter, A. E.: The anatomy of a limb replantation failure. Arch. Surg. **91**:211, 1965.
41. Mehl, R. L., Paul, H. A., Shorey, W., Schneewind, J., and Beattie, E. J.: Treatment of "toxemia" after extremity replantation. Arch. Surg. **89**:871, 1964.
42. Shaw, R. S.: Treatment of the extremity suffering near or total severance with special consideration of the vascular problem. Clin. Orthop. **29**:56, 1963.
43. Snyder, C. C., Knowles, R. P., Mayer, P. W., and Hobbs, J. C.: Extremity replantation. Plast. Reconstr. Surg. **26**:251, 1960.
44. Kohama, A.: Changes following recirculation of ischemic leg. Cent. Jpn. Orthop. Trauma **12**:555, 1969.
45. Meer, D. C., Valkenburg, P. W., Ariens, A. T., and Benthem, R. V.: Cause of death in tourniquet shock in rats. Am. J. Physiol. **21**:513, 1966.
46. Onji, Y., Kohama, A., Tamai, S., Fukunishi, H., and Komtsui, S.: Metabolic alteration following replantation of an amputated extremity. J. Jpn. Orthop. Assoc. **41**:55, 1967.

Sports and Overuse Injuries to the Elbow

• CHAPTER 39 •

Arthroscopy

Portals in Elbow Arthroscopy

• FELIX H. SAVOIE, III, and LARRY D. FIELD

As noted in the following, arthroscopy of the elbow may be hazardous to important nearby nerves and vessels. The portals described for the elbow are based on avoiding these neurovascular structures. Proper portal placement and careful technique can significantly diminish the risk to these structures.[1]

Patient positioning for elbow arthroscopy can be supine, prone, or lateral decubitus, based on the surgeon's experience and preference. Supine positioning provides for easier administration of anesthesia, better anterior compartment access, and easier conversion to open procedures. The drawbacks to supine positioning include limited access to the posterior compartment and the need for special equipment to hold the arm or for an assistant. The prone position allows improved access to the posterior compartment compared to the supine position, and an assistant is not required. However, this position may not be tolerated by some patients undergoing regional anesthesia, and conversion to an open anterior procedure may require repositioning. The advantages of the lateral decubitus position are similar to those of prone positioning, and anesthesia access is improved. A special arm bolster is needed for this position, and as with prone positioning the patient may require repositioning for open procedures other than posterior procedures.

A tourniquet is usually used in elbow arthroscopy. Once inflated, sterile preparation and draping is accomplished. The external anatomy is drawn on the arm. Portals should be created with a fully distended joint, and the elbow flexed to 90 degrees, especially while one creates anterior portals, to provide maximum clearance of neurovascular structures.[2] Posterior portal placement may require slight extension. All incisions are made through the skin, followed by blunt dissection with a hemostat and the use of a blunt trochar to enter the joint capsule.

The preferred starting portal continues to be a subject of controversy. Some authors believe starting at the proximal anteromedial portal decreases the risk to the radial nerve[3]; however, others have promoted a lateral starting position with success, especially with the description and use of the proximal lateral portal.[4] The surgeon's preference, based on knowledge of the local anatomy and his or her experience, should determine the starting point.

PROXIMAL PORTALS

Anteromedial Portal

The proximal anteromedial portal was first described by Poehling and colleagues[5] and is used primarily in the prone or lateral decubitus position. It is located 2 cm proximal to the medial epicondyle and immediately anterior to the intermuscular septum (Fig. 39–1). The ulnar nerve, which is the primary structure at risk, is approximately 4 mm from this site.[6] Other structures that are at risk include the medial antebrachial cutaneous nerve, median nerve, and brachial artery. This portal allows visualization of the anterior compartment, which includes the trochlea, medial gutter, coronoid process, medial condyle, radial head, capitellum, and annular ligament. We agree with others that this portal is more safe than the standard anteromedial portal, as it is farther from the median nerve, rather parallel to it, and the nerve is protected by the substance of the brachialis muscle.[7]

Anterolateral Portal

The proximal anterolateral portal is located 2 cm proximal and 1 cm anterior to the lateral epicondyle (Fig. 39–2). This portal is significantly farther (average 13.7 mm) from the radial nerve than other anterolateral portal sites as demonstrated by Field and associates.[4] Through this portal, excellent visualization of the anterior radiohumeral and ulnohumeral joints, and anterior capsular margin can be achieved.

Posterolateral Portal

Anatomically, this portal boasts the largest area of safety. Traditionally, this portal is placed 3 cm proximal to the olecranon, lateral to the triceps tendon, and posterior to the

505

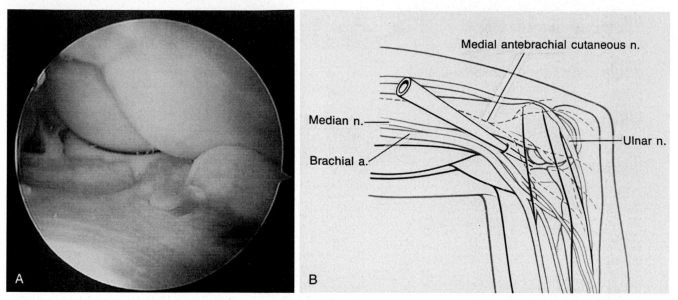

FIGURE 39–1 • Proximal anteromedial portal. *A,* Anterosuperior medial portal (proximal anteromedial portal). *B,* Illustration of gross anatomy.

lateral epicondylar ridge (Fig. 39–3). The elbow is held in 20 degrees to 30 degrees of flexion while this portal is established in order to relax the triceps and posterior capsule. Structures at risk when this incision is made include the posterior antebrachial cutaneous and the lateral brachial cutaneous nerves as well as the triceps tendon itself.

The posterolateral portal provides access to the olecranon fossa, medial and lateral gutters, and the posterior radiocapitellar joint. As an operative portal, its primary uses are for posterolateral plica excision and lateral osteophyte débridement. It can also be useful in initiating ulnohumeral arthroplasty and excision of the olecranon tip. If necessary, the entire posterolateral side of the elbow is accessible for portal placement from the soft spot to the standard posterolateral portal.[8]

Posterocentral Portal

This portal has also been called the transtriceps and straight posterior portal. It is located midline through the triceps 3 cm proximal to the olecranon tip (see Fig. 39–3). The entire posterior aspect of the elbow, including the medial and lateral gutters, olecranon fossa, and olecranon, can be visualized and instrumented. This portal is used as a working portal for loose body removal, osteophyte resection, posterior synovectomy, and ulnohumeral arthroplasty.

DISTAL PORTALS

Straight Lateral Portal

The straight lateral portal is created by an incision directly over the radiocapitellar joint. Visualization is limited owing to the acute nature of the portal; however, the portal can be shifted anteriorly to visualize the anterior joint or posteriorly to assess the posterolateral gutter, posterolateral radial head, capitellum, trochlear notch, and olecranon. As a working portal, it is useful around the lateral epicondyle

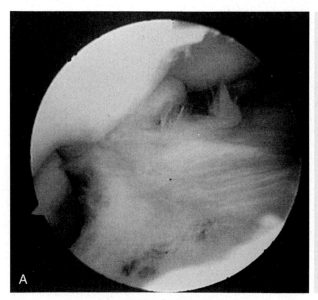

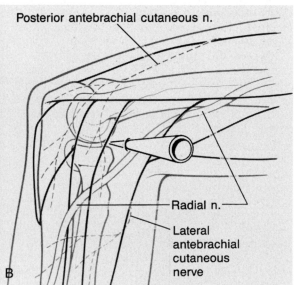

FIGURE 39–2 • Proximal anterolateral portal. *A,* Arthroscopic view from the anterolateral portal. *B,* Illustration of gross anatomy.

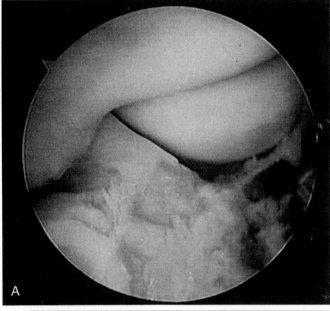

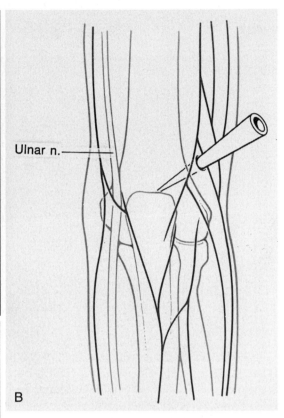

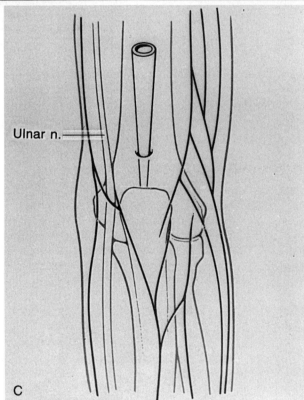

FIGURE 39–3 • Posterolateral/posterocentral portals. *A*, Arthroscopic view of the lateral gutter from the posterolateral portals. *B*, Illustration of gross anatomy. *C*, Illustration of gross anatomy.

and posterolateral gutter. The primary structure at risk here is the radiocapitellar joint itself.

Soft Spot

The soft spot is a variation of the straight lateral portal (Fig. 39–4). As discussed previously, the entire posterolateral aspect of the elbow can be accessed via a portal for visualization of the lateral gutter and posterior radiocapitellar joint. This portal allows evaluation of posterolateral rotatory instability, osteochondritis dessicans of the capitellum, radial head pathology, and posterior meniscoid liai-

sons, as well as posterolateral synovial plicae. The primary structures at risk here include the radiocapitellar joint and the ulnohumeral joint.

Anteromedial Portal

The anteromedial portal is located 2 cm distal and 2 cm lateral to the medial epicondyle (Fig. 39–5). This portal provides a view of the anterior compartment, as described for the proximal anteromedial portal. The structures at risk with this portal include the medial antebrachial cutaneous nerve, the median nerve, and the brachial artery. Stothers

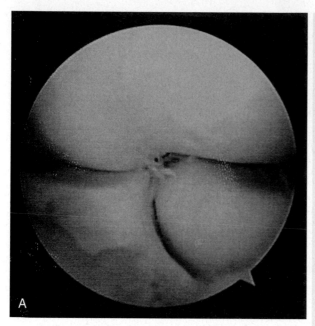

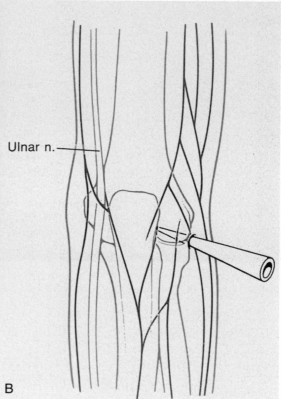

FIGURE 39–4 • Soft spot portal. A, Arthroscopic view from the soft spot portal revealing the posterior aspect of the radiocapitellar joint and proximal radioulnar articulation. B, Illustration of gross anatomy.

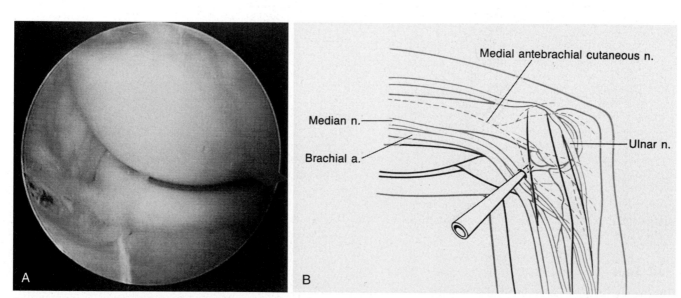

FIGURE 39–5 • Anteromedial portal. A, Arthroscopic view from the anteromedial portal showing the anterior aspect of the radiocapitellar joint. B, Illustration of gross anatomy.

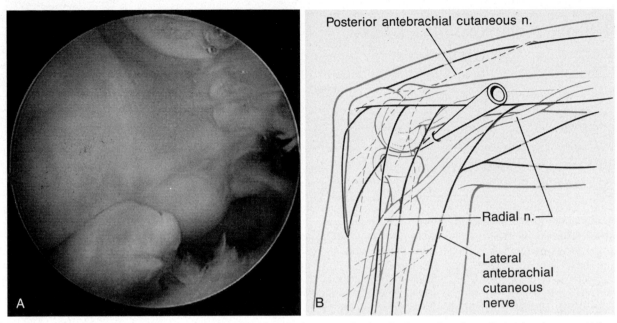

FIGURE 39–6 • Anterolateral portal. *A,* Arthroscopic view from the anterosuperior (proximal anterolateral portal) showing the coronoid fossa, coronoid process, and trochlea. *B,* Illustration of gross anatomy.

and associates[9] recorded an average distance 7 mm to the median nerve with the joint distended and flexed. Therefore, to increase the margin of safety, use of the proximal medial portal is preferred in most situations.

Anterolateral Portal

Originally described by Andrews and Carson,[1] the anterolateral portal is located 3 cm distal and 1 cm anterior to the lateral epicondyle (Fig. 39–6). Most surgeons stay more proximal because the original description places perilous risk to the radial nerve.[2] It is located 4 to 7 mm[1, 2] from the radial nerve and 1 to 14 mm from the posterior interosseous nerve.[10] Other at-risk structures include the anterior branch of the posterior antebrachial cutaneous nerve and the lateral antebrachial cutaneous nerve.

This portal allows visualization of the medial elbow joint, including the coronoid process, the trochlea, the coronoid fossa, and the brachialis insertion. The anterior radioulnar joint and the medial aspect of the radial head may also be seen.

Transhumeral Portal

The transhumeral portal is rarely used, but it provides an additional access to the anterior compartment. A posterocentral portal is created, followed by a fenestration technique through the distal humerus. If the medial and lateral columns of the humerus remain intact, the structural integrity of the humerus will not be compromised. This portal is most commonly useful for débriding those patients with primary arthritis and is sometimes used for restricted anteromedial access because of ulnar nerve transposition.[9]

Summary

Recent advances in elbow arthroscopy have made numerous elbow conditions more readily treatable through the use of elbow arthroscopy. However, the primary risks of this procedure continue to involve damage to surrounding neurovascular structures. In order to minimize these risks and maximize success, a thorough understanding of the pertinent anatomy is mandatory and a specific routine of set-up, portal placement, and arthroscopic examination should be followed. Doing so will ensure the safe and effective use of elbow arthroscopy and provide a rewarding experience to both the patient and the surgeon.

REFERENCES

1. Andrews, J., and Carson, W.: Arthroscopy of the elbow. Arthroscopy **1**:97, 1985.
2. Lynch, G., Meyers, J. F., Whipple, T. L., and Caspari, R. B.: Neurovascular anatomy and elbow arthroscopy: Inherent risks. Arthroscopy **2**:191, 1986.
3. Verhaar, J., van Mameren, H., and Brandsma, A.: Risks of neurovascular injury in elbow arthroscopy: Starting anteromedially or anterolaterally? Arthroscopy **7**:287, 1991.
4. Field, L., Altchek, D. W., Warren, R. F., O'Brien, S. J., Skyhar, M. J., and Wickiewicz, T. L.: Arthroscopic anatomy of the lateral elbow: A comparison of three portals. Arthroscopy **10**:602, 1994.
5. Poehling, G.C., Goldman, B., Sisco, L., and Whipple, T. L.: Elbow arthroscopy: A new technique. Arthroscopy **5**:222, 1989.
6. Adolfsson, L.: Arthroscopy of the elbow joint: A cadaveric study of portal placement. J. Shoulder Elbow Surg. **3**:53, 1994.
7. Plancher, K. D., Peterson, R. K., and Brezenhoff, L.: Diagnostic arthroscopy of the elbow: Set-up, portals and technique. Operative Techniques Sports Med. **6**:2, 1998.
8. Savoie, F. H., and Field, L. D.: Arthroscopy of the Elbow. New York, Churchill Livingstone, 1996.
9. Stothers, K., Day, B., and Reagan, W. R.: Arthroscopy of the elbow: Anatomy, portal sites, and description of the proximal lateral portal. Arthroscopy **11**:449, 1995.
10. Marshall, P., Day, B., and Reagan, W. R.: Avoiding nerve damage during elbow arthroscopy. J. Bone Joint Surg. **75B**:129, 1993.

ACKNOWLEDGMENT • Malcolm Stubbs, M.D., Fellow in Sports Medicine, Mississippi Sports Medicine and Orthopaedic Center, Jackson, Mississippi.

Elbow Arthroscopy: Loose Bodies

• SHAWN W. O'DRISCOLL

PREOPERATIVE DIAGNOSIS AND EVALUATION

The most common, and perhaps the most useful indication for elbow arthroscopy is for the removal of suspected or diagnosed loose bodies.[4, 15, 18, 19] We must realize that our patients are becoming increasingly conscious of the expanding role of arthroscopy of the elbow, as with arthroscopy of other areas; thus, familiarity with it as a diagnostic and therapeutic tool is valuable.[1, 2, 4, 5, 7, 8, 10–17, 19, 22, 24–26, 30] Although some patients will indeed undergo elbow arthroscopy for diagnostic reasons, we must realize that the history and physical and radiographic examination determine whether the procedure is indicated. Loose bodies are to be suspected in a patient with mechanical symptoms, including locking, catching, or snapping, and are often seen in association with degenerative changes, such as osteophytes on the olecranon and coronoid, and in their respective fossae. In other words, loose bodies often signify something more important and general. They rarely *cause* flexion contractures—patients with such contractures almost always have associated posterior impinging osteophytes on the olecranon and in the olecranon fossa, as part of an early degenerative process. This can be further assessed by lateral tomography.

Standard anteroposterior and lateral radiographs are obtained routinely, and oblique views are sometimes helpful. Unfortunately, as many as 30 percent of loose bodies are not detected on plain radiographs.[18, 19, 23, 29] O'Driscoll and Morrey reported 23 patients with loose bodies, of whom 7 were not diagnosed by the preoperative anteroposterior and lateral radiographs.[20] All of these loose bodies were in the posterior compartment of the elbow. A total of 5 of the 23 patients had multiple loose bodies, the number ranging from 2 to 4. In 4 of the 5 patients, more loose bodies were demonstrated by arthroscopy than were seen on the preoperative radiographs. In 2 patients, loose bodies were found in both the anterior and the posterior compartments, in 7 patients they were in the anterior compartment only, and 14 patients had loose bodies only in the posterior compartment. Thus, it is wise to thoroughly evaluate the entire elbow at the time of arthroscopy so that none are missed. All patients undergoing arthroscopy for the removal of anterior loose bodies should also undergo the procedure in the posterior compartment as well. Especially in degenerative conditions, one will often find loose bodies "that are not loose"; that is, that are stuck in the soft tissues and only minimally mobile (Fig. 39–7). However, these are prone to painful impingement in the olecranon or coronoid fossae.

Magnetic resonance imaging and computed tomographic arthrography occasionally are indicated and can be helpful in establishing the diagnosis of loose bodies or synovial diseases. Ward and co-workers[29] correlated preoperative plain radiographs and arthrotomograms with arthroscopic findings in 37 elbows and found that arthrotomograms were 100 percent sensitive and 71 percent specific. In clinical practice, however, it is useful to determine whether the patient is experiencing symptoms of a severity sufficient to justify arthroscopic intervention, because, if so, it may be more appropriate to proceed straight to the ultimate imaging modality—the arthroscope.

Preoperatively, one must ascertain whether the ulnar nerve subluxates or dislocates anteriorly. If it does—which has been found to be the case in 16 percent of the population[6]—it may be at risk for injury when the anterior medial portal is established.

SURGICAL TECHNIQUE

In addition to standard equipment, one should use a sheath that fits inside the plastic cannulae for two reasons. First, this permits one to move the scope into the portals occupied by the plastic cannulae. More importantly, when a portal is "lost"—that is, when a cannula slips out or is pulled out with an instrument or during loose body removal—it takes but a few seconds to re-establish it by passing the scope out through the portal, reinserting the cannula into the joint over that scope, and drawing the scope back into the joint. This technique is extremely important in elbow arthroscopy. A variety of hand-held graspers, power shaver blades and burrs, and even osteotomes are used. A sharp 4-mm Steinmann pin that has been smoothed off to a blunted conical tip at the end is useful for the switch-stick technique. Additional plastic cannulae are necessary. I prefer smooth ones (versus those with threads on the outer surface) because they can be moved in and out readily, which is necessary for certain maneuvers, although they have the disadvantage of sometimes slipping out.

Ideal portal location for removing posterior compartment loose bodies can be confirmed by placement of a needle prior to their removal (Fig. 39–8). Loose bodies are removed with various-sized graspers that have teeth. Those that are smooth on their outside surface, without irregular surfaces or corners, work best, as they do not catch on the soft tissues as they exit the elbow. Always grasp loose bodies so that they can be pulled out longitudinally, rather than obliquely or transversely, which often requires that they be rotated into position for the grasper. Grasp them *very* firmly if possible. Some are quite soft and will be crushed if one is not careful. Rotate them fully so as to confirm that they are not still attached to soft tissue prior to extraction. Observe the fragment until it exits the capsule so that it can be recovered if lost from the jaws of the grasper. Check each one after extraction, to confirm that a fragment has not broken off in the soft tissues. Rotate the loose body in the soft tissues to "work it out." A large loose body in the anterior elbow can be pushed out with the sheath of the scope (uncouple and back the scope itself out of the sheath a few millimeters to avoid damaging the lens) while it is pulled with the grasper (Fig. 39–9). Finally,

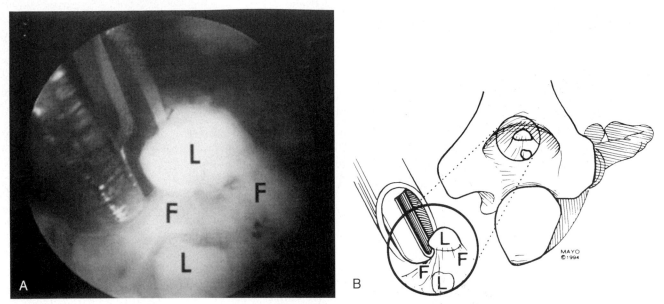

FIGURE 39–7 • *A* and *B,* Loose bodies (L) "that are not loose." Often, loose bodies can be found embedded in the synovium and fibrous scar tissue (F), such as in the olecranon fossa. It is necessary to clear such tissue to ensure no loose bodies are present.

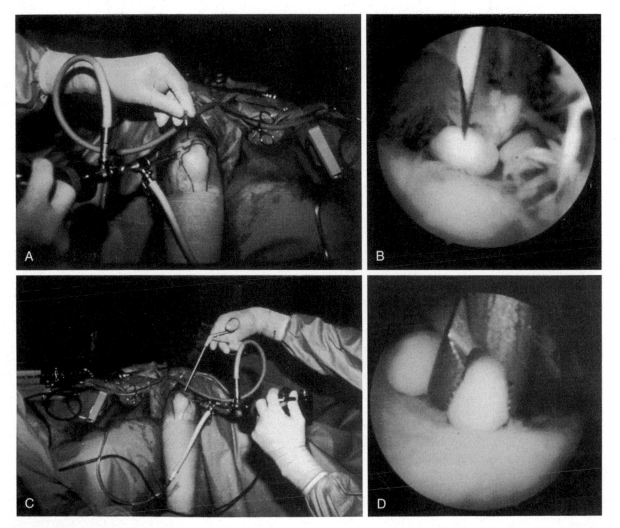

FIGURE 39–8 • Locating and removing posterior loose bodies. *A* and *B,* A needle is inserted into the joint under direct vision to confirm ideal portal placement. *C* and *D,* The grasper is inserted through the portal at the same site.

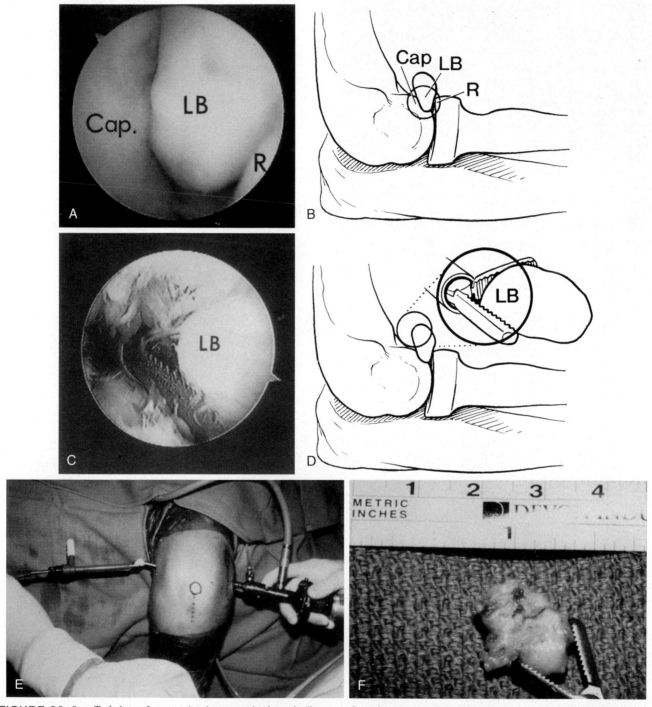

FIGURE 39–9 • Techniques for removing large anterior loose bodies up to 2 centimeters. *A* and *B,* Very large loose body (LB), from osteochondritis dissecans, between the capitellum (Cap.) and radial head (R). *C* and *D,* A grasper (preferably large, with teeth) is inserted from the medial side. *E,* As the grasper is withdrawn against the cannula, the scope is advanced against the loose body, uncoupled from the sheath, and the scope sheath used to *push* the loose body out while it pulled by the grasper. The cannula of course exits with the loose body, but is simply reinserted over the scope sheath. *F,* The cannula acts as a dilator ahead of the loose body, and also helps to prevent prominences such as those seen on this loose body from catching up in the soft tissues.

do not hesitate to enlarge the portal somewhat. Otherwise, the fragment could be lost in the soft tissues.

RESULTS

The procedure can be said to be of therapeutic benefit to the patient if it is (1) completely successful and obviates the need for any further surgery; (2) partially successful, in that the patient is clinically improved and needs no further surgery; or (3) adjunctive, in that an important part of the operation is performed arthroscopically *and* the arthroscopy directs the surgical intervention in an important manner.

In a risk-to-benefit analysis of 71 consecutive arthroscopies, we found that 70 percent were therapeutically beneficial.[19] Loose body removal was the most successful. All patients with isolated loose bodies benefited from the procedure.

Removal of loose bodies has been found by all authors to prove successful in 90 percent or more of patients.[4, 15, 18-23, 28] Ogilvie-Harris and Schemitsch[23] reported successful outcomes in 89 percent of 34 patients with loose bodies. It is important to recognize that removal of loose bodies alone does not help patients with osteoarthritis.[18, 19, 23]

Arthroscopic treatment of osteochondritis dissecans can be very successful if the symptoms are related primarily to loose bodies.[1, 2, 4, 9, 11] Jackson and associates[11] found, however, that a return to full painless elbow function is unlikely in high-level female gymnasts once the main fragment became detached. Long-term follow-up will be required to confirm the results, as Bauer and colleagues[3] have demonstrated in a 23-year follow-up report of 321 patients with osteochondritis dissecans of the ankle that 50 percent had arthritic changes.

Redden and Stanley[27] reported that 12 of 12 patients with osteoarthritis and loose bodies benefited from arthroscopic removal of osteophytes and loose bodies. They performed their procedure in a manner similar to the open Outerbridge-Kashiwagi procedure, with fenestration of the distal humerus through the olecranon fossa to the coronoid fossa. They did not notice any improvement in elbow range of motion, presumably because they did not release the capsular contractures present.

TIPS

- If the reason for arthroscopy is removal of a loose body, go for it first. Spending too much time with multiple diagnostic portals can cause edema that obscures the field.
- Large anterior loose bodies (up to 2 cm) can best be removed through arthroscopic portals after being firmly grasped by uncoupling the scope and retracting it a few millimeters into the sheath, advancing the scope sheath up against the loose body, and *pushing* the loose body out through the opposite portal, together with the plastic cannula in that portal, while pulling with the grasper. This prevents loss of the loose body in the soft tissues. The cannula is then reinserted over the scope sheath, and the scope is coupled in the sheath and redrawn back into

the joint. The presence of the cannula is helpful because it keeps the soft tissue track "dilated" ahead of the loose body during its removal.

- If one loses an anterior portal by withdrawing an instrument too far, advance the instrument in the opposite portal across the elbow and out the empty portal, and then insert a cannula over it, or a blunt Steinmann pin inside it to allow reinsertion of the appropriate instrument.
- Removal of loose bodies without excision of osteophytes does not help patients with osteoarthritis.
- There are usually more loose bodies than seen on the x-ray.
- Learn to *work fast*. Elapsed time is a handicap, as it means more intra-articular edema and periarticular soft tissue swelling, both of which make the work more difficult.

REFERENCES

1. Andrews, J. R., and Carson, W. G.: Arthroscopy of the elbow. Arthroscopy. **1:**97, 1985.
2. Andrews, J. R., St. Pierre, R. K., and Carson, W. G.: Arthroscopy of the elbow. Clin. Sport Med. **5:**653, 1986.
3. Bauer, M., Jonsson, K., and Linden, B.: Osteochondritis dissecans of the ankle: A 20-year follow-up study. J. Bone Joint Surg. **69B:**93, 1987.
4. Boe, S.: Arthroscopy of the elbow: Diagnosis and extraction of loose bodies. Acta Orthop Scand. **57:**52, 1986.
5. Carson, W.: Arthroscopy of the elbow. Instr. Course Lect. **37:**195, 1988.
6. Childress, H. M.: Recurrent ulnar nerve dislocation at the elbow. Clin. Orthop. **108:**168, 1975.
7. Clarke, R.: Symptomatic, lateral synovial fringe (plica) of the elbow joint. Arthroscopy **4:**112, 1988.
8. Commandre, F., Taillan, B., Benezis, C., Follacci, F., and Hammou, J.: Plica synovialis (synovial fold) of the elbow: Report on one case. J. Sports Med. Phys. Fit. **28:**209, 1988.
9. Fixsen, J. A., and Maffulli, N.: Bilateral intra-articular loose bodies of the elbow in an adolescent BMX rider. Injury **20:**303, 1989.
10. Guhl, J.: Arthroscopy and arthroscopic surgery of the elbow. Orthopedics **8:**1290, 1985.
11. Jackson, D., Silvino, N., and Reiman, P.: Osteochondritis in the female gymnast's elbow. Arthroscopy **5:**129, 1989.
12. Johnson, L. L.: Arthroscopic Surgery: Principles and Practice. St. Louis, CV Mosby, 1986, pp. 1451–1475.
13. Lindenfeld, T. N.: Medial approach in elbow arthroscopy. Am. J. Sports Med. **18:**413, 1990.
14. Lynch, G., Meyers, J., Whipple, T., and Caspari, R.: Neurovascular anatomy and elbow arthroscopy: Inherent risks. Arthroscopy **2:**191, 1986.
15. McGinty, J.: Arthroscopic removal of loose bodies. Orthop. Clin. North Am. **13:**313, 1982.
16. Morrey, B. F.: Arthroscopy of the elbow. *In* Morrey, B. F. (ed.): The Elbow and Its Disorders. Philadelphia, W. B. Saunders, 1985, pp. 114–121.
17. Morrey, B. F.: Arthroscopy of the elbow. Instr. Course Lec. **35:**102, 1986.
18. O'Driscoll, S. W.: Elbow arthroscopy for loose bodies. Orthopedics **15:**855, 1992.
19. O'Driscoll, S. W., and Morrey, B. F.: Arthroscopy of the elbow: Diagnostic and therapeutic benefits and hazards. J. Bone Joint Surg. **74A:**84, 1992.
20. O'Driscoll, S. W., and Morrey, B. F.: Loose bodies of the elbow: Diagnostic and therapeutic roles of arthroscopy (Abstract). J. Bone Joint Surg. **74B(suppl III):**290, 1992.
21. O'Driscoll, S. W., and Morrey, B. F.: Arthroscopy of the elbow. *In* Morrey, B. F. (ed.): The Elbow and Its Disorders. Philadelphia, W. B. Saunders,1993, pp. 120–130.
22. O'Driscoll, S. W., and Morrey, B. F.: Arthroscopy of the elbow: Master techniques in orthopedic surgery. *In* Morrey, B. F. (ed.): The Elbow. New York, Raven Press, 1994, pp. 21–34.

23. Ogilvie-Harris, D. J., and Schemitsch, E.: Arthroscopy of the elbow for removal of loose bodies. Arthroscopy **9**:5, 1993.
24. Papilion, J., Neff, R., and Shall, L.: Compression neuropathy of the radial nerve as a complication of elbow arthroscopy: A case report and review of the literaturel. Arthroscopy **4**:284, 1988.
25. Poehling, G., Whipple, T., Sisco, L., and Goldman, B.: Elbow arthroscopy: A new technique. Arthroscopy **5**:222, 1989.
26. Poehling, G. G., and Ekman, E. F.: Arthroscopy of the elbow. J. Bone Joint Surg. **76A**:1265, 1994.
27. Redden, J. F., and Stanley, D.: Arthroscopic fenestration of the olecranon fossa in the treatment of osteoarthritis of the elbow. Arthroscopy **9**:14, 1993.
28. Ward, W. G., and Anderson, T. E.: Elbow arthroscopy in a mostly athletic population. J. Hand Surg. **18A**:220, 1993.
29. Ward, W. G., Belhobek, G. H., and Anderson, T. E.: Arthroscopic elbow findings: Correlation with preoperative radiographic studies. Arthroscopy **8**:498, 1992.
30. Woods, G.: Elbow arthroscopy. Clin. Sports Med. **6**:557, 1987.

Arthroscopy: Débridement

• EVAN F. EKMAN and NEIL S. ELATTRACHE

Débridement during elbow arthroscopy is useful in many pathologic conditions. This section of the chapter will focus on débridement specifically as it pertains to issues not discussed in "loose bodies" or "capsular release."

TECHNIQUE

Original work in elbow arthroscopy was done with the patient in the supine position.[1] In the recent past, a prone technique, and a lateral decubitis modification of the prone technique, have been described.[12] Each technique has its advantages (and advocates who espouse them). Common to all techniques is the following: an elbow arthroscopist needs an intimate knowledge of the anatomy of the elbow, as well as regional neurovascular anatomy, surface anatomy, and compartment anatomy.[11] Perhaps more than in other joints, drawing local anatomic landmarks, neurovascular structures, and portal positions is of use in safeguarding against neurovascular injury.[10] Pre-insufflation of the joint with fluid, and flexing the elbow during portal placement moves neurovascular structures away from articular surfaces, also decreasing the chance of morbidity from portal placement.[9] This maneuver does not, however, separate the capsule from the neural structures.

Indications for Arthroscopic Débridement

The indications for arthroscopic débridement are evolving, since this procedure is still a relatively new technique. As its role in some pathologic conditions is being established investigators are assessing other conditions in which arthroscopic débridement may have a role. Specifically, arthroscopic débridement is effective in treating situations in which cartilage and bone are débrided (osteophytosis, osteochondritis dessicans, Panner's disease, post-traumatic osteoarthritis) and in situations where tissue of synovial

origin is primarily débrided (rheumatoid arthritis,[8] pigmented villonodular synovitis, synovial chondromatosis).[4] Arthroscopic débridement is also effective in sepsis of the elbow joint.

OSTEOPHYTOSIS

Osteophytes occur in a variety of elbow conditions, creating pain and sometimes limiting motion.

Olecranon osteophytosis can occur in the overhead and, specifically, the throwing athlete from posterior compartment extension overload.[15] During the deceleration phase of the throw, the forearm must be halted. While the elbow flexors and extensors are primarily responsible for this,[13] the articulation between the olecranon and the olecranon fossa often becomes the final decelerator. This process can create a spectrum of injuries, which includes posteromedial olecranon osteophytosis, loose bodies, and fibrosis in the olecranon fossa.[7, 15] Posteromedial olecranon osteophyte débridement (Fig. 39–10), as well as débridement of scar in the olecranon fossa, can decrease pains, and sometimes improve motion (Figs. 39–11 and 39–12). Keep in mind the following three notes of caution: First, posterior compartment extension overload is often a part of the syndrome of valgus extension overload,[7, 15] with concomitant injury to the medial collateral ligament (MCL). In a series of 72 baseball players who underwent elbow surgery, patients who underwent only arthroscopic removal of posteromedial olecranon osteophytes had the highest rate of reoperation, often requiring a later MCL reconstruction.[2] This suggests that MCL injury was probably underdiagnosed at the index operation. In this case, if treatment does not address MCL insufficiency, failure is likely. Second, throwing generates compressive forces in the lateral aspect of the joint. The possibility of osteochondral injury to the radiocapitellar joint is real; hence, one should not ignore the anterior part of the joint. As a rule, the authors routinely perform a complete diagnostic arthroscopy in all cases, inspecting the entire anterior and posterior aspect of the joint. Third, it is

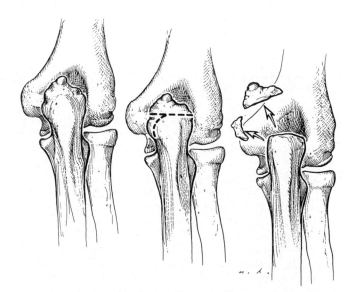

FIGURE 39–10 • Drawing of a hyperextension overload osteophyte formation and its surgical correction with decompression osteotomy of the olecranon tip.

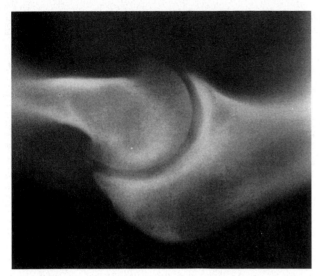

FIGURE 39–11 • Tomogram demonstrating olecranon osteophyte.

noid and fossa osteophytes are present, and (3) the contracted capsule may need to be addressed.

OSTEOCHONDRITIS DESSICANS

Elbow arthroscopy can be useful in the diagnosis and treatment of osteochondritis dessicans of the capitellum (see Chapters 20 and 45). If nonoperative management fails after an appropriate time period and limitations in motion persist, arthroscopy can be used to definitively diagnose and assess the condition of the lesion. If separation of the lesion has occurred, the lesion can be arthroscopically débrided. Alternatively, a variety of fixation techniques have been described, sometimes requiring an arthrotomy.[5] The principles of treatment of osteochondritis dessicans of the radial head are similar.[3] Although large series of arthroscopically treated osteochondritis dessicans of the radial head have not been reported, the arthroscope's role in treating separated or displaced injuries parallels that seen in osteochondritis dessicans of the capitellum.

POST-TRAUMATIC OSTEOARTHRITIS

The role of arthroscopic débridement in the treatment of post-traumatic osteoarthritis has been noted earlier but has not been fully elucidated. Débridement of spurs or osteophytes and removal of loose bodies may provide symptomatic relief of pain and mechanical symptoms. Additionally, successful excision of the radial head can be

not known how much the olecranon can be débrided without creating instability. While further study is needed, we try to resect only pathologic osteophytes, leaving native olecranon intact. In this context, when the osteophytes develop as a result of primary degenerative arthritis, a similar therapeutic approach is followed. However, there are several differences, including the following: (1) loose bodies are more frequently encountered, (2) anterior coro-

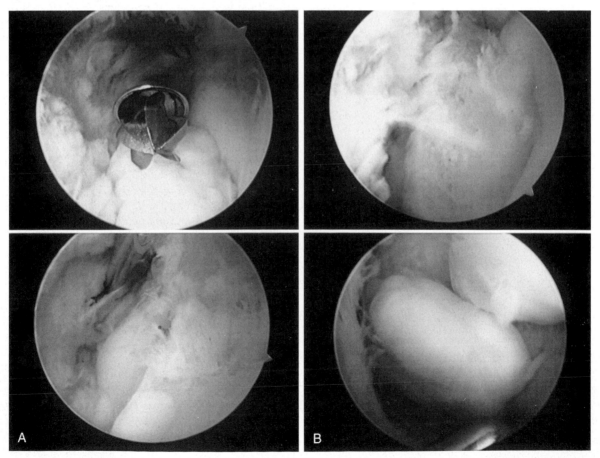

FIGURE 39–12 • *A* and *B,* Arthroscopic débridement of posteromedial olecranon osteophytosis.

performed arthroscopically.[6, 11] In addition to the radial head, as much as 1 cm of the radial neck can be removed. Although uncommonly indicated with the use of standard anterior portals and a midlateral portal (situated in the middle of the anconeous triangle), an adequate excision of the radial head can be performed, without violating the integrity of the annular ligament.

SYNOVIAL DISORDERS

A partial or nearly total synovectomy can be performed arthroscopically for maladies of the synovium, such as rheumatoid arthritis[8] and joint sepsis.[4] Two technical considerations: First, synovectomy can result in a significant hemarthrosis. Consider using a drain, or leaving the portals open postoperatively. Second, beware of "inside-out" injury to regional neurovascular structures.[9] In other words, keep in mind the relative proximity of the median, radial, and ulnar nerves on the extra-articular side of the capsule. The radial nerve is at particular risk.

INVESTIGATIONAL APPLICATIONS

In a relative sense, elbow arthroscopy is a very new procedure. The role of arthroscopic débridement in the injured athlete continues to be defined and expanded. Some are exploring the role of arthroscopic débridement in the treatment of tennis elbow. Owing to the lack of information regarding long-term outcome, arthroscopic débridement for tennis elbow would, at this point, be thought experimental.

REFERENCES

1. Andrews, J. R., and Carson, W. G.: Arthroscopy of the elbow. Arthroscopy 1:97, 1985.
2. Andrews, J. R., and Timmerman, L. A.: Outcome of elbow surgery in professional baseball players. Am. J. Sports Med. 23:407, 1995.
3. Bennett, J. B.: Articular injuries in the athlete. In Morrey, B. (ed.): The Elbow and Its Disorders, 2nd ed. Philadelphia, W. B. Saunders, 1993, pp. 581–595.
4. Ekman, E. F., Cory J. W., and Poehling, G. G.: Pigmented villonodular synovitis and synovial chondromatosis arthroscopically diagnosed and treated in the same elbow. Arthroscopy 13:114, 1997.
5. Indelicato, P. A., Jobe, F. W., Kerlin, R. K., et al.: Correctable elbow lesions in professional baseball players. Am. J. Sports Med. 7:72, 1979.
6. Kim, S. J., Kim, H. K., and Lee, J. W.: Arthroscopy for limitation of motion of the elbow. Arthroscopy 11:680, 1995.
7. Kvitne, R. S., and Jobe, F. W.: Ligamentous and posterior compartment injuries. In Jobe, F. W. (ed.): Operative Techniques in Upper Extremity Sports Injuries. St. Louis, Mosby, 1996, pp. 411–430.
8. Lee, B. P. H., and Morrey, B. F.: Arthroscopic synovectomy of the elbow for rheumatoid arthritis. J. Bone Joint Surg. 79B:770, 1997.
9. Miller, C. D., Jobe, C. M., and Wright, M. H.: Neuroanatomy in elbow arthroscopy. J. Shoulder Elbow Surg. 4:168, 1995.
10. Poehling, G. G., and Ekman, E. F.: Arthroscopy of the elbow. In Jackson, D (ed.): Instructional Course Lectures, Volume 44. Chicago, IL, AAOS, 1994, pp. 214–223.
11. Poehling, G. G., and Ekman, E. F.: Elbow arthroscopy: Introduction and overview. In Poehling, G. G., Koman, L. A., and Pope, T. (eds.): Arthroscopy of the Wrist and Elbow. New York, Raven Press, 1994, pp. 129–136.
12. Poehling, G. G., Whipple, T. L., and Cisco, L., et al.: Elbow arthroscopy: A new technique. Arthroscopy 5:222, 1989.
13. Sisto, D. J., Jobe, F. W., Moynes, D. R., and Antonelli, D. J.: An electromyographic analysis of the elbow in pitching. Am. J. Sports Med. 15:260, 1987.
14. Timmerman, L. A., and Andrews, J. R.: Arthroscopic treatment of post-traumatic elbow pain and stiffness. Am. J. Sports Med. 22:230, 1994.
15. Wilson, F. D., Andrews, J. R., Blackburn, T. A., and McCluskey, G.: Valgus extension overload in the pitching elbow. Am. J. Sports Med. 11:83, 1983.

Arthroscopic Capsular Release

• FELIX H. SAVOIE, III, and LARRY D. FIELD

Arthrofibrosis or pathologic contracture of the elbow may result from a variety of causes. Fractures, dislocations, arthritic or osteochondritic conditions, head injury, burns, and neurologic injury all can cause dysfunction and stiffness of the elbow.[1, 2, 3, 5, 6, 9] Conditions such as intra-articular fractures, loose bodies, and synovitis would be considered intrinsic causes, whereas extrinsic causes would be conditions including capsular contracture, collateral ligament contracture, musculotendinous contracture, and heterotopic bone. Certainly, not all elbow flexion contractures are amenable to arthroscopic treatment; however, those with intrinsic etiologies and certain extrinsic causes may be treated arthroscopically with new advances in the technology of elbow arthroscopy.

INDICATIONS

The American Academy of Orthopaedic Surgeons defines normal elbow motion as 0 to 146 degrees of flexion.[11] Morrey and colleagues[4] in 1981 determined the functional range of elbow motion to be 30 degrees to 130 degrees of elbow flexion. However, no sports or work activities were used in these determinations, and certain occupations and activities such as shoe tying require more than 30 degrees of elbow extension. Therefore, treatment is indicated for contractures in patients whose functional demands require more than 30 degrees of elbow extension. Those patients with a lesser contracture who also have mechanical symptoms suggestive of intra-articular pathology may also be candidates for surgical treatment as well as those patients who have failed nonoperative measures.

SURGICAL TECHNIQUE (Table 39–1)

The arthroscopic setup for surgical release of elbow flexion contracture is that of standard prone elbow arthroscopy. The 4.5 or 5.0 mm arthroscope and shaver are used, along with a standard camera and video recording equipment. The arm is elevated on a 4-inch block placed on a standard arm board oriented parallel to the operating room table, or an arthroscopic elbow holder is used. Either device functions to allow adequate portal access and elbow mobility. The limb is then exsanguinated, and the tourniquet inflated to a pressure usually between 250 and 300 mm Hg. The

• TABLE 39–1 • **Steps in Arthroscopic Treatment of the Contracted Elbow**

1. Diagnostic arthroscopy of the anterior elbow
2. Anterior débridement
   a. Removal of loose bodies
   b. Excision of coronoid spurs
   c. Radiocapitellar débridement
3. Anterior capsular release with excision
4. Diagnostic arthroscopy of the posterior elbow
5. Olecranon fossa débridement
6. Excision of the olecranon tip
7. Medial gutter débridement
8. Lateral gutter débridement
9. Release capsule beneath the triceps
10. Ulnohumeral arthroplasty

limb is prepped and draped in the usual sterile fashion. After draping, a compressive wrapping material, such as Coban, is wrapped around the forearm distal to the elbow joint. This decreases the space for fluid extravasation during the procedure. Examination under anesthesia is then performed, with elbow motion checked in forearm pronation, neutral rotation, and supination.

The joint is insufflated with normal saline through a standard soft spot portal. Initially, a proximal anteromedial portal is established after careful palpation of the ulnar nerve and intermuscular septum. A blunt trochar is used to palpate the intermuscular septum and is then directed anteriorly through muscular tissue to the capsule of the elbow joint. The arthroscope is inserted, and the anterior compartment of the elbow is evaluated.

A proximal anterolateral portal is then established. If the tissues are relatively free, this portal may be established by an outside-in technique with a spinal needle. Often, the capsular contracture will require an inside-out technique with a Wissinger rod. This portal then becomes a working portal, and the anterior joint is débrided.

Once débridement and definition of intra-articular pathology is accomplished, anterior capsulectomy is begun.

The arthroscope is positioned in the proximal medial portal and the shaver in the proximal anterolateral portal. The capsule is then released from the humerus, beginning at the coronoid fossa and proceeding laterally to the lateral intermuscular septum (Fig. 39–13). The arthroscope is then switched to the proximal lateral portal, and the shaver brought in from the medial portal. In similar fashion, release is performed from the middle portion of the humerus medially to the medial intermuscular septum, but not beyond this point because of the potential risk to the ulnar nerve. Excision of the proximal 1 to 2 cm of capsule is accomplished from septum to septum until brachialis fibers are visualized. Capsular resection is continued anteriorly until there is no anterior restriction or brachialis fibers are visualized across the complete anterior aspect, or until a posterior extension block is encountered. To prevent neurovascular complications, it is crucial to confirm that the arthroscope and shaver remain in the joint as well as maintain the shaver in proximity to the humeral cortex at all times.[10] It is important to note that the posterior interosseous nerve lies adjacent to the anterolateral capsule distal to the radiocapitellar joint and is at risk during capsular resection.[10] This area must be strictly avoided during elbow arthroscopy.

On completion of the capsular resection from septum to septum, extension is evaluated while the anterior elbow is visualized. The instruments are removed from the anterior portals and a posterocentral (straight posterior) portal is established. A posterolateral portal is created under direct visualization with the arthroscope in the posterocentral portal. The shaver is inserted in the posterolateral portal, and the olecranon fossa is débrided. At this point, the instruments are switched, with the arthroscope introduced through the posterolateral portal and the posterocentral portal used for instrumentation. A pilot hole is drilled with a 3.5- to 4.5-mm drill bit in the center of the olecranon fossa, connecting it to the coronoid fossa. This hole is then enlarged to accommodate the coronoid process in elbow flexion (Fig. 39–14). The burr is then used to resect the

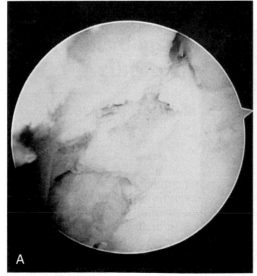
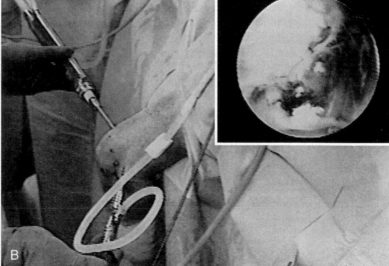

FIGURE 39–13 • Release at the anterior capsule. *A*, Beginning capsular release. *B*, Completed release. Note brachialis fibers.

referable to the portal site. However, a distended joint in no way protects either of these nerves from an intra-articular procedure.[13] As a matter of fact, the distended capsule may theoretically render these nerves more—rather than less—vulnerable. In general, it has been shown that the most vulnerable nerve anatomically is the radial. This nerve may typically be 5 to 10 mm from an anterior lateral portal. However, there is significant variation, and in some instances the nerve can be as close as 2 to 3 mm to the capsule. Similarly, the median nerve demonstrates a variation of approximately 5 mm between the distended and the nondistended capsule referable to the anteromedial portal. However, once again, the distended capsule approximates the nerve—it does not separate the nerve. Finally, the ulnar nerve is only a matter of millimeters from the medial capsule.[25] The vulnerability is to the posteromedial portal site, but its greatest risk consists of procedures performed in the posteromedial corner of the elbow.

In general, these nerves are not at risk from portal insertion if the portal sites are accurately defined and the joint is distended. The risk of nerve injury is as follows: radial > ulnar > median.

Pathology

The risk of arthroscopy is dependent to some extent on the pathology being treated[15] (Table 39–3).

Rheumatoid Arthritis. The most common reason for arthroscopy of an elbow involved with rheumatoid arthritis is arthroscopic synovectomy. The capsule is extremely thin, and the nerves are therefore at significant risk of injury with this procedure. We have had one patient develop an ulnar nerve paresthesia owing to the instability associated with rheumatoid synovitis and the vulnerability of the nerve referable to a thin capsule covered by proliferative synovium.

Loose Body. The removal of loose bodies is still probably the best indication for elbow arthroscopy in both the degenerative and the post-traumatic elbow.[4, 17, 18, 21] The complications are uncommon unless the portal site strays from the recommended positions or débridement is required. Both generally places the radial nerve at risk.

Degenerative Arthritis. Primary degenerative arthritis is a good indication for elbow arthroscopy.[4, 7] The selection of a procedure may include removal of loose bodies, débridement of the coronoid and olecranon osteophytes, and, in some instances, anterior and posterior capsular release. The anterior capsular release places the median and, particularly, the radial nerve at risk. The posterior release may place the ulnar nerve at risk. In addition, the multiple portal

sites necessary for effectively carrying out this procedure may further add an element of vulnerability to these nerves. In addition to the degenerative as well as the post-traumatic elbow, the capsular capacity is very limited,[16] making even a diagnostic procedure something of a risk particularly for articular scuffing.

Post-traumatic Elbow. The potential risks of this are similar to those with primary degenerative arthritis. Contracture and altered anatomy make the procedure technically difficult. The articular structures as well as the neural and even the vascular ones may be at risk, depending on the aggressiveness of the procedure, which is typically débridement.

SURGICAL PROCEDURE

In addition to variation in pathology as implied previously, different risks are also associated with varying complexities of surgical procedures (Table 39–4).[15]

Loose Body. The procedure that has the lowest risk is that of loose body removal. However, attention must be paid to the location of the portal with the distended joint.

Osteophyte Removal. Removal of an osteophyte can predispose to articular scuffing, but removal of an olecranon space places the ulnar nerve at particular risk, as this osteophyte frequently forms and is the offending pathology. This osteophyte may approximate the ulnar nerve. Certainly, any medial osteophytic removal from the humerus should be performed with extreme care, since the ulnar nerve frequently rests on or very near this medial osteophytic process.

Capsular Release. A capsular release may be the most dangerous arthroscopic procedure.[7, 15] The capsule is usually thick, and the joint capacity limited. Some débridement may be required to obtain adequate visualization. The radial nerve is at particular risk, as it is often closely applied to the anterior capsule at the radial head. However, injury to the median nerve may also occur, but at a lower risk.

Synovectomy. Complication from synovectomy is a function of the aggressiveness of the procedure.[10] Multiple portals do place the nerves at some risk, even for the diagnostic component. In addition, the thin capsule generally present in the rheumatoid patient may unknowingly be violated, thus immediately placing the anterior nerves at risk. Furthermore, use of low suction may draw the nerve into the débriding instrument. Finally, the pathology itself frequently makes visualization difficult, and débridement to attain better visualization may violate the capsule, thus increasing the vulnerability to nerve injury.

• TABLE 39–3 • **Authors' View of the Relative Risk of Complication by Diagnosis***

| Diagnosis | Articular Scuff | Neural | | | Infection | Vascular |
		Radial	Median	Ulnar		
Rheumatoid	NA	◐	◐	◐	●*	◐
P. trauma	◐	◑	◐	◐	◐	◐
Primary OA	◐	◑	◐	◑	○	◐
Post. u. nerve transfer	NA	NA	NA	●*	○	NA

*If anterior medial portal used.
Risk: NA = Not applicable; very low = ○; low = ◐; intermediate = ◑; high = ●.

• TABLE 39–4 • Authors' View of the Relative Risk of Complication by Procedure

Procedure	Articular Scuff	Neural Radial	Medial	Ulnar	Infection	Vascular
Diagnostic (portal)	◐?	●	◐?	◐?	NA	○
Loose body	○	◐	◐	◐	◐	◐
Osteophyte	◐	◐	○	●	◐	NA
Capsular release	◐	●	◐	◐	◐	◐
Synovectomy	◐	●	◐	◐	◐	◐

Risk: Not applicable = NA; very low = ○; low = ◑; intermediate = ◐; high = ●.

Vascular Insult

To date, we were unable to identify any documentation of vascular injury or compartment syndrome after elbow arthroscopy. The marked swelling that may occur quickly resolves. It has been shown that infusion systems that control both pressure and flow cause less extravasation than systems that control pressure alone.[19]

INCIDENCE

The incidence of complications has been poorly documented. In 1986, the Arthroscopic Association of North America conducted a survey of almost 1600 procedures, and only one radial nerve injury was reported, along with two instances of infection. Obviously, this complication rate (0.2 percent) grossly understates the actual incidence of these injuries.

A review of the literature reveals that the greatest focus is placed on neural injury, documented in about 1 percent, although this is usually transient (Table 39–5). Infection and all other problems are not commonly reported. Overall, a review of about 500 procedures reveals some form of complication in 5 percent.[4, 6, 9, 12, 17, 18, 23, 28] We consider this an inaccurate estimate of the reality.[8]

Mayo Clinic Experience. Because the potential risk is high and owing to a lack of information in the literature regarding the true incidence of elbow arthroscopy complications, we have reviewed our experience with elbow arthroscopy.[8] A preliminary assessment reveals that of more than 400 procedures, 1 percent of individuals have a significant complication requiring treatment or altering outcome. Further, 10 percent have a nonpermanent "problem" associated with the procedure.

PREVENTION

The recommendations for avoiding complications of elbow arthroscopy are generally well recognized: (1) define landmarks before distention; (2) recognize that distention protects the nerve from portal injury, but not from capsular procedures; (3) portals more proximal to the joint tend to be safer[25]; (4) keep the elbow flexed 90 degrees to increase the distance between the nerves and the capsule; (5) do not use pressurized infusion[19]; (6) débriding with radius pronated protects the posterior interosseous nerve; (7) always visualize the instrument tip; (8) avoid suction around a nerve; (9) capsular "retraction" may be useful; and (10) use local anesthesia judiciously since this can cause neural anesthesia, which confuses the postoperative status.

REFERENCES

1. Adolfsson, L.: Arthroscopy of the elbow joint: A cadaveric study of portal placement. J. Shoulder Elbow Surg. **3:**53, 1994.
2. Andrews, R. J., and Carson, W. G.: Arthroscopy of the elbow. Arthroscopy **1:**97, 1985.
3. Angelo, R. L.: Advances in elbow arthroscopy. Orthopedics **16:**1037, 1993.
4. Baker, C. L., and Brooks, A. A.: Arthroscopy of the elbow. Clin. Sports Med. **15:**261, 1996.
5. Drescher, H., Schwering, L., Jerosch, J., and Herzig, M.: The risk of neurovascular damage in elbow joint arthroscopy: Which approach is better: Anteromedial or anterolateral? Z. Orthop. Ihre Grenzgeb. **132:**120, 1994.
6. Guhl, J. F.: Arthroscopy and arthroscopic surgery of the elbow. Orthopedics **8:**1290, 1985.

• TABLE 39–5 • Complications Reported with Elbow Arthroscopy

Author	Year	Procedures	Nerve (Transient)	Infection (Drainage)	Other
Guhl	1985	45	1	0	0
Lynch	1986	21	3(2)	0	0
O'Driscoll	1992	71	3(3)	(4)	0
Ward	1993	35	0	1	3
Ogilvie-Harris	1993	34	2(2)	0	0
Schneider	1994	67	7(7)	0	0
Kim	1995	25	2(2)	0	1
Baker	1996	200	0	0	1
Totals		498	18 (4%)	1 (.20%)	5 (1%)
Complications		24/498 (5%)			

 7. Jones, G. S., and Savoie, F. H.: Arthroscopic capsular release of flexion contractures (arthrofibrosis) of the elbow. Arthroscopy **9**:277, 1993.
 8. Kelly, E., O'Driscoll, S., and Morrey, B. F.: Complications of Elbow Arthroscopy (in press).
 9. Kim, S. J., Kim, H. K., and Lee, J. W.: Arthroscopy for limitation of motion of the elbow. Arthroscopy **11**:680, 1995.
10. Lee, B. P. H., and Morrey, B. F.: Arthroscopic synovectomy of the elbow for rheumatoid arthritis. J. Bone Joint Surg. **79B**:770, 1997.
11. Lindenfeld, T. N.: Medial approach in elbow arthroscopy. Am. J. Sports Med. **18**:413, 1990.
12. Lynch, G. J., Myers, J. F., Whipple, T. L., and Caspari, R. B.: Neurovascular anatomy and elbow arthroscopy: Inherent risks. Arthroscopy **2**:191, 1986.
13. Marshall, P. D., Fairclough, J. A., Johnson, S. R., and Evans, E. J.: Avoiding nerve damage during elbow arthroscopy. J. Bone Joint Surg. **75B**:129, 1993.
14. Miller, C. D., Jobe, C. M., and Wright, M. H.: Neuroanatomy in elbow arthroscopy. J. Shoulder Elbow Surg. **4**:168, 1995.
15. Morrey, B. F.: Complications of Elbow Arthroscopy. Instr. Course Lect. **48**:405, 1999.
16. O'Driscoll, S. W., Morrey, B. F., and An, K. N.: Intraarticular pressure and capacity of the elbow. Arthroscopy **6**:100, 1990.
17. O'Driscoll, S. W., and Morrey, B. F.: Arthroscopy of the elbow: Diagnostic and therapeutic benefits and hazards. J. Bone Joint Surg. **74A**:84, 1992.
18. Ogilvie-Harris, D. J., and Schemitsch, E.: Arthroscopy of the elbow for removal of loose bodies. Arthroscopy **9**:5, 1993.
19. Ogilvie-Harris, D. J., and Weisleder, L.: Fluid pump systems for arthroscopy: A comparison of pressure control versus pressure and flow control. Arthroscopy **11**:591, 1995.
20. Papilion, J. D., Neff, R. S., and Shall, L. M.: Compression neuropathy of the radial nerve as a complication of elbow arthroscopy. Arthroscopy **4**:284, 1988.
21. Poehling, G. G., and Ekman, E. F.: Arthroscopy of the elbow. Instr. Course Lect. **44**:217, 1995.
22. Ruch, D.S., and Poehling, G.G.: Anterior interosseous nerve injury following elbow arthroscopy. Arthroscopy **13**:756, 1997.
23. Schneider, T., Hoffstetter, I., Finnk, B., and Jerosch, J.: Long-term results of elbow arthroscopy in 67 patients. Acta Orthop. Belg. **60**:378, 1994.
24. Small, N.: Complications in arthroscopy: The knee and other joints. Committee on Complications of the Arthroscopy Association of North America. Arthroscopy **2**:253, 1986.
25. Stothers, K., Day, B., and Regan, W. R.: Arthroscopy of the elbow: Anatomy, portal sites, and a description of the proximal lateral portal. Arthroscopy **11**:449, 1995.
26. Thomas, M. A., Fast, A., and Shapiro, D.: Radial nerve damage as a complication of elbow arthroscopy. Clin. Orthop. **215**:131, 1987.
27. Verhaar, J., van-Mameren, H., and Brandsma, A.: Risks of neurovascular injury in elbow arthroscopy: Starting anteromedially or anterolaterally? Arthroscopy **7**:287, 1991.
28. Ward, W. G., and Anderson, T. E.: Elbow arthroscopy in a mostly athletic population. J. Hand Surg. **18**:220, 1993.

Elbow Arthroscopy: The Future

• SHAWN W. O'DRISCOLL

As we look to the future, we must consider the direction and origins from which we have come. It was not that long ago that world-renowned surgeons were heard to comment on the futility and waste of time involved in attempting to perform partial meniscectomies arthroscopically, or more recently to reconstruct the anterior cruciate ligament with these techniques. In the shoulder, subacromial arthroscopy was thought to be "ridiculous" by many, and of course "you can't see anything anyway." We do not practice orthopedics the way we did 30 years ago, and it would make no sense to assume that in the next 30 years the status quo would remain unchanged. Therefore, we might stop to ponder the question, "What am I doing today that might be improved upon in the future?"

One can address this concern by considering the problems we are currently facing that have not been solved, the treatments we provide that still yield less than optimal results, and where "the marketplace" is driving us to go.

It is easy to consider these, starting with the last. Two factors are driving orthopedics in the direction of arthroscopic intervention. First, patients place a high priority on minimally invasive surgery. This is true regardless of the body part, and certainly is true for the elbow. Second, there is a generation of surgeons who have been trained in the use of the arthroscope, which has now become a standard tool in the armamentarium, just as the desktop computer has. In fact, some consider arthroscopy as much a lifestyle as a tool. These are the individuals who have driven the advances in shoulder surgery in the area of arthroscopy, and will do the same in the elbow, regardless of whether or not they have substantial experience with traditional elbow surgery. Of course, there are surgical risks in the elbow, particularly serious nerve injuries.

Current open surgery of the elbow results in considerable swelling and pain, which make the postoperative recovery not only difficult but often incomplete. It is not as difficult to eliminate a contracture in the operating room as it is to maintain that range of motion postoperatively. To the extent that such swelling and pain can be reduced by percutaneous surgery, the latter will be preferable. We are already recognizing this in treating contractures, although the safety is yet to be confirmed.

Finally, there are clinical problems that have not been solved, such as the treatment of young patients with arthritis. Synovectomy for rheumatoid arthritis can now be performed in a manner that is virtually complete, and the contracted capsule can also be excised. With this thorough approach, patients may respond better than has been traditionally found. Similarly, the removal of osteophytes and the release of capsular contractures in patients with osteoarthritis can eliminate the impingement pain in these patients.

Fractures of the elbow can be difficult to treat because of the small size of the fragments and the challenge of exposure. Fractures of the radial head and coronoid and distal humerus have already been treated arthroscopically by some, and as instrumentation improves, we anticipate finding that there will be a role for such an approach, just as in other joints.

The limiting factors will relate to the ability of individual surgeons to practice these techniques safely, the development of suitable instruments, and the accumulation and dissemination of collective experience and knowledge in this rapidly expanding field.

CHAPTER 40

Muscle and Tendon Trauma: Tennis Elbow Tendinosis

• ROBERT P. NIRSCHL

*T*ennis elbow, which was originally coined as *lawn tennis elbow* in 1883,[34] is a popular term. Over the years, it has been used to describe a variety of maladies that occur in and about the elbow.[6, 10, 11, 13, 18] To eliminate confusion, it is important to define terms accurately. On the basis of clinical and surgical experience,[16, 24, 33, 47, 48] it can be stated with confidence that the pathology of classic tennis elbow resides primarily in tendon tissue. However, recent arthroscopic data demonstrate that additional capsular involvement is present in some patients.[1] Some controversy exists concerning the histology of tennis elbow. The traditional term *tendinitis* has been used in the past, but inflammatory cells are usually not noted, and I have introduced an alternative term *(angiofibroblastic tendinosis).*[33, 48] Others have also demonstrated degenerative changes as the principal histologic finding.[56]

INCIDENCE

A random study of 200 tennis players in three tennis clubs revealed that half of the players older than 30 years of age had experienced symptoms of characteristic tennis elbow at one time or another.[41] Of this group, half noted minor symptoms with a duration of less than 6 months, and the rest had had major symptoms with an average duration of 2½ years. A larger statistical analysis of 2500 patients performed by Priest at the Vic Braden Tennis Camps revealed similar data.[54, 55] Not restricted to tennis, the malady is commonly seen in other sports, including baseball, and other field events involving throwing, fencing, and swimming. Occupational activity that requires stressful use of the forearm, such as computer keyboard, carpentry, plumbing, meat cutting, textile production, and constant handshaking (e.g., politicians) is also related to the occurrence of tennis elbow.

CLASSIFICATION

Elbow tendinosis may be simply classified on an anatomic basis.

Lateral Tennis Elbow. Lateral tendinosis involves primarily the origin of the extensor carpi radialis brevis. It is seen less commonly in the anteromedial edges of the extensor communis; less commonly still in the underside of the extensor carpi radialis longus; and, rarely, in the origin of the extensor carpi ulnaris.

Medial Tennis Elbow. Medial tennis elbow involves primarily the flexor pronator origin at the medial epicondyle. An additional complicating factor of medial tennis elbow is the commonly associated finding of compression neurapraxia of the ulnar nerve (see Chapter 41).

Posterior Tennis Elbow. Tendinosis of the triceps at its attachment to the olecranon is relatively uncommon as an isolated event, but it has been noted in throwers (e.g., baseball players, javelin athletes) in association with olecranon compartment abnormalities, such as synovitis and loose bodies.

Combinations. It is quite common to have combined signs and symptoms of both lateral and medial tennis elbow tendinosis occurring simultaneously.

ASSOCIATED ABNORMALITIES AND DIFFERENTIAL DIAGNOSIS

Associated problems can and do appear either independently or in combination with tennis elbow tendinosis. The most common examples include the following.

Ulnar Nerve Neurapraxia. Ulnar nerve neurapraxia is commonly associated with medial tennis elbow and has an impact on the prognosis (see Chapter 41).

Carpal Tunnel Syndrome. In my experience, about 10 percent of surgical patients have signs and symptoms of carpal tunnel syndrome.[40] This association, as well as the association of rotator cuff tendinosis and bilateral tennis elbow, has led to the conclusion that a constitutional factor may play a significant role in certain patients with tennis elbow.[40, 45]

Radial Nerve Entrapment. Entrapment of the motor branch of the radial nerve in the radial tunnel can cause symptoms similar to those seen with lateral tennis elbow tendinosis. Roles and Maudsley[57] reported a surgical experience with 33 cases in 1972. Specific care was taken to decompress the radial tunnel by releasing the origin of the extensor carpi radialis brevis. Thus, the success of the reported operation may be due to an alteration of the origin of the extensor brevis. Entrapment of the posterior interosseous nerve has also been implicated as the cause of lateral elbow pain by Werner,[67] Dobyns,* and others (see Chapter 42). A random sample of 20 electromyographic studies in patients with the classic signs of clinical lateral tennis elbow, however, failed to reveal any radial nerve abnormality.[44] In my opinion, although radial nerve entrapment may occur, it is not associated in a major statistical way with classic lateral tennis elbow. Werner[67] demonstrated that the two coexist in about 5 percent of patients. When, on occasion, entrapment of the posterior interosseous nerve does occur, it may be an entirely separate entity with vague aching symptoms that are more diffuse and felt more distally over the extensor muscle mass, tenderness in the same area, and a provocative handshake stress test that elicits symptoms in forced supination. As noted, electromyographic studies tend to be normal.

Rotator Cuff Tendinosis. As noted, multiple tendinosis areas often occur in association with tennis elbow.[45] I have coined the term *mesenchymal syndrome* to identify this

---

*Personal communication.

subset of fairly common patient presentation.[40] It is the author's current hypothesis that this entity is hereditary and probably represents a slight collagen distortion—perhaps cross-linkage—as it relates to tendons. The practical ramifications of this entity include the necessity of rehabilitative exercise dedicated to the shoulder as well as the elbow when one formulates a treatment plan.

Cervical Osteoarthritis and Nerve Root Compression. Gunn and Milbrandt[28] have reported the achievement of pain relief in tennis elbow in 53 cases by directing treatment to osteoarthritis of the cervical spine. The greatest incidence of tennis elbow occurs in individuals in the fourth and fifth decades of life. Because the findings of lateral tennis elbow are usually specific, including response to local elbow tendon injections, it is unlikely that osteoarthritis in the cervical spine is anything but a coincidental finding.

Intra-articular Abnormalities and Joint Laxity. Individuals who use the arm with high torque and shearing forces, as in the aggressive activities of baseball or javelin throwing, are vulnerable to associated intra-articular problems. These generally take the form of synovitis, traumatic osteoarthritis,[39] and osteocartilaginous loose bodies present in the lateral or, more rarely, medial elbow compartments, as well as in the posterior olecranon fossa. When associated with ligamentous laxity of the medial ulnar collateral ligamentous structures, ulnar nerve neuropathy may also complicate the clinical picture. Appropriate history and physical and imaging examinations identify this subset of patients, and treatment should be adjusted accordingly. In a review, Baker and Cummings[1] demonstrated that in some patients arthroscopic evidence of capsular degeneration coexists with degeneration of the extensor carpi radialis brevis.[1]

ETIOLOGY

Age and Sex. The characteristic age at onset of classic uncomplicated tennis elbow is between 35 and 50 years, with a median of 41 years.[38, 40, 41, 44, 45] Although the condition is most common in the third, fourth, and fifth decades, the author has diagnosed tennis elbow in patients as young as 12 and as old as 80 years. Depending on a given patient population, the overall male/female ratio is usually equal.

Overuse. The overall intensity and duration of arm use is the ultimate inciter of symptoms and the major cause of this tendinosis. In this regard, younger patients such as competitive tennis players and professional baseball athletes characteristically place high demands on the upper extremities. An inadequate, marginal, or compromised musculoskeletal condition also appears to play a role in the etiology of medial or lateral elbow tendinosis.

Lateral tennis elbow is directly related to activities that increase the tension, and hence the stress, of the wrist and finger extensors and, possibly, the supinator muscles. Funk and associates[21] revealed that the extensor carpi radialis brevis is active with flexion, extension, varus, or valgus stress; hence, supporting the notion of overuse or overexertion.

Medial tennis elbow characteristically occurs with wrist flexor activity and active pronation, as in baseball pitching,

the tennis serve and overhead strokes, and the pull-through strokes of swimming.

Posterior tennis elbow consists of overload of the triceps attachment that occurs in sports such as javelin throwing and baseball pitching, which initiate a sudden snap into elbow extension.

The primary overload abuse in tendinosis is caused by intrinsic muscular contraction (see Chapter 5). These muscular contractile overloads may occur concentrically or eccentrically. Tensile extrinsic overload (e.g., valgus instability or macrotrauma) is more likely to cause excessive joint torque forces, leading to ligamentous rupture and traumatic osteoarthritis. In sports activities, both intrinsic and extrinsic factors are likely to be factors.

Traumatic Etiology. Excessive forearm use is clearly associated with the development of tennis elbow.[45, 48] A typical patient is an active recreational tennis player who plays at least three or four times per week.[45, 46, 54] Less commonly, acute onset may be associated with a direct blow to one of the epicondylar areas or a sudden extreme effort or activity.

Constitutional Factors. I have observed that the etiologic factors of tennis elbow also involve a distinct, albeit small, subgroup of patients who have a tendency to develop generalized tendinosis. This observation was initially reported in 1969 and termed *mesenchymal syndrome.*[40] In the extreme case, the mesenchymal abnormalities may include bilateral rotator cuff tendinosis, medial and lateral tennis elbow, carpal tunnel syndrome, triggering tenosynovitis of the finger flexors, and De Quervain's syndrome all in the same patient. In almost all instances, the routine rheumatologic evaluation is normal. These observations have led to the conclusion that some individuals have a heritable constitutional factor that predisposes them to such profuse or generalized tendinosis.

PATHOLOGY

Gross Abnormalities

Before 1960, some confusion existed about the precise pathologic anatomy of this condition. In 1922 Osgood,[51] and in 1932 Carp,[13] related the condition to radiohumeral bursitis. Goldie, in his classic 1964 report, was the first to describe pathology adjacent to the lateral elbow (the term used at the time).[24] Goldie used longitudinal incisions and binocular magnification for more thorough assessment of the tissues.[24] Previous release techniques described by Bosworth[8] and Hohmann[29] are characterized by the failure to observe pathologic abnormalities.

Careful gross surgical inspection of the abnormal specimen reveals a characteristically grayish color and homogeneous and generally edematous tissue (Fig. 40–1). This typical gross pathologic appearance is present in lateral, medial, and posterior tendinosis. Indeed, similar visual characteristics are present in tendinosis involving the rotator cuff, and patellar and Achilles tendons, and even in plantar fasciosis (old term *fasciitis*). In my original surgical series of lateral tennis elbow, 97 percent of cases demonstrated varying degrees of this pathologic tissue at the origin of the extensor brevis tendon (which was ruptured

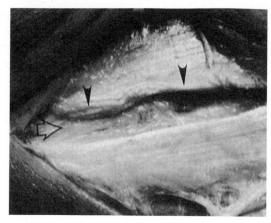

FIGURE 40–1 • Gross pathologic appearance. The brevis origin is exposed by retracting the extensor longus anteriorly *(closed arrows)*. The characteristic visual appearance of angiofibroblastic hyperplasia *(open arrow)* is a grayish, homogeneous, edematous, and friable tissue. This appearance has led us to coin the phrase *thick unhappy gray tendon, weeping with edema.*

in some degree in 35 percent).[48] Observations in these and subsequent surgical cases also revealed that approximately 35 percent of cases also had associated tendinosis changes in the anteromedial edge (usually 10 to 20 percent of edge) of the tendon of the extensor digitorum communis or extensor aponeurosis.[46, 47] Radiographic examination revealed that 22 percent of patients had some form of bony exostosis at the tip of the lateral epicondyle.[46, 47] Calcification in the substance of the tendon occurs much less commonly.

Microscopic Pathology

An understanding of the dense connective tissue that makes up the fibrous portion of the tendon is necessary for a better appreciation and definition of the pathologic process that is present in tennis elbow.* In tendons, collagen fibers and primary tendon bundles run parallel courses. In normal tendons, nerves and blood vessels extend through the major connective tissue septa but do not invade the fascicles.[62] On gross examination, the tendon appears firm, taut, and yellowish white or beige.[46, 47]

In tendinosis, the abnormal tissue ordinarily can be identified easily by its appearance and is distinct from the normal tendon. Visual examination usually reveals, gray, dull, sometimes edematous and friable, immature-appearing tissue that grossly resembles firm granulation tissue.[42, 46–48] Microscopically, the normal orderly tendon fibers are disrupted by a characteristic invasion of fibroblasts and vascular granulation-like tissue, which may be described as an angiofibroblastic hyperplasia-tendinosis[33, 46, 48, 62] (Fig. 40–2). Adjacent to this early proliferating vascular reparative tissue, the tendon appears hypercellular, degenerative, and microfragmented. The degree of angiofibroblastic infiltration appears to correlate generally with the duration of symptoms.[45, 46] In advanced lesions, fibroadipose, connective, and even musculoskeletal tissue can reveal infiltration by this pathologic proliferative tissue.[33]

*Stay, E.: Personal communication.

The microscopic appearance of this tissue was considered by Sarkar and Uhthoff.[59] These investigators were also impressed with the neovascular channels but emphasized that the mesenchymal cell proliferation indicated that the appearance was one of a healing process. On the other hand, Regan and colleagues[56] compared 12 patients having surgery for lateral epicondylitis with 12 control patients. The unequivocal changes of hyaline degeneration were interpreted as demonstrating that the basic pathologic lesion was one of degeneration, although the increased vascularity noted by others also was reported. These investigators emphasized the fact that there is no microscopic evidence of inflammation associated with tennis elbow (Fig. 40–3).[56] It is highly unusual to detect inflammatory cells in the tendinous tissue itself, even in cases of long duration. Evidence of acute inflammation is virtually absent in all cases.

In cases treated with corticosteroid injection, nonpolarizable amorphous eosinophilic material can be identified, often without any foreign body response and usually without evidence of calcification (Fig. 40–4). Indeed, the proliferating vascular reparative tissue often insinuates itself between normal and abnormal tissues in regions close to the injection site.[62]

Immunohistology and Electron Microscopy of Tendinosis

In 1999, Kraushaar and Nirschl[33] reported a study of the histology, immunohistochemistry, and electron microscopy of tennis elbow tendinosis in nine surgical resection specimens. The origin of the extensor carpi radialis brevis was compared to 10 cadaveric specimens of the same anatomic region. Electron microscopy clearly defined major disruption of collagen, and distortion of fibroblasts and nonfunc-

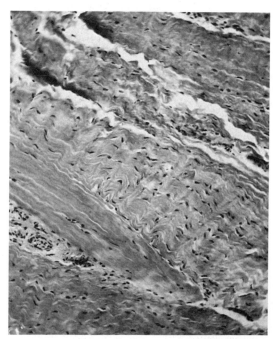

FIGURE 40–2 • Angiofibroblastic hyperplasia. The absence of inflammatory cells has resulted in the term *tendinosis* replacing *tendinitis.*

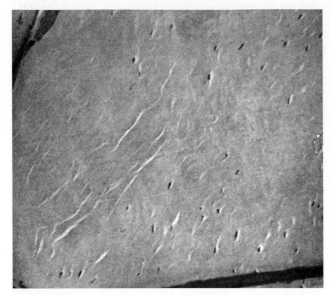

FIGURE 40–3 • Microscopic appearance on hematoxylin and eosin stains may reveal hyaline degeneration as a feature of the surgical pathology of tennis elbow.

tional vascular elements. Immunohistochemical stains for neurofilaments, smooth muscle antigen, factor 8, protein S-100, and vimentin provided insight into the neural, vascular, ground substance, and cartilaginous composition of tendinosis material. These studies revealed that myofibroblasts are present in tendinosis material, a cell type with contractive properties not usually found in healthy tendons. Tendinosis material therefore contains hyperplasia of nonfunctional vascular elements, active distorted fibroblasts, and a lack of lymphocyte or neutrophilic populations that is clearly distinct from inflammatory tendinitis and/or normal

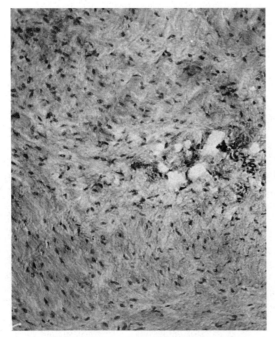

FIGURE 40–4 • Cortisone injection site. Microscopic photograph demonstrates nonpolarizable amorphous eosinophilic material.

tendon.[33] This study reinforces the prior original hematoxylin and eosin (H&E) stain microscopic observations that tendinosis, rather tendinitis, is the histopathologic lesion in tendon overuse.[48, 62]

CLINICAL CORRELATIONS OF PATHOLOGY

As noted in my 1992 report, the following pathologic categories, with corresponding clinical and therapeutic implications, are suggested.[46]

Category I

Pathology. Acute, reversible inflammation is likely, but no angiofibroblastic invasion is seen.

Clinical Signs. Minor aching pain is evident, usually after heavy activity.

Treatment. There is a quick response to simple anti-inflammatory measures followed by rehabilitative exercise and future avoidance of force overload or overuse.

Category II

Pathology. There is a partial angiofibroblastic invasion. The pathology is permanent, but some healing response may occur, depending on the biologic maturation of the pathologic process and the extent of involvement.

Clinical Signs. Often, there is intense pain with activity as well as symptoms at rest. After periods of rest, however, most routine activities can be accomplished without significant discomfort.

Treatment. If less than half of the tendon diameter is involved, treatment concepts that promote healing gradually bring about resolution, and this process can be managed nonoperatively. Occasionally, however, these patients must undergo surgery for a more complete resolution of symptoms.

Category III

Pathology. Extensive angiofibroblastic invasion with or without partial or complete rupture of the tendon is present.

Clinical Signs. Significant functional defects that include pain at rest as well as night pain make routine daily activities difficult or impossible. At this stage, the complete lesion can be observed arthroscopically (Fig. 40–5).

Treatment. The condition invariably requires surgery for pain relief, as this advanced stage usually does not respond to nonoperative measures.

NONSURGICAL TREATMENT

The general concepts of elbow rehabilitation are covered in detail in Chapter 10. A brief overview, however, is appropriate at this time.[42, 45, 46, 49] The patient with tennis elbow most commonly presents for evaluation and treatment because of pain, rather than impairment of mechanical functional. Therefore, it is important to control pain,

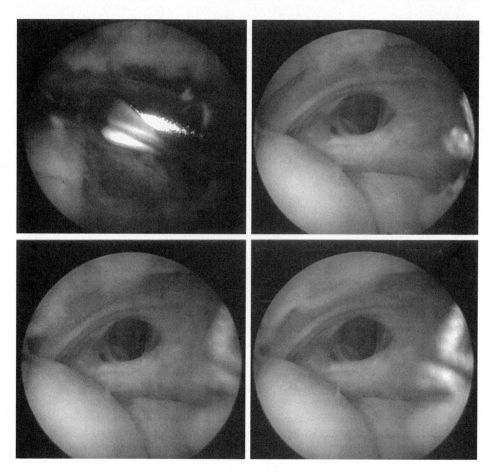

FIGURE 40–5 • Arthroscopic inspection of the lateral capsule reveals a full-thickness tear, including the capsule in a patient with chronic epicondylitis/tendinosis.

but this, in itself, does not necessarily imply enhancement of healing. The time-honored modalities of relative rest (not absence of activity but abstinence from abuse) and application of cold are appropriate. Activity that aggravates the condition should be eliminated. The use of aspirin as an anti-inflammatory agent is the first choice, but nonsteroidal anti-inflammatory medications, including indomethacin, seem to be helpful in some patients. The former popularity of dimethyl sulfoxide (DMSO) among the lay population has prompted one prospective, double-blind study of its effectiveness in tennis elbow. Surprisingly, the relief offered by this topical medication was no greater than that of a placebo.[52] The physical therapy modality of high-voltage electrical stimulation has been helpful in relieving pain, and the author's anecdotal observations suggest the possibility of enhancing a biologic healing response.[44]

If the malady does not respond to this treatment program and the patient is incapable of doing the prescribed rehabilitative exercises, a cortisone injection is appropriate. The author uses 2.5 ml of 0.5 percent lidocaine (Xylocaine) mixed with 20 mg of triamcinolone, instilled below the extensor brevis just anterior and slightly distal to the lateral epicondyle into a triangular fatty recess that occupies this area. If the injection is too superficial or is done on a repetitive basis, subdermal atrophy may occur.[44] The repeated use of cortisone injections (more than a total of three) is inappropriate and probably harmful, secondary to the causation of tenocyte cellular death and the potential

weakening of the surrounding normal tissues.[63] Indeed, some patients are extremely sensitive to local instillation of cortisone; subcutaneous atrophy (Fig. 40–6), occasionally after only one injection, may be noted when the injection is placed superficial to the tendon. Thus, no more than three injections should be instilled in any one area, and direct intratendinous injections should be avoided.[44]

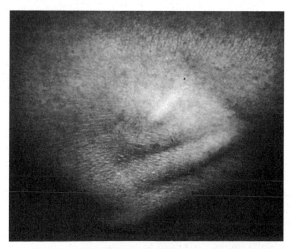

FIGURE 40–6 • Subcutaneous atrophy from a subdermal cortisone injection.

Promotion of Healing

A biologic healing response includes infiltration of healthy neovascular and fibroblastic elements, collagen production, and collagen maturation at the cellular level in addition to the restoration of strength, endurance, and flexibility to the entire extremity, including the upper back, neck, and shoulder. The healing process may be hastened by three general measures: relative rest, high-voltage electrical stimulation, and, most importantly, rehabilitation exercises.[42, 49]

RELATIVE REST

The injured part may be rested through the use of (1) immobilizing devices to avoid abuse, (2) alteration of inappropriate technique or activity, (3) selection of proper equipment, and (4) counterforce bracing.

Abstinence of Abuse. Rest attained by casting often weakens the affected area and has not been effective in controlling pain when activities are resumed. Partial immobilization by wrist extension splints has the limited value of casting except in the early, fully reversible inflammatory phase of category I injuries. Overall, therefore, modification or elimination of abusive activities is a more appropriate and useful interpretation of the term *relative rest* than is formal immobilization. A graduated activity program for the injured part, coupled with an aggressive activity program for the adjacent normal, uninjured tissues, should be emphasized.

Alteration of Training Technique. Careful history taking and observation are fundamental to the identification of faulty technique. Evidence is accumulating that the correct technique of a sport not only enhances activity performance but also is less likely to cause injury.[42, 45, 49] The sports most likely to be causally related to either lateral or medial tennis elbow include tennis, golf, baseball throwing, squash, racquetball, weightlifting, fly and cast fishing, swimming, and track and field events. The occupational activities commonly associated with tennis elbow include meat cutting and handling, carpentry, plumbing, repetitive assembly line activity, computer keyboard and mouse activity, typing, writing, and handshaking (e.g., politicians at campaign time).[42]

Alteration of Equipment. Equipment (especially in the racquet sports) may play an important role in imparting forces that can result in tendon overuse injury.[6, 41, 42, 49, 54, 55] Biomechanically, in tennis as well as other implement ball sports it is most appropriate to strike the ball at the center of percussion ("sweet spot") because the increased torsion of off-center hits increases the stresses at musculotendon units, especially at or near tendon epicondylar attachment areas.[26, 41, 42, 54, 55]

Activities that cause forearm impact or stress necessitate equipment of the proper size, weight, balance, and grip to avoid excessive forces.[35, 37, 40] In general, the larger the handle of the device, the greater the leverage for torsion control, but the handle must be molded to hand size.[6, 41, 42]

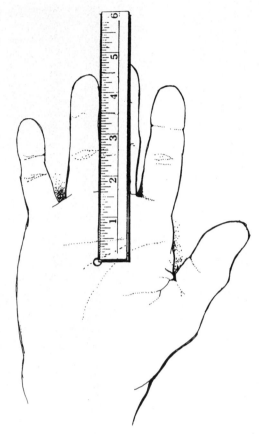

FIGURE 40–7 • Author's method of determining proper racket grip diameter (see text).

The distance from the midpalmar crease to the ring finger is helpful in selecting the proper handle size[41, 42, 45, 46, 49] (Fig. 40–7).

Finally, the weight, dimension, and flexibility of the equipment should match the available strength of the individual. It is better to use a device that is somewhat lighter to ensure proper positioning of the equipment at the time of impact.[42]

Counterforce Bracing. The concepts of functional elbow bracing for tennis elbow were initially introduced by Ilfeld and Field in 1965,[30] and by Froimson in 1971.[19] The term counterforce, introduced by this author in 1973, describes a wide nonelastic support curved for better fit and support of the conical shape of the forearm.[41] Simply stated, the counterforce concept constrains full muscular expansion, thereby decreasing intrinsic muscular force to sensitive or vulnerable areas—the forearm extensors for lateral tennis elbow and the forearm flexors for medial tennis elbow (Fig. 40–8). Studies have shown objective improvement in wrist extension and grip strength or positive biomechanical effects with the counterforce brace.[26, 66] In medial tennis elbow, an additional support just distal to the medial epicondyle is sometimes helpful.[45, 46]

More recent focused compression braces (either air or gel pads) offer no observed advantage and may have a theoretical disadvantage if balanced forearm muscle strength is disturbed.

As noted previously, rigid types of immobilization at the

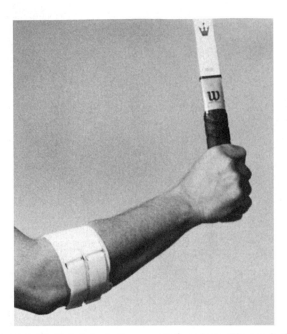

FIGURE 40–8 • Lateral elbow counterforce brace. The nonelastic support is curved to fit the conical forearm shape. Dual tension straps extend the width of the brace and allow full brace tension control. Wide balanced support appears to be most effective for clinical pain control.

elbow or wrist relieve pain, but at the price of atrophy and immobility, and thus are not recommended.

HIGH-VOLTAGE ELECTRICAL STIMULATION

It has been the practice of the sports medicine rehabilitation unit in the author's institution to use high-voltage electrical stimulation in the treatment of both acute and chronic tendinosis. In the author's experience, this modality diminishes pain (chemical inflammation) and may promote healing. This observation certainly parallels reports of enhancement of the bone healing through the electrical stimulation.[3, 4] Our standard practice for tendinosis is to employ four to six sessions of high-voltage electrical stimulation during a 2- to 3-week period.[42, 49]

REHABILITATIVE EXERCISE PROGRAM

This topic is discussed in detail in Chapter 10. It is important to emphasize, again, that rehabilitation should include not only the cardinal forearm exercises but also those for the upper back and shoulder.[42, 49] Once the probable initial adjacent inflammatory response and the pain have been controlled, an orderly progression of the graduated strength and endurance exercise is started.[27, 42, 49] The patient is protected in the early going by the use of the appropriate lateral or medial elbow counterforce brace. Counterforce bracing is generally eliminated after the patient has obtained about 60 percent of the exercise goals.[42, 49]

Graduated Exercise and Full Strength Training. After the patient has reached the early rehabilitative strength and flexibility goals, these functions are monitored by objective testing until strength, endurance, and flexibility have returned to nearly normal levels.

Continuation of the strength and endurance exercise program beyond the preinjury level includes either isokinetic or isotonic exercise, interspaced with isoflex exercises.[27, 42, 49] Before a final return to a sport or an occupational activity, the patient should be capable of anaerobic sprint repetitions to fatigue without major activity pain.[42]

SURGICAL TREATMENT

Historical Review

The popular literature concerning the surgical treatment of tennis elbow is considered to have begun in 1927 with Hohmann,[29] who described release of the extensor aponeurosis at the level of the lateral epicondyle. The technique, now commonly referred to as a muscle slide or release procedure,[36] does not identify the offending pathology.[8, 29, 36, 67]

In 1936, Cyriax[17] was the first to correctly identify the origin of the extensor carpi radialis brevis as the major site of pathology. Cyriax theorized that the extensor brevis origin was often partially torn, and reported treatment by closed manipulation of passive forceful elbow extension and forearm supination, thereby presumably converting a partial tear to a complete tear.

Wadsworth[65] described a similar approach in 1972. Those that include manipulation in treatment relate that the approximately 50 percent success rate is related to the audible or palpable snap or popping associated with the maneuver. This is thought to represent completion of the tear.

In 1955, Bosworth[8] reported on the treatment of a series of 27 elbows, in which four different techniques were used. He suggested that his third technique, which included a release of the extensor aponeurosis as well as the orbicular ligament in and about the radial head, was seemingly curative, although only four patients had been so treated. Bosworth also correctly observed the intimate relationship between the orbicular ligament and the subtendinous layers of the finger and wrist extensors. With release of the extensor aponeurosis and generous removal of the orbicular ligament, he undoubtedly released or removed the origin of the extensor brevis. Curiously, Bosworth[8] performed the Hohmann-type operation in 17 instances, but "all" still had some complaints. In addition to the concepts of tendon release as advanced by Hohmann and Bosworth, a companion intervention of resection of a portion of the lateral epicondyle has been undertaken by some authors.[38, 53] This approach undoubtedly was based on the erroneous premise that the pathology was an inflammation of the lateral epicondyle secondary to the misnomer *lateral epicondylitis*.

In a fascinating application of the conviction that the origin of the extensor carpi radialis brevis was the source of pathology, Garden[22] reported 50 instances in which the extensor brevis tendon was lengthened in the *distal forearm*. He concluded, as had others,[16] that active muscular contraction of the tendons, including the extensor carpi radialis brevis, causes pain. In 44 cases treated with open Z-plasty lengthening at the musculotendinous junction, Garden noted full pain relief was apparently obtained in all cases. However, in 20 cases (40 percent) strength had not returned to normal. Stovall and Beinfeld[61] has also reported success with extensor carpi radialis lengthening.

Surgical Options

As noted, historical open-surgical options have focused predominantly on the release of the extensor aponeurosis, as originally proposed by Hohmann. More recent versions of this approach have included percutaneous release.[60, 68] The reports to date, although limited, do suggest that this procedure can be effective in as many as 90 percent or more of patients and has a relatively low complication rate.[60, 68] As an adjunct to the surgical release of the common extensor tendon, Cabot[11] also recommends the release of the anterior capsule for patients who have flexion contracture. He indicates an 87 percent success rate among the 47 cases in whom this adjunctive approach was included. In my observation, adhesive capsulitis does occur, but usually not in association with the classic tennis elbow presentation; thus, capsular release is not a typical feature of my preferred surgical procedure.

Several surgical options are available besides release of the extensor aponeurosis from the lateral epicondyle. In 1964, Goldie[24] presented a comprehensive thesis that for the first time detailed pathologic changes in the subtendinous tissue in and about the lateral epicondyle in 49 patients. He described tendinous tissue that was invaded in many places by cellular infiltration of round and fibroblastic cells as well as vascular infiltrates.

Kaplan[32] reported three cases of resection of the radial nerve branches to the lateral epicondyle and lateral articular areas with no attempt to identify or remove pathologic tissues. He noted excellent pain relief, but denervation of a motor branch to the extensor brevis probably occurred with this technique. Interestingly, his three patients were hospitalized postoperatively for an average of 7 days. Roles and Maudsley[57] described 33 patients who responded to surgical decompression of the radial nerve. The surgery was performed by 11 different surgeons over a 10-year period. Review of this paper suggests that the extensor brevis was released as part of the decompression. Posterior interosseous nerve compression continues to be recognized as an entity, with recent reports emphasizing the association of compression of the nerve at the arcade of Frohse.[12, 31] The significance of this entity is still unclear, at least from a statistical standpoint. In one study, 5 percent of patients were noted to have nerve entrapment in association with tendinosis.[67]

More recently, Baker and Cummings[1] introduced an arthroscopic approach as a surgical option for lateral tennis elbow. They describe débridement of the extensor brevis as well as occasional intra-articular synovitis when present. The approach identifies tendon pathology but results in the increased costs and risks of intra-articular transgression for a problem which is primarily extra-articular. It is consistent, however, with the recommendations of Bosworth,[8] which include an intra-articular component to the procedure.

Surgical Pathology

A basic principle of any orthopedic surgery is that a clear definition of the pathology is essential for a well-conceived surgical procedure. Because the extensor brevis origin is largely covered by the muscle of the extensor carpi radialis longus, release operations have not visualized the ten-

dinosis pathology. Release of the common extensor origin, however, may alter the attachment of the brevis, since a significant segment of its origin is derived from the extensor aponeurosis.[10, 20, 25, 46–48] This helps to explain the instances of success of release techniques, including percutanous procedures.[5, 20, 60, 68]

Coonrad and Hooper[16] described gross pathologic changes (including tears) in and about the tendinous structures in both medial and lateral tennis elbow, but did not comment on histologic changes. Blazina and colleagues[7] suggested that the major pathologic tendon changes in chronic patellar tendinosis occur by moderate but repetitive overload that results in microrupture of the normal tendinous tissue and secondary replacement by the resulting pathologic healing process. Although this theory is attractive, I believe that a more likely hypothesis is related to vascular supply and follows a sequence of events similar to that described by McNab in the rotator cuff region of the shoulder[35, 37]; namely, vascular compromise, an altered nutritional state, and intrinsic mechanical failure that results from force overload. In any event, actual gross disruption of the extensor carpi radialis brevis tendon, usually incomplete, occurs in approximately 35 percent of my surgical cases. Overall, the extensor carpi radialis brevis is involved by tendinosis in 100 percent of cases with additional involvement of the anteromedial aspects of the extensor digitorum communis tendon (e.g., extensor aponeurosis) also in approximately 35 percent.

Historical Surgical Results

The literature suggests that for lateral tennis elbow approximately 85 to 90 percent of patients can expect some pain relief success with the varied surgical techniques discussed.[8, 9, 16, 29, 36, 53] Most articles, however, are limited or silent regarding the logistics and speed of postoperative recovery. Utilizing this author's preferred technique, 97 percent of patients can expect pain improvement.[46–48] In 85 percent, full return to all prior activities without pain can be expected. In 12 percent, improvement has occurred, with some pain during aggressive activities, but often patients are able to participate in their usual sports, including the racquet and throwing sports. In about 3 percent, no improvement is obtained, and the surgery is considered a failure. The reasons for failure of the preferred technique are not always clear, but possibilities include misdiagnosis, such as entrapment of the posterior interosseous nerve and nonphysical or secondary gain factors.[50] Failure of the biologic healing response has been noted in one primary case of the authors's reported series of salvage procedures.[50]

AUTHOR'S PREFERRED SURGICAL TREATMENT METHOD

Selection Factors For Surgery

Failure of Rehabilitation and Duration of Symptoms. Patients who have undergone a high-quality rehabilitation and resistance-exercise conservative treatment program but have symptoms that linger for more than 1 year are more likely to have category III pathologic changes.[42, 46, 49]

Multiple Cortisone Injections. The success of cortisone injections or the delivery of corticosteroids by other mechanisms generally has been accepted clinically. Clarke and Woodland[15] confirmed this clinical impression but emphasize that the improvement is short-lived and recurrence is the rule. Patients who have received three or more cortisone injections in or about the same area are likely surgical candidates.[46] There are two considerations in this group of candidates. First, the patient's symptoms were of such severity that cortisone injection was warranted and may have indicated a higher pathologic category at the time the patient sought clinical help. Second, the studies of Unverferth and Olix[63] and others[2] suggest that large amounts of cortisone infiltration have a deleterious effect on the quality of the tendon.

Lateral Epicondylar Bony Exostosis. In the author's observations, bony exostosis at the anteromedial area of the lateral epicondyle is present in approximately 20 percent of those undergoing surgery and suggests a refractory process.

Pain (Constant) Without Activity. Pain at rest and that which alters routine daily function invariably reflects category III tendon pathology, suggesting the need for surgery.[42, 46]

Ease of Injection Flow. It has been the author's experience that easy injection flow into the triangular recess under the extensor brevis origin, just distal and anterior to the lateral epicondyle, invariably indicates loosened friable, edematous tendinosis tissue. This injection "feel" is a clear indication that category III pathologic changes are present.

Tendon Calcification. Calcification in the body of the common extensor tendon (extensor aponeurosis) just distal to the lateral epicondyle has been noted on rare occasions. This form of presentation represents a pathologic tendon and is separate and distinct from lateral epicondylar exostosis (Fig. 40–9).

Associated Intra-articular Pathology. In the author's experience, approximately 5 percent of lateral tennis elbow cases have associated intra-articular signs and symptoms (e.g., synovial entrapment, chondromalacia, occasional loose bodies). Combined tendinosis and intra-articular pathologies should be evident after appropraiate preoperative evaluation. Such combined pathologies warrant resection and repair of the tendinosis and a miniarthrotomy to resolve the intra-articular pathology.

Patient Frustration. Those unable or unwilling to modify their activity level are likely candidates for surgical intervention when the process is a major limitation to the activities of daily living as well as appropriate sports and occupational activities.

Technique

Identification of Pathology. Identification and excision of all pathologic tendinosis tissue generally includes most of, if not the entire, origin of the extensor carpi radialis brevis (Fig. 40–10). On occasion, this also includes the anteromedial aspects of the extensor digitorum communis aponeurosis and, rarely, the removal of pathologic tissue from the underside of the extensor longus. When the extensor brevis origin is excised, the intimate and firm attachments between the fascia of the extensor brevis and the orbicular ligament and insertion into the distal aponeurosis

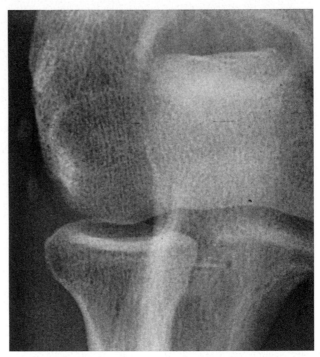

FIGURE 40–9 • Calcification in and about the lateral epicondyle occurs in 22 percent of surgical cases.

eliminate any distal extensor brevis retraction beyond 1 to 2 mm. Maintenance of normal muscle length ensures normal leverage of the remainder of the musculotendinous unit of the extensor brevis; therefore, return to nearly normal forearm extensor strength can be anticipated with the preferred surgical technique.

Healing. Once the pathologic tissue has been removed, a tissue defect is present in varying degrees. It is appropriate to attempt to enhance the blood supply to this area by drilling two or three small holes through the cortical bone into the cancellous area, thereby encouraging hematoma formation, followed by ingrowth of vascular and fibrotendinosis healthy replacement tissue for the extensor carpi radialis brevis origin[46, 47] (see Fig. 40–10).

Tissue Repair. Imbrication of the extensor longus over the anterior edge of the extensor aponeurosis or sewing remaining extensor brevis is unnecessary and tends to block full elbow extension. Restoration of the normal anatomic position, by sewing the posterolateral edge of the extensor longus to the anterior edge of the extensor aponeurosis, has been successful without causing loss of motion and is the repair technique of choice.[46, 47]

Because all the incisions are made longitudinally and, in most cases, do not disturb the extensor aponeurosis attachment to the lateral epicondyle, the surgery provides a firm anchoring point for prompt initiation of the postoperative rehabilitative exercises.

Postoperative Rehabilitation

The postoperative rehabilitation of either lateral or medial tennis elbow for the author's preferred techniques follows the treatment principles outlined for conservative care[42, 49] and detailed in Chapter 10. The elbow is maintained in

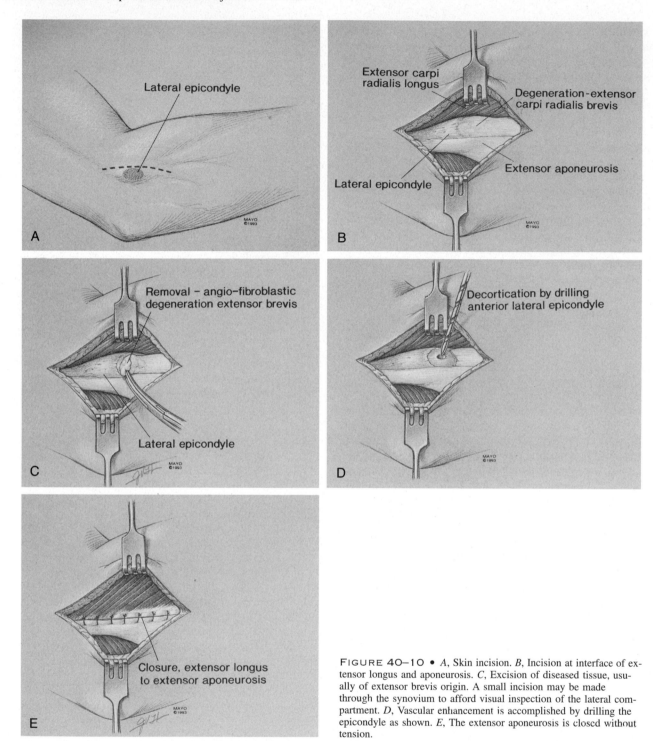

FIGURE 40–10 • *A*, Skin incision. *B*, Incision at interface of extensor longus and aponeurosis. *C*, Excision of diseased tissue, usually of extensor brevis origin. A small incision may be made through the synovium to afford visual inspection of the lateral compartment. *D*, Vascular enhancement is accomplished by drilling the epicondyle as shown. *E*, The extensor aponeurosis is closed without tension.

an easily removable elbow immobilizer in the immediate postoperative period for approximately 6 days.[46, 47] Limbering activities are undertaken, however, on days 2 to 3, generally by working the arm actively in a warm shower for 1 week, followed by a gradual return to strength training exercises without resistance for the first 3 weeks postoperatively. Gradual isotonic and isoflex resistances are then implemented, starting at 3 weeks postoperatively with protection by a medial or lateral counterforce brace. Coun-

terforce bracing usually persists for 2 to 3 months for activities of daily living (ADLs) and thereafter for sports or occupational activity. Strength training and discretionary use of the arm for other activities are individualized to patient needs.[41, 46, 49] For recreational tennis, it is usual to start easy strokes about 6 weeks from the time of surgery. For return to competitive athletics or occupational activities, the increase in intensity should be gradual and gentle, with counterforce brace protection until full strength has

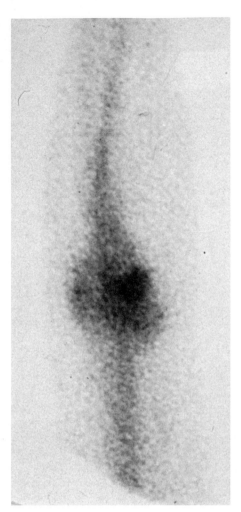

FIGURE 40–11 • A positive ⁹⁹Tc bone scan in a patient who had in-tra- and extra-articular lateral joint symptoms of 2 years' duration.

Associated Considerations

In about 20 percent of cases, bony exostosis is noted at the tip of the lateral epicondyle. This abnormality is often caused by a direct blow to the lateral epicondyle. On these occasions, a partial peel-back of the origin of the extensor aponeurosis and removal of the exostosis or calcification are undertaken. Routine reattachment of the anteromedial aponeurosis to the posterior edge of the extensor longus is then instituted. It is rarely necessary to retract more than 25 percent of the aponeurosis from the lateral epicondyle or excise more than 50 percent of the epicondylar tip.

As noted, in the author's experience intra-articular patho-logic changes in the lateral compartment without additional unrelated trauma or disease (e.g., osteochondritis dissecans, primary or traumatic arthritis, osteocartilaginous loose bod-ies) is uncommon (5 percent).

However, partial and, on occasion, complete tears with penetration through the synovium into the lateral joint compartment may occur in 35 percent of cases. In the performance of the operation, if preoperative evaluation suggests an intra-articular problem, it is recommended to make a small opening in the synovium to inspect the lateral articular compartment. On occasion, during this inspection of the lateral compartment, the author has noted synovitis, scar plicae, or chondromalacic change. Intra-articular changes, including a small erosion of the hyaline cartilagi-nous surface on the radial head, have also been observed by others.[1, 39, 60] In these circumstances, the author performs an intra-articular débridement. When symptoms suggest an intra-articular component, a preoperative bone scan is often ordered (Fig. 40–11). If positive or if intra-articular analge-sia relieves the pain, an arthroscopy rather than limited arthrotomy might be considered to address intra-articular pathology. My experience with limited arthrotomy, how-ever, closely reduplicates the postoperative morbidity of arthroscopy (Fig. 40–12).

returned to the extremity as measured by Cybex or dyna-mometer tests and circumferential forearm girth.[42] Satisfac-tory completion of the rehabilitative process includes tran-sitional exercise programs for a return to sports activities. A return to full-strength use of the arm in competitive athletics, including the world class level, averages 5 to 6 months for lateral elbow tendinosis and 6 to 8 months for medial elbow tendinosis.

SUMMARY

The key issue in tennis elbow, whether lateral or medial, is understanding and identification of the tendinosis histo-pathology that is devoid of inflammatory cells. The goals of treatment focus on revitalization of the area of tendinosis by rehabilitation. If the rehabilitative process fails, surgical

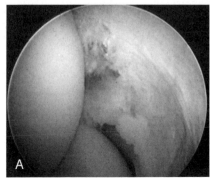
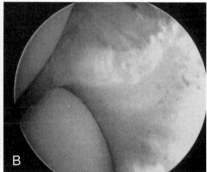

FIGURE 40–12 • A, Arthroscopy of the patient in Figure 40–11 shows moderate capsular degenera-tion. B, After the degenerated capsule was removed arthroscopically, the pain decreased.

resection and repair is an appropriate and highly successful option.

ACKNOWLEDGMENT • Appreciation is expressed to E. Russell Stay, M.D., Department of Pathology, Arlington Hospital, for his initial and original histopathologic evaluation and description of tennis elbow (Angio-Fibroblastic Hyperplasia).[62]

REFERENCES

1. Baker, C., and Cummings, P.: Arthroscopic management of miscellaneous elbow disorders. Operative Techniques Sportsmed. **6**:16, 1998.
2. Balasubramaniam, P., and Prathap, K.: The effect of injection of hydrocortisone into rabbit calcaneal tendons. J. Bone Joint Surg. **54B**:729, 1972.
3. Bassett, C. A. L.: Pulsing electromagnetic fields: A new method to modify cell behavior in calcified and noncalcified tissues. Calcif. Tissue Int. **34**:1, 1982.
4. Bassett, C. A. L., Choksh, H. R., Hernandez, E., Pawlik, R. J., and Strap, M.: The effect of pulsing electromagnetic fields on cellular calcium and calcification of nonunions. In Brighton, C. T., Black, J., and Pollack, S. R. (eds.): Electrical Properties of Bone and Cartilage: Experimental Effects and Clinical Applications. New York, Grune & Stratton, 1979.
5. Baumgard, S. H., and Schwartz, D. R.: Percutaneous release of the epicondylar muscles for humeral epicondylitis. Am. J. Sports Med. **10**:233, 1982.
6. Bernhang, A. M.: The many causes of tennis elbow. N. Y. State J. Med. **79**:1363, 1979.
7. Blazina, H. E., Kerlan, R. K., Jobe, F. W., Carter, J. S., and Carlson, G. J.: Jumper's knee. Orthop. Clin. North Am. **413**:665, 1973.
8. Bosworth, D. H.: The role of the orbicular ligament in tennis elbow. J. Bone Joint Surg. **37A**:527, 1955.
9. Boyd, H. B., and McLeod, A. C.: Tennis elbow. J. Bone Joint Surg. **55A**:1183, 1973.
10. Briggs, C. A., and Elliott, B. G.: Lateral epicondylitis: A review of structures associated with tennis elbow. Anat. Clin. **7**:149, 1985.
11. Cabot, A.: Tennis elbow, a curable affliction. Orthop. Rev. **16**:69, 1987.
12. Capener, N.: The vulnerability of the posterior interosseous nerve of the forearm: A case report and an anatomical study. J. Bone Joint Surg. **48B**:770, 1966.
13. Carp, L.: Tennis elbow caused by radiohumeral bursitis. Arch. Surg. **24**:905, 1932.
14. Carroll, R. E.: Personal communication.
15. Clarke, A. K., and Woodland, J.: Comparison of two steroid preparations used to treat tennis elbow, using the hypospray. Rheum. Rehabil. **14**:47, 1975.
16. Coonrad, R. W., and Hooper, W. R.: Tennis elbow: Its course, natural history, conservative and surgical management. J. Bone Joint Surg. **55A**:1177, 1973.
17. Cyriax, J. H.: The pathology and treatment of tennis elbow. J. Bone Joint Surg. **18**:921, 1936.
18. Emery, S. E., and Gifford, J. F.: 100 years of tennis elbow. Contemp. Orthop. **12**:53, 1986.
19. Froimson, A. I.: Treatment of tennis elbow with forearm support band. J. Bone Joint Surg. **53A**:183, 1971.
20. Field, L., Altchek, D., Warren, R., O'Brien, S., Shyhar, M., and Wickiewicz, T.: Arthroscopic anatomy of the lateral elbow. Arthroscopy **10**:602, 1994.
21. Funk, D. A., An, K. N., Morrey, B. F., and Daube, J. R.: Electromyographic analysis of muscles across the elbow joint. J. Orthop. Res. **5**:529, 1987.
22. Garden, R. S.: Tennis elbow. J. Bone Joint Surg. **43B**:100, 1961.
23. Gardner, R. C.: Tennis elbow: Diagnosis, pathology and treatment: Nine severe cases treated by a new reconstructive operation. Clin. Orthop. Rel. Res. **72**:248, 1970.
24. Goldie, I.: Epicondylitis lateralis humeri (epicondylalgia or tennis elbow): A pathogenetical study. Acta Chir. Scand. Suppl. 339, 1964.
25. Greenbaum, B., and Vangsness, T.: Extensor carpi radialis brevis: An anatomic analysis of its origin. Presented to the Interim Meeting, American Orthopedic Society for Sportsmedicine. New Orleans, March 22, 1998.
26. Groppel, J. L., Nirschl, R. P., Pfantsch, E., and Greer, N.: A mechanical and electromyographical analysis of the effects of various joint counterforce braces on the tennis player. Am. J. Sports Med. **14**:195, 1986.
27. Groppel, J. L., Nirschl, R. P., Sholes, J., and Sobel, J.: A mechanical comparison of an isoflex exercise device to the use of free weights. Unpublished data, 1984.
28. Gunn, C. C., and Milbrandt, W. E.: Tennis elbow and the cervical spine. Can. Med. Assoc. J. **114**:803, 1976.
29. Hohmann, G.: Das Wesen und die Behandlung des Sogenannten tennissellenbogens. Munch. Med. Wochenschr. **80**:250, 1933.
30. Ilfeld, F. W., and Field, S. M.: Treatment of tennis elbow: Use of special brace. J.A.M.A. **195**:67, 1966.
31. Jalovaara, P., and Lindholm, R. V.: Decompression of the posterior interosseous nerve for tennis elbow. Arch. Orthop. Trauma Surg. **108**:243, 1989.
32. Kaplan, E. B.: Treatment of tennis elbow (epicondylitis) by denervation. J. Bone Joint Surg. **41A**:147, 1959.
33. Kraushaar, B., and Nirschl, R.: Tendinosis of the elbow (tennis elbow): Clinical features and findings of histological, immunohistochemical, and electron microscopy studies. J. Bone Joint Surg. **81A**:259, 1999.
34. Major, H. P.: Lawntennis elbow. B.M.J. **2**:557, 1883.
35. McNab, I.: Rotator cuff tendinosis. Ann. R. Coll. Surg. Engl. **53**:271, 1973.
36. Michele, A. A., and Krueger, F. J.: Lateral epicondylitis of the elbow treated by fasciotomy. Surgery **39**:277, 1956.
37. Moseley, H. F., and Goldie, I.: The arterial pattern of the rotator cuff of the shoulder. J. Bone Joint Surg. **45B**:780, 1963.
38. Neviaser, T. J., Neviaser, R. J., Neviaser, J. S., and Ain, B. R.: Lateral epicondylitis: Results of outpatient surgery and immediate motion. Contemp. Orthop. **11**:43, 1985.
39. Newman, J. H., and Goodfellow, J. W.: Fibrillation of the head of the radius: One cause of tennis elbow. J. Bone Joint Surg. **57B**:115, 1975.
40. Nirschl, R. P.: Mesenchymal syndrome. Virginia Med. M. **96**:659, 1969.
41. Nirschl, R. P.: Tennis elbow. Orthop. Clin. North Am. **4**:787, 1973.
42. Nirschl, R. P.: Arm care. Arlington, VA, Med. Sports Pub., 1983.
43. Nirschl, R. P.: Isoflex exercise system. Arlington, VA, Med. Sports Pub., 1983.
44. Nirschl, R. P.: Unpublished data.
45. Nirschl, R. P.: Prevention and treatment of elbow and shoulder injuries in the tennis player. Clin. Sportsmed. **7**:289, 1998.
46. Nirschl, R. P.: Elbow tendinosis/tennis elbow. Clin. Sportsmed. **2**:851, 1992.
47. Nirschl, R. P.: Lateral and medial epicondyltis. In Morrey, B. (ed.): Master Techniques in Orthopedic Surgery: The Elbow. New York, Raven Press, 1994, pp. 129–148.
48. Nirschl, R. P., and Pettrone, F.: Tennis elbow: The surgical treatment of lateral epicondylitis. J. Bone Joint Surg. **61A**:832, 1979.
49. Nirschl, R. P., and Sobel, J.: Conservative treatment of tennis elbow. Phys. Sports Med. **9**:42, 1981.
50. Organ, S., Nirschl, R., Kraushaar, B., and Guidi, E.: Salvage surgery for lateral tennis elbow. Am. J. Sportsmed. **25**:746, 1997.
51. Osgood, R. B.: Radiohumeral bursitis, epicondylitis, epicondylalgia (tennis elbow): A personal experience. Arch. Surg. **4**:420, 1922.
52. Percy, C., and Carson, J. D.: Use of DMSO in tennis elbow and rotator cuff tendinosis: Double-blind study. Med. Sci. Sports Exer. **13**:215, 1981.
53. Posch, J. N., Goldberg, V. M., and Larrey, R.: Extensor fasciotomy for tennis elbow: A long-term follow-up study. Clin. Orthop. **135**:179, 1978.
54. Priest, J. D., Braden, V., and Gerberich, J. G.: The elbow and tennis (part I). Phys. Sports Med. **8**:80, 1980.
55. Priest, J. D., Braden, V., and Gerberich, J. G.: The elbow and tennis (part II). Phys. Sports Med. **8**:77, 1980.
56. Regan, W., Wold, L. E., Coonrad, R., and Morrey, B. F.: Microscopic histopathology of lateral epicondylitis. Am. J. Sports Med. **20**:746, 1992.
57. Roles, N. C., and Maudsley, R. H.: Radial tunnel syndrome, resistant tennis elbow as a nerve entrapment. J. Bone Joint Surg. **54B**:499, 1972.
58. Runge, F.: Zur Genese und Behandlung des Schreibekrampfes. Berl. Klin. Wochenschr. **10**:245, 1873.

59. Sarkar, K., and Uhthoff, H. K.: Ultrastructure of the common extensor tendon in tennis elbow. Virchows Arch. Pathol. Anat. Histol. **386**:317, 1980.

60. Savoie, F.: Percutaneous release in the release on the surgical treatment of lateral epicondylitis. Presented to the 3rd International Meeting of the Society for Tennis Medicine. New Haven, Conn., June 1997.

61. Stovall, P. B., and Beinfield, M. S.: Treatment of resistant lateral epicondylitis of the elbow by lengthening of the extensor carpi radialis brevis tendon. Surg. Gynecol. Obstet. **149**:526, 1979.

62. Stay, E. R.: Personal communication.

63. Unverferth, L. J., and Olix, M. L.: The effect of local steroid injection on tendon. J. Sports Med. **1**:31, 1973.

64. Vangsness, T., and Jobe, F.: The surgical treatment of medial epicondylitis. American Shoulder and Elbow Surgeons Interim Meeting, Atlanta, Feb. 7, 1988.

65. Wadsworth, T. G.: Lateral epicondylitis. Lancet **1**:959, 1972.

66. Wadsworth, C. T., Nielsen, D. H., Burns, L. T., Krull, J. D., and Thompson, C. G.: The effect of the counterforce armband on wrist extension and grip strength and pain in subjects with tennis elbow. J. Orthop. Sports Phys. Ther. **11**:192, 1989.

67. Werner, C. O.: Lateral elbow pain and posterior interosseous nerve entrapment. Acta Orthop. Scand. Suppl. **174**:1, 1979.

68. Yerger, B., and Turner, T.: Percutaneous extensor tenotomy for chronic tennis elbow: An office procedure. Orthopaedics **8**:1261, 1985.

CHAPTER 41

Medial Epicondylitis

- GERARD T. GABEL and
  BERNARD F. MORREY

Medial epicondylitis is the most common cause of medial elbow pain but is only 15 to 20 percent as common as lateral epicondylitis. The relative infrequency of medial epicondylitis has resulted in a paucity of information on medial epicondylitis until the last 10 years. Work by Vangsness and Jobe,[21] Gabel and Morrey,[5] Ollivierre and associates,[16] and Kurvers and Verhaar[10] has clarified the pathology, treatment, and outcomes in medial epicondylitis. The significance of associated ulnar neuropathy at the elbow has also been assessed and is the primary component of the classification of medial epicondylitis. The results of nonoperative management, including corticosteroid injections, have been reported by Stahl and Kaufman.[20] The compilation of information in these studies[6] has resulted in a clearer understanding of medial epicondylitis and its management, allowing more appropriate patient care.

ANATOMY

The anatomy of medial epicondylitis involves musculotendinous, neural, and ligamentous concerns. The flexor pronator origin at the anterior medial epicondyle is the central focus of medial epicondylitis. The pronator teres originates in part off the superoanterior medial epicondyle, but its primary origin is from an intramuscular tendon (the medial conjoint tendon [MCT]) that has been previously described as the accessory anterior oblique ligament or anisometropic anterior oblique ligament. Although it has been demonstrated to be a weak valgus stabilizer in near full extension, it is expendable and plays no role in valgus stability in the presence of an intact anterior oblique ligament (AOL). (The only clinical circumstance in which this structure plays a role in valgus stability is in elbow dislocations such that if the flexor pronator mass is minimally disrupted the accessory anterior oblique ligament may prevent gross instability.)

The pronator teres origin off the MCT occupies the proximoradial side of this vertically oriented septum (Fig. 41–1). The flexor carpi radialis, which also has a very small direct muscular epicondylar origin, finds its primary origin off the distoulnar aspect of the MCT. Although additional muscular or tendinous origins off the epicondyle are seen, the critical lesion of medial epicondylitis consists of this medial conjoint tendon and its associated pronator teres and flexor carpi radialis origins.

Although it plays a central mechanical role in medial epicondylitis, the MCT serves surgically as a landmark for the pathology of medial epicondylitis as well as a means of identification and avoidance of the anterior oblique ligament proper. The MCT rises off the anterior inferior epicondyle with an oblique parasagittal orientation extending approximately 12 cm into the proximal forearm. Immediately posterior to the proximal 3 to 4 cm of the MCT is the AOL (see Fig. 41–1). There is a surgical interval between the MCT and AOL, but anatomically they are contiguous throughout the length of the AOL. Any surgical elevation off the medial epicondyle posterior to the MCT necessarily violates the origin of the AOL.

The neural concerns in medial epicondylitis consist of the medial antebrachial cutaneous nerve (MABCN) and the ulnar nerve. The MABCN courses in the subcutaneous tissue in the anteromedial arm[12] until just proximal to the medial epicondyle, where it divides into an anterior branch, which travels distally, and a posterior branch,[2] which travels directly over the flexor pronator mass to the posterior medial forearm. The ulnar nerve rests on the posterior aspect of the medial intermuscular septum in the arm. As it approaches the medial epicondyle, it is covered by a retinaculum,[15] which maintains its position preventing subluxation. It enters the forearm through the two heads of the flexor carpi ulnaris at the cubital tunnel. At entry into the cubital tunnel, the ulnar nerve lies immediately adjacent to the posterior margin of the flexor pronator mass.

PRESENTATION

Medial epicondylitis presents with medial elbow pain, activity-related, especially repetitive or forceful pronation. It has a peak incidence in the third through fifth decade with a 2:1 male/female ratio. It occurs in the dominant elbow in 60 percent of cases and is associated with an acute injury

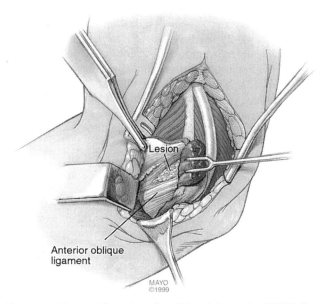

FIGURE 41–1 • Illustration of medial conjoint tendon (MCT). Forceps are on the vertically oriented MCT. Note that the anterior oblique ligament (AOL) lies on the posterior margin of the MCT. Elevation of the MCT should be performed carefully to avoid injury to the AOL.

537

11. Martin, C. D., and Schweitzer, M. E.: MR imaging of epicondylitis. Skel. Radiol. **27**:133, 1998.
12. Masear, V. R., Meyer, R. D., Pichora, D. R.: Surgical anatomy of the medial antebrachial cutaneous nerve. J. Hand Surg. Am. **14**:267, 1989.
13. Molsberger, A., and Hille, E.: The analgesic effect of acupuncture in chronic tennis elbow pain. Br. J. Rheum. **33**:1162, 1994.
14. O'Driscoll, S. W., Horii, E., and Morrey, B. F.: Anatomy of the attachment of the medial ulnar collateral ligament. J. Bone Joint Surg. **17**:164, 1992.
15. O'Driscoll, S. W., Horii, G., Carmichael, S. W., and Morrey, B. F.: The cubital tunnel and ulnar neuropathy. J. Bone Joint Surg. **73B**:613, 1991.
16. Ollivierre, C. O., Nirschl, R. P., and Pettrone, F. A.: Resection and repair for medial tennis elbow. A prospective analysis. Am. J. Sports Medicine. **23**:214, 1995.
17. Potter, H. G., Hannafin, J. A., Morwessel, R. M., Dicarlo, E. F., O'Brien, S. J., and Altchek, D. W.: Lateral epicondylitis: correlation of MR imaging, surgical, and histopathologic findings. Radiology **196**:43, 1995.
18. Rompe, J. D., Hope, C., Kullmer, K., Heine, J., and Burger, R.: Analgesic effect of extracorporeal shock wave therapy on chronic tennis elbow. J. Bone Joint Surg. **78B**:233, 1996.
19. Schwab, G. H., Bennett J. B., Woods, G. W., and Tullos, M. S.: Biomechanics of elbow instability. The role of the medial collateral ligament. Clin. Orthop. **146**:42, 1980.
20. Stahl, S., and Kaufman, T.: Ulnar nerve injury at the elbow after steroid injection for medial epicondylitis. J. Hand Surg. Br. **21**:69, 1997.
21. Vangsness, C. T., and Jobe, F. W.: Surgical management of medial epicondylitis. J. Bone Joint Surg. **73B**:409, 1991.
22. Vassellen, O., Jr., Hoeg, N., Kjeldstad, B., et al.: Low level laser versus placebo in the treatment of tennis elbow. Scand. J. Rehabil. Med. **24**:37, 1992.

•CHAPTER 42•

Surgical Failure of Tennis Elbow

• BERNARD F. MORREY

Lateral epicondylitis is the most common elbow affliction in adults. Failures after surgery are recognized, but the cause and the means of re-evaluation are seldom addressed. Initially, the most frequent explanation for residual symptoms is too brief a period after surgery or inadequate rehabilitation. The latter may be due to noncompliance or an inadequate program of strengthening and stretching exercises.[16] This type of problem is readily determined with a careful interview. The reliability of surgical procedures for lateral epicondylitis makes the need for reoperation uncommon. For this reason, few surgeons have extensive experience with the management of patients after failed intervention for epicondylitis, and reports of such experience in the literature are lacking. The intent of this chapter is to share our experience with this problem and to provide a basis for determining the cause of failure and a basis for further management. Specific focus is on determining which patients might benefit from a second surgical procedure.

ETIOLOGY AND PATHOLOGY

Because the treatment of surgical failure in large measure relates to the etiology and pathology, analysis of treatment failure logically begins with a brief consideration of the pathoanatomy of lateral epicondylitis. This is discussed in detail in Chapter 40. Consensus major opinion in recent years has placed the pathology at the origin of the common extensor muscle tendon,[4, 6, 10, 12, 16] specifically the extensor carpi radialis brevis tendon.[19] This is an important point in the subsequent evaluation of residual pain after surgery.

Although lateral epicondylitis is generally considered an inflammatory lesion, the precise pathology of the condition is debated, with as many as 14 pathologic features being reported in the literature (Table 42–1).[20] A careful blinded study of pathologic and control material reported by Regan and colleagues[20] demonstrated a histopathologic picture as one of hyaline degeneration with neovasculature. In essence, the material removed at surgery reveals an aborted effort of healing and hyaline degeneration, but not of inflammation, an observation that is now generally accepted.

Regardless of the etiology or underlying pathology, nonoperative management is reported successful in as many as 90 percent of patients.[16] Similarly, when surgery is performed, a 90 percent success rate is typical. The interesting feature of these data is that the success of surgery seems independent of the surgical technique.[2, 3, 6, 11, 15, 16, 19, 22, 26] On the other hand, when surgical intervention is not successful, there has been but a single description of the causes of failure, the method of assessment, and the results of reoperation.[13]

PATIENT EVALUATION

History

The first step in the evaluation process is to critically assess the patient and motives. Next, determine whether an adequate period has elapsed since surgery, including whether the patient has exhibited adequate compliance to the rehabilitation program. If concern exists about either point, the patient is treated for symptoms and reassessed. If at least 6 to 9 months has passed since surgery and there are no worrisome personality features or litigation or compensation issues, the problem may be further studied.

The patient is carefully interviewed to determine whether the symptom complex is identical to or different from that for which the original surgery was performed. This allows the failure to be classified as one of two types, which serves as a basis to direct the subsequent examination and treatment plan.

Classification

TYPE I FAILURE

A type I failure is one in which the patient indicates that the location and character of symptoms are identical to those for which the original surgery was performed. Type I failure consists of three basic types: improper patient selection, incomplete or improper diagnosis, and inadequate or incomplete surgical procedure.

Improper Patient Selection. Patient selection issues include adequate motivation, compliance, and consideration of secondary gain.[23] The same factors that resulted in a failure of nonoperative treatment obtain in the patient undergoing surgery. The best solution for this difficult problem is obvious: avoid the initial surgical procedure in patients known to be at risk for secondary gain.

• TABLE 42–1 • **Histopathologic Features Reported to Be Associated with Lateral Epicondylitis**

Hemorrhage
   Recent (i.e., pooled red blood cells)
   Old (i.e., hemosiderin-laden macrophages)
Fibrinoid degeneration
Hyaline degeneration
Vascular proliferation
Fibroblastic proliferation
Granulation tissue in subtendinous space
Necrosis of tendon fascicles
Calcific debris
Crystalline debris
Cellular infiltrate
Polymorphonuclear leukocytes
Histiocytes
Lipid-laden histiocytes
Lymphocytes

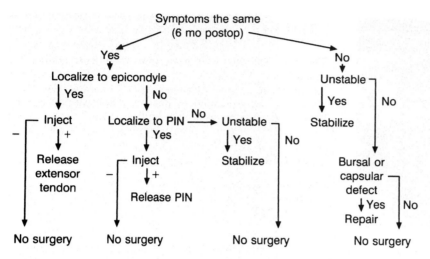

FIGURE 42–8 • A logical sequence of assessment for patients with surgical failure for lateral epicondylitis. Notice that the majority of categories indicate that no surgical intervention is necessary. Also note the major distinction between symptoms that are the same (type I) and those that are different (type II).

correct initial diagnosis, or persistence of the original pathologic condition not corrected by surgery. Type II failure—altered symptoms—may represent a condition associated with the surgical procedure. A careful history leading to studies directed at a specific cause generally isolates the basis of persistent symptoms. In patients with type I failure, if the assessment suggests residual pain at the epicondyle, further release of the extensor tendon at the lateral epicondyle is generally successful. If pain does not localize well to the lateral epicondyle, however, PIN entrapment should be considered. In a patient with a type II failure, either instability or bursal or capsular pathology must be considered. The pivot shift test and arthroscopy are useful in revealing ligamentous insufficiency in the former instance. Arthrography is helpful in identifying capsular and bursal conditions. A satisfactory reoperation may be anticipated in as many as 85 percent of properly selected patients if the reoperation procedure has been well planned.

REFERENCES

1. Abrahamsson, S. O., Sollerman, C., Söderberg, T., Lundborg, G., Rydholm, U., and Pettersson, H.: Lateral elbow pain caused by anconeus compartment syndrome: a case report. Acta Orthop. Scand. **58**:589, 1987.
2. Bosworth, D. M.: The role of the orbicular ligament in tennis elbow. J. Bone Joint Surg. **37A**:527, 1955.
3. Boyd, H. B., and McLeod, A. C.: Tennis elbow. J. Bone Joint Surg. **55A**:1183, 1973.
4. Briggs, C. A., and Elliott, B. G.: Lateral epicondylitis: A review of structures associated with tennis elbow. Anat. Clin. **7**:149, 1985.
5. Capener, N.: The vulnerability of the posterior interosseous nerve of the forearm: a case report and an anatomical study. J. Bone Joint Surg. **48B**:770, 1966.
6. Coonrad, R. W., and Hooper, W. R.: Tennis elbow: its course, natural history, conservative and surgical management. J. Bone Joint Surg. **55A**:1177, 1973.
7. Cyriax, J. H.: The pathology and treatment of tennis elbow. J. Bone Joint Surg. **18**:921, 1936.
8. Dewey, P.: The posterior interosseous nerve and resistant tennis elbow. J. Bone Joint Surg. **55B**:435, 1973.
9. Emery, S. E., and Gifford, J. F.: 100 years of tennis elbow. Contemp. Orthop. **12**:53, 1986.
10. Garden, R. S.: Tennis elbow. J. Bone Joint Surg. **43B**:100, 1961.
11. Gardner, R. C.: Tennis elbow: Diagnosis, pathology and treatment. Nine severe cases treated by a new reconstructive operation. Clin. Orthop. Rel. Res. **72**:248, 1970.
12. Goldie, I.: Epicondylitis lateralis humeri. Acta Chir. Scand. **339(Suppl)**:7, 1964.
13. Morrey, B. F.: Reoperation for failed surgical treatment of refractory lateral epicondylitis. J. Shoulder Elbow Surg. **1**:47, 1992.
14. Morrison, D. L.: Tennis elbow and radial tunnel syndrome: differential diagnosis and treatment. J. Aust. Orthop. Assoc. **80**:823, 1981.
15. Neviaser, T. J., Neviaser, R. J., Neviaser, J. S., and Ain, B. R.: Lateral epicondylitis: results of outpatient surgery and immediate motion. Contemp. Orthop. **11**:43, 1985.
16. Nirschl, R. P., and Pettrone, F. A.: Tennis elbow and the surgical treatment of lateral epicondylitis. J. Bone Joint Surg. **61A**:832, 1979.
17. Organ, S. W., Nirschl, R. P., Kraushaar, B. S., and Guidi, E. J.: Salvage surgery for lateral tennis elbow. Am. J. Sports Med. **25**:746, 1997.
18. O'Driscoll, S. W., Bell, D. F., and Morrey, B. F.: Posterolateral rotatory instability of the elbow. J. Bone Joint Surg. **73A**:440, 1991.
19. Posch, J. N., Goldberg, V. M., and Larrey, R.: Extensor fasciotomy for tennis elbow: a long-term follow-up study. Clin. Orthop. **135**:179, 1978.
20. Regan, W., Wold, L. E., Coonrad, R., and Morrey, B. F.: Microscopic histopathology of lateral epicondylitis. Presented at the Annual Meeting of the Canadian Orthopaedic Association, Toronto, Ontario, June 3, 1989.
21. Roles, N. C., and Maudsley, R. H.: Radial tunnel syndrome: resistant tennis elbow as a nerve entrapment. J. Bone Joint Surg. **54B**:499, 1972.
22. Rossum, J. V., Buruma, J. S., Kamphuisen, H. A. C., and Onvlee, G. J.: Tennis elbow: a radial tunnel syndrome? J. Bone Joint Surg. **60B**:197, 1978.
23. Stovall, P. B., and Beinfield, M. S.: Treatment of resistant lateral epicondylitis of the elbow by lengthening of the extensor carpi radialis brevis tendon. Surg. Gynecol. Obstet. **149**:526, 1979.
24. Volz, R., and Morrey, B. F.: Physical examination of the elbow. In Morrey, B. F. (ed.): The Elbow and Its Disorders. New York, W. B. Saunders Co., 1985.
25. Werner, C. O.: Lateral elbow pain and posterior interosseous nerve entrapment. Acta Orthop. Scand. **114(Suppl)**:174, 1979.
26. Yerger, B., and Turner, T. Percutaneous extensor tenotomy for chronic tennis elbow: an office procedure. Orthopedics **8**:1261, 1985.

CHAPTER 43

Diagnosis and Treatment of Ulnar Collateral Ligament Injuries in Athletes

• FRANK W. JOBE and NEAL S. ELATTRACHE

The ulnar collateral ligament is the primary structure resisting valgus stress at the elbow (see Chapters 3 and 30) (Fig. 43–1).[22, 26] Although trauma to this ligament rarely leads to symptomatic instability of the elbow,[8, 17, 18, 20, 22, 24, 26] throwing sports place repetitive high valgus stress on the medial aspect of the elbow joint.[10, 23] This may result in symptomatic valgus instability caused by ulnar collateral ligament injury, occasionally requiring operative treatment to restore overhead athletic function. Of the complex, the anterior bundle is the major component resisting valgus stress (see Fig. 43–1).

PATHOPHYSIOLOGY

With throwing, the acceleration phase of the arm begins with the elbow in a flexed position between 90 degrees and 120 degrees, followed by rapid extension over 30 to 40 msec to 25 degrees of flexion at ball release. Average angular velocity over this arc of motion can exceed 5000 degrees per second, with peak elbow accelerations of 500,000 degrees/sec^2.[23] This produces concentrated force in a position stabilized nearly exclusively by the anterior band of the ulnar collateral ligament. The articulation contributes little to joint stability over this arc of motion.[11, 21, 22, 26, 28, 30] These forces may exceed the tensile strength of the ligament, producing microscopic tears.[16] Continued throwing can lead to attenuation or rupture of the weakened ligament, preventing a throwing athlete from competing at the highest level.

That few activities expose the ulnar collateral ligament to forces of this magnitude explains the relative paucity of symptomatic elbow instability in the general population. However, many throwers and overhead athletes are incapacitated by ulnar collateral ligament insufficiency.[15]

This ligamentous insufficiency can lead to degenerative or traumatic arthritis, with the formation of osteophytes and loose bodies posteriorly and medially. Calcifications within the injured ligament are also common. Also, developmental cubitus valgus and hypertrophy of the humeral condyles, coronoid process, and posteromedial olecranon can occur.[3, 19, 31] Elbow flexion deformities are often found but usually do not adversely affect performance because the throwing motion involves elbow positions between 120 and 20 degrees of flexion.[23]

Symptoms of ulnar nerve irritation are present in over 40 percent of patients with ulnar collateral ligament insufficiency.[4] Inflammation involving the ulnar collateral ligament, traction, friction, and compression[7, 15] can secondarily affect the ulnar nerve as it crosses the elbow.[14] Medial joint instability under valgus loading and the cubitus valgus deformity lead to traction injury, while friction injuries result from recurrent subluxation of the nerve or abrasion by posteromedial osteophytes. Ulnar nerve compression can result from entrapment by thickened or inflamed tissue in the cubital tunnel and by hypertrophied musculature in the brachium and forearm.

DIAGNOSIS

The keys to making the correct diagnosis of ulnar collateral ligament insufficiency are a detailed history and physical examination. Previous elbow injuries and treatment are noted. A history of repetitive overhand throwing activities is common. Pain is localized to the medial side of the elbow, especially during the late cocking or acceleration phases of the throwing motion (Fig. 43–2). The history typically is further characterized by one of three scenarios: (1) an acute "pop" or sharp pain on the medial aspect of the elbow with the inability to continue to throw; (2) the gradual onset of medial elbow pain over time with throwing; or (3) pain following an episode of throwing with the inability on successive attempts to throw above 50 to 75 percent of full function. The patient may report associated recurrent pain or paresthesia radiating into the ulnar aspect of the forearm, the hand, and the fourth and fifth fingers, especially with throwing.

Examination

Tenderness to palpation over the ulnar collateral ligament complex at the distal insertion is most commonly observed, depending on the degree of inflammation at the time of examination. Such inflammation also may irritate or compress the ulnar nerve locally as it traverses the cubital tunnel.[14] A positive Tinel sign along the cubital tunnel is an

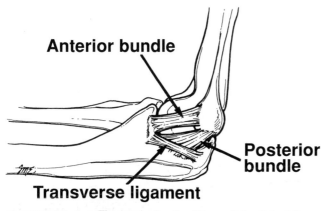

Anterior bundle

Posterior bundle

Transverse ligament

FIGURE 43–1 • The anterior bundle of the medial collateral ligament is the major stabilizer of the elbow to resist valgus stress. The reconstruction is directed at restoring the function of this structure.

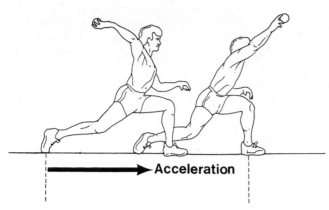

FIGURE 43–2 • Symptoms of ulnar collateral ligament insufficiency are noted primarily during the late cocking and early acceleration phases of the throwing motion.

indication of ulnar nerve irritability, and careful neurologic examination is performed.

Valgus stability of the elbow is best examined with the patient seated and the hand and wrist held securely between the examiner's forearm and trunk (Fig. 43–3). The patient's elbow is flexed beyond 25 degrees to unlock the olecranon from its fossa and minimize the bony contribution to joint stability. The ulnar collateral ligament is palpated while a valgus stress is applied simultaneously. Local pain, tenderness, and end point laxity are characterized with this maneuver. For patients with tears in continuity, these maneuvers are not diagnostic. O'Brien has described the milking test to help diagnose the tear in continuity (Fig. 43–4). The examiner grasps the thumb and fully flexes the elbow, which places a valgus stress on the ligament, causing pain with full flexion.[13] Although these injuries can occur together, especially in throwers,[4] an attempt should be made to differentiate flexor-pronator tendinitis or conjoined tendon rupture from ulnar collateral ligament injury (see

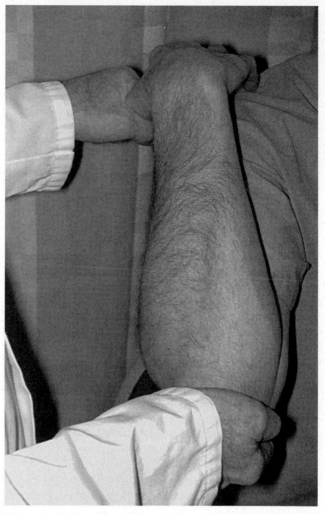

FIGURE 43–4 • The milking test diagnoses tears in continuity without gross instability. It is performed by hyperflexing the elbow with a valgus stress imparted by grabbing the thumb and fully flexing the joint.

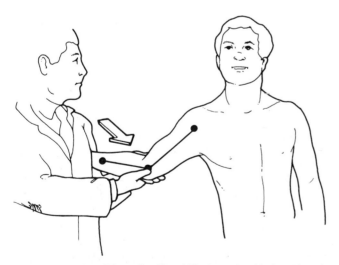

FIGURE 43–3 • Diagnosis of instability is made with the patient sitting and the hand supported in the axilla of the examiner. While one hand of the examiner supports the elbow, valgus stress is applied with the elbow in 25 degrees of flexion. The ulnar collateral ligament is palpated while applying valgus stress. Tenderness and laxity both are assessed during this maneuver.

Chapter 4). With a flexor-pronator tendon injury, resisted volar flexion of the wrist, resisted pronation of the forearm, or a tightly clenched fist elicits pain near the medial epicondyle.

Motion loss or crepitus may also be present, but this is common in throwers and is not specific for medial collateral ligament injury.

Imaging

Radiographic tests, if negative, do not rule out the diagnosis of ulnar collateral ligament insufficiency. Standard radiographs may identify ossification within the ulnar collateral ligament, loose bodies in the posterior compartment, olecranon and condylar hypertrophy, or osteochondrotic lesions of the capitellum. Stress radiographs can show excessive medial joint line opening, indicating ligament laxity (Fig. 43–5). The most important finding is that of a medial ulnohumeral olecranon osteophyte.[1]

Recently, we have found magnetic resonance imaging to be useful as an investigational tool in studying the collateral ligaments. However, as Cotten and associates have

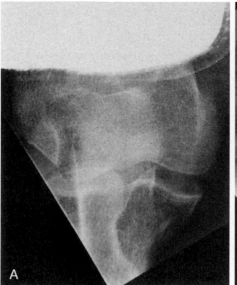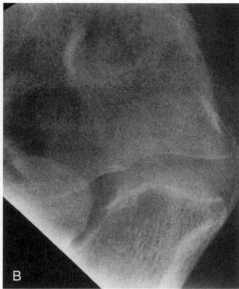

FIGURE 43–5 • Fluoroscopically localized anteroposterior view of the right dominant elbow without *(A)* and with valgus stress *(B)*. Note the opening of the medial joint.

demonstrated, the posterior oblique coronal plane image with gadolinium enhancement improves the accuracy of the diagnosis.[5] Although inflammation or disruption of the ulnar collateral ligament often can be demonstrated, more experience is needed to determine the true sensitivity and specificity of magnetic resonance imaging with regard to this injury. We and others[6] have not found arthrography to be useful, owing to frequent false-negative findings, especially in cases of chronic ulnar collateral ligament insufficiency.

TREATMENT

Rest and nonoperative management, including nonsteroidal anti-inflammatory medications, alternating ice and heat, and other physical therapy modalities applied in the early symptomatic period, may arrest the progression of instability and allow return to full function.[2] We have not found steroid injection to be helpful over the long term. Rest periods with rehabilitation of up to 3 months should be attempted and repeated at least once, especially in those patients who have not experienced an acute rupture.

If relief of pain is the main goal, nonoperative treatment may suffice. Efforts to stabilize by rehabilitating the flexor pronator muscle group are not successful. Hamilton and co-workers,[9] from our laboratory, have shown by electro-myelographic study that the flexor-pronator group cannot compensate for a deficient ligament. Hence, if the patient desires to return to highly competitive overhead or throwing sports and has failed to improve despite a formal nonoperative treatment program, surgical intervention is indicated. Occasionally, a highly motivated patient with an acute rupture of the ligament causing inability to compete may be a candidate for early surgical treatment.

There are two surgical options: repair of the ligament and reconstruction using tendon graft. In our experience, the indications for repair of the ulnar collateral ligament are limited. This technique is reserved for those patients with an acute proximal avulsion of the ulnar collateral ligament from its humeral attachment. The avulsed ligament should be of good quality and without calcifications within it. In this uncommon case, repair may be attempted.[2]

Since 1987, we have avoided repair and performed a reconstruction using free autologous tendon graft in all patients with ulnar collateral ligament insufficiency who have symptomatic valgus instability unresponsive to nonoperative treatment. If the ipsilateral palmaris longus tendon for the free graft is not available, the contralateral tendon, the plantaris tendon, a 3- to 5-mm medial strip of Achilles tendon, or tendons from lesser toe extensors may be used. The palmaris longus tendon has been shown to fail at higher loads with nearly four times the ultimate strength as compared with the anterior band of the ulnar collateral ligament.[25] In our experience, the removal of palmaris tendon for reconstruction of the ulnar collateral ligament causes minimal morbidity with superior overall results as compared with repair of the ulnar collateral ligament. The frequency of postoperative ulnar nerve symptoms is similar following repair or reconstruction, and the recommended rehabilitation times are the same.[4] Therefore, reconstruction of the insufficient ulnar collateral ligament with free autologous tendon graft is our surgical treatment of choice whether acute or chronic.

AUTHORS' PREFERRED SURGICAL TECHNIQUE

In the supine position, the tourniquet is inflated and the arm is abducted, and a 10-cm incision centered over the medial epicondyle is used to expose the myofascia and aponeurosis of the flexor pronator muscle mass, the medial epicondyle, and the medial intermuscular septum in the brachium. Care is taken to protect the medial antebrachial cutaneous nerve as it passes through the medial aspect of the forearm across the surgical field (Fig. 43–6). If there has been a previous anterior transposition of the ulnar nerve, the nerve should be identified and protected prior to exposure of the ulnar collateral ligament. To expose the

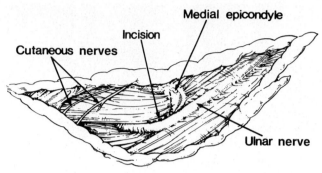

FIGURE 43–6 • Exposure of the medial aspect of the elbow, with particular care to preserve the medial antebrachiocutaneous nerve as it emerges in the distal portion of the surgical field.

ulnar collateral ligament, a longitudinal split is made in the myofascia, the underlying flexor pronator aponeurosis, and the muscle mass at its more anterior origin from the medial epicondyle. Retraction of the flexor mass to both sides provides access and exposure to the anterior portion of the ulnar collateral ligament. Elevation of the common flexor origin from the epicondyle is not necessary for simple repair of the ligament.

Repair

A longitudinal incision is made into the ligament itself to inspect the medial aspect of the elbow joint. The elbow is flexed to 20 to 30 degrees, and a valgus stress is applied. With insufficiency of the medial collateral ligament, the medial joint should easily open several millimeters. However, micro-tears may not reveal any gross insufficiency. A primary repair may be performed in a few patients with adequate ligamentous tissue remaining after débridement of calcific deposits from the ligament or in those with an acute injury causing an avulsion of the ligament from the medial epicondyle. However, we believe that this is the exception and not the rule, especially in overhead and throwing athletes. Usually, it is necessary to reconstruct the ligament. If the ligament does permit primary repair, it

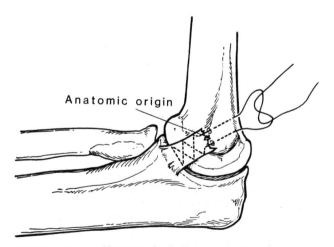

FIGURE 43–7 • Uncommonly, the ligament may be repaired with a Bunnell-type suture placed through holes in the anatomic origin in the humerus.

should be débrided and reattached to the periosteum of the medial epicondyle or any substantial proximal remnant of ligamentous tissue. Slack in the ligament can be imbricated and tightened by using a figure-of-eight suture on each side of the longitudinal split, and then suturing the two halves of the ligament together. An avulsion of the ligament from its attachment to the medial epicondyle can be repaired by placing a Bunnell-type stitch through the body of the ligament and then through drill holes in the medial epicondyle (Fig. 43–7). The reattachment site should be prepared well with a rongeur to provide a good base for healing; the sutures are then tied, with care taken to protect the ulnar nerve.

Reconstruction

In the majority of patients, reconstruction of the ligament is necessary. In the past, exposure was obtained by transection of the tendinous origin of the flexor pronator muscle bundle 1 cm distal to the attachment of the aponeurosis on the medial epicondyle, leaving a stump of tendon for reattachment. The tendon and muscles were then reflected distally, leaving a thin layer of muscle fibers attached to their bed of origin on the ulnar collateral ligament itself. This provided excellent exposure of the entire ulnar collateral ligament as well as its attachment to the tubercle on the medial aspect of the coronoid process. More recently, we[13] and others[27] have found that the flexor pronator mass may be split and not detached, while still allowing adequate exposure with less morbidity. Any calcification within the remaining ligament and soft tissues is removed.

We currently direct the tunnels in the medial epicondyle anteriorly so that the ulnar nerve is not exposed unless it is symptomatic. Convergent 3.2-mm drill holes are made in the ulna located at the level of the tubercle on the medial aspect of the coronoid process. These holes are separated by approximately 1 cm (Fig. 43–8). After the isometric point of origin has been identified, a tunnel is formed that originates from the isometric origin of the ligament. Proximally, the tunnel exits anteriorly on the medial column, one exit site 5 to 10 mm proximal to the other. In this way, the nerve is observed and protected but not translocated (see Fig. 43–8).

At this point, attention is turned to harvesting suitable tendon for autologous graft tissue. The presence of a palmaris longus tendon should be documented preoperatively. If absent, alternative autologous graft tissue may be used, as mentioned earlier.

The palmaris longus tendon is harvested by first creating a 2-cm transverse skin incision at the level of the distal flexor crease of the wrist. The median nerve and its palmar cutaneous branch are protected by isolating the tendon and identifying the tendinous insertion into the palmar fascia. A second transverse skin incision is made 10 cm proximal to the wrist at the level of the palmaris longus musculotendinous junction. The tendon is then transected distally and brought out through the proximal incision. It is divided at or proximal to the musculotendinous junction, providing a free autogenous graft approximately 15 cm in length. These incisions are irrigated and closed routinely. A 1-0 nonabsorbable braided suture is placed in one end of the graft, and a flexible suture passer is used to thread the tendon

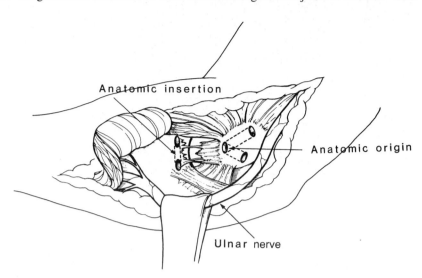

FIGURE 43-8 • The humeral drill hole originates at the anatomic origin of the ligament and exits at two sites anterior on the lateral column.

through the bone tunnels in a figure-of-eight fashion. With the elbow held in 45 degrees of flexion and neutral varus-valgus position, the graft is pulled taut and sutured to itself. An effort is made to pull the ends into the drill holes for better fixation (Fig. 43–9). The graft also is sutured to the tough fascial tissue near the intermuscular septum and to any remnants of the ulnar collateral ligament. The elbow is then brought through a full passive range of motion to verify isometricity and is checked for abrasion of the graft on the joint line. A gentle valgus stress is applied with the elbow in 20 to 30 degrees of flexion to test stability. A stable reconstruction will prevent medial joint line opening.

The flexor-pronator muscle group is reattached to the medial epicondyle. A surgical drain is also placed beneath the flexor-pronator mass.

The tourniquet is then released, hemostasis is obtained with electrocautery, and the wound is closed in routine

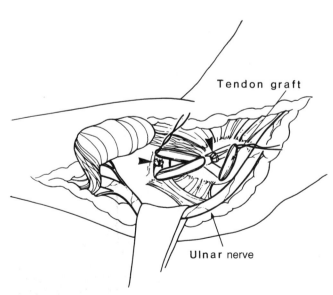

FIGURE 43-9 • The palmaris longus tendon is passed through both bone tunnels in a figure-of-eight fashion and secured with the elbow in 45 degrees of flexion. A suture on the end of the tendon facilitates this maneuver. Care is taken to pull the ends of the graft into the osseous tunnels for better fixation.

fashion. A long-arm posterior plaster splint is used to immobilize the elbow in 90 degrees of flexion and neutral rotation, leaving the wrist and hand free.

POSTOPERATIVE REHABILITATION

The patient is discharged from the hospital on the second postoperative day. Immobilization is discontinued at 10 days, at which time active elbow and shoulder and wrist range of motion exercises are started. The same postoperative regimen is used following repair and reconstruction of the ulnar collateral ligament (Fig. 43–10). The patient begins gentle hand grip exercises, squeezing a sponge or a soft ball on the first postoperative day or as soon as it is comfortable to do so. After 4 to 6 weeks, muscle strengthening exercises of the wrist and forearm are initiated, including flexion, extension, pronation, and supination of the hand and wrist. Also at 6 weeks, elbow-strengthening exercises are begun; valgus stress is avoided until 4 months postoperatively. Shoulder exercises, including those for strengthening and maintaining the rotator cuff, are continued throughout the rehabilitative period.

At 3 to 4 months after surgery, the patient may toss a ball without a windup motion for a distance of 30 to 40 feet two or three times per week for about 10 to 15 minutes per session. At 5 months, the patient may increase the tossing distance to 60 feet, and at 6 months, he or she may use an easy windup. Thereafter, the patient may perform exercises and tossing on alternative days. Ice is used following all workouts to decrease swelling and inflammation.

At 7 months, a graduated program of range of motion and strengthening exercises, as well as total body conditioning, is performed. Throwers and pitchers are carefully supervised, limiting throwing to half speed while gradually increasing the duration of their sessions to 25 to 30 minutes. Pitchers are permitted to return to the mound and progress to 75 percent of maximum velocity during the eighth or ninth month.

Over the next 2 months, careful attention is focused on the body mechanics of throwing, including the lower extremities and torso. Duration of throwing sessions and

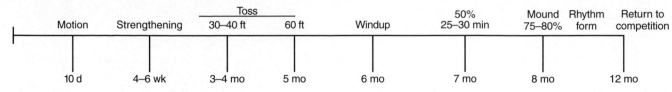

FIGURE 43–10 • Typical rehabilitation schedule for pitchers.

velocity are slowly increased to eventually simulate a game situation. Throwing in competition is permitted at 1 year if the shoulder, the elbow, and the forearm are pain-free during throwing and have returned to normal strength and range of motion. Rhythm, proprioception, and accuracy are the last skills to be regained in overhead athletes following reconstruction of the ulnar collateral ligament of the elbow. In a professional pitcher, over 18 months may be required to regain preoperative ability and competitive level, [15, 16] with relatively shorter periods required for other player positions or overhead sports.

RESULTS

Reconstruction of the ulnar collateral ligament in overhead or throwing athletes unable to compete owing to valgus instability of the elbow has been successful in returning the majority of patients to their previous level of participation.[4, 16] Of 70 operations on 68 patients with valgus instability of the elbow treated at the Kerlan-Jobe Orthopaedic Clinic, 14 had direct repair, and 56 had a reconstruction of the torn or incomplete ligament using a free tendon graft.[4] These patients were followed for 6.3 years postoperatively. Fifty percent of the repair group and 68 percent of the reconstruction group returned to their previous levels of participation. The mean time to return to competition was 9 months in the repair group and 12 months in the reconstruction group. Twelve of 16 major league baseball players who underwent reconstruction without previous elbow surgery returned to playing in the major leagues. Two of seven major league players who had a direct repair as their primary procedure returned to that level. Previous operations on the elbow are shown to decrease patients' chances of returning to their preinjury level of participation in their sport.

If specific sport participation and player position are considered, it appears that baseball pitchers are the most difficult patients to return to their previous competitive level, with 62 percent excellent results in the reconstruction group and 46 percent excellent results in the repair group. On the other hand, of 72 professional baseball players having a surgical procedure on the elbow, one third required two or more procedures.[1] Patients with posterior medial ligaments had a high incidence of ulnar collateral ligament injury but also had a higher rate of return to competition.

In our experience, the length of time from onset of symptoms to operation, the mode of onset of symptoms (acute vs. insidious), and the type of ligament injury (avulsion vs. attenuation) did not affect the postoperative outcome. Also, postoperative flexion deformities of the elbow up to 25 degrees may not decrease a thrower's perfor-

mance, especially if present preoperatively. A series of five patients from Japan revealed acute injuries of the muscle ligament complex that could be reliably fixed with a spiked washer technique.[12] We have no experience with this.

Postoperative problems involving the cutaneous nerves or the ulnar nerve itself account for the major complications following ulnar collateral ligament repair or reconstruction and may occur in up to 25 percent of patients.[4] Although some may require surgery or translocation, all but 3 percent of our series of patients had recovered by the time of final assessment. Careful subcutaneous dissection may prevent inadvertent transection of cutaneous nerves, causing local paresthesia or painful neuroma formation.

We have had little problem with the ulnar nerve since employing the current technique whereby the nerve is not translocated or distracted.[29] We have found that the flexor pronator mass could be split without being detached proximally. This approach further protects the nerve and is performed routinely by us at this time, as noted previously.

SUMMARY

Since the prior edition of this book, new diagnostic techniques such as the "milking maneuver" and magnetic resonance imaging in the oblique plane have increased diagnostic accuracy.[5] Appreciation of the stable tear in continuity has emerged. Modifications of the exposure and the tunnel placement in the humerus have resulted in less need to translocate the ulnar nerve.

Reconstruction of the ulnar collateral ligament is indicated for the treatment of symptomatic valgus instability of the elbow, which is unresponsive to nonoperative treatment. In the well-motivated overhand and throwing athlete, this procedure has been successful in allowing return to the previous level of athletic participation.

REFERENCES

1. Andrews, J. R., and Timmerman, L. A.: Outcome of elbow surgery in professional baseball players. Am. J. Sports Med. 23:407, 1995.
2. Barnes, P. A., and Tullaos, H. S.: An analysis of 100 symptomatic baseball players. Am. J. Sports Med. 6:63, 1978.
3. Bennett, J. B., and Tullos, H. S.: Ligamentous and articular injuries in the athlete. In Morrey, B. F. (ed.): The Elbow and Its Disorders. Philadelphia, W. B. Saunders Co., 1975, p. 502.
4. Conway, J. E., Jobe, F. W., Glousman, R. E., and Pink, M.: Medial instability of the elbow in throwing athletes: Surgical treatment by ulnar collateral ligament repair or reconstruction. J. Bone Joint Surg. 74A:67, 1992.
5. Cotten, A., Jacobson, J., Brossmann, J., Pedowitz, R., Haghighi, P., Trudell, D., and Resnick, D.: Collateral ligaments of the elbow: Conventional MR imaging and MR arthrography with coronal oblique plane and elbow flexion. Radiology 204:806, 1997.

6. Field, L. D., Callaway, G. H., O'Brien, S. J., and Altchek, D. W.: Arthroscopic assessment of the medial collateral ligament complex of the elbow. Am. J. Sports Med. 23:396, 1995.

7. Glousman, R. E.: Ulnar nerve problems in the athlete's elbow. Clin. Sports Med. 9:365, 1990.

8. Habernek, H., and Ortner, F.: The influence of anatomic factors in elbow joint dislocation. Clin. Orthop. 274:266, 1992.

9. Hamilton, C. D., Glousman, R. E., Jobe, F. W., Brault, J., Pink, M., and Perry, J.: Dynamic stability of the elbow: Electromyographic analysis of the flexor pronator group and the extensor group in pitchers with valgus instability. J. Shoulder Elbow Surg. 5:347, 1996.

10. Hang, Y. S., Lippert, G. F., III, and Spolek, G. A.: Biomechanical study of the pitching elbow. Int. Orthop. 3:217, 1979.

11. Hotchkiss, R. N., and Weiland, A. J.: Valgus instability of the elbow. J. Orthop. Res. 5:372, 1987.

12. Inoue, G., and Kuwahata, Y.: Surgical repair of traumatic medial disruption of the elbow in competitive athletes. Br. J. Sports Med. 29:139, 1995.

13. Jobe, F., and Elattrache, N.: Reconstruction of the MCL. In Morrey BF (ed.): Masters Techniques: The Elbow. Philadelphia, Raven Press, 1994.

14. Jobe, F. W., and Kvitne, R. S.: Elbow instability in the athlete. Inst. Course Lect. 40:17, 1991.

15. Jobe, F. W., and Nuber, G.: Throwing injuries of the elbow. Clin. Sports Med. 5:521, 1986.

16. Jobe, F. W., Stark, H., and Lombardo, S. F.: Reconstruction of the ulnar collateral ligament in athletes. J. Bone Joint Surg. 68:1158, 1986.

17. Josefsson, P. O., Gentz, C. F., Johnell, O., and Wenderberg, B.: Surgical vs nonsurgical treatment of ligamentous injuries following dislocation of the elbow joint. J. Bone Joint Surg. 69A:605, 1987.

18. Josefsson, P. O., Johnell, O., and Gentz, C. F.: Long-term sequelae of simple dislocations of the elbow. J. Bone Joint Surg. 66A:927, 1984.

19. King, J. W., Brelsford, J. H., and Tullos, H. S.: Analysis of the pitching arm of the professional baseball pitcher. Clin. Orthop. 67:116, 1969.

20. Kuroda, S., and Sakamaki, K.: Ulnar collateral ligament tears of the elbow joint. Clin. Orthop. 208:266, 1986.

21. Morrey, B. F.: Applied anatomy and biomechanics of the elbow joint. Instr. Course Lect. 35:39, 1986.

22. Morrey, B. F., and An, K. N.: Articular and ligamentous contributions to the stability of the elbow joint. Am. J. Sports Med. 11:315, 1983.

23. Pappas, A. M., Zawacki, R. M., and Sullivan, T. J.: Biomechanics of baseball pitching: A preliminary report. Am. J. Sports Med. 13:216, 1985.

24. Protzman, R. R.: Dislocation of the elbow joint. J. Bone Joint Surg. 60A:539, 1978.

25. Regan, W. D., Korinek, S. F., Morrey, B. F., and An, K. N.: Biomechanical study of ligaments around the elbow joint. Clin. Orthop. 271:170, 1991.

26. Schwab, G. H., Bennet, J. B., Woods, G. W., et al.: Biomechanics of elbow instability: The role of the medial collateral ligament. Clin. Orthop. 146:42, 1980.

27. Smith, G. R., Altchek, D. W., Pagnani, M. J., and Keeley, J. R.: A muscle-splitting approach to the ulnar collateral ligament of the elbow. Neuroanatomy and operative technique. Am. J. Sports Med. 24:575, 1996.

28. Sojbjerg, J. O., Oveson, J., and Nielsen, S.: Experimental elbow instability after transection of the medial collateral ligament. Clin. Orthop. 218:186, 1987.

29. Starkweather, R. J., Nevaiser, R. J., Adams, J. P., and Parson, D. B.: The effect of devascularization on the regeneration of lacerated peripheral nerves. An experimental study. J. Hand Surg. 3:163, 1978.

30. Tullos, J. S., Schwab, G., Bennett, J. B., and Woods, G. W.: Factors influencing elbow instability. Instr. Course Lect. 30:185, 1981.

31. Wilson, F. D., Andrews, J. R., Blackburn, T. A., and McCluskey, G.: Valgus extension overload in the pitching elbow. Am. J. Sports Med. 11:83, 1983.

CHAPTER 44

Lateral Collateral Ligament Injury

• BERNARD F. MORREY and
SHAWN W. O'DRISCOLL

Injury and treatment of the lateral collateral ligament has only recently been described. Although lateral joint stabilization procedures have been described for recurrent dislocation, isolated lateral collateral ligament deficiency has been poorly understood and described. Recognition of the ulnar part of the lateral collateral ligament complex, known as the lateral ulnar collateral ligament, and diagnosis of posterolateral rotatory instability by the posterolateral rotatory subluxation test (or lateral pivot-shift test) have expanded our understanding of this problem. The cause as well as the presentation of this condition is different from that of medial collateral ligament insufficiency.[8] Yet the surgical procedure for correcting this ligamentous deficiency is, not surprisingly, analogous to that for correction of the medial deficiency.

ETIOLOGY

Unlike the medial ligament injury, which can occur from pure valgus stress, lateral collateral ligament injury rarely occurs after isolated varus stress to the elbow, as few mechanisms deliver such a load.[2] Complete elbow dislocation is the most recognized cause of chronic deficiency of this ligament.[6, 9, 11] It also occurs with elbow subluxations and sprains that may or may not be associated with fractures about the elbow, such as those of the radial head. A less common cause is an iatrogenic development subsequent to the release of the common extensor tendon for lateral epicondylitis[16] or radial head excision, due to inadvertent violation of the ulnar part of the lateral collateral ligament complex or inadequate repair or healing of this structure.

Varus Injury

Varus stress as a cause of lateral collateral ligament disruption does occur with acute injury, but this is not a common problem.[17] Because repetitive varus stress, unlike the stress associated with throwing injuries, rarely occurs at the elbow, chronic lateral collateral ligament injury is distinctly uncommon and to date has been recognized only in long-term crutch-walkers such as post-polio patients. We have observed lateral instability after a discrete varus injury to the elbow,[17] but this is much less common than after complete dislocation.

Posterior Dislocation of the Elbow

Posterior dislocation of the elbow uncommonly results in recurrent instability. In 1980, Malkawi[13] reviewed the world's literature, documenting 63 patients with recurrent instability recorded in a 100-year period after the condition was first described in 1881. When residual instability does result from a complete elbow dislocation, it is often not recognized as such. The symptoms have been interpreted as radial head dislocation,[3, 5] recurrent locking,[10] recurrent subluxation,[18] and frank recurrent dislocation.[7] The cause of this complication is becoming better understood, most often representing an "incomplete healing of the initial trauma."[4, 27]

Iatrogenic

Release or repair of the common extensor tendon for lateral epicondylitis must be done with care, to ensure that the lateral collateral ligament is left intact. Our experience has revealed that approximately 25 percent of cases of failed tennis elbow surgery are associated with lateral collateral ligament insufficiency.[15] Rarely, lateral ulnar collateral ligament deficiency might be diagnosed as epicondylitis. If radial head excision is performed through an incision that is too posterior or is perpendicular to the lines of the fibers, the lateral ulnar collateral ligament might also be disrupted.

PRESENTATION

As suggested from the different etiologies, the presentation of patients with lateral collateral ligament insufficiency varies considerably, from an obvious recurrent dislocation to minor subluxations to pain of questionable etiology. Our patients have ranged in age from 2 to 74, but they tend to be in the second or third decade of life. Malkawi[13] indicates that 80 percent of all patients with recurrent dislocation reported in the literature from 1888 through 1980 consisted of those in whom the initial dislocation occurred prior to the age of 15. The majority, 84 percent, were males. Nonunion of the lateral epicondyle was common.

Recurrent frank posterior displacement of the ulna referable to the humerus is the most common *recognized* form of elbow instability. However, O'Driscoll and associates[19] have suggested a global entity that includes rotatory subluxation caused by partial incompetence of the lateral collateral ligament to frank recurrent posterior dislocation with complete insufficiency of the lateral collateral ligament complex (see Chapter 29). This explanation helps us to understand the protean presentation of patients with lateral complex deficiency. Patients who have recurrent subluxations rather than dislocations are most often mistakenly thought to have recurrent dislocation of the radial head.[3] These patients may complain of recurrent snapping, clicking, or locking commonly noted when the elbow is supinated and extended. Symptoms noted with flexion and pronation are really those of the reduction that occurs from the supinated extended position.

The history is characteristic and classic. The patient has usually had a dislocation or fracture to the elbow or has had surgery involving the lateral collateral ligament. Symptoms of recurrent subluxation—clicking, catching, snapping, locking, or the sensation of the bones "slipping out of joint"—are then noted. The diagnosis is usually apparent from the history, although the details might need to be carefully elicited. If the patient has had a previous elbow dislocation or another significant injury, any of these events should alert the physician to the possibility of residual incompetence of the lateral collateral ligament complex.

PHYSICAL EXAMINATION

A diagnosis may be made even if a documented recurrent dislocation is not reproduced on examination, because the history is usually adequate and specific for diagnosing this entity. Patients complaining of pain, locking, catching, or intermittent slipping of the elbow pose a more difficult diagnostic challenge. Motion is usually normal, but the patient may be apprehensive with the elbow supinated and in full extension. In our experience, the lateral pivot-shift maneuver is a reliable means of demonstrating marked but not subtle instability.[18] The most sensitive test is the lateral pivot-shift apprehension test.

Posterolateral Rotatory Instability Test (Lateral Pivot-Shift Test of the Elbow)

The patient lies supine on the examining table, the shoulder is flexed with the arm overhead, and the examination is performed from the head of the table (Fig. 44–1). In this position, the examination is almost identical to the pivot-shift assessment of the knee. The elbow is supinated with a mild force at the wrist, and a valgus moment is applied to the elbow during flexion. This results in a typical apprehension response, with reproduction of the patient's symptoms (a sense that the elbow is about to dislocate). Reproducing the actual subluxation and the clunk that occurs with reduction usually can be accomplished only with the patient under general anesthesia or, occasionally, after injection of local anesthetic into the elbow joint. Subluxation of the radius and the ulna off the humerus causes a prominence posterolaterally over the radial head and a dimple between the radial head and the capitellum. As the elbow is flexed to approximately 40 degrees or more, reduction of the ulna occurs suddenly, with a palpable, visible clunk. The pivot-shift test may fail to cause apprehension in patients with severe instability because it is not very uncomfortable.

Other Assessments

POSTEROLATERAL ROTATORY DRAWER TEST

We have found that in some instances a test similar to the anterior drawer or Lachman maneuver of the knee will demonstrate subtle posterolateral rotatory translation. With the elbow flexed 90 or 30 degrees, respectively, the lateral forearm is grasped and anteroposterior translation force is

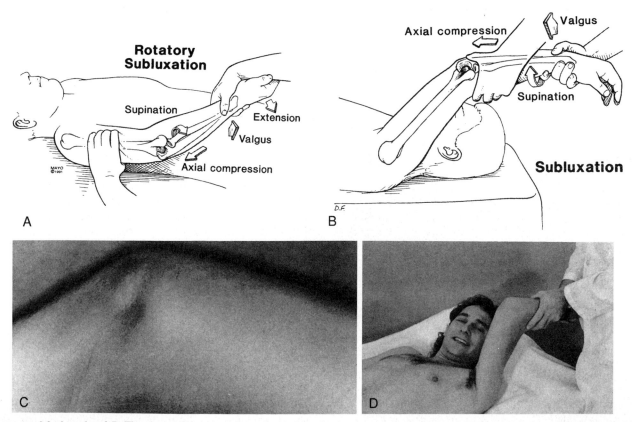

FIGURE 44–1 • A and D, The pivot-shift test is performed with the patient's arm over the head (B and D). Full external rotation of the shoulder provides a counterforce for the supination of the forearm and leaves one hand of the examiner free to control valgus moments (A). The subluxation produces a prominence over the radial head and a dimple in the skin behind it (C). Further flexion causes a reduction to occur with a palpable, audible clunk (B). (From O'Driscoll, S. W., Bell, D. F., and Morrey, B. F.: Posterolateral rotatory instability of the elbow. J. Bone Joint Surg. **73A**:440, 1991.)

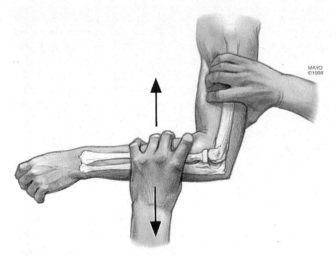

FIGURE 44–2 • Lateral translation, which consists of superior and inferior stress to the lateral aspect of the flexed elbow while the forearm is fully supinated.

applied referable to the distal humerus (Fig. 44–2). The lateral forearm pivots around the intact medial side. If the test result is positive, a sense of instability is perceived both by the examiner and by the patient.

IMAGING

Varus Stress. Varus stress to the elbow may reveal the insufficiency. If a varus stress test is conducted, we prefer that this be done under fluoroscopic control, centering the x-ray beam on the olecranon fossa and observing for subtle changes (Fig. 44–3). It should be recognized, however, that results of varus stress tests may be entirely normal in the presence of a positive pivot-shift maneuver finding and clinically significant lateral ligament insufficiency.

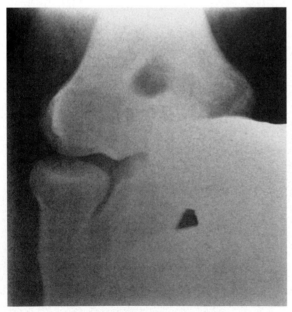

FIGURE 44–3 • Mild to moderate varus instability shown on varus stress view in a professional football player. Gross varus instability is rare.

Magnetic Resonance Imaging. Potter and colleagues[23] recently demonstrated that properly performed magnetic resonance imaging is quite accurate, in both sensitivity and specificity, to demonstrate and localize the lateral ligament pathology.

PATHOPHYSIOLOGY

As may be obvious from this discussion, the basic pathology of recurrent elbow instability consists of deficiency of the lateral collateral ligament complex. Until recently, it was believed that this ligament consisted principally of the radial collateral and annular ligaments.[1] However, since the identification of the lateral ulnar collateral ligament,[12, 15] the structure has been well characterized in the basic anatomy literature,[20] and identified and studied in other reports.[21, 24] Recent descriptions have attempted to further refine the components of the lateral complex. Regardless of the terminology, the essential lesion is deficiency of the essential lateral stabilizer, which is the component that inserts onto the ulna. It is now known that damage to this structure is the essential lesion for posterolateral rotatory subluxation and, in some or even most instances, recurrent dislocation of the elbow.[19] This ligament and its function are described and discussed in detail in Chapters 2 and 3. The rotatory subluxation occurs from supination of the ulna to allow the radial head to slide below the capitellum. This may not be apparent from the anteroposterior radiograph (Fig. 44–4). Although the clinical presentation may suggest radial head dislocation, in fact, the entire radioulnar joint is rotated referable to the humerus, which is the phenomenon occurring with the pivot-shift maneuver and is observed on the lateral radiograph (Fig. 44–5). This is secondary to deficiency of the ulnohumeral stabilizer, that is, the lateral ulnohumeral ligament (Fig. 44–6). In our experience, the ligament and the remainder of the lateral complex are attenuated or even avulsed from the lateral epicondyle. It is probably for this reason that recurrent dislocations have been long recognized and effectively treated, even without knowledge of the precise characterization or role of the lateral ulnar collateral ligament. The fact that the lateral ligament may be considered the "essential lesion" for both dislocation and subluxation is suggested by the basic investigations conducted in our laboratory as well as by the excellent clinical results reported after reconstruction or repair of the lateral part of the joint for most recurrent symptoms of elbow instability.[7, 13, 14, 17, 22, 25, 26]

Patient Selection

With lateral collateral ligament deficiency, the presentation may be subtle, and the need or justification for surgery may be a matter of careful judgment. Recurrent elbow instability associated with lateral collateral ligament insufficiency does not, in our experience, resolve with time. Furthermore, the condition may markedly interfere with daily function. Therefore, once the diagnosis has been made, serious consideration of repair or reconstruction should be entertained. Alternatively, less active patients may have learned to modify activities and thus accommodate.

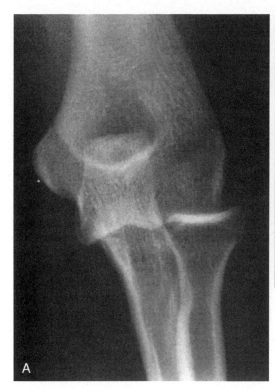

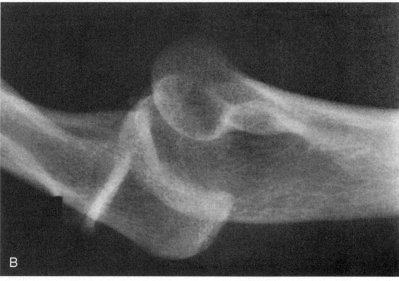

FIGURE 44–4 • *A*, Despite a long history of instability, there is little change in the anteroposterior radiograph of this elbow. Rotatory instability is observed on the lateral radiograph, as the radial head is inferior to the capitellum. *B*, The ulnohumeral joint, however, appears to be reasonably well aligned.

SURGICAL TECHNIQUE

Reconstruction of the Lateral Ulnar Collateral Ligament (Mayo)

POSITION

The patient is placed supine on the operating table, and the arm is draped free and brought across the chest. The joint capsule is exposed through Kocher's interval, reflecting the anconeus posteriorly (see Fig. 4–6A). The ulnar attachment of the lateral ulnar collateral ligament may be palpated at the tubercle of the supinator crest deep to the fascia over the extensor carpi ulnaris and the supinator muscles. The triceps and anconeus are reflected from the posterior margin of the lateral column, and the common extensor tendon is elevated sufficiently to allow exposure of a portion of the anterior capsule as well (see Fig. 44–6B). The common

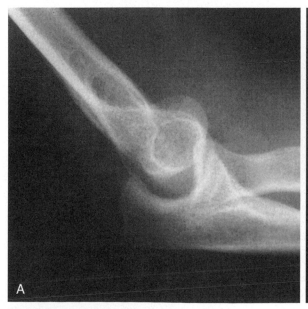

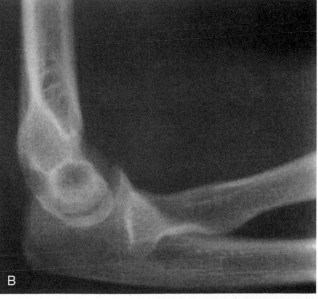

FIGURE 44–5 • Posterolateral rotatory instability test shown radiographically. The ulna is rotated off the humerus, and the radial head has rotated with the ulna so that it now rests posterior to the capitellum *(A)*. This is contrasted with an elbow with true posterior radial head subluxation; while the radial head is inferior, the ulnohumeral joint is normal *(B)*.

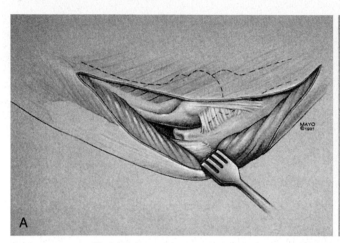
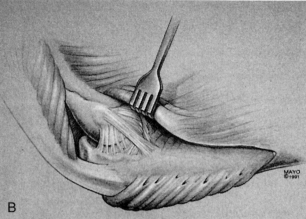

FIGURE 44-6 • Kocher's interval is entered and the anconeus is reflected dorsally *(A)*. The common extensor tendon is then elevated from the collateral ligament and the capsular complex. Care is taken to ensure preservation of the collateral attachment at the humerus *(B)*.

extensor tendon is carefully reflected from the epicondyle, with care taken to preserve the capsule and the lateral ulnar collateral ligament. The pivot-shift or flexed translation maneuver is repeated. This reveals that the radial head slides inferior to the capitellum into the redundant portion of the posterior capsule. The entire lateral ulnar collateral ligament complex can be noted to be either stretched or detached from the humerus. The anterior capsule on the radial side is also stretched and allows the radial head to assume its posterior position.

LIGAMENT REPAIR

After assessment of the pathology has been carefully made, a transverse incision is made in the anterior capsule at the radiohumeral joint, and a similar incision is made posteriorly behind the collateral complex (Fig. 44-7A). If the lateral collateral ligament has become detached from the humerus, this is elevated. Two nonabsorbable sutures (No. 2 or No. 5) are placed according to the choice of the

surgeon in the lateral ligament complex, including both the radial collateral ligament and the lateral ulnar collateral ligament. These sutures are then brought through drill holes placed in the anatomic origin of the ligament at the midportion of the lateral epicondyle, thus tightening the lateral complex (see Fig. 44-7B). Capsular redundancy is eliminated by plicating the anterior and posterior capsules.

LIGAMENT RECONSTRUCTION

In general, adults require ligament reconstruction, whereas children are treated by repair of an avulsed ligament origin. Should the lateral ligamentous complex appear to be thin, attenuated, and insufficient, the repair is reinforced with a tendon graft, typically the palmaris longus. If the palmaris longus is not available, the split-semitendinosus, fascia lata, a toe extensor tendon, or an allograft may be used. Through a small incision at the wrist crease, the palmaris longus is obtained using a tendon stripper. A length of tendon, ideally at least 20 cm, is required for the reconstruction. The

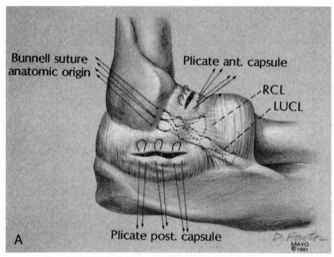
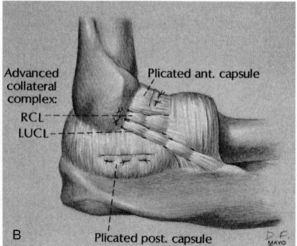

FIGURE 44-7 • The anterior and posterior capsules are incised *(A)*. If the collateral ligament substance is of adequate quality, sutures are placed in the radioulnar lateral collateral ligaments, and these structures are reattached to their anatomic origin at the lateral epicondyle *(B)*. The anterior and posterior capsules are plicated.

insertion site of the lateral ulnar collateral ligament on the tubercle of the supinator crest is identified by palpation while stressing the elbow with supination or varus. One hole, 3 to 4 mm, is made in the ulna with a burr just posterior to this point. Another is made proximally, near the annular ligament, so that a bridge of bone 1 to 1.25 cm spans the two holes. A tunnel to connect them (Fig. 44–8) is created with a curved awl from the Bankart set of shoulder instruments. A No. 1 suture is passed through the holes and tied to itself. The free end is passed up toward the lateral epicondyle and grasped with a snap and moved until the isometric point on the epicondyle is identified (see Fig. 44–8). It is held tight against that spot while the elbow is flexed and extended to confirm its isometricity. This point is generally more anterior and proximal than might be apparent. To create the entry site on the humerus, a burr hole is made at the isometric point, with care taken to reconfirm it after a slight depression is made and not removing bone distally or anteriorly. That is, the hole should be placed eccentrically in a posterior and proximal orientation with reference to where the snap was placed (Fig. 44–9). An exit site is created with the burr just posterior to the supracondylar ridge, about 2 cm proximally, and a tunnel is created between the two with the curved and straight awls. A re-entry site is created with the burr distally so that a bridge of bone 1.25 cm wide spans the two holes, and a tunnel is created from this site to the original entry site at the epicondyle, where the tendon will exit again.

The suture used to determine the isometric point is removed. The tendon graft is passed through the tunnel in the ulna and sutured to itself at a length that enters the humeral origin point. The suture to attach the tendon is pulled through the tunnel along with the tendon. Tension on the suture assists in tensioning the graft. The elbow is kept in full pronation at about 40 degrees of flexion, where it is normally most lax. No sutures are placed directly over the joint margin. The tendon origin sutured to itself pro-

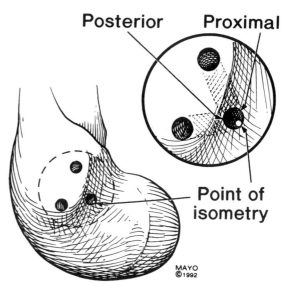

FIGURE 44–9 • The humeral graft origin site is developed posteriorly and superiorly from the point of isometry. Tunnels directed posterosuperiorly and posteroinferiorly emerge on the back side of the epicondyle.

vides a three-ply reconstruction. The capsule is closed so that the tendon does not rub directly on the lateral margin of the capitellum (Fig. 44–10). A No. 2 polydioxanone suture can be placed through the same course, woven through the lateral tissues, to protect the reconstruction for the first few weeks of healing.

AFTERCARE

Postoperatively, the limb is immobilized at 90 degrees flexion for 10 to 14 days. A brace with a 30-degree extension block with the forearm in full pronation is used an additional 4 weeks. In a patient with soft tissue laxity or previous failed surgery, the limb is sometimes kept immobilized for 3 to 6 weeks. After 3 months, the elbow is allowed free flexion-extension without protection, but varus stress and extension or supination maneuvers are avoided. Forearm flexor and extensor muscle-building exercises are initiated in the cast and are continued in the splint and subsequently for 6 months after surgery. At 6 months, the patient is allowed activity as tolerated but is to avoid varus stress. At 9 to 12 months, all restrictions are lifted.

RESULTS

There are limited data about the long-term results for the treatment of posterolateral rotatory instability. O'Driscoll and associates briefly reported on five patients at the time this entity was described. Nestor and associates[17] reviewed our experience with 11 cases at the Mayo Clinic that were followed a minimum of 1 year. Using an objective rating system, the results of these 11 cases were graded with respect to both objective and subjective features, including motion, pain, and stability. For an excellent result, all these features were considered normal, and the patient perceived the elbow to be normal. A good result consisted of no objective or subjective elements of instability; mild pain or

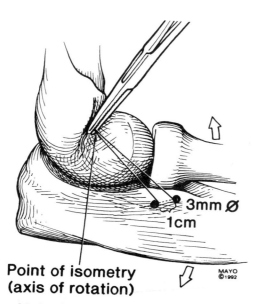

Point of isometry (axis of rotation)

FIGURE 44–8 • Reconstructive procedures use a tunnel placed in the ulna at the anatomic insertion of the lateral ulnar collateral ligament. Isometry is determined by a suture placed through this tunnel and held at the humeral origin of the lateral ulnar collateral ligament.

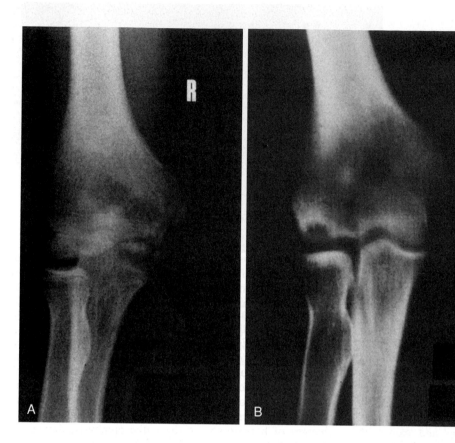

FIGURE 45–11 • A, In a 13-year-old Little League pitcher with pain at the lateral aspect of the right elbow, the radiograph appears reasonably normal, although a vague lucency may be detected on careful inspection. B, Tomogram shows a focal but definite lucent area of the capitellum, indicating limited involvement with osteochondritis dissecans.

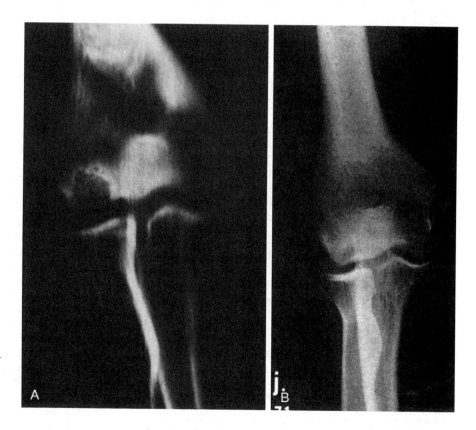

FIGURE 45–12 • Tomogram of a 15-year-old boy showing a generalized involvement of the capitellum with osteochondritis dissecans. Ten years later, a reasonably well-healed lesion of the capitellum is demonstrated.

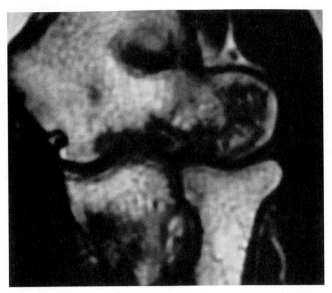

FIGURE 45–13 • Magnetic resonance imaging is extremely helpful in revealing the presence of osteochondritis dissecans when the radiograph shows no abnormality and in demonstrating the extent of involvement.

merus may be considered. When the osteochondritis dissecans involves the anterior and proximal aspect of the capitellum, arthroscopic instrumentation can be easily delivered to the defect through the anterolateral and anteromedial portals. However, more posterior portions of the capitellum may be more difficult to view and to operate. The direct lateral (soft spot) portal typically provides the best view. Accessory portals may be required for subchondral drilling and microfracture at the base of the defect. It is recommended that the perforations should be approximately 2 mm apart and penetrate to the level of cancellous bone, to encourage the formation of a fibrocartilage to fill the defect. Synovectomy at the radiocapitellar joint and removal of any loose fragments will improve the mechanical symptoms.

Osteochondritis Dissecans of the Radial Head

This curious lesion was recognized and described over 30 years ago.[1, 80] It is believed to be a less common expression of the lateral overload from repetitive throwing (Fig. 45–

• TABLE 45–2 • Characteristics of Osteochondritis

	Osteochondritis Dissecans	Panner's Disease
Age	Teens	~10 years
Onset	Insidious	Acute
Radiographic Finding	Island of subchondral bone demarcated by a rarefied zone	Fragmentation of entire capitellar ossific nucleus
Loose Bodies	Present	Absent
Residual Deformity of Capitellum	Present	Minimal

14). An additional manifestation of lateral joint compression is radial neck angulation, which was reported by Ellman.[18] Treatment is the same as that for osteochondritis dissecans of the capitellum. Radial head resection is to be avoided in the young throwing athlete.[17, 71] One of the most interesting features of this condition is disappearance of the lesion in recent years, attributed to the rule changes that limit the number of pitches thrown by Little League pitchers.

Flexion-Extension Stress

Flexion-extension stress in adolescents may result in avulsion of the olecranon apophysis, olecranon traction apophysitis, or medial epicondylar apophysitis.[25] Coronoid and olecranon hypertrophy and cartilage proliferation may occur. Classic changes of primary osteoarthritis (Fig. 45–15) are discussed in depth in Chapter 67.

ACUTE INSTABILITY IN ADULTS

Elbow Dislocation with Comminuted Radial Head Fracture

In about 10 percent of cases, elbow dislocation may be associated with a displaced or comminuted fracture of the radial head.[74, 82] If the radial head is removed, stability has been further compromised. In some instances, the elbow

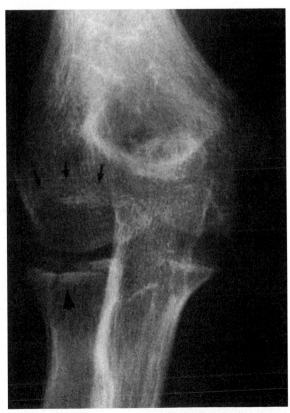

FIGURE 45–14 • Repetitive stress of throwing can cause changes in the proximal radial growth center consistent with osteochondritis dissecans. (From Silvino, N. J., and Jackson, D. W.: Osteochondritis dissecans in the gymnast elbow. Surg. Rounds Orthop. **53**:62, 1989.)

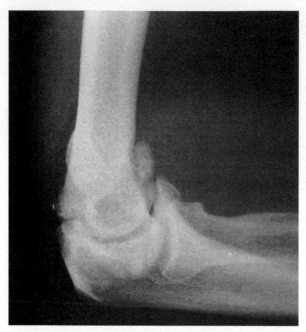

FIGURE 45–15 • Coronoid and olecranon hypertrophy from repetitive stress. Anterior coronoid fossa loose body. These are classic changes of primary osteoarthritis.

may be unstable clinically and radiographically, even in 90 degrees of flexion or in plaster. Collateral ligament insufficiency or osteochondral fracture fragment interposition in the joint must be considered.

In our opinion, stabilization of this type of elbow dislocation in the athlete requires surgery. The demands of valgus stress on the elbow for the athlete will require direct repair of the medial collateral ligament. Reconstructive restoration of the radial head alone may be sufficient to restore stability in the non-athlete and allow the ligament to heal. For Mason type IV radial head fractures that necessitate excision, the use of a radial head prosthesis or spacer may be required[30, 51, 52] (see Chapters 25 and 30).

Elbow Arthroscopy in Acute Trauma

Although it is discussed in detail in Chapter 39, some comment regarding arthroscopy is appropriate here and subsequently. Subtle elbow fractures and articular injuries are certainly amenable to arthroscopic diagnosis and possibly even to treatment. Contraindications to the use of arthroscopy for acute trauma may be severe soft tissue swelling, severely displaced intra-articular fractures that may distort anatomic landmarks, or a previous history of ulnar nerve transposition.

RADIAL HEAD FRACTURES

Some nondisplaced fractures of the radial head may offer an excellent opportunity for arthroscopic evaluation and management, if the athlete remains persistently symptomatic after injury.[35] More attention is recently being given to the long-term sequelae for nondisplaced Mason type I radial head fractures. Recognition of associated soft tissue injuries is imperative, such as medial collateral ligament

disruption, annular ligament or lateral collateral ligament disruption, or the interosseous membrane disruption of the Essex-Lopresti lesion.

Continued complaints of locking or pain despite radiographic healing of a nondisplaced radial head fracture may merit arthroscopic intervention. In a series of 34 Mason type I radial head fractures, diagnostic elbow arthroscopy in two patients allowed identification of a significant osteochondral defect in the capitellum and loose bodies.[36] Identification of a symptomatic lateral plica band at the radiocapitellar joint may be possible only with arthroscopic evaluation, and the band can be resected with good relief of symptoms.[13]

Capitellum Fractures

Capitellum fractures have been acceptably classified and are discussed in Chapter 23.[41] Sleeve osteochondral fractures of the capitellum are usually best excised. Complete fractures of the capitellum in a coronal plane are best treated with anatomic reduction and stable internal fixation, usually using several Herbert screws (Fig. 45–16). Anatomic restoration can at times be very difficult. If lateral stability of the joint is lost by fragment resection, then direct suture or reconstruction of a disrupted medial collateral ligament is mandatory to prevent valgus instability.[67, 69]

Coronoid Fractures

Coronoid fractures, as classified and discussed by Regan and Morrey,[63] are stable if type I or type II. Chip fractures of the coronoid process (type I) usually are contained by the joint capsule and do not require excision as a loose body. Type III coronoid fractures require open reduction and stable internal fixation of the large fracture fragment to (1) restore the integrity of the medial collateral ligament and (2) retain the anterior bone support for stability of the elbow joint. If necessary, an elbow hinged external fixator may be required to maintain a congruent elbow joint during soft tissue and bony healing (Fig. 45–17). Excision of a coronoid fracture may result in anteroposterior instability, which is exaggerated if the medial collateral ligament has been disrupted. This is discussed in detail in Chapter 28.

Heterotopic Ossification

Ossification is commonly observed in the medial collateral ligament, the lateral collateral ligament, and the anterior and posterior capsules after injury.[28] It remains within the confines of the ligament or capsule and does not become intra-articular or form loose bodies.

Acute Rupture of the Medial Collateral Ligament

Isolated tears of the anterior oblique ligament of the elbow can occur, and were described initially in javelin throwers.[80, 84] Although early reports suggested that this injury was rare, during the past 5 to 6 years, increasing awareness has made the diagnosis much more common.[31, 34, 53]

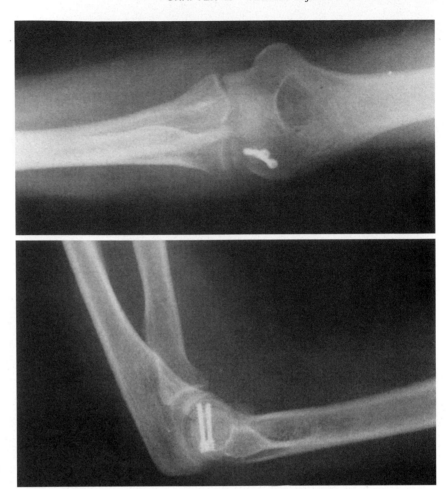

FIGURE 45–16 • Radiograph of a Herbert screw fixation of a large osteochondral fracture of the capitellum.

CHRONIC VALGUS INSUFFICIENCY IN ADULTS

Throwing Injuries

It has been shown that repetitive throwing can be detrimental to the integrity of the elbow joint in the pitching arm.[15, 23, 29, 33] The data presented in Table 45–3 demonstrate that both pain and radiographic findings of joint pathology are common in professional throwers. These findings do increase and the symptoms worsen with advancing age. In one series, approximately 50 percent of athletes were successfully returned to throwing with conservative treatment such as rest, physical therapy, and anti-inflammatory measures.[7] The other 50 percent required surgery.[7]

Slocum has classified throwing injuries of the elbow into three groups: (1) medial tension injuries, (2) lateral compression injuries, and (3) extensor overload injuries.[72] Characteristic lesions have been described in the elbows of throwing athletes.[39, 79, 80] Baseball players, especially pitchers, are susceptible to developing these conditions because of repetitive high forces generated on a highly congruous elbow joint while throwing (Fig. 45–18). Common medial tension injuries include ulnar collateral ligament tears, flexor-pronator tendinitis, and ulnar nerve traction injuries. The lateral compartment sustains compression shear force between the radial head and the capitellum, resulting in articular cartilage chondromalacia and loose body forma-

tion. The posterior compartment also experiences shear forces, commonly referred to as hyperextension valgus overload syndrome.

Loose Bodies

Shear forces to the athlete's elbow may result in loose bodies in the anterior compartment. Extension overload causes posterior loose body formation (Fig. 45–19).

Symptoms of catching and intermittent locking in the athlete's elbow are suggestive of a loose body. Following a locking episode, swelling and limited motion is typical for several days, followed by improved motion.

Plain radiographs often confirm a loose body, but non-calcified osteochondral fragments will not be evident on a plain radiograph. A computed tomographic arthrogram of the elbow can identify loose bodies to a size of 3 mm, but has potential for problems with interpretation due to synovial folds or bone spurs. MRI will miss a loose body if no marrow elements are present in the fragment.[62]

The removal of loose bodies from the elbow is one of the most common indications for elbow arthroscopy (see Chapter 39). Surgical results with arthroscopy or arthrotomy for removal of loose bodies are good, with less pain and locking reported in 85 to 90 percent of athletes.[4, 44, 56, 70] With reasonable surgical discretion, accurate diagnosis, and arthroscopic or muscle-splitting approaches when necessary, return to throwing can be anticipated. In our experi-

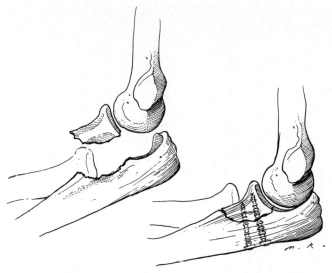

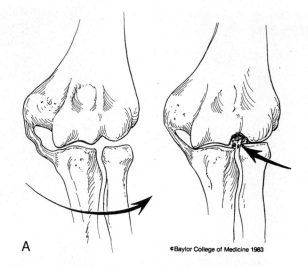

©Baylor College of Medicine 1983

FIGURE 45–17 • Illustration of a type III coronoid fracture with dislocation. Screw fixation for stabilization and reduction of dislocation.

ence, the average professional pitcher has continued to throw effectively for 3 or more years, with a range of 2 to 11 years, after loose body removal.

Hyperextension Valgus Overload Syndrome

Medial elbow laxity with repetitive hyperextension stress results in impingement of the posteromedial olecranon tip into the olecranon fossa, resulting in osteophyte formation and subsequent posterior fossa loose bodies. Bennett and associates[10] first described the posterior compartment bone and cartilage lesions seen in throwing athletes. Wilson and associates[87] emphasized the importance of recognizing osteophyte formation on the posteromedial aspect of the olecranon process, as well as in the posterior compartment. Similar osteophyte and loose body formation may occur at the coronoid process with repetitive hyperflexion and traction syndromes. Surgical excision of loose bodies (Fig. 45–20) and olecranon osteotomy may be indicated to decompress the posterior compartment, either arthroscopically or by open procedure (Fig. 45–21).[4, 5, 87]

Nonoperative treatment of hyperextension valgus overload syndrome includes rest, nonsteroidal anti-inflammatory medication, and correction of throwing mechanics, as well as a supervised rehabilitation program emphasizing the strengthening of the flexor-pronator mass. A gradual return to sports and throwing will be necessary.

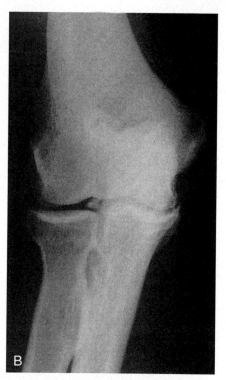

FIGURE 45–18 • A, Chronic instability of the elbow with resulting fragmentation and degenerative changes at the lateral aspect of the ulno-humeral joint. B, Radiograph of a radiocapitellar loose body and a medial coronoid tubercle spur.

• TABLE 45–3 • Pitchers with Radiographic Evidence of Joint Pathology			
Age	Pitchers	Pathology	Percent
26–33	17	14	83
25–27	21	13	62
18–21	12	5	42
Total	50	32	

If nonoperative treatment fails, arthroscopic débridement or limited incision arthrotomy is of particular benefit to decompress the posterior compartment when mechanical symptoms are a predominant feature. A small loose body and mild hypertrophic osteophytes on the olecranon tip are particularly amenable to arthroscopic débridement. Visualization of the posterior compartment is usually best through the posterolateral portal, with use of the straight posterior portal as the working portal. Removal of loose bodies is performed first, followed by synovectomy. A burr may then be introduced into the posterior portal, resecting the olecranon tip. Motorized resectors must be carefully used

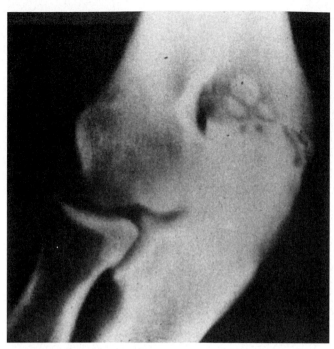

FIGURE 45–19 • Loose bodies of the olecranon fossa from repetitive impingement. (From King, J. W., et al: Analysis of the pitching arm of the professional baseball pitcher. Clin. Orthop. **67**:116, 1969.)

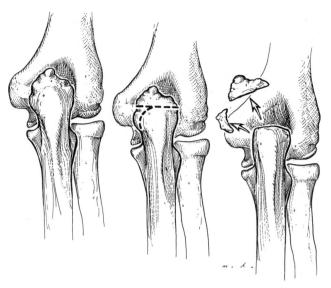

FIGURE 45–21 • Drawing of a hyperextension overload osteophyte formation and its surgical correction with decompression osteotomy of the olecranon tip. This may be done by arthrotomy or arthroscopy, but the medial corner must be included in the decompression.

when in the medial gutter to minimize risk of injury to the ulnar nerve.

During arthroscopic examination, degenerative or post-traumatic chondromalacia changes may be seen on the capitellum, radial head, or ulnohumeral joint as well. Chondromalacia on the anterior margin of the supinated radial head may be a sign of an occult posterolateral rotatory instability.[55] Widespread chondromalacia and arthritic changes have a less favorable prognosis for return to pitching.[6]

Open removal of the large olecranon osteophytes in the posterior compartment with a biplane osteotomy has been described by Wilson and colleagues[87] for the treatment of valgus extension overload syndrome. Approximately 1.0 cm of the olecranon tip is excised, followed by a portion of

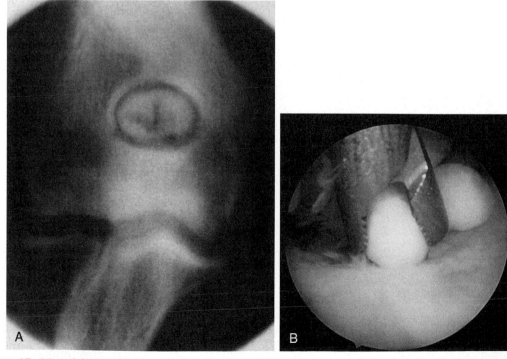

FIGURE 45–20 • A large ossified loose body in the olecranon fossa *(A)* represents the best indication for elbow arthroscopy *(B)*.

the posteromedial olecranon. The rehabilitation following a limited incision arthrotomy with the triceps splitting approach is quite similar to that of the arthroscopic surgery. Professional major league baseball players have been able to return to pitching at 6 weeks following surgery.

Synovial Lesions

Repetitive trauma to an athlete's elbow may result in a localized reactive synovitis. Several case reports have described findings of a lateral synovial plica band, symptomatic with lateral elbow pain, clicking or popping suggestive of loose body symptoms, and swelling that was activity related.[13] Two types of lateral synovial plica bands have been appreciated in our experience, a lateral synovial plica in the lateral gutter that pops over the olecranon process, and a plica near the radiocapitellar joint folding over the margins of the radial head and capitellum. The lateral gutter plica presents as a hypertrophic palpable band at the lateral ulnohumeral joint, symptomatic particularly with extension. The radiocapitellar joint plica protrudes onto the radial head and elicits a popping or snap with forearm rotation while the elbow is in flexion.

Nonoperative management includes an elbow pad, nonsteroidal anti-inflammatory medication, and modification of the training technique. In selected cases, steroid injection is helpful to decrease the synovial reaction. If recalcitrant, arthroscopy of the elbow will permit synovectomy and resection of the plica band, with fairly dramatic relief of symptoms.

Chronic Elbow Instability

Secondary soft tissue and bone changes can result in chronic medial or lateral instability for the athlete. These instabilities, such as chronic valgus instability or posterolateral rotatory instability, may be difficult to appreciate on clinical examination (see Chapters 43 and 44).

The arthroscope may play a role in diagnosing and treating chronic instability in the athlete. An arthroscopic valgus instability test has been described.[21, 22, 77] During arthroscopic examination, the medial ulnohumeral joint should not open with an intact anterior oblique ligament. A 2-mm opening of the ulnohumeral joint could be demonstrated in cadavers with complete transection of the anterior oblique ligament.[77] Arthroscopy may also be useful in diagnosis of posterolateral rotatory instability.[55]

RECURRENT ELBOW DISLOCATIONS

Perhaps the most interesting and one of the least common elbow lesions is that of recurrent dislocation. Few surgeons have personally seen more than one case in their lifetime. This accounts for the fact that reports discussing repair of this entity are both plentiful and inventive.[19, 37, 46, 57, 65, 75, 83] The topic is thoroughly addressed in Chapters 29 through 31, 43, and 44. Emphasis here is on the articular causes for recurrent elbow dislocations.

Recurrent Dislocations Secondary to Coronoid Insufficiency

Gartsman and others discussing olecranon fractures have indicated that significant amounts of the olecranon process can be excised without essentially compromising joint stability.[2, 17, 20, 24, 45] Excision of more than 50 percent must be done very judiciously in the athlete, as excessive articular deficiency places increased stress on the collateral ligaments.[64]

Recurrent Elbow Dislocations Secondary to Neglected Medial Epicondyle Fracture

A common cause of recurrent elbow dislocation is the neglected medial epicondylar fracture.[42, 61, 66] The injury occurs in both children and adults, and the displaced fragment frequently heals with a fibrous union. When this occurs, a functionally elongated medial collateral ligament may result. If recognized early, replacement of the fragment with pins or a screw provides predictable results (Fig. 45–22). More commonly, the displaced fragment has been present for many years. Yet it is usually possible to restore length and tension to the anterior oblique ligament through surgical repair even though anatomic restitution of the osseous anatomy is less than optimal.[46]

REHABILITATION

A rehabilitation program should be established in all cases of elbow ligamentous and articular injuries (see Chapters 10 and 12). A comprehensive approach will include the patient, the surgeon, the therapist, and the trainer. The use of splints, orthoses, and various strengthening modalities of rehabilitation should be integrated into the patient's activity program. Early motion is encouraged, and usually begins 7 to 10 days after injury or reconstruction unless otherwise specified. A protective hinge cast brace to prevent varus, valgus, or extension stress can be used.

Flexion contracture of the elbow and a resulting loss of motion is common following intra-articular injury to the elbow. Morrey has defined a functional arc of motion for the elbow as 30 to 130 degrees of flexion.[39] Most activities of daily living can be performed through this 100-degree arc of motion. However, 30 degrees of flexion contracture of the elbow may not be satisfactory for the demands of an athlete.

Treatment may be indicated for those contractures greater than 30 degrees in athletes whose sport demands more extension from the elbow. If recalcitrant to therapy and serial static splinting, contracture of the elbow may be successfully managed by arthroscopic techniques.[36] Jones and Savoie[36] have reported good results with complete anterior capsular release, medial and lateral gutter débridement, and removal of excessive bone when needed, to restore near-normal motion to a majority of patients. Fifty-three patients managed by this technique improved their range of motion from a flexion contracture of 46 degrees to one of 5 degrees. One patient sustained an injury to the posterior interosseous nerve. Arthroscopic release of the

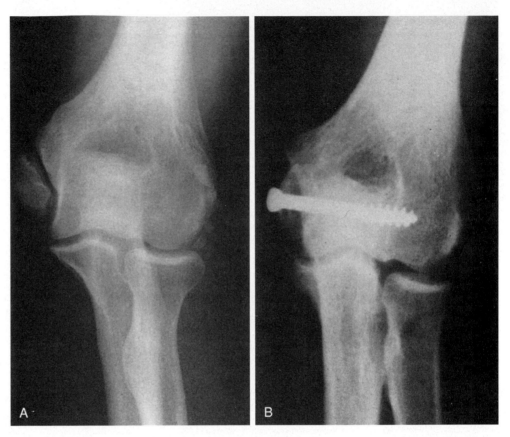

FIGURE 45–22 • *A*, Large medial epicondyle fracture nonunion with medial collateral ligament instability. This can be managed with screw fixation *(B)*. Postoperatively, large nonunited medial epicondyle has been repaired with a cancellous screw.

contracture is technically demanding, but may provide satisfactory results with less morbidity for the athlete.

REFERENCES

1. Adams, J. E.: Injury to the throwing arm: A study of traumatic changes in the elbow joints of boy baseball players. Calif. Med. **102**:127, 1965.
2. Adler, S., Fay, G. F., and MacAusland, W. R.: Treatment of olecranon fracture, indications, for excision of the olecranon fracture, repair of the triceps tendon. J. Trauma **2**:597, 1962.
3. Anderson, L.: Fractures. *In* Crenshaw, S. H. (ed.): Campbell's Operative Orthopedics, 5th ed. St. Louis, C. V. Mosby Co., 1971.
4. Andrews, J. R., and Carson, W. G.: Arthroscopy of the elbow. Arthroscopy **1**:97, 1985.
5. Andrews, J. R., and Craven, W. M.: Lesions of the posterior compartment of the elbow. Clin. Sports Med. **10**:637, 1991.
6. Baker, C. L., Peterson, W. W., DaSilva, R: Operative elbow arthroscopy: Long-term follow-up. Presented at the Annual Meeting of the Arthroscopy Association of North America. San Diego, California, April 14–27, 1991.
7. Barnes, D. A., and Tullos, H. S.: An analysis of 100 symptomatic baseball players. Am. J. Sports Med. **6**:62, 1978.
8. Bennett, G. E.: Elbow and shoulder lesions of the professional baseball pitcher. J.A.M.A. **117**:510, 1941.
9. Bennett, G. E.: Shoulder and elbow lesions distinctive of baseball players. Ann. Surg. **126**:107, 1947.
10. Bennett, J. B., Green, M. S., and Tullos, H. S.: Surgical management of chronic medial elbow instability. Clin. Orthop. **278**:62, 1992.
11. Boe, S.: Arthroscopy of the elbow: Diagnosis and extraction of loose bodies. Acta Orthop. Scand. **57**:52, 1986
12. Brodgon, B. G., and Crow, N. F.: Little Leaguer's elbow. Am. J. Roentgenol. **8**:671, 1960.
13. Clarke, R. P.: Symptomatic lateral synovial fringe (plica) of the elbow joint. Arthroscopy **4**:112, 1988.
14. Conn, J., and Wade, P.: Injuries of the elbow: A ten-year review. J. Trauma **1**:248, 1961.
15. DeHaven, K. E., and Evarts, C. M.: Throwing injuries of the elbow in athletes. Orthop. Clin. North Am. **1**:801, 1973.
16. DeHaven, K. E., Ferguson, A. B., Hale, C. J., Larson, R. L., and Tullos, H. S.: Symposium: throwing injuries to the adolescent elbow. Contemp. Surg. **9**:65, 1976.
17. Dunn, N.: Operation for fracture of the olecranon. B.M.J. **1**:214, 1939.
18. Ellman, H.: Anterior angulation deformity of the radial head. J. Bone Joint Surg. **57A**:776, 1975.
19. Eppright, R. H., and Wilkins, K. E.: Fractures and dislocations of the elbow. *In* Rockwood, C. A., Jr., and Green, D. P. (eds.): Fractures. Philadelphia, J. B. Lippincott Co., 1975.
20. Eriksson, E., Sahlin, O., and Sandah, U.: Late results of conservative and surgical treatment of fracture of the olecranon. Acta Chir. Scand. **113**:153, 1957.
21. Field, L. D., Callaway, G. H., O'Brien, J. S.: Arthroscopic assessment of the medial collateral ligament complex of the elbow. Am. J. Sports Med. **23**:396, 1995.
22. Field, L. D., and Altchek, D. W.: Evaluation of the arthroscopic valgus instability test of the elbow. Am. J. Sports Med. **24**:177, 1996.
23. Gainor, B. J., Piotrowski, G., Puhl, J., Allen, W. C., and Hagen, R.: The throw: biomechanics and acute injury. Am. J. Sports. Med. **8**:114, 1980.
24. Gartsman, G. M., Sculco, T. P., and Otis, J. C.: Operative treatment of olecranon fractures: excision or open reduction with internal fixation. J. Bone Joint Surg. **63A**:718, 1981.
25. Gore, R. M., Rogers, L. F., Bowerman, J., Suker, J., and Conpere, C. L.: Osseous manifestations of elbow stress associated with sports pitchers. AJR Am. J. Roentgenol. **134**:971, 1980.
26. Gudmundsen, T. E., and Ostensen, H.: Accessory ossicles in the elbow. Acta Orthop. Scand. **58**:130, 1987.
27. Gugenheim, J. J., Stanley, R. F., Woods, G. W., and Tullos, H. S.: Little League survey: the Houston study. Am. J. Sports Med. **4**:189, 1976.
28. Hait, G., Boswick, J. A., and Stone, N. H.: Heterotopic bone formation secondary to trauma (myositis ossificans traumatica). J. Trauma **10**:405, 1970.
29. Hang, V. S., Lippert, F. G., Spolek, G. A., Frankel, V. H., and Harrington, R. M.: Biomechanical study of the pitching elbow. Int. Orthop. **3**:217, 1979.

30. Harrington, I. J., and Tountas, A. A.: Replacement of the radial head and the treatment of unstable elbow fractures. Injury 12:405, 1980.
31. Indelicato, P. A., Jobe, F. W., Kerlin, R. K., Carter, V. S., Shields, C. L., and Lombardo, S. J.: Correctable elbow lesions in professional baseball players. Am. J. Sports Med. 7:72, 1979.
32. Jackson, D. W., Silvino, N., Reiman, P.: Osteochondritis in the female gymnast elbow. Arthroscopy 5:129, 1989.
33. James, S.: Discussion of the Pitching Act. Presented at the Committee on Sports Medicine, American Academy of Orthopaedic Surgeons Post Graduate Course, San Francisco, 1971.
34. Jobe, F., and Stark, H.: Reconstruction of the ulnar collateral ligament in athletes. J. Bone Joint Surg. 68:1158, 1986.
35. Jones, G. S., and Geissler, W. B.: Complications of minimally displaced radial head fractures. Annual Meeting of the American Academy of Orthopoaedic Surgeons, Seattle, February, 1993.
36. Jones, G. S., and Savoie, F. H.: Arthroscopic capsular release of flexion contractures (arthrofibrosis) of the elbow. Arthroscopy 9:277, 1993.
37. Kapel, O.: Operation for habitual dislocation of the elbow. J. Bone Joint Surg. 33A:707, 1951.
38. Kerin, R.: Elbow dislocation and its association with vascular disruption. J. Bone Joint Surg. 51A:756, 1969.
39. King, J. W., Brelsford, H. J., and Tullos, H. S.: Analysis of the pitching arm of the professional baseball pitcher. Clin. Orthop. 67:116, 1969.
40. Larson, R. L., and McMahan, R. O.: The epiphysis and the childhood athlete. J.A.M.A. 196:607, 1966.
41. Lee, W. E., and Summey, T. J.: Fracture of the capitellum of the humerus. Am. Surg. 99:497, 1934.
42. Linscheid, R. L., and Wheeler, D. K.: Elbow dislocations. J.A.M.A. 194:1171, 1965.
43. Mains, D. B., and Freeark, R. J.: Report of compound dislocations of the elbow with entrapment of brachial artery. Clin. Orthop. 106:180, 1975.
44. McGinty, J. F.: Arthroscopic removal of loose bodies. Orthop. Clin. North Am. 13:313, 1982.
45. McKeever, F. M., and Buck, R. M.: Fracture of the olecranon process of the ulna: treatment by excision of fragment and repair of triceps tendon. JAMA 135:1, 1947.
46. Milch, H.: Bilateral recurrent dislocation of the ulna at the elbow. J. Bone Joint Surg. 18:777, 1936.
47. Milgram, J. W.: The classification of loose bodies in human joints. Clin. Orthop. 124:282, 1977.
48. Milgram, J. W.: Surgical osteochondromatosis. J. Bone Joint Surg. 59B:492, 1977.
49. Mink, J. H., Eckardt, J. J., and Grant, T. T.: Arthrography in recurrent dislocation of the elbow. AJR Am. J. Roentgenol. 136:1242, 1981.
50. Morrey, B. F., and An, K. N.: Articular and ligamentous contributions to the stability of the elbow joint. Am. J. Sports Med. 11:315, 1983.
51. Morrey, B. F., Tanaka, S., and An, K. N.: Valgus stability of the elbow. Definition of primary and secondary constraints. Clin. Orthop. 265:187, 1991.
52. Morrey, B. F., Askew, L., and Chao, E. Y.: Silastic prosthesis replacement for the radial head. J. Bone Joint Surg. 63A:454, 1981.
53. Norwood, L. A., Shook, J. A., and Andrews, J. R.: Acute medial elbow ruptures. Am. J. Sports Med. 9:16, 1981.
54. O'Driscoll, S. W., and Morrey, B. F.: Arthroscopy of the elbow. J. Bone Joint Surg. 74A:84, 1991.
55. O'Driscoll, S. W., Bell, D. F., Morrey, B. F.: Posterolateral rotatory instability of the elbow. J. Bone Joint Surg. 73A:440, 1991.
56. Ogilvie-Harris, D. J., Shemitsch, E.: Arthroscopy of the elbow for removal of loose bodies. Arthroscopy 9:5, 1993.
57. Osborne, G., and Cotterill, P.: Recurrent dislocation of the elbow. J. Bone Joint Surg. 48B:340, 1966.
58. Panner, H. J.: A peculiar affection of the capitulum humeri resembling Calve-Perthes' disease of the hip. Acta. Radiol. 10:234, 1928.
59. Pappas, A. M.: Osteochondritis dissecans. Clin. Orthop. 158:59, 1981.
60. Pappas, A. M.: Elbow problems associated with baseball during childhood and adolescence. Clin. Orthop. 164:30, 1982.
61. Pritchard, D. J., Linscheid, R. L., and Svien, H. J.: Intra-articular median nerve entrapment with dislocation of the elbow. Clin. Orthop. 90:100, 1973.

62. Quinn, S. F., Haberman, J. J., Fitzgerald, S. W.: Evaluation of loose bodies in the elbow with MR Imaging. J. Magn. Reson. Imag. 4:169, 1994.
63. Regan, W., and Morrey, B. F.: Fracture of the coronoid process of the ulna. J. Bone Joint Surg. 71A:1348, 1989.
64. Regan, N. M., and Morrey, B. F.: Classification and treatment of coronoid process fractures. Orthopaedics 15:345, 1992.
65. Reichenheim, P. P.: Transplantation of the biceps tendon as a treatment for recurrent dislocation of the elbow. Br. J. Surg. 35:201, 1947.
66. Roberts, A. W.: Displacement of the internal epicondyle into the elbow joint. Lancet 2:78, 1934.
67. Roberts, P. H.: Dislocation of the elbow. Br. J. Surg. 46:806, 1969.
68. Ruch, D. S., and Poehling, G. G.: Arthroscopic treatment of Panner's disease. Clin. Sports Med. 10:629, 1991.
69. Schwab, G. H., Bennett, J. B., Woods, G. W., and Tullos, H. S.: Biomechanics of elbow instability: the role of the medial collateral ligament. Clin. Orthop. 146:42, 1980.
70. Shepherd, C. W., and Andrews, J. R.: Surgical Correction of Pitching Injuries of the Elbow. Presented at The Sports Medicine Society, Williamsburg, Virginia, 1983.
71. Silvino, N. H., and Jackson, D. W.: Osteochondritis dissecans in the gymnast elbow. Surg. Rounds Orthop. 53:62, 1989.
72. Slocum, D. B.: Classification of elbow injuries from baseball pitching. Texas Med. 64:48, 1968.
73. Smith, F. M.: Surgery of the Elbow, 2nd ed. Philadelphia, W. B. Saunders Co., 1972.
74. Sneed, J. S., and Boyd, H. B.: Fractures about the elbow. Am. J. Surg. 38:727, 1937.
75. Soring, W. E.: Report of a case of recurrent dislocation of the elbow. J. Bone Joint Surg. 35B:55, 1953.
76. Tachdijan, M. O.: Pediatric Orthopedics. Philadelphia, W. B. Saunders Co., 1972, p. 1597.
77. Timmerman, L.A., Andrews, J.R.: Histology and arthroscopic anatomy of the ulnar collateral ligament of the elbow. Am. J. Sports Med. 22:667, 1994.
78. Trias, A., and Comeau, Y.: Recurrent dislocations of the elbow in children. Clin. Orthop. 100:74, 1974.
79. Tullos, H. S., Erwin, W., Woods, G. W., Wukasch, D. C., Cooley, D. A., and King, J. W.: Unusual lesions of the pitching arm. Clin. Orthop. 88:169, 1972.
80. Tullos, H. S., and King, J. W.: Lesions of the pitching arm in adolescents. J.A.M.A. 220:264. 1972.
81. Tullos, H. S., Schwab, G. H., Bennett, J. B., and Woods, G. W.: Factors influencing elbow instability. In American Academy of Orthopedic Surgeons, Instructional Course Lectures, Vol. 8. St. Louis, C. V. Mosby Co., 1982, p. 185.
82. Wadsworth, T. G.: The Elbow. Edinburgh, Churchill Livingstone, 1982.
83. Wainwright, D.: Recurrent dislocation of the elbow joint. Proc. R. Soc. Med. 40:885, 1947.
84. Waris, W.: Elbow injuries in javelin throwers. Acta Chir. Scand. 93:563, 1946.
85. Warwick, R., and Williams, P. L. (eds.): Gray's Anatomy, 35th ed. (Brit.), Philadelphia, W. B. Saunders Co., 1973, pp. 324, 429.
86. Wheeler, D. K., and Linscheid, R. L.: Fracture dislocations of the elbow. Clin. Orthop. 50:95, 1967.
87. Wilson, F. D., Andrews, J. R., Blackburn, T. A., and McClusky, G.: Valgus extension overload in the pitching elbow. Am. J. Sports Med. 2:83, 1983.
88. Wilson, J. N.: The treatment of fractures of the medial epicondyle of the humerus. J. Bone Joint Surg. 42B:778, 1960.
89. Wilson, P. D.: Fractures and dislocations in the region of the elbow. Surg. Gynecol. Obstet. 56:335, 1933.
90. Woods, G. W., and Tullos, H. S.: Elbow instability and medial epicondyle fractures. Am. J. Sports Med. 5:23, 1977.
91. Woods, G. W., Tullos, H. S., and King, J. W.: The throwing arm: elbow injuries. Am. J. Sports Med. (Sports Safety Supplement) 1:4, 1973.
92. Woodward, A. H., and Bianco, A. J.: Osteochondritis dissecans of the elbow. Clin. Orthop. 110:35, 1975.
93. Zertlin, A.: The traumatic origin of accessory bone at the elbow. J. Bone Joint Surg. 17:933, 1935.

• CHAPTER 46 •

Overuse Syndrome

• RICHARD A. BERGER

Although many tissues are subject to fatigue injury, especially those of the immature skeleton,[16] the concept of "overuse syndrome" has a broader definition. "No pain, no gain," a cliché promoted in athletic circles for decades, expresses the underlying attitude that the advancement of one's physical abilities may depend on exceeding the body's limits far enough to cause pain and that less vigorous activity constitutes suboptimal performance. The pain that results from these activities may be transient, representing little more than a focal accumulation of muscle metabolic byproducts, or it may be longer lasting, indicating tissue injury. One dilemma is where to draw the line between the two extremes. Others are when it is safe to resume the activities that initially led to the noxious episode, whether or not adjustments in those activities are indicated, and at what point persistent pain no longer represents an acute injury state but signals a more ominous and less understood condition of chronic pain. These are only a few of the unknowns that are associated with overuse syndromes.

DEFINITIONS AND SYNONYMS

Usually thought to affect muscle or nerve, the overuse syndromes are imprecisely defined and go by a variety of names—repetitive strain injury, repetitive stress syndrome, chronic pain syndrome, cumulative trauma disorder, pain dysfunction syndrome (see Chapter 72), cervicobrachial occupational disorder, fibromyalgia, transepidermal nerve stimulator (TENS), and a variety of activity-specific conditions such as writer's cramp and tennis elbow, among others.[5, 11, 15, 17, 32, 40] The multiplicity of terms reflects the fact that the pathophysiologic mechanisms are, at best, poorly understood. It also contributes to confusion in classification, which in turn interferes with our learning from outcome studies. Overall, however, the term *overuse syndrome* is generally understood to reflect a painful condition, and all tissue types are at risk (Table 46–1). In this text, the term applies to a painful condition of the elbow region that results from excessive activity and whose symptoms have been present for an extended period of time.[14]

Overuse syndrome is a diagnosis of exclusion. No clear history of injury or date of onset is reported. Conditions that involve injury to specific structures, such as lateral epicondylitis and nerve entrapment syndromes (discussed in other chapters), must be ruled out before overuse conditions are considered. Chronicity also plays a role in the diagnosis of overuse syndrome. Pain of traceable onset less than 3 months before presentation for evaluation may be more likely to signify actual tissue injury related to a specific set of circumstances and to respond more favorably to conventional medical intervention. Conversely, pain of more than 6 months' duration is much more likely (1) to have been affected by numerous nonorganic factors, (2) to present as a regional complaint, and (3) to display resistance to conventional medical intervention.[5]

EPIDEMIOLOGY

The overuse syndromes are most prominent in two groups of patients, performers and workers.[4, 6, 7, 10, 14, 19, 26, 33, 39] Among the former are athletes and musicians, whose professions demand exceptional physical performance and arduous practice sessions. The tissues most often involved in athletes are the musculotendinous units, the ulnar nerve, and the collateral ligaments.[38] In practice sessions, an activity is repeated to improve the performance level, often for extended periods. When the performers are called on to use the skills so perfected, an alteration in the performance level caused by pain may be noticeable and possibly may threaten their ability to continue. Any pre-existing injury can further increase the risk of developing an overuse condition.

Workers who daily are expected to perform certain job tasks are also at risk. Occupations reported to carry increased risk for overuse syndromes include typist, telephone operator, cash register operator, interpreter for the deaf, and packing plant worker.[7, 13, 18, 32] In the most common scenario, workers are stationed for long periods, during which they perform repetitive tasks. The actual number of workers who suffer from overuse syndrome is difficult to determine. Four percent of noninstitutionalized adults could recall at least 1 month of musculoskeletal pain and the nature of the impact of that pain.[8] When specific jobs are evaluated, however, the incidence of upper extremity pain related to overuse may approach 30 percent.[28]

In both groups, psychosocial influences may play a major role in determining the pattern of functional recovery once a change in performance level is detected. Such fac-

• TABLE 46–1 • Overuse-Induced Lesions at the Elbow and Affected Tissue Types	
Involved Tissue	**Manifestations**
Bone	Angular change, hypertrophy
Joint	Degenerative arthrosis, loose body, spur, osteophyte (olecranon), osteochondritis dissecans
Synovium	Reactive synovitis, effusion
Ligament	Collateral ligament tear, stretch, calcification
Tendon	Epicondylitis, distal biceps, triceps detachment
Muscle	Myofasciitis, hypertrophy, compartment syndrome (anconeus)
Bursa	Inflammation, radiobicipital, olecranon
Nerve	Entrapment, cubital tunnel, arcade of Frohse

tors actually may influence the manner in which the painful condition is presented to the treating physician, which, in turn, may alter the diagnosis and generate a self-perpetuating cycle of pain and reinforcement behaviors. It also must be understood that the worker's condition is not static and that new stresses may enter into the situation over time. Often, the patience of both employee and employer evaporates and mutual mistrust develops. This may prompt the patient subconsciously to exaggerate reports of pain and limitation of function, further frustrating the care of the condition and often ending in confrontation and litigation.

ETIOLOGY

The causes of overuse syndrome have been the subject of speculation in many publications and studies.[9, 23, 30, 34, 37] One of the earliest observations of pain in a worker subjected to "irregular motions and unnatural postures" dates to the early 18th century.[37] Generally, overuse conditions are believed to arise from a combination of static and dynamic loads applied to postural muscles beyond the tolerable contraction level or duration.[30] Isometric contraction greater than 10 percent of the maximum contraction level is not recommended[34] because circulation in the contracting muscle, may be compromised enough to cause tissue ischemia and accumulation of noxious metabolites.[23] The noxious stimulus may prompt recruitment of other muscle groups which, however, may be at a mechanical disadvantage for assuming such a role and may likewise, in the end, suffer muscle strain. The Japanese Association of Industrial Health identified several risk factors for the development of overuse syndrome, including dynamic muscle recruitment for repetitive tasks, static muscle recruitment for postural support, uncomfortable postures, mental stress, and ergonomic factors such as unpleasant working conditions (Fig. 46–1).[2] Continued engagement in high-load activities other than occupational tasks, including hobbies, domestic chores, and recreational activities, may perpetuate the condition by reducing recovery time.

Psychological Factors

Historically, the involvement of psychological factors in the initiation and perpetuation of overuse syndrome has been recognized.[22, 25] For example, stress has been reported to be a pertinent risk in visual display operators.[42] Stress, in this instance, may be related to high expectations on the part of the employee and the employer for accuracy and productivity in the face of monotonous tasks, equipment failure, static posture, and so on. Stress also may result from variables in physical surroundings such as lighting, noise, and coworker distractions. Athletes' competitive bent may mean that stress plays a more prominent role in the development of overuse syndrome, and the unwillingness to rest the affected body part merely exacerbates the condition. Although it is important to identify the psychological and social factors that may contribute to overuse syndrome, it is equally important to avoid the common tendency to ascribe the entire problem to these factors.

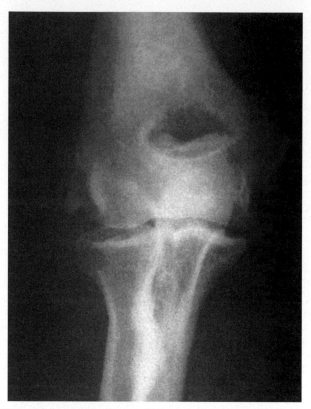

FIGURE 46–1 • A 32-year-old carpenter had pain on elbow motion of 40 to 110 degrees. Primary arthrosis prompted a career change.

HISTORY AND PHYSICAL EXAMINATION

History taking is a most important and time-consuming component of the assessment. At first evaluation, several features commonly are evident. First, the degree of perceived impairment from the discomfort is significant, and the patient's description of the discomfort may be dramatic and graphic.[1, 5] Some objective measure of pain may be useful, such as a pain thermometer to establish a baseline for future comparisons. Second, the patient typically has received many—and often conflicting—"other opinions" from family members, the popular press, coworkers, trainers, employers, and other physicians. Early in the first meeting, it is important tactfully to direct the patient's attention away from previous opinions, to minimize learned behavior and bias and to maximize the effectiveness of future treatments. Finally, the patient may have learned to distort or exaggerate the severity and the area of involvement in an attempt to engage medical attention, this being a reaction to earlier incidents when the painful condition was trivialized by supervisors or industrial health care workers. It is critical, while establishing rapport, to assure the patient that all symptoms are important and that an accurate report of those symptoms greatly enhances the process.

A complete description of the patient's condition and the activities he was involved in before and after the onset of symptoms is important to record. For the worker, each job and its duration and a description of its specific tasks should also be recorded. Each task should be thoroughly understood, and the record should note the height of the working station, the frequency of repetitions, the loads applied, the ambient temperature, the job rotation, the frequency of breaks, and any other relevant conditions. For athletes and musicians, a careful history of practice schedules and conditions is desirable. Next, a chronology of painful trends since the onset of symptoms, evaluations by physicians and chiropractors, and all treatments instituted and the patient's response to those treatments should be recorded. The examiner seeks to gain thorough understanding of the nature of the presenting complaint, in terms of severity, duration, type of pain, exacerbating and relieving factors, sleep patterns, and resultant functional limitations. Finally, in consultation with the worker, it is important to gain insight into his relationship with the employer, whether legal counsel has been obtained, and especially whether the patient is currently receiving worker's compensation benefits.

During the physical examination, the key objective is to rule out all other possible causes of similar pain, including nerve entrapment syndromes, tendinitis, arthritis, bursitis, fracture, sprain, and other conditions such as tennis elbow. A systematic examination of the extremity, including musculoskeletal and neurologic function, circulation, and integument, is standard. After the more common processes have been ruled out, the diagnosis of overuse syndrome or of a similar condition begins to emerge.[21, 44] Generally, the patient has a relatively diffuse region of discomfort, and "trigger points" are not uncommon. One condition that may present as an unexplained overuse syndrome is fibromyalgia, which may demonstrate trigger points just distal to the medial or lateral epicondyle.[17] Weakness may be a prominent complaint in overuse syndrome, but specific testing of muscles will likely demonstrate neurologically intact neuromuscular pathways and "breakaway" weakness secondary to pain. It is critical to be mindful of the possible existence of the manifestations of pain dysfunction syndrome, because the treatment modalities are unique to that disorder, which generally does not respond to the therapies recommended for overuse syndrome.[1, 12] It may be useful to observe the athlete performing the activities that produce the discomfort in the field or the musician playing an instrument. An ergonomic evaluation of the worker's environment, by either the physician or a qualified ergonomist, may be useful for understanding the circumstances surrounding the patient's complaints. Finally, serial examination to determine the reproduceability of physical findings and to determine whether the nature of the condition "evolves" is extremely informative and useful.

LABORATORY EVALUATION

If there is concern that the patient may be describing signs and symptoms of an early inflammatory condition, the erythrocyte sedimentation rate, white blood count with differential, electrolyte assays, rheumatoid factor, and antinuclear antibody levels should be determined. The serum levels of the muscle enzymes creatine phosphokinase and aldolase have been reported to be elevated in some workers with upper extremity overuse syndrome, but it is believed that further investigation is necessary before widespread use of these determinations can be justified.[4] Serologic testing for Lyme disease may be considered, especially if exposure risk factors are suggestive, because in the early clinical phases this disease can mimic overuse syndrome.[36]

Standard radiographs of the elbow are necessary to evaluate the skeletal integrity of the humerus, the radius, and the ulna. It may be necessary to obtain special oblique views such as a radial head view or tomogram, if a specific lesion is suspected. Magnetic resonance imaging is useful as a means of excluding obvious derangements or pathologic conditions. The usefulness of three-phase bone scintigraphy in the diagnosis of reflex sympathetic dystrophy has been largely accepted, and this study should be considered when evaluating for overuse syndrome.[31] In fact, the technetium Tc 99m bone scan is a useful screen for suspected inflammatory conditions with minimal findings (Fig. 46-2). Thermography, electromyography, quantitative sudomotor and autonomic reflex testing, and plethysmography all require substantially more investigation before they can be recommended for general use.[32, 35, 45]

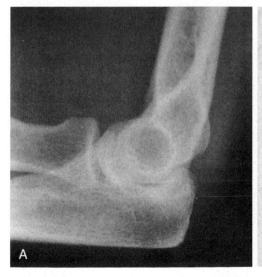
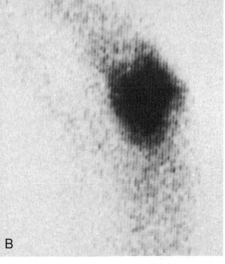

FIGURE 46-2 • A patient with chronic elbow pain had normal ("negative") radiographs *(A)* but a positive ^{99}Tc bone scan *(B)*.

TREATMENT

There is no simple or standard treatment for overuse syndrome. Treatment must take into consideration not only improvement of the immediate painful condition but also prevention of future exacerbations. The treatment modalities for acute pain are different from those for chronic symptoms.

In the acute setting, standard techniques of pain management are appropriate—rest, thermal therapy (cold versus heat), ultrasound and phonophoresis, friction massage, oral nonsteroidal anti-inflammatory medication, and occasional injections of corticosteroid solutions into regions that are particularly tender and troublesome (see Chapter 10). Rest may be provided by temporary splint immobilization, but full-time immobilization causes stiffness and deconditioning that can quickly compound the original problem. Gentle, progressive, well-supervised physical therapy often enhances the rehabilitation process and maintains the strength and conditioning of body parts not affected by the overuse syndrome.[41] The patient should continue to work when that is at all possible. To that end, the surgeon can define tolerable limits for tasks that will allow the patient to progress to recovery while maintaining a productive posture with the employer. Keeping the patient away from the workplace can affect the patient's perception of the degree of impairment that the condition may be generating and could constitute negative reinforcement for recovery (see Chapter 40). On the other hand, some conditions are markedly correlated with occupation, and changing jobs may be an important treatment measure (see Fig. 46–1).

Treatment of chronic pain, regardless of the cause, is a difficult process that requires a multidisciplinary approach. Generally speaking, the conventional therapeutic approach described earlier is ineffective and in certain circumstances may be counterproductive. Attempts to treat the symptoms with splints, medications, or injections should cease. It must be made clear that the condition will not respond to medical or surgical intervention. This is not to say that it will not improve with some types of therapy; it merely underscores the need for the patient to stop searching for a medical answer to the problem. A survey of 116 therapists revealed that many common educational themes are employed, especially the nature of the disease process, normal and abnormal anatomy, and job modification.[24]

The patient should have a functional capacity evaluation, which is useful for determining impairment levels and constructing a work-hardening program.[41] Referral to a pain management clinic may avail the patient of unconventional modalities such as transcutaneous electrical nerve stimulation and biofeedback. Stellate ganglion block, contrast baths, and massage may benefit patients who are believed to have autonomic dysfunction. If the patient has retained legal counsel or is pursuing workmen's compensation independently, the treating physician becomes an important source of information and will be asked to determine if the workplace was responsible for, or substantially contributed to, the onset of symptoms, what level of impairment due to the symptoms has been established, and what if any permanent restrictions will be necessary as a result of these findings. An independent impairment evaluation center can be very helpful in these circumstances.

Prevention at the workplace and preconditioning of workers are critical to combating the overuse syndrome epidemic. Reasonable employers are evaluating workplaces with ergonomists to determine what modifications in the workplace and in task rotations will reduce the incidence of overuse syndromes.[3, 29, 43] Additionally, implementation of ergonomic exercise programs, better employee education and orientation, and soliciting employees' feedback seem to have salutary effects on reducing overuse syndrome.[29]

SUMMARY

Overuse syndrome of the upper extremity is a poorly understood condition that, by some measures, is reaching nearly epidemic proportions. Clear guidelines for classification, diagnosis, and treatment are needed. Until they are established, the physician carries the responsibility of educating patients, employers, and the community at large and the burden of studying the process to educate fellow physicians.[20]

REFERENCES

1. Amadio, P. C.: Pain dysfunction syndromes: current concept reviews. J. Bone Joint Surg. **70A**:944, 1988.
2. Aoyama, H., Ohara, H., Oze, Y., and Itani, T.: Recent trends in research on occupational cervicobrachial disorder. J. Hum. Ergol. (Tokyo) **8**:39, 1979.
3. Armstrong, T. J.: Ergonomics and cumulative trauma disorders. Hand Clin. **2**:553, 1986.
4. Bjelle, A., Hagberg, M., and Michaelsson, G.: Clinical and ergonomic factors in prolonged shoulder pain among industrial workers. Scand. J. Work Environ. Health **5**(Suppl.):205, 1979.
5. Blair, W. F.: Cumulative trauma disorder in the upper extremity. Iowa Orthopedics J. **11**:103, 1990.
6. Brooks, P. M.: Occupational pain syndromes. Med. J. Austral. **144**:170, 1986.
7. Cohn, L., Lowry, R. M., and Hart, S.: Overuse syndromes of the upper extremity in interpreters for the deaf. Orthopedics **13**:207, 1990.
8. Cunningham, L. S., and Kelsey, J. L.: Epidemiology of musculoskeletal impairments and associated disability. Am. J. Public Health **74**:574, 1984.
9. Dennett, X.: Overuse syndrome: a muscle biopsy study. Lancet **23**:905, 1988.
10. Dimberg, L., Olafsson, A., Stefansson, E., Aagaard, H., Oden, A., Anderson, G. B., Hansson, T., and Hagert, C. G.: The correlation between work environment and the occurrence of cervicobrachial symptoms. J. Occup. Med. **31**:447, 1989.
11. Dobyns, J. H.: Cumulative trauma disorder of the upper limb. Hand Clin. **7**:587, 1991.
12. Dobyns, J. H.: Pain dysfunction syndrome. In Gelberman, R. H. (ed.): Operative Nerve Repair and Reconstruction, 2nd ed. Philadelphia, J. B. Lippincott Co., 1991, p. 1489.
13. Ferguson, D.: The "new" industrial epidemic. Med. J. Austral. **142**:318, 1984.
14. Fry, H. J. H.: Overuse syndrome of the upper limb in musicians. Med. J. Austral. **144**:182, 1986.
15. Fry, H. J. H.: Overuse syndrome, alias tenosynovitis/tendinitis: the terminology hoax. J. Plast. Reconstr. Surg. **78**:414, 1986.
16. Gill T. J. 4th, and Micheli, L. J.: The immature athlete. Common injuries and overuse syndromes of the elbow and wrist. Clin. Sports Med. **15**:401–423, 1996.
17. Goldenberg, D. L.: Fibromyalgia syndrome (fibrositis). Mediguide Inflam. Dis. **7**:1, 1988.
18. Hadler, N. M.: Work-related disorders of the upper extremity. Part I: Cumulative trauma disorders—a critical review. Occup. Prob. Med. Prac. **4**:1, 1989.
19. Hadler, N. M.: Industrial rheumatology: the Australian and New Zealand experiences with arm pain and backache in the work-place. Med. J. Austral. **144**:191, 1986.

20. Hadler, N. M.: Cumulative trauma disorders: an iatrogenic concept. J. Occup. Med. 32:38, 1990.

21. Howard, N. J.: Peritendinitis crepitans. J. Bone Joint Surg. 19:447, 1937.

22. Ireland, D. C. R.: Psychological and physical aspects of occupational arm pain. J. Hand Surg. 13B:5, 1988.

23. Karlsson, J., and Ollander, B.: Muscle metabolites with exhaustive static exercises of different durations. Acta Physiol. Scand. 86:309, 1972.

24. Lawler, A. L., James, A. B., and Tomlin G.: Educational techniques used in occupational therapy treatment of cumulative trauma disorders of the elbow, wrist and hand. Am. J. Occup. Ther. 51:113–118, 1997.

25. Linton, S. J., and Kamwendo, K.: Risk factors in the psychosocial work environment for neck and shoulder pain in secretaries. J. Occup. Med. 31:609, 1989.

26. Louis, D. S.: Cumulative trauma disorders. J. Hand Surg. 5:823, 1987.

27. Louis, D. S.: Evolving concerns relating to occupational disorders of the upper extremity. Clin. Orthop. 254:140, 1990.

28. Luopajarvi, T., Kuorinka, I., Virolainen, M., and Holmberg, M.: Prevalence of tenosynovitis and other injuries of the upper extremities in repetitive work. Scand. J. Work Environ. Health 5(Suppl.):48, 1979.

29. Lutz, G., and Hansford, T.: Cumulative trauma disorder controls: the ergonomic program at Ethicon, Inc. J. Hand Surg. 12A:863, 1987.

30. Maeda, K., Hunting, W., and Grandjean, E.: Factor analysis of localized fatigue complaints of accounting machine operators. J. Hum. Ergol. (Tokyo) 11:37, 1982.

31. Mackinnon, S. E., and Holder, L. E.: The use of three-phase radionuclide bone scanning in the diagnosis of reflex sympathetic dystrophy. J. Hand Surg. 9:556, 1984.

32. McDermott, F. T.: Repetition strain injury: a review of current understanding. Med. J. Austral. 144:196, 1986.

33. McPhee, B., and Worth, D. R.: Neck and upper extremity pain in the work-place. In Grant, R. (ed.): Physical Therapy of the Cervical and Thoracic Spine. New York, Churchill Livingstone, 1988, p. 291.

34. Onishi, N., Sakai, K., and Kogi, K.: Arm and shoulder muscle load in various keyboard operating jobs of women. J. Hum. Ergol. (Tokyo) 11:89, 1982.

35. Pochachevskyl, R.: Thermography in post-traumatic pain. Am. J. Sports Med. 15:243, 1987.

36. Arthritis Foundation: Primer on the Rheumatic Diseases, 9th ed. Atlanta, Arthritis Foundation, 1988, p. 188.

37. Ramazinni, B.: In Wright, W. (trans.): The Diseases of Workers. Chicago, University of Chicago Press, 1940, p. 1717.

38. Rettig AC: Elbow, forearm and wrist injuries in the athlete. Sports Med. 25:115–130, 1998.

39. Ryan, G. A., and Hampton, M.: Comparison of data process operators with and without upper limb symptoms. Comm. Health Stud. 12:63, 1988.

40. Semple, J. C.: Tenosynovitis, repetitive strain injury, cumulative trauma disorder, and overuse syndrome, et cetera (Editorial). J. Bone Joint Surg. 73B:536, 1991.

41. Schultz-Johnson, K.: Work hardening: a mandate for hand therapy. Hand Clin. 7:597, 1991.

42 Smith, M. J., Cohen, B. G., and Stammerjohn, L. W.: An investigation of health complaints and job stress in visual display operations. Hum. Factors 23:387, 1981.

43. Stock, S. R.: Work-place ergonomic factors and the development of musculoskeletal disorders of the neck and upper limbs: a meta-analysis. Am. J. Indust. Med. 19:87, 1991.

44. Thompson, A. R., Plewes, L. W., and Shaw, E. G.: Peritendinitis crepitans and simple tenosynovitis: a clinical study of 544 cases in industry. Br. J. Industr. Med. 8:150, 1951.

45. Uematsu, S., Hendler, N., Hungerford, D., Long, D., and Ono, N.: Thermography and electromyography in the differential diagnosis of chronic pain syndromes and reflex sympathetic dystrophy. Electromyogr. Clin. Neurophysiol. 21:165, 1981.

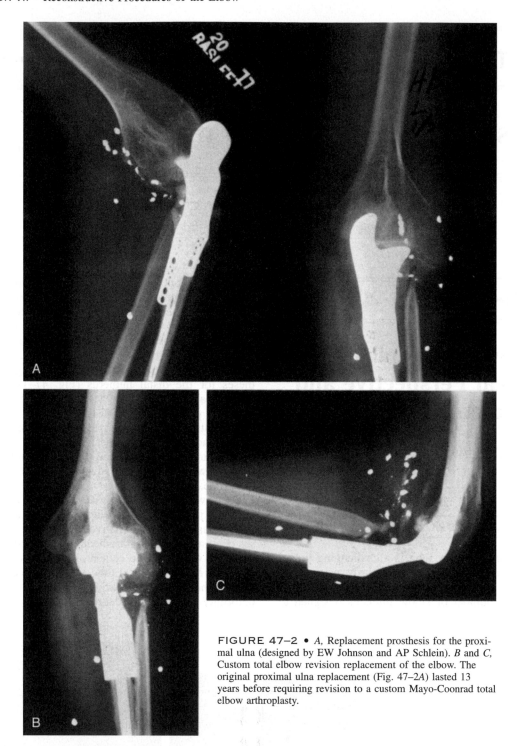

FIGURE 47–2 • *A,* Replacement prosthesis for the proximal ulna (designed by EW Johnson and AP Schlein). *B* and *C,* Custom total elbow revision replacement of the elbow. The original proximal ulna replacement (Fig. 47–2A) lasted 13 years before requiring revision to a custom Mayo-Coonrad total elbow arthroplasty.

subsequent efforts at hinge elbow prosthesis, either custom-designed or general manufactured implants, were metal on polyethylene or were metal-metal with polyethylene interface.

The final effort before a true total elbow replacement involved a joint articular resurfacing prosthesis. Several attempts were made to replace just the proximal ulna or distal humerus. For example in 1971, L.F.A. Peterson,[58] along with William Bickel at Mayo, designed a vitallium "saddle" for the proximal ulna (Fig. 47–3), and Street

and Stevens[72] reported the use of a convex trochlea and capitellum replacement of the distal humerus (Fig. 47–4). The goal of these implants was a hemiarthroplasty that required less bone resection and, hopefully, preservation of the collateral ligaments. A few long-term successes were reported; but in general, joint function was limited and the clinical experience consisted of only 8 to 10 patients.

The era of total elbow joint prosthetic replacement followed the limited success with custom-designed and resurfacing hemiarthroplasty. In addition to the initial design of

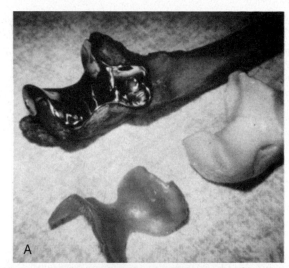

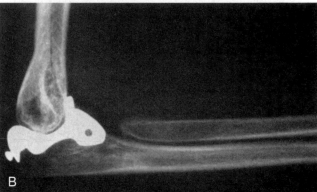

FIGURE 47–3 • *A,* A vitallium saddle designed by Bickel and Peterson to resurface the proximal ulna. *B,* Fifteen-year follow-up of a patient with post-traumatic arthritis treated with a vitallium interposition ("saddle") arthroplasty. There was motion of extension to 80 degrees and flexion to 135 degrees. (From Peterson, L.F.A., and Jones, J.M.: Surgery of the rheumatoid elbow. Orthop. Clin. North Am. **2:**667, 1971.)

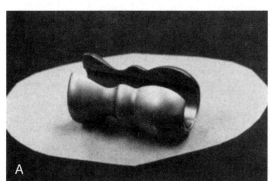

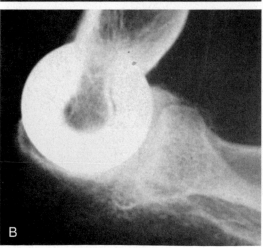

FIGURE 47–4 • *A,* Distal humerus resurfacing prosthesis designed by Street and Stevens. *B,* Three-year follow-up of a Stevens-Street prosthesis. Note the new cortical bone growth around the prosthesis. (From Street, D. M., and Stevens, P. A.: A humeral replacement prosthesis for the elbow: Results in ten elbows. J. Bone Joint Surg. **56A:**1147, 1974.)

Dee, there followed a number of hinged elbow arthroplasties[9, 12, 29, 32, 60, 66, 71] (Figs. 47–5 and 47–6). These prostheses almost uniformly provided pain relief and a reasonable range of elbow motion (20 degrees of extension, to 110 to 120 degrees of flexion). Unfortunately, complication rates proved too high, including loosening, component fracture, and infection leading to a rate of reoperation of 22 to 30 percent. Our experience at the Mayo Clinic began in 1973 with the development of a semiconstrained, hinged ulno-humeral prosthesis, including a radial head–capitellum articulation (Mayo type I) (Fig. 47–7). A metal encasement of the polyethylene ulnar component was added in 1975. We also had an experience with the original design of the Coonrad hinged prosthesis, which was metal-to-metal humeral and ulna components separated by a high-density polyethylene bushing (Fig. 47–8).[48] Patient selection included both rheumatoid arthritis and post-traumatic arthritis. The Coonrad design was used more frequently in the post-traumatic patient than the Mayo design, with equal amounts of experience with both designs in patients with rheumatoid arthritis. In 1981, Morrey and colleagues[49] reported the results of 80 Mayo or Coonrad prostheses in 72 patients. The results were good in 60 percent, fair in 16 percent, and poor in 24 percent.[49] Revisions were not infrequent, however, and were related to initial experience in elbow joint design and limited knowledge of elbow biomechanics. The complication rate was 55 percent, including loosening, infection, triceps rupture, ulnar neuropathy, and medial or lateral condyle fracture. Nevertheless, pain relief and reasonably good motion (24 to 129 degrees, Coonrad design) were noted and encouraged our group toward further development of a total elbow joint prosthesis.

Two major developments in the redesign of the Coonrad prosthesis, along with an improved surgical approach and cementing techniques, led to the continued pursuit of the ideal total elbow joint arthroplasty. Under the direction of Dr. Richard Bryan, now deceased, a study group of Mayo investigators examined the issue of prosthetic loosening and implant failure. It was concluded that the Mayo snap-fit relatively unconstrained implant was potentially too unstable, especially in the rheumatoid patient, and this finding was sufficient to defer further implantation. With the Coonrad design, we combined increased biomechanical knowledge of elbow kinematics[47a] and clinical experience to determine that the addition of an extracortical anterior

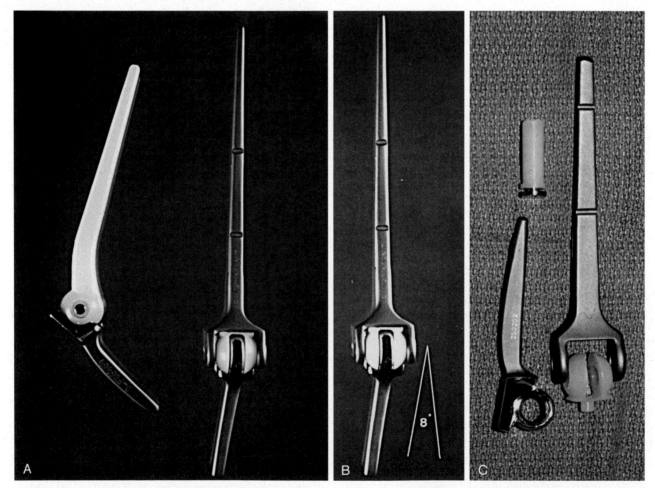

FIGURE 47–5 • Hinged total elbow arthroplasty. A, Pritchard-Walker semiconstrained ulnohumeral prosthesis. (*Left,* original design, polyethylene on metal; *right,* second-generation metal stems with polyethylene interface). B, Pritchard-Walker articulated generation II provided an 8-degree valgus carrying angle and 8 to 10 degrees of varus-valgus angulation. C, Disarticulation, Pritchard-Walker design with polyethylene bushing and articular surface interface.

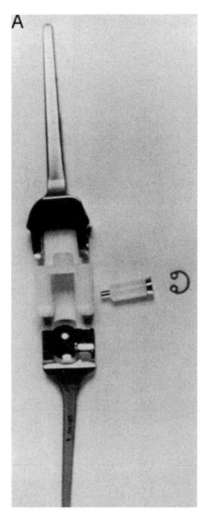

FIGURE 47–6 • Hinged total elbow. Inglis design triaxial total elbow arthroplasty with three-component interface of two metallic stems
and a polyethylene interface and bushing. (From Inglis, A. E., and Pellicci, P. M.: Total elbow replacement. J. Bone Joint Surg. **62A**:1252,
1980; and Inglis, A.E., et al. Total elbow arthroplasty for flail and unstable elbow. J. Shoulder Elbow Surg. **6**:29, 1997.)

rior flange in 1981 with the surface preparation to the
proximal ulna, and distal humerus, to provide further improvement in prosthetic fixation and overall stability. The
complications related to total elbow replacement have significantly diminished, and this procedure now rewards the
patient and surgeon with a very safe, functional, and long-
term satisfactory outcome to the multiple types of arthritic
deformity that affect the elbow. The history of total elbow
arthroplasty still has not been fully told, as better materials,
biomechanical analysis of forces, prosthetic designs, liga-

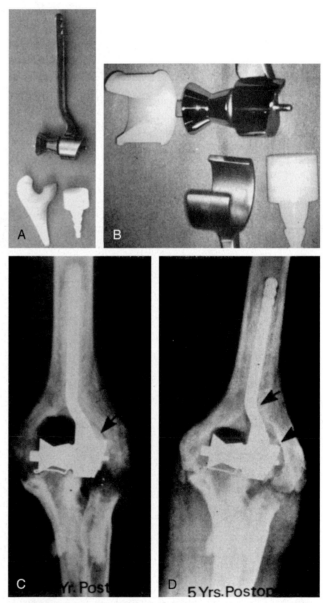

FIGURE 47–7 • Mayo prosthesis (Mark I and II) semiconstrained
ulnohumeral joint with radial head replacement. *A*, Original Mayo prosthesis with polyethylene radial head and proximal ulna components articulated with a metal humeral stem and articulation. *B*, Revision Mayo
prosthesis with metal-encased ulna and metal humeral components and
polyethylene articulation. *C*, One year postoperatively; the Mayo implant is stable but with evidence of a radiolucent line *(arrow)* of 2 mm
in a patient with rheumatoid arthritis. *D*, After 5 years, there is progression of the radiolucent zone *(double arrow)*. (From Morrey, B. F., et al.:
Total elbow arthroplasty: A five-year experience. J. Bone Joint Surg.
63A:1050, 1981.)

flange plus a slightly forgiving loose-hinged prosthetic interface would be beneficial to our patients in the prevention
of implant loosening (Fig. 47–9). Biomechanical studies
suggested that the humeral loosening, in particular, might
be prevented by better force transfer across what clearly
was evidence of forces equal to a "weight-bearing" joint.
The addition of the anterior flange significantly reduced
the problems of the "windshield wiper" effect of stem
loosening within the distal humerus (see Fig. 47–8C and
D). Better intramedullary cavity bone preparation plus cementing techniques provided more secure fixation of both
proximal ulna and distal humerus. As a consequence of
these changes, implantation of the Mayo-modified Coonrad
prosthesis, the Coonrad-Morrey, became the procedure of
choice at our institution for the majority of patients requiring total elbow arthroplasty. We applied this design not
only in advanced rheumatoid disease but also in osteoarthritis, post-traumatic arthritis, distal humerus nonunion,
and supracondylar fractures. The final design change suggested by Morrey and Bryan was the addition of the ante-

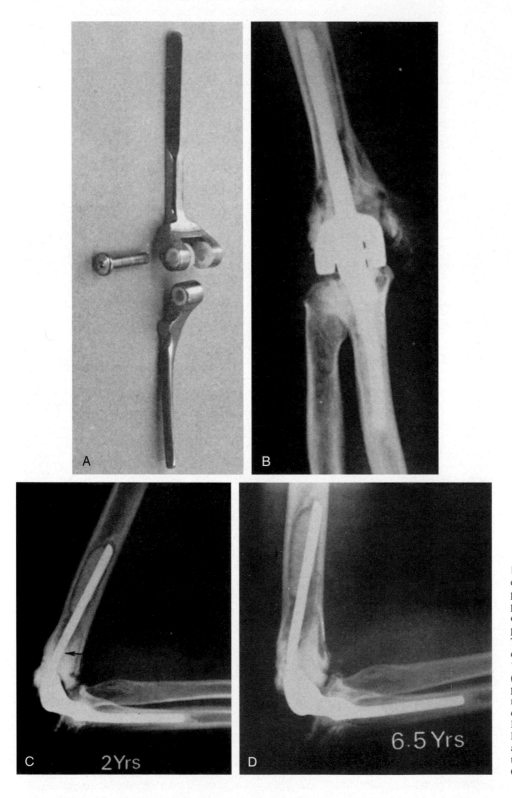

FIGURE 47–8 • Coonrad total elbow prosthesis. *A,* Original Coonrad prosthesis. Polyethylene bushing and polyethylene insert. *B,* Two-year postoperative replacement with Coonrad prosthesis; note radiolucent lines. *C,* Two-year postoperative lateral with radiolucent line and anteroposterior "toggle" of the humeral stem *(arrow). D,* Six and one-half years postoperative with stable asymptomatic lucent line about the humeral component. (From Morrey, B. F., Bryan, R. S., Dobyns, J. H., and Linscheid, R. L.: Total elbow arthroplasty: A five-year experience at the Mayo Clinic. J. Bone Joint Surg. **63A:**1050, 1981.)

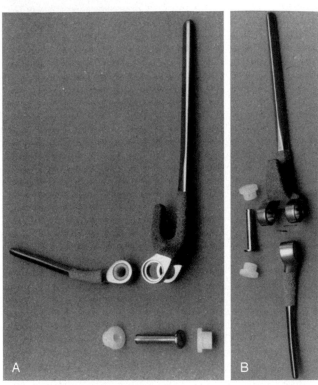

FIGURE 47–9 • Mayo modified Coonrad implant (Coonrad-Morrey). *A,* Disarticulated lateral view of the prosthesis demonstrating changes from the original design, which include sintered proximal ulna and distal humerus components, anterior flange with the humeral component, and polyethylene bushing. *B,* Anterior view with humeral and ulnar components shown and polyethylene bushings.

ment reconstructions, and protection against infection are developed by interested clinical and basic researchers in the years to come. The story, to date, has been an interesting and challenging effort of combining anatomy, mechanics, and surgical know-how to produce very good options for total elbow replacement.

ELBOW ARTHROPLASTY: INDICATIONS AND IMPLANT SELECTION

Replacement of the elbow can be a formidable surgical procedure, and specific indications are necessary so that the risk-benefit ratio is clear to both the patient and the surgeon. Over time and with increasing experience, surgical indications and patient selection have changed. Selection of a total joint arthroplasty has clearly emerged as both a primary and a secondary salvage procedure for the damaged elbow, as other reconstructive procedures have had less reliable success. Faced with the choice of elbow fusion, for example, resection arthroplasty or total joint arthroplasty is almost always preferred. In general, interposition arthroplasty is preferred in the younger patient, and total elbow arthroplasty in the older patient. In many cases of post-traumatic arthritis[67] or comminuted distal humeral fractures[8] or nonunions,[56] previously treated conservatively, total elbow arthroplasty is considered the treatment of

choice. It is considered optimal in the older patient, in nearly all patients with rheumatoid arthritis, and in most patients with post-traumatic fracture or nonunion. Based on historical perspectives, the optimum selection of a reconstructive procedure still favors total joint replacement, although interposition arthroplasty is gaining specific favor as experience increases.[52]

CHOICE OF JOINT IMPLANT REPLACEMENT (Table 47–1)

The choice of a joint implant for elbow reconstructive surgery is usually based on three factors: (1) the extent and the etiology of the disease process (post-traumatic, degenerative, or rheumatoid process),[31, 54] (2) the specific needs of the patient, and (3) the experience of the surgeon.[54] The disease process is influenced most significantly by the degree of pain, the amount of joint instability, and the limitation of motion that affects the elbow. Relief of pain is clearly the primary goal of implant arthroplasty.[8, 16, 19, 20] In general, with all the current elbow prostheses, relief of pain can and should be anticipated in 90 to 95 percent of all patients. The difference between the resurfacing and the semiconstrained implants is related to the spectrum of pathology that can be successfully addressed by the design. The potential for instability is greater with the resurfacing implant, whereas loosening and wear are the concerns associated with semiconstrained devices. Otherwise, the complications related to neuropathy (ulnar), surgical approach (triceps weakness), and implant fracture are not dissimilar.

Joint stability, by definition, is greater with semiconstrained[4, 12, 48, 53–57, 60] than with unconstrained implants.[20, 26, 61] The original customed-designed hinged implants were fully constrained and provided immediate stability. Loosening at bone-cement interfaces, however, was the serious price paid for rigid constraint of these prostheses.[9, 16, 27] Concomitant with the development of the low-friction metal and high-density polyethylene total hip and knee prostheses came improvement in semiconstrained elbow joint implants. Many of the changes occurred following extensive clinical and basic research studies and the trend toward relatively unconstrained (Fig. 47–10) anatomic elbow resurfacing procedures. New designs in semiconstrained prostheses[32, 49, 53, 60] (Fig. 47–11; see Fig. 47–9) provided almost the same degree of stability as the hinged fully constrained implants, yet allowed a "toggle," or play,

• TABLE 47–1 • Current Elbow Prosthetic Implants	
Resurfacing	**Semiconstrained**
Capitellocondylar[19, 20]	Mayo or Morrey-Coonrad[48, 53–56]
Roper-Tuke[2]	Trispherical[32]
London[43]	Norway[63, 64]
Souter[71]	Pritchard[60]
Sorbie*	Arizona[74]
Kudo[38]	GSB III (Gschwend)[29, 30]
Pritchard II[61]	

*Personal communication.

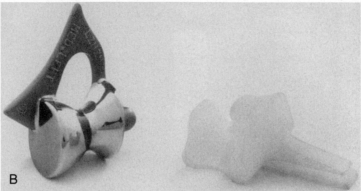
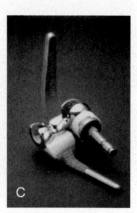
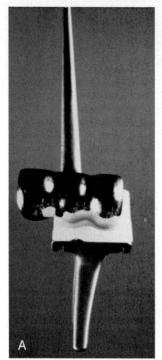

FIGURE 47–10 • Unconstrained "anatomic" total elbow prosthesis. *A,* Capitellocondylar prosthesis with ulnar humeral resurfacing articulation with an articulation for radial head component. *B,* Souter-Strathclyde metal humeral and polyethylene ulnar component. *C,* Pritchard unconstrained ulnohumeral, with radial head humeral articulation.

of 8 to 10 degrees for varus-valgus and axial rotation. Resurfacing designs[20, 26, 38, 71] (Figs. 47–12 and 47–13) and semiconstrained designs lessen the stresses on the bone-cement interface, allowing the soft tissue capsule and ligaments to transmit forces and decrease the risk of mechanical loosening. These theoretical advantages have proved to be effective in the clinical experience of many, and moreover the new designs did not have the problems of both loosening and instability.[55]

Elbow surgeons have learned to select different implants based on the primary pathology and potential soft tissue supports requiring treatment. Different elbow prostheses had better results in rheumatoid arthritis, for example, than in post-traumatic arthritis. Resurfacing implants were quite satisfactory for both juvenile- and adult-onset rheumatoid disease, provided that collateral ligament stability was reasonably present or could be obtained by implant insertion.[1, 10, 20, 22, 38, 65, 68, 75] After failed synovectomy and radial head resection in the rheumatoid elbow, for example, the resurfacing implants have proved to be a good salvage alternative.[69] In primary and post-traumatic arthritis, semiconstrained implants are generally preferred, as there is more clinical experience with their use than with resurfacing implants.[53] In post-traumatic arthritis cases with bone loss,[36] in particular either the original or the custom-designed semiconstrained implants, loose-hinged implants of the Mayo-modified Coonrad design provide the best option—if not the only solution. With most of these designs, the surgeon and the patient can rely on pain relief and a reasonable degree of movement.

Improved motion following elbow arthroplasty is important because after relief of pain, what the patient needs most is the ability to flex the elbow to touch the face and the head and to extend the elbow forward to reach and grasp objects. Unlike the case with the hip or the knee, improved motion at the elbow may be a primary indication for joint replacement. Motion is particularly relevant in patients with concomitant shoulder and wrist disease. Current studies suggest that 30 to 130 degrees will provide a functional arc of motion.[50] Resurfacing implants[21, 38, 71] reportedly have less extension, 25 to 40 degrees, as a consequence of longer postoperative immobilization to prevent instability. Semiconstrained implants average 20 to 130 degrees of motion.[28, 32, 49, 55] It is for this reason that a semiconstrained, loose-hinge implant is preferred when the goal is improved motion and stability for the elbow. The resurfacing arthroplasty is more preferred by some in the younger patient in whom pain relief is desired and collateral ligaments and joint stability are close to normal, with motion being a secondary consideration.

In addition to motion, associated strength in elbow extension and flexion is beneficial. Loss of extension strength can follow triceps scarring or adhesions,[5, 16] limiting the patient's ability to rise from a chair or to reach out for a phone or hold a stack of dishes. Improvement of strength alone is not an indication for elbow replacement. The absence of strength in the triceps and biceps, in itself, is a contraindication to elbow arthroplasty unless muscle transfer (see contraindications) can replace them. Improvement in the surgical approach to the elbow, resulting from a triceps-sparing Bryan muscle reflection procedure, has resulted in fewer difficulties with the function and strength of elbow extension.

RHEUMATOID DISEASE

Elbow implants were first used for rheumatoid arthritis.[9, 12, 34, 72] The hemiarthroplasty was first attempted with a concept similar to a cup arthroplasty of the hip.[43] The ineffi-

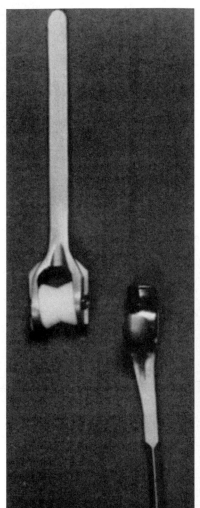

FIGURE 47–11 • Norway total elbow—semi-constrained system. *A,* The jaw-like end of the ulnar component *(lower right)* wraps around the humeral articulation *(upper left).* This provides both angular and rotational play. *B,* Articulated Norway elbow (posterior view). *C,* Components of Norway semiconstrained elbow consist of humeral component stem metal bushing and polyethylene articulations *(to the left)* and ulnar component stem *(side view),* polyethylene articulation, and connecting band.

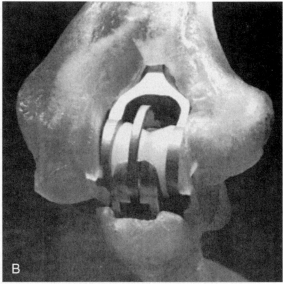

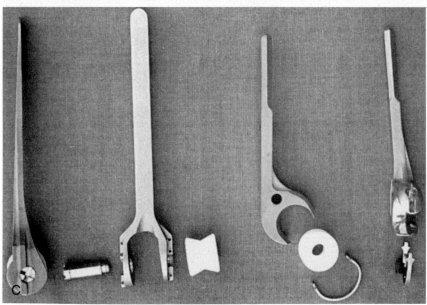

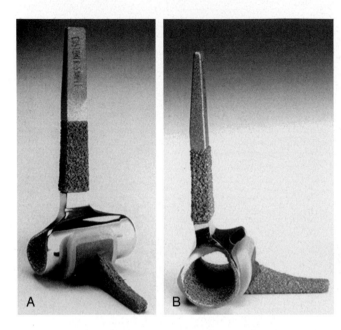

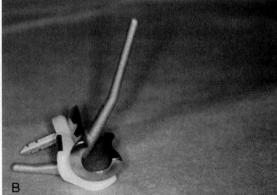

FIGURE 47–12 • Kudo Elbow System resurfacing design. Cobalt-chrome alloy humeral component articulated with a polyethylene bearing titanium alloy ulnar component. *A,* Anteroposterior view and *(B)* lateral-side view. Stems finished for enhanced cement fixation.

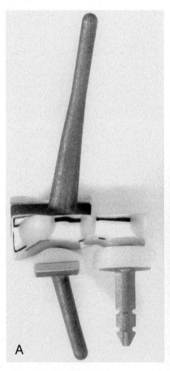

FIGURE 47–13 • Unconstrained Sorbie total elbow prosthesis. *A,* Anteroposterior view showing ulnohumeral articulation and radiohumeral articulation, both components cobalt chrome alloy with metal polyethylene articulation. *B,* Lateral view showing ulno-humeral articulation.

	• TABLE 47-2 • **Stages of Rheumatoid Disease**		
Stage	Pathology	Radiograph	Operative Rx and Prosthesis Choice
I	Pathology, mild synovitis	Normal joint surface, osteoporosis	None
II	Moderate synovitis	Joint space narrowed, joint contour maintained	Synovectomy (resurfacing?)
III	Moderate to severe synovitis; mechanical joint contact; loss of joint cartilage	Loss of joint space; mild instability, collateral ligaments intact	Resurfacing implant
IV	Mechanical instability, bone-bone articulation	Complete loss of joint space	Semiconstrained implant

ciencies of hemiarthroplasty in controlling pain led to the development of humeral and ulnar replacement, discussed earlier. In many rheumatoid arthritic elbows, instability as well as loss of the joint articular surface was present, and for that reason a hinged design[4, 12, 13, 18] to replace the elbow became popular. While conceptually attractive and representative of elbow anatomy, the initial hinge design concept proved unsuccessful and led to modified loose-hinged semiconstrained designs. Today, there are several choices for elbow arthroplasties in rheumatoid arthritis, depending on the stage of disease both clinically and radiographically (Table 47-2). In earlier stages of disease, the implantation of an unconstrained elbow prosthesis, with the goal of resurfacing the diseased joint surface, has been beneficial and is usually successful, while in the later stages of disease a semiconstrained or full constrained hinged elbow (Fig. 47-14) would be required. Ligament and capsule laxity may be present, with instability a major concern. Each of the total elbow implants has differences in design or degree of constraint, amounts of polyethylene on metal articulation, and variation of intramedullary fixation related to the prosthesis stem size and length. With the more constrained prosthesis, greater polyethylene wear can be anticipated; the degree of wear is generally related to the stress and load activities of the patient and the length of time from initial implantation. Revision of the implant must always be considered, as the age and lifestyle of the implant recipient are taken into consideration. At variable

periods of 8 to 15 years,[22, 28, 29] implant revision of the joint articular surfaces or the polyethylene bushing of the loose-hinged implants may be necessary.

Not all patients with rheumatoid arthritis of the elbow joint require total elbow arthroplasty. The indications for implant arthroplasty in rheumatoid arthritis are based primarily on pain when more conservative options are not available. A secondary indication is loss of motion. Occasionally, instability combined with either loss of motion or some degree of pain is a third indication. Radiographic criteria are very important in the decision-making process (see Table 47-2).[55] For radiographic stage I or II (retained joint space), synovectomy with or without radial head excision can be recommended.[15, 31] Arthroscopic synovectomy has replaced open synovectomy as the procedure of choice for most early stages of the rheumatoid elbow. If there is isolated radial head–to–capitellar joint involvement, radial head resection combined with synovectomy should be considered. Removing the radial head in a potentially unstable elbow with rheumatoid disease would tend to exacerbate the joint cartilage wear and increase lateral laxity and instability. The radial head is a very important constraint to valgus instability and should be preserved. For radiographic stage III (loss of joint cartilage) or stage IV (significant resorptive arthropathy), total joint replacement is advised.[20, 38, 39, 49, 71] The choice of elbow implant is a balance of surgeon choice and experience combined with patient needs. Either an unconstrained elbow prosthesis or a semiconstrained prosthesis is the consideration. The surgeon's experience, combined with careful patient assessment of ligament laxity (potential joint instability), is needed to make the decision for each patient. In general, in the rheumatoid patient, we prefer the semiconstrained loose hinge in all but the most stable elbow. This is particularly true when the disease is progressive, and further ligament laxity might be anticipated. Similarly, when joint ankylosis is present in association with destructive rheumatoid arthritis (so-called arthritis mutilans), the semiconstrained joint replacement is the best alternative.

Finally, implant selection in rheumatoid arthritis should be based on factors related to the degree of rheumatoid disease (the wet synovitis type versus the dry cartilage-destructive type), patient expectations of motion and activity load, functional use, bone stock, and the potential for later revision or component replacement (Fig. 47-15). In stage III rheumatoid disease, a resurfacing implant may not be satisfactory because the supracondylar columns are erosive, and ligament stability may be lost. In late stage III or stage IV disease, a semiconstrained implant is almost always required (Fig. 47-16). The semiconstrained implant

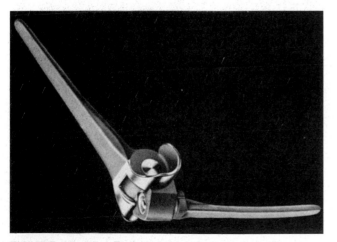

FIGURE 47-14 • Total constrained elbow prosthesis. The Gschwend prosthesis. Mach III design with low-friction hinge and large flanges resting on anterior and and lower surfaces of the humeral condyles.

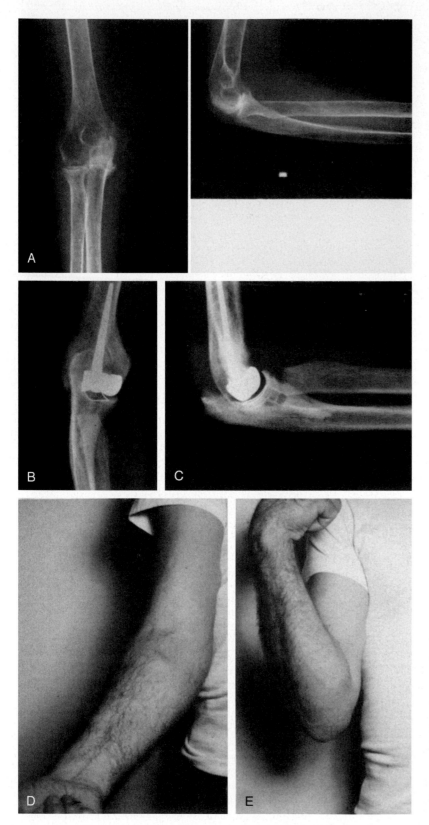

FIGURE 47–15 • Unconstrained total elbow arthroplasty stage II–III rheumatoid arthritis. *A,* Loss of joint cartilage radiocapitellar joint and ulnohumeral joint. Intact collateral ligaments, moderate synovitis. *B,* Posterolateral radiograph. Capitellocondylar prosthesis replacement. Elbow in extension (lacks 20 degrees full extension). *C,* Lateral radiograph. Elbow flexion 90 degrees, with stable joint articulation. *D,* Clinical appearance of elbow extension (lacks 30 degrees full extension). No instability. *E,* Flexion of elbow to 135 degrees. Good strength and stability.

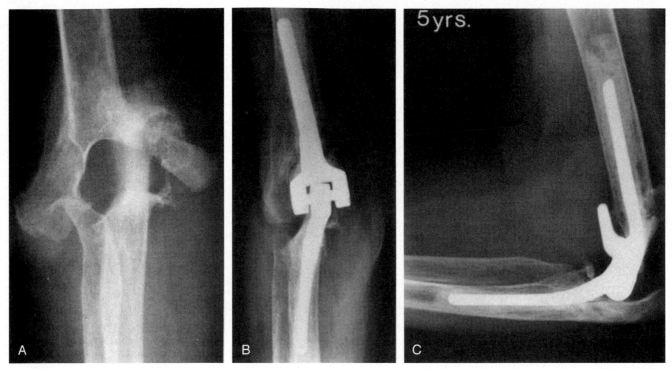

FIGURE 47–16 • Semiconstrained elbow prosthesis in stage IV. Rheumatoid arthritis. *A,* Resorptive (wet-type) rheumatoid arthritis with unstable elbow. *B,* (Anteroposterior view) Mayo-Coonrad prostheses; absent medial condyle. *C,* (Lateral view) Coonrad-Morrey at 5-year follow-up. No loosening; stable.

has been our preference in the majority of rheumatoid patients, since it provides the inherent stability that the resurfacing implant may lack, without the need for reconstruction of soft tissue support. In the older patient, the semiconstrained implant gives immediate stability and uncomplicated rehabilitation, which again is preferred. In general, older patients have fewer expectations with respect to strength, and a resurfacing implant may have advantages.[6, 19, 20, 22, 26, 32, 39, 59] While the orthopedic literature supports the choice of unconstrained elbow arthroplasty in these patients, our experience suggests that the semiconstrained implant is actually preferred.[28, 49] The older patient often has weak bone stock related to osteoporosis and thereby a poor structural foundation on which to support a unconstrained elbow implant.

Those who favor an unconstrained prosthesis for the rheumatoid elbow point out that the advantages of such an implant are that less bone removal is needed, fixation with methyl methacrylate is more easily performed, and support collateral ligaments are preserved. Indeed, if the patients' activity levels are less, elbow surgeons may prefer a resurfacing implant. If occupation or avocation requires more strength and stability, it is then that a loose-hinged hemiconstrained arthroplasty is used. I tend to recommend the resurfacing implant only in stage II or early stage III rheumatoid disease, in which there is good bone stock and ligament stability. I would recommend the semiconstrained arthroplasty in the rheumatoid individual with osteoporosis in whom condylar bone stock is deficient, in the arthritis mutilans patient, in younger patients (less than 40 years) with increased extremity demands, and in most late stage III and all stage IV disease presentations. The exception to

this is the young juvenile rheumatoid arthritis patient in the second or third decade of life with a destroyed joint. A resurfacing implant is preferred in these patients because revision may be needed 10 to 15 years later. To date, there does not appear to be any specific advantage to a semiconstrained joint system that retains or replaces the radial head. We concentrate on ulnohumeral replacements with radial head excision and have not observed untoward results with this approach.[55]

In the final analysis, that design found most effective and reliable for each specific patient is the best determinant of the device selection.

POST-TRAUMATIC ARTHRITIS

Post-traumatic arthritis typically has been treated with non-implant techniques because of the possibility of implant failure.[1, 47] This philosophy has changed, however, over the last several years with improvements in elbow implant design and patient selection. Recent reports suggest quite satisfactory outcomes for the patient with post-traumatic arthritis.[53] In fact, some of the first hemiarthroplasty prostheses and custom prostheses were designed for post-traumatic bone loss,[3, 43, 72] but experience was usually limited to a few cases. Allograft replacement of the distal humerus, the proximal ulna, and, most recently, both joint surfaces has been used in post-traumatic conditions.[10, 25] The experience is, however, quite limited. The occurrence of late neurotrophic arthritis and secondary instability has dampened enthusiasm for allografts, and only a few cases of complete elbow joint replacement with an allograft have been reported. Our personal experience with allografts is with tumor resection or for revision of failed total elbow arthroplasty where the allograft is used to replace lost bone stock as part of a revision elbow joint replacement.

Implant selection in post-traumatic arthritis is dependent on patient selection and is much different from that with rheumatoid arthritis. More attention is paid to factors such as patient age, occupation, avocations, and importantly the degree of intra-articular versus extra-articular bone reaction related to the arthritis. If there is, for example, considerable extra-articular heterotopic bone formation with involvement of the collateral ligaments, then the more stable semiconstrained, loose-hinged implant would generally be preferred. Appropriate resection of the heterotopic bone and release of ligaments to re-establish motion can be performed, such as a semiconstrained elbow implant. However, if joint resurfacing only is needed, related to the degree of post-traumatic arthritis, and if on examination the collateral ligaments are strong and stable, then a resurfacing procedure should be satisfactory.[73]

There have been several studies that report successful use with semiconstrained implants and occasional unconstrained implants, but patient selection once again must be carefully considered.[53] Many traumatic arthritic cases can be managed with joint débridement and capsular releases alone to improve motion. There are also improved results reported with interpositional arthroplasty and application of the new models of hinged distraction. However, when joint surfaces are destroyed and motion is not only limited but also quite painful, joint replacement should be considered.[53] The age for selection of any implant arthroplasty has been proposed in post-traumatic arthritis as around 60 years. We believe that younger patients should still be treated with distraction arthroplasty.[52] In older patients needing joint replacement, our preference has been the Mayo-modified Coonrad semiconstrained implant. In a recent study published in August 1997, Schneeberger and associates reported on 41 patients with osteoarthrosis managed by the semiconstrained Mayo-Coonrad implant design. With 5 years of follow-up (average), the results were 16 patients excellent (39 percent), 18 patients good (44 percent), and 5 patients fair (12 percent), with only two patients (5 percent) having poor results.[67] While mechanical failure was a concern related to implant fracture and polyethylene bushing wear, the series reported that 95 percent of patients had a functioning implant at the time of follow-up with a satisfactory outcome. My personal experience is reflected in that series with mainly good to excellent results, the fair results in those patients with periarticular bone formation or fibrosis.

Resurfacing implants can be considered in post-traumatic arthritis of the elbow when the arthritic process is confined to the joint surface. Based on my review of the English scientific literature, there has been little experience with resurfacing implants in this condition. The resurfacing designs may have specific advantages with respect to implant life expectancy, provided that the collateral ligaments are sound and are not in need of reconstruction. The addition of a radial head component when one considers surface replacement implants should be an added consideration. Improved stress sharing between the radial head implant and the capitellar surface should reduce the ulnohumeral loads and potentially reduce the risk of implant loosening.[57] However, only the Sorbie implant (see Fig. 47–13A) and ERS (elbow-resurfacing implant designed by Pritchard) have included a radial head component, and the experience with these implants has been limited. Both humeral, ulnar, and radial stem designs have replaced the initial attempts of condylar replacement with stemless articular designs. Pain relief with these implants has been excellent and motion reasonable, but implant loosening and failure of the prosthetic components are reported. The largest experience in the United States has been with the capitellocondylar implant.[22] With current improved surgical techniques, this is reported to be quite a reliable implant replacement with generally good to excellent result.[10, 26, 65]

With all of the resurfacing designs, there have been continued reports primarily of joint instability, including frank dislocation, intermittent subluxation (notably the capitellocondylar), and malposition of the ulna on the humeral component.[2, 40, 65, 73] This suggests that soft tissue reconstruction remains difficult. Long-term instability would be expected in 20 to 28 percent of patients at follow-up intervals of 3 to 5 years, requiring revision surgery for either the implant or soft tissue balance, or both, based on recent reports.[73]

SUPRACONDYLAR FRACTURES AND NONUNION OF THE HUMERUS

Further indications for elbow implants following post-traumatic conditions are malunion and nonunion of the distal humerus[24, 33, 56] and selected comminuted fractures in the elderly.[7] Displaced or poorly reduced supracondylar or T-condylar fractures in the elderly often are not amenable to open reduction and internal fixation as a result of poor bone stock and excessive fracture comminution. When these fractures cannot be treated conservatively by closed reduction and casting and when the patient has both persistent pain and severely restricted motion, the patient may benefit from implant replacement of the elbow. Our experience in the elderly population with distal humeral fracture demonstrated that in 20 patients (mean age of 72 years) with 2 years' review or more, all implants remained intact and in place without evidence of loosening. This was true except for one patient who had a fracture of the ulnar component following a fall. All patients had good to excellent results, as measured by the Mayo elbow score, and none had a poor or fair result.[7]

Similarly, in the treatment of the elderly patient with a distal humerus nonunion, our experience in 36 consecutive patients (average age of 68 years) is that 31 patients (86 percent) had good to excellent results, three patients (8 percent) had a fair result, and only two patients (6 percent) had poor results.[56] Five flail elbows were stable at 4-plus years of follow-up. As some of these patients were younger than in the supracondylar fracture group, there were complications of particulate synovitis and bushing wear, leading to an overall complication rate of 18 percent and reoperation rate of 13 percent. I believe that in selected patients (especially the elderly), total elbow arthroplasty can be a better alternative than osteosynthesis, particularly after a failed primary procedure. Resection of the pseudarthrosis or comminuted distal humerus replaced by elbow joint arthroplasty can return patients rapidly to their former lifestyle with a low risk of complications.[24, 54, 56]

While there is controversy related to the use of a total elbow in acute fractures and nonunion of the humerus, my experience in these selected groups of patients with painful supracondylar or intercondylar fractures and nonunions suggests that despite the concern of firm implant fixation in osteoporotic bone and a primary goal of retention of bone stock a semiconstrained hinged elbow implant can provide very satisfactory immediate and long-term results (Fig. 47–17).

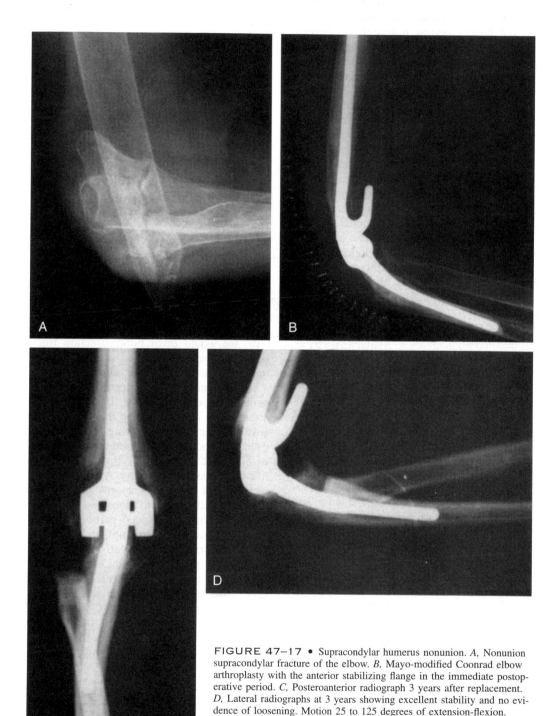

FIGURE 47–17 • Supracondylar humerus nonunion. *A,* Nonunion supracondylar fracture of the elbow. *B,* Mayo-modified Coonrad elbow arthroplasty with the anterior stabilizing flange in the immediate postoperative period. *C,* Posteroanterior radiograph 3 years after replacement. *D,* Lateral radiographs at 3 years showing excellent stability and no evidence of loosening. Motion 25 to 125 degrees of extension-flexion.

presentation, a semiconstrained elbow prosthesis is preferred. In my experience, many more patients require the semiconstrained arthroplasty than resurface arthroplasty, and the results of comparative series favor the semiconstrained prosthesis because motion is greater and the incidence of prosthetic loosening and perioperative complications is less.[28, 55] Our preference for rheumatoid arthritic conditions is demonstrated in the treatment algorithm (Fig. 47–18).

In the treatment of post-traumatic arthritis, there are several options for improved motion and relief of pain. I prefer interposition arthroplasty or joint contracture release (see Chapter 60) to free capsule and muscle and to excise heterotopic bone. Therefore, with patients under the age of 50 years, a distraction arthroplasty is preferred. In patients between the ages of 50 and 60 years, judgment is required regarding joint replacement versus distraction arthroplasty versus excision of heterotopic bone and early continuous passive motion (CPM). More recent experience has demonstrated successful outcomes of total elbow arthroplasty that are superior to resection procedures. After the age of 60 years, joint replacement arthroplasty is recommended. Our experience with this procedure suggests excellent results with semiconstrained implants. In addition, as there are few reliable alternatives for the treatment of established supracondylar or T-condylar fracture malunions and nonunions in the elderly patient, my preference is for a semiconstrained total elbow arthroplasty. My preference for post-traumatic conditions is demonstrated in the treatment algorithm (Fig. 47–19).

REFERENCES

1. Ackerman, G., and Jupiter, J. B.: Nonunion of fractures of the distal end of the humerus. J. Bone Joint Surg. **70A**:75, 1988.
2. Allieu, Y., Meyer, zu Reckendorf G., and Daude O: Long-term results of unconstrained Roper-Tuke total hip arthroplasty in patients with rheumatoid arthritis. J. Shoulder Elbow Surg. **7**:560, 1998.
3. Barr, J. S., and Eaton, R. G.: Elbow reconstruction with a new prosthesis to replace the distal end of the humerus: A case report. J. Bone Joint Surg. **47A**:1408, 1965.
4. Bell, S., Gschwend, N., and Steiger, U.: Arthroplasty of the elbow. Experience with the mark III GSB prosthesis. Aust. N.Z. J. Surg. **56**:823, 1986.
5. Bryan, R. S., and Morrey, B. F.: Extensive posterior exposure of the elbow: Triceps sparing approach. Clin. Orthop. **166**:199, 1982.
6. Chantelot, C., Fontaine, C., Migaud, H., and Duquennoy, A.: Complete elbow prosthesis for inflammatory and hemophiliac arthropathy: A retrospective analysis of 22 cases (Kudo and GSB III prostheses). Ann. Chir. Main. Membr. Super. **16**:49, 1997.
7. Cobb, T. K., and Morrey, B. F.: Total elbow arthroplasty as primary treatment for distal humeral fractures in elderly patients. J. Bone Joint Surg. **79**:826, 1997.
8. Connor, P. M., and Morrey, B. F.: Total elbow arthroplasty in patients who have juvenile rheumatoid arthritis. J. Bone Joint Surg. **80A**:678, 1998.
9. Coonrad, R. W.: History of total elbow arthroplasty. In Inglis, A. E. (ed.): Upper Extremity Joint Replacement (Symposium on Total Joint Replacement of the Upper Extremity, 1979). St. Louis, C. V. Mosby Co., 1982.
10. Davis, R. F., Weiland, A. J., Hungerford, D. S., Moore, J. R., and Volenec-Dowling, S.: Nonconstrained total elbow arthroplasty. Clin. Orthop. **171**:156, 1982.
11. Dean, G. S., Holliger, E. H., 4th, and Urbaniak, J. R.: Elbow allograft for reconstruction of the elbow with massive bone loss: Long-term results. Clin. Orthop. **(341)**:12, 1997.
12. Dee, R.: Total replacement arthroplasty of the elbow for rheumatoid arthritis. J. Bone Joint Surg. **54B**:88, 1972.
13. Dee, R.: Total replacement of the elbow joint. Orthop. Clin. North Am. **4**:415, 1973.
14. Dent, C. M., Hoy, G., and Stanley, J. K.: Revision of failed total elbow arthroplasty. J. Bone Joint Surg. **77**:691, 1995.
15. Dickson, R. A., Stein, H., and Bentley, G.: Excision arthroplasty of the elbow in rheumatoid disease. J. Bone Joint Surg. **58B**:227, 1976.
16. Dobyns, J. H., Bryan, R. S., Linscheid, R. L., and Peterson, L. F. A.: The special problems of total elbow arthroplasty. Geriatrics **31**:57, 1976.
17. Dunn, W. A.: A distal humeral prosthesis. Clin. Orthop. **77**:199, 1971.
18. Engelbrecht, E., Bucholz, H. W., Rottger, J., and Siegal, A.: Total elbow replacement with a hinge and a nonblocked system. In Joint Replacement of the Upper Limb. London, Mechanical Engineering Publications, 1978.
19. Ewald, F. C.: Total elbow replacement. Orthop. Clin. North Am. **6**:685, 1975.
20. Ewald, F. C., Scheinberg, R. D., Poss, R., Thomas, W. H., Scott, R. D., and Sledge, C. B.: Capitellocondylar total elbow arthroplasty: Two- to five-year follow-up in rheumatoid arthritis. J. Bone Joint Surg. **62A**:1259, 1980.
21. Ewald, F. C.: Nonconstrained metal to plastic total elbow arthroplasty. In Inglis, A. E. (ed.): Symposium on Total Joint Replacement of the Upper Extremity. St. Louis, C.V. Mosby Co., 1982, p. 141.
22. Ewald, F. C., Simmons, E. D., Sullivan, J. A., et al.: Capitellocondylar total elbow replacement in rheumatoid arthritis: Long-term results. J. Bone Joint Surg. **75**:498, 1993.
23. Ferlic, D. C., and Clayton, M. L.: Salvage of failed total elbow arthroplasty. J. Shoulder Elbow Surg. **4**:290, 1995.
24. Figgie, M. P., Inglis, A. E., Mow, C. S., and Figgie, H. E., III: Salvage of nonunion of supracondylar fracture of the humerus by total elbow arthroplasty. J. Bone Joint Surg. **71A**:1058, 1989.
25. Faulkes, G. D., and Mitsunago, M. M.: Allograft salvage of failed total elbow arthroplasty: A report of two cases. Clin. Orthop. **296**:113, 1993.
26. Friedman, R. J., Lee, D. E., and Ewald, F. C.: Nonconstrained total elbow arthroplasty. J. Arthroplasty **4**:31, 1989.
27. Garrett, J. C., Ewald, F. C., Thomas, W. H., and Sledge, C. B.: Loosening associated with GSB hinge total elbow replacement in patients with rheumatoid arthritis. Clin. Orthop. **127**:170, 1977.
28. Gill, D. R., and Morrey, B. F.: The Coonrad-Morrey total elbow arthroplasty in patients who have rheumatoid arthritis: A 10 to 15 year follow-up study. J. Bone Joint Surg. **80A**:1327, 1998.
29. Gschwend, N., Loehr, J., Ivosevic-Radovanovic, D., and Scheler, H.: Semiconstrained elbow prostheses with special reference ot the GBS III prosthesis. Clin. Orthop. **232**:104, 1988.
30. Gschwend, N., Simmen, B. R., Matejovsky, Z.: Late complications in elbow arthroplasty. J. Shoulder Elbow Surg. **5**(2 Pt 1):86, 1996.
31. Inglis, A. E., Ranawat, C. S., and Straub, L. R.: Synovectomy and débridement of the elbow in rheumatoid arthritis. J. Bone Joint Surg. **53A**:652, 1971.
32. Inglis, A. E., and Pellicci, P. M.: Total elbow replacement. J. Bone Joint Surg. **62A**:1252, 1980.
33. Inglis, A. E., Inglis, A. E., Jr., Figgie, M. M., and Asnis, L.: Total elbow arthroplasty for flail and unstable elbows. J. Shoulder Elbow Surg. **6**:29, 1997.
34. Johnson, E. W., Jr., and Schlein, A. P.: Vitallium prosthesis for the olecranon and proximal part of the ulna: Case report with thirteen-year follow-up. J. Bone Joint Surg. **52A**:721, 1970.
35. Kozak, T. K., Adams, R. A., and Morrey, B. F.: Total elbow arthroplasty in primary osteoarthritis of the elbow. J. Arthroplasty **13**:837, 1998.
36. King, G. J., Itoi, E., Niebur, G. L., Morrey, B. F., and An, K. N.: Kinematics and stability of the Norway elbow. Acta Orthop. Scand. **64**:657, 1993.
37. King, G. J., Adams, R. A., and Morrey, B. F.: Total elbow arthroplasty: Revision with use of a non-custom semiconstrained prosthesis. J. Bone Joint Surg. **79A**:394, 1997.
38. Kudo, H., Iwano, K., and Watanabe, S.: Total replacement of the rheumatoid elbow with a hingeless prosthesis. J. Bone Joint Surg. **62A**:277, 1980.
39. Kudo, H., and Kunio, I.: Total elbow arthroplasty with a nonconstrained surface replacement prosthesis in patients who have rheumatoid arthritis: A long-term follow-up study. J. Bone Joint Surg. **72A**:355, 1990.
40. Kudo, H., Iwano, K., and Nishino, J.: Cementless or hybrid total

elbow arthroplasty with titanium alloy implants. J. Arthroplasty **9:**269, 1994.

41. Kudo, H.: Non-constrained elbow arthroplasty for mutilans deformity in rheumatoid arthritis: A report of six cases. J Bone Joint Surg **80B:**234, 1998.

42. Ljung, P., Jonsson, K., and Rydholm, U.: Short-term complications of the lateral approach for non-constrained elbow replacement: Follow-up of 50 rheumatoid elbows. J. Bone Joint Surg. **77B:**937, 1995.

43. London, J. T.: Endoprosthetic prosthetic replacement of the elbow. *In* Morrey, B. F. (ed.): The Elbow and Its Disorders. Philadelphia, W. B. Saunders, 1985.

44. MacAusland, W. R.: Replacement of the distal end of the humerus with a prosthesis: Report of four cases. West. J. Surg. **65:**557, 1954.

45. Madsen, F., Gudmundson, G. H., Sojbjerg, J. O., and Sneppen, O.: The Pritchard Mark II elbow prosthesis in rheumatoid arthritis. Acta Orthop. Scand. **60:**249, 1989.

46. Mellen, R. H., and Phalen, G. S.: Arthroplasty of the elbow by replacement of the distal end of the humerus with an acrylic prosthesis. J. Bone Joint Surg. **29:**348, 1947.

47. Mitsunaga, M. S., Bryan, R. S., and Linscheid, R. L.: Condylar nonunions of the elbow. J. Trauma **22:**787, 1982.

47a. Morrey, B. F., and Chao, E. Y.: Passive motion of the elbow joint. J. Bone Joint Surg. **58A:**501, 1976.

48. Morrey, B. F., and Bryan, R. S.: Total joint arthroplasty: The Elbow. Mayo Clin. Proc. **54:**507, 1979.

49. Morrey, B. F., Bryan, R. S., Dobyns, J. H., and Linscheid, R. L.: Total elbow arthroplasty: A five-year experience at the Mayo Clinic. J. Bone Joint Surg. **63A:**1050, 1981.

50. Morrey, B. F., Askew, L. J., An, K. N., and Chao, E. Y.: A biomechanical study of normal functional elbow motion. J. Bone Joint Surg. **63A:**87, 1981.

51. Morrey, B. F., and Bryan, R. S.: Complications of total elbow arthroplasty. Clin. Orthop. **170:**204, 1982.

52. Morrey, B. F.: Treatment of the stiff elbow: Distraction arthroplasty. J. Bone Joint Surg. **72A:**601, 1990.

53. Morrey, B. F., Adams, R. A., and Bryan, R. S.: Total replacement for post-traumatic arthritis of the elbow. J. Bone Joint Surg. **73B:**607, 1991.

54. Morrey, B. F.: Elbow replacement arthroplasty: Indications and patient selection. *In* Morrey, B. F. (ed.): Joint Replacement Arthroplasty. New York, Churchill Livingstone, 1991.

55. Morrey, B. F., and Adams, R. A.: Semiconstrained total elbow arthroplasty for rheumatoid arthritis. J. Bone Joint Surg. **74A:**479, 1992.

56. Morrey, B. F., and Adams, R. A.: Semiconstrained elbow replacement for distal humeral nonunion. J. Bone Joint Surg. **77B:**67, 1995.

57. O'Driscoll, S. W., Tanaka, S., An, K. N., and Morrey, B. F.: The semiconstrained total elbow replacement: A biomechanical analysis. J. Bone Joint Surg. **74B:**297, 1992.

58. Peterson, L. F. A., and James, J. A.: Surgery of the rheumatoid elbow. Orthoped. Clin. North Am. **2:**667, 1971.

59. Poll, R. G., and Rozing, P. M.: Use of the Sauter-Strathclyde total elbow prosthesis in patients who have rheumatoid arthritis. J. Bone Joint Surg. **73A:**1227, 1991.

60. Pritchard, R. W.: Long-term follow-up study: Semiconstrained elbow prosthesis. Orthopedics **4:**151, 1981.

61. Pritchard, R. W.: Anatomic surface elbow arthroplasty: A preliminary report. Clin. Orthop. **179:**223, 1983.

62. Ramsey, M. L., Adams, R. A., and Morrey, B. F.: Instability of the elbow treated with semiconstrained total elbow arthroplasty. J. Bone Joint Surg. **81:**38, 1999.

63. Risung, F.: The Norway elbow prosthesis system: Six years experience. Presented at the 1993 European Rheumatoid Arthritis Surgery Society, Oslo, Norway.

64. Risung, F.: The Norway elbow replacement: Design, technique and results after nine years. J. Bone Joint Surg. **79B:**394, 1997.

65. Ruth, J. T., and Welde, A. H.: Capitellocondylar total elbow arthroplasty. J. Bone Joint Surg. **74A:**95, 1992.

66. Schlein, A. P.: Semiconstrained total elbow arthroplasty. Clin. Orthop. **121:**222, 1976.

67. Schneeberger, A. G., Adams, R., and Morrey, B. F.: Semiconstrained total elbow replacement for the treatment of post-traumatic osteoarthrosis. J. Bone Joint Surg. **78A:**1211, 1997.

68. Schwyzer, H. K., Simmen, B. F., and Gschwend, N.: Infekt nach Schulter-und Ellbogenarthroplastik. Diagnostik Therapie. Orthopade **24:**367, 1995.

69. Schemitsch, E. H., Ewald, F. C., and Thornhill, T. S.: Results of total elbow arthroplasty after excision of the radial head and synovectomy in patients who had rheumatoid arthritis. J. Bone Joint Surg. **78:**1541, 1996.

70. Sjoden, G. O., Lundberg, A., and Blomgren, G. A.: Late results of the Souter-Strathclyde total elbow prosthesis in rheumatoid arthritis: 6/19 implants loose after 5 years. Acta Orthop. Scand. **66:**391, 1995.

71. Souter, W. A.: Arthroplasty of the elbow: With particular reference to metallic hinge arthroplasty in rheumatoid patients. Orthop. Clin. North Am. **4:**395, 1973.

72. Street, D. M., and Stevens, P. S.: A humeral replacement prosthesis for the elbow: Results in ten elbows. J. Bone Joint Surg. **56A:**1147, 1974.

73. Trancik, T., Wilde, A. H., and Borden, L. S.: Capitellocondylar total elbow arthroplasty: Two to eight-year experience. Clin. Orthop. **223:**175, 1987.

73a. Venable C. S.: An elbow and an elbow prosthesis: Case of complete loss of the lower third of the humerus. Am. J. Surg. **83:**271, 1952.

74. Volz, R. G.: Development and clinical analysis of a new semiconstrained total elbow prosthesis. *In* Inglis, A. E. (ed.): Upper Extremity Joint Replacement Symposium on Total Elbow Joint Replacement of the Upper Extremity, 1979. St. Louis, C. V. Mosby Co., 1982.

75. Weiland, A. J., Weirs, A. P. C., Wells, R. P., and Moore, J. R.: Capitellocondylar total elbow replacement. J. Bone Joint Surg. **71A:**217, 1989.

76. Yamaguchi, K., Adams, R. A., and Morrey, B. F.: Infection after total elbow arthroplasty. J. Bone Joint Surg. **80A:**481, 1998.

CHAPTER 48

Resurfacing Elbow Replacement Arthroplasty

Rationale, Technique, and Results

• RONALD L. LINSCHEID

INTRODUCTION

The dysfunctional elbow may be treated by a variety of surgical procedures once it has reached the pain or functional tolerance of the patient. Early attempts with various types of resection and tissue interposition arthroplasties[5, 22] and custom-designed hemiarthroplasty devices[1, 5, 8, 22, 34, 37, 56] have not shown reliable results. Subsidence, loosening, and dislocation often followed an initial period of pain relief.[2, 8, 10, 40] The success of the cemented low-friction metal/high-density polyethylene (HDPE) arthroplasty concept rapidly succeeded a brief period of cemented but constrained metal-metal elbow devices, which developed corrosive metal deposition throughout the joint as well as the complications of loosening.[7, 8, 19] Although the complication rate for total elbow arthroplasties (TEAs) has remained higher than that for comparable designs for the hip and knee, the overall results are beginning to approach these procedures for reliability and longevity. The decision as to whether to choose a constrained or nonconstrained—that is, a surface replacement prosthesis (SRP)—does not follow rigid guidelines but is, to some extent, dictated by the preference of the surgeon and the adequacy of the remaining joint.

DESIGN IMPLICATIONS

The basic premise of the resurfacing design is that the skeletal structures and the fixation interface will tolerate the stresses passing through the joint better if these are attenuated by the ligaments and the muscles that surround the joint. The broader contact area afforded in the coronal plane by the trochlea and capitellum, as well as the tensile constraints of the collateral ligaments, tends to dissipate the mechanical loads through the medial and lateral metaphyseal cortical columns for the SRP (Figs. 48–1 to 48–3). It goes without saying that there must be sufficient bone stock, capsular integrity, and muscle strength to validate the concept of resurfacing arthroplasty.

Modified from Linscheid, R. L.: Resurfacing elbow replacement arthroplasty: rationale, technique, and results. *In* Morrey, B. F. (ed.): The Elbow and Its Disorders, 2nd ed. Philadelphia, W. B. Saunders Co., 1993, pp. 638–647.

DESIGN CONSIDERATIONS

The unconstrained or resurfacing implants replicate the condylar and sigmoid notch surface and contours. Most designs originally lacked stems for easier insertion but now have stem fixation and usually do not require a radial head replacement.[20, 24, 30, 33, 48, 55, 59] Kudo reports 5 of 37 with posterior displacement of the nonstemmed humeral implant.[28]

A variety of design strategies have been used to cope with the complex anatomy of the elbow.[12] The simplest is to align the ulnar and humeral shafts with straight stems of the components.[21, 23] This is based on the assumption that the radial head has been or will be excised. Most designs have made the metal component convex to replicate the humerus and the HDPE concave to accommodate the sigmoid notch. This produces less wear. The normal valgus inclination of the trochlea relative to the anatomic axis of the humerus approximates 6 degrees.[12, 15, 31] It is internally rotated with respect to the interepicondylar axis by a similar amount. The evolution of the ulnar design has increasingly reflected a preference for a metallic backing or "tray" to aid implantation and inhibit cold flow deformation of the softer material.[15, 45] Several early designs, and even a recent design,[51] that favored a stemless humeral articular surface that fit on a central buttress of corticocancellous bone required precise carpentry to obtain a good fit (Figs. 48–4 and 48–5). The SRP design universally recognized that the condylar replacement needed to be angled anteriorly approximately 30 to 45 degrees.[15, 19, 20, 21, 30, 32, 34, 45, 46, 50, 51] Most have come to recognize the need for a stem to further stabilize the device (see Figs. 48–4 and 48–5).

The joint reactive force, which is directed obliquely posteriorly and proximally, often caused bony erosion of the chamfered central strut and eventual posterior displacement of the prosthesis[28, 33, 35] (Fig. 48–6). While a stem resists this stress, if one is to maintain an anatomic relationship, it is necessary to offset the ulnar component medially from the anatomic axis of the humerus. This often necessitates introducing a valgus torque because of the slight eccentricity of the elbow flexors with regard to the contact

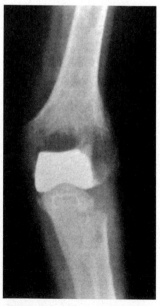

FIGURE 48–1 • Most resurfacing implants do not include a radial head implant as with the early London design.

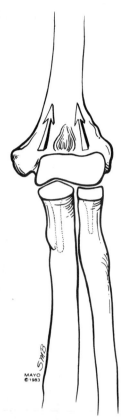

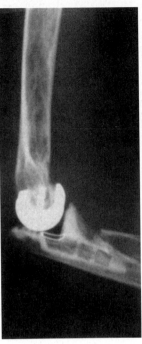

FIGURE 48–4 • Early resurfacing design of London implant, similar to the uncemented Stevens and Street implant, was inserted without a stem.

FIGURE 48–2 • The theoretical advantages of distributing forces across the ulnohumeral and both columns of the humerus are obvious.

area of the ulnohumeral articulation. It is therefore logical to direct flexion-extension force vectors within the coronal plane contact area of the elbow by including a radiocapitellar articulation. This, however, introduces additional complexity to the system. Stringent technique considera-

tions are necessary to ensure alignment and accurate component length in all three planes. Eccentric motions that would impose additional shear across the bone prosthetic interfaces, especially during pronosupination, are thus avoided. In addition, there are recent studies suggesting that radiocapitellar loading is variable with both angulation and imposed load. This makes accurate determination of

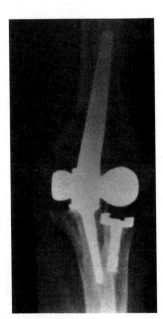

FIGURE 48–3 • The ERS implant does provide for the optional replacement of the radial head if it is thought to be useful for stability or to lessen the stresses across the prosthetic interface.

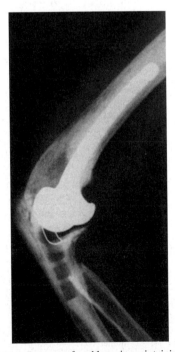

FIGURE 48–5 • Because of problems in maintaining fixation across the condyle, as with most resurfacing devices, a stem was eventually added to the implant.

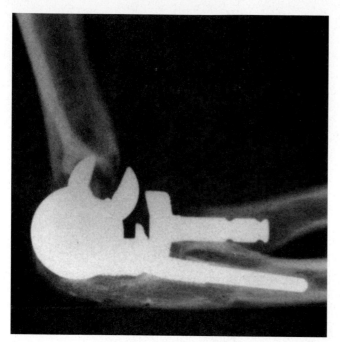

FIGURE 48–6 • Five-and-a-half years after insertion, a fracture has occurred across the distal humeral condyles at the site of fixation of a 39-year-old patient with rheumatoid arthritis. (By permission of Mayo Foundation.)

the correct prosthetic height of the radial component difficult.[17, 58]

MAYO EXPERIENCE

Our experience has been primarily with two surface replacement systems. The first was with the capitellocondylar (Codman and Shurtleff, Cintor Division, Randolf, MA), designed by F. C. Ewald[13–15] (Fig. 48–7). This is a well-designed and -sized cobalt chrome metal and HDPE prosthesis that comes with three humeral valgus angulations of 5, 10, and 15 degrees to accord with anatomic variations. The ulnar component has a metal backing in its latest model. The other model is the Surface Replacement System (ERS, Depuy Manufacturing Co., Warsaw, IN), designed by Pritchard (Fig. 48–8).[45] This is a three-component system with a metal humeral component and metal-backed ulnar and radial components that have snap-fit HDPE inserts for articulation with the humerus. The capitellocondylar was used at our institution from 1977 to 1984, after which the SRS was substituted because of its apparent greater stability.

SURGICAL TECHNIQUE

A variety of surgical exposures have been used, and each has its drawbacks and advantages. The triceps-reflecting approach gives the best overall view of the joint and allows the ulnar nerve to be protected.

The preferred exposure for the capitellocondylar prosthesis is a Kocher approach that preserves the triceps mechanism. This exposure may be modified by reflecting the triceps in continuity with the anconeus. In this respect, it

approximates the concept of Bryan and Morrey with the Mayo approach.[3] The ulnar nerve is also at greater risk during joint manipulation and is not routinely anteriorly displaced.[15, 41] Earlier motion is possible with this approach. Repair of the ulnar collateral ligament, which must be released from the medial condylar in either approach, is more difficult.

Author's Preferred Technique

The technique of the capitellocondylar has been presented by Ewald. The following description is that which I use for the ERS implant.

The surgical approach is similar to that described for the semiconstrained device.[3] The ulnar nerve is identified and dissected free so that it may be protected. The triceps, its tendon, and the periosteum are then reflected laterally, exposing the posterior aspect of the joint (see Chapter 8). The capsule is dissected from the humeral condyles and the epicondyles in continuity, so that the joint may be dislocated. Tagging the collateral ligaments will facilitate their later repair.

The ulnar alignment jig is then placed on the subcutane-

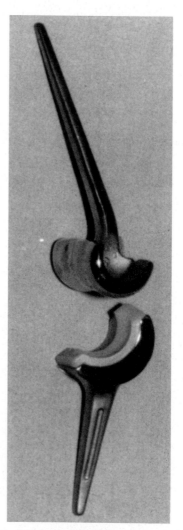

FIGURE 48–7 • The capitellocondylar implant employs several thicknesses of the high-density polyethylene with varying humeral and ulnar angles to accommodate anatomic variation.

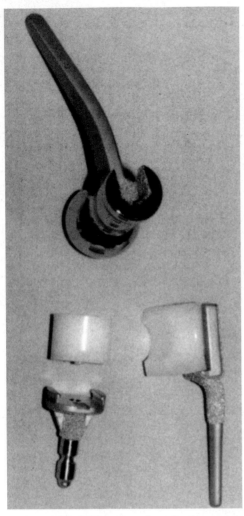

FIGURE 48-8 • The ERS implant allows for the replacement of the radial head with a modular system providing for some flexibility with regard to thickness of the implants.

ous surface, and a mark is made on the olecranon level with the depth of the sigmoid notch. A sagittal saw is then used to cut the tip of the olecranon parallel with the subcutaneous surface. Additional marks are then made on the medial surface of the ulna separated by the length of the metal tray of the ulnar component 3 mm below the previous cut. A 3-mm bit is then drilled through the ulna perpendicularly. The sagittal saw removes the sigmoid notch. A high-speed burr is introduced into the angle below the coronoid process and directed distally, posteriorly, and slightly radially. A close tolerance for the bone ingrowth area should be maintained. A trial fitting of the metal component may require several adjustments before it fits flush with the flattened olecranon surface. Avoid too vertical an orientation of the ulnar implant.

The humeral jig is then aligned with the longitudinal axis of the humerus, and 5 mm of the distal articular surface is removed on the plane of the jig. The saw guide is then placed on the center of the newly created surface, and the double saw blade is placed on a reciprocating power tool to perform the chamfer and the vertical cuts. A sagittal saw removes the anterior and posterior bone remnants without undercutting the central bone block. The

intramedullary cavity is opened through the olecranon fossa. Using the humeral trial as a template, vertical cuts in the sagittal plane align the removed section of the humeral condyles. A small broach is usually sufficient to ream the medullary cavity. Several introductions of the humeral trial and revision may be necessary to ensure a snig fit without damaging the now vulnerable humerus.

In the rheumatoid patient, a thorough synovectomy typically is carried out. The sagittal saw is placed perpendicularly, and the proximal aspect of the radial head is removed. Careful centering of graduated awls should be checked under the image intensifier in two planes before completing the enlargement for the radial stem. Good axial alignment of the radial component should prevent eccentric rotation of the radius during pronosupination.

The three trial components may then be inserted after placing the plastic inserts for the radial and ulnar metal components in place. Some trial-and-error fitting is usually necessary, starting with the smallest of the four sizes. Axial rotation of the humeral component may be the most sensitive variable that controls stability.[25] This is a good time to carefully check the alignment and fit under the image intensifier as the elbow is being moved through a full range of motion. The appropriately sized radial head and olecranon articular surfaces are assembled.

The raw bone is irrigated with saline by pulsed lavage followed by irrigation with 0.1 percent neomycin by bulb syringe. The medullary cavities are dried with suction. Because the openings are small, the use of appropriately sized suction tubing or large-bore intravenous catheters to gain sufficient depth for the introduction of antibiotic-impregnated methylmethacrylate is recommended. A preliminary plug of cement in the humeral cavity is optional. The positioning can be accomplished more accurately if the humeral and forearm components are inserted sequentially. We have avoided uncemented application.

After preparing the collateral ligaments for repair, the tourniquet is deflated and hemostasis is obtained. Persistent oozing requires a suction drain. If necessary, small drill holes in the bone to anchor the collateral ligaments are made before the sutures are tied.

Drill holes for sutures anchor the triceps to the olecranon, but the knots are buried to avoid wound irritation and possible wound-stitch infection. The remaining closure technique is optional. A postoperative radiograph to ensure that the joint is located in both planes is a necessity.

POSTOPERATIVE MANAGEMENT

Positioning the elbow at 20 to 45 degrees of flexion is preferred because the elbow tends to be unstable near extension. A compressive dressing with a plaster splint to hold the position is recommended for 4 days. After this, a cast is applied with the elbow still in relative extension for 3 to 4 weeks to allow adequate healing of the triceps and the posterior capsule. Gentle, active, assisted extension is encouraged prior to active flexion. A thermoplastic splint for use during rehabilitation and for nocturnal protection is desirable. After 6 weeks, the elbow should be allowed to regain full flexion and extension.

RESULTS

Earlier Experience. The experience of various surface replacement for rheumatoid arthritis reveals that pain relief and range of motion have been very acceptable. The complication rates for these and most designs have been relatively high.[2, 4, 9, 14, 16, 17, 19–21, 23, 28, 29, 33, 39, 47, 62] Because of bone resorption, several stemless articular designs have been superseded largely by stemmed varieties.[29, 30, 45, 53] Reports from England reveal that most patients (98 percent) had rheumatoid arthritis.[29, 43, 53] Although pain relief was unusually good, sepsis and loosening occurred at the non-stemmed humeral component in 8 of 13 Wadsworth implants, on average at 5.7 years after surgery.[29] A loose component also was observed in 2 of 22 nonstemmed Liverpool implants.[53] A comprehensive review from the Netherlands of the Souter implant reported instability in 3 of 34 implants (9 percent). Again, pain relief was marked in those avoiding surgical complications.[43] Kudo recently reported an overall satisfactory result in 29 of 37 implants (78 percent), an average of 9.5 years after resurfacing arthroplasty. The most common problem was posterior displacement of the articulation (14 percent) due to the lack of a stem on the humeral device.[28]

The largest experience of resurfacing elbow arthroplasty in this country is with the capitellocondylar prosthesis. The results have been categorized into three series: (1) 69 cases with an all-plastic ulnar component inserted through a posterior approach; (2) 31 cases with a metal-backed ulnar component inserted posteriorly; and (3) 54 cases through a Kocher midlateral approach. In the last part of this series, the results are recorded as good or excellent in 90 percent[13] (Figs. 48–9 and 48–10). Complications have included dislocation (7 percent); malalignment, loosening, triceps rupture, ulnar nerve palsy (4 percent); and wound dehiscence and infection (4 percent). Less serious complications were transient ulnar nerve palsies, subluxations, and burns or

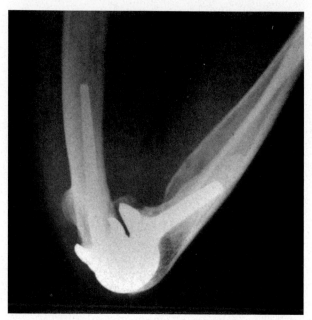

FIGURE 48–10 • Excellent function with a quiet bone-cement interface 2 years after surgery (same patient as in Fig. 48–9).

blisters, for an overall complication rate of 15 percent. Other complications include loosening of the humeral component, triceps rupture, and infection.[7, 14, 20, 24, 28, 29, 43, 48] Weiland and associates[62] noted malposition of the ulna on the humeral component as it displaced into the groove between the trochlea and the capitellar condyles in 20 percent of patients in their series. The European and the Asian experiences are similar, with a comparable or a higher incidence of instability.[24, 29, 33, 35, 43, 49, 52, 53, 60]

Mayo Clinic Results

The experience with these devices has been restricted to the capitellocondylar and SRS prostheses (see Figs. 48–7 and 48–8). Fifty-two of the former prostheses and 35 of the latter were inserted for rheumatoid arthritis in all but two instances. Pain, crepitus, and decreased range of motion were indications for surgery when there was adequate bone stock apparent by radiograph. Moderate erosive changes with the previous excision of the radial head were present in 15 percent.

CAPITELLOCONDYLAR IMPLANT

Overall relief of pain and restoration of elbow flexion were reliably obtained with this implant. Unfortunately, with the capitellocondylar prosthesis, postoperative dislocation was a disconcerting problem that did not easily resolve with relocation and immobilization in several instances. Of a total of 52 cases, posterior dislocation occurred in 6 (Fig. 48–11). Three of these prostheses were eventually replaced with hinged prostheses, and 2 became secondarily infected with wound dehiscence. This experience prompted us to use the three-component system designed by Roland Pritchard.

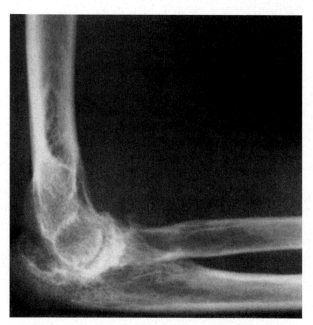

FIGURE 48–9 • Patient with grade IIA rheumatoid involvement of the elbow.

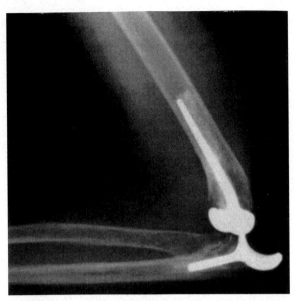

FIGURE 48–11 • The capitellocondylar implant was associated with posterior dislocation or translatory instability in 11 percent of the 52 patients operated on at Mayo.

ERS EXPERIENCE

In the ERS series of 35 elbows, follow-up ranged from 6 to 67 months, with an average of 40 months. The range of motion improved from 39 to 124 degrees, average flexion-extension to 24 to 135 degrees. Pronosupination improved moderately from preoperative values.

The results were based on the 100 point scale (Ewald), with pain assigned 50; function, 30; motion, 10; flexion-contracture, 5; and deformity, 5 points. Based on this standard, there were 24 (69 percent) good results, 8 (23 percent) fair, and 3 (9 percent) poor (Figs. 48–12 and 48–13).

Infection. There were 4 infections: 2 superficial and 2 deep. Each was associated with a partial triceps disruption. Two infections responded to débridement, reconstitution of the triceps, immobilization for 6 weeks, and prolonged antibiotic coverage. One infection eventually was revised to a hinged prosthesis, and one was converted to a fibrous arthroplasty.

Neuropathy. Ulnar paresthesias occurred in 5 patients, 1 of whom required release of the nerve at 24 hours. The others recovered rapidly without further treatment.

Loosening. Malalignment of an ulnar or humeral component required intraoperative revision in five instances. Loosening occurred in two early noncemented humeral components that required later revision to a cemented state. A lucent line on either side of the bone-cement junction of 1 mm or more was noted on follow-up radiographs around 2 ulnar, 1 humeral, and 2 radial components (Figs. 48–14 to 48–16).

Instability. There was one immediate dislocation associated with a brachial plexopathy that required 4 weeks of external fixator support. There was eventual recovery of muscle function and a good result. There were two subluxations that required manipulations and casting. One dislocated at 10 months, and a hinged prosthetic replacement was performed (Figs. 48–17 and 48–18).

The probability of revision becoming necessary with the use of the Kaplan-Meier method of estimation was 8 percent at 1 year and 28 percent at 3 years.

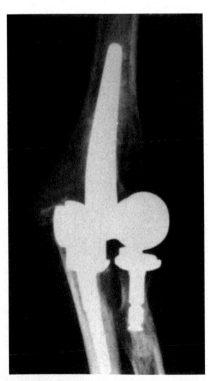

FIGURE 48–12 • A 44-year-old female with rheumatoid involvement of the left elbow 1 year after replacement demonstrated no pain and almost normal range of motion after an ERS implant. (With permission, Linscheid, Mayo Foundation.)

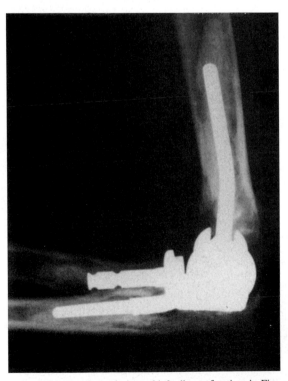

FIGURE 48–13 • Lateral view of left elbow of patient in Figure 48–12. (With permission, Linscheid, Mayo Foundation.)

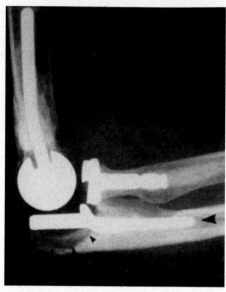

FIGURE 48–14 • One month following resurfacing replacement, the components are well aligned, but deficiency in the support of the proximal ulna is noted *(arrowheads)*.

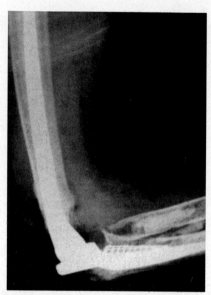

FIGURE 48–16 • Same patient as in Figures 48–14 and 48–15: The implant was converted to a semiconstrained Pritchard device at another institution. (With permission, Linscheid, Mayo Foundation.)

ALTERNATIVE PROCEDURES

Alternative procedures for rheumatoid arthritis include synovectomy, synovectomy with radial head resection, fibrous arthroplasty, and cadaveric alloplasty and have been discussed elsewhere (see Chapters 47, 49, and 65).

COMPLICATIONS—GENERAL DISCUSSION

Complications in TEAs have been higher than in other major joints (see Chapter 55).

Predisposing factors besides those inherent in total joint

arthroplasty are attributable to the idiosyncrasies of the elbow. The joint itself lies in a shallow sleeve of soft tissue that offers less protection to the joint. Dislocation or subluxation is also a consequence of the relatively flimsy capsule of the joint and the necessity of releasing the collateral ligaments during the exposure. Motion of the joint postoperatively puts these structures at risk. The shallow contours of the joint provide modest resistance to the joint reactive forces, which are competent to induce a dislocation.[12] The complicated kinematics of the joint make accurate positioning and alignment of the prosthetic com-

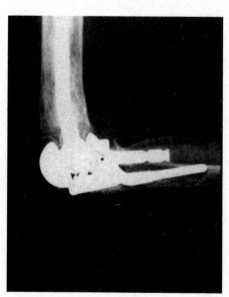

FIGURE 48–15 • Same patient as in Figure 48–14: 2 years later, the ulnar implant has become loose and rotated in the ulnar canal.

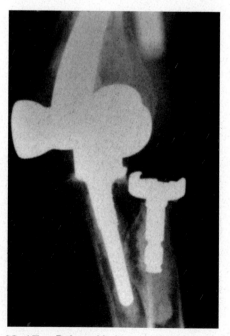

FIGURE 48–17 • Patient with rheumatoid arthritis and previous radial head resection demonstrated instability in the postoperative period while still in a cast. (With permission, Mayo Foundation.)

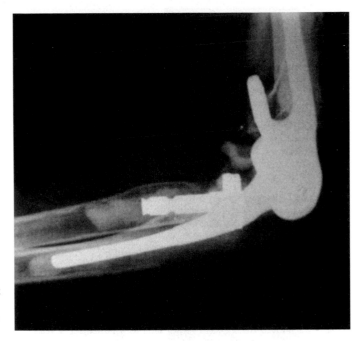

FIGURE 48–18 • The same patient as in Figure 48–17 underwent a Mayo modified Coonrad semiconstrained revision procedure. Because the radial head implant was not causing symptoms it was left in place. (With permission, Mayo Foundation.)

ponents a difficult task.[25] Preparation of the intramedullary cavities is sometimes difficult owing to small bone, residual deformity, or fragility. The openings to the medullary cavities are usually small, rendering cement injection difficult and cortex violation a constant risk.

Avoidance of complications is best achieved by careful planning and meticulous technique. Exposure and gentle retraction of the ulnar nerve will help prevent postoperative palsies. Identifying and tagging the collateral ligaments will improve the ability to restore stability during closure.[14, 45] Completion of the synovectomy aids exposure. A clear understanding of the radiographic appearance and gentle technique during a bone contouring will prevent inadvertent fractures. Examination of the position and movement of the components under the image intensifier before cementing allows identification and correction of malposition. Injection tubing with a cement gun improves cement technique. The triceps insertion should be kept moist during the procedure and repaired accurately onto the ulna if a posterior approach is used. Immobilization of the elbow for 4 weeks in slight flexion allows the triceps to heal and helps prevent late disruption with unhurried mobilization.[36]

The treatment of the more severe complications can be very challenging for both the patient and the surgeon. For this reason, the topic is discussed at length in Chapter 55.

THE FUTURE

Total elbow arthroplasty improvements will likely result from incremental improvements in design and instrumentation for the near term. At longer range, new materials, methods of fixation, and customizing features will doubtless follow the overall trends in arthroplasty.

REFERENCES

1. Barr, J. S., and Eaton, R. G.: Elbow reconstruction with a new prosthesis to replace the distal end of the humerus. J. Bone Joint Surg. 47A:1408, 1965.
2. Bayley, J. I. L.: Elbow replacement in rheumatoid arthritis. Reconstr. Surg. Traumatol. 18:70, 1981.
3. Bryan, R. S., and Morrey, B. F.: Extensive posterior exposure of the elbow: triceps sparing approach. Clin. Orthop. 166:19, 1982.
4. Brumfield, R. H., Jr., Volz, R. G., and Green, J. F.: Total elbow arthroplasty: a clinical review of 30 cases employing the Mayo and AHSC prosthesis. Clin. Orthop. 158:137, 1981.
5. Coonrad, R. W.: History of total elbow arthroplasty. In Inglis, A. E. (ed.): Symposium on Total Joint Replacement in the Upper Extremity. St. Louis, C.V. Mosby Co., 1982, p. 76.
6. Czitrom, A. A., Dobyns, J. H., and Linscheid, R. L.: Ulnar variance in carpal instability. J. Hand Surg. 12A:205, 1987.
7. Davis, R. F., Weiland, A. J., Hungerford, D. S., Moore, J. R., and Volnec-Dowling, S.: Nonconstrained total elbow arthroplasty. Clin. Orthop. 171:156, 1982.
8. Dee, R.: Total replacement arthroplasty of the elbow for rheumatoid arthritis of the elbow. J. Bone Joint Surg. 54B:88, 1972.
9. Dobyns, J. H., Bryan, R. S., Linscheid, R. L., and Peterson, L. F. A.: The special problems of total elbow arthroplasty. Geriatrics 31:57, 1976.
10. Dunn, W. A.: A distal humeral prosthesis. Clin. Orthop. 77:199, 1971.
11. Engelbrecht, E., Bucholz, H. W., Rottger, J., and Siegal, A.: Total elbow replacement with a hinge and a nonblocked system. In Joint Replacement of the Upper Limb. London, Mechanical Engineering Publications, 1978.
12. Evans, B. G., Daniels, A. U., Serbousek, J. C., and Mann, R. J.: A comparison of the mechanical designs of articulating total elbow prostheses. Clin. Materials 3:235, 1988.
13. Ewald, F. C.: Nonconstrained metal to plastic total elbow arthroplasty. In Inglis, A. E. (ed.): Symposium on Total Joint Replacement of the Upper Extremity. St. Louis, C. V. Mosby Co., 1982, p. 141.
14. Ewald, F. C., and Jacobs, M. A.: Total elbow arthroplasty. Clin. Orthop. 182:137, 1984.
15. Ewald, F. C., Scheinberg, R. D., Poss, R., Thomas, W. H., Scott, R. D., and Sledge, C. B.: Capitellocondylar total elbow arthroplasty: two to five year follow-up in rheumatoid arthritis. J. Bone Joint Surg. 63A:1259, 1980.
16. Ferlic, D. C., Clayton, M. L., and Parr, C. L.: Surgery of the elbow in rheumatoid arthritis. Proceedings of the American Academy of Orthopedic Surgeons. J. Bone Joint Surg. 58A:726, 1976.
17. Friedman, R. J., Lee, D. E., and Ewald, F. C.: Nonconstrained total elbow arthroplasty. J. Arthroplasty, 4:31, 1989.
18. Friedman, R. J., and Ewald, F. C.: Arthroplasty of the ipsilateral shoulder and elbow in patients who have rheumatoid arthritis. J. Bone Joint Surg. 69A(5):661, 1987.
19. Garret, J. C., Ewald, F. C., Thomas, W. H., and Sledge, C. B.: Loosening associated with the GSB hinge total elbow replacement in patients with rheumatoid arthritis. Clin. Orthop. 127:170, 1977.

Painful stiffness is present if elbow movement is painful and if the elbow cannot be flexed beyond 100 degrees. This invariably makes it difficult for patients to bring their hand to their face.

Painful instability occurs if despite adequate passive range of movement, the elbow cannot be actively moved while carrying any weight.

RADIOLOGIC ASSESSMENT

Patients for whom the Kudo total elbow replacement is appropriate usually lie between grades III and V of the Larsen, Dale, and Eek classification.[3] Professor Kudo has also on occasion used the implant for mutilans deformity in rheumatoid arthritis.[4] In this group of patients, bone grafting is necessary at the time of insertion of the implant.

OPERATIVE TECHNIQUE

Either the patient can be placed in the semilateral position with the arm across the chest and with the posterior aspect of the elbow facing superiorly (as is Professor Kudo's preferred operative position) or the patient can be put in the full lateral position with the upper arm horizontal and the forearm hanging vertically. This is the operative position that I personally prefer. A high tourniquet is applied and a straight midline skin incision is made centered at the tip of the olecranon.

The ulnar nerve should then be identified and protected. The exact surgical exposure that is used depends on the surgeon's preference, but the Campbell,[5] Gschwend,[6] Bryan and Morrey,[7] and Wolfe and Ranawat[8] techniques all give good exposure to the elbow joint.

The radial head should be excised, and the ulnar collateral ligament, including the tight anterior band, should be released from the humerus, enabling dislocation of the elbow joint. This gives adequate access to both the distal humerus and the proximal ulna.

The distal humerus is first prepared (Fig. 48–22), and as can be seen by the diagrams the preparation preserves bone. Following this, the proximal ulna is prepared (Fig. 48–23).

The trial humeral and ulnar components are then inserted, and a trial reduction is performed. If extension is markedly limited, some improvement can be achieved by removing the ulnar trial component and preparing the ulnar bone surface so as to allow slight distal advancement of the ulnar component.

Once a satisfactory trial reduction has been achieved, the trial components are removed. Professor Kudo has found that a press fit of the humeral component can be achieved in almost 95 percent of cases, whereas he has found it necessary to cement the ulnar component in 70 percent of cases. In my own practice, both the humeral and the ulnar components are always cemented.

The extensor mechanism is then repaired, as determined by the initial surgical approach. The wound is closed over suction drainage in order to reduce the risk of postoperative hematoma formation. A plaster slab is applied, maintaining the arm in as much extension as possible. The plaster slab is removed after 48 hours, and the patient is permitted to begin mobilization of the elbow.

RESULTS OF USING THE KUDO TOTAL ELBOW ARTHROPLASTY

The Kudo total elbow arthroplasty will give good or excellent results in up to 90 percent of patients, provided that the indications for surgery were appropriate. Pain relief is frequently significantly improved,[9] as is the patient's ability to undertake activities of daily living.

Professor Kudo has shown an average increase in flexion postoperatively of 25 degrees (average, preoperative 106 degrees to postoperative 131 degrees). No improvement in extension occurred.[9] Improvement in rotation movements has also been noted, with pronation increasing from 30 to 46 degrees while supination has increased from 40 to 61 degrees postoperatively.[9] All of the aforementioned improvements in movement that Professor Kudo has shown are statistically significant.

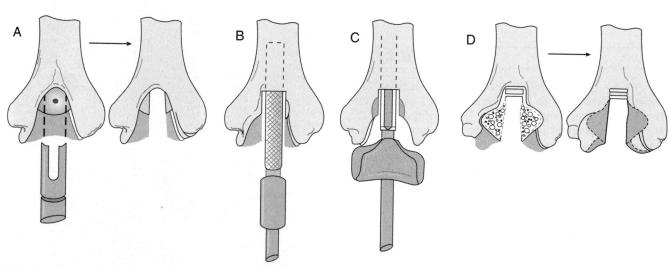

FIGURE 48–22 • Humeral preparation for insertion of the Kudo total elbow arthroplasty. Cutting the distal humerus with a double-bladed chisel (A), preparing the humeral canal (B), insertion of the trial implant (C), the extent of the humeral bone resection (D).

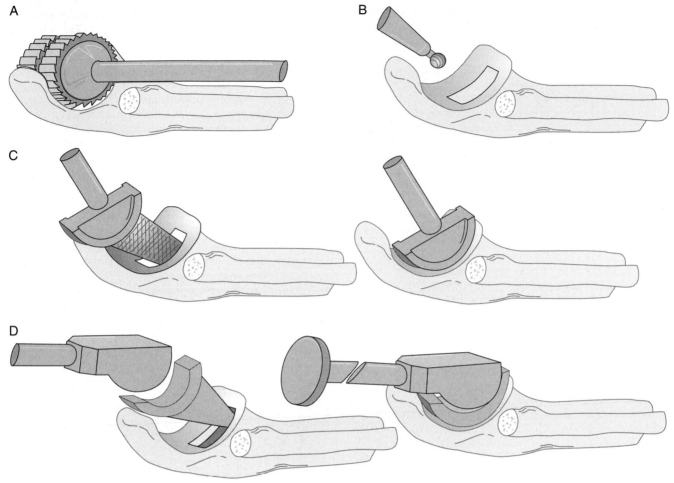

A

B

C

D

FIGURE 48-23 • Ulna preparation using the implant instruments (A), (B), and (C). Insertion of the implant (D). (With permission D. Stanley.)

COMPLICATIONS

The complication that distinguishes unlinked surface replacement implants, such as the Kudo elbow arthroplasty, from linked implants is the potential for a dislocation. In my own practice, of 86 Kudo elbow arthroplasties inserted since 1992, I have had three dislocations. The first dislocation occurred early in my clinical experience, and in hindsight it was not an appropriate joint to insert into the patient. The level of instability present preoperatively was gross. Of the other two dislocations, one required soft tissue tensioning and the other required revision, owing to a poorly positioned ulnar component.

REFERENCES

1. Kudo, H., Iwano, K., and Watanabe, S.: Total replacement of the rheumatoid elbow with a hingeless prosthesis. J. Bone Joint Surg. 62A:277, 1980.
2. Kudo, H., and Iwano, K.: Total elbow arthroplasty with a non-constrained surface replacement prosthesis in patients who have rheumatoid arthritis. J. Bone Joint Surg. 72A:355, 1990.
3. Larsen, A., Dale, K., and Eek, M.: Radiographic evaluation of rheumatoid arthritis and related conditions by standard reference films. Acta Rad. Diagn. 18:481, 1977.
4. Kudo, H., Non-constrained elbow arthroplasty for mutilans deformity in rheumatoid arthritis. J. Bone Joint Surg. 80B:234, 1998.
5. Campbell, W. C.: Incision for exposure of the elbow joint. Am. J. Surg. 15:65, 1932.
6. Gschwend, N.: Our operative approach to the elbow joint. Arch. Orthop. Trauma Surg. 98:143, 1981.
7. Bryan, R. S., and Morrey, B. F.: Extensive posterior exposure of the elbow: A triceps-sparing approach. Clin. Orthop. 166:188, 1982.
8. Wolfe, S. W., and Ranawat, C. S.: The osteo-anconeus flap. J. Bone Joint Surg. 72-A: 684, 1990.
9. Kudo, H., Iwano, K., and Nishino, J.: Cementless or hybrid total elbow arthroplasty with titanium-alloy implants: A study of interim clinical results and specific complications. J. Arthroplasty 9:269, 1994.

Souter-Strathclyde Elbow Arthroplasty

• IAN A. TRAIL and JOHN K. STANLEY

DESIGN CONSIDERATIONS

The Souter-Strathclyde arthroplasty of the elbow was initially developed in 1973, and the first prototype was inserted in 1977. The fundamental principles in the initial design were as follows: (1) an anatomic replacement should resemble the trochlea of the humerus and the trochlear notch of the ulna; (2) the articular surfaces, although not linked, are closely congruent; (3) the stability of the elbow is maintained by retention of the normal ligaments; and (4) both components are cemented and fixed into the epicondyles and epicondylar ridges, giving resistance to both flexion and extension and rotational stresses.

The humeral component is fashioned from vitallium and consists of a trochlea modeled as closely as possible on the contours and alignment of the normal anatomic trochlea. In addition, there are two side flanges for insertion into the medial and lateral epicondylar ridges and a stirrup closely molded to the contours of the medullary cavity (Fig. 48–24). There are three sizes of component available, allowing an implant to be inserted into any size distal humerus. The capitellar flange consists of a stout circular peg projecting from the middle of the lateral aspect of the metal trochlea. The aim of this is to obtain a good fit on the lateral side, although in practice it can be difficult to insert. Once inserted, the valgus-varus alignment is usually satisfactory, as a result of the fit of the component into the supracondylar ridges. However, care must be taken to align the stem in the lateral plane; as with the standard posterior approach, in difficult cases there is a tendency to tilt the tip of the implant anteriorly.

The ulnar component is fashioned from high-density polyethylene, and, again, its articular surface is modeled on the contours of the normal ulna (see Fig. 48–24). Its dorsal surface carries a dovetail keel for insertion into the excavated olecranon. This keel is continued distally into the medullary cavity of the ulna, terminating in a short 2.5-cm stem, which is set slightly obliquely in order to take account of the 5 degrees of radial deviation of the proximal ulna shaft. In view of this design feature, both right and left varieties of the component are required.

INDICATIONS

The indications for this arthroplasty are principally in patients with rheumatoid arthritis suffering with severe inflammatory arthritis of the elbow. Involvement should be such that the patients are experiencing significant pain and discomfort both at rest or with activity. Typically, the shoulder, hand, and wrist are less severely involved. There should be sufficient bone so that the components can be supported and adequate ligament integrity can be maintained. In this type of patient, age and sex do not appear to be an important contraindication, and certainly the implant has been inserted into a number of patients younger than the age of 50 years with good results. The implant is not generally recommended for post-traumatic or osteoarthritic cases.

TECHNIQUE

The operative technique involves a posterior approach through a virtually straight midline incision. A distally based triceps tongue is fashioned, the muscle then being split longitudinally and dissected out to both epicondylar ridges. It is usual at this stage to identify the ulnar nerve, although it is left in its bed in the cubital tunnel. In the author's experience, the incidence of ulnar nerve problems is greater following transposition, rather than simple decompression. The capsular incision is prolonged on the radial side to allow excision of the radial head. As a consequence of this, the posterior half of the radial collateral ligament is divided. On the ulnar side, however, great care is taken to preserve the medial collateral ligament. Once exposed, the bones of the distal humerus and proximal ulna are resected to accept the trial components. Originally, a set of hand-held guides was provided, although more recently the author has developed his own intramedullary devices, which have helped with alignment. Ultimately, the aim is to insert the largest component that the bone will accept on each side of the joint. As might be expected, the usual combination is a small humerus and a small ulna, medium humerus and/or medium ulna. However, occasionally, sizes are mixed so that a medium humerus is inserted with a small ulna. A trial reduction assesses stability. In an unlinked implant, the integrity of the collateral ligaments is crucial, and following cementation an accurate and sound repair of the collateral ligaments is essential. Fortunately, in the vast majority of patients, instability has not been a problem. Postoperative care in a routine case involves immobilization, generally about 5 days. Subsequent to this, the elbow is mobilized in a supervised manner.

Apart from instability, the complications of this arthroplasty are similar to those of other elbow implants. Initially, the skin incision was to the lateral side, resulting in considerable undermining of the soft tissue, to obtain exposure of the medial structures. With this approach, there was a small but defined incidence of skin necrosis, particularly at the tip of the flap. With the modified longitudinal approach, the incidence of skin problems in primary replacements has disappeared. As stated previously, simple decompression of the ulnar nerve has dramatically diminished the incidence of postoperative ulnar nerve problems. Returning to the subject of instability, obviously this type of unlinked replacement is unsuitable for any arthritic elbow that is grossly unstable. In this scenario, a linked implant is the only option. Similarly, if it is found during

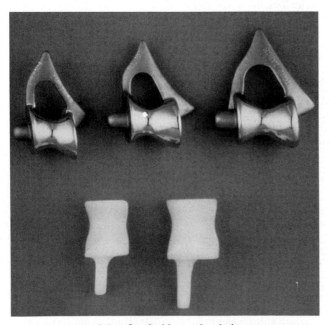

FIGURE 48–24 • Standard humeral and ulnar components.

surgery that the elbow is unstable despite satisfactory soft tissue repair, conversion to a linked implant would seem sensible. Finally, as with all implants, there is a small but defined risk of infection or fracture.

RESULTS

In 1989, the effectiveness of this implant was published by Souter, based on his personal experience with 250 cases. He reported pain relief in 92 percent and an improvement in flexion from 127 to 135 degrees, with similar improvements in pronation and supination. Unfortunately, there was often little gain in extension. He noted ulnar neuritis in 15 percent, infection in 2 percent, instability in 3.5 percent, and finally radiologic evidence of loosening in 11 to 12 percent. Pöll and Rozing[5] reported the results of 33 patients following a mean of 4 years. Five (15 percent) were revised, three for dislocation, one for loosening, and one for infection. The mean arc of flexion was 31 to 138 degrees. A similar experience was reported by Chiu and co-workers.[4] Of 20 replacements followed a mean of 43 months, only one had instability and one required revision. The complication rate was 45 percent, and the loss of extension averaged 7 degrees but the flexion arc increased a mean of 14 degrees.

At Wrightington, this implant has been used for 15 years. The long-term results of 186 procedures in patients with

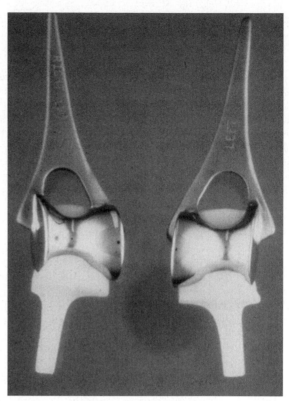

FIGURE 48–26 • Long-stemmed humeral component.

rheumatoid arthritis have been analyzed. This has revealed a long-term survivorship at 12 years of 87 percent if revision is taken as the end point. If asymptomatic yet complete radiologic loosening is added, the figure drops to 80 percent. The causes of failure include infection and instability, but aseptic loosening of the humeral component is the main cause of failure, accounting for 75 percent of all revisions. Also of interest was the fact that the direction of loosening was identical to that described for other elbow devices. The proximal tip of the implant tilted anteriorly abutting, and on occasion perforating, the anterior humeral cortex (Fig. 48–25). Indeed, a gradual increase in this tilt, as seen on the lateral radiograph, is a good indicator of loosening. The exact reasons for this are unclear.

FAILURE ANALYSIS

In an attempt to identify any preoperative, perioperative, and subsequent factors that may lead to loosening, a thorough clinical and radiologic assessment of the 23 revisions undertaken at our institution over the last 10 years has been performed and compared with the unrevised group as a control. The revised group of patients were often not highly dependent and did not have severe generalized rheumatoid involvement, but had disease principally in the elbow. Also a number of this group had had extensive surgery of their lower limbs, necessitating a period on crutches, which placed increased stress on the joint. Finally, it was also noted that in the patients who had undergone revision, the range of motion, particularly extension, was less than that in the normal group. The exact reason for this remains unclear. We hypothesized that in the elbow in

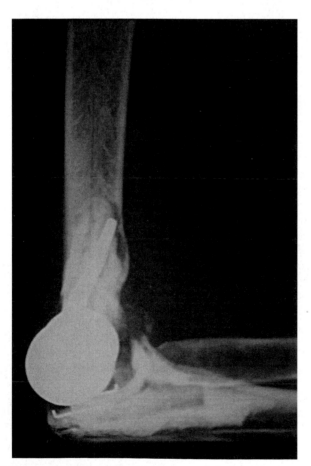

FIGURE 48–25 • Aseptic loosening around the humeral component.

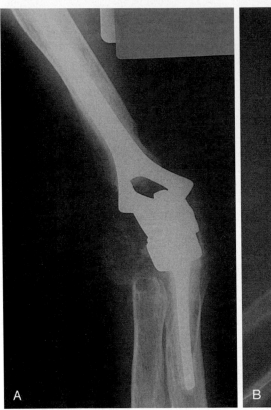
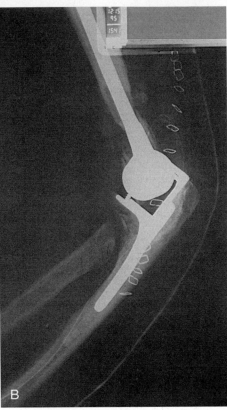

FIGURE 48–27 • Revision components.

extension and with an extension contracture of, for example, 50 or 60 degrees, much of the load is transmitted through the implant itself.

Of the perioperative factors, any fracture had an extremely detrimental effect on long-term survival. Otherwise, at least radiologically, the alignment of the humerus or ulna, or indeed the quality of cement mantle, did not appear to have a significant effect.

Having identified the mode of failure in certain cases approximately 4 years ago, the authors changed the humeral component used from a standard 3.5-cm short stem to the longer 7.5-cm stem (Fig. 48–26). The latter was initially designed for revision or difficult cases; however, in the authors' view the shape of this implant undoubtedly makes it easier to insert and align. It is also our view that the longer stem will improve stability in the anteroposterior plane, thus counteracting the flexion-extension forces. In the initial phase, the results with this longer stemmed humeral component appear better than those with the shorter stemmed one. It should be noted, however, that the implant remains unlinked. Furthermore, a set of intramedullary alignment jigs were introduced with second-generation cementation techniques, specifically the use of bone plugs and cement guns.

REVISION

The range of standard Souter-Strathclyde implants has now been supplemented by additional devices (Fig. 48–27).

Effectively, all these have longer stems. In addition, in the case of the humeral component, a number are augmented to replace bone loss. Further, apart from increased length, there are facilities for metal backing to the ulnar component, triceps ligament reattachment and, finally, "snap-fit," that allow the implant to be linked when there are concerns about stability. At this time, the authors have some experience with the use of these implants. Undoubtedly, revision surgery is complex, and at times arduous. However, the results can often be quite gratifying in that patients regain a painless, stable elbow, with a functional range of motion. The long-term survivorship of these implants is unknown, although at this time the number of further revisions is extremely low.

REFERENCES

1. Souter, W. A.: Surgery for rheumatoid arthritis: Upper limb surgery of the elbow. Curr. Orthopaed. 3:9, 1989.
2. Trail, I. A., Nuttall, D., and Stanley, J. K.: Survivorship and radiographic analysis of the standard Souter-Strathclyde total elbow arthroplasty. J. Bone Joint Surg. 81B:80, 1999.
3. Dent, C. M., Hoy, G., and Stanley, J. K.: Revision of failed total elbow arthroplasty. J. Bone Joint Surg. 5:691, 1995.
4. Chiu, K. Y., Luk, K. D. K., and Pan, W. K.: Souter-Strathclyde elbow replacement for severe rheumatoid arthritis. J. Orthop. Rheum. 9:194, 1996.
5. Pöll, R. G., and Rozing, P. M.: Use of the Souter-Strathclyde total elbow prosthesis in patients who have rheumatoid arthritis. J. Bone Joint Surg. 73A:1227, 1991.

• CHAPTER 49 •

Semiconstrained Elbow Replacement Arthroplasty: Rationale and Surgical Technique

• BERNARD F. MORREY

As noted in Chapter 48 and as described in Chapters 50 through 54, the results of total elbow arthroplasty are improving with increased basic knowledge of elbow mechanics,[20] better designs, and greater surgical experience.[18] The general principles of the surgical technique and improved designs[2, 6, 11, 17, 20] and a detailed description of my specific method of inserting the Coonrad-Morrey implant are presented. The results of semiconstrained joint replacement arthroplasty emphasize the Mayo Clinic experience with the modified Coonrad device.

RATIONALE

The selection and the rationale for elbow replacement are described in Chapter 47 and the rationale and the results of the use of resurfacing implants in Chapter 48. Our rationale for continuing to use a semiconstrained implant is simple: the current design works and can address a broad spectrum of lesions. The Coonrad-Morrey device and similar implants are distinctly different, both conceptually and clinically, from the original, fully constrained articulated implants. The one feature in common is that the ulnar and humeral components are coupled but have out-of-plane angular laxity of 5 to 10 degrees (Fig. 49–1). The theoretical advantage has been confirmed by O'Driscoll and colleagues, who showed that the articulation tracks within the limits of its tolerance (Fig. 49–2). This decreases stresses on the bone-cement interface.[20] Markedly improved clinical results attest to the effectiveness of semiconstrained implants.[3, 10, 11, 13, 17, 19] Of equal significance in my practice is the fact that the articulated implant dramatically broadens the indications for reconstructive surgery of the elbow. Whereas resurfacing devices may be very effective for rheumatoid arthritis, it is well known that this approach is limited by the amount of bone and the integrity of soft tissue constraints. The semiconstrained implant, on the other hand, may be used with equal effectiveness in patients with rheumatoid arthritis or[19] post-traumatic arthrosis,[18] and for revision surgery.[17] The enhanced stability supplied by this and similar designs is provided without transmission of stress to the bone-cement interface.[20]

PRINCIPLES OF SURGICAL TECHNIQUE

In my opinion, one of the most important factors in the improved results with all elbow joint replacements, but particularly with those of semiconstrained implants, is the improved surgical technique.

Positioning

The patient is placed in the position of the surgeon's preference. I place the patient supine with sandbags under the hip and the scapula. The arm is draped free, a nonsterile tourniquet is used, and the extremity is brought across the chest.

Surgical Exposure

A straight posterior skin incision is preferred. If a previous incision is present it is employed when possible. If more than 4 or 5 years old, it may be repaired if it cannot be incorporated. The incision need not and should not be curved.

The Ulnar Nerve

We always elevate a medial flap and first address the ulnar nerve. Opinions are divided with respect to the management of the ulnar nerve. Some surgeons believe that it should not be exposed,[5, 9, 13, 22] whereas others feel that the ulnar nerve should be directly visualized and moved as an

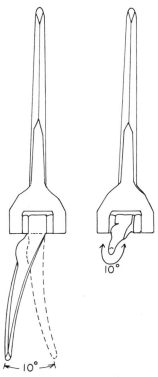

FIGURE 49–1 • A semiconstrained implant, whether it be of an axle or a snap-fit design, is characterized by varus-valgus and axial rotation tolerances of several degrees at the articulation.

617

NORMAL KINEMATICS

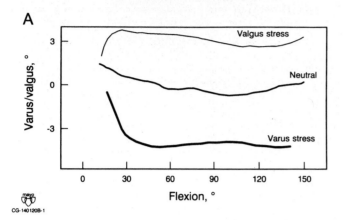

CG-140120B-1

TEA KINEMATICS

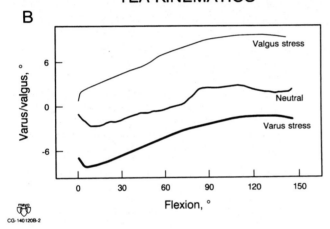

CG-140120B-2

FIGURE 49–2 • The semiconstrained articulation provides flexion motion that replicates normal kinematics *(A)* and constraints of the design and thus reduces stress at the bone-cement interface *(B)*. TEA, total elbow arthroplasty.

integral part of the surgical approach and procedure.[3, 7, 12, 14] We favor the latter approach.

The Triceps

The fascial tongue exposure of Campbell (Van Gorder) causes a good deal of soft tissue dissection, with a significant amount of dead tissue that provides an environment favorable to infection, which may result in weakness.[4, 16] Splitting the triceps in the midline, in our experience, tends to cause detachment of the medial insertion. Therefore, I prefer the Mayo technique of reflecting the triceps in continuity with the ulnar periosteum and forearm fascia described by Bryan and Morrey.[4]

Exposure

Regardless of the means of exposure, adequate visualization of the joint and of the proximal ulnar and distal humeral shafts should be obtained. This should prevent

supracondylar column fracture or cortical perforation for routine—and especially for revision—operations when cement must be removed. Reliable orientation of the stemmed implant requires an intramedullary alignment system.

Trial Reduction

Trial reduction is an essential step for a reliable elbow joint replacement of any design. This is particularly important for semiconstrained devices in persons who have a moderate or severe flexion contracture. It is the only way to determine if the implant has been adequately seated and to assess whether sufficient soft tissue has been released.

Cementing Technique

The cement should be introduced down the medullary canal for stemmed implants with an injection system. Generally speaking, the injector systems have dramatically improved the radiographic appearance of the bone-cement interface. It was shown in our early experience that the quality of the cementing technique is inversely related to the presence of lucent lines, and, ultimately, to implant loosening (Fig. 49–3).[14, 19]

Triceps Reattachment

Whenever the triceps is reflected from its attachment, it must be reattached to the olecranon by nonabsorbable sutures placed through bone. The sutures should be tied with the elbow in 90 degrees of flexion but knots are avoided over the subcutaneous border of the ulna. It is not acceptable simply to allow the triceps to resume its position over the tip of the olecranon, because this communicates with the joint and motion will allow the synovial fluid to become interposed between the triceps and the olecranon, which prevents healing. To enhance strength and ensure continuity, we also tend to displace the mechanism slightly medially if possible, bringing the anconeus over the proximal ulna.

Postoperative Dressing

We have had virtually no incision problems because we have been routinely placing the elbow in full extension

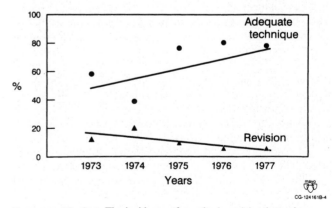

CG-124161B-4

FIGURE 49–3 • The incidence of prosthesis revision loosening shows an inverse relationship to the technical quality of the cementing.

with an anterior splint and elevating the arm for approximately 24 hours. We see no advantage to allowing the elbow to assume 90 degrees of flexion immediately after surgery. Because of continued concern for the variable swelling and occasional blistering that may occur after surgery, I no longer use the Steri-Drape on most patients, and I avoid Betadine solution if the barrier drape is used. A prospective, randomized study recently revealed statistically measurable decreases in swelling after surgery with the use of a compression Cryocuff (Aircast Co.).[1]

The Semiconstrained Implant

Today, in the United States, several semiconstrained elbow replacements are commercially available, including the Pritchard III, Triaxial, and Coonrad-Morrey. The GSB III has evolved through the years and is frequently used in Europe (Fig. 49–4). Limited long-term data are available on the Pritchard device. Experience with the Triaxial and the GSB III devices is discussed under the appropriate indications in subsequent chapters. Risung[21] has also reported quite favorable outcomes with a rather novel implant designed termed the *Norway elbow*.

THE COONRAD-MORREY DEVICE

The Mayo modified Coonrad total elbow prosthesis (Coonrad-Morrey) is a semiconstrained device manufactured from Tivanium Ti-6Al-4V alloy. The current prosthesis was manufactured and released on a restricted prescription basis in 1981 by Zimmer Company (Warsaw, Ind.). It currently has a basic hinge articulation with a hollow cobalt chrome pin that passes through the ultra-high–molecular weight polyethylene bushings to capture the ulnar component. A second pin is inserted from the opposite side to secure the articulation (Fig. 49–5). The prosthesis is easily disassembled if desired.

Right and left specificity is attained from the contoured quadrangular ulnar stem. The triangular humeral stem is interchangeable right or left. In 1978, the initial design (Coonrad I) was modified by the Mayo Clinic to permit 7 to 10 degrees of hinge laxity, or toggle (Coonrad II), which is consistent with the average laxity of the normal elbow joint. This change accounts for the semiconstrained designation applied to the device. The effect of this design concept is discussed above (see Figs. 49–1 and 49–2). The implant was designed for use with methylmethacrylate and is manufactured in two sizes: a regular and a small size (15 percent reduction).

The prosthesis was further modified in 1981 by adding a band of porous coating of the distal humeral and proximal ulnar stems to permit better fixation (Table 49–1). An anterior flange was also added to the lower humeral stem, to permit the insertion of a bone graft anteriorly to enhance fixation at the point maximum stress. This implant is intended to be used with bone cement for both immediate and long-term fixation. The humeral stem comes in 10-, 15-, and 20-cm stem lengths (Fig. 49–6). The 15-cm stem is most often used in nonrheumatoid patients to ensure adequate mechanical resistance to rotation in the humerus. The 4-inch stem is used when a shoulder involved by

• TABLE 49–1 • Coonrad-Morrey Implant Modifications 1981–1998		
Device	Year	Feature/Modification
Coonrad	1971	Rigid hinge
Coonrad II	1978	Semiconstrained loose hinge
Coonrad-Morrey	1981	Flange, surface treatment
	1984	Plasma spray replaced with beads
	1991	Beads on ulna replaced with polymethyl methacrylate precoat
	1993	Titanium articular pin replaced by cobalt-chromium pin
	1998	C ring replaced by pin within a pin

rheumatoid arthritis has been or may be replaced with a humeral prosthesis.[8, 10] The 8-inch stem is used for revision procedures requiring the device to bypass the prior stem tip (see Chapter 57). The ulna implant is made in standard and small dimensions. The small dimension also comes in an extra long size. Finally, for the patient with juvenile rheumatoid arthritis or a very small canal, a special extra-small implant is available (Fig. 49–7).

Surgical Technique for Coonrad-Morrey Total Elbow Arthroplasty

EXPOSURE

The patient is positioned supine with a sandbag under the scapula, and the arm is draped free with a nonsterile tourniquet and brought across the chest (Fig. 49–8). The Mayo (Bryan-Morrey) approach is used exclusively for this procedure.[4] A straight 15-cm incision is centered just lateral to the medial epicondyle and just medial to the tip of the olecranon. The medial aspect of the triceps is identified, and the ulnar nerve is carefully isolated and translocated using ocular magnification and a bipolar cautery. It is gently protected throughout the remainder of the procedure.

An incision is made over the medial aspect of the proximal ulna, and the ulnar periosteum is elevated along with the forearm fascia (Fig. 49–9). The medial aspect of the triceps is then elevated along with the posterior capsule. The triceps is elevated from the proximal ulna by transecting Sharpey's fibers at the site of insertion. The extensor mechanism, including the anconeus, is reflected laterally, allowing complete exposure of the distal humerus, the proximal ulna, and the radial head. The radial and ulnar collateral ligament complexes are released from the anconeus in persons with rheumatoid arthritis (Fig. 49–10). Failure to do this may allow the ligament to fracture the medial column as the forearm is manipulated.

The tip of the olecranon is removed. The humerus is externally rotated, and the forearm is brought lateral to the humeral shaft.

HUMERAL PREPARATION

After the ulna and the radius have been rotated out of the way, the midportion of the trochlea is removed with a rongeur or a saw, depending on the softness of the bone. The medullary canal of the humerus is identified by entering it with a rongeur or a burr at the roof of the olecranon

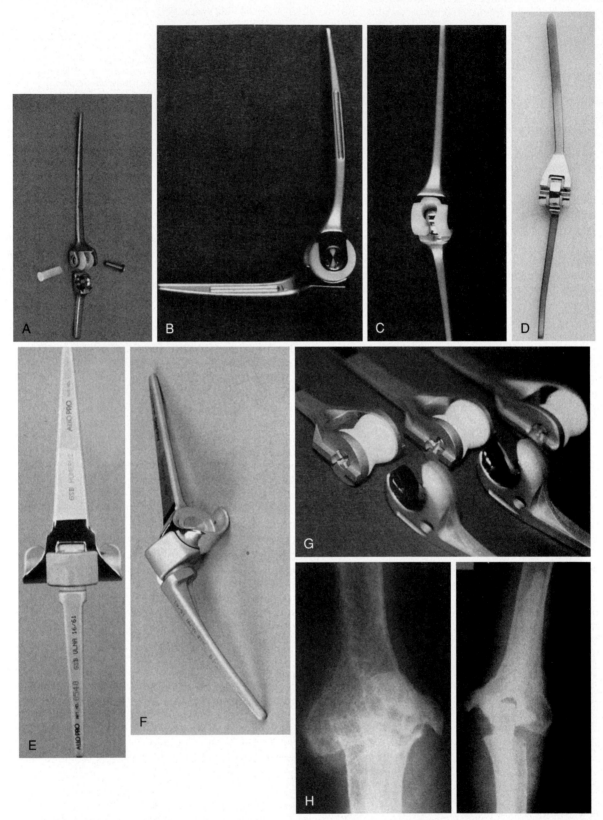

FIGURE 49–4 • *(A)* The Pritchard II was an early and widely used semiconstrained elbow replacement. *B* and *C,* The coupling mechanism of the triaxial device *(B* and *C)* has been modified several times. The triaxial began as a snap-fit design to provide joint stability, as does the English Stanmore prosthesis *(D).* *E* and *F,* The GSB III is a popular semiconstrained device used in Europe. *G,* The Norway elbow designed by Risung is a type of snap-fit design, but with a spool-type snap-fit trochlear design. *H,* Clinical results have been excellent.

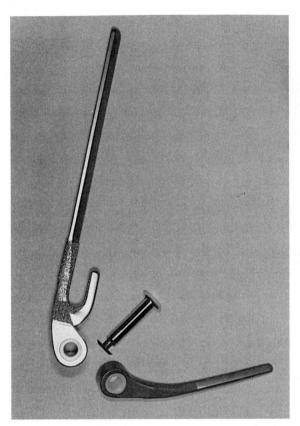

FIGURE 49–5 • The current Coonrad-Morrey semiconstrained implant. Note redesigned articulation locking pin.

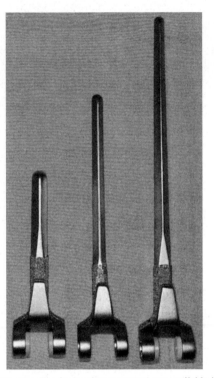

FIGURE 49–6 • The humeral components are available in 10-, 15-, and 20-cm lengths and in small and standard sizes.

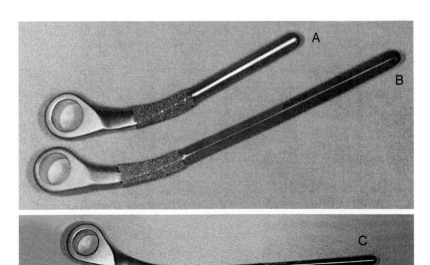

FIGURE 49–7 • The ulnar component is available in small (A) and standard sizes. A longer small implant, also available, is commonly used for revision (B). An extra-small, long device is available and can be shortened for very small canals, as in patients with juvenile rheumatoid arthritis (C).

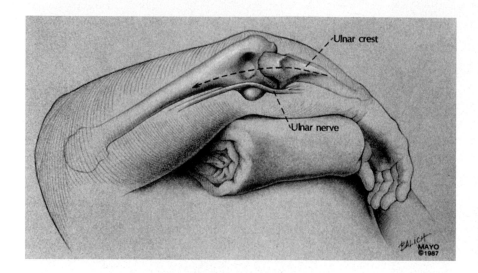

FIGURE 49–8 • The preferred supine position with a sandbag under the patient's shoulder and the arm lying across the chest. (With permission from the Mayo Foundation.)

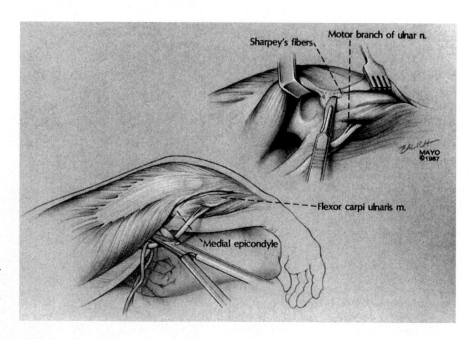

FIGURE 49–9 • In the Mayo approach used for the semiconstrained implant, the ulnar nerve is identified and the triceps is released from the tip of the olecranon in continuity with the forearm fascia and periosteum. (With permission from the Mayo Foundation.)

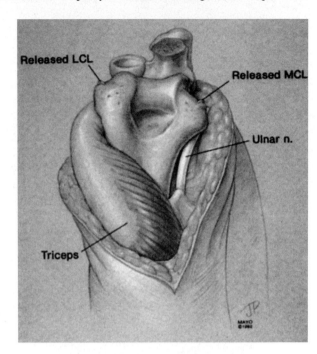

FIGURE 49–10 • The tip of the olecranon is removed along with the medial collateral ligament (MCL) and the lateral collateral ligament (LCL). The ulna is flexed and rotated to expose the humerus. The radial head is resected or débrided, depending on the extent of disease. (With permission from the Mayo Foundation.)

fossa (Fig. 49–11). The medullary canal of the humerus is entered with a twist reamer. The medial and lateral aspects of the supracondylar columns should be identified and visualized throughout the preparation of the distal humerus to ensure proper alignment and orientation.

The alignment stem is placed down the canal (Fig. 49–12). The handle is removed, and a cutting block is attached, which allows accurate removal of the appropriate amount of the articular surface of the distal humerus.

The interchangeable side arm of the cutting block is attached laterally to rest on the capitellum and to provide the appropriate depth of cut (Fig. 49–13). The flat of the template rests on the posterior columns to ensure accurate rotatory alignment. With an oscillating saw, the trochlea is removed according to the dimensions of the appropriate cutting block that corresponds to the sizes of the humeral component. Care should be taken to avoid violating either supracondylar bony column because such disruption may cause a stress riser, leading to a fracture.

The humerus involved by rheumatoid arthritis is easily prepared with a rasp in such a way as to receive the appropriately sized humeral component. In younger pa-

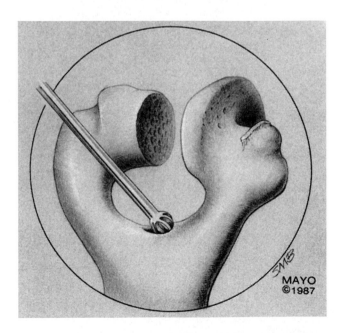

FIGURE 49–11 • The medullary canal is identified by perforating the roof of the olecranon fossa with a burr or a rongeur. (With permission from the Mayo Foundation.)

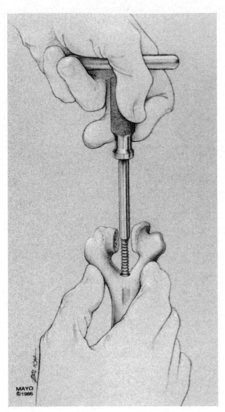

FIGURE 49–12 • Sufficient exposure is required to identify the medial and lateral columns. An alignment stem is placed down the canal. (With permission from the Mayo Foundation.)

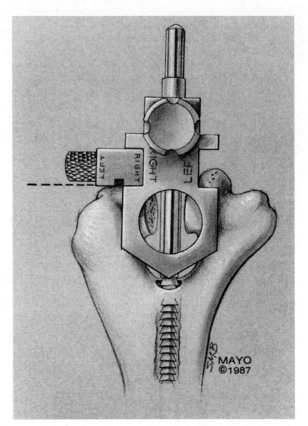

FIGURE 49–13 • The appropriate cutting block depth is adjusted by the outrigger, which rests over the capitellum and allows accurate removal of bone to receive an implant of a given size. (With permission from the Mayo Foundation.)

tients and those with post-traumatic conditions, the canal may be tight, or the anterior humeral bow may make preparation more difficult.

ULNAR PREPARATION

The medullary canal of the ulna is identified by using a high-speed burr at about a 45-degree angle to the base of the coronoid (Fig. 49–14). The tip of the olecranon is removed, notched, or both, to allow identification of the canal by a small reamer. An appropriately sized rasp is then used, and a mallet is generally required to remove the subchondral bone around the coronoid (Fig. 49–15).

TRIAL REDUCTION

A trial reduction allows assessment of depth of insertion and soft tissue restriction to extension.

IMPLANT INSERTION

The medullary cavities of both bones are cleansed with a pulsating lavage irrigation system and dried. Medullary plugs are not routinely utilized but are useful for restricting cement flow to the proximal humerus in patients with rheumatoid arthritis. We occasionally use a medullary plug of bone graft fragments to avoid excess cement when a shoulder replacement is performed or is being contemplated. The orifice of the humeral opening is smaller than the medullary canal, making insertion of an intramedullary

plug difficult. Insertion of the device may be accomplished by cementing the components individually or coupled. In the first instance, cement is injected down the medullary canal of the ulna first with an intramedullary injection system designed to fit even the small canal. The component is inserted distally so that the center of the ulnar component

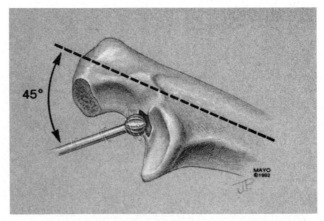

FIGURE 49–14 • The subcutaneous border of the proximal ulna is visualized and palpated so that the medullary canal may be safely entered with a burr oriented at about a 45-degree angle at the base of the coronoid. The olecranon is notched to allow direct entry down the canal. (With permission from the Mayo Foundation.)

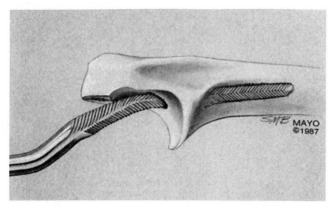

FIGURE 49–15 • The proximal canal is prepared with an appropriately sized ulnar rasp. (With permission from the Mayo Foundation.)

aligns with the projected center of the greater sigmoid fossa (Fig. 49–16).

The cement is now injected down the humeral medullary canal to a depth determined by the length of the humeral stem (Fig. 49–17). A bone graft is prepared from the excised trochlea or from the bone bank for revision surgery. The graft should measure about 3 to 4 mm in thickness and should be about 2 cm long and 1.5 cm wide. The bone graft is placed anterior to the anterior cortex of the distal humerus, and the humeral component is inserted down the canal to a point that allows articulation of the device at a level where the bone graft is partially covered by the flange as well (Fig. 49–18). If the canal is tight, the anterior bow of the humerus is accommodated by making a slight bow in the humeral stem with the plate bender (Fig. 49–19).

The ulnar component is articulated with the humeral device by placing the hollow axis through the humerus and ulna and securing it with the solid pin inserted from the opposite direction (Fig. 49–20). After the prosthesis has been coupled, the ulna is placed at a 90-degree angle, and the humeral component is impacted down the medullary canal (Fig. 49–21). In general, the device is inserted to a point at which the axis of rotation of the prosthesis is at the level of the normal anatomic axis of rotation. This is approximated when the base of the flange is flush to the anterior bone of the olecranon fossa and the distal aspect

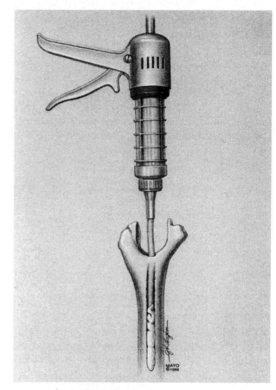

FIGURE 49–17 • The humeral canal is filled with the intramedullary cement injector system to accommodate a 4-, 6-, or 8-inch humeral component.

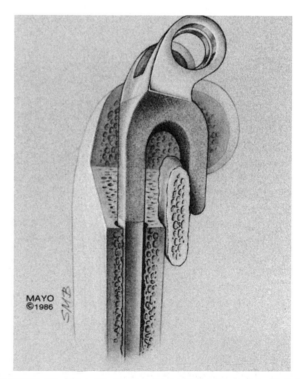

FIGURE 49–18 • The bone graft placed simultaneously behind the distal humerus engages the flange before the joint is articulated. This ensures that the bone graft will be positioned accurately when the humeral component is finally seated. (With permission from the Mayo Foundation.)

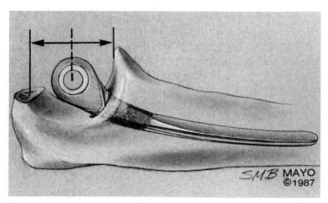

FIGURE 49–16 • The ulna is inserted until the center of the ulnar component coincides with the center of the greater sigmoid fossa. (With permission from the Mayo Foundation.)

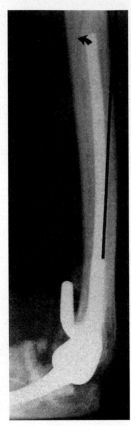

FIGURE 49–19 • When the canal is small, the normal slight anterior bow may require that the 15- or 20-cm implant be bent slightly anteriorly with a plate bender.

of the humeral component is flush or slightly proximal to the distal aspect of the capitellum.

ALTERNATIVE INSERTION TECHNIQUE

Coonrad prefers to insert the implant with the components articulated. In this case, the elbow must be acutely flexed. The cementing technique is similar to that described earlier. I have no experience with this technique, but when it is used, it is essential that a reduction be performed with the trial implants before injecting methacrylate. This ensures adequate exposure for insertion.

The cement is permitted to harden with the elbow in full extension. The range of motion is evaluated again, and excess bone and cement are removed as needed, ensuring that none is left anteriorly that might limit flexion.

THE TRICEPS

If the triceps has been reflected, it is secured to the ulna with a heavy (No. 5) nonabsorbable suture. The stitch is criss-crossed through the tendon and the olecranon. An additional transverse suture holds the tendon in place (Fig. 49–22). Sutures are tied beneath the tendon because were they subcutaneous, they might irritate or cause stitch abscess.

CLOSURE

The arm is elevated and compressed for 4 to 5 minutes. The tourniquet is deflated, and hemostasis is obtained.

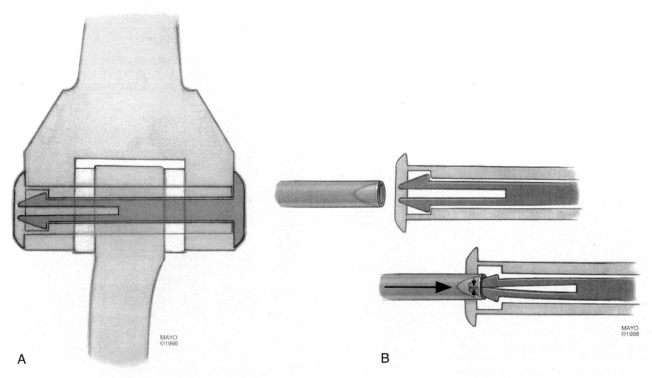

A   B

FIGURE 49–20 • The articulation is coupled by a pin-within-a-pin mechanism (A) that is very easy to apply. Removal is equally easily done with a special device (B).

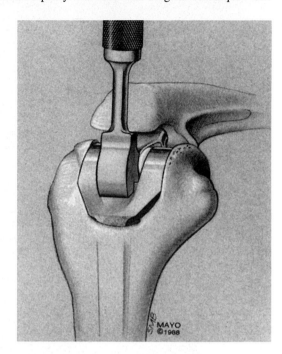

FIGURE 49–21 • A specially designed instrument allows impaction of the humeral implant down the canal. (With permission from the Mayo Foundation.)

Drains are optional and the wound is closed in layers. A suture closes the subcutaneous tissue over the translocated ulnar nerve at the medial epicondyle. The rest of the closure is routine.

A compressive dressing is applied with the elbow in full extension. The plaster splint is no longer used.

Postoperative Management

The arm is elevated postoperatively for 24 hours with the elbow above shoulder level. If drains are used, they are removed after approximately 24 hours, and the compressive dressing is removed 24 hours later. A light dressing is

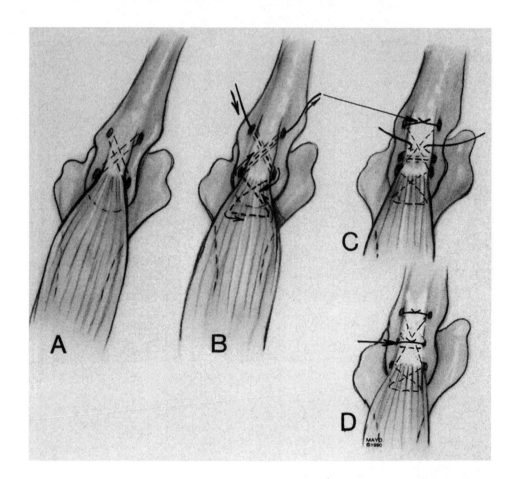

FIGURE 49–22 • A, The triceps is reattached with a suture that goes through the forearm and the periosteal sleeve and then through one of the diagonal holes placed in the proximal ulna. A criss-cross suture is placed on the triceps. B, The suture is then brought through a second diagonal hole in the forearm and the ulnar periosteum and is tied. A second suture is placed through the tip of the olecranon and through the triceps (C) to ensure firm apposition of the triceps at the site of its previous insertion (D). (With permission from the Mayo Foundation.)

applied, and elbow flexion and extension are allowed, as tolerated. A collar and cuff are used, and the patient is allowed to begin activities of daily living. No formal physical therapy is required or indicated. Strength exercises are avoided. Currently, the patient leaves the hospital on the third or fourth day and is advised not to lift more than 1 pound over the next 3 months. We typically recommend that the patient not lift more than 10 pounds with the operated arm as a single event, or more than 2 pounds

repeatedly. If a flexion contracture greater than 45 degrees existed before surgery, an extension turnbuckle splint is regularly used at night for 4 to 12 weeks.

RESULTS

Experience with this device for several conditions is discussed in subsequent chapters. Long-term experience, how-

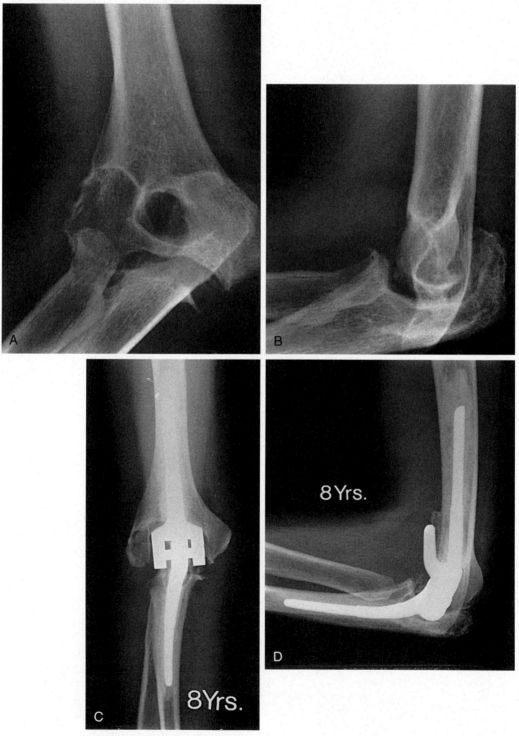

FIGURE 49-23 • A and B, Patient with severe grade III rheumatoid arthritis. C and D, Excellent result after replacement.

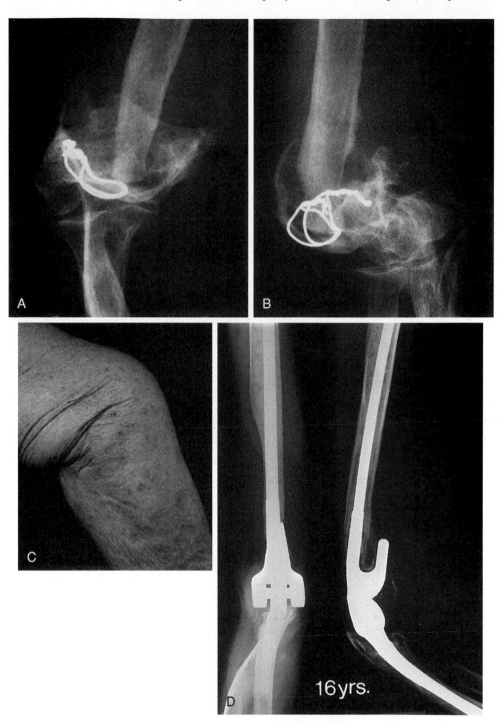

FIGURE 49–24 • Two years after sustaining a supracondylar fracture, the patient had painful nonunion and tapering of the distal humeral shaft, as shown on the anteroposterior *(A)* and lateral *(B)* radiographs. *C,* Gross instability is evidenced by 45 degrees of varus angulation against gravity. The patient was treated with the newer design of elbow arthroplasty that incorporates an anterior flange to control the rotational and posterior displacement stresses. *D,* Anteroposterior and lateral views 16 years after replacement.

ever, is emerging for those with rheumatoid arthritis (Fig. 49–23) and for post-traumatic conditions (Fig. 49–24). The results have been gratifying.

REFERENCES

1. Adams, R.A., and Morrey, B.F.: The effectiveness of a compressive Cryocuff after elbow surgery. A prospective randomized study. Presented at the annual meeting of the AAOS, Anaheim, CA, Feb. 1999.
2. Bell, S., Gschwend, N., and Steiger, U.: Arthroplasty of the elbow. Experience with the Mark III GSB prosthesis. Aust. N.Z. J. Surg. **56:**823, 1986.
3. Brumfield, R.H., Kuschner, S.H., Gellman, H., Redix, L., and Stevenson, D.V.: Total elbow arthroplasty. J. Arthr. **5:**359, 1990.
4. Bryan, R.S., and Morrey, B.F.: Extensive posterior exposure of the elbow. A triceps-sparing approach. Clin. Orthop. **166:**188, 1982.
5. Ewald, F.C., Scheinberg, R.D., Poss, R., Thomas, W.H., Scott, R.D., and Sledge, C.B.: Capitellocondylar total elbow arthroplasty: 2- to 5-year follow-up in rheumatoid arthritis. J. Bone Joint Surg. **62A:**125, 1980.
6. Figgie, M.P., Inglis, A.E., Mow, C.S., and Figgie, H.E., III: Salvage of nonunion of supracondylar fracture of the humerus by total elbow arthroplasty. J. Bone Joint Surg. **3:**235, 1988.
7. Figgie, H.E., III, Inglis, A.E., Ranawat, C.S., and Rosenberg, G.M.: Results of total elbow arthroplasty as a salvage procedure for failed elbow reconstructive operations. Clin. Orthop. **219:**185, 1987.
8. Friedman, R.J., and Ewald, F.C.: Arthroplasty of the ipsilateral shoulder and elbow in patients who have rheumatoid arthritis. J. Bone Joint Surg. **69A:**661, 1987.

9. Friedman, R.J., Lee, D.E., and Ewald, F.C.: Nonconstrained total elbow arthroplasty: development and results in patients with functional class IV rheumatoid arthritis. J. Arthr. **4**:31, 1989.
10. Gill, D., and Morrey, B.F.: The Coonrad-Morrey total elbow arthroplasty in patients with rheumatoid arthritis: a 10–15 year follow-up study. J. Bone Joint Surg. **80A**:1327–1335, 1998.
11. Gschwend, N., Loehr, J., Ivosevic-Radovanovic, D., Scheier, H., and Munzinger, U.: Semiconstrained elbow prostheses with special reference to the GSB III prosthesis. Clin. Orthop. **232**:104, 1988.
12. Johnson, J.R., Getty, C.J.M., and Lettin, A.W.F.: The Stanmore total elbow replacement for rheumatoid arthritis. J. Bone Joint Surg. **66B**:732, 1984.
13. Madsen, F., Gudmundson, G.H., Søjbjerg, J.O., and Sneppen, O.: The Pritchard-Mark II elbow prosthesis in rheumatoid arthritis. Acta Orthop. Scand. **60**:249, 1989.
14. Morrey, B.F., Bryan, R.S., Dobyns, J.H., and Linscheid, R.L.: Total elbow arthroplasty: a five-year experience at the Mayo Clinic. J. Bone Joint Surg. **63A**:1050, 1981.
15. Morrey, B.F.: The Elbow and Its Disorders. Philadelphia, W. B. Saunders Co., 1985.
16. Morrey, B.F., Askew, L.J., and An, K.N.: Strength function after elbow arthroplasty. Clin. Orthop. **234**:43, 1988.
17. Morrey, B. F.: Semi-constrained total elbow arthroplasty. In Morrey, B.F. (ed.): Joint Replacement Arthroplasty. New York, Churchill Livingstone, 1991.
18. Morrey, B.F., Adams, R.A., and Bryan, R.S.: Total replacement for posttraumatic arthritis of the elbow. J. Bone Joint Surg. **73B**:607, 1991.
19. Morrey, B.F., and Adams, R.A.: Semiconstrained elbow replacement for rheumatoid arthritis. J. Bone Joint Surg. **74A**:479, 1992.
20. O'Driscoll, S., An, K., and Morrey, B.F.: The kinematics of elbow semiconstrained joint replacement. J. Bone Joint Surg. **74B**:297, 1992.
21. Risung, F.: Characteristics, design and preliminary results of the Norway Elbow System. In Hämäläinen, M., and Hagena, F.-W. (eds.): Rheumatoid Arthritis Surgery of the Elbow. Rheumatology. Vol 15. Basel, Karger, 1991, p. 68.
22. Wolfe, S.W., and Ranawat, C.S.: The osteo-anconeus flap. J. Bone Joint Surg. **72A**:684, 1990.

CHAPTER 50

Total Elbow Arthroplasty in Patients with Rheumatoid Arthritis

• DAVID R. J. GILL, BERNARD F. MORREY, and ROBERT A. ADAMS

PRESENTATION: INDICATIONS AND SURGICAL CONSIDERATIONS

The coupled (semiconstrained) and the uncoupled (unconstrained) elbow replacement prostheses are the predominant configurations for total elbow arthroplasty. This chapter reviews the results of several semiconstrained total elbow arthroplasties characterized by laxity of the ulnohumeral articulation as demonstrated by the Coonrad-Morrey implant in patients with rheumatoid arthritis (Fig. 50–1). As noted previously in this text, the clinical and radiologic presentation of rheumatoid arthritis varies considerably (Fig. 50–2). The semiconstrained implant is especially useful in the type III and IV presentations (Fig. 50–3).

When considering the outcome of total elbow arthroplasty, it is useful to define the important components of outcome:

1. Relief of pain
2. Range of motion, flexion, extension, and supination pronation
3. Stability
4. Measure of function

To date, several evaluation systems exist that allow a critical assessment of the semiconstrained device in the patient with rheumatoid arthritis. We employ the Mayo Elbow Performance Score (MEPS) as defined in Table 50–1.[26]

Review of the literature reveals improving and encouraging results with several semiconstrained designs (Table 50–2). In this chapter, we review several of these experiences in detail, then focus on Mayo's experience.

THE PRITCHARD II PROSTHESIS

The Pritchard II prosthesis (Fig. 50–4) was an early design but has been used to a limited extent in recent years.[24, 31, 32] Pritchard surveyed the results in 92 patients with Mark II prostheses in 1981, among whom 60 percent had rheumatoid arthritis. The mean follow-up was 2.5 years. Although the range of motion, stability, and measure of function were not reported, relief of pain was reported as 98 percent.[31] A 15 percent complication rate and 2 percent loosening requiring revision were recorded.

Subsequently, Madsen and associates[24] followed 25 consecutive Pritchard II implants for a mean of 3 years. Twenty-three of 25 patients had relief of pain. The flexion arc averaged 28 to 130 degrees and pronation-supination was 65 to 62 degrees, respectively. Stability was not discussed, but the mean assessment score[17] improved from 40 to 82. However, radiographic loosening occurred in 6 of 24 elbows, and 2 necessitated revision.

These initial reports of the Pritchard II implant are of small numbers, and their findings may be regarded as preliminary. Although the initial outcome was encouraging, the design has largely been replicated by other implants, so this particular device is not frequently used today.

THE TRIAXIAL DEVICE

The articulation of the Triaxial Device has undergone numerous modifications but basically is that of a snap fit, which allows several degrees of varus-valgus and axial rotation "play" (Fig. 50–5). There has been a tendency for wear and dislocation over time, however. The device has been used for patients with rheumatoid arthritis and also frequently in a customized version for various pathologic states.

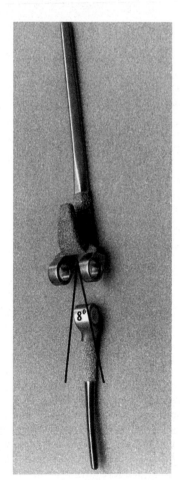

FIGURE 50–1 • The concept of the semiconstrained implant allows some "play" or laxity at the articulation.

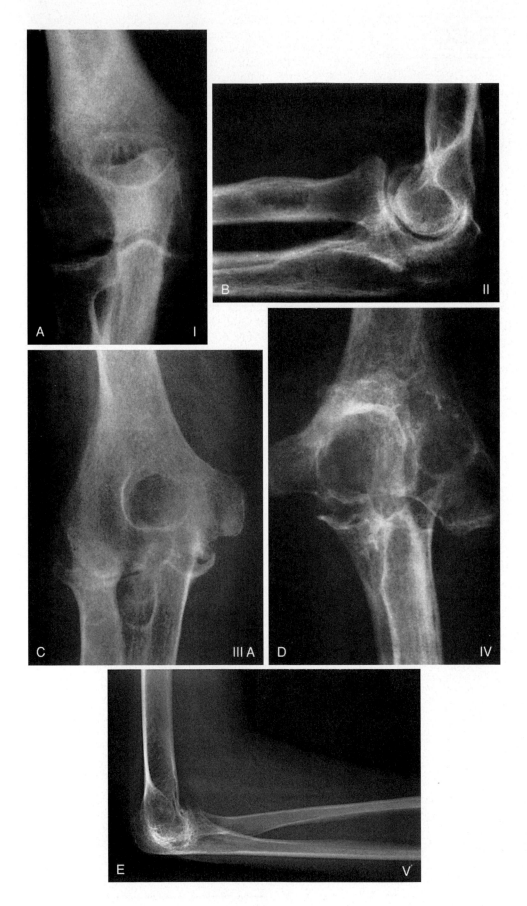

FIGURE 50–2 • The spectrum of radiographic presentation from grades I to V in patients with rheumatoid arthritis after Connor and Morrey[7] and Morrey.[25]

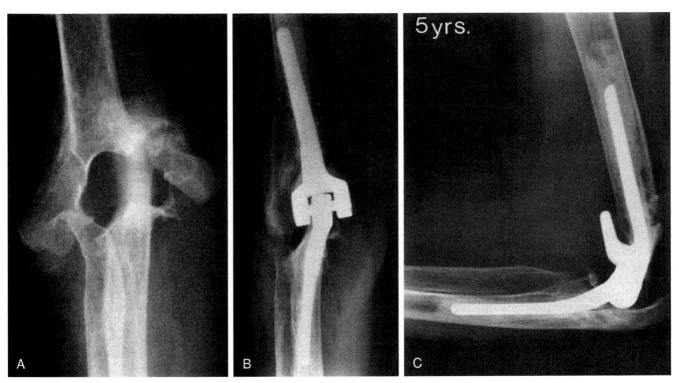

FIGURE 50–3 • Severe type IV involvement (A) is unpredictably treated by resurfacing implants but readily managed with a semiconstrained device (B and C).

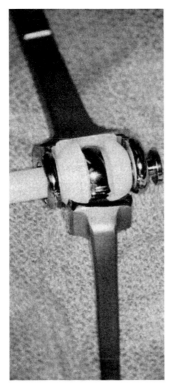

FIGURE 50–4 • The Pritchard II semiconstrained implant.

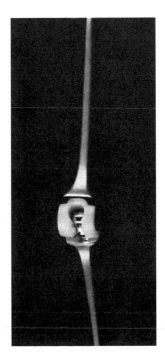

FIGURE 50–5 • The Triaxial Device.

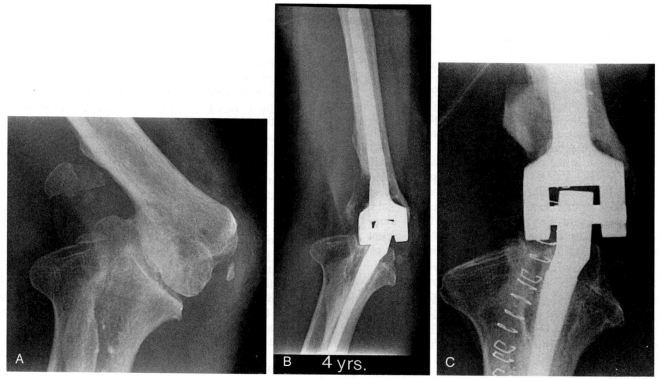

FIGURE 52–2 • *A,* Preoperative radiograph showing marked osseous deformity in a 41-year-old man who had sustained a supracondylar fracture in his childhood. He had severe pain and moderate instability. *B,* Anteroposterior radiograph, made 4 years postoperatively, showing worn bushings with recurrence of the valgus deformity. The patient had returned to his previous job as a construction worker, which involved lifting as much as 150 kg on a regular basis, against the advice of the surgeon. *C,* Postoperative anteroposterior radiograph made after exchange of the bushings. Both the humeral and the ulnar components were found to be solidly fixed.

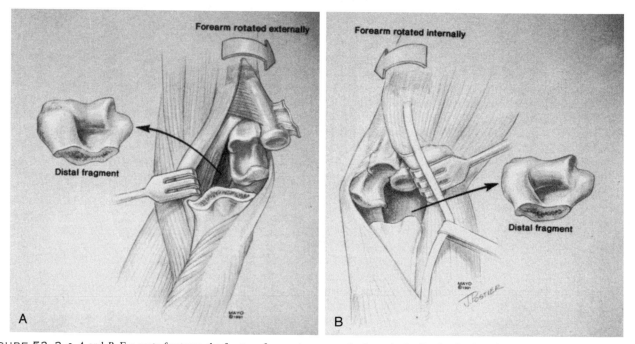

FIGURE 52–3 • *A* and *B,* For acute fractures, the fracture fragments are completely excised, allowing implantation without removal of the triceps.

semiconstrained prostheses have the major advantage of being able to correct deformity, this correction may be at the expense of persistent or increased asymmetrical loads imparted by the distorted soft tissues, causing an increased wear of the prosthesis. Overall, in our experience, a marked preoperative deformity of the elbows was associated with a significantly higher rate of complications ($P = .02$).[37]

TECHNIQUE: TRAUMATIC CONDITIONS

The operative technique for the implantation of the semiconstrained Coonrad-Morrey prosthesis is described in Chapter 49.[32] However, some features are unique to this type of prosthesis and should be emphasized. A type II or III compound fracture should first be irrigated and débrided to avoid wound infection. Total elbow replacement is then performed in a second stage. A type I wound may be treated in a single stage after careful and thorough débridement.

A posterior midline incision is used, including posterior scars from previous procedures. The ulnar nerve is always identified and transposed anteriorly in a subcutaneous pocket, if the procedure has not already been performed. If condyles are present, the recommended operative technique includes a triceps-sparing approach, which is accomplished by the release and lateral reflection of the triceps from the olecranon in continuity with the ulnar periosteum and the fascia of the forearm, along with the anconeus, as described by Bryan and Morrey.[3] Alternatively, particularly in acute fractures involving the condyles, the triceps insertion is left intact.

If contracted soft tissue persists, the humeral component is inserted more proximally after removal of additional humeral bone. All soft tissues are released from the humeral fragments, which are then excised (Fig. 52–3). Cultures are taken if there has been prior surgery. The collateral ligaments are detached from the epicondyles, which allows complete exposure of the elbow joint. The repair of the collateral ligaments is not necessary.

An intramedullary injecting system is used for optimal insertion of cement to which 1 gm of vancomycin has been added for every 40 gm of cement. An important element is the placement of a bone graft between the anterior flange and the distal part of the humerus to resist, after ingrowth, posterior displacement and rotational stresses on the humeral component. Ingrowth of this bone graft is consistently observed, confirming its role in absorbing mechanical loads.[37]

Significant bone stock deficiencies with the lack of one or both epicondyles do not change or complicate the implantation of the humeral component. This device requires only the humeral diaphysis to obtain secure fixation. Therefore, the reconstruction of the condyles is not required.

The device offers three lengths of humeral component: 10, 15, and 20 cm in standard and small sizes (Fig. 52–4). In cases of post-traumatic osteoarthrosis, we normally use the 15-cm stem. If the patient needs or may need a shoulder replacement, the shorter 10-cm stem for the elbow prosthesis may be a more appropriate choice to avoid a conflict of the elbow and shoulder implants within the humeral

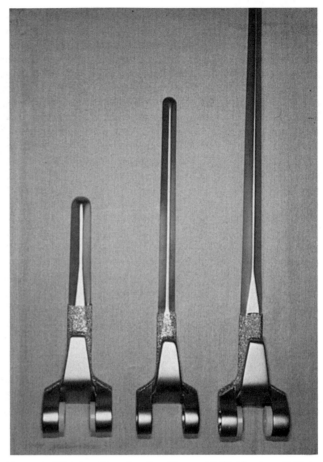

FIGURE 52–4 • Three lengths of humeral implants are available. The short stem illustrates the standard diameter, the median and long stems are of the small diameter. Both sizes are available for all three lengths.

diaphysis. Variable lengths and diameters of the ulna are also available.

At the end of the procedure if the triceps has been reflected, it is reattached to the olecranon with two No. 5 nonabsorbable sutures, allowing the immediate use of the joint. Compression dressings and elevation of the extremity are recommended for about 2 days, followed by gentle range-of-motion exercises as tolerated. Formal physical therapy is not necessary.

RESULTS

Literature Review

The results of total elbow replacements with highly constrained designs in the 1970s were disappointing because of high rates of loosening.[6, 12, 27] Although less loosening was reported after the introduction of semiconstrained and unconstrained replacement devices,[5, 9, 13, 33, 36] those reports dealt almost exclusively with the treatment of rheumatoid arthritis. There is very little information regarding total elbow replacement with an unconstrained or a semiconstrained device for the treatment of post-traumatic osteoarthrosis.[2, 10, 13, 18, 21, 23, 24, 30, 38] Most of what has been reported showed unfavorable results.[21, 23, 24, 38] In 1980,

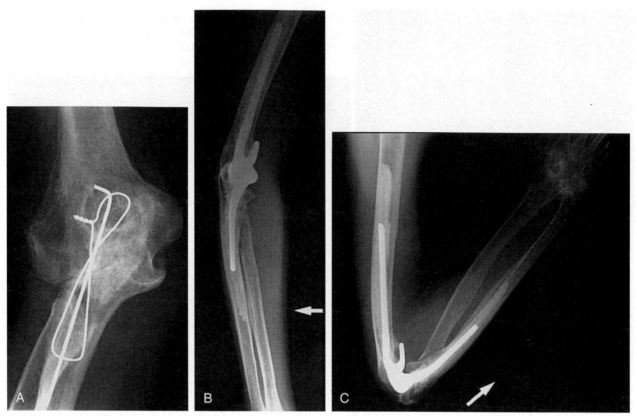

FIGURE 52–7 • *A,* Valgus deformity of 20 degrees, and stiffness (50 to 100 degrees) after two procedures. *B* and *C,* Excellent pain relief and motion after replacement.

group. This contrasts with the report of Gschwend and colleagues,[15] who in 1996 described a complication rate of 43 percent from a meta-analysis of 22 publications of total elbow replacement. Most of these procedures were performed for rheumatoid arthritis; such cases are usually associated with fewer complications than those in post-traumatic osteoarthrosis cases.

The majority of the complications were of a mechanical cause. Fracture of the ulnar component occurred in one prosthesis in the acute fracture group and in five elbows in

---

• TABLE 52–1 • **Major Complications with Total Elbow Arthroplasty After Acute Fracture and Traumatic Arthrosis**

Orthopedic Complication	Acute* n = 21	Arthrosis† n = 41
Loosening	0	0
Infection	0	2‡
Wear	0	2‡
Fracture		
Ulnar component	1‡	5‡
Other	1	4

* Cobb, T. K., and Morrey, B. F.: Total elbow replacement as primary treatment for distal humeral fractures in elderly patients. J. Bone Joint Surg. **79A:**826, 1997.

† Schneeberger, A. G., Adams, R., and Morrey, B. F.: Semiconstrained total elbow replacement for the treatment of post-traumatic osteoarthrosis. J. Bone Joint Surg. **79A:**1211, 1997.

‡ Required revision or reoperation.

the post-traumatic group 2 to 9 years (average, 4.3 years) postoperatively. Before breakage, all six patients had an excellent result, with an asymptomatic, essentially normal elbow. The cause of failure was severe noncompliance, such as regular lifting of weights of more than 50 kg in two patients (Fig. 52–8). The revisions involved an average of less than 70 minutes of tourniquet time. There were no operative or delayed complications from the reoperation.

The fractures of the ulnar component always occurred at the site of sintered beads. Hence, in 1991, the beads were replaced by a precoat of methylmethacrylate. No fractures of such precoated ulnar components have been observed to date.

Two patients of the group of post-traumatic osteoarthrosis presented with a particulate synovitis associated with worn bushings. Both cases also had a significant preoperative deformity, and one excessive use. Treatment of the worn bushing consisted of synovectomy and exchange of the bushings, resulting in a satisfactory outcome.

Despite the use of semiconstrained devices, most other series of post-traumatic osteoarthrosis are still complicated by a certain rate of loosening.[23] However, no loosening was observed by Figgie and colleagues[10] in their series of 9 semiconstrained triaxial prostheses with custom-designed stems. Gschwend and associates[14] reported that after a mean of 4.3 years (maximum, 14 years), loosening had occurred in 2 of 26 patients. That few of the 62 cases reported here have loosened indicates the great improvement in total elbow replacement, particularly in this very difficult group of patients.

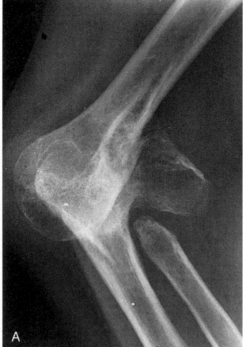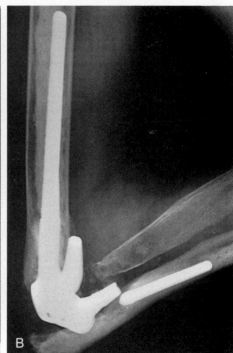

FIGURE 52–8 • *A,* A 58-year-old farmer showing extensive preoperative osseous deformity owing to a malunited supracondylar fracture from age 10. The patient had moderate pain and marked loss of motion. *B,* Fracture of the ulnar component 9 years after implantation of the prosthesis. The patient had had no pain and had full function during these 9 years, and he had returned to his previous strenuous activities, regularly lifting weights of more than 50 kg, against the advice of the surgeon.

REFERENCES

1. Askew, L. J., An, K. -N., Morrey, B. F., and Chao, E. Y. S.: Isometric elbow strength in normal individuals. Clin. Orthop. **222:**261, 1987.
2. Brumfield, R. H., Jr., Kuschner, S. H., Gellman, H., Redix, L., and Stevenson, D. V.: Total elbow arthroplasty. J. Arthroplasty **5:**359, 1990.
3. Bryan, R. S., and Morrey, B. F.: Extensive posterior exposure of the elbow: A triceps-sparing approach. Clin. Orthop. **166:**188, 1982.
4. Cobb T. K., and Morrey, B. F.: Total elbow replacement as primary treatment for distal humeral fractures in elderly patients. J. Bone Joint Surg. **79A:**826, 1997.
5. Davis, R. F., Weiland, A. J., Hungerford, D. S., Moore, J. R., and Volenec-Dowling, S.: Nonconstrained total elbow arthroplasty. Clin. Orthop **171:**156, 1982.
6. Dee, R.: Total replacement arthroplasty of the elbow for rheumatoid arthritis. J. Bone Joint Surg. **54B:**88, 1972.
7. Dee, R.: Nonimplantation salvage of failed reconstructive procedures of the elbow. *In* Morrey, B. F. (ed.): The Elbow and Its Disorders, 2nd ed. Philadelphia, W. B. Saunders Co., 1993, pp. 690–695.
8. DeLee, J. C.: Fractures and dislocations of the hip. *In* Rockwoood, C. A., Jr., Green, D. P., Bucholz, R. W., and Heckman, J. D. (eds.): Rookwood and Green's Fractures in Adults, 4th ed. Philadelphia, Lippincott-Raven, 1996, p. 1687.
9. Ewald, F. C., and Jacobs, M. A.: Total elbow arthroplasty. Clin. Orthop. **182:**137, 1984.
10. Figgie, H. E., III, Inglis, A. E., Ranawat, C. S., and Rosenberg, G. M.: Results of total elbow arthroplasty as a salvage procedure for failed elbow reconstructive operations. Clin. Orthop. **219:**185, 1987.
11. Froimson, A. I., Silva, J. E., and Richey, D.: Cutis arthroplasty of the elbow joint. J. Bone Joint Surg. **58A:**863, 1976.
12. Garrett, J. C., Ewald, F. C., Thomas W. H., and Sledge, C. B.: Loosening associated with GSB hinge total elbow replacement in patients with rheumatoid arthritis. Clin. Orthop. **127:**170, 1977.
13. Gschwend, N., Loehr, J., Ivosevic-Radovanovic, D., Scheier, H., and Munzinger, U.: Semi-constrained elbow prosthesis with special reference to the GSB III prosthesis. Clin. Orthop. **232:**104, 1988.
14. Gschwend, N., Scheier, H., Bähler, A., and Simmen, B.: GSB III elbow. *In* Ruther, W. (ed.): The Elbow, Endoprosthetic Replacement and Non-endoprosthetic Procedures. Berlin, Springer Verlag, 1996, pp. 83–98.
15. Gschwend, N., Simmen, B. R., and Matejovsky, Z.: Late complications in elbow arthroplasty. J. Shoulder Elbow Surg. **5:**86, 1996.
16. Helfet, D. L., and Schmerling, G. J.: Bicondylar intra-articular fractures of the distal humerus in adults. Clin. Orthop. **292:**26, 1993.
17. Hughes, R. E., Schneeberger, A. G., An, K.-N., Morrey, B. F., and O'Driscoll, S.: Reduction of triceps muscle force after shortening of the distal humerus: A computational model. J. Shoulder Elbow Surg. **6:**444, 1997.
18. Inglis, A. E., and Pellicci, P. M.: Total elbow replacement. J. Bone Joint Surg. **62A:**1252, 1980.
19. John, H., Rosso, R., Neff, U., Bodoky, A., Regazzoni, P., and Harder, F.: Operative treatment of distal humeral fractures in the elderly. J. Bone Joint Surg. **76B:**793, 1994.
20. Jupiter, J. B., Neff, U., Holzach, P., and Allgöwer, M.: Intercondylar fractures of the humerus. J. Bone Joint Surg. **67-A:**226, 1985.
21. Kasten, M. D., and Skinner, H. B.: Total elbow arthroplasty. Clin. Orthop. **290:**177, 1993.
22. Knight, R. A., and Zandt, L. V.: Arthroplasty of the elbow. J. Bone Joint Surg. **34A:**610, 1952.
23. Kraay, M. J., Figgie, M. P., Inglis, A. E., Wolfe, S. W., and Ranawat, C. S.: Primary semiconstrained total elbow arthroplasty. J. Bone Joint Surg. **76B:**636, 1994.
24. Lowe, L. W., Miller, A. J., Allum, R. L., and Higginson, D. W.: The development of an unconstrained elbow arthroplasty. J. Bone Joint Surg. **66B:**243, 1984.
25. McAuliffe, J. A., Burkhalter, W. E., Ouellette, E. A., and Carneiro, R. S.: Compression plate arthrodesis of the elbow. J. Bone Joint Surg. **74B:**300, 1992.
26. Morrey, B. F., Askew, L. J., An, K.-N., and Chao, E. Y.: A biomechanical study of normal functional elbow motion. J. Bone Joint Surg. **63A:**872, 1981.
27. Morrey, B. F., Bryan, R. S., Dobyns, J. H., and Linscheid, R. L.: Total elbow arthroplasty: A five-year experience at the Mayo Clinic. J. Bone Joint Surg. **63A:**1050, 1981.
28. Morrey, B. F., Askew, L. J., and An, K.-N.: Strength function after elbow arthroplasty. Clin. Orthop. **234:**43, 1988.
29. Morrey, B. F.: Post-traumatic contracture of the elbow: Operative treatment including distraction arthroplasty. J. Bone Joint Surg. **72A:**601, 1990.
30. Morrey, B. F., Adams, R. A., and Bryan, R. S.: Total replacement for post-traumatic arthritis of the elbow. J. Bone Joint Surg. **73B:**607, 1991.
31. Morrey, B. F., and Adams, R. A.: Semi-constrained arthroplasty for the treatment of rheumatoid arthritis of the elbow. J. Bone Joint Surg. **74A:**479, 1992.

32. Morrey, B. F., and Adams, R. A.: Semi-constrained elbow replacement arthroplasty: Rationale, technique, and results. *In* Morrey, B. F. (ed.): The Elbow and Its Disorders, 2nd ed. Philadelphia, W. B. Saunders Co., 1993, pp. 648–664.

33. Morrey, B. F., and Adams, R. A.: Semi-constrained elbow replacement for distal humeral nonunion. J. Bone Joint Surg. **77B:**67, 1995.

34. O'Driscoll, S. W., An, K.-N., Korinek, S., and Morrey, B. F.: Kinematics of semiconstrained total elbow arthroplasty. J. Bone Joint Surg. **74B:** 297, 1992.

35. O'Neill, O. R., Morrey, B. F., Tanaka, S., and An, K.-N.: Compensatory motion in the upper extremity after elbow arthrodesis. Clin. Orthop. **281:**89, 1992.

36. Pritchard, R.W.: Anatomic surface elbow arthroplasty: A preliminary report. Clin. Orthop. **179:**223, 1979.

37. Schneeberger, A. G., Adams, R., and Morrey, B. F.: Semiconstrained total elbow replacement for the treatment of post-traumatic osteoarthrosis. J. Bone Joint Surg. **79A:**1211, 1997.

38. Soni, R. K., and Cavendish, M. E.: A review of the Liverpool elbow prosthesis from 1974 to 1982. J. Bone Joint Surg. **66B:**248, 1984.

39. Souter, W. A., Nicol, A. C., and Paul, J. P.: Anatomical trochlear stirrup arthroplasty of the rheumatoid elbow. J. Bone Joint Surg. **67B:**676, 1985.

40. Tsuge, K., Murakami, T., Yasunaga, Y., and Kanaujia, R. R.: Arthroplasty of the elbow. J. Bone Joint Surg. **69B:**116, 1987.

41. Urbaniak, J. R., and Black K. E., Jr.: Cadaveric elbow allografts: A six-year experience. Clin. Orthop. **197:**131, 1985.

42. Zuckerman, J. D., and Lubliner, J. A.: Arm, elbow and forearm injuries. *In* Zuckerman, J. D. (ed.): Orthopaedic Injuries in the Elderly. Baltimore, Urban & Schwarzenberg, 1990, pp. 345–407.

• CHAPTER 53 •

Total Elbow Arthroplasty for Nonunion and Dysfunctional Instability

• MATTHEW L. RAMSEY and
BERNARD F. MORREY

A stable, freely mobile elbow joint is required for normal upper extremity function. The unique architecture of the elbow and surrounding soft tissues is responsible for joint stability. Mobility of the elbow requires a functional joint to act as a fulcrum for motion and the power provided by the muscles crossing the elbow joint. Disruption of the elements that confer mobility and stability on the elbow joint limits the ability to position the hand in space for functional activities.

Destruction of the fulcrum typically results from severe rheumatoid arthritis, nonunion of the distal humerus, traumatic bone loss, or surgical management of infection. In the most extreme circumstance the forearm is dissociated from the upper arm, resulting in a flail extremity and loss of angular and longitudinal stability of the extremity. Less severe joint destruction allows some degree of elbow motion with the arm splinted against the side; however, for activities for which the arm is held away from the body the fulcrum is insufficient for effective function. Total elbow arthroplasty for patients with dysfunctional instability has evolved over the past decade into a reliable treatment option for certain carefully selected patients.

PRESENTATION

Destruction of the fulcrum necessary for stable elbow motion results in varying degrees of elbow instability, depending on the degree of joint involvement. Patients considered for total elbow arthroplasty have instability that precludes useful function of the extremity. The defining feature in this group of patients is the inability to position the arm in space because of instability or dissociation of the elbow. At the most extreme end of the spectrum are patients whose forearm and arm are dissociated and pistoning of the forearm proximally on the arm with attempted motion results (Fig. 53–1). Over time, the soft tissues about the elbow may be contracted. These patients have a flail extremity. A second group of patients with dysfunctional instability have enough of a fulcrum remaining so that they are capable of active motion with the arm adducted against the side. When a load is applied to the arm or activities away from the body are attempted, however, the fulcrum for elbow motion is insufficient to maintain stability (Fig.

53–2). These patients have gross instability of the elbow. The underlying causes for dysfunctional instability vary considerably but can include rheumatoid destruction of the elbow, traumatic bone loss, surgical resection of the humerus, and nonunion of the distal humerus.

INDICATIONS

The indications for total elbow arthroplasty have changed dramatically over the past decade. The increasing documentation of success of total elbow arthroplasty as a primary or a secondary reconstructive procedure has resulted in its being applied to more demanding lesions, especially when other reconstructive procedures have proven less reliable. The options for treatment of dysfunctional instability include external bracing, open reduction and internal fixation for nonunion of the distal humerus,[1, 3, 10, 11] resection

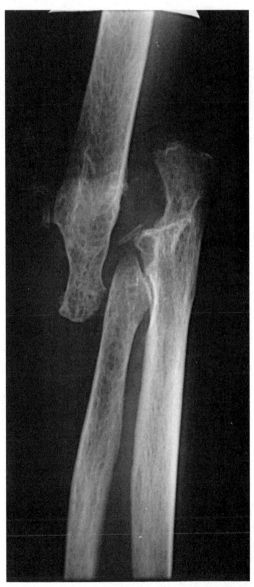

FIGURE 53–1 • Dysfunctional instability with loss of the fulcrum owing to gross malalignment of the forearm with the humerus.

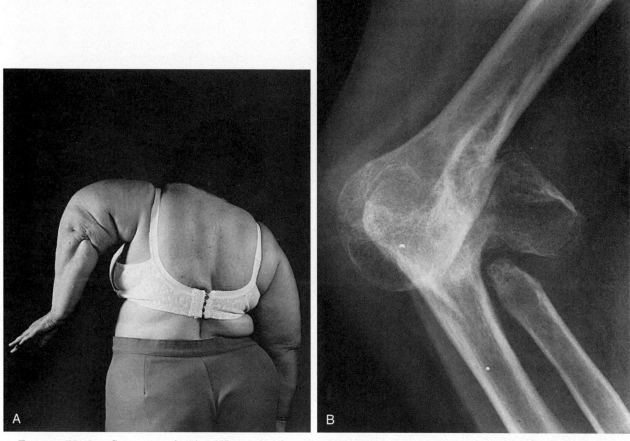

FIGURE 53–2 • Gross varus-valgus instability resulted from distal humeral nonunion (A), but some flexion function is preserved (B).

arthroplasty, arthrodesis,[9] allograft reconstruction,[1, 19] and total elbow arthroplasty.[4, 6, 11, 13, 14] External bracing is poorly tolerated and does not restore mobility or stability to the elbow joint. Open reduction and internal fixation with autogenous bone grafting, contracture release, and ulnar neurolysis remains the treatment of choice for established nonunion of the distal humerus.[10] Exclusion criteria for further attempts to obtain union include age older than 60 years, patients whose activity is limited, bone loss, poor bone quality of the ununited fragment, and irreversible articular damage.[10, 14] The goal of arthrodesis of the elbow joint is to obtain a stable, immobile joint. While elbow fusion can be achieved successfully in the face of bone loss, fusion limits the ability to perform activities of daily living.[16] Allograft reconstruction of the elbow joint has been used in patients considered too young for arthroplasty and for traumatic conditions about the elbow. Serious complications reported limit widespread use of this method.[19] Given the option of resection arthroplasty, arthrodesis, allograft reconstruction, or total elbow arthroplasty, the latter is often preferred because it provides the best functional results with the least morbidity.[14, 17]

The primary indication for total elbow arthroplasty is instability that prevents useful function of the arm because of inability to position the hand in space.[2, 16, 21] The typical patient is older than 60 years and has low functional demands; however, younger patients for whom other options are unfeasible and who are willing to cooperate with the activity restrictions are considered for total elbow arthroplasty. Pain is a variable complaint in patients with dysfunctional instability, but it tends to be mild to moderate and rarely is the principal indication for surgery.

Aside from active infection, there are few absolute contraindications to total elbow arthroplasty for dysfunctional instability of the elbow. A history of infection is a relative contraindication to joint replacement and the infection must be demonstrated to have been completely eradicated before joint replacement is undertaken. Young, active patients are at risk for mechanical failure of the implant because of demanding work and recreational activities, so youth and an active lifestyle are relative contraindications.

CONSIDERATIONS

Selecting patients for whom this method is appropriate is critical to its success. Careful consideration of the patient's expectations and the underlying lesion and detailed preoperative planning avoid the potential pitfalls inherent in treating this group of patients. The dissociated elbow is realigned by the implant. This extreme demand places the implant at risk for mechanical failure.

Many patients considered for total elbow arthroplasty have had multiple previous surgeries, a fact that further increases the concern for a possible low-grade infection. If possible infection is a concern, a staged procedure is considered, the initial intervention being débridement and collection of specimens for histologic and microbiologic evaluation. Component implantation is a second procedure performed after all cultures are negative and histologic evaluation excludes infection.

Careful neurologic evaluation is mandatory. The ulnar nerve may have been repeatedly manipulated during other operations or scarred at the nonunion site. Documentation of nerve function by physical examination, and in some cases electrodiagnostic studies, will direct appropriate treatment of the nerve.

The choice of implants is critical to the success of treatment. Unlinked resurfacing implants have no role in this clinical circumstance. Linked, semiconstrained implants provide stability through the coupled articulation of the ulnar and humeral components.[2, 7, 16, 21] Several different semiconstrained implants are available.[2, 7, 21] The Coonrad-Morrey device was specifically designed in consideration of this type of lesion.[16] The position of the humeral yoke distal to the level of humeral insertion restores the anatomic axis of rotation even when bone loss extends up to the level of the roof of the olecranon fossa (Fig. 53–3). Shortening of the humerus up to 2 cm proximal to the olecranon fossa is

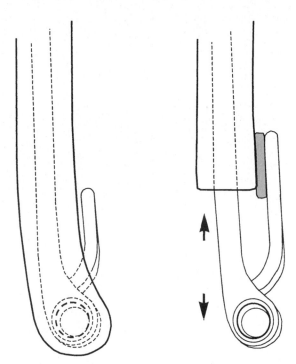

FIGURE 53–4 • An extended flange provides greater flexibility for depth of insertion and allows even severe deficiencies to be managed without a custom implant.

permitted and eliminates the need for custom implants.[7, 16, 19] Bone loss greater than 2 cm can be managed with an implant with an extended anterior humeral flange (soon to be a standard feature of the device; Fig. 53–4). This allows the humeral length to be restored while it provides the stabilizing effect of the anterior flange in preventing the forces that tend to both rotate and displace the implant posteriorly.

TECHNIQUE

The technique for total elbow arthroplasty for dysfunctional instability of the elbow is similar to that for conventional total elbow arthroplasty (see Chapter 49) with a few important differences similar to that for the acute fracture (see Chapter 52).[14, 16, 17] The patient is placed supine on the operating room table, and a tourniquet is applied high on the arm before preparation and draping of the extremity, or a sterile Esmarch tourniquet is useful if the humerus is shortened. The previous skin incision or a posterior one is utilized, as appropriate. Medial subcutaneous dissection allows identification and protection of the ulnar nerve in all patients. In those who previously had ulnar nerve transposition and who have no symptoms dissection of the entire nerve is not necessary and only its location need be determined. For symptomatic elbows, re-exploration and decompression are carried out.

A triceps-sparing approach is the favored method of surgical exposure in these cases, as the distal humeral bone stock is absent or will be resected. The triceps insertion is not released from the olecranon but is left intact. A triceps-reflecting (Bryan-Morrey) approach[15] that is used for most

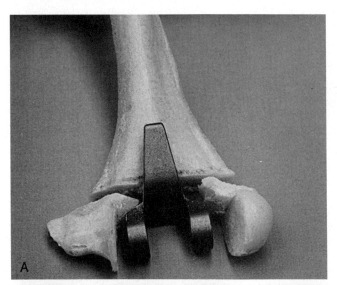

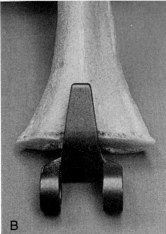

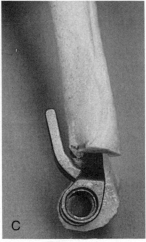

FIGURE 53–3 • The ideal depth of insertion of the Coonrad-Morrey implant places the flange at the level of the roof of the olecranon fossa in front of the anterior cortex (A). This position is attainable even when bone is missing from the distal humerus (B and C).

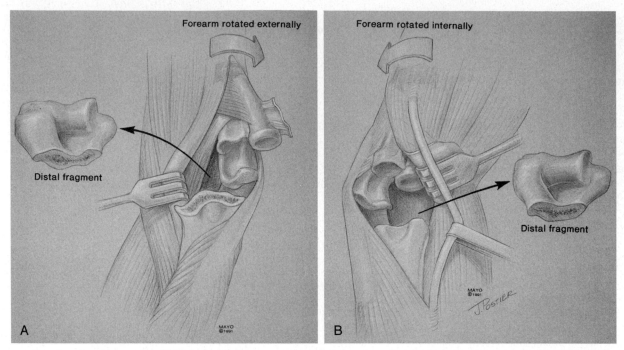

Forearm rotated externally

Distal fragment

A

Forearm rotated internally

Distal fragment

B

FIGURE 53–5 • The absence of the distal humerus allows exposure of the humeral canal, either laterally (A) or medially (B), without releasing the triceps from the olecranon.

problems is not necessary in the majority of these cases[14] (Fig. 53–5).

The medial and lateral aspects of the triceps tendon are developed, exposing the distal humerus. For nonunion, any retained hardware is removed from the medial and lateral aspects of the distal humerus. The collateral ligaments and the common extensor and common flexor muscle masses are released from their epicondylar attachments. The distal humeral fragment is excised to allow ready exposure to implant the prosthesis.

The ulna is delivered through the medial aspect of the triceps with a supination motion exposing the intramedullary canal for component insertion. The subcutaneous border of the ulna is exposed and is an important maneuver to ensure that the ulna is not violated during preparation.

Trial reduction of the components is very useful in patients with a long-standing fixed dissociation of the elbow, as the limb could be shortened and malaligned owing to rigid soft tissue contracture. Forced articulation of a shortened extremity limits postoperative motion, risks neurovascular injury, and increases stress transfer to the bone-cement interface. In this situation, shortening of the humerus up to 2 cm can be undertaken with only mild triceps weakness.[8]

The implants are cemented with tobramycin-impregnated polymethylmethacrylate. The tourniquet is regularly released at this point to achieve hemostasis due to the usual extensive dissection. Obtaining hemostasis of the anterior compartment of the elbow is particularly difficult when the components are in place.

The common extensor and common flexor muscle masses are sutured to the lateral and medial triceps fascia, respectively. There is no need to preserve the epicondylar attachment of these muscle masses or to reconstruct the epicondyles to the remainder of the humeral shaft.

Since the triceps tendon is not released from its attachment, immediate postoperative motion is permitted. If a triceps-reflecting approach is utilized, active motion is allowed in a couple of days or delayed, according to the surgeon's judgment.

RESULTS

The goal of total elbow arthroplasty for dysfunctional instability of the elbow is to restore a stable fulcrum for elbow motion that allows useful function. The early experience with total elbow arthroplasty for instability using constrained or custom implants proved disappointing: high complication rates were associated with component loosening, articular dissociation, and deep infection that necessitated component removal.[7, 13] When successful, however, the early total elbow arthroplasty for dysfunctional instability produced remarkable return of function.[2, 16, 19, 21] Because of the high rate of infection, little experience was gained specifically addressing the issue of total elbow arthroplasty in patients with dysfunctional instability of the elbow; however, recent reports on total elbow arthroplasty in patients with this condition have highlighted the advances made in their treatment.[2, 19, 21] Overall, objective satisfactory results with medium- to long-term follow-up range from 76 to 84 percent and subjective satisfaction approaches 90 percent.[19] Stability is restored by utilizing a linked, semiconstrained implant. Postoperative instability due to uncoupling of the humeral and ulnar components is a risk with this type of lesion and has been reported to be related to snap-fit–type designs.[7, 9] Even custom designs have proven unreliable, often owing to the inadequacy of the articulation.[5, 7, 9]

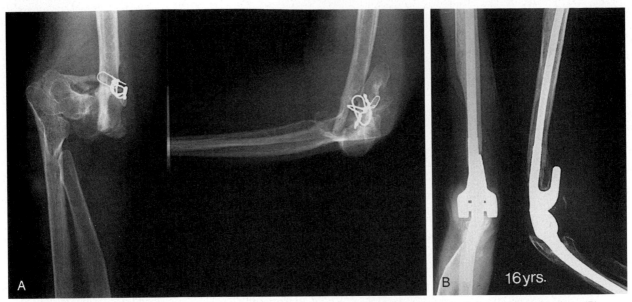

FIGURE 53–6 • Gross instability from nonunion (A) was treated successfully for 16 years with total elbow arthroplasty (B).

The Mayo Experience

Experience with 39 distal humeral nonunions was reported with a mean surveillance of more than 4 years after the Coonrad-Morrey replacement. Of these, 86 percent were rated by the Mayo Elbow Performance Score (MEPS) as satisfactory (Fig. 53–6).[16] Ramsey and coworkers recently reported the intermediate- to long-term results of Coonrad-Morrey prosthetic replacement for gross instability.[19] With surveillance between 2 and 12 years, 16 of 19 patients (84 percent) had a satisfactory outcome based on the MEPS (Fig. 53–7). Most problems were "mechanical" ones, more

than half of them related to wear debris and ulnar nerve irritation (the latter the second most frequent untoward event). The complication rate for their similar group was 21 and 18%, respectively. Reoperation was required for eight of the combined group of 58 (14%).

Improvement in useful elbow motion is marked after surgery, whereas before surgery, instability prevents useful motion. Patients who have limited elbow motion have instability for activities for which the arm is held away from the body. Postoperatively, functional range of motion is re-established with an average flexion arc of approximately 100 degrees.[16, 19] The limitations of a patient with

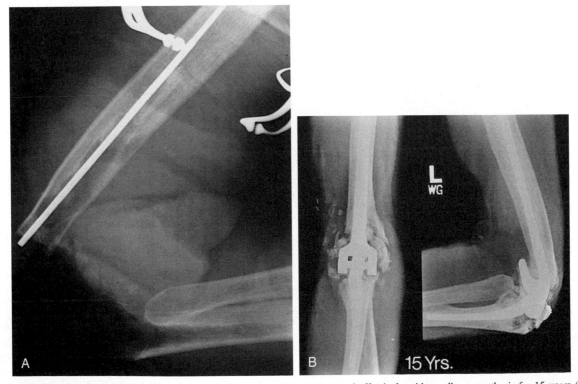

FIGURE 53–7 • A flail extremity, the result of joint resection (A), was treated effectively with an elbow prosthesis for 15 years (B).

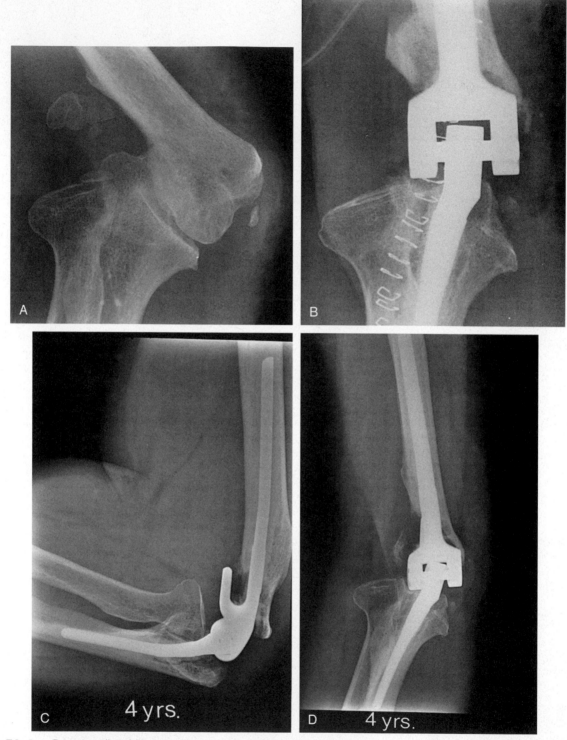

FIGURE 53–8 • Gross nonunion of 20 years' duration *(A)* was treated by total elbow arthroplasty *(B)*. Persistent forearm malalignment is seen on the lateral view *(C)*, and excessive use caused worn bushings at 4 years *(D)*.

dysfunctional instability are obvious. The inability to position the hand in space compromises the ability to perform daily activities. Re-establishing a stable fulcrum for elbow motion significantly improves functional activities.

COMPLICATIONS

The complications related to implant design and surgical technique have been largely eliminated through better de-

signs and modification of the surgical technique. Currently, the most serious issue in patients with dysfunctional instability is the long-term mechanical integrity of the implant. Realignment of the extremity through the implant and the application of this technique to younger active patients places tremendous stress on the implant. In this setting, mechanical problems such as loosening, component fracture, and bushing wear might be expected and have been reported in these patients (Fig. 53–8).[5, 7, 9, 16, 19] While the ability of these patients to engage in activities that require physical strength attests to the success of the operation, there will no doubt be an increase in the need for revision surgery in the future.

Other complications encountered in this patient population include deep infections, ulnar nerve dysfunction, and wound problems. The causes of these complications are not related to this unique clinical situation and the incidence is no higher than that in the general population undergoing total elbow arthroplasty.

The early use of constrained implants resulted in humeral loosening that has been reduced with semiconstrained devices; however, loosening of semiconstrained implants has been reported. Surface delamination has been proposed to contribute to humeral loosening and has prompted design modifications.[20] Humeral loosening has also been reported with press-fit humeral stems and fluted humeral components.[12] Dissociation of the humeral and ulnar components has been reported with shaft implants. Design modifications have eliminated or markedly reduced component uncoupling as a cause of failure. The mechanical performance of the implant is particularly relevant in this patient population. Polyethylene bushings may wear and cause wear debris, instability, or both, necessitating bushing replacement. Revision of the bushings to a more captured bushing has been necessary for component dissociation of the snap-fit design. The coupled Coonrad-Morrey implant has required bushing exchange for excessive wear.

REFERENCES

1. Ackerman, G., and Jupiter, J. B.: Non-union of fractures of the distal end of the humerus. J. Bone Joint Surg. **70A:**75–83, 1988.
2. Baksi, D. P.: Sloppy hinge prosthetic elbow replacement for post-traumatic ankylosis or instability. J. Bone Joint Surg. **80B:**614–619, 1998.
3. Breen, T., Gelberman, R. H., Leffert, R., and Botte, M.: Massive allograft replacement of hemiarticular traumatic defects of the elbow [published erratum appears in J. Hand Surg (Am) 14:582, 1989]. J. Hand Surg. **13A:**900–907, 1988.
4. Cobb, T. K., and Linscheid, R. L.: Late correction of malunited intercondylar humeral fractures. Intra-articular osteotomy and tricortical bone grafting. J. Bone Joint Surg. **76B:**622–626, 1994.
5. Figgie, H. E., III, Inglis, A. E., and Mow, C.: Total elbow arthroplasty in the face of significant bone stock or soft tissue losses. Preliminary results of custom-fit arthroplasty. J. Arthroplasty **1:**71–81, 1986.
6. Figgie, H. E., III, Inglis, A. E., Ranawat, C. S., and Rosenberg, G. M.: Results of total elbow arthroplasty as a salvage procedure for failed elbow reconstructive operations. Clin. Orthop. **Jun(219):**185–193, 1987.
7. Figgie, M. P., Inglis, A. E., Mow, C. S., and Figgie, H. E., III: Salvage of non-union of supracondylar fracture of the humerus by total elbow arthroplasty. J. Bone Joint Surg. **71A:**1058–1065, 1989.
8. Hughes, R. E., Schneeberger, A. G., An, K. N., Morrey, B. F., and O'Driscoll, S. W.: Reduction of triceps muscle force after shortening of the distal humerus: A computational model. J. Shoulder Elbow Surg. **6:**444–448, 1997.
9. Inglis, A. E., Inglis, A. E., Jr., Figgie, M. M., and Asnis, L.: Total elbow arthroplasty for flail and unstable elbows. J. Shoulder Elbow Surg. **6:**29–36, 1997.
10. Jupiter, J. B.: Complex fractures of the distal part of the humerus and associated complications. Instructional Course Lectures. **44:**187–198, 1995.
11. McAuliffe, J. A., Burkhalter, W. E., Ouellette, E. A., and Carneiro, R. S.: Compression plate arthrodesis of the elbow. J. Bone Joint Surg. **74B:**300–304, 1992.
12. McKee, M., Jupiter, J., Toh, C. L., Wilson, L., Colton, C., and Karras, K. K.: Reconstruction after malunion and nonunion of intra-articular fractures of the distal humerus. Methods and results in 13 adults. J. Bone Joint Surg. **76B:**614–621, 1994.
13. Mitsunaga, M. M., Bryan, R. S., and Linscheid, R. L.: Condylar nonunions of the elbow. J. Trauma **22:**787–791, 1982.
14. Morrey, B. F.: Surgical exposures of the elbow. *In* Morrey, B. F. (ed.): The Elbow and Its Disorders, 2nd ed. Philadelphia, W. B. Saunders, 1993, pp. 139–166.
15. Morrey, B. F., and Adams, R. A.: Semiconstrained arthroplasty for the treatment of rheumatoid arthritis of the elbow. J. Bone Joint Surg. **74A:**479–490, 1992.
16. Morrey, B. F., and Adams, R. A.: Semiconstrained elbow replacement for distal humeral nonunion [see Comments]. J Bone Joint Surg. **77B:**67–72, 1995.
17. O'Driscoll, S. W.: Prosthetic elbow replacement for distal humeral fractures and nonunions. Op. Tech. Orthop. **4:**54–57, 1994.
18. O'Neill, O. R., Morrey, B. F., Tanaka, S., and An, K. N.: Compensatory motion in the upper extremity after elbow arthrodesis. Clin. Orthop. **Aug(281):**89–96, 1992.
19. Ramsey, M., Adams, R., and Morrey, B.: Instability of the elbow treated with semi-constrained total elbow arthroplasty. J. Bone Joint Surg. **81A:**38–47, 1999.
20. Ross, A. C., Sneath, R. S., and Scales, J. T.: Endoprosthetic replacement of the humerus and elbow joint. J. Bone Joint Surg. **69B:**652–655, 1987.
21. Tonino, A. J.: Total elbow arthroplasty in the salvage of pseudarthrosis of a supracondylar humerus fracture. Ztschr. Orthop. Grenzgebiete **133:**328–329, 1995.
22. Urbaniak, J. R., and Aitken, M.: Clinical use of bone allografts in the elbow. Orthop. Clin. North Am. **18:**311–321, 1987.

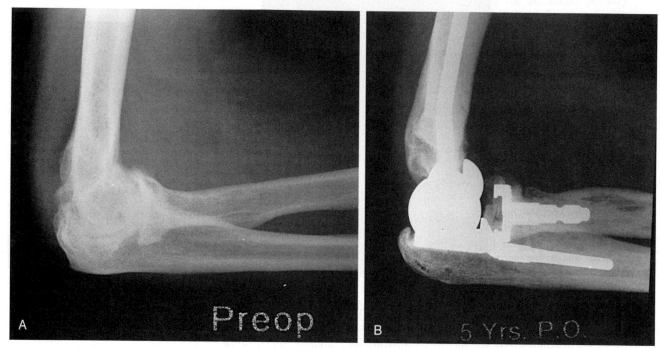

FIGURE 54–3 • Before (*A*) and five years after (*B*) resurfacing implant for primary osteoarthritis of the elbow.

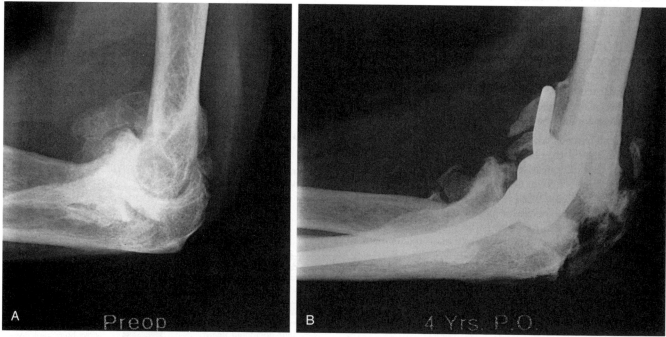

FIGURE 54–4 • *A*, Preoperative lateral radiograph shows marked hypertrophic osteophyte formation as a feature of the degenerative process. *B*, At 41 months review, a lateral radiograph shows heterotopic ossification anteriorly and posteriorly. There is marked involvement in the triceps tendon insertion, but the Mayo Elbow Performance Score is 95.

Chapter 12 and according to the specific features. Postoperatively, motion is encouraged as tolerated and according to swelling and pain. The patient is usually discharged on day 3.

RESULTS

Little has been published on joint replacement for osteoarthritis. Our limited experience with a series of cases was recently reported.[8] With surveillance of more than 5 years, the mean age of the four men and one woman was 68 years (range 61 to 72). The mean postoperative arc was 37 to 122 degrees, less than that reported for other diagnoses but better by an average of 20 degrees than the mean 40- to 105-degree arc preoperatively. One of two treated with a resurfacing device had an unsatisfactory result, and results in all three of those with the semiconstrained device were graded satisfactory (Fig. 54–3).

COMPLICATIONS

Complications may be surprisingly frequent. There were four major and two minor complications in four elbows, including fracture of the humeral component with particulate synovitis, implant subluxation, heterotopic ossification, and ulnar neuropathy (Fig. 53–4). Two of these elbows required revision of one of the components. This is a higher rate than that reported at our institution during the same period for total elbow arthroplasty for rheumatoid arthritis (9 percent),[13] post-traumatic arthritis (18 percent),[15] nonunion of the distal humerus (13 percent),[14] and even revision total arthroplasty (17 percent).[7] The problems encountered, however, are consistent with the relatively high level of activity typical of persons with this diagnosis.

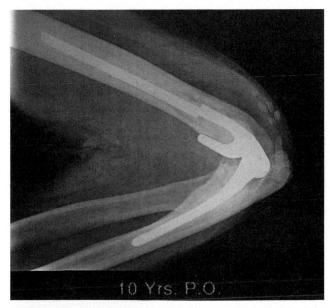

FIGURE 54–5 • At 10 years after total elbow arthroplasty, the lateral radiograph shows transverse fracture of the humeral component with surrounding lysis of the bone in a patient who continuously engaged in heavy work during those 10 years.

Patients with primary degenerative arthritis of the elbow tend to be active, and most are involved in manual occupations that place greater demands on the prosthesis. One patient returned to his former occupation of carpentry, heavy lifting, and stonework. The humeral component fractured from overuse (Fig. 54–5). Two of the patients had transient postoperative ulnar neuropathy with altered sensation; both cases resolved spontaneously. Ulnar nerve irritation is associated with the development of primary osteoarthritis of the elbow joint.

SUMMARY

Primary joint replacement is not usually indicated for osteoarthritis; yet, if the patient is older than 65 years and has aching discomfort most of the time, through the entire arc, and at night that also is worse during use, replacement may be considered. Careful attention to technique and limited postoperative use, however, must be emphasized.

REFERENCES

1. Bryan, R.S., and Morrey, B.F.: Extensive posterior exposure of the elbow. A triceps-sparing approach. Clin. Orthop. **166:**188–192, 1982.
2. Coonrad, R.W.: Comments on the historical milestones in the development of elbow arthroplasty: indications and complications. AAOS Instructional Course Lectures **40:**51–55, 1991.
3. Dennis, D.A., Clayton, M.L., Ferlic, D.C., Stringer, E.A., and Bramlett, K.W.: Capitello-condylar total elbow arthroplasty for rheumatoid arthritis. J. Arthroplasty **5:**(Suppl):S83–S88, 1990.
4. Ewald, F.C., Scheinberg, R.D., Poss, R., Thomas, W.H., Scott, R.D., and Sledge, C.B.: Capitellocondylar total elbow arthroplasty. J. Bone Joint Surg. **62A:**1259–1263, 1980.
5. Goldberg, V.M., Figgie, H.E., III., Inglis, A.E., and Figgie, M.P.: Total elbow arthroplasty, current concepts review. J. Bone Joint Surg. **70A:**778–783, 1988.
6. Kashiwagi, D.: Intraarticular changes of the osteoarthritic elbow, especially about the fossa olecrani. J. Jpn. Orthop. Assn. **52:**1367–1382, 1978.
7. King, G., Morrey, B.F., and Adams, R.A.: Revision of aseptic failure of total elbow arthroplasty using a semi-constrained prosthesis. Unpublished data, 1995.
8. Kozak, T.K.W., Adams, R.A., and Morrey, B.F.: Total elbow arthroplasty in primary osteoarthritis of the elbow. J. Arthroplasty. **13:**837–842, 1998.
9. Minami, M., Kato, S., and Kashiwagi, D.: Outerbridge-Kashiwagi's method for arthroplasty of osteoarthritis of the elbow. 44 elbows followed for 8–16 years. J. Orthop. Sci. **1:**11–15, 1996.
10. Morrey, B.F.: Primary degenerative arthritis of the elbow. J. Bone Joint Surg. **74B:**409–413, 1992.
11. Morrey, B.F.: Degenerative arthritis of the elbow. *In* (ed.): Reconstructive Surgery of the Joints, 2nd ed. New York, Churchill Livingstone, 1996.
12. Morrey, B.F.: The future of elbow joint replacement. *In* Joint Replacement Arthroplasty. New York, Churchill Livingstone, 1991, pp. 375–382.
13. Morrey, B.F., and Adams, R.A.: Semiconstrained arthroplasty for the treatment of rheumatoid arthritis of the elbow. J. Bone Joint Surg. **74A:**479–490, 1992.
14. Morrey, B.F., and Adams, R.A.: Semiconstrained elbow replacement arthroplasty for distal humeral nonunion. J. Bone Joint Surg. **77B:**67–72, 1995.
15. Morrey, B.F., Adams, R.A., and Bryan, R.S.: Total replacement for post-traumatic arthritis of the elbow. J. Bone Joint Surg. **73B:**607–612, 1991.
16. Stanley, D.: Prevalence and etiology of symptomatic elbow osteoarthritis. J. Shoulder Elbow Surg. **3:**386–389, 1994.
17. Tsuge, K., and Mizuseki, T.: Debridement arthroplasty for advanced primary osteoarthritis of the elbow. J. Bone Joint Surg. **76B:**641–646, 1994.

CHAPTER 55

Complications of Elbow Replacement Surgery

• BERNARD F. MORREY

Complications after total elbow arthroplasty have been widely publicized and are well recognized. An explanation for the high incidence of complications rests on the fact that the elbow is a complex joint that is poorly covered by soft tissue, is intimately transversed by a major nerve, and is vulnerable to host-compromising conditions, such as rheumatoid arthritis and previously operated-on post-traumatic arthritis.

The majority of these complications neither require surgery nor adversely influence the ultimate result. Thus, these problems might best be discussed according to their management and significance: (1) those that increase the morbidity but do not influence the outcome by requiring additional surgery, removal, or replacement of the implant; and (2) those requiring additional surgery, including revision of the implant. Gschwend and colleagues,[21] in a recent review of the world's literature from 1986 to 1992, discussed 828 procedures. Of these, 43 percent had complications (Table 55–1). In this edition, the treatment of infection is discussed in detail in Chapter 56, and loosening and periprosthetic fractures are dealt with in the chapter on revision, Chapter 57. A detailed summary of the current literature regarding complications is given in Table 55–1.

COMPLICATIONS NOT USUALLY REQUIRING SURGERY

Motion Restriction

The goal of elbow replacement surgery is to obtain the functional arc of 30 to 130 degrees of flexion.[34] Those

• TABLE 55–1 • Complications of Elbow Replacement, 1986–1992

Complication	Incidence (%)*
Aseptic loosening	
Radiologic	17.2
Clinical	6.4
Infections	8.1
Ulnar nerve lesions	10.4
Instability	7 to 19
Disassembly	—
Dislocation	4.3
Subluxation	2.2–6.5
Intraoperative fractures	3.2
Fractures of prosthesis	0.6
Ectopic bone formation	—

*Total number of cases = 8.28.

rheumatoid arthritic patients who have the ankylosing type of disease tend not to obtain the typical 30 to 130 degrees of flexion-extension after surgery.[7] We therefore attempt to treat this motion restriction with an aggressive capsular resection at the time of the implantation. If the anterior capsule is contracted, sufficient depth of insertion is most important. A trial reduction is essential to identify this potential problem so that it can be avoided. Often, a static adjustable splint is used to gain or maintain motion. Further, a slight but consistently greater flexion contracture is observed with resurfacing designs (see Chapter 48).

Wounds

Wounds are much less a problem today[19] than the 5% incidence previously reported.[9, 13, 23, 36, 46]

Management. Wound healing problems are best avoided. At the Mayo Clinic, we avoid the use of the steri-drape after skin preparation with iodinated solutions, especially in patients with rheumatoid arthritis. I also use a straight incision just medial to the tip of the olecranon and carefully cauterize vessels during surgery. The elbow is placed in full extension with a compression/cryotherapy (Cryocuff Aircast) device, now used routinely.[1] If the wound remains tenuous at 1 week or 10 days, we do not hesitate to place the patient in a cast or anterior splint for 10 to 14 days and then reassess.[33] If severe wound necrosis occurs, surgical treatment may involve special soft tissue coverage, discussed in Chapter 37.

Neuritis

In patients with rheumatoid arthritis or in a joint that has been subjected to previous surgery, the ulnar nerve is particularly vulnerable. The incidence of ulnar nerve involvement has been reported in 2 percent[3] to 26[54] percent[13] of patients and varies in severity from profound neuropathy in less than 5 percent[9, 31, 49, 52] to transient paresthesias in as many as 25 percent.[21] Implicated causes are excessive traction, perineural or epineural hematoma, direct mechanical pressure during the procedure, and irritation by the bandage or from swelling. The possibility of thermal damage from juxtaposed methylmethacrylate may be considered, as well as devitalization during the translocation procedure. Review of the last 10 years' experience in the literature reveals an incidence of approximately 10 percent after almost 900 procedures.[21] We have found 3 percent subjective symptoms after 700 procedures. No patient has motor weakness.

Management. If profound motor weakness is present immediately after surgery and uncertainty about the neural status exists, the nerve should be explored. We have not yet had to do this. Our technique translocates the nerve; thus, little might be gained by another procedure. Sensory defects, especially if they are incomplete, usually will resolve spontaneously, and therefore re-exploration is not warranted.

Triceps Insufficiency

Triceps insufficiency is probably common, but it is not reported very often. The poor quality of the triceps tendon in patients with rheumatoid arthritis is well recognized, but only about 4 percent of rheumatoid patients have been recognized as having significant triceps insufficiency.[38, 39] The Mayo approach was developed because of this problem.[5] We have documented 13 of 700 (2 percent) since 1981.

Treatment. Triceps weakness is expected after any exposure that violates the extensor mechanism.[39] Today, most exposures reflect rather than transect the attachment. Reattachment is with heavy nonabsorbable No. 2 or No. 5 suture (Fig. 55–1).

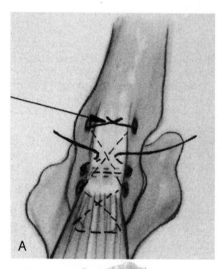

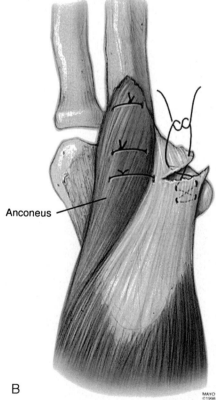

Anconeus

A

B

FIGURE 55–1 • *A,* Triceps reattachment technique used for both primary and reoperation procedures. *B,* An anconeus slide is used if the triceps attachment is deficient.

Ectopic Bone

Ectopic bone has been reported after total elbow arthroplasty.[15] Although some heterotopic ossification may be seen following elbow replacement, in our experience and opinion, this is a very rare complication that occurs only under unusual circumstances, such as in patients with severe degenerative arthritis.[26] We have observed only three cases of this problem after approximately 700 primary and revision total elbow replacements using several implant designs and exposures. In one patient, marked hypertrophic changes existed before surgery, extensive bleeding occurred after surgery, and moderate ectopic bone developed (Fig. 55–2).

Fracture

As greater experience is gained with elbow replacement, an increased incidence of fracture associated with elbow replacement is being observed. These may be classified in several ways, but for consistency the topic will be discussed in the next section.

COMPLICATIONS REQUIRING REOPERATION

As with all prostheses, reoperations may or may not require implant revision.

Nonreimplantation Revision Procedures

COMPONENT FAILURE

Stem. At the Mayo Clinic, we have observed an increasing frequency of ulnar component stem fracture, especially associated with traumatic arthritis in which near-normal activity is conducted after replacement (Fig. 55–3).[51] An incidence of approximately 1.8 percent has been observed at the ulna and less than 0.5 percent at the humerus. The cause of these fractures is due to the success of the initial replacement, which allows heavy use of the arm, and to the stress riser effect or to sintered titanium. Few cases of this kind of failure have been reported except with use of the Coonrad-Morrey component. Since 1994, this problem has not been observed, since the beaded surface finish has been removed from the ulnar component.

Articulation. Bushing wear has been a major problem with the GSB and triaxial device, occurring in frequencies of 12 percent with the Pritchard II prosthesis,[32] and in 5 percent of 173 GSB implants.[21] This is attributed primarily to instability and less to osteolysis. Recent modifications in both designs are hoped to decrease or eliminate this problem. At Mayo, we have had an increasing incidence of displacement of the locking ring (Fig. 55–4), but it is unusual to have the pin back out. A modification of a pin within a pin (see Chapter 49), approved by the Food and Drug Administration, should eliminate this problem.

Inglis and Pellicci reported 2 of 36 articular bushing failures in the early design of the triaxial semiconstrained prosthesis.[23] Pin backout had been a relatively common problem with the Pritchard-Walker implant in up to 5 percent.[36, 46] This is less a problem with the current Pritchard III design and has not occurred with the Coonrad device.

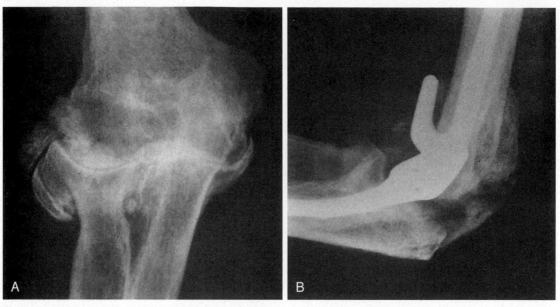

FIGURE 55–2 • A patient with hypertrophic osteoarthritis and motion from 60 to 90 degrees before surgery *(A)* developed marked hematoma and significant posterior ectopic bone *(B)*.

Component failure is rare in resurfacing implants, usually occurring as deformity, wear, or subluxation of the polyethylene.

Treatment. Articulation failure is treated by replacement of the bushing. The technique is usually not too demanding because the stable, remaining elements are left intact.[14] Replacement of a fractured stem requiring techniques used

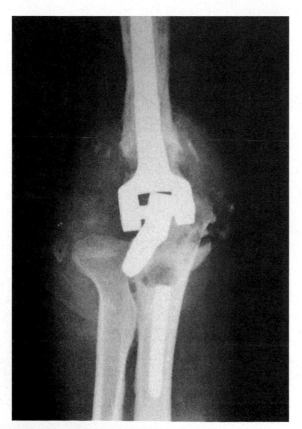

FIGURE 55–3 • Fracture of the ulnar component a full 3 years after surgery.

for failed femoral devices, while difficult, is usually successful (see Chapter 57).

WEAR

Until recently, total elbow implants have not been associated with excessive high-density polyethylene debris. The radial head has shown deformity and subluxation in the Mayo design and, more recently, in the resurfacing device designed by Pritchard. We noted significant problems due to metallic synovitis in the early design of the Mayo-modified Coonrad device. This is caused by particulate titanium being freed from the plasma spray surface as it is exposed to the local environment.

With increased longevity, an increased incidence of polyethylene wear was noted, at least for the Coonrad-Morrey device. This can be measured radiographically (Fig. 55–5). It has been observed in patients with survival in excess of 10 years[19] and in those with greater stress of the articulation, as with arthritis and instability underlying the process.[44, 57]

Treatment. The treatment for excessive wear of the articulation is simply to remove and replace the articulation. The goal is a complete cleansing of the joint of the particulate debris that elicits the adverse response. If the implant is loose and must be removed, care is taken that the intramedullary pseudomembrane is completely removed. The hallmark of the treatment of such a circumstance is to meticulously débride all of the metal- or polyethylene-laden soft tissues. Implant exchange is usually not required.

Complications Treated by Implant Removal

INFECTION

Sepsis after total elbow arthroplasty is more common than after any other replacement procedure.[37] A review of the

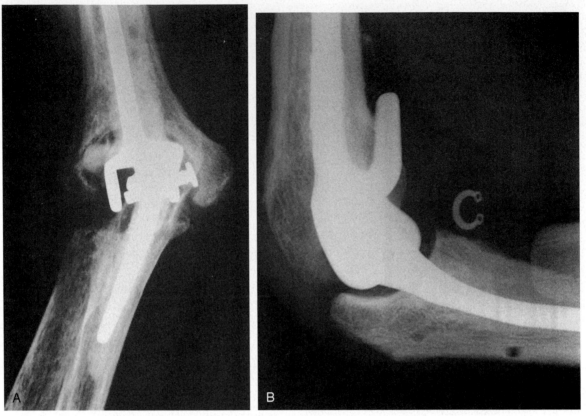

FIGURE 55–4 • Pritchard Mark II with pin failure *(A)*; "C" ring displaced with Coonrad-Morrey *(B)*.

literature suggests that infection with total elbow arthroplasty occurs in about 7 percent of cases for both types of implant design. Thus, 22 of 332 (7 percent) resurfacing implants have been reported as infected[9, 13, 31, 45, 49, 52, 54]; semiconstrained implants have developed this complication.[3, 4, 23, 37, 43] However, this is changing. Souter reported only one infection after over 100 procedures using antibiotic-impregnated cement (Souter, personal communication, 1980). Our infection rate decreased from about 8 percent[37] to less than 2 percent over the last 10 years. Although the diagnosis is not difficult (Fig. 55–6), the treatment is more challenging. This topic is a major one and is dealt with in a focused manner in Chapter 56.

REIMPLANTATION

Reimplantation is required for loosening and implant fracture and in some cases following deep sepsis.[57] If a resection arthroplasty is painful or if resection causes significant functional insufficiency due to gross instability (Fig. 55–7), then reimplantation may be considered. If performed for infection, the technique used is similar to those recommended for reimplantation of the septic knee and hip implant. If an implant fractures, we make no effort to remove all cement, but rather leave the cement mantle, if intact, and enlarge with a burr to remove the new device. Patients who have had resected joints may show significant shortening and must be prepared to accept this shortening. With the new longer flanged device, this should be less of an issue in the future. Also, patients should be advised that

their extensor mechanism may not actively extend the elbow.

Results. We have reimplanted eight fractured ulnar components; all are still functioning without loosening. Experience with the infected joint is discussed in Chapter 56.[57]

INSTABILITY

Instability after total elbow arthroplasty is a problem that is basically limited to resurfacing-type implants (see Chapter 48). Elbow instability following the use of resurfacing implants, either as frank dislocation or subluxation, occurs in approximately 10 percent of cases.[9, 12, 31, 49, 52, 54] All designs are valuable for treating this problem (Fig. 55–8). Subluxation occurs about twice as frequently as frank dislocation. Only about 20 percent of patients with instability will require surgical revision. Thus, instability requiring revision is seen in approximately 1 to 5 percent of the resurfacing devices.

Attempts have been made to improve the design and the surgical technique and, hence, to minimize this complication. It is disappointing to realize that even current reports continue to relate an instability rate of 7 to 8 percent.[9, 54] At Mayo we had 7 of 49 (14 percent) instability with the Capitello-condylar device (Johnson and Johnson). Attaining the proper balance of the soft tissue envelope is technically very difficult, and it requires a thorough understanding of the anatomy and biomechanics[25] and a meticulous surgical technique that preserves or restores the function and balance of both ligaments and muscles. Axial

Text continued on page 675

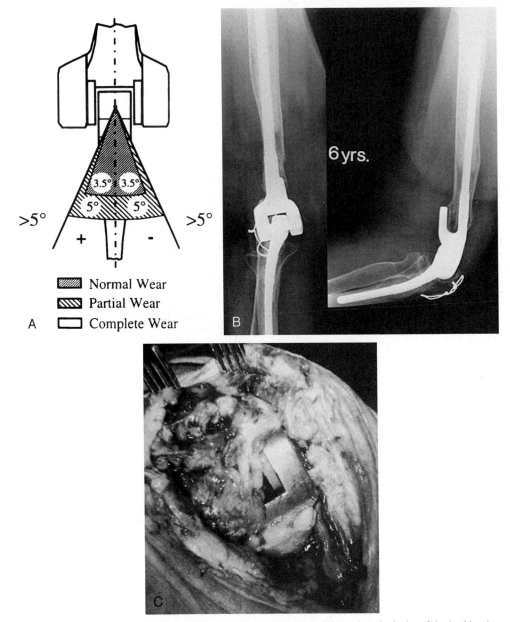

FIGURE 55-5 • Wear can be measured in semiconstrained total elbow arthroplasty (TEA) when the laxity of the bushing is excluded (A). High demand in male with resected distal humerus at 6 years (B). Particulate synovitis from both metal and ultrahigh molecular-weight polyethylene (UHMWPE) (C).

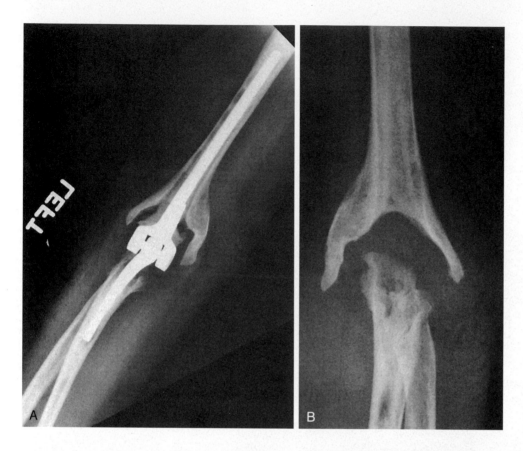

FIGURE 55–6 • Infected elbow (A). Reasonable function of the resection (B).

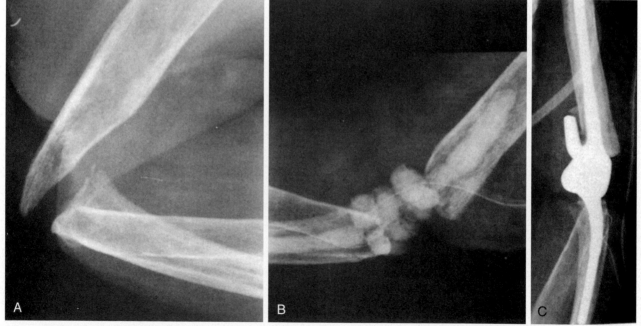

FIGURE 55–7 • A patient with infected total elbow arthroplasty underwent resection 8 years previously (A). Because of persistent and significant dysfunction, revision was performed first by using antibiotic-impregnated methylmethacrylate as a spacer and to treat the local tissues and medullary canal (B). Reimplantation was effectively accomplished (C).

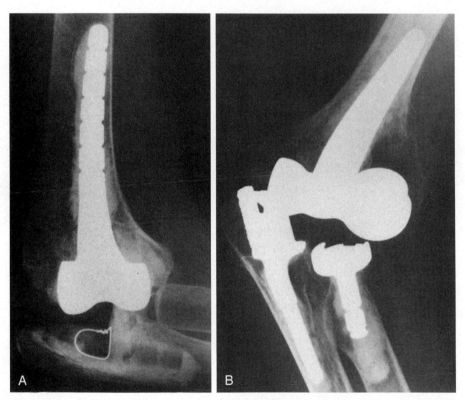

FIGURE 55–8 • Instability is seen with all resurfacing implants of a London device *(A)*, the three-part ERS device *(B)*, the Capitello-condylar device *(C)*, and Souter Strathclyde *(D)* and Kudo *(E)* devices.

Illustration continued on following page

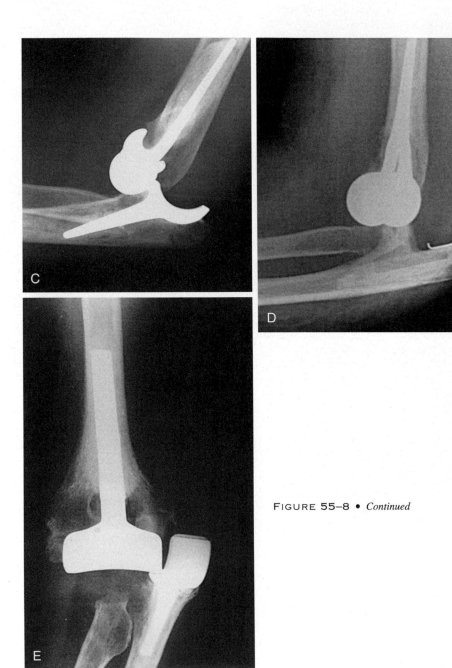

FIGURE 55–8 • *Continued*

malrotation of either the humerus or the ulna appears to be a crucial pitfall of the surgical technique.[25]

Treatment. A period of immobilization to avoid full extension may help eliminate or decrease the frequency of this problem.[45, 52] If the elbow has dislocated, immobilization in flexion of 90 degrees or more for 3 to 6 weeks is the most common treatment. If this does not render the joint stable, translatory instability is generally well tolerated. If symptomatic, soft tissue revision is usually not successful, and revision to a semiconstrained device is required in my practice.

LOOSENING

Loosening after total elbow arthroplasty is a well-publicized complication.[2, 4, 18, 20, 24, 35, 47] Our initial experience reveals that approximately 25 percent of the constrained hinged total elbow arthroplasties will loosen within 5 years.[35]

The three factors that have been identified to account for nonseptic loosening are joint mechanics, implant design, and surgical technique.

Biomechanics. The resultant force vector of up to three times body weight is directed anteriorly during dynamic flexion and posteriorly during extension of the joint.[22, 42] A cyclic compression-distraction loading pattern occurs up to 1 million cycles per year[8] (Fig. 55–9).

Prosthetic Design. Today, all devices are low friction metal and polyethylene. In addition, the semiconstrained design includes some play or laxity at the bushing, which has dramatically lessened the rate of loosening of total elbow arthroplasty.[3, 14, 32, 38, 43, 46, 50] The anterior flange of the Mayo-modified Coonrad device absorbs the load applied to the humerus (Fig. 55–10).

Surgical Technique. From the early experience, it is known that the cementing technique is directly correlated to the incidence of radiolucent lines. A stable interface is now reliably attained with intramedullary injecting systems (Fig. 55–11).

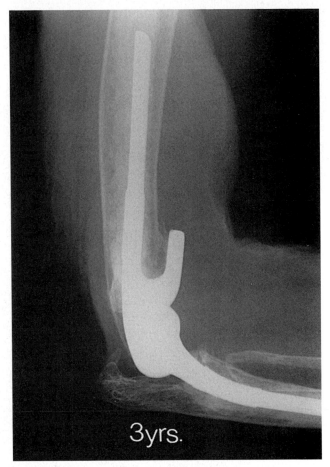

FIGURE 55–10 • The anterior flange absorbs the forces that otherwise cause loosening.

Current Data. As noted earlier, Gschwend and colleagues[41] reviewed the literature from 1986 to 1992, collecting 828 cases. From this sample, a loosening rate was defined as radiographic 17 percent, clinical 6 percent. Our own experience constitutes a group of approximately 500 semiconstrained implants, of which 60 percent were for rheumatoid arthritis. The loosening rate at 5 years is, surprisingly, less than 2 percent. Others have reported similar and improved loosening rates as well.[2, 3, 20, 23, 32, 43, 46] There is little question that loosening does not appear to be a major problem with the current generation of semiconstrained or resurfacing procedures in the rheumatoid population.[41]

Following trauma, we have reported a rate of loosening of less than 2 percent after 101 procedures followed for 5 years.[6, 40, 51] Gschwend and colleagues[21] note a loosening rate of 3 percent for rheumatoid arthritis and a radiographic rate of 6 percent for post-trauma arthritis.

Treatment. Loosening is less a problem, but the treatment remains a challenge (see Chapter 57). With aseptic loosening and bone resorption, revision should be offered. Options include removal of the implant, leaving a resection arthroplasty; revision to a different type of prosthetic replacement; fusion of the resected joint; and possibly cadaveric replacement of the resected elbow (see Chapter 58).

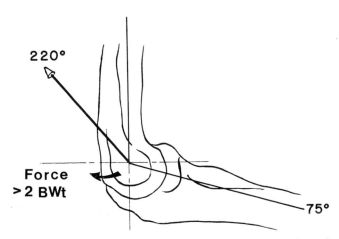

FIGURE 55–9 • Flexion-extension causes a cyclic compression and distraction load directed anteriorly, superiorly, and posteriorly. This severe loading condition accounts for loosening of the early, more constrained elbow replacement.

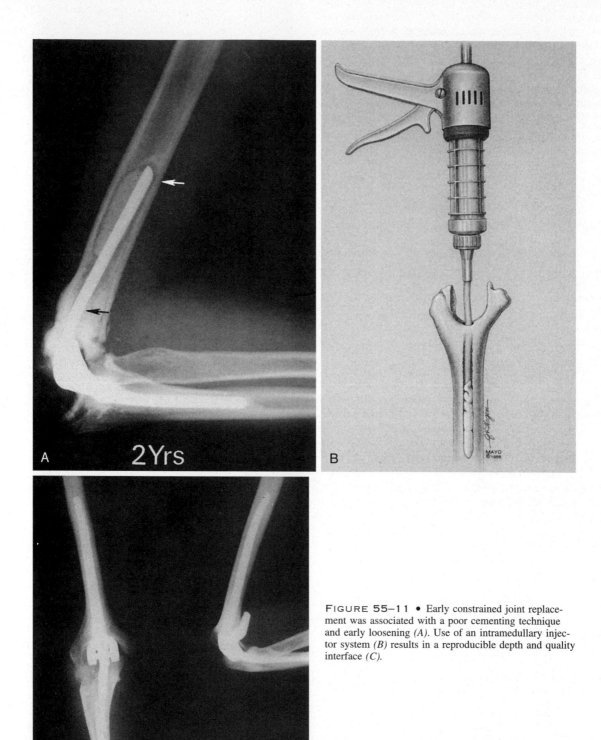

FIGURE 55–11 • Early constrained joint replacement was associated with a poor cementing technique and early loosening (A). Use of an intramedullary injector system (B) results in a reproducible depth and quality interface (C).

REFERENCES

1. Adams, R., Morrey, B. F.: The effect of cold compressive dressings after elbow surgery. AAOS Annual Meeting, Anaheim, CA, Feb. 4–8, 1999.
2. Bayley, J. I. L.: Elbow replacement in rheumatoid arthritis. Reconstr. Surg. Traumatol. 18:70, 1981.
3. Bell, S., Gschwend, N., and Steiger, U.: Arthroplasty of the elbow. Experience with the Mark III GSB prosthesis. Aust. N. Z. J. Surg. 56:823, 1986.
4. Brumfield, R. H., Volz, R. G., and Green, J. F.: Total elbow arthroplasty: a clinical review of 30 cases employing the Mayo and AHSC prostheses. Clin. Orthop. 158:137, 1981.
5. Bryan, R. S., and Morrey, B. F.: Extensive posterior exposure of the elbow: a triceps-sparing approach. Clin. Orthop. 166:188, 1982.
6. Cobb, T. K., and Morrey, B.F.: Use of distraction arthroplasty in unstable fracture dislocations of the elbow. Clin. Orthop. 312:201, 1995.
7. Conner P. M., Morrey, B. F.: Total elbow arthroplasty in patients who have juvenile rheumatoid arthritis. J. Bone Joint Surg. 80A(5):678, 1998.
8. Davis, P. R.: Some Significant Aspects of Normal Upper Limb Functions. Conference on Joint Replacement of the Upper Extremity. London, Institute of Mechanical Engineers, 1977.
9. Davis, R. F., Weiland, A. J., Hungerford, D. S., Moore, J. R., and Dowling, S. V.: Nonconstrained total elbow arthroplasty. Clin. Orthop. 171:156, 1982.
10. Dennis, D. A., Clayton, M. L., Ferlic, D. C., Stringer, E. A., Bramlett, K. W.: Capitello-condylar total elbow arthroplasty for rheumatoid arthritis. J. Arthroplasty 5(Suppl):S83, 1990.
11. Dee R.: Total replacement arthroplasty of the elbow for rheumatoid arthritis. J. Bone Joint Surg. 54B:88, 1972.
12. Ewald, F. C., and Jacobs, M. A.: Total elbow arthroplasty. Clin. Orthop. 182:137, 1984.
13. Ewald, F. C., Scheinberg, R. D., Poss, R., Thomas, W. H., Scott, R. D., and Sledge, C. B.: Capitellocondylar total elbow arthroplasty: two- to five-year follow-up in rheumatoid arthritis. J. Bone Joint Surg. 62A:125, 1980.
14. Figgie, H. E., III, Inglis, A. E., and Mow, C.: Total elbow arthroplasty in the face of significant bone stock or soft tissue losses. J. Arthroplasty 1:71, 1986.
15. Figgie, M. P., Inglis, A. E., Mow, C. S., and Figgie, H. E., III: Salvage of nonunion of supracondylar fracture of the humerus by total elbow arthroplasty. J. Bone Joint Surg. 71A:1058, 1989.
16. Fitzgerald, R. H., Jr., Nolan, D. R., Ilstrup, D. M., Van Scoy, R. E., Washington, J. A., II, and Coventry, M. B.: Deep wound sepsis following total hip arthroplasty. J. Bone Joint Surg. 59A:847, 1977.
17. Friedman, R. J., Lee, D. E., and Ewald, F. C.: Nonconstrained total elbow arthroplasty. Development and results in patients with functional class IV rheumatoid arthritis. J. Arthroplasty 4:31, 1989.
18. Garrett, J. C., Ewald, F. C., Thomas, W. H., and Sledge, C. B.: Loosening associated with GSB hinge total elbow replacement in patients with rheumatoid arthritis. Clin. Orthop. 127:170, 1977.
19. Gill DRJ, Morrey BF: The Coonrad-Morrey total elbow arthroplasty in patients who have rheumatoid arthritis. A ten to fifteen year follow-up study. J. Bone Joint Surg. 80A(9):1327, 1998.
20. Goldberg, V. M., Figgie, H. E., III, Inglis, A. F., and Figgie, M. P.: Total elbow arthroplasty. J. Bone Joint Surg. 70A:778, 1988.
21. Gschwend, N., Simmen, B. R., Matejovsky, Z.: Late complications in elbow arthroplasty. J. Shoulder Elbow Surg. 5(2)Part 1:86, 1996.
22. Hui, F. C., Chao, E. Y., and An, K. N.: Muscle and joint forces at the elbow during isometric lifting. [Abstract.] Orthop. Trans. 2:169, 1978.
23. Inglis, A. E., and Pellicci, P. M.: Total elbow replacement. J. Bone Joint Surg. 62A:1252, 1980.
24. Johnsson, J. R., Getty, C. J. M., Lettin, A. W. F., and Glasgow, M. M. S.: The Stanmore total elbow replacement for rheumatoid arthritis. J. Bone Joint Surg. 66B:732, 1984.
25. King, G., Itoi, E., Morrey, B. F., et al.: Motion and laxity of the capitellocondylar total elbow prosthesis. J. Bone Joint Surg. 76A:1000–1008, 1994.
26. Kozak, T. K. W.: Total elbow arthroplasty in primary osteoarthritis of the elbow: a brief report. J. Arthroplasty 13:837, 1998.
27. Kudo, H., Iwano, K., and Watanabe, S.: Total replacement of the rheumatoid elbow with a hingeless prosthesis. J. Bone Joint Surg. 62A:277, 1980.
28. Linscheid, R. L.: Resurfacing elbow joint replacement. In Morrey, B. F. (ed.): Joint Replacement Arthroplasty. New York, Churchill Livingstone, 1991.
29. Ljung, P. Lidgren, L., Rydholm, U.: Failure of the Wadsworth elbow:

19 cases of rheumatoid arthritis followed for 5 years. Acta Orthop. Scand. 60:254, 1989.
30. London, J. T.: Resurfacing Total Elbow Arthroplasty. Presentation. AAOS Annual Meeting, Atlanta, Georgia, February, 1980.
31. Lowe, L. W., Miller, A. J., Allum, R. L., and Higginson, D. W.: The development of an unconstrained elbow arthroplasty: a clinical review. J. Bone Joint Surg. 66B:243, 1984.
32. Madsen, F., Gudmundson, G. H., Sojbjerg, J. O., and Sneppen, O.: The Pritchard Mark II elbow prosthesis in rheumatoid arthritis. Acta Orthop. Scand. 60:249, 1989.
33. Maloney, W. J., and Schurman, D. J.: Cast immobilization after total elbow arthroplasty. A safe cost-effective method of initial postoperative care. Clin. Orthop. 245:117, 1989.
34. Morrey, B. F., Askew, L. J., An, K. N., and Chao, E. Y.: A biomechanical study of normal functional elbow motion. J. Bone Joint Surg. 63A:872, 1981.
35. Morrey, B. F., Bryan, R. S., Dobyns, J. H., and Linscheid, R. L.: Total elbow arthroplasty: a five-year experience at the Mayo Clinic. J. Bone Joint Surg. 63A:1050, 1981.
36. Morrey, B. F.: Complications of total elbow arthroplasty. In Morrey, B. B. (ed.) The Elbow and Its Disorders, 2nd ed. Philadelphia, W. B. Saunders Co., 1993.
37. Morrey, B. F., and Bryan, R. S.: Infection after total elbow arthroplasty. J. Bone Joint Surg. 65A:330, 1983.
38. Morrey, B. F.: The Elbow and Its Disorders. Philadelphia, W. B. Saunders Co., 1985.
39. Morrey, B. F., Askew, L. J., and An, K. N.: Strength function after total elbow arthroplasty. Clin. Orthop. 234:43, 1988.
40. Morrey, B. F., Adams, R. A.: Semiconstrained joint replacement arthroplasty for distal humeral nonunion. J. Bone Joint Surg. 77B(1):67, 1995.
41. Morrey, B. F., and Adams, R.: Semiconstrained total elbow arthroplasty for rheumatoid arthritis. J. Bone Joint Surg. 74A:479, 1992. My 103
42. Pearson, J. R., McGinley, D. R., and Butzel, L. M.: A dynamic analysis of the upper extremity: planar motions. Hum. Factors 5:59, 1963.
43. Pritchard, R. W.: Long-term follow-up study: semiconstrained elbow prosthesis. Orthopedics 4:151, 1981.
44. Ramsey, M. L., Morrey, B. F.: Instability of the elbow treated with semiconstrained total elbow arthroplasty. J. Bone Joint Surg. 81A:38, 1998.
45. Roper, B. A., Tuke, M., O'Riordan, S. M., and Bulstrode, C. J.: A new constrained elbow. A prospective review of 60 replacements. J. Bone Joint Surg. 68B:566, 1986.
46. Rosenfeld, S. R., and Ansel, S. H.: Evaluation of the Pritchard total elbow arthroplasty. Orthopedics 5:713, 1982.
47. Ross, A. C., Sneath, R. S., and Scales, J. T.: Endoprosthetic replacement of the humerus and elbow joint. J. Bone Joint Surg. 69B(4):652, 1987.
48. Rozing, P. M., Poll, R. G.: Use of the Souter-Strathclyde total elbow prosthesis in patients who have rheumatoid arthritis. J. Bone Joint Surg. 73A:1227, 1991.
49. Rydholm, U., Tjornstrand, B., Pettersson, H., and Lidgren, L.: Surface replacement of the elbow in rheumatoid arthritis. J. Bone Joint Surg. 66B:737, 1984.
50. Schlein, A. P.: Semiconstrained total elbow arthroplasty. Clin. Orthop. 121:222, 1976.
51. Schneeberger, A. G., Adams, R., Morrey, B. F.: Semiconstrained total elbow replacement for the treatment of posttraumatic arthritis and dysfunction. J. Bone Joint Surg. 79A:1211–1222, 1997.
52. Soni, R. K., and Cavendish, M. E.: A review of the Liverpool elbow prosthesis. J. Bone Joint Surg. 66B:248, 1984.
53. Souter, W. A.: Arthroplasty of the elbow: with particular reference to metallic hinge arthroplasty in rheumatoid patients. Orthop. Clin. North Am. 4:395, 1973.
54. Trancik, T., Wilde, A. H., and Borden, L. S.: Capitellocondylar total elbow arthroplasty. Two- to eight-year experience. Clin. Orthop. 223:175, 1987.
55. Trepman, E., Vella, I. M., and Ewald, F. C.: Radial head replacement in capitellocondylar total elbow arthroplasty. Two- to six-year follow-up evaluation in rheumatoid arthritis. J. Arthroplasty 6(1):67, 1991.
56. Wolfe, S. W., and Ranawat, C. S.: The osteoanconeus flap. An approach for total elbow arthroplasty. J. Bone Joint Surg. 72A(5):684, 1990.
57. Yamaguchi K. K., Adams R. A., Morrey B. F.: Infection after total elbow arthroplasty. J. Bone Joint Surg. 80A(4):481, 1998.

CHAPTER 56

Treatment of the Infected Total Elbow Arthroplasty

• KEN YAMAGUCHI and
BERNARD F. MORREY

Despite multiple improvements in total elbow arthroplasty, infection has remained a relatively common and potentially catastrophic complication with reported rates as high as 11 percent.[2, 4–6, 8–14, 18, 19, 22, 24, 25] The rate has decreased considerably, however, and is currently less than 2 percent in our practice.[12] Until recently, most reports have focused only on identification and characterization of infections.[9, 13, 14, 25] With little information on which to base treatment decisions, poorly functioning and sometimes painful excisional arthroplasty has been the procedure of choice.[9, 14, 25] More recently, treatment options that have allowed concurrent eradication of the infection with either prosthetic retention or reimplantation have been explored with relatively good results, especially at the knee and hip. The objective of this chapter is to review the evaluation and treatment of the infected total elbow arthroplasty. In particular, patient presentation including health profile, duration of symptoms, fixation of components, and bacteriology are discussed in relation to indications for various treatment strategies for the infected elbow arthroplasty (Fig. 56–1).

ETIOLOGY AND INCIDENCE

Since the initial reports on infections of total elbow arthroplasties the clinical presentation of these prosthetic infections has changed. Increased awareness of this complication has led to a high index of suspicion and hence earlier recognition.[9] However, even at 2 percent, the rate of infection for elbow arthroplasties remains well above that for the lower extremity arthroplasties, in part because of the high prevalence of severe rheumatoid arthritis or post-traumatic arthritis.[9, 14, 25] In addition to being immunocompromised, patients with rheumatoid arthritis often place a great deal of direct pressure on this subcutaneous joint. Those with post-traumatic arthritis frequently have undergone multiple operations that compromise the vascularity of the soft-tissues and thus increase the risk of wound healing complications.[9, 25] Risk factors for total elbow infections include rheumatoid arthritis, previous surgical procedures,[14] and previous local infections.[25] Delayed wound healing, wound drainage longer than 10 days postoperatively, and re-operation are prognostic factors associated with increased infection rates.[25]

The incidence of infections following total elbow arthroplasties appears to have declined with improvements in surgical techniques. Experience at the Mayo Clinic has shown a decrease in infection rate from initial report of 8 percent to a more recent incidence of about 2 percent.[12, 14, 26] In one recently reported long-term series of total elbow arthroplasty, there was no reported infections after the institution of routine use of antibiotic impregnated cement.[24] It appears that the use of antibiotic impregnated cement to implant the components as well as meticulous postoperative hematoma control has been helpful in lowering the incidence of infections. By protocol at the Mayo Clinic, postoperative elbows are kept in full extension for a period of 2 days with the arm elevated prior to the institution of range of motion exercises.

PATIENT PROFILE

Perhaps the most important consideration in treating a patient with an infected total elbow arthroplasty is the overall health status. The health status comprises both the patient's medical condition and his or her functional needs and expectations. Many patients with rheumatoid arthritis are medically debilitated owing to immunosuppressive medications, anemia of chronic disease, previous surgery, and, sometimes, poor nutrition. For these patients, the only

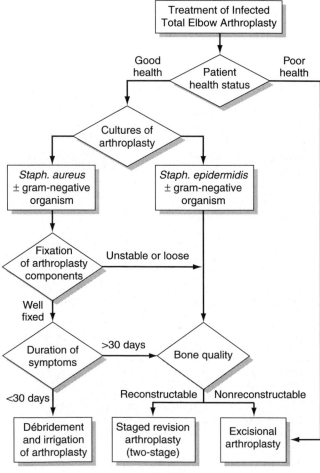

FIGURE 56–1 • Treatment algorithm for the infected total elbow.

goal for surgery may be a noninfected, pain-free elbow. The most appropriate treatment for these people may be resection arthroplasty. For others in relatively good health, preservation of function remains an important goal. Treatment of infection with arthroplasty preservation requires multiple surgical procedures and aggressive treatment associated with a high risk of complications. Thus, any treatment plan should be placed in the context of the patient's needs and abilities to withstand this treatment.

The clinical presentation of an infected total elbow arthroplasty may be subtle and only recognized by maintaining a high index of suspicion.[25] Systemic signs of sepsis (fever and tachycardia) may be absent,[14] with the patient complaining of increased pain or pain at rest. Acute inflammation is usually detectable by local signs such as the presence of warmth, erythema, and tenderness. In some patients, there may be drainage from the wound or soft tissues.[9, 14, 25] Those with an obvious infected bursa should be assumed to have a deep infection unless proven otherwise. These points become important in determining the onset and thus chronicity of an infection.

Preoperative evaluation is critical to establish range of motion, stability of the elbow, neurologic status, and function of the biceps and triceps muscles. Laboratory data may be of limited value, with most patients having a normal leukocyte count but an elevated neutrophil count on differential analysis.[14] The erythrocyte sedimentation rate (ESR) is often elevated but not specific, as many have systemic inflammatory disease. The definite step is to aspirate the joint (Fig. 56–2). Patients are considered infected when there are positive cultures or strong clinical suspicion (based on high white blood cell count, erythro-cyte sedimentation rate, operative observations, and so on) in the context of supportive microscopic pathology.

DURATION OF SYMPTOMS

Traditionally, infections have been classified according to length of time from surgery. An infection is considered acute if developed within 3 months of operation, subacute if presentation was between 3 months and 1 year, and late if recognition was after 1 year from surgery.[14, 25] The time interval from the index procedure to the development of infection has not been shown to correlate with infection results, however.[16] The duration of symptoms, as in the experience with total knee arthroplasty, has demonstrated a correlation with successful treatment by irrigation and débridement.[20] Therefore, delineating the onset of symptoms has correlated better with the onset of infection and has direct implications on the treatment strategy.

FIXATION OF COMPONENTS

The determination of component fixation in the context of infection is based on the initial radiographic assessment in conjunction with intraoperative findings. The quality of the fixation has been enhanced in recent years, and this is critical to the treatment protocol undertaken. High-quality and comparison radiographs are necessary for the detection of radiolucent lines, cortical erosions and osteolysis consistent with septic loosening of the prosthesis. Loose or poorly fixed components obviate treatment with component retention.

BACTERIOLOGY

As opposed to soft tissue infections, the microorganisms of implant infections are often difficult to eradicate and continue to be a significant problem. This has been demonstrated in total elbow infections in which the type of organism has had a profound impact on the treatment methods.[26] Organisms vary in virulence, adherence, and the elaboration of extracellular components. Many factors influence the adherence of bacteria to the prosthesis, including alterations in host immune competence and the ability of bacteria to produce an extracellular matrix.[3, 8] Studies of infected orthopedic implants have shown that up to 76 percent of the infectious microorganisms produce a significant biofilm extracellular matrix to improve adherence to the implant.[3] Of these, coagulase-negative staphylococci have been the most common and the most problematic biofilm producers.[8, 23] Unlike total hip and total knee replacements, the infection rate of elbow replacements with gram-negative microorganisms has been low.[26]

Coagulase-positive staphylococci (i.e., *Staphylococcus aureus*), which are more virulent microorganisms with the capacity to invade and infect healthy tissues, have a lesser ability to form a significant biofilm. Coagulase-negative staphylococcal organisms, particularly *Staphylococcus epidermidis*, has been recognized as the primary pathogen of orthopedic device infections owing to its unusual capac-

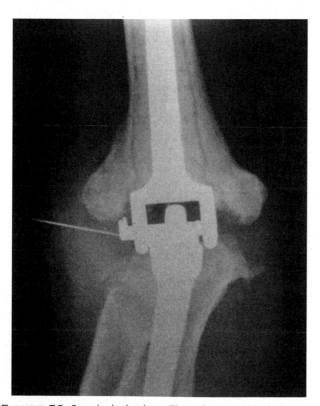

FIGURE 56–2 • Aspiration is readily performed and is the best method of providing an early diagnosis.

ity to attach to and to colonize orthopedic implants.[1, 8] Although a relatively nonvirulent pathogen that normally exists on the skin, it can form a tenacious bacterial biofilm ("slime")—a polysaccharide glycocalyx (protein plus carbohydrate) that envelopes the bacteria. This promotes colonization and adherence and protects the bacteria from desiccation and host defense mechanisms.[3] It also protects from antibiotic penetration and can even permit adherence to antibiotic-impregnated cement. This accounts for the persistence of *S. epidermidis* and its resistance to treatment.[8] Not surprisingly, the presence of *S. epidermidis* has thus been associated with high incidence of failure with attempted prosthetic retention with irrigation and débridement.[26]

TREATMENT OPTIONS

Once the diagnosis of an infected total elbow arthroplasty is suspected or confirmed, treatment is focused on the surgical intervention. In choosing a particular treatment plan, strong consideration must be given to (1) duration of symptoms, (2) the component fixation, (3) the bacteriology, and (4) the patient's health status (see Fig. 56–1). Debilitated patients unable to withstand the rigors of multiple surgical procedures are best served with an excisional arthroplasty. Irrespective of treatment chosen, the primary objective of treatment remains a long-term infection cure, which is dependent on the complete removal of the bacteria and its glycocalyx. A secondary concern is restoration of function. All treatment plans require a minimum 6-week course of intravenous antibiotics.

Irrigation and Débridement with Retention of the Components

The initial experience with irrigation and débridement with retention of the components resulted in poor outcomes, with most patients failing this treatment. Wolfe and coworkers[25] reported 8 failures in 11 patients with this technique, with the other 3 elbows deemed successes despite intermittent wound drainage. The Mayo Clinic's initial experience was similar, with only one of nine patients treated successfully. However, with increased awareness and earlier detection of infection, patients are often now seen acutely with well fixed components without apparent bone involvement. In the series by Wolfe and associates,[25] three of eight patients sustained fractures of the humerus or ulna with component removal.[25] In aseptic revisions, Morrey and Bryan[15] noted fractures in 11 of 33 subjects. These results exemplify the difficulty in removal of the components without compromising the bone structure and have renewed interest in component retention. Experience with infected total knee arthroplasty has demonstrated a high correlation between the duration of symptoms of infection (21 days or less) and outcome with component retention.[20] Using this principle of symptom duration less than 30 days, a recent study reports a 50 percent long term success rate (at a mean 71-month follow-up).[26] Further, bacteriology played a significant role, with all four patients infected by *S. epidermidis* failing this treatment protocol while six of eight were successfully eradicated of the *S.*

aureus infection.[26] Therefore, treatment with débridement and component retention is dependent upon both the duration of symptoms and the bacteriologic findings.

The indications for this treatment include (1) the presence of well fixed surgical components by both radiographic and intraoperative examination, (2) bacteriology suggests *S. aureus* or other pathogen amenable to this form of treatment, (3) a suitable soft tissue envelope with or without the use of flaps, (4) the patient medically fit to withstand the required multiple surgical procedures, and (5) duration of symptoms less than 30 days. A contraindication to component retention is an infection caused *S. epidermidis*.

The technique for irrigation and débridement with component retention is through a posterior approach utilizing the previous incisions.[26] The stability of the components is confirmed, followed by complete disarticulation of the components including removal of the bushings (Fig. 56–3). This is an essential component of the procedure. The joint is débrided of all necrotic debris and copiously irrigated with pulsatile saline lavage. Antibiotic-impregnated polymethyl methacrylate (PMMA) beads, with a concentration of 1 g tobramycin per package of cement, are placed in the wound prior to wound closure. Patients return to the operating room every fourth day for repeat irrigation and débridement with antibiotic PMMA bead exchange. The number of repeat irrigation and débridement procedures is variable but usually three or four required. The patient concurrently receives bacteria-sensitive intravenous antibiotics for a minimum period of 6 weeks (based on serum minimal inhibitory and bactericidal concentrations).[26] The use of chronic suppressive antibiotics is controversial and surgeon-dependent.

The overall success rate of the Mayo series reported by Yamaguchi and coworkers[26] was 50 percent but increased to 70 percent when those patients infected with *S. epidermidis* were eliminated. Outcomes produced good functional results but carried a 43 percent incidence of complication, including 21 percent incidence of wound breakdown or triceps avulsion and 21 percent with peripheral nerve injury.

Staged Exchange Arthroplasty

With the success of staged exchange arthroplasty for lower extremity infections,[17] this technique has been successfully used for infected total elbow arthroplasties. Yamaguchi and associates[26] report an 80 percent success rate at the Mayo Clinic with staged revision, with the only failures occurring in patients infected with *S. epidermidis*. Moreover, the mean increase in Mayo Elbow score was from 21 to 79, demonstrating good functional improvement. The procedure's success is dependent upon the complete eradication of the pathogenic microorganism necessitating the complete removal of all prosthetic components including PMMA.[27]

Although not yet well defined, the most common indications for staged exchange arthroplasty are (1) radiographic or intraoperative evidence of loose components with sufficient bone stock for reconstruction, (2) duration of symptoms longer than 30 days, and (3) a medically fit patient.

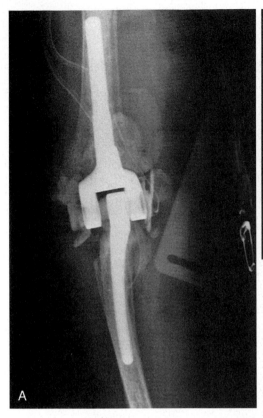

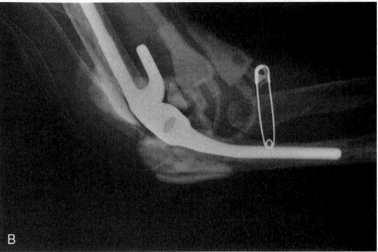

FIGURE 56–3 • *A* and *B*, Intraoperative radiograph from a representative patient who underwent successful irrigation and débridement. The patient presented with well-fixed components and symptoms of infection of 1 day's duration. The component was disarticulated with bushings and pin removal as an essential portion of the débridement procedure.

A relative contra-indication, dependent on the surgeon and the patient, is an infection caused by *S. epidermidis.*

Surgical technique utilizes the previous posterior incision to expose the joint, with considerations to flaps for soft tissue coverage (Fig. 56–4).[15, 26] Arthroplasty components along with all bone cement are meticulously débrided while preserving bone stock. Antibiotic-impregnated PMMA (tobramycin 1 g per package of PMMA) is then used as a spacer between the humerus and ulna to maintain soft tissue tension. The wound is closed and the limb is placed in a cast or hinged orthosis for 4 weeks. A concurrent 6-week treatment with sensitivity-specific intravenous antibiotics is initiated. Repeat irrigation, débridement, and biopsies of the tissues are performed as necessary. Consideration to longer staging intervals and repeat irrigation and débridement may be given to more resistant infections such as *S. epidermidis.* Arthroplasty reconstruction is performed at some point after 6 weeks using a long-stem semiconstrained arthroplasty with antibiotic-impregnated PMMA.[26]

Immediate Exchange Arthroplasty

There has been very minimal information regarding immediate exchange for infected total elbows. To date, only one case has been reported.[26] This case resulted in a failure to eradicate the infection.

The majority of the lower extremity experience has occurred in Europe with only anecdotal and early reports in North America. Success rates with immediate exchange arthroplasty for infected total knee replacements vary from 35 to 75 percent, with suggested improved results with gram-positive non–glycocalyx-producing organisms.[7, 21]

The indications for immediate exchange arthroplasty are probably very limited and at this time undetermined. The principles of the surgical treatment are similar to those of the staged revision with aggressive débridement with removal of all foreign material, antibiotic-impregnated cement fixation, and concomitant 6 to 12 weeks of intravenous antibiotics.

Resection Arthroplasty

Resection arthroplasty has been the standard of treatment for infected elbow arthroplasty and constitutes the largest treatment experience. Functional results are usually limited but can be associated with a high satisfaction rate. Moreover, with many of these patients debilitated, it is considered the treatment of choice for those medically frail and unfit for extensive or multiple surgical procedures. If successful, if often provides a relatively pain-free satisfactory range of active motion with reasonable stability (Fig. 56–5). This will more likely occur when the medial and lateral columns of the distal humerus are intact. If the elbow is flail or grossly unstable, the elbow is usually nonfunctional and often painful.

The technique of elbow resection arthroplasty involves removal of the implant components through the previous incision followed by complete removal of the PMMA. All necrotic and contaminated tissue is excised. If remaining intact, the condyles of the distal humerus are then contoured and deepened to encircle the ulna, The soft tissue coverage is established by primary closure or local rotation flaps. Concurrent treatment with 4 to 6 weeks of appropriate antibiotic therapy is used. The limb is placed in a

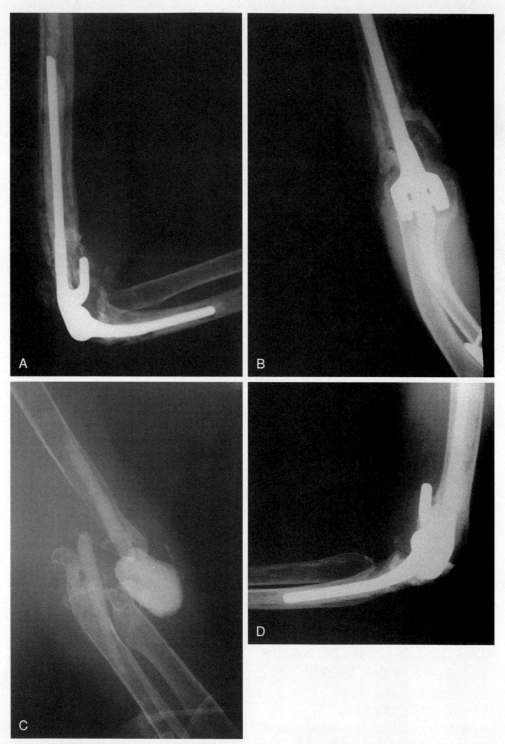

FIGURE 56–4 • Radiographs from a representative patient who underwent staged exchange arthroplasty. This 45-year-old male presented with a *Staphylococcus aureus* infection 68 months from the primary procedure. He had had 56 days of symptoms prior to presentation. *A* and *B,* AP and lateral radiographs of the elbow with scalloping of the cortical bone and prosthetic loosening consistent with infection. *C,* The component was removed, and antibiotic-impregnated cement placed. Seven weeks later, the patient underwent a reimplantation of a semiconstrained prosthesis with antibiotic-impregnated cement. *D,* At 64 months of follow-up, there are no signs of persistent infection.

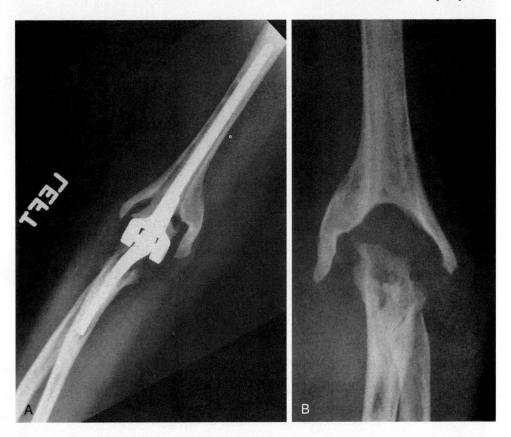

FIGURE 56–5 • A chronically infected joint *(A)* successfully managed by resection arthroplasty *(B)*.

cast or external fixator for 3 to 4 weeks to obtain soft tissue stability.

COMPLICATIONS

Treatment of the infected elbow requires multiple irrigation and débridement and hence the complications are as expected: fracture, triceps insufficiency, nerve injury, and skin or wound breakdown. Thus, special attention should be given to protect surrounding neurovascular structures as well as the triceps insertion and operative wound. Hence, special consideration should be taken using triceps-on approaches and proactive planning for possible soft tissue coverage procedures. Of course, the high risk of complications and the associated morbidity are significant considerations that have to be discussed with the patient before any prosthetic salvage strategy is attempted in the context of infected elbow arthroplasty.

CONCLUSION

Infection remains a significant and severe complication of total elbow arthroplasty with an incidence above that of lower extremity joint replacements. Previously, the only method of treatment option was excisional arthroplasty. Recent reports of this problem suggest that both irrigation and débridement and staged exchange arthroplasty can be successful treatment modalities given the appropriate indications (see Fig. 56–1). As such, selected treatment meth-

ods may improve both the functional and satisfaction rate of this most devastating complication.

REFERENCES

1. Blanchard, C. R., Sanford, B. A., Lankford, J., and Railsback, R.: *Staphylococcus epidermidis* biofilm formation on orthopaedic implant materials. Orthop. Trans. In press.
2. Brumfield, R. H., Jr., Kuschner, S. H., Gellman, H., Redix, L., and Stevenson, D. V.: Total elbow arthroplasty. J. Arthroplasty **5**:359, 1990.
3. Christensen, G. D., Baldassarri, L., and Simpson, W. A.: Colonization of medical devices. *In* Bisno, A. L., and Waldvogel, F. A. (eds.): Infections Associated with Indwelling Medical Devices, 2nd ed. Washington DC, American Society for Microbiology, 1994, pp 45–78.
4. Davis, R. F., Weiland, A. J., Hungerford, D. S., Moore, J. R., and Volenec-Dowling, O. T. R.: Nonconstrained total elbow arthroplasty. Clin. Orthop. Related Res. **171**:156, 1982.
5. Ewald, F. C., Simmons, E. D., Jr., Sullivan, J. A., Thomas, W. H., Scott, R. D., Poss, R., Thornhill, T. S., and Sledge, C. B.: Capitellocondylar total elbow replacement in rheumatoid arthritis: Long-term results. J. Bone Joint Surg. **75A**:498, 1993.
6. Figgie, M. P., Gerwin, M., and Weiland, A. J.: Revision total elbow replacement. Hand Clin. **10**:507, 1994.
7. Fitzgerald, R. H., and Nasser, S.: Infections following total hip arthroplasty. *In* Callaghan, J. J., Dennis, D. A., Paprosky, W. G., Rosenberg, A. G. (eds.): Hip and Knee Reconstruction. Rosemont, IL, American Academy of Orthopaedic Surgeons, 1995, pp 157–62.
8. Gristina, A. G.: Biomaterial-centred infection: Microbial adhesion versus tissue integration. Science **237**:1588, 1987.
9. Gutow, A. P., and Wolfe, S. W. Infection following total elbow arthroplasty. Hand Clin. **10**:521, 1994.
10. Kasten, M. D., and Skinner, H. B.: Total elbow arthroplasty: An 18-year experience. Clin. Orthop. Rel. Res. **290**:177, 1993.
11. Kraay, M. J., Figgie, M. P., Inglis, A. E., Wolfe, S. W., and Ranawat, C. S.: Primary semiconstrained total elbow arthroplasty. J. Bone Joint Surg. **76B**:636, 1994.

12. Morrey, B. F., and Adams, R. A.: Semiconstrained arthroplasty for the treatment of rheumatoid arthritis of the elbow. J. Bone Joint Surg. **74A:**479, 1992.

13. Morrey, B. F., and Bryan, R. S.: Complications of total elbow arthroplasty. Clin. Orthop. Rel. Res. **170:**204, 1982.

14. Morrey, B. F., and Bryan, R. S.: Infection after total elbow arthroplasty. J. Bone Joint Surg. **65A:**330, 1983.

15. Morrey, B. F., and Bryan, R. S. Revision total elbow arthroplasty. J. Bone Join Surg. **69A:**523, 1987.

16. Poss, R., Thornhill, T. S., Ewald, F. C., Thomas, W. H., Batte, N. J., and Sledge, C. B.: Factors influencing the incidence and outcome of infection following total joint arthroplasty. Clin. Orthop. Rel. Res. **182:**117, 1984.

17. Rand, J. A., Morrey, B. F., and Bryan, R. S.: Management of the infected total joint arthroplasty: Symposium on musculoskeletal sepsis. Orthop. Clin. North Am. **15:**491, 1984.

18. Rosenberg, G. M., and Turner, R. H.: Nonconstrained total elbow arthroplasty. Clin. Orthop. Rel. Res. **187:**154, 1984.

19. Ruth, J. T., and Wilde, A. H.: Capitellocondylar total elbow replacement: A long-term follow-up study. J. Bone Joint Surg. **74A:**95, 1992.

20. Schoifet, S. D., and Morrey, B. F.: Treatment of infection after total knee arthroplasty by débridement with retention of the components. J. Bone Joint Surg. **72A:**1383, 1990.

21. Thornhill, T. S.: Total knee infections. *In* Callaghan, J. J., Dennis, D. A., Paprosky, W. G., Rosenberg, A. G. (eds.): Hip and Knee Reconstruction. Rosemont, IL, American Academy of Orthopaedic Surgeons, 1995, pp. 297–300.

22. Trancik, T., Wilde, A. H., and Borden, L. S.: Capitellocondylar total elbow arthroplasty. Clin. Orthop. Rel. Res. **223:**175, 1987.

23. Van Pett, K., Schurman, D. J., and Smith, R. L.: Quantitation and relative distribution of extracellular matrix in staphylococcus epidermidis biofilm. J. Orthop. Res. **8:**321, 1990.

24. Weiland, A. J., Weiss, A. P. C., Wills, R. P., and Moore, J. R.: Capitellocondylar total elbow replacement. A long-term follow-up study. J. Bone Joint Surg. **71A:**217, 1989.

25. Wolfe, S. W., Figgie, M. P., Inglis, A. E., Bohn, W. M., and Ranawat, C. S.: Management of infection about total elbow prostheses. J. Bone Joint Surg. **72A:**198, 1990.

26. Yamaguchi, K., Adams, R. A., and Morrey, B. F.: Infection after total elbow arthroplasty. *J. Bone Joint Surg.* **80A:**481, 1998.

27. Yamaguchi, K., Adams, R. A., and Morrey, B. F.: Semiconstrained total elbow arthroplasty in the context of treated previous infection. J. Shoulder Elbow Surg. **8:**461, 1999.

CHAPTER 57

Revision of Failed Total Elbow Arthroplasty

• BERNARD F. MORREY and GRAHAM J. KING

A number of surgical options are available to treat failed elbow arthroplasty. In this chapter we emphasize the indications and the surgical techniques for prosthetic reimplantation of the joint. Allograft revision is also discussed. The general problems of failed elbow arthroplasty are first placed in perspective, and mention is made of other treatment possibilities that are more thoroughly reviewed elsewhere in this book (see Chapters 58 and 61).

FAILURE MODE

There are several ways of categorizing failed elbow arthroplasty, and they have markedly different implications for treatment. The first is failure of a nonimplantation procedure such as interposition or resection arthroplasty. This is a straightforward matter, and the treatment and characteristics are no different from those of a severe fracture with bone loss (see Chapters 23 and 24). In this chapter, we deal with failed total elbow arthroplasty, a condition of several causes: septic failure, device failure, instability, and loosening. The clinical presentation is a function of the type of failure, and factors that should be considered in both the assessment and the treatment decision process are highlighted in the following discussion.

Septic Failure

The real importance of this diagnosis is to exclude a septic process as the cause of implant failure. Radiolucency of the bone-cement interface may be due to either mechanical failure or sepsis, but implant loosening is not usually associated with a septic joint unless the process is a chronic one.[23] Infection of a well-fixed device is particularly bothersome, because removing the prosthesis may result in fracture of bone that poses major reconstructive problems for the surgeon. This topic was reviewed recently by Yamaguchi and colleagues[33] and is discussed in detail in Chapter 56.

Device Failure

Device failure may involve the stem or the articular coupling elements of the device. High-density polyethylene articular components have shown some tendency to fracture, but design changes have made this less of a problem

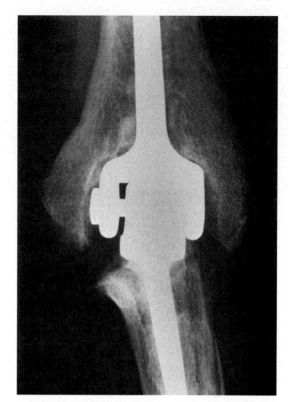

FIGURE 57–1 • Articular coupling mechanism failure with backing out of the transhumeral pin.

today. The articulation may dislocate in the snap-fit designs,[17, 28, 31] and the axis pin has backed out in a number of the devices (Fig. 57–1). Since the semiconstrained implant is being used for broader indications and loosening is much less of a problem, articular wear may well emerge as a major consideration over long-term follow-up.[15] Implant fracture is a rare complication that usually follows excessive activity or a single significant trauma. This has occurred with the Coonrad-Morrey device owing to the stress-riser effect of the surface treatment of the titanium implant and in patients with excessive physical demands (Fig. 57–2).[30]

Instability

With resurfacing prostheses, instability is not uncommon (see Chapter 55). Delayed or chronic subluxation is associ-

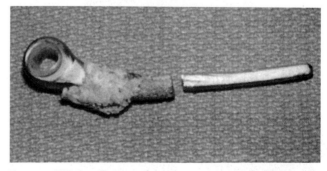

FIGURE 57–2 • Fracture of the ulnar component of a Mayo modified Coonrad device removed from a patient who repeatedly lifted more than 50 pounds.

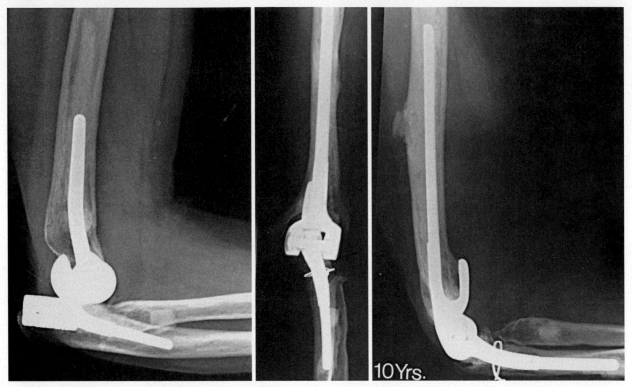

FIGURE 57–3 • Failure of the articulation due to instability of a resurfacing implant, as seen on lateral *(left)* and anteroposterior *(middle)* radiographs. The 10-year revision is asymptomatic *(right)*.

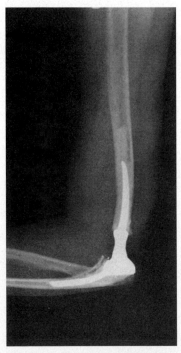

FIGURE 57–4 • The patient developed pain 18 years after a Dee total elbow arthroplasty. The radiograph did not suggest loosening of the bone-cement interface; however, at revision gross loosening was observed at the humeral prosthesis–cement interface.

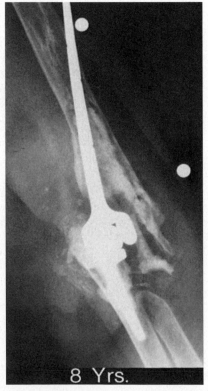

FIGURE 57–5 • Because the grossly loose Pritchard-Walker II implant was not painful, the patient continued to use it, but marked osseous resorption was due to the foreign body wear.

ated with either specific activities or simply flexion and extension of the elbow.[9, 23]

If acute instability of a resurfacing implant is due to excessive motion, revision may not be necessary. The elbow may be splinted or casted, and with periarticular scarring it becomes stable. If acute instability is due to ligament insufficiency and does not respond to a period of immobilization, revision with a semiconstrained implant should be considered. If early dislocation is due to malpositioning of the components, revision must be done. In questionable cases, examination under fluoroscopy may show the cause of the instability and allow the diagnosis to be made with ease (Fig. 57–3). Frank dislocation is usually posterior and is considerably more disabling than mediolateral translocation. Dislocation may or may not be painful; it often occurs early in the postoperative or perioperative period; and occasionally general anesthesia is required for reduction.

Loosening

The early experience with total elbow arthroplasty demonstrated loosening of the humeral component about twice as often as loosening of the ulnar component.[13, 18, 23] This difference is less obvious with the Coonrad-Morrey device: loosening occurs as often at the ulna as at the humerus.[15] Pain is a typical but not a universal feature. Three forms of presentation are recognized. One is a loose implant with pain but few or no x-ray changes and no bone resorption (Fig. 57–4). The second is gross instability and obvious loosening due to bone destruction, with minimal pain and sometimes none (Fig. 57–5). When particulate debris results in cortical thinning or "ballooning" of the humerus or the ulna, the prosthesis should be removed, even if it is not painful. Resorption of a significant amount of bone can pose major problems with the reconstructive procedure, especially when the bone loss is complicated by fracture (Fig. 57–6). The third presentation is acute fracture. Fractures that are not caused by loosening, such as those of the humeral condyle or the ulnar shaft, tend to heal and are not an indication for implant revision.

TREATMENT OPTIONS AND INDICATIONS

If the failure requires removal of the components, treatment possibilities may be categorized according to reimplantation and nonreimplantation types. A nonreimplantation option depends largely on the amount of bone present (Fig. 57–7 and Table 57–1); however, the amount of distal bone present is relatively unimportant if reimplantation is to occur.

Nonreimplantation Salvage Procedures

ARTHRODESIS

In our judgment, arthrodesis is rarely indicated for the elbow under any circumstances, because there is really no optimal position for a stiff elbow (see Chapter 5).[20, 27] Furthermore, if bone stock is adequate to allow the

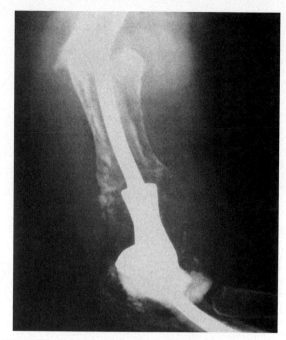

FIGURE 57–6 • A loose Dee implant remained reasonably functional and caused minimal pain; however, the osseous resorption allowed fracture of the proximal aspect of the humeral stem.

arthrodesis, a simple resection arthroplasty probably would also be effective and would provide a functional result.[10, 16] On the other hand, with gross bone loss, arthrodesis is technically more difficult than reimplantation. Elbow arthrodesis is discussed in detail in Chapter 61.

INTERPOSITION ARTHROPLASTY

Several types of interposition arthroplasty are described and may be indicated, depending on the amount of available bone and the presence of sepsis.[4] Chapter 60 discusses interposition arthroplasty, and Chapter 58 reviews nonimplantation salvage procedures for failed elbow replacement.

RESECTION ARTHROPLASTY

Resection arthroplasty is indicated in the presence of a septic prosthesis (see Chapter 68). If the articular substrate is present, resection and distraction arthroplasty may be considered.[10] If bone columns are preserved, a "tongue-and-groove"–type salvage procedure might be considered. Resection arthroplasty is otherwise a devastating event

• TABLE 57–1 • Revision Options as a Function of Bone Stock	
Bone Stock	**Options**
Adequate	Arthrodesis, resection, interposition, total elbow arthroplasty, semiconstrained prosthesis
Inadequate	Resection, allograft, total elbow arthroplasty, semiconstrained (long-flanged) prosthesis composite (total elbow arthroplasty with allograft), custom-made prosthesis

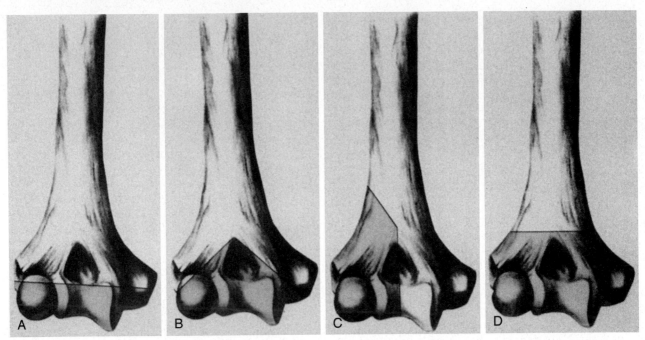

FIGURE 57–7 • A useful classification of bone loss. *A,* Type I involves the articulation, but excellent bone stock remains. *B,* In type II, both supracondylar columns are intact. *C,* In type III, one or the other supracondylar column and articular surface are gone. *D,* In type IV, the entire articulation and supracondylar columns are deficient at the level of or above the olecranon fossa. (From Morrey, B. F., Adams, R. A., and Bryan, R. S.: Total elbow replacement for post-traumatic arthritis. J. Bone Joint Surg. **73B**:607, 1991.)

because of the resultant dysfunctional instability, even in the absence of pain, and the need for an indefinite period of bracing.

Reimplantation Options

Three reconstructive options preserve or restore elbow joint function: prosthetic and allograft replacement and a combination of the two.

PROSTHETIC REIMPLANTATION

In most practices, the vast majority of loose-stemmed implants are revised by implant reinsertion. The Coonrad-Morrey implant has is made with 6- and 8-inch humeral stems, either of which may be used for this purpose, depending on the amount of available bone and the need for long-stemmed fixation (Fig. 57–8). An extended ulnar component is available for problems of proximal ulnar bone deficiency (Fig. 57–9).

Indications. Reimplantation is indicated for removal of a resurfacing or semiconstrained prosthesis in a nonseptic joint, ideally in an older patient who has some bone stock with which the surgeon can work. The majority of our patients fall into this category.

Considerations. Revision strategies can be predicated according to the characteristics of the failure mode. We have found the thought process used for failed femoral components to be helpful in this regard. In addition to age, diagnosis, and anticipated use level, the factors that determine the pertinent strategy include these:

• Humeral: (1) presence of distal humerus referable to the olecranon fossa; (2) quality of periprosthetic bone; (3)

presence and location of the fracture; (4) presence of a shoulder lesion.
• Ulnar: (1) presence of olecranon; (2) quality of periprosthetic bone; (3) presence and location of the fracture.

Furthermore, the revision must overcome the shortcomings of the first prosthesis or technique and the effect of the loose implant noted earlier. This usually demands a stem that bypasses any cortical weakness or fracture, provisions for adequate distal humeral or ulnar fixation, and a reliable articulation. Bone grafting of any cortical defect and biologic fixation of the revision device are also desirable features in a revision design as dictated by the presentation factors. Unless these measures are taken, reimplantation will not be successful. It must be re-emphasized that, if reimplantation is to be considered a viable option, the mechanical or biologic causes of the initial failure must be addressed and solved by the new design and technique.

Semiconstrained Revision Implant Design. The Coonrad-Morrey elbow replacement has in our practice been an ideal option for the resected joint after failed total elbow arthroplasty or after trauma. The range of sizes and lengths of the humeral (see Fig. 57–8) and ulnar (see Fig. 57–9) components is a most useful feature. Furthermore, the anatomic axis of rotation is restored even with resection at the level of the roof of the olecranon fossa (Fig. 57–10). Shortening of the humerus of up to 2 cm proximal to the olecranon fossa is accepted without resorting to allograft augmentation or the need for a custom implant.[12, 17, 28] Long-flanged implants have been very valuable as they allow various depths of insertion. If the bone loss is greater than the long flange can accommodate, either a custom implant or a component reconstruction with an interposed distal humeral allograft may be considered. The particular

fo
na
is

R
g
th
n
a
c
o
d
c
5
i
p
l

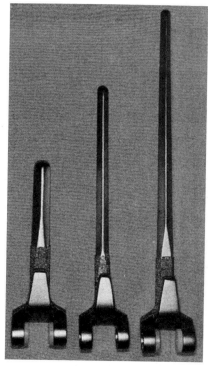

FIGURE 57–8 • Morrey-Coonrad implants are made with 10-, 15-, and 20-cm humeral stems, so routine use of custom implants is unnecessary.

value of the design of the Coonrad-Morrey device is that the intramedullary cement fixation is enhanced by an extramedullary bone graft placed behind the flange. This flange design resists forces that tend to displace the implant posteriorly as well as rotatory forces (Fig. 57–11). For most applications, we have resorted to using a longer flange, grafting bone behind the flange, and inserting the implant to less than its full depth (Fig. 57–12).

Preoperative Planning

The factors noted above should be specifically considered before reimplantation revision of failed total elbow arthroplasty. Successful intervention requires careful planning to address deficiencies, to anticipate potential complications, and to make available all the options that may be required at the time of surgery. The broad scope of preoperative planning includes these considerations:

1. Assessment of bone quality, the potential for injury to the bone at the time of revision, and the contribution of the native bone to fixation of the revised device. We have classified distal humeral osseous deficiency according to involvement of the columns (see Fig. 57–7). This is important as a consideration of the viability of a resection salvage procedure; however, more important is the quality of the periprosthetic bone and the presence or absence of fracture.

2. Ensuring availability of the appropriate array of tools necessary to remove both the components and the cement, especially if the device was inserted at another institution.

3. Preparation of the iliac crest or availability of banked bone if bone supplementation is required.

4. Ensuring that external fixation or distraction devices are available if needed.

5. Having the prosthesis available in several sizes if reimplantation is considered. A long-stemmed device is desirable for many revisions.[3, 23]

6. Assessing the possible need for special soft tissue coverage.

Technique

The technique of revision is next discussed in detail, with an overview that considers the pitfalls of the surgical procedure.

SKIN EXPOSURE

Skin coverage in this group of patients is sometimes compromised, even at the time of the initial procedure. Use of the previous incision is recommended, if possible. Skin flaps should be kept to a minimum (see Chapter 37). A local or a remote pedicle flap may be necessary to ensure adequate wound healing. In certain cases, preoperative discussion with a microsurgeon or a plastic surgeon is particularly helpful.

ULNAR AND RADIAL NERVES

In our opinion, the ulnar nerve must routinely be identified in the revision procedure. In many instances, it will already have been transferred anteriorly; nevertheless, it must be properly identified and protected during the procedure. If ulnar neuropathy is already present and is a significant problem, decompressing the nerve and freeing it of scar

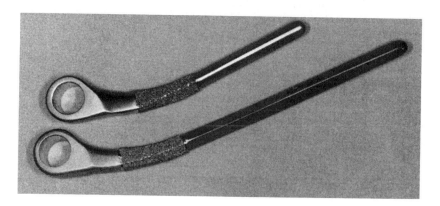

FIGURE 57–9 • A special long-stemmed ulnar component is used as an intramedullary rod when the ulna has fractured.

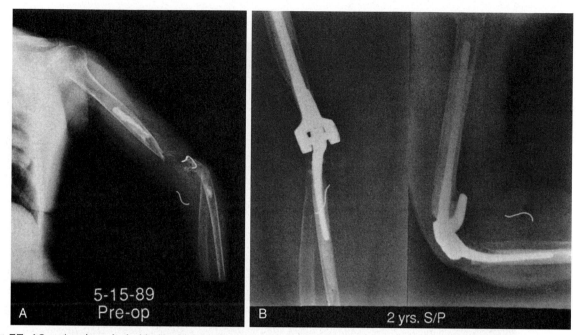

FIGURE 57–18 • A patient who had had multiple surgical procedures had a flail extremity for more than a year. *A,* The soft tissues were mark-edly contracted, making an augmentation procedure not only difficult but of questionable functional value. *B,* Shortening was accepted, and the elbow was replaced with the flange device without bone augmentation. The patient has had an excellent result and an arc of motion from 0 to 140 degrees. Note incorporation of bone graft behind the flange.

COMPOSITE ALLOGRAFT AND IMPLANT RECONSTRUCTION

Nothing has been published on composite allograft and implant reconstruction, but we have had several occasions to employ the semiconstrained implant with an allograft to salvage joints with marked bone deficiency. Humeral bone loss of 2 to 3 cm above the olecranon fossa is treated with reinsertion without augmentation. Greater shortening can be accepted if the soft tissues have contracted (Fig. 57–18). Composite allograft replacement (Fig. 57–19) is preferable

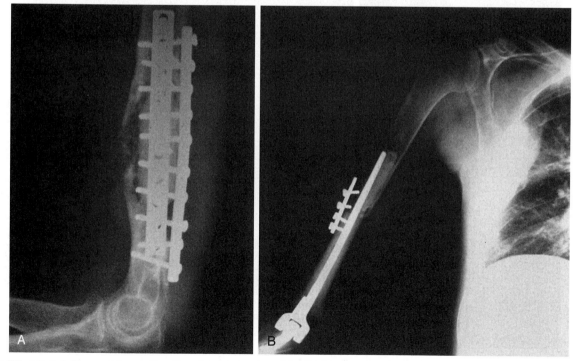

FIGURE 57–19 • *A,* Recurrent tumor after allograft reconstruction of the distal humerus. *B,* Resection of the distal two thirds of the humerus was accommodated by an allograft composite with a 20-cm humeral stem. Note plate used to control rotation until the allograft heals to the host bone.

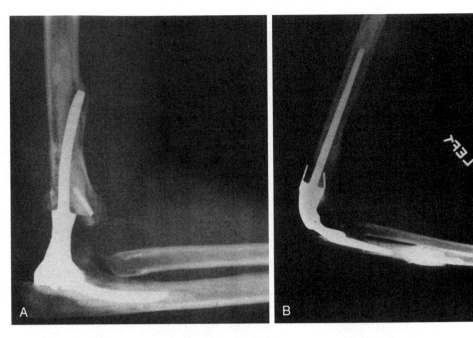

FIGURE 57–20 • Early failed Dee implant (*A*) was treated with a custom implant employing a long stem and flange (*B*). The revision was successful for 10 years.

if the shortening will have marked functional or cosmetic consequences. The technique is the same as at the hip with cement fixation in the allograft; however, we also cement proximally because otherwise rigid fixation is not possible. A plate with single cortical screws placed into the cement and a bone graft are essential (see Fig. 57–19). Our results to date are encouraging, although this procedure is problematic in that biologic fixation of the flange to the allograft probably does not occur. Thus, resistance to torsional stress is reduced. Success is predicated on the ultimate healing of the allograft–host bone interface. Nonetheless, in extreme cases, this is a very viable procedure that can be performed in a single session or as a staged procedure.

CUSTOM IMPLANT REPLACEMENT

When extensive bone loss either cannot be restored by allograft or composite allograft augmentation or when that option is not appealing, custom implant replacement is indicated. Even when carefully planned and designed, the custom implant often does not fit as well as might be desired, its fabrication is difficult to arrange from a timing perspective, and the device is expensive (Fig. 57–20).

Since a custom implant has been used mainly to compensate for marked bone loss,[12, 29] this option is less attractive today because a partially seated long-flanged device or allograft reconstruction in conjunction with the joint replacement is more often performed (see Fig. 57–20). Nonetheless, some excellent long-term successes have been reported in the past.[29]

The acceptance of custom implants is limited by the extremely high cost and delay in manufacture. The uncertainty of success, as a result of the occasional misfit, sometimes renders them unattractive in our practice. Currently, in my judgment, the only use for a custom or special design relates to length-bridging defects in the ulna caused by the loose stem of an earlier implant (Fig. 57–21).

Results

Ross and associates reported on 26 patients with significant bone loss from malignancy or trauma, three of whom had failed total elbow arthroplasties. Custom implants with a rigid articulation were associated with an infection rate of 11 percent and a loosening rate of 11 percent.[29] The implant

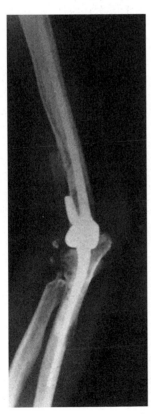

FIGURE 57–21 • Fracture of the ulna at the tip of the previous ulnar component was stabilized with a special long-stemmed ulnar device.

reconstruction of the elbow with massive bone loss. Long term results. Clin Orthop **341**:12–22, 1997.

5. Dee, R.: Revision surgery after failed elbow endoprosthesis. *In* Inglis, A.E. (ed.): Upper Extremity Joint Replacement (Symposium on Total Joint Replacement of the Upper Extremity, 1979). St. Louis, C.V. Mosby Co., 1982.

6. Dee, R.: Reconstructive surgery following total elbow endoprosthesis. Clin. Orthop. **170**:196, 1982.

7. Dee, R., and Ries, M.: Nonprosthetic elbow reconstruction. Contemp. Orthop. **14**:37, 1987.

8. Dent, C.M., Hoy, G., and Stanley, J.K.: Revision of failed total elbow arthroplasty. Adv. Orthop. Surg. **20**:172–173, 1996.

9. Ewald, F.C., Scheinberg, R.D., Poss, R., Thomas, W.H., Scott, R.D., and Sledge, C.B.: Capitellocondylar total elbow arthroplasty: two- to five-year follow-up in rheumatoid arthritis. J. Bone Joint Surg. **62A**:1259, 1980.

10. Ewald, F.C.: Distraction arthroplasty. Presented at the Annual Meeting of the Society of Shoulder and Elbow Surgeons, Rochester, NY, November 1983.

11. Ferlic, D.C., and Clayton, M.L.: Salvage of failed total elbow arthroplasty. J. Shoulder Elbow Surg. **4**:290–297, 1995.

12. Figgie, H.E., Inglis, A.E., and Mow, C.: Total elbow arthroplasty in the face of significant bone stock or soft tissue losses: preliminary results of custom-fit arthroplasty. J. Arthroplasty **1**:71, 1986.

13. Figgie, H.E., Inglis, A.E., Ranawat, C.S., and Rosenberg, G.M.: Results of total elbow arthroplasty as a salvage procedure for failed elbow reconstructive operations. Clin. Orthop. **219**:185, 1987.

14. Figgie, M.P., Inglis, A.E., Mow, C.S., Wolfe, S.W., Sculco, T.P., and Figgie H.E., III: Results of reconstruction for failed total elbow arthroplasty. Clin Orthop **253**:123–132, 1990.

15. Gill, D., and Morrey, B.F.: The Coonrad-Morrey total elbow arthroplasty in patients who have rheumatoid arthritis: A 10- to 15-year follow-up study. J. Bone Joint Surg. **80**:1327–1335, 1998.

16. Gschwend, N.: Salvage procedure in failed elbow prosthesis. Arch. Orthop. Trauma Surg. **101**:95, 1983.

17. Inglis, A.E., and Pellicci, P.M.: Total elbow replacement. J. Bone Joint Surg. **62A**:1252, 1980.

18. Inglis, A.E.: Revision surgery following a failed total elbow arthroplasty. Clin. Orthop. **170**:213, 1982.

19. King, G.J.W., Adams, R.A., and Morrey, B.F.: Total elbow arthroplasty: revision with use of a non-custom semiconstrained prosthesis. J. Bone Joint Surg. **79A**:394–400, 1997.

20. Koch, M., and Lipscomb, P.R.: Arthrodesis of the elbow. Clin. Orthop. **50**:151, 1967.

21. Mankin, H.J., Doppelt, S., and Tomford, W.: Clinical experience with allograft implantation: the first ten years. Clin. Orthop. **174**:69, 1983.

22. Morrey, B.F., Adams, R.A., and Bryan, R.S.: Total elbow replacement for post-traumatic arthritis. J. Bone Joint Surg. **73B**:607, 1991.

23. Morrey, B.F., and Bryan, R.S.: Complications of total elbow arthroplasty. Clin. Orthop. **170**:204, 1982.

24. Morrey, B.F., and Bryan, R.S.: Prosthetic arthroplasty of the elbow. *In* Chapman, M. (ed.): Surgery of the Musculoskeletal System. Vol. 3, No. 2. New York, Churchill Livingstone, 1983, p. 273.

25. Morrey, B.F., and Bryan, R.S.: Revision total elbow arthroplasty. J. Bone Joint Surg. **69A**:523, 1987.

26. O'Driscoll, S., and Morrey, B.F.: Periprosthetic fractures about the elbow. Orthop. Clin. North Am. **30**:319–325, 1999.

27. O'Neill, O.R., Morrey, B.F., Tanaka, S., and An, K.N.: Compensatory motion in the upper extremity after elbow arthrodesis. Clin. Orthop. Aug **(281)**:89–96, 1992.

28. Rosenfeld, S.R., and Anzel, S.H.: Evaluation of the Pritchard total elbow arthroplasty. Orthopedics **5**:713, 1982.

29. Ross, A.C., Sneath, R.S., and Scales, J.T.: Endoprosthetic replacement of the humerus and elbow joint. J. Bone Joint Surg. **69B**:652, 1987.

30. Schneeberger, A.G., Adams, R., and Morrey, B.F.: Semiconstrained total elbow replacement for the treatment of posttraumatic arthritis and dysfunction. J. Bone Joint Surg. **79A**:1211–1222, 1997.

31. Urbaniak, J.R., and Black, K.E., Jr.: Cadaveric elbow allografts: a six-year experience. Clin. Orthop. **197**:131, 1985.

32. Volz, R.G.: Total elbow arthroplasty. *In* American Academy of Orthopedic Surgeons Continuing Education Course. The Upper Extremity. Tucson, February 1983.

33. Yamaguchi, K., Adams R. A., and Morrey, B.F.: Infection after total elbow arthroplasty. J Bone Joint Surg. **80A**:481–491, 1998.

CHAPTER 58

Nonimplantation Salvage of Failed Reconstructive Procedures of the Elbow

• ROGER DEE

Refinement of the technical methods of open reduction and internal fixation of severe intra-articular fragments involving the elbow joint has continued to improve the prognostic expectations of patient and surgeon. Secure and accurate surgical reconstruction of the shattered fragments of the articulation in such fractures permits early motion and better functional outcomes (see Chapter 23).

Two common residual problems may follow such injuries. The first of these is dysfunctional stiffness and the second is instability associated with major bone loss.

THE STIFF ELBOW

As noted in Chapter 33, the stiff elbow can result from a technical error, such as failure to correct articular incongruity. It may follow an injury in which there was extensive shearing or a crushing-type injury to the periarticular soft tissues. Other causes include the development of joint infection and an extended period of joint immobilization. Myositis ossificans or ectopic bone formation may occur around the joint in such conditions as severe burns or prolonged coma (see Chapter 32).

Provided that the articular surfaces are congruous and the cartilage is healthy, there are well-described soft tissue procedures to restore motion in these joints.[30, 36] When the elbow has been stiff for a period exceeding several months or years and is completely ankylosed or when there is loss of articular cartilage, some kind of interpositional arthroplasty is recommended (see Chapter 60).

Interpositional Arthroplasty

Interpositional arthroplasty has a long history, and numerous materials—such as fascia,[21, 23] muscle,[3] fat,[17, 34] silicone rubber,[31] and even animal membrane[1] have been used with some success. My own preference is for cutis arthroplasty. This technique is described elsewhere in this book (see Chapter 66). I have modified the technique described by Froimsen and colleagues.[12] My surgical approach is to utilize a transolecranon osteotomy after carefully dissecting the ulnar nerve out of harm's way from above the medial humeral condyle as far distally as the coronoid. This provides good access to the front and back of the humerus, which is particularly important when it is necessary to remove ectopic bone.

Old hardware, particularly that which impinges on the articular surface, must be removed. Nonunion of humeral condyles requires stabilization by internal fixation prior to the application of the graft.

We skim off a thin epidermal layer from the donor site, which is usually in the groin, and then utilize the underlying thick dermal graft, which is defatted and then harvested. The epidermis is discarded and the donor area sutured back as a linear scar after the surrounding soft tissues are mobilized. The cutis graft is applied with its deep surface facing the bone. It is sutured under light tension to the front and back of the distal humerus with through-and-through drill holes. If the radiocapitellar joint is normal, it is not resurfaced, and care is then taken to preserve the lateral ligamentous complex and the annular ligament. The skin graft in such cases is attached to the humerus at the margins of the capitellum. Usually, however, both components of the joint require resurfacing.

BONY FUSION

In some patients, the joint space is preserved and is easily detected when ectopic bone is removed (see Chapter 32). When taking down a bony fusion of long standing in which the articular surfaces have fused, it is important to have a good three-dimensional knowledge of the normal articular anatomy so that by using gouges and osteotomies, some resemblance to the normal sculptured shape of the lower humerus and ulna can be restored. In many elbows, no recognizable ligamentous structures can be preserved despite careful subperiosteal dissection. In these cases, it is critically important to make sure that the insertion of brachialis into the ulna is intact. Otherwise, after taking down the arthrodesis, there will be absolutely no stability within the arthroplasty. Preoperative magnetic resonance imaging scans are useful in making this evaluation, as well as careful clinical examination. Occasionally, the distal inch or so of the insertion of the brachialis will be ossified, and when removing ectopic bone to mobilize the joint it is important not to remove that bone which represents the functional insertion of this important elbow stabilizer (Fig. 58-1). If it is found that the brachialis attachment is not present, anteroposterior stability may be restored by transplanting the biceps tendon into the region of the coronoid. If this is not done, there is the possibility of posterior dislocation. Although Dr. Morrey, the editor of this book, routinely reconstructs the collateral ligaments, I have not found it necessary to perform formal reconstruction of the medial collateral ligament (MCL) or the lateral collateral ligament (LLC) after cutis arthroplasty for any reason.

RESULTS

I have achieved a range of motion in a useful arc of at least 90 degrees in 22 cases using cutis arthroplasty. All these elbows have been functionally stable despite the fact that often the lateral and medial ligaments of necessity were compromised, either as a result of the trauma or due to their needing to be divided to gain access during surgery. None have required bracing. There have been no neurovascular complications. The use of a postoperative continuous

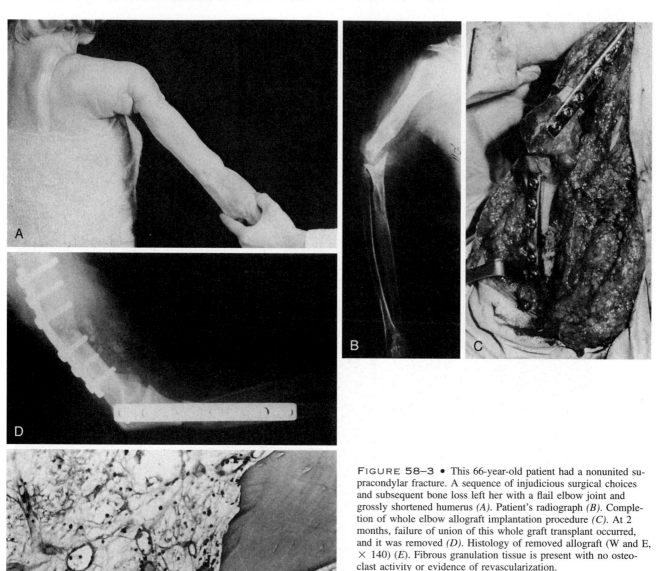

FIGURE 58–3 • This 66-year-old patient had a nonunited supracondylar fracture. A sequence of injudicious surgical choices and subsequent bone loss left her with a flail elbow joint and grossly shortened humerus (A). Patient's radiograph (B). Completion of whole elbow allograft implantation procedure (C). At 2 months, failure of union of this whole graft transplant occurred, and it was removed (D). Histology of removed allograft (W and E, × 140) (E). Fibrous granulation tissue is present with no osteoclast activity or evidence of revascularization.

Allograft Replacement

For the younger patient at this time, allograft replacement of the missing bone segment should be considered. Autografts such as vascularized fibula[39] and iliac crest[16] have been used in the upper limb, but lack of articular surface and donor site morbidity limit their application. Lexer is credited with the first use of allograft transplantation.[19] Renewed interest sparked in a series of publications in the late 1960s and 1970s.[25, 29, 30] Ottolenghi[29] believed that partial joint transplantation gave better results than replacement of the whole joint with allograft. Urbaniak[35] found whole joint transplantation to be successful in six of eight cases, with a follow-up period of up to 6 years, but subsequent surveillance has tempered this enthusiasm. I have attempted whole elbow transplantation only twice, with nonunion and failure in both cases (Fig. 58–3C to E) but have had considerable success in replacing isolated segments of the humerus.[7] Animal studies indicate that a major cause of failure in whole joint replacement is delayed or incomplete union and failure of revascularization.[13] Allograft reconstruction is a viable choice for short-term restoration of function in this difficult group of patients (Fig. 58–4). It provides a stable joint without a requirement for associated complex soft tissue reconstruction. It is important, if good stability and function are to be achieved, that the allograft match as nearly as possible the size of the lost segment of bone and its articular contour.[7, 35] Radiographs of the normal side are valuable for planning purposes. When inserting the allograft, we take care to

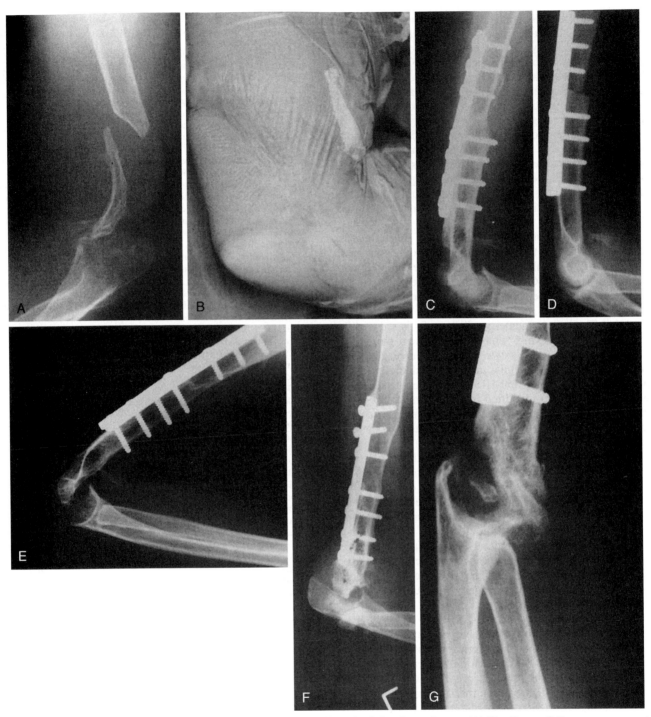

FIGURE 58–4 • Radiograph of a 20-year-old female with flail elbow following infected open fracture *(A)*. The elbow soft tissues were augmented with free vascularized skin flap 6 months before elbow reconstruction (here, seen immediately prior to allograft implantation surgery) *(B)*. Radiograph immediately following the procedure. In this case, fresh-frozen graft was used *(C)*. Eight months postoperatively, union has occurred *(D)*. The patient is doing office work. The arm is not braced and the joint is stable (no soft tissue reconstruction or ligamentous support of any kind). Three years postoperatively *(E)*. Five years postoperatively *(F* and *G)*. Note progressive bone loss. The elbow is braced but fulcrum is maintained and the arm is functional. No dislocation is present, but there is some posterior subluxation in extension.

achieve the correct degree of muscle tension. These measures not only guarantee good functional restoration but also improve joint stability, and ligamentous reconstruction is unnecessary. Before any reconstructive procedure, there must be a careful assessment of the quality of all soft tissues, including the muscle as well as skin and soft tissues. The soft tissues must be able to accommodate a large allograft and still permit closure. Vascularized free flaps of soft tissue may be required (see Chapter 37).

The fate of implanted allograft material depends on many factors, some of which are not fully understood. Large segmental allografts must unite with host bone (by a process of osteoconduction) if they are to succeed.[15] This union occurs frequently, provided that the fixation to the

• CHAPTER 59 •

Synovectomy of the Elbow

• BRIAN P. H. LEE and BERNARD F. MORREY

Synovectomy of the elbow performed for rheumatoid arthritis is a well-recognized and accepted form of treatment. With the increasing use and success of total joint replacement for patients with advanced rheumatoid arthritis involving the elbow, the role of synovectomy has been more clearly defined and is the initial interventive procedure considered for patients with early stages of rheumatoid arthritis (Fig. 59–1). In Finland, operative synovectomy of the elbow constitutes about 40 percent of elbow operations for rheumatoid arthritis.[31] Despite this, some controversies still remain as to its role and method of execution, particularly with regard to patients with instability and stiffness. The issues of open versus arthroscopic techniques and preservation of the radial head are also less clearly defined at present.

INDICATIONS AND PATIENT SELECTION

Patients who present with uncontrolled, painful synovitis of the elbow and limitation of function are considered for synovectomy. A period of nonsurgical treatment including medications and physical therapy for at least 6 months should be attempted before surgery is considered.[5] Clinically, the synovitis is most easily detected by a bulge in the lateral compartment posterior to the radial head with the elbow in extension, indicating an effusion or synovitis.

We have classified involvement of rheumatoid arthritis of the elbow radiologically into four categories (Fig. 59–2).[26] This has proven helpful in providing a basis for treatment options.

Type I: Synovitis with a normal-appearing joint.
Type II: Loss of joint space but maintenance of the subchondral architecture.
Type IIIA: Alteration of the subchondral architecture.
Type IIIB: Alteration of the architecture with deformity.
Type IV: Gross deformity. Recently, the radiographic appearance of anklyosis was described by Connor and Morrey[5a] as a Type V presentation (Fig. 59–3).

The procedure therefore is ideally reserved for the early stages of the disease (type I, type II, and early type IIIA) (Fig. 59–4).

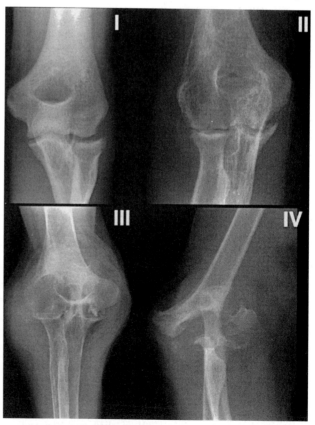

FIGURE 59–2 • Mayo radiographic classification of rheumatoid involvement of the elbow considers synovitis, articular involvement, and joint distraction (see text).

RHEUMATOID SURGERY OF THE ELBOW

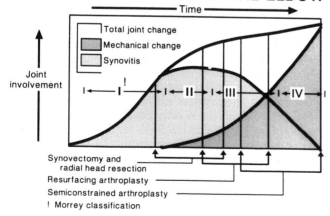

FIGURE 59–1 • Scheme depicting the relationship of synovitis and joint distraction to treatment options.

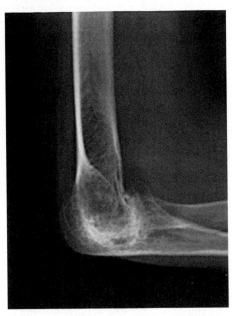

FIGURE 59–3 • A type V radiographic presentation is one of ankylosis as reported by Connor and associates.[5a]

Synovectomy is not effective or reliable in restoring motion. A functional arc should ideally be present[27] (30 to 130 degrees of flexion), but a total arc of at least 80 degrees of flexion ought to be present before the procedure is considered. Some patients may, however, benefit from a combined capsulectomy and synovectomy, and these criteria only provide guidelines for selection.

Although debate is still ongoing as to the role of synovectomy in the more advanced stages of disease in which instability of the elbow is present, the success of total elbow replacement has limited the role of synovectomy in the case with significant architectural erosion of the radial head or deficiency of the medial collateral ligament, both of which render the elbow unstable.[5, 26, 36] Although some reports indicate that the results are not as good in later stages,[9] others suggest that it does not preclude synovectomy.[3, 4, 6, 22, 33, 40] Currently, such support is mainly from centers and countries in which total elbow replacement is not as readily available, or experience with it is limited. In general, those experienced with the techniques of total elbow replacement as well as synovectomy, and familiar with the results of both, favor total elbow replacement over synovectomy in the later stages of disease. Under these circumstances, patients are much more satisfied and the functional improvement is much greater.[26]

CONTRAINDICATIONS

The major contraindications to synovectomy are gross instability and severe stiffness of the elbow. Gross instability indicates severe joint destruction. Synovectomy performed in this situation will not resolve problems related to instability, and débridement of the joint may actually aggravate these symptoms, particularly where radial head excision is performed.[33]

Severe joint stiffness resulting from inflammatory fibroarthrosis is more commonly seen in juvenile rheumatoid arthritis, and synovectomy is unable to predictably improve function in patients with this condition. As a matter of fact, Connor and colleagues[5a] suggest a type V radiographic presentation: complete ankylosis (see Fig. 59–3). Radiographic involvement of joint architecture with deformity (type IIIB) is also a relative contraindication.

TECHNIQUES

Several methods of synovectomy are available. These include chemical or radiation synovectomy[7, 10, 29, 37] and surgical synovectomy, which can be performed open or by an arthroscopic technique.[10, 16, 18–20, 22, 24, 28, 42]

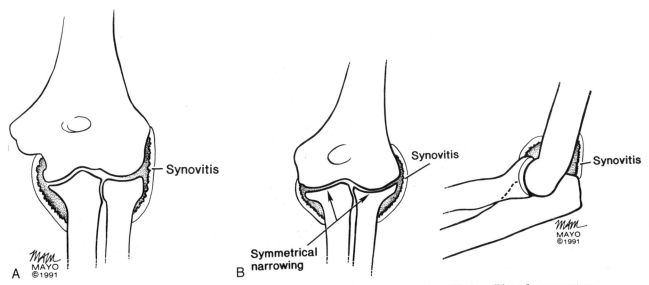

FIGURE 59–4 • Only type I, II (A and B), and early IIIA involvement are considered ideal candidates for synovectomy.

NONSURGICAL SYNOVECTOMY

Chemical and radiation synovectomy has been advocated for the knee as a noninvasive procedure.[32] Agents used include osmic acid and radioactive yttrium. Little information on outcome is available in the literature. Oka and associates[29] reported that an intra-articular injection of osmic acid is effective in coagulating the superficial layer of synovium but that remnants of the agents can exist for 9 months after injection. The potential for cartilage necrosis has limited the use of these agents in the United States.[5, 14, 25] In addition, radial head excision, if needed, is not possible. However, these techniques can be considered as a more conservative treatment option to surgical synovectomy.

SURGICAL SYNOVECTOMY

Arthrotomy

Open surgery remains the most commonly performed procedure for elbow synovectomy. It is well established and requires less technical expertise than arthroscopic synovectomy, particularly when radial head excision is performed.

TECHNIQUE

An extensile Kocher approach provides excellent visualization of the lateral joint and preserves the medial collateral ligament (Fig. 59–5). The radial head is removed if there are significant symptoms with pronation and supination or marked radiohumeral joint pain with flexion and extension.

The synovitis typically involves the sacriform recess of the radial neck, and a thorough synovectomy of this region is required. If the radial head is removed, a very thorough synovectomy can be carried out.[3, 30, 38, 41] If the radial head is preserved, anterior compartment exposure is more difficult but can still be adequately achieved. Our preference has been to leave the radial head whenever possible. The posterior capsule is also readily exposed through the Kocher approach, and a second medial exposure is not necessary in our experience and that of most investigators.[6, 35, 39] The triceps is elevated from the lateral column and the joint is extended. The posterior compartment synovectomy can then be carried out.

AFTERCARE

Following synovectomy, the joint is injected with bupivacaine with epinephrine and a corticosteroid at a 4:1 ratio. Closure of the lateral soft tissue and capsule is carried out with a suction drain in situ. The elbow is extended and a padded Jones dressing with anterior plaster slab is applied. The extremity is elevated by being suspended in a stockinette. The plaster, dressing, and drain are removed the next day. The brachial plexus block is removed after 48 hours, and the patient is discharged the following day. A portable continuous passive motion machine is used for 3 weeks. The sutures are then removed and the patient is allowed to resume activity as tolerated. Static night splinting is used if there are concerns about maintaining motion. Alternatively, an immediate continuous passive motion machine can be started postoperatively under brachial plexus anesthetic block.

The use of the Mayo posteromedial triceps reflecting

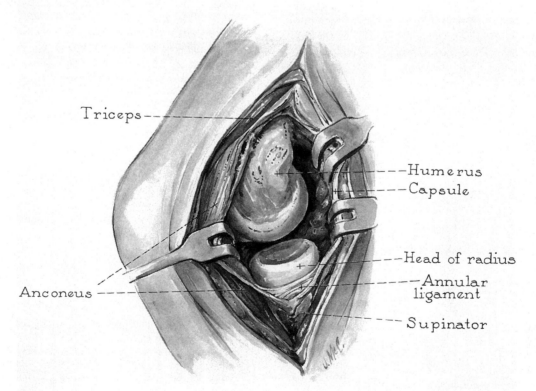

FIGURE 59–5 • A Kocher incision is the preferred arthrotomy and allows posterior capsule exposure as well.

exposure has also been advocated for synovectomy of the elbow.[15] It provides for identification of the ulnar nerve and facilitates subsequent skin incisions for total elbow replacement. However, surgery is more extensive than the extensile Kocher approach with the added potential for extensor mechanism complications, and we have not found it necessary to use this approach for routine synovectomy. Synovectomy and débridement through a transolecranon approach has been used in the past but is rarely performed today in view of the problem with healing of the osteotomy in these patients.[16]

Arthroscopic Synovectomy

Arthroscopic synovectomy is technically very demanding, with associated risks of neurovascular injury. One must be constantly aware of the fact that the neurovascular structures can be within 2 mm of the shaving instruments in the anterior compartment of the joint.[23] The risks can be minimized with observation of certain safety precautions. In experienced hands, the advantages of arthroscopic over open synovectomy are obvious. It can be done on an outpatient basis, causes minimal morbidity, results in rapid return of motion, and shortens the recovery period. With improved technique and greater experience, a complete synovectomy including excision of the radial head, if necessary, is possible (Fig. 59–6).

TECHNIQUE

Several strategies can be used, but our technique of elbow arthroscopy has been described elsewhere.[28] The patient is placed in the lateral decubitus position with the arm on a padded support. The joint is evaluated through an initial

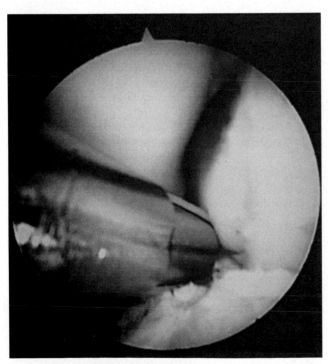

FIGURE 59–6 • Arthroscopic synovectomy is less invasive but the effectiveness compared with arthrotomy is yet to be demonstrated.

midlateral portal. Typically, the joint is lax enough to allow visualization of the mid-anterior and lateral capsule. The débriding instrument, a 4-mm reciprocating device with a vacuum control adjusted to the low setting to draw tissue into its teeth, is inserted through an anterolateral portal and a subtotal synovectomy carried out (Fig. 59–7A). Synovitis can be extensive, and visualization improves as removal of synovium proceeds. The tip of the resecter must be in view at all times and closed immediately if muscle fibers are seen. The shaver blades should always point inward and away from the capsule. A switch stick is used and an anteromedial portal is established to complete the anterior synovectomy (Fig. 59–7B). More recently, we have begun the procedure by visualization through the anterior medial portal initially. The anterior lateral portal is then used to begin the synovectomy.

Considerable visualization of the posterior compartment can usually be achieved through the mid-lateral portal. A posterior synovectomy is completed by inserting the débriding instrument through a posterolateral portal (Fig. 59–7C) The instruments can then be switched (with the arthroscope in the posterolateral and shaver in the mid-lateral portals) to facilitate removal of synovium in the sacriform recess and removal of the radial head when indicated (Fig. 59–7D). A mid-posterior portal is also useful to clean the medial recess. This is done in a limited fashion to avoid injury to the ulnar nerve. This is justified by the fact that the results of subtotal synovectomy are comparable to those of a complete synovectomy. An arthroscopic burr is used for removal of the radial head if necessary. The radial head can also be removed with the instruments in the anterior portals (see Fig. 59–7B).

As each portal is established, extreme caution is necessary to avoid damage to the nearby vessels and nerves, since the radial nerve may be only 2 mm from the capsule in some patients.[1, 12, 23] An 18-gauge needle helps determine the optimal site for the portal.

After completion of the synovectomy, the joint is injected with 10 ml of bupivicaine with epinephrine and a steroid. If several puncture sites are used, the possibility of anesthetizing the radial as well as the ulnar and median nerves must be considered when evaluating the patient after surgery. The wounds are sutured; a drain is optional. Neurovascular status is checked as soon as the patient is awake.

POSTOPERATIVE MANAGEMENT

The patient is given an axillary block and placed in a continuous passive motion machine. The block is discontinued after 48 hours. The patient is encouraged to move the joint and discharged on the second or third day to carry on with daily activities. Physiotherapy is not necessary.

Results

OPEN SYNOVECTOMY

The long-term results of open elbow synovectomy are summarized in Table 59–1. Taking into account recognized inconsistencies inherent in summarizing diverse reports using different evaluation standards, 70 to 90 percent of the

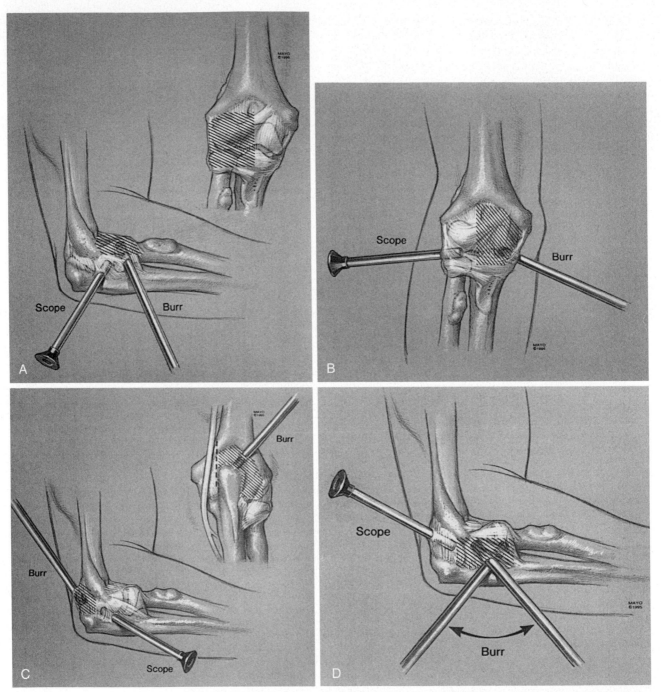

FIGURE 59–7 • *A*, The arthroscope is introduced into the mid-lateral portal while the resecting instrument is placed through an anterolateral portal. In rheumatoid arthritis, accurate visualization can be obtained by removing the synovium over the radial head and in the lateral compartment. *B*, The arthroscope is now placed in the anterolateral portal. Using a switch stick, the resecting instrument is introduced through an anteromedial portal. This allows removal of the remainder of the synovium in the anterior compartment. The portals for the arthroscope and the burr may be interchanged. *C*, After the arthroscope is placed in the mid-lateal portal again, the resecting instrument is inserted through a posterolateral site. The posterior synovium is removed, with special care taken to avoid the medial gutter and the ulnar nerve. *D*, The instruments are now changed, the arthroscope being placed in the posterolateral portal and the resecting instrument in the mid-lateral portal. This allows resection of the synovium in the sacriform recess. The radial head may be removed at this stage or at stage 2 with the instruments in the anterior portals. (By permission, Mayo Foundation.)

procedures can be considered to have a satisfactory outcome within the first 3 to 5 years.[4, 6, 11, 20, 22, 40] The need for radial head removal continues to be debated. Although most series report radial head excision in the majority of cases,[4, 8, 11, 34, 42] more recent results suggest that preservation of the radial head can reliably achieve comparable results with pain relief in almost 80 percent of patients at about 5 years.[35]

The majority of patients maintain or regain a functional arc of motion, with approximately 50 percent improving flexion and extension, 30 to 35 percent remaining unchanged, and 15 percent losing a small amount of motion.

• TABLE 59–1 • Results of Elbow Synovectomy for Rheumatoid Arthritis (Open Procedures, Average Follow-Up > 5 Years)

Author	Year	No. of Procedures	No. of Radial Heads Removed	Recommended Approach	Pain Relief No.	Pain Relief %	Motion (%) Gained	Motion (%) No Change	Motion (%) Lost	% Satisfactory	Follow-Up (Mo) Mean	Follow-Up (Mo) Range
Taylor et al.[38]	1976	44	44	Lateral	38	86	0	0	11	91	60	6–96
Eichenblat et al.[8]	1982	25	25	Lateral	22	88	80	0	20	100	60	24–132
Rymaszewski et al.[33]	1984	40	40	Lateral	20	50	21	—	—	55	72	12–180
Brumfield & Resnic[4]	1985	42	42	Lateral, medial, transolecranon	27	64	64	14	17	78	84	24–204
Ferlic et al.[11]	1987	57	57	Lateral	—	—	76	9	15	77	86	12–240
Tulp & Winia[40]	1989	61	41	Lateral, bilateral	—	—	—	—	—	70	78	48–120
Alexiades et al.[2]	1990	21	21	Lateral, transolecranon	14	67	54	18	28	67	173	120–252
Vahvanen et al.[41]	1991	70	66	Lateral and medial	55	79	64	—	—	71	90	18–264
Smith et al.[35]	1993	85	0	Lateral	67	79	64	—	—	<75	108	60–240
Herold & Schroder[17]	1995	12	11	Lateral	10	83	—	—	—	83	168	144–180
Lonner & Stuchin[21]	1997	12	12	Lateral (with anterior, capsular release)	10	83	83	—	17	100	73	24–132
Gendi et al.[13]	1997	115	113	—	60	54	—	—	—	54	78	60–288

Improvement in pronation and supination is consistently noted, particularly with radial head excision.[11, 31, 33, 41] Lonner and Stuchin,[21] combining anterior capsule release with synovectomy, noted improvement of the flexion arc from a mean of 93 degrees to 116 degrees, with an average 13 degrees improvement in the flexion contracture.

Some reports suggest that results deteriorate minimally with time.[6, 40] In a recent study by Herold and Schroder[17] in 11 patients (12 elbows) at 14 years after surgery, 83 percent maintained satisfactory pain relief (Fig. 59–8). However, radiographic progression was noted and reoperation was required in two elbows. Vahvanen amd colleagues[41] and Smith and colleagues,[35] reporting at follow-ups averaging 7 to 8 years, showed that initial satisfactory results of 90 percent had decreased to less than 75 percent at final assessment. In a long-term study at 10 to 20 years after surgery, only 67 percent of 21 patients were satisfied with the procedure.[2] Gendi and associates[13] reported on

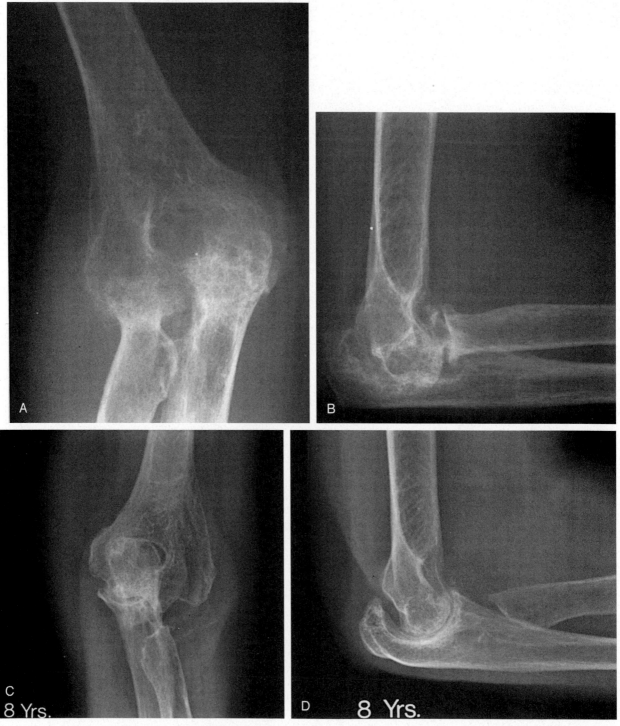

FIGURE 59–8 • A 43-year-old female with late type II changes (A and B), still functioning without pain at 8 years (C and D). Note remodeling on the lateral radiograph (D).

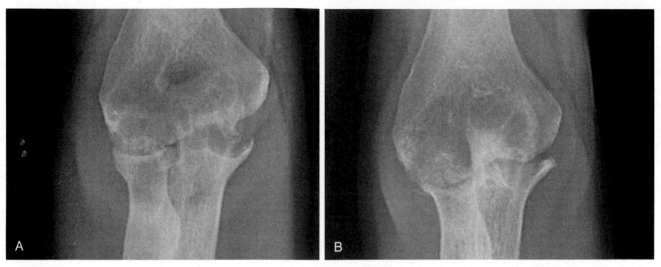

FIGURE 59–9 • Type IIIA involvement (A). Three years after arthroscopic synovectomy, the patient has less pain and has maintained a 100 degree arc of motion (B).

113 elbows 5 to 20 years after synovectomy and noted a cumulative survival rate of 81 percent at 1 year, decreasing at 2.6 percent per year. By final follow-up, 46 percent of the procedures had failed. It does appear that results deteriorate with time and patients develop recurrent synovitis in addition to radiographic progression. It cannot be assumed, nor has it been demonstrated, that synovectomy arrests the progress of the disease process.

ARTHROSCOPIC SYNOVECTOMY

The reported experience with arthroscopic synovectomy is too limited to offer firm conclusions on its long-term effectiveness. Our experience with 14 procedures in 11 patients has been reported.[19] An initial benefit was recorded in 93 percent at 6 months after surgery, after an average follow-up of 3.5 years (Fig. 59–9). However, at the final assessment, only 57 percent maintained excellent or good ratings by the Mayo Elbow Performance Index (Fig. 59–10). Four patients had already gone on to elbow replace-

ment. There are no reports in the literature regarding the long-term benefits of arthroscopic synovectomy of the elbow.

Although a more complete synovectomy can theoretically be achieved arthroscopically with better visualization of all compartments of the elbow, the risk of neurovascular injury is always a concern and a significant disadvantage (see Chapter 39). With increasing experience and expertise, these risks may be minimized, but the dangers of neurovascular injury cannot be overemphasized.[27a] We currently perform arthroscopic synovectomy if the patient is under 45 to 50 years of age with more than 90 degrees of movement and radiologic changes of early grade IIIA or less.

CONTROVERSIES

Radial Head Excision and Stage of Involvement

The role of radial head excision remains unclear. There is no obvious distinction in the results between radial head preservation and excision. Typically, articular cartilage damage is more severe in the ulnohumeral articulation than in the radiohumeral or radioulnar articulation. Rymaszewski and associates[33] noted progressive destruction following synovectomy and radial head excision in 40 elbows after an average of 6 years. Although they suggested that radial excision caused biomechanical changes leading to this destruction, the selection process included some patients with more extensive (IIIB) involvement. Therefore, our indication for radial excision is clinical evidence of painful involvement of the radiohumeral or radioulnar joint. Otherwise it is preserved, as its role in instability is greater in the rheumatoid elbow with bone loss and soft tissue damage. This is supported by observations that the radial head need not always be removed in total elbow arthroplasties and leaving it does not yield worse results.

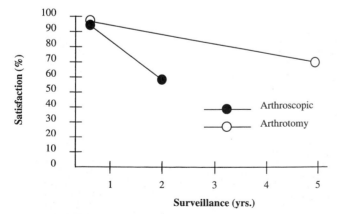

FIGURE 59–10 • The Mayo experience reported by Lee and Morrey suggests that the success of the open synovectomy is superior to that of the arthroscopic procedure. However, results should improve with better arthroscopic techniques.

Repeat Synovectomy

Repeat synovectomy following an initial failed procedure has been rarely recommended or reported. The frequency of performing repeat synovectomy has been variably reported between 7 and 20 percent.[6, 35, 39] Smith and colleagues[35] have the most carefully analyzed data on repeat synovectomy. They reported that 10 of 18 patients who underwent a repeat synovectomy did so 3 years or less after the first procedure, indicating the lack of an initial satisfactory response. Hence, a repeat synovectomy following a recurrence of symptoms is not to be generally recommended, particularly with the success of total elbow replacement that is now being reported (Fig. 59–11).[9, 26, 36] The results of a repeat procedure are also less predictable with only 55 percent of patients continuing to have significant pain relief.

Complications

Recurrence. Recurrence of pain and synovitis is the most common complication following synovectomy. It was discussed earlier.

Motion Loss. In addition, loss of motion as noted earlier can occur in 10 to 20 percent of patients. These problems are less commonly seen in those with clear indications for the procedure initially. Early aggressive motion is essential to prevent loss of motion.

Instability. Instability is not uncommonly seen as a complication following a synovectomy. Residual instability has been reported in about 15 percent of patients.[39] The incidence is higher in patients with more advanced disease and significant instability prior to synovectomy, as noted by Rymaszewski and associates,[33] who reported up to 50 percent incidence of instability following synovectomy. This is particularly true if radial head excision is performed in patients with instability prior to the procedure. Instability is not a common problem, even with radial head excision, if the ulnohumeral joint is reasonably intact and if the medial collateral ligament is also competent.

Neuropathy. Nerve injury is rare after open synovectomy but is a significant risk with arthroscopic synovectomy given the fact that the neurovascular structures are related very closely to the joint capsule.[27a] Ulnar nerve injury and dysfunction can occur and temporary ulnar nerve neurapraxia occurred in one patient (7 percent) in our series on arthroscopic synovectomy.[19] We are also aware of median and radial nerve injuries that have occurred following arthroscopic synovectomy but have not ourselves found permanent nerve complications.

SUMMARY

Although traditionally some have reported satisfactory results in patients with significant joint involvement,[11, 33, 38, 40] more recent results suggest that the best outcome is seen when less extensive joint involvement has occurred.[35, 41] The current recommendation to avoid synovectomy in those patients with severe (type IIIB) disease is based on predictable outcomes with total elbow arthroplasty and unpredictable results with synovectomy in this type of patient.[9, 26, 36] A capsulectomy performed together with synovectomy may facilitate improvement in motion.[21] Im-

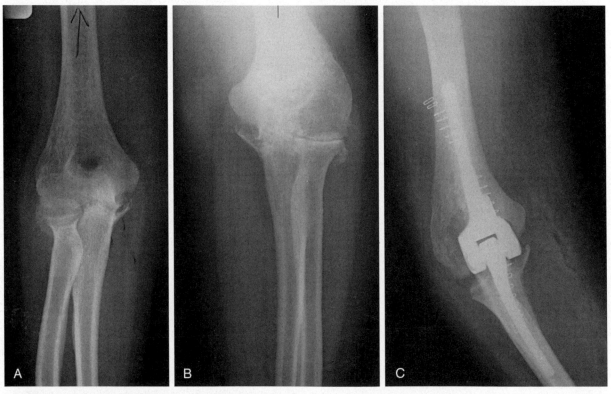

FIGURE 59–11 • Late type II involvement *(A)*. Mild progression 4 years after arthroscopic synovectomy *(B)*. Patient successfully treated with Coonrad-Morrey elbow replacement *(C)*.

proved outcome with arthroscopic synovectomy is to be expected as the surgical techniques improve, with continued caution regarding the potential for nerve injury.

REFERENCES

1. Adolfsson, L.: Arthroscopy of the elbow joint: a cadaveric study of portal placement. J. Shoulder Elbow Surg. **3**:53, 1994.
2. Alexiades, M. M., Stanwyck, T. S., Figgie, M. P., and Inglis, A. E.: Minimum ten-year follow-up of elbow synovectomy for rheumatoid arthritis. Orthop. Trans. **14**:255, 1990.
3. Brattstrom, H., and Khudairy, H. A.: Synovectomy of the elbow in rheumatoid arthritis. Acta Orthop. Scand. **46**:744, 1975.
4. Brumfield, R. H., and Resnic, C. T.: Synovectomy of the elbow in rheumatoid arthritis. J. Bone Joint Surg. **67A**:16, 1985.
5. Bryan, R. S., and Morrey, B. F.: Rheumatoid arthritis of the elbow. *In* Evarts, C. M. (ed.): Surgery of the Musculoskeletal System, Vol. 2, 2nd ed. London, Churchill Livingstone, 1990, p. 1759.
5a. Connor, P. M., and Morrey, B. F.: Total elbow arthroplasty in patients who have juvenile rheumatoid arthritis. J. Bone Joint Surg. **80A**:678, 1998.
6. Copeland, S. A., and Taylor, J. G.: Synovectomy of the elbow in rheumatoid arthritis: the place of excision of the head of the radius. J. Bone Joint Surg. **61B**:69, 1979.
7. Dawson, T. M., Ryan, P. F., Street, A. M., et al.: Yttrium synovectomy in haemophilic arthropathy. Br. J. Rheumatol. **33**:351, 1994.
8. Eichenblat, M., Hass, A., and Kessler, L.: Synovectomy of the elbow in rheumatoid arthritis. J. Bone Joint Surg. **64A**:1074, 1982.
9. Ewald, F. C.: Capitellocondylar total elbow replacement in rheumatoid arthritis: long-term results. J. Bone Joint Surg. **75**:498, 1993.
10. Eyring, E. J., Longert, A., and Bass, J.: Synovectomy in juvenile rheumatoid arthritis: indications and short-term results. J. Bone Joint Surg. **53A**:638, 1971.
11. Ferlic, D. C., Patchett, C. E., Clayton, M. L., and Freeman, A. C.: Elbow synovectomy in rheumatoid arthritis. Clin. Orthop. **220**:119, 1987.
12. Field, L. D., Altchek, D. W., Warren, R. F., et al.: Arthroscopic anatomy of the lateral elbow: a comparison of three portals. Arthroscopy **10**:602, 1994.
13. Gendi, N. S. T., Axon, J. M. C., Carr, A. J., et al.: Synovectomy of the elbow and radial head excision in rheumatoid arthritis. J. Bone Joint Surg. **79B**:918, 1997.
14. Goldberg, V. M., Rashbaum, R., and Zika, J.: The role of osmic acid in the treatment of immune synovitis. Arthritis Rheum. **19**:737, 1976.
15. Inglis, A. E., and Figgie, M. P.: Septic and non-traumatic conditions of the elbow. *In* Morrey, B. F. (ed.): The Elbow and Its Disorders, 2nd ed. Philadelphia, WB Saunders Co., 1993, p. 759.
16. Inglis, A. E., Ranawat, C. S., and Straub, L. R.: Synovectomy and debridement of the elbow in rheumatoid arthritis. J. Bone Joint Surg. **53A**:652, 1971.
17. Herold, N., and Schroder, H. A.: Synovectomy and radial head excision in rheumatoid arthritis: 11 patients followed for 14 years. Acta Orthop. Scand. **66**(3):252, 1995.
18. Kay, L., Stainsby, D., Buzzard, B., et al.: The role of synovectomy in the management of recurrent haemarthroses in haemophilia. Br. J. Haematol. **49**:53, 1981.
19. Lee, B. P. H., and Morrey, B. F.: Arthroscopic synovectomy of the elbow for rheumatoid arthritis: a prospective study. J. Bone Joint Surg. **79B**:770, 1997.
20. Linclau, L. A., Winia, W. P. C. A., and Korst, J. K.: Synovectomy of the elbow in rheumatoid arthritis. Acta Orthop. Scand. **54**:935, 1983.
21. Lonner, J. H., and Stuchin, S. A.: Synovectomy, radial head excision, and anterior capsular release in stage III inflammatory arthritis of the elbow. J. Hand [Am.] **22**(2):279, 1997.
22. Low, W. G., and Evans, J. P.: Synovectomy and rehabilitation in rheumatoid arthritis. J. Bone Joint Surg. **53A**:621, 1971.
23. Lynch, G., Meyers, J., Whipple, T., and Caspari, R.: Neurovascular anatomy and elbow arthroscopy: inherent risks. Arthroscopy **2**:191, 1986.
24. McEwen, C.: Synovectomy and rehabilitation in rheumatoid arthritis. J. Bone Joint Surg. **53A**:621, 1971.
25. Mitchel, N., Laurin, C., and Shepard, N.: The effect of osmium tetroxide and nitrogen mustard on normal articular cartilage. J. Bone Joint Surg. **55B**:814, 1973.
26. Morrey, B. F., and Adams, R. A.: Semiconstrained arthroplasty for the treatment of rheumatoid arthritis of the elbow. J. Bone Joint Surg. **74A**:479, 1992.
27. Morrey, B. F., Askew, L. J., An, K. N., and Chao, E. Y.: A biomechanical study of normal functional elbow motion. J. Bone Joint Surg. **63A**:872, 1981.
27a. Morrey, B. F.: Complications of elbow arthroscopy. AAOS Instruction Course Lecture, 1999.
28. O'Driscoll, S. W., and Morrey, B. F.: Arthroscopy of the elbow: diagnostic and therapeutic benefits and hazards. J. Bone Joint Surg. **74A**:84, 1992.
29. Oka, M., Rekonen, A., and Ruotsi, A.: The fate and distribution of intra-articularly injected osmium tetroxide (Os-191). Acta Rheum. Scand. **15**:35, 1969.
30. Porter, B. B., Park, N., Richardson, C., et al.: Rheumatoid arthritis of the elbow: the results of synovectomy. J. Bone Joint Surg. **56B**:427, 1974.
31. Raunio, P.: Synovectomy of the elbow in rheumatoid arthritis. Reconstr. Surg. Traumatol. **18**:673, 1981.
32. Rivard, G.-E., Girard, M., Belanger, R., et al.: Synoviorthesis with colloidal ³²P chromic phosphate for the treatment of hemophilic arthropathy. J. Bone Joint Surg. **76A**:482, 1994.
33. Rymaszewski, L. A., MacKay, I., Ames, A. A., and Miller, J. H.: Long-term effects of excision of the radial head in rheumatoid arthritis. J. Bone Joint Surg. **66B**:109, 1984.
34. Saito, T., Koshine, T., Okamoto, R., and Horiuchi, S.: Radical synovectomy with muscle release for the rheumatoid elbow. Acta Orthop. Scand. **57**:71, 1986.
35. Smith, S. R., Pinder, I. M., and Ang, S. C.: Elbow synovectomy in rheumatoid arthritis: present role and value of repeat synovectomy. J. Orthop. Rheum. **6**:155, 1993.
36. Souter, W. A.: Surgery of the rheumatoid elbow [review]. Ann. Rheum. Dis. **49**(Suppl 2):871, 1990.
37. Stucki, G., Bozzone, P., Treuer, E., et al.: Efficacy and safety of radiation synovectomy with yttrium-90: a retrospective long-term analysis of 164 applications in 82 patients. Br. J. Rheumatol. **32**:383, 1993.
38. Taylor, A. R., Mukerjea, S. K., and Rana, N. A.: Excision of the head of the radius in rheumatoid arthritis. J. Bone Joint Surg. **58B**:485, 1976.
39. Torgerson, W. R., and Leach, R. E.: Synovectomy of the elbow in rheumatoid arthritis. J. Bone Joint Surg. **52A**:371, 1970.
40. Tulp, N. J. A., and Winia, W. P. C. A.: Synovectomy of the elbow in rheumatoid arthritis: long-term results. J. Bone Joint Surg. **71B**:664, 1989.
41. Vahvanen, V., Eskola, A., and Peltonen, J.: Results of elbow synovectomy in rheumatoid arthritis. Arch. Orthop. Trauma Surg. **110**:151, 1991.
42. Wilson, D. W., Arden, G. P., and Ansell, B. M.: Synovectomy of the elbow in rheumatoid arthritis. J. Bone Joint Surg. **55B**:106, 1973.

• CHAPTER 60 •

Interposition Arthroplasty of the Elbow

• PHILLIP E. WRIGHT, II, AVRUM I. FROIMSON,
and BERNARD F. MORREY

HISTORICAL ASPECTS

The predecessor of interposition arthroplasty is the so-called functional arthroplasty, popularized by Hass (1944).[21] This is actually a variety of resection arthroplasty, except that the distal humerus is fashioned in the shape of a wedge and various interposed tissues have been used (Fig. 60–1). Hass reported the long-term results of functional arthroplasty in 15 patients with an average follow-up period of 5.5 years. A satisfactory result was observed in 73 percent, and a tendency for the bone to remodel according to its functional demands was noted. Because this is a type of resection arthroplasty, it is not surprising that 13 of the 15 procedures were in patients with previous infection.

Interposition arthroplasty has been used for treatment of arthritis involving the temporomandibular, shoulder, wrist, knee, and hip joints. Of these, the elbow has been reported as second only to the temporomandibular as the joint most amenable to the technique.[22] In Europe, arthroplasty was popularized by Putti[40] and by Payr.[38] Schüller was the first

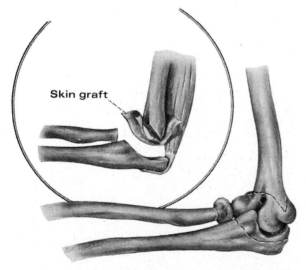

FIGURE 60–1 • The so-called functional or anatomic arthroplasty resects variable amounts of distal humerus but fashions the bone as a fulcrum against which the proximal ulna pivots. Skin and other substances can be used to cover the humerus and create a new articular surface, hence the term *interposition arthroplasty*.

to recommend the procedure for patients with rheumatoid arthritis.[44] Various muscle flaps, pig bladder,[4] fascia-fat transplants, skin, and other materials have been used as the interposing agent. In 1902, Murphy introduced and popularized arthroplasty in the United States.[34, 35] Lexer,[29] in 1909, emphasized the value of autogenous tissue and confirmed the impression of Murphy[35] that fat and fascia were the best substances for interposition arthroplasty. He reported that fascia remained viable and was replaced by fibrous and fibrocartilaginous tissue. The mechanism of the transformation to the new articulation was also studied by Phemister and Miller.[39] Little histologic difference was noted after cartilage resection with or without interposition materials.

Shahriaree and colleagues[45] reported that of 30 patients, 90 percent returned to their previous occupations after excisional arthroplasty with Gelfoam interposition. Smith and associates[48] successfully used silicone sheets as interposition material in six patients with hemophilic arthropathy.

Autogenous or xenograft cutis has been used as an interposing membrane in resection arthroplasties (cutis arthroplasty) of various joints since 1913, and its successful use in the elbow has been reported by several authors.[16, 25, 32] Cutis is the thick dermal layer of skin that remains after the superficial epidermal layer has been removed. It is a tough, durable, elastic membrane, and it closely adheres to the cut surface of the distal humerus.

Fascia lata is easy to harvest and conforms readily to the bony surfaces, but the donor site leaves variable morbidity. Efforts to enhance its effect have been reported by Kita[27] using chromicized fascia lata, the so-called J-K membrane. The concept has been reassessed after the addition of two important elements to the technique—distraction and motion.

INDICATIONS

Basic Concepts

For the young individual who has lost the use of the elbow, avoidance of arthroplasty is desirable. Alternative recommendations include (1) no surgical treatment and altered activity, (2) orthotics for the unstable elbow, (3) arthrodesis, and (4) interposition (distraction) arthroplasty. Resection arthroplasty is rarely if ever indicated at this time, the only indication being uncontrollable infection.

If the elbow is ankylosed in a functional position, no treatment may be required. If it is ankylosed in a poor position, osteotomy with correction of the position may be adequate treatment. If the patient has painful motion or an unstable elbow, an orthotic fitting may allow continuation of regular activities indefinitely or until the pain demands other treatment. The individual who is required to carry out strenuous activities such as heavy labor may not be a suitable candidate for any type of arthroplasty.

Interposition

SPECIFIC INDICATIONS

The basic indications for interposition arthroplasty are either incapacitating pain or loss of motion in an individual less than 30 years of age with rheumatoid arthritis, and less than 60 years of age with traumatic arthritis. Loss of motion may follow trauma, sepsis, burns, or degenerative or inflammatory arthritis. However, the most compelling indication for arthroplasty of the elbow is incapacitating pain. If the loss of motion and pain are postinfectious, careful evaluation must be done to ensure that the patient has been free of the infection for at least 6 months and preferably 1 year. The best indication for this procedure is post-traumatic, painful loss of motion not complicated by sepsis in an individual who does not require long-term heavy demand on the joint.[33]

Selection of the proper candidate for interposition arthroplasty involves assessment of the type and nature of the pathology and the type of patient under consideration. Regardless of the etiology, the integrity of the soft tissue is of paramount importance for a successful outcome. Extensive scarring with adherence of skin to bone may lead to an unsatisfactory result. Of great importance is the condition of the musculature about the arm and forearm because dynamic stability is important for the success of the operation.

CONTRAINDICATIONS

If recent sepsis has occurred, no reconstruction should be considered. If epiphyseal closure has not occurred, arthroplasty should be delayed until growth is complete. In the past, a major contradiction to interposition arthroplasty was inadequate bone stock. Grishin and colleagues,[17] however, have reported using interposition arthroplasty in conjunction with reconstructive bone grafts for marked osseous deficiency. The patient with a grossly unstable elbow from rheumatoid or post-traumatic arthritis cannot be adequately stabilized by an interposition procedure. Congenital ankylosis of the elbow joint that lacks the necessary ligamentous support may be treated with interposition and ligamentous reconstruction. However, the absence of flexion motor power is an absolute contraindication to this procedure. The need to use the upper extremity in ambulation or for transfer from bed to chair is a relative contraindication because excessive loading of the elbow will destabilize the joint.

If the patient is a heavy laborer, interposition arthroplasty may not be as satisfactory as a painless arthrodesis of the elbow in a functional position. Although interposition arthroplasty offers the patient a painless, durable joint, it cannot guarantee enough stability to allow for the activities of heavy labor.

If multiple joints in the same extremity have become ankylosed, it will be more difficult to secure a satisfactory result.

Finally, it is of utmost importance that the patient have the motivation and fortitude to participate in a preopcrative and postoperative rehabilitation program for proper rehabilitation of the musculature of the upper extremity.

PREFERRED TISSUE

In general, autogenous skin and fascia and Achilles tendon allografts are currently favored by the authors. The cutis is very durable and thick, rapidly adheres to the bone, and has been quite successful in early[7, 11] and more recently reported experiences.[16] The harvest techniques are attractive in those patients in whom primary closure may be carried out. Cutis tissue without the epidermis is somewhat more difficult to harvest. Fascia is also commonly used.[28, 33] It is readily available from the thigh and can be overlapped to ensure adequate bulk. The Achilles tendon allograft is attractive for its ready availability, absence of donor site morbidity, large size and thickness, and sufficient material for ligament reconstruction if necessary.

PREFERRED TECHNIQUES

Fascia Lata Interposition Arthroplasty*

TECHNIQUE

With few modifications, the fascial arthroplasty technique is similar to that advocated by Campbell in 1939.[10] Two teams of surgeons expedite the procedure. While one team approaches the elbow, the other harvests the fascia lata graft, usually from the contralateral thigh (Fig. 60–2).

Exposure. Start the elbow incision about 7 or 8 cm proximal to the joint on the posterior aspect of the arm. Continue the incision distally 15 to 20 cm onto the forearm, curving lateral to the olecranon, and then back to the midline of the limb. Elevate the deep fascia laterally 2 to 3 cm to expose the triceps aponeurosis. In the method described by Campbell, the distal humerus and the elbow joint are approached by making a longitudinal incision in the midline through the aponeurosis, the triceps muscle, and the periosteum.

Preparation. Using a periosteal elevator, strip the periosteum from the distal third of the posterior surface of the humerus. Retract the periosteum medially and laterally, exposing the radial head and olecranon. If there is osseous ankylosis of the elbow joint, use an osteotome to disrupt any fusion between the humerus and the olecranon and between the radial head and the humerus. Care should be taken at all times to isolate and protect the ulnar nerve as well as all structures in the antecubital fossa. Anterior transplantation of the ulnar nerve usually is not required. After releasing any bony or fibrous ankylosis, flex the elbow and displace the radius and ulna medially. Using a motorized saw, osteotome, rongeur, and rasp, contour the distal end of the humerus into one condyle, convex distally from anterior to posterior. At times it may be helpful to fashion an inverted, shallow V-shaped notch in the humeral condyle. This should not be made into an excessively deep notch, however. Use a curved chisel or gouge to deepen and lengthen the trochlear notch of the ulna. Excise the head of the radius to the level of the distal portion of the trochlear notch. Smooth all bony surfaces with a rasp, and close the periosteum or a portion of fascia over the cut end of the radius.

Harvest and Application. On the lateral aspect of the thigh, make the skin incision long enough to allow removal of sufficient fascia lata to cover the exposed bone. A portion of fascia lata measuring about 8 to 9 cm by 20 to

---

*P. E. Wright.

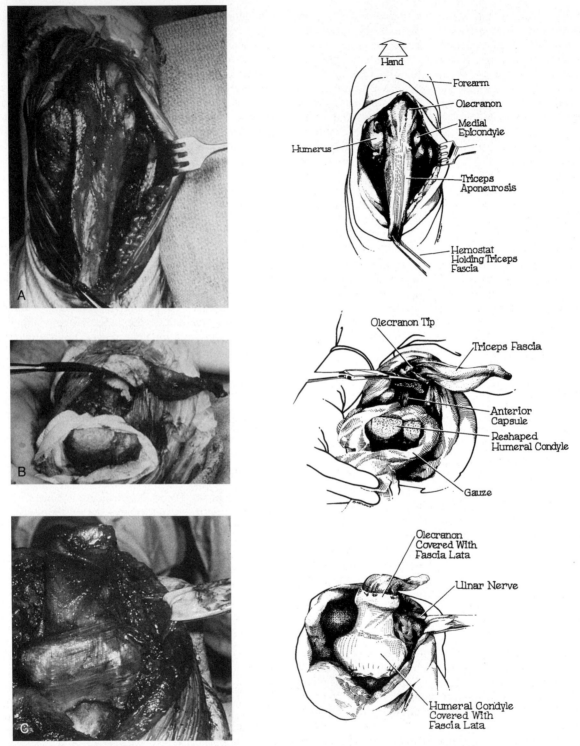

FIGURE 60–2 • Operative technique of fascial arthroplasty. *A,* Flap of triceps aponeurosis released with incisions on each side. The humerus is at the bottom, the ulna at the top, and the retractor on the medial side of the elbow. *B,* After the humerus has been exposed, bone is removed from the olecranon notch with a curved gouge. The triceps aponeurosis is at the right. The distal humeral articular surface has been removed (wrapped in sponge). *C,* The fascia lata has been loosely laid over olecranon *(top)* and distal humerus *(bottom).* The retractor is medial to elbow. The Penrose drain is protecting the ulnar nerve.

25 cm is usually sufficient. Always dissect the fascia from proximal to distal. Fold the fascia in half longitudinally with the raw surface that was stripped from the muscle turned toward the bone and the smooth outer surface turned to face itself. Anchor the folded edge to the anterior capsule with three interrupted absorbable sutures, one on each side and one in the middle. Place the proximal half of the fascia with interrupted sutures to the soft tissues proximal to the condyles. Use drill holes in the distal humerus to pass these sutures if the soft tissues are insufficient. Now place

the distal half of the fascia over the trochlear notch and suture this portion in place. Insert a fold of fascia between the radius and ulna, cover the radial neck, and fix it with a pursestring suture (see Fig. 60–2).

Reduce the joint and hold the elbow flexed to 90 degrees. Insert suction drainage catheters as needed. Close the capsule, usually from distally to proximally. If a flap of triceps aponeurosis has been raised, suture it a bit more distally to allow elbow flexion to occur more freely. If there is a tendency for instability, this can be avoided by placing a Steinmann pin across the joint at 90 degrees. This pin is removed in 2 to 3 weeks.

POSTOPERATIVE CARE

A cast or posterior elbow splint is applied, holding the elbow immobilized at 90 degrees for 2 to 3 weeks. The arm may be placed on an abduction humeral splint to prevent rotation. The abduction humeral splint is worn for 7 to 10 days. If a pin has been used for stability, it is removed at this time as well. The posterior arm splint is removed for 1 to 2 hours three or four times daily to allow active exercises to develop the elbow flexors and extensors. Three weeks after surgery, the posterior arm splint is discontinued except for night wear until a useful range of elbow motion and good muscle strength have been regained. A sling may be worn for support as needed for about 8 weeks. It is important to warn the patient that motion will be lost at this time and that there will be considerable tightening of the elbow for the next 2 or 3 months. However, if the patient works at building up the musculatures, motion gradually returns. At about 5 to 6 months after surgery, motion usually returns and improves rapidly. Active exercises should continue for at least 12 months. About 2 years are required to regain maximum strength and motion.

Cutis Arthroplasty*

TECHNIQUE

A supine position is used as noted for the previous technique.

Exposure. A posterior approach is made to the elbow. Split the extensor musculature between the extensor carpi radialis brevis and the extensor carpi ulnaris. Subperiosteally, dissect all soft tissues off the distal humerus (Fig. 60–3).

Dislocate the elbow joint and section the medial collateral ligaments from inside. Exposure or transposition of the ulnar nerve usually is not performed with a lateral approach.

Harvest and Application. Preparation of the distal humerus is similar to that described previously. After joint preparation, the size of the graft is determined. If pronation and supination are satisfactory, do not remove the radial head because its presence improves medial-lateral stability.

Using a hand-held or motorized dermatome, remove a thin split-thickness skin graft from the patient's lower abdomen, leaving a standard split-thickness donor site with punctate bleeding. With a sharp knife, remove this deep dermal layer with minimal subcutaneous fat (Fig. 60–4). Secure hemostasis with electrocautery and use the split-thickness graft to cover the donor site. Dr. Morrey has used an alternative method to harvest the cutis graft (see Fig. 60–4). This has the advantage of being relatively quick with a more pleasing scar at the donor site.

Attach the cutis graft to the prepared end of the distal humerus by drilling small holes along the medial and lateral epicondylar ridges. An additional one or two holes are placed between the medial and lateral margins of the humeral articulation. Suture the graft over the distal end of the humerus with the superficial cut dermal surface placed

---

*A. I. Froimson.

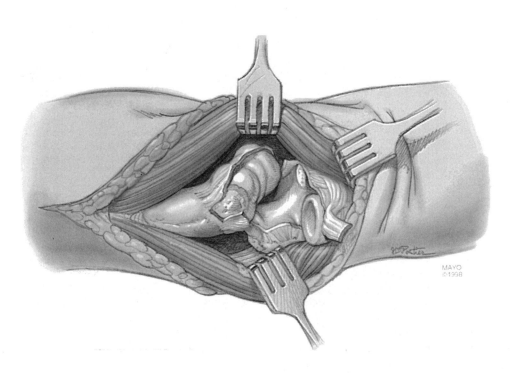

FIGURE 60–3 • An extensile Kocher approach is performed, sometimes removing a portion of the triceps attachment as necessary for adequate exposure. The collateral ligament must be released.

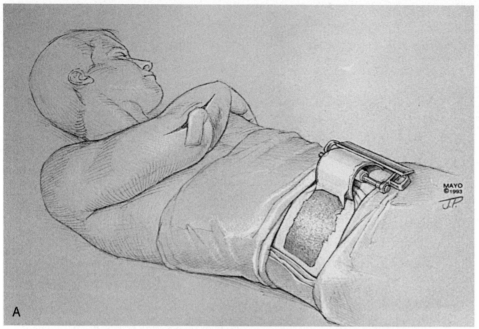

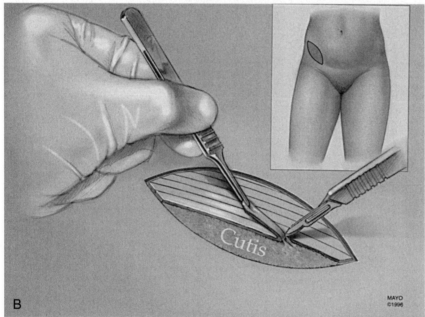

FIGURE 60–4 • *A*, Froimson technique for harvesting cutis from low abdomen. *B*, Morrey technique to harvest cutis from groin region. in a manner to allow primary closure.

against the bone and the fat facing the new joint space (Fig. 60–5). Reduce the elbow, approximate the extensor musculature with nonabsorbable sutures, and apply a compression dressing and a posterior plaster splint with the elbow in 90 degrees of flexion.

POSTOPERATIVE CARE

The splint is removed at approximately 2 weeks, and gentle, active exercises are begun under supervision. The splint is worn at all times, except for exercise periods. At 1 month after surgery, a functional range of flexion and extension usually is possible, and splinting can be discontinued in most patients. Resistive flexion exercises are begun, and at 6 weeks, resistive extension exercises are added. External bracing occasionally is used during the

second and third months if the patient must participate in heavy manual activities.

Achilles Tendon Allograft*

Position. The patient is supine and the arm brought across the chest.

Exposure and Preparation. We prefer a posterior incision, as we always expose the ulnar nerve. The elbow is then exposed as described previously with an extensile Kocher, occasionally releasing a small portion of the lateral triceps attachment to improve the exposure (see Fig. 60–3). The radial head is preserved if at all possible. Care is taken to remove the ridge (incisura) of the olecranon to allow a

---

*B. F. Morrey.

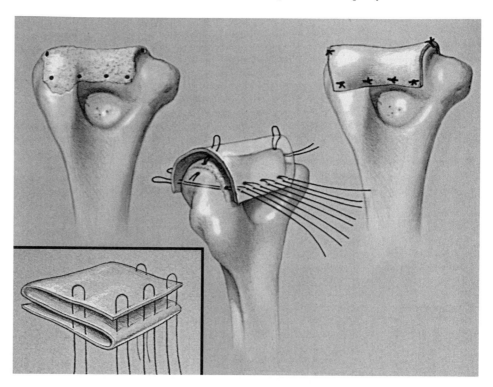

FIGURE 60–5 • The tissue is attached by through-and-through sutures across the distal humerus. If fascia is used, a three-ply composite is used and is attached as shown.

flat articulation on the humerus. Care is taken to remove enough bone for the trochlea and capitellum to accommodate the tendon graft, allowing a few millimeters of laxity to ensure adequate motion (Fig. 60–6). If the collateral ligament is deficient, one or both are reconstructed with remnants of the Achilles tendon graft.

Closure is as previously described. Care is taken to ensure stability. We routinely apply the dynamic joint distractor (DJD, Rutherford, NJ) external fixator to allow early motion and preserve stability (see Chapter 34).

Aftercare. Motion is begun on the first day with a continuous motion machine and maintained for 3 to 4 weeks. The fixator is removed under anesthesia and elbow motion and stability examined. Activity is begun, and, if the joint is stiff, static splints are prescribed (Chapter 12).

RESULTS

Early reports of fascial arthroplasty by Campbell,[9, 10] Henderson,[22, 23] and MacAusland and MacAusland[31] showed that excellent or good pain relief and improvements in motion and function were obtained in about 75 percent of patients. In 1940, Speed and Smith[49] noted that the best results could be obtained in patients between the ages of 18 and 40 years. In 1952, Knight and Van Zandt[28] reported 56 percent good and 22 percent fair results in 45 patients an average of 14 years after fascial arthroplasty. Their best results were obtained in patients between the ages of 20 and 50 years. Most patients regained motion between 6 months and 6 years after surgery, and maximum strength was obtained at about 1 year. Vainio,[53] in 1967, reported that over half of 131 patients undergoing fascial

arthroplasty were free of pain and had more than 90 degrees of flexion.

Subsequent reports have supported the value of fascial arthroplasty of the elbow in well selected patients.[16, 25, 32, 52] Although the technique is favored for rheumatoid arthritis in Europe, both rheumatoid and traumatic conditions are available to interposition arthroplasty if the proper indications are met (Figs. 60–7 and 60–8).

Little correlation between the final radiographic appearance of the elbow and the functional result is accepted. Range of motion and stability of the arthroplasty are best in patients with good periarticular structures and good elbow flexor and extensor musculature.

Uuspaa[52] reported improved range of motion and decreased contractures after 51 cutis arthroplasties in 48 patients with rheumatoid arthritis; these patients ranged in age from 25 to 69 years. In a recent review of cutis arthroplasties in 14 patients ranging in age from 26 to 51 years, motion and medial-lateral stability were satisfactory in all.[29]

A more recent review of 37 fascial arthroplasties of the elbow revealed that 26 patients (70 percent) had excellent or good results (see Fig 60–7).[30] There was one fair result, and seven had poor results. Three patients were lost to follow-up. Most of the patients with excellent or good results had a functional range of motion and were able to return to their activities of daily living with little or no pain. The fair and poor results were due to persistent pain, loss of motion, and excessive instability. Kita[27] reported the use of a chromicized fascial interposition material in 31 patients in an attempt to reduce the inflammatory response initiated by fascia lata. At 19-year follow-up, half of his patients had excellent or good results and 20 percent had poor results. Since the last edition, there have been four reports of this procedure that have markedly increased our years (range, 2–12) after surgery. It is of note that those without pre-existing instability revealed 80 percent satisfactory outcomes.

COMPLICATIONS

Complications of this procedure included bone resorption, heterotopic bone formation, triceps rupture, medial and lateral subluxation, infection, and seroma formation in the fascial graft donor site, and long-term failure.

Bone resorption occasionally occurs at the distal humeral condyles. It may cause no difficulty, or it may contribute to instability, especially if resorption occurs more on one side than on the other. Subluxation and instability may occur from resorption or because of technical difficulties, yet the joint may function reasonably well in spite of medial or lateral subluxation. If the tendency to subluxate is apparent at the time the arthroplasty is performed, the elbow may be stabilized with a transarticular Steinmann pin, which is removed in about 3 weeks or before motion is begun. If significant instability develops as a late sequela, ligamentous reconstruction may be beneficial. We have successfully avoided instability by repairing or reconstructing the collateral ligaments and applying a distraction device.[17]

Prominent spurs rarely impair function after elbow arthroplasty unless it is sufficiently extensive to limit functional motion. Triceps rupture is an uncommon complication that is related to the surgical exposure rather than to the procedure itself. This can be minimized by using the exposure described subsequently or by elevating the triceps in continuity.

Infection following fascial arthroplasty should be managed promptly and aggressively. For superficial infections and cellulitis, the part should be placed at rest, elevated, and immobilized in a long arm posterior splint while appropriate antibiotics are administered. If the infection involves the deep structures, open drainage and excision of the fascial graft may be required. If bony infection occurs, removal of the implant and osseous débridement is required. Although this will leave the elbow more unstable, a useful limb often can be salvaged. Salvage with prosthetic replacement is out of the question.

If a hematoma or seroma forms at the fascial donor, it will usually resolve over a period of weeks. These collections rarely require drainage. If such an accumulation persists or is unusually large, drainage, if undertaken, must be done with strict aseptic technique. Needle aspiration should be attempted first.

Failure of the procedure due to pain, reankylosis, or instability may occur. The result can deteriorate with time, especially in the active individual. Additional surgery may not be offered because frequently little more can be done to modify the symptoms or attain the expectations of the patient. If the precise cause of failure can be identified, revision is occasionally helpful. Typically, prosthetic replacement is the salvage procedure of choice and is readily performed (Fig. 60–9).

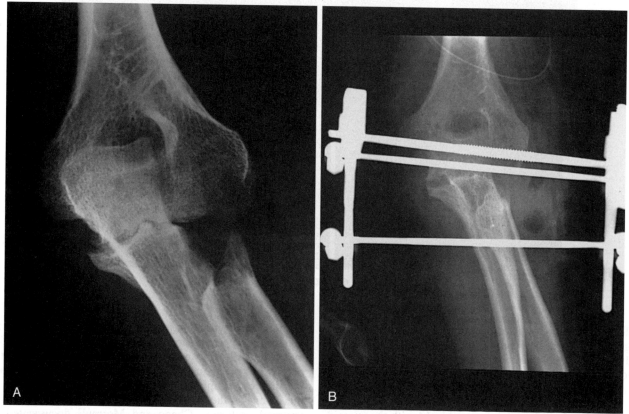

FIGURE 60–9 • Rheumatoid arthritis in 34-year-old female (A) treated with fascial interposition arthroplasty using the distractor as discussed in the text (B). At 3 years, the patient complained of severe pain (C). Three years after elbow replacement, she is again pain-free (D).

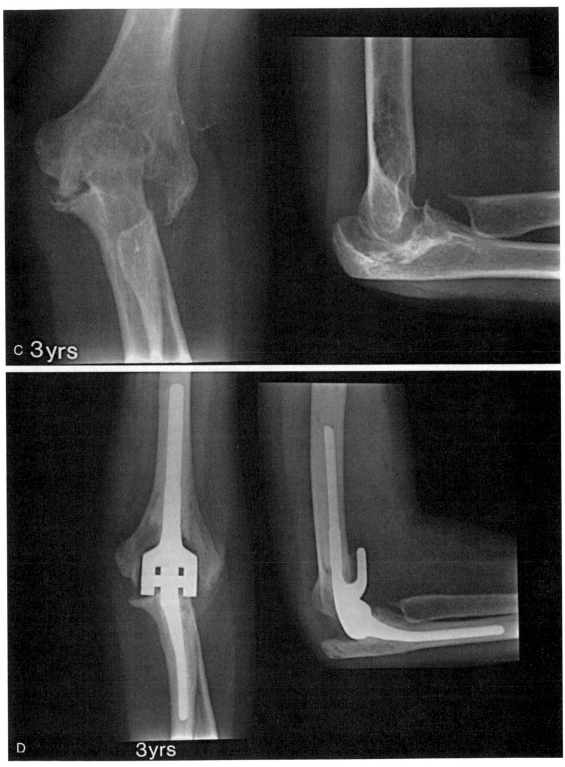

FIGURE 60–9C AND D • *Continued*

internal fixation (screws), with or without bone grafts.[9] If significant instability or deformity is present preoperatively, internal fixation with screws and supplemented with external skeletal fixation or plates should be used.

Early Surgical Techniques

Steindler described a single posterior tibial cortical graft keyed into the olecranon for fusion (Fig. 61-2A).[20] Brittain developed a technique of crossed grafts through the elbow joint[4, 6] (see Fig. 61-2B). Noting that gravitational forces tended to compress the ends of the graft, he believed that the crossing of the grafts was important. Koch and Lipscomb have described a modification of this technique in which a tibial graft is placed through a large drill hole in the humerus and ulna and other cancellous bone grafts are added to the joint.[10]

Staples uses a corticocancellous iliac graft through the posterior portion of the elbow and oblique humeral and olecranon intra-articular resection (see Fig. 61-2C).[19]

Recent Surgical Techniques

Today fusion is achieved through rigid plate fixation, transfusion fixation screws, an external fixator, or a combination of the last two.

PLATE FIXATION

Spier[18] and Plank[15] have described a compression arthrodesis that makes use of a bent plate and an external compression device (Fig. 61-3). This is also the method favored by Burkhalter.[11]

COMPRESSION SCREWS

For post-traumatic arthrosis of the elbow with minimal motion that causes significant pain, we have used compression fixation of the elbow with screws. The procedure involves partial débridement of remaining articular surfaces and compression screw fixation without grafts (Fig. 61-4). Irvine and Gregg recently reported on a similar technique in conjunction with bone grafting.[9]

For active draining sinuses with tuberculosis of the elbow, Arafiles has described a technique that locks the olecranon in the humeral fossa and stabilizes it by screw fixation.[1] In 13 patients with tuberculosis, he achieved healing of the arthrodesis within 3 months.

A straight longitudinal incision is made over the posterior elbow. The triceps tendon is split longitudinally and detached distally for 5 cm with medial and lateral periosteal sleeves. The ulnar nerve is freed and retracted, and the distal humerus is freed subperiosteally, elevating the soft tissues off the condyles, including the flexor and extensor origins. The radial head and both humeral condyles are resected. Complete synovectomy and removal of the articular cartilage is performed. The proximal ulna and the olecranon fossa are shaped into matching triangular sets (Fig. 61-5A). After the olecranon is inserted into the trochlea, a single cortical screw is placed from the posterior

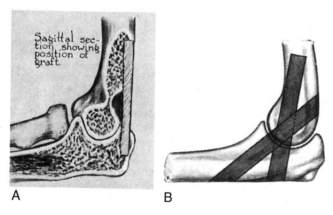

A   B

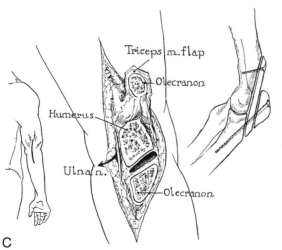

C

FIGURE 61-2 • *A*, Steindler technique of elbow fusion. *B*, Crossed tibial graft technique of Brittain. *C*, Staples' technique of elbow arthrodesis. (*A* from Steindler, A.: Reconstructive Surgery of the Upper Extremity. New York, D. Appleton & Co., 1923; *B* from Brittain, H. A.: Architectural Principles in Arthrodesis, 2nd ed. Edinburgh, E. & S. Livingstone, Ltd., 1952; *C* from Staples, O. S.: Arthrodesis of the elbow joint. J. Bone Surg. **34A**:207, 1952.)

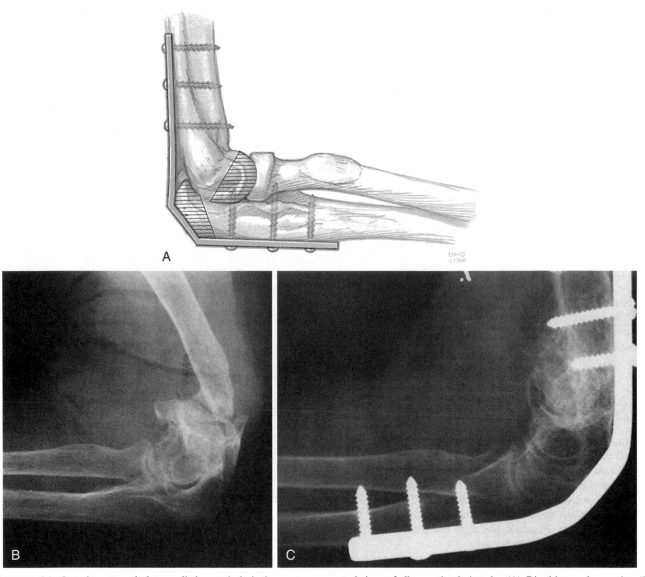

FIGURE 61–3 • A contoured plate applied posteriorly is the most common technique of elbow arthrodesis today *(A)*. Distal humeral nonunion *(B)* treated with the posterior plate (Spier's technique) *(C)*. (*B* and *C* from Spier, W.: Beitrag zur Technik der Druckarthrodese des Ellenbogengelenks. Monatsschr. Unfallheilkd. **76**:274, 1973.)

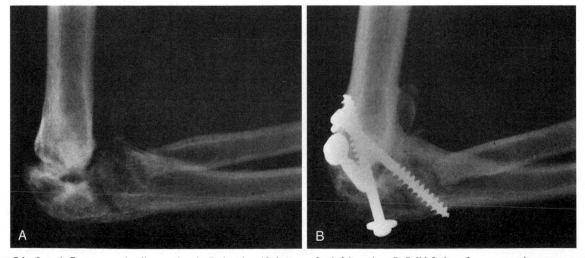

FIGURE 61–4 • *A*, Post-traumatic elbow arthrosis. Patient has 10 degrees of painful motion. *B*, Solid fusion after compression screw application across elbow without bone graft.

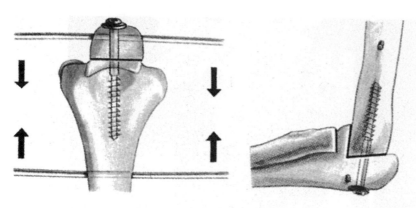

FIGURE 61–9 • The AO technique of axial fixation and external skeletal fixation for arthrodesis of the elbow. (From Muller, M. E., et al.: Manual of Internal Fixation: Techniques Recommended by the AO-Group, 2nd ed. Berlin, Springer-Verlag, 1979.)

grafting, if necessary. This, in conjunction with cast fixation, should produce simplified and more rapid union.

With Infection. In the presence of infection and an unstable elbow, however, I prefer to use simple external skeletal fixation with cancellous grafting if necessary. There is often a hypertrophic bony response to infection. Thus, external skeletal fixation with the bilateral or unilateral triangular configuration can achieve compression and good immobilization and allow the wounds to be left open and to close gradually in anticipation of spontaneous union (see Fig. 61–7).

For Stable Elbows

For a stable elbow without infection, internal fixation with cancellous compression screws is a very simple method that promotes more rapid union and earlier mobilization. Grafts generally are not necessary, and minimal débridement of cortical surfaces is required to allow the fusion to mature. Again, in the presence of infection, external skeletal fixation with articular débridement and open wound packing promotes union. In some instances when good bone stock is available, the compression screw may be supplemented by the dynamic joint distractor (DJD; Havmedica, Rutherford, NJ) external fixator (Fig. 61–8).

COMPLICATIONS

Nonunion. Few data are available about success rates for primary arthrodesis. Koch and Lipscomb reported that primary arthrodesis failed in nine of 17 patients treated at the Mayo Clinic.[10] Six of 11 elbows treated for tuberculosis failed to unite. Extensive joint destruction and unavailability of chemotherapy were cited as contributory factors to this poor rate of fusion. A recent updating of the Mayo Clinic experience has demonstrated a significant decrease in nonunion rates with internal fixation.

Fracture. The long lever arm created by elbow fusion increases stress along the entire extremity. Fracture through or proximal to the fused or ankylosed joint is not uncommon and was reported in four of 17 patients by Koch and Lipscomb.[10] Conservative treatment, however, usually results in union (Fig. 61–10).

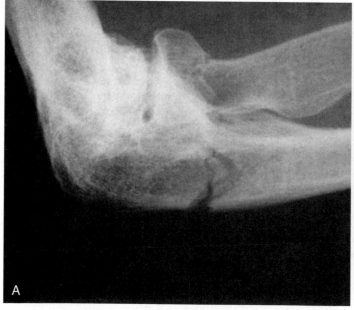
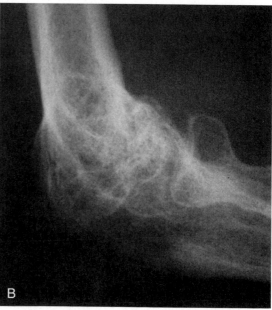

FIGURE 61–10 • A, Fracture below elbow arthrodesis. B, Rapid healing with simple immobilization.

REFERENCES

1. Arafiles, R. P.: A new technique of fusion for tuberculous arthritis of the elbow. J. Bone Joint Surg. **63A**:1396, 1981.

2. Bonnel, F.: Technique d'arthrodese du coude par fixateur externe. J. Chir. (Paris) **107**:79, 1974.

3. Boyd, A. D. Jr., and Thornhill, T. S.: Surgical treatment of the elbow in rheumatoid arthritis. Hand Clin. **5**:645, 1989.

4. Brittain, H. A.: Architectural Principles in Arthrodesis, 2nd ed. Edinburgh, E. & S. Livingstone, 1952, p. 161.

5. Connes, H.: Hoffmann's External Anchorage: Techniques, Indications and Results. Paris, Editions GEAD, 1977, p. 118.

6. Crenshaw, A. H. (ed.): Campbell's Operative Orthopaedics, 5th ed. St. Louis, C. V. Mosby Co., 1971, p. 1191.

7. Dahl, H. K.: AO Metoden ved Osteotomi og Arthrodese. Nord. Med. **85**:599, 1971.

8. Figgie, M. P., Inglis, A. E., Mow, C. S., Wolfe, S. W., Sculco, T. P., and Figgie, H. E., III: Results of reconstruction for failed total elbow arthroplasty. Clin. Orthop. **253**:123, 1990.

9. Irvine, G. B., and Gregg, P. J.: A method of elbow arthrodesis: brief report. J. Bone Joint Surg. **71B**:145, 1989.

10. Koch, M., and Lipscomb, P. R.: Arthrodesis of the elbow. Clin. Orthop. **50**:151, 1967.

11. McAuliffe, J., and Burkhalter, W.: Post-traumatic elbow infection and fixation failure. Orthop. Consultation **12**:1, 1991.

12. Morrey, B. F., Askew, L. J., An, K. N., and Chao, E. Y.: A biomechanical study of normal functional elbow motion. J. Bone Joint Surg. **63A**:872, 1981.

13. Muller, M. E., Allgower, M., Schneider, R., and Willenegger, H.: Manual of Internal Fixation: Techniques Recommended by the AO-Group, 2nd ed. Berlin, Springer-Verlag, 1979, p. 387.

14. O'Neill, O.R., Morrey, B.F., Tanaka, S., and An, K.N.: Compensatory motion in the upper extremity after elbow arthrodesis. Clin. Orthop. **281**:89–96, 1992.

15. Plank, E., and Spier, W.: Die Arthrodese des Ellenbogens. Aktuel Probl. Chir. Orthop. **2**:41, 1977.

16. Rashkoff, E., and Burkhalter, W. E.: Arthrodesis of the salvaged elbow. Orthopedics **9**:733, 1986.

17. Snider, W. J., and De Witt, H. J.: Functional study for optimum position for elbow arthrodesis or ankylosis. *In* Proceedings of the American Academy of Orthopedic Surgeons. J. Bone Joint Surg. **55A**:1305, 1973.

18. Spier, W.: Beitrag zur Technik der Druckarthrodese des Ellenbogengelenks. Monatsschr. Unfallheilkd. **76**:274, 1973.

19. Staples, O. S.: Arthrodesis of the elbow joint. J. Bone Joint Surg. **34A**:207, 1952.

20. Steindler, A.: Reconstructive Surgery of the Upper Extremity. New York, D. Appleton & Co., 1923.

21. Wolfe, S. W., Figgie, M. P., Inglis, A. E., Bohn, W. W., and Ranawat, C. S.: Management of infection about total elbow prostheses. J. Bone Joint Surg. **72A**:198, 1990.

insertion of some muscles can be transferred: triceps,[21] pectoralis major,[15] and sternocleidomastoid.[19] All or part of the origin of a muscle or muscle group can be transferred: forearm flexor-pronator,[103] sternocostal portion of pectoralis major,[29] latissimus dorsi,[55] and pectoralis minor.[100] The entire muscle can be located on its neurovascular pedicle—latissimus dorsi[91] and pectoralis major.[25] Finally, a muscle can be transplanted using a microneurovascular anastomosis, as with the gracilis.[44]

Steindler's Flexorplasty

Steindler first described his simple but ingenious concept of proximally shifting the origin of the flexor-pronator muscle group to increase its lever arm in flexing the elbow in 1918.[101, 102] His technique consisted of the subperiosteal dissection of the origin of the flexor-pronator muscles of the forearm from the medial epicondyle. The muscle flap was then transposed proximally between the brachialis and the triceps and was sutured to the medial epicondylar ridge through two drill holes 2 inches above the epicondyle. Steindler recommended the procedure only if the wrist flexors were normal or only slightly weakened.

Subsequent authors differed on the prerequisites for Steindler's flexorplasty. Mayer and Green believed that the epicondylar muscle group strength should be grade 3 or better, and they re-emphasized the need for strong wrist flexors if the operation is to succeed.[70] They described this simple test:

The arm is abducted to 90 degrees to eliminate gravity. Any patient who can flex the elbow in this position (using the epicondylar muscle group) is a candidate for the operation. Nyholm believed that the criteria for forearm muscle strength should be liberalized because all his patients achieved 90 degrees of elbow flexion, even though a relatively large number had forearm muscles that were "primarily paretic."[83] Dutton and Dawson performed the operation if the strength of the forearm flexor-pronator group was rated fair or better.[37] Alnot[4] believed that the shoulder flexorplasty was most indicated to reinforce a biceps that had recovered to M2 strength. It seems that there is considerable variability in the preoperative muscle strength needed for active flexion, and the axiom that the muscle loses a grade in transferring it does not necessarily apply in this particular situation.

Others have modified and refined Steindler's original concept to increase flexor strength and decrease the tendency toward development of a pronation deformity. Bunnell described extending the common tendon of origin with a fascia lata graft that would reach 2 inches up the lateral border of the humerus.[19] This resulted in moderate but not complete correction of the pronation tendency. Mayer and Green detached the flexor-pronator origin with a portion of the medial epicondyle and attached it through a window cut in the anterior cortex of the humerus 5 to 7.5 cm proximal to the joint.[70] Their description of the technical details of the Steindler flexorplasty, which includes careful dissection of the ulnar and median motor branches, is the best in the literature. Lindholm and Einola used a screw to fix the epicondylar fragment to the humerus in two cases.[65] Eyler advocated omitting the flexor carpi ulnaris to allow the surgeon to work in the "internervous plane" between

the flexor sublimis, anteriorly, and the flexor profundus and flexor carpi ulnaris, dorsally.[39]

Efforts have been made to augment the strength of elbow flexion, especially in patients who have weakness of the flexor-pronator muscle group. Initially, Steindler recommended proximal transfer of the radial wrist extensor muscle origins off the lateral epicondyle in conjunction with the medial transfer, but he did not comment on it in his later communications.[103] Mayer and Green reported having difficulty mobilizing the lateral epicondylar muscle group without damaging the nerve supply[70] and gave up the procedure after two unsatisfactory results. Lindholm and Einola were unable to detect any increase in flexion strength in the six patients who had the additional lateral transfer.[65]

ANATOMY

The pronator teres arises from two heads. The humeral head originates from the medial supracondylar ridge, the medial intermuscular septum, and the common flexor tendon. The smaller ulnar head arises from the coronoid process of the ulna. The median nerve enters the forearm between the two heads of the pronator teres. The flexor carpi radialis, palmaris longus, and humeral head of the flexor superficialis all originate from the common flexor tendon. The flexor carpi ulnaris arises from two heads: the humeral head originates from the common flexor tendon, and the ulnar head originates along the medial border of the olecranon and posterior border of the upper three fifths of the ulna. Branches originating from the medial surface of the median nerve supply the pronator teres (C6, C7), the flexor carpi radialis (C6, C7), the palmaris longus (C7, C8), and the humeral head of the flexor superficialis (C8 and T1). The flexor carpi ulnaris (C8 and T1) is innervated by two or three branches of the ulnar nerve, the first of which usually leaves the nerve just as it passes between the two heads of the muscle.

TECHNIQUE (MODIFIED FROM MAYER AND GREEN)

A sandbag is placed under the opposite hip (Fig. 62–2). A tourniquet usually is not used. The incision begins on the anterior aspect of the arm about 7.5 cm above the elbow and swings gently in a medial direction. At the elbow, it runs just posterior to the epicondyle. It then curves anteriorly, following the direction of the pronator teres, ending about 10 cm below the elbow. The ulnar nerve is isolated and freed distally to the branches of the flexor carpi ulnaris. Preserving these motor branches, the surgeon continues the dissection distally for 5 cm. The lacertus fibrosus is divided, and the median nerve is exposed above the elbow and dissected distally, exposing the motor branches (all of which leave the medial aspect of the nerve) to the common flexor-pronator muscle group. The common flexor-pronator muscle origin is then detached with a flake of epicondyle (cartilage in children and bone in adults). The flake of bone or cartilage is then grasped with a clamp, and, while traction is exerted in distal and anterior directions, the muscles are stripped from the anterior surface of the joint and from the coronoid process of the ulna. As the ulnar

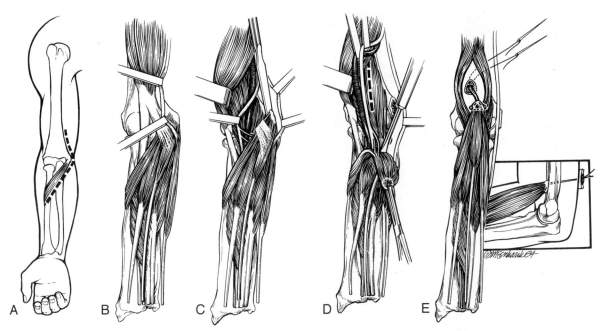

FIGURE 62-2 • Steindler's flexorplasty. *A*, The incision. *B*, The ulnar nerve is mobilized proximally and distally, and its motor branches to the flexor carpi ulnaris are identified and protected. *C*, The common flexor-pronator origin is detached with a flake of medial epicondyle. The motor branches of the median nerve to the flexor-pronator group are identified and protected. *D*, The detached flexor-pronator group is mobilized distally as far as the motor branches of the medial and ulnar nerves will permit. The brachialis muscle is divided. *E*, The distal humerus is prepared, and a Prolene pull-out suture is used to anchor the transferred muscles to the anterolateral surface of the humerus 5 to 7.5 cm above the elbow. (After Mayer and Green.)

head of the flexor carpi ulnaris is detached from the ulna with an elevator, the assistant puts gentle traction on the median and ulnar nerves, demonstrating the motor twigs that must be carefully avoided. Dissection is continued distally as far as the anatomic distribution of the nerves permits. The common tendon is then transfixed with a modified pull-out suture of No. 1 prolene. The elbow is flexed to 120 degrees, and traction is exerted on the transfer to determine how far above the elbow the transfer will reach. This is usually between 5 and 7.5 cm. The ulnar nerve often seems to have less tension on it if it is transferred anterior to the epicondyle. The atrophic fibers of the brachialis are slit longitudinally, the periosteum is incised, and the anterior humerus is exposed subperiosteally. An opening in the anterior cortex of the humerus nearer to the lateral than to the medial border is made at the point to which the transplant reaches when the elbow is flexed. Two small drill holes are made from anterior to posterior through this cortical window. The prolene suture ends are then threaded through the holes and out through the triceps muscle and skin. To be sure that they are not subjected to undue tension on twisting, the nerves are inspected as the transfer is pulled into the cortical window. The distal portion of the wound is closed, up to the bend in the elbow. The sutured ends are drawn tight with the elbow in maximal flexion and tied over a button under which a thick piece of felt has been placed. Several auxiliary sutures between the periosteum and the transplanted epicondylar tissues are placed, and the wound is closed with a drain.

A posterior splint is then applied with the elbow in about 120 degrees' flexion and the forearm in full supination. Four weeks after surgery, the pull-out suture is removed. A removable orthoplast splint is applied, and active flexion

and supination and extension exercises are begun. No special retraining is required because the muscles transferred functioned as an accessory elbow flexor before transfer.[28] Splinting is discontinued 6 to 8 weeks after surgery, the longer time being necessary for patients with normal triceps function. A dynamic extension splint is often useful if the patient has no triceps function (Fig. 62-3).

RESULTS

Published results of the Steindler flexorplasty reflect a high degree of success in achieving a functional range of elbow flexion against gravity. Most transfers reported have been performed for poliomyelitis. Steindler achieved 79.5 percent good results (flexion against gravity of not less than 90 degrees) in 39 cases.[105] Fifteen good results (useful range of flexion with good to fair power) in 27 flexorplasties were reported by Carroll and Gartland.[23] Using strict criteria for success, including subtracting from the total score for flexion contracture over 15 degrees and for supination of less than 45 degrees, Mayer and Green recorded 11 excellent results, 5 good, 4 fair, and 2 poor results among the 22 flexorplasties they followed up.[70] Segal and associates compared the results of 13 Steindler flexorplasties (transplantation of both flexor and extensor origins) and 17 Clark pectoralis major transfers.[97] The flexorplasty results were better than the pectoralis transfers, but the average flexion contracture in the flexorplasty group was 60 degrees, whereas it rarely exceeded 15 degrees in the Clark transfer group. Kettelkamp and Larson, evaluating 15 flexorplasties using Mayer and Green's scoring system, noted 8 excellent or good results, 6 fair results, and 1 poor one.[58] They also measured the carry-lift strength (flexion slips from the lower four ribs. It inserts into the medial wall and floor of the intertubercular groove of the humerus. The major vascular pedicle of the muscle is the thoracodorsal artery, a terminal branch of the subscapular artery. In 94 percent of the 114 specimens, a bifurcation of the common neurovascular trunk into lateral (parallel to the lateral border of the muscle) and medial (parallel to the upper border) branches has been documented.[111] Bartlett and co-workers studied 50 latissimus dorsi muscles and noted the same bifurcation in 56 percent of the dissections.[8] These studies provide the anatomic basis for the clinical findings noted by Axer and colleagues.[7] The thoracodorsal nerve (C6–8) is derived from the posterior cord and enters the muscle with the artery and its vein on its deep surface about 10 cm from its insertion. There are one to three branches from the thoracodorsal artery to the serratus muscle that have to be ligated to allow complete mobilization of the latissimus during a bipolar transfer. In the study by Bartlett and co-workers, the vascular pedicle to the latissimus dorsi had an average length of 11 cm and the thoracodorsal nerve a mean length of 12.3 cm.[8]

TECHNIQUE

The bipolar transplantation is preferable to the unipolar transfer for several reasons. The mechanical efficiency of the transplant is increased by the more anterior placement of the origin into the coracoid process, the proper length is easier to determine when the distal insertion is completed first, and there is less chance for kinking the neurovascular pedicle.

Bipolar Transplantation

This description follows that of Zancolli and Mitre (Fig. 62–5).[123] The operation is carried out in four steps:

1. Division of the latissimus dorsi muscle origin and insertion while preserving its neurovascular pedicle.

2. Exposure of both ends of the biceps muscle through separate incisions.

3. Transplantation of the latissimus dorsi muscle under a cutaneous bridge in the axilla to the bed of the paralyzed biceps and brachialis, resecting the biceps muscle, if need be, to provide room for the latissimus dorsi.

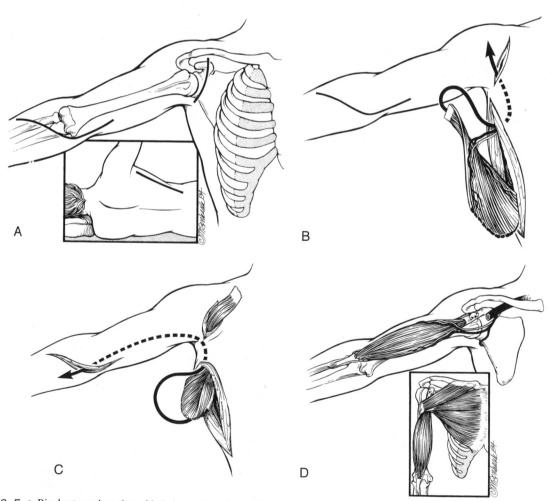

FIGURE 62–5 • Bipolar transplantation of latissimus dorsi. *A*, Incisions used for this procedure. *B*, The origin and insertion of the latissimus dorsi are divided, and the muscle is mobilized on its neurovascular pedicle. *C*, Transplantation of the muscle under a cutaneous bridge in the axilla; the origin is redirected through a subcutaneous tunnel in the arm to the biceps tendon. *D*, The distal anastomosis is completed first, and the proximal attachment to the coracoid process and its conjoined tendon is used to set the tension. (After Zancolli, E., and Mitre, H.: Latissimus dorsi transfer to restore elbow flexion. J. Bone Joint Surg. **55A**:1265, 1973.)

4. Fixation of the transposed muscle to the coracoid process and biceps tendon.

The patient is in the lateral position, and the upper extremity is draped free. A longitudinal incision is made parallel to the lateral border of the latissimus dorsi muscle, extending from the posterior border of the axilla to the iliac crest. The dissection of the muscle is begun along its lateral border and leads from distal to proximal. The neurovascular pedicle must be freed up to its origin in the axilla, and this requires the ligation of any branches of the thoracodorsal artery that enter the serratus anterior. Once the neurovascular pedicle is freed, the origin and insertion of the latissimus dorsi are sectioned. When the muscle is small, it is transplanted completely, but when it is entirely normal, it may be necessary to transplant only its lateral half. It is also possible to fold over the vertebral border of the muscle to make it more tubular in shape.

A deltopectoral incision is used to expose the coracoid process and free the tendon of the pectoralis major, behind which the transposed latissimus dorsi will be routed. The insertion of the biceps is then exposed through a bayonet incision over the anterior aspect of the elbow. If the paralyzed biceps is to be resected, the resection is carried out through these two incisions and care is taken to protect the neurovascular bundle of the arm and to preserve a long segment of distal biceps tendon. The latissimus dorsi muscle is then passed under the skin bridge of the axilla, protecting its neurovascular pedicle from any kinking or tension. The insertion of the transposed muscle is passed deep to the pectoralis major tendon and up to the coracoid process while its distal end is passed downward toward the elbow beneath the skin of the arm. It is convenient at this time to close the thoracic incision over several drains. The distal biceps aponeurosis is opened up and spread out so that it can be wrapped around the distal end of the latissimus dorsi. A significant amount of distal latissimus muscle usually has to be excised because it is too long. After the distal anastomosis is completed, the distal skin incision is closed. The proximal end is then fixed at the junction of the conjoined tendon with the coracoid process, the length of the transplant being adjusted so that the elbow remains spontaneously at 90 to 100 degrees of flexion with some trial sutures in place. When the proper length has been determined, the final suturing of the proximal end is carried out and the shoulder wound is closed. A plaster Velpeau bandage is then applied with the elbow flexed and the forearm supinated.

The drains are removed at 48 hours. Postoperative immobilization is maintained for 6 weeks. Flexion exercises are then permitted (with gravity eliminated) with gradually decreasing extension block splinting over the next 2 weeks. At 8 weeks, flexion against gravity begins. Four to 6 months is required before the transplant attains maximum strength.

Myocutaneous transplantation of the latissimus dorsi is performed using the same technique, except that an appropriately sized segment of skin is left attached to the muscle (Fig. 62–6).

Unipolar Transfer

This description is based on that of Hovnanian (Fig. 62–7). The patient is positioned as for the bipolar transfer. The

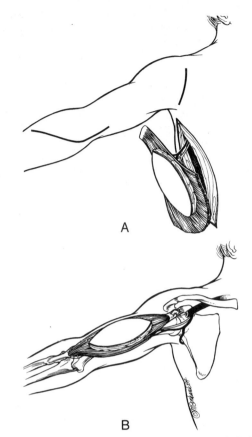

FIGURE 62–6 • Technique used for a myocutaneous latissimus dorsi transplantation.

incision begins in the loin, extends along the lateral margin of the latissimus to the posterior axillary fold, and continues across the axilla and downward along the medial arm to the elbow. The muscle is detached from its origin, preserving part of the aponeurosis with it, and is freed up proximally. Branches from the thoracodorsal artery to the serratus anterior muscle are ligated. The muscle is then transferred to the anterior arm, where it is attached to the biceps tendon and periosteal tissues of the bicipital tuberosity. The arm is bandaged to the thorax for 3 to 4 weeks, at which time active and passive exercises are started.

RESULTS

Experience is with small patient samples.[7, 10, 55] Zancolli and Mitre observed eight patients who had had bipolar transplantation of the latissimus dorsi for more than 4 years.[123] Active range of flexion was 105 to 140 degrees, and flexion strength varied from 0.7 to 5 kg. Flexion contractures of 10 degrees and 15 degrees occurred in two, and active supination of 20 to 50 degrees was achieved in six. Takami and others[109] reported on two patients. One obtained elbow motion from 0 to 125 degrees and supination of 30 degrees and could lift 3 kg; the other had motion from 0 to 130 degrees with 60 degrees of supination and could lift 2 kg. Moneim and Omer[77] achieved satisfactory flexion (100 degrees or more) in three of five patients. The two others achieved 65 to 70 degrees of flexion and initially

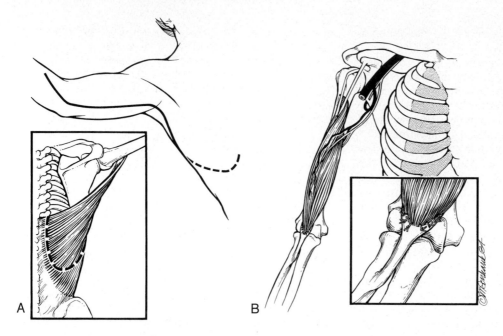

FIGURE 62–7 • Unipolar transfer of the latissimus dorsi for elbow flexion. *A*, Incisions employed. *B*, The detached origin, rotated on its neurovascular pedicle, is attached to the biceps tendon and aponeurosis.

had paralysis of the latissimus dorsi, so they were advised that the procedure should not be done unless the muscle was normal. Preoperative EMG evaluation of the muscle was recommended. Hirayama and associates[51] reported four excellent results, three good results, and one failure among eight patients who had transfers of the latissimus dorsi. Botte and Wood[11] noted satisfactory function in four of five patients treated with unipolar or bipolar latissimus dorsi transfer, and flexion that averaged 87 degrees (range 35 to 130). Chen[27] achieved satisfactory function with average motion from 32 degrees of extension to 126 degrees of flexion in six patients who had bipolar transfers of the latissimus dorsi. They could lift only 1.5 to 2.5 kg, which was sufficient for most activities of daily living but not for heavy manual work. Concurrent skin coverage with restoration of elbow flexion is accomplished nicely with a latissimus dorsi myocutaneous flap.[14, 52, 89, 107] Clinical evidence of a functional deficit after transfer or transplantation of the latissimus dorsi is unusual. Russell and co-workers[90] did document some minimal changes in shoulder strength and range of motion after transfer or transplantation of the latissimus dorsi in 24 patients.

Pectoralis Muscle Transfer

HISTORY

The first use of the pectoralis major muscle to restore elbow flexion was reported in the European literature in 1917 by Schulze-Berge, who transferred its tendon of insertion directly into the belly of the biceps.[93] Subsequent modifications of the method of insertion of the pectoralis major included the use of fascia lata or strands of silk to form tendons of insertion, either into the biceps tendon or directly into the ulna.[53, 62, 63, 88] Clark reported the first really successful physiologic transfer of the pectoralis major in 1946.[29] In his procedure, the sternocostal origin of the muscle with its separate nerve (medial pectoral) and blood supply was mobilized, passed subcutaneously down the

upper arm, and attached to the biceps tendon. Seddon modified Clark's operation by elevating a segment of rectus abdominis sheath in continuity with the distal end of the transplant to act as a tendon.[94]

Brooks and Seddon described a unipolar transfer of the entire pectoralis major muscle, employing the devascularized long head of the biceps as its tendon of insertion.[15] They recommended this operation instead of a Clark transfer when either the lower part of the pectoralis major was paralyzed but the clavicular head strong, or the whole muscle was weak.[97]

In 1955, Schottstaedt and others first reported bipolar transplantation of the chondrosternal portion (lower two thirds) of the pectoralis major on its neurovascular pedicle to restore elbow flexion.[91] The humeral insertion was detached and shifted to the coracoid process, and the origin was transplanted to the biceps tendon. Carroll and Kleinman transplanted the entire pectoralis major muscle on both of its neurovascular pedicles.[25] The muscle origin with its attached anterior rectus abdominis sheath was attached to the biceps tendon, and its tendon of insertion was secured to the anterior aspect of the acromion. With bipolar transplantation of the entire muscle, they noted increased shoulder stability, which obviated shoulder arthrodesis and improved mechanical efficiency for elbow flexion as compared with the unipolar transfer. Matory and co-workers[69] transferred the lower sternocostal portion of the muscle with a 4-cm portion of rectus sheath mobilized with the medial and lateral pectoral nerves and accompanying vessels. The muscle was "tubularized" and woven through the biceps tendon and the transverse aponeurosis was repaired to restore a pulley. Separate midline and deltopectoral incisions were used to avoid the undesirable scar from the standard pectoralis transfer approach.

Tsai and associates added unipolar transfer of the pectoralis minor muscle to a bipolar pectoralis major transplant, noting excellent strength of elbow flexion without endangering the two muscles' common neurovascular bundles.[113]

The lateral half of the clavicular origin of the pectoralis major was left intact to preserve shoulder adduction.

The first transfer of the pectoralis minor to the paralyzed biceps to restore elbow flexion was done in 1910 by Bradford.[12] Spira reported on one patient who had complete paralysis of the pectoralis major secondary to poliomyelitis who enjoyed excellent function after the transfer of the origin of the pectoralis minor into the distal biceps.[100] Alnot[4] recommended transferring the pectoralis minor to the biceps at the time of plexus exploration and nerve repair.

ANATOMY

Phylogenetically, the pectoralis major muscle evolved from three separate ones, and today it has a segmental configuration with an independent neurovascular supply (Fig. 62–8A). The pectoralis major muscle has two constant (clavicular and sternocostal) subunits and, in about half of humans, an abdominal subunit.[110] The clavicular portion of the muscle originates from the medial third of the clavicle. The sternocostal portion arises from the anterior surface of the manubrium and the body of the sternum and cartilage of the first six ribs. The abdominal portion, when present, arises from the aponeurosis of the external oblique muscle and is found posterior to the axillary border of the sternocostal portion. The lateral pectoral nerve, derived from the lateral cord and containing fibers from nerve roots C5, C6, and C7, supplies the clavicular and upper portions of the sternocostal parts of the muscle. The medial pectoral nerve, derived from the medial cord and containing fibers from C8 and T1, innervates the lower sternocostal and abdominal parts of the pectoralis major after piercing the pectoralis minor or passing around its lateral edge as it also innervates this muscle. The clavicular and upper sternocostal portions of the pectoralis major are supplied by the pectoral branch of the thoracoacromial artery. The lower sternocostal portion, and the abdominal portion when present, receive their blood supply from the lateral thoracic artery.

TECHNIQUE

Unipolar Transfer

The unipolar transfer approach is based on that of Clark[29] and Holtmann and associates[54] (Fig. 62–8B–D). The patient is supine with a sandbag behind the shoulder. The arm is draped free and supported on a hand table or Mayo stand. An incision is made parallel to the lateral border of the pectoralis major muscle from the axilla to the seventh rib. The origin of the lower third of the muscle is detached from the sternum and fifth and sixth costal cartilages in continuity with a 6-cm segment of anterior rectus abdominis sheath. The sternocostal segment is carefully freed from the rest of the pectoralis major muscle to protect its nerve (medial pectoral) and vascular (lateral thoracic branches) supplies.

The biceps tendon is exposed through an oblique incision over the anterior aspect of the distal arm and elbow. Large forceps are then thrust upward from this distal incision to create a subcutaneous tunnel continuous with the upper end of the other incision. The muscle is pulled through the

tunnel, and its rectus sheath segment is woven through the biceps tendon with the elbow in 125 degrees' flexion and the forearm fully supinated. With the shoulder in adduction and internally rotated, the elbow and forearm are immobilized in acute flexion and supination for 6 weeks. Isometric contractions are begun at 3 weeks, followed by active elbow flexion from an initial position of 90 degrees of elbow flexion.

Partial Bipolar Transplantation of Pectoralis Major

This description follows that of Schottstaedt and colleagues.[91] The muscle is exposed through an incision extending from 2.5 cm distal to the margin of the axilla along the lateral border of the pectoralis major muscle to within 5 cm of the midline. The lower half of the pectoralis major muscle is detached from its sternocostal origin and separated from the underlying pectoralis minor, care being taken to protect its nerve (medial pectoral) and vascular supply (lateral thoracic arterial branches).

Through a separate 10-cm deltopectoral incision, the pectoralis major tendon of insertion is detached. The clavicular fibers of insertion should be detached from the freed tendon. The lower portion of the muscle is detached from the upper portion in line with its fibers; it is now completely free on its neurovascular pedicle. The biceps tendon is exposed in the distal arm and antecubital space through an oblique 12-cm incision extending from the proximal medial to the distal lateral aspect. A subcutaneous tunnel is created upward to the deltopectoral incision, and the sternocostal origin of the muscle is drawn through the tunnel so that it overlies the paralyzed biceps. The pectoralis muscle is then sewn to the biceps tendon and the aponeurosis is closed with heavy, nonabsorbable sutures. The distal wound is closed, and the pectoralis major insertion is attached to the conjoined tendon at the coracoid by weaving it through several times. While the proximal suturing is performed, the muscle tension should be maximal with the elbow in about 125 degrees of flexion. At this point, it can be noticed that the pedicle is made more lax by relieving some of the downward pull placed on it initially when the muscle was sutured to the distal biceps. According to Schottstaedt and others, an extension of length using rectus abdominis sheath is usually unnecessary.

The postoperative position of immobilization and the exercise program are as described above.

Complete Bipolar Transplantation of Pectoralis Major

This procedure is based on that of Carroll and Kleinman[25] (Fig. 62–9). The patient is placed in the supine position with a flat bolster under the blade of the scapula and the upper extremity draped free. A long, curvilinear incision is made from the seventh sternocostal joint proximally to two fingerbreadths inferior to the clavicle. The incision continues laterally to the coracoid process, then distally along the anteromedial aspect of the arm to the level of the axilla.

With the acromion and the entire pectoralis major muscle

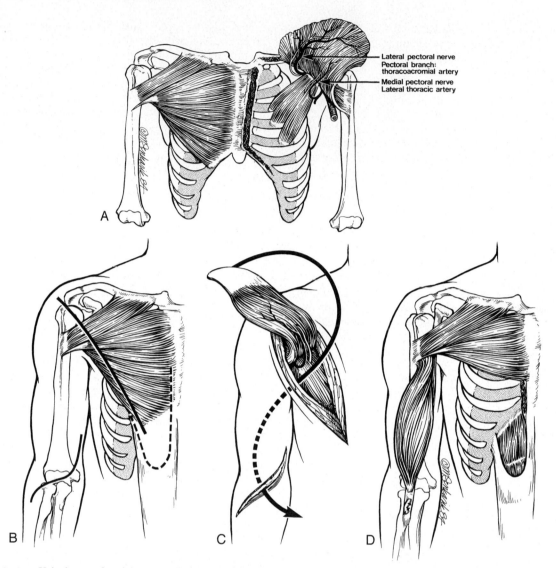

Lateral pectoral nerve
Pectoral branch: thoracoacromial artery
Medial pectoral nerve
Lateral thoracic artery

A

B   C   D

FIGURE 62–8 • Unipolar transfer of the pectoralis major for elbow flexion. *A*, The anatomy of the pectoralis major muscle. The lateral pectoral nerve and pectoral branch of the thoracoacromial artery supply the clavicular portion and the upper part of the sternocostal portion of the muscle. The medial pectoral nerve and branches from the lateral thoracic artery supply the lower part of the sternocostal portion and the abdominal portion (when present) of the pectoralis major. *B*, Incisions employed in performing a unipolar transfer of the lower sternocostal portion of the pectoralis major (Clark's transfer). *C*, The lower third of the pectoralis major, detached with a 6-cm segment of anterior rectus abdominis sheath, is mobilized proximally on its neurovascular pedicle. *D*, The detached origin with the attached rectus abdominis sheath is passed through a subcutaneous tunnel and attached to the biceps tendon.

exposed, a second curvilinear incision is made over the antecubital fossa with its transverse limb across the fossa and the longitudinal limb extending medially and distally 6 cm. The entire pectoralis major muscle is then detached from its origin along the medial half of the clavicle and its sternocostal border with a 10- by 4-cm strip of attached rectus abdominis fascia. In the process of freeing the pectoralis major from the chest wall and the underlying pectoralis minor, meticulous care is given to preserving its two neurovascular pedicles. The entire muscle mass is then rotated 90 degrees on its two neurovascular pedicles. The clavicular and sternocostal origins with the attached rectus sheath are rolled into a tube and directed through the subcutaneous tunnel, exiting through the second incision. With the elbow flexed 135 degrees, the fascial tube is enclosed under maximal tension to the biceps tendon with

nonabsorbable sutures, including a transcutaneous stay suture tied over a bolster. The tendon of insertion is then detached, directed proximally, and anchored securely to the anterior acromion by nonabsorbable sutures through drill holes. Before exercises are commenced, the elbow is immobilized for 6 weeks with the joint flexed 135 degrees using a collar and cuff with a swathe.

RESULTS

The original description was of only one patient, who had flexion limited by only 15 degrees, extension limited by 5 degrees, and flexion power 40 percent of normal 16 weeks after a partial bipolar transfer of the pectoralis major.[29] Seddon noted excellent results (powerful flexion against gravity and resistance) in 7 of 16 Clark's transfer patients

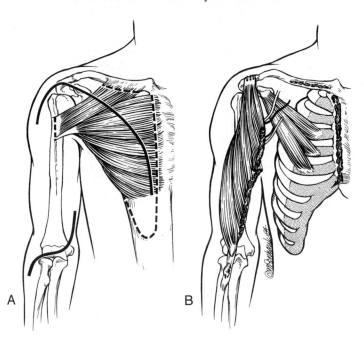

FIGURE 62–9 • Bipolar transplantation of the pectoralis major muscle for elbow flexion. *A*, The incisions. Solid lines indicate skin incisions and dotted lines indicate the extent of detachment of the pectoralis major and rectus abdominis sheath. *B*, The completely detached pectoralis major is rotated on its two neurovascular pedicles. Its origin is attached to the biceps tendon, and its insertion is attached to the acromion through drill holes.

A   B

on whom he reported.[94] In the remainder, the elbow could be flexed against gravity and slight resistance. Seven patients regained supination against resistance (from 10 to 90 degrees). In 4 cases in which the pectoralis major power was subnormal, the pectoralis minor was used in addition. D'Aubigne reported excellent active flexion, independent of shoulder adduction, in 2 patients who had Clark's transfer.[31] Using the unipolar transfer of the pectoralis major into the devascularized long head of the biceps, Brooks and Seddon achieved three excellent, three good, and two fair results (less active flexion than passive or flexion against gravity but not against resistance), and two complete failures.[15] Two of the good results, however, required second operations (triceps to biceps) because of simultaneous action of the pectoralis major and the triceps, a phenomenon they ascribed to axonal confusion during regeneration after brachial plexus lesions. Holtmann and associates noted useful active elbow flexion through a mean range of 96 degrees, accompanied by supination of the forearm, in all seven of Clark's transfers on which they reported.[54] Four of the patients had arthrogryposis, and, in all cases, the transfer was extended with a 6-cm segment of anterior rectus sheath. Leffert and Pess[64] reported the results of 15 pectoralis transfers: good result in 8, improvement in 4, and no improvement in 3 cases. They recommended that shoulder fusion be carried out several months before the transfer in patients who have a paralyzed shoulder.

Botte and Wood[11] recorded satisfactory results in all five patients who had bipolar pectoralis major transfers but cautioned against using it in women because of the cosmetic disfigurement. Matory and associates[69] transferred the lower sternocostal segment of the pectoralis major in seven patients and achieved a functional range of elbow flexion (mean 98 degrees) in all. Extension loss was only 15 to 25 degrees, and sustained flexion strength averaged 8 pounds. Tsai and others used modified bipolar transplantation of the pectoralis major (leaving the lateral half of the clavicular origin intact), supplemented with a unipolar transfer of the pectoralis minor, in four patients.[113] Three of the four achieved excellent results (full extension with at least 60 degrees of flexion), and the other patient required a secondary Steindler's flexorplasty.

Spira achieved strong flexion through a range of 135 degrees with virtually full extension in a patient with total paralysis of the pectoralis major and elbow flexors secondary to poliomyelitis whose pectoralis minor origin he transferred to the biceps tendon.[100]

Arthrogryposis

In arthrogrypotic children, Lloyd-Roberts and Lettin observed that preliminary posterior release and triceps lengthening may be necessary to secure passive flexion.[66] They modified Clark's transfer by obtaining a longer anterior rectus abdominis sheath and inserting the transfer into the ulna, because the biceps tendon frequently is absent. All seven patients who had the modified transfer could get their hands to their mouth against gravity and some resistance. Atkins and co-workers[6] transferred the pectoralis major by detaching its clavicular origin to allow its insertion to be tied into the biceps tendon remnant in six children, five of whom were arthrogrypotic. The operations achieved good results in three, three others were fair, and one was poor. Doyle and co-workers reported on seven cases of arthrogryposis in which a bipolar transfer of the entire sternal head of the pectoralis major with a generous tongue of anterior rectus abdominis sheath was performed.[34] All seven patients achieved improved elbow motion, and six were able to feed themselves using only one hand. Three of the four patients reported on by Carroll and Kleinman who had bipolar transfers of the entire pectoralis major muscle achieved excellent results.[25] Because of the increased shoulder stability achieved with this operation, shoulder arthrodesis was not necessary.

Comparative Studies

Segal and associates, using combined objective and subjective evaluations, compared the results of 13 flexorplasties, 3 triceps transfers, 17 Clark's transfers, and 8 Brooks-Seddon transfers.[97] Fifty-three percent of Clark's transfers and 75 percent of Brooks-Seddon transfers either had fair results or failed, whereas only 31 percent of the flexorplasties had a fair result and there were no failures. The decreased flexion contracture of the elbow, simultaneous contraction of the triceps when the pectoralis transfer flexed the elbow, and undesirable shoulder adduction and internal rotation movements accompanying elbow flexion all contributed to less satisfactory results in the pectoralis transfer group. These authors, and Clark himself, advised against using the pectoralis transfer when some biceps activity was present or could be anticipated.[30]

COMPLICATIONS

Doyle and associates reported on two patients who developed transient nerve palsy, one medial and one radial, after pectoralis major transfer.[34] Both problems resolved completely after several weeks. Simultaneous contraction of the triceps when the elbow is flexed by the transfixed pectoralis major was noted in three cases by Segal and co-workers.[97] All three had brachial plexus injuries and initially had had paralysis of the triceps and elbow flexors. Axonal confusion after regeneration seems to be the likely explanation, but the complication cannot be predicted, because in six other cases in which the triceps initially was paralyzed and later recovered, no simultaneous flexor-extensor action developed.

Triceps Transfer

HISTORY

Use of the triceps muscle to restore elbow flexion was condemned by Steindler in 1939 because, he felt, "Loss of the normal function of the triceps is too great a sacrifice."[104] Bunnell, however, described a successful triceps transfer.[18] In his opinion, "It is more important to flex than to extend the elbow."[19] In 1955, Carroll described the technical details[21] and in 1970 reported the results of triceps transfer in 15 patients.[24] They advised against performing triceps transfer bilaterally or in a patient who uses crutches. Botte and Wood[11] also advised against the procedure in patients who use a cane or a wheelchair and those who have to work with their hands overhead. Several authors have recommended triceps to biceps transfer with poorly functioning biceps when there is co-contraction of a reinnervated triceps.[4, 11]

ANATOMY

The triceps muscle arises from three heads—one from the scapula (long head) and two from the posterior humerus (lateral and medial heads). The medial head has an extensive origin from the posterior shaft of the humerus, extending from the insertion of the teres major to within 2.5 cm of the trochlea of the humerus. The muscle is supplied by the radial nerve (C7 and C8, with a smaller contribution from C6) through branches that arise above the spiral groove, except the posterior branch to the medial head, which leaves the radial nerve just as it enters the groove.[13]

TECHNIQUE

This description is based on that of Carroll (Fig. 62–10). The patient is placed in the distal decubitus position and the extremity is draped free. A posterior midline incision is made that extends over the distal two thirds of the arm and then curves laterally to the olecranon, extending distally over the subcutaneous border of the ulna for 5 cm. The skin flaps are widely undermined so that the ulnar nerve can be exposed medially and the lateral intermuscular septum laterally. A tail of periosteum as long as possible is raised from the ulna in continuity with the triceps insertion, and the medial head is mobilized from the distal third of the shaft of the humerus. The radial motor nerves enter the muscle in the interval between the lateral and medial heads as the radial nerve enters the spiral groove. The raw surface of the stripped medial head is then covered by suturing its two edges together into a tube.

The biceps tendon is exposed through a curvilinear incision in the antecubital fossa, and the tendon is dissected free to its insertion onto the radius. The biceps tendon is split longitudinally. The triceps tendon is passed through a laterally placed subcutaneous tunnel between the two incisions, superficial to the radial nerve. The triceps tendon is then passed through the split biceps tendon and sutured in place under maximum tension with the elbow at 90 degrees of flexion and the forearm in full supination. As an alternative, the triceps tendon can be attached to the radial tuberosity using a pull-out wire technique, as described by Bunnell.[19] The elbow is immobilized in a posterior splint at 90 degrees of flexion and full supination for 4 weeks, at which time active exercises are begun.

RESULTS

Carroll and Hill recorded the results of 15 triceps transfers.[24] Five successes (flexion against gravity with ability

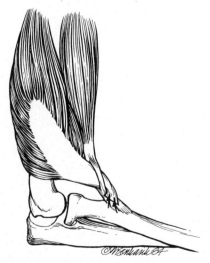

FIGURE 62–10 • Transfer of triceps insertion around the lateral side of the elbow to the biceps tendon.

to bring the hand to the mouth), 1 limited result, and 1 failure were noted in the 7 trauma or paralysis patients. Among the 8 patients with arthrogryposis, there were 5 successes, 1 limited result, and 2 failures. The average range of motion was 116 degrees and average flexion contracture 24 degrees in the first group, whereas in the arthrogrypotic group motion averaged only 43 degrees and the average fixed flexion deformity was 59 degrees. Seven of the eight arthrogrypotic patients required adjunctive procedures such as excision of a dislocated radial head or modified elbow arthroplasty to achieve an acceptable passive range of motion before triceps transfer. Williams reported improvement measured by flexion against gravity in all 19 arthrogrypotic elbows submitted to triceps transfer, and he did not hesitate to perform the procedure bilaterally.[118] However, extension was usually restricted to approximately a right angle because of the tenodesis effect of the triceps. Other authors have reported variable improvement, if any, after triceps transfer in arthrogrypotic patients.[34, 46, 72] Leffert and Pess[64] recorded four good and three improved results in seven patients who underwent triceps-to-biceps transfers. Botte and Wood[11] reported mean flexion of 125 degrees in three patients who had triceps-to-biceps transfers. No effort was made to mobilize elbow extension past a 30-degree flexion contracture, since this was thought to be mechanically advantageous for elbow flexion. Alnot[4] achieved 10 good and 1 acceptable result in 11 triceps-to-biceps transfers. Three were done after spontaneous triceps recovery, 2 in patients with co-contraction, and 8 after nerve grafting. The investigators noted that 36 percent of their patients had a dominant triceps innervation from C8 and T1, making it available for transfer in C5, C6, and C7 lesions in these patients. Complications have not been reported for any of these series.

Miscellaneous Transfers for Elbow Flexion

STERNOCLEIDOMASTOID TRANSFER

In 1951, Bunnell reported on a single patient with a paralyzed upper extremity secondary to poliomyelitis who gained elbow flexion from transfer of the insertion of the sternocleidomastoid muscle, extended with a strip of fascia lata, into the bicipital tuberosity.[19] Carroll reported 80 percent satisfactory results in 15 cases with this technique.[22]

FLEXOR CARPI ULNARIS TRANSFER

In 1975, Ahmad published a single case report of a patient with a brachial plexus palsy who achieved 130 degrees of elbow flexion after the transfer of the insertion of the flexor carpi ulnaris, turned back on itself, into the distal humerus.[1] No subsequent reports of this transfer have appeared in the literature.

FREE MUSCLE TRANSPLANTS

Gilbert reported an excellent result in a 5-year-old child treated with free transplantation of the gracilis, using the musculocutaneous nerve as the recipient nerve, after traumatic destruction of the biceps muscle.[44] Five other patients (two with poliomyelitis and three with brachial plexus palsies), however, achieved no useful flexion after a gracilis transplantation that was innervated through a long nerve graft connected to the sternocleidomastoid nerve. O'Brien and colleagues also recorded a failure in one patient 8 years after a free gracilis transplant that was innervated by the second and third intercostal nerves.[85] Hirayama and others[51] used a free latissimus dorsi muscle flap innervated by the intercostal nerve in a 35-year-old man with a complete brachial plexus palsy and disuse atrophy of the biceps. Three years later, he had 90 degrees of flexion and a 30-degree flexion contracture. Botte and Wood[11] achieved no useful flexion in three patients who had free latissimus dorsi transfers (two had distant neurotization) and recommended against the procedure. Manktelow[67] reported on one patient who had a free gracilis transfer that was innervated by the musculocutaneous nerve to replace crushed biceps and brachialis muscles. Eighteen months after surgery, the patient could flex to 120 degrees from the fully extended position with a 15-pound weight. Dumontier and Gilbert[35] achieved 4+ muscle function in a 6-year-old girl who had neurotization of a free gracilis transfer for elbow flexion using the contralateral medial pectoral nerve. Friedman and colleagues[42] achieved good elbow flexion in two of four patients who had free gracilis transplants, neurotized with intercostal nerves, to replace atrophic biceps. By far the greatest experience in free muscle transplants for brachial plexus injuries has been accumulated by Akasaka and associates.[2] If more than 6 months has elapsed since injury, they perform a free biceps femoris transplant neurotized with the third and fourth intercostal nerves, without an interposition graft. Eleven of 17 patients have been observed for more than 1 year, and 8 of them have recovered M3 or better elbow flexion power, flexion of 80 degrees or more, and the ability to lift 2 to 4 kg.

RESTORATION OF ELBOW EXTENSION

Latissimus Dorsi Transfer or Transplant

HISTORY

Several authors have proposed unipolar transfer of the latissimus dorsi insertion into the extensor mechanism to restore elbow extension.[47, 53, 62] Harmon added the teres major to the latissimus dorsi transfer in one case report.[47] Hovnanian devised a unipolar transfer of the latissimus dorsi in which its origin was transferred to the triceps tendon.[55] Myocutaneous unipolar transfer of the latissimus dorsi was reported by Landra to provide skin coverage and elbow extension at the same time.[61] Tobin and associates performed a similar procedure but used only the lateral segment of the latissimus dorsi with an attached island of skin.[111]

Bipolar transplantation of the latissimus dorsi was first reported by Schottstaedt and co-workers in 1955.[91] The origin was sutured to the triceps tendon, and the insertion was moved to the acromion. DuToit and Levy emphasized the necessity for discarding the distal 3 inches of the latissimus dorsi to get the transplant tight enough.[36]

TECHNIQUE

Unipolar Transfer

This description is based on that of Hovnanian (Fig. 62–11). The patient is placed on the side with the arm draped

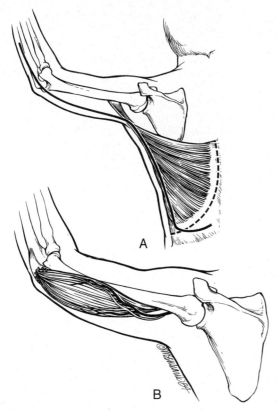

FIGURE 62–11 • Unipolar transfer of the latissimus dorsi for elbow extension. *A*, The incisions. The solid line indicates skin incisions, and the dotted line indicates the muscle incision. *B*, The insertion is undisturbed, and the muscle is rotated on its long neurovascular pedicle. Its origin (after appropriate shortening) is attached to the triceps tendon and olecranon periosteum under maximum tension with the elbow fully extended.

free. The technique of exposing, detaching, and mobilizing the latissimus dorsi on its neurovascular pedicle is the same as that described for flexor replacement. The incision on the arm, however, is carried over from the posterior axillary fold onto the posteromedial aspect without crossing the neurovascular bundle. Distally, the incision is carried over the medial epicondyle onto the posterior aspect of the proximal ulna. The aponeurotic fascia at the free end of the latissimus dorsi muscle is then sutured under tension to the triceps tendon, the periosteum over the olecranon, and the connective tissue and muscle septa on the extensor surface of the forearm, keeping the elbow in full extension. A considerable amount of muscle usually has to be excised to make the transfer as tight as possible.

The elbow is immobilized in extension and bandaged to the side of the body. Passive and active elbow movements are begun after 3 to 4 weeks.

Bipolar Transplantation

This description is based on the technique of Schottstaedt and co-workers (Fig. 62–12). The latissimus dorsi muscle is exposed, freed, and completely detached on its neurovascular pedicle through an incision extending from the posterior axillary fold along the muscle's lateral margin to within 5 to 7.5 cm of the iliac crest. The lower triceps and olec-

ranon are exposed through a posterior incision. A subcutaneous tunnel is then created between this incision and the dorsolateral incision, and the origin of the latissimus dorsi is drawn through it. This portion of the muscle is then attached to the triceps tendon and adjacent soft tissue around the olecranon. The acromion is exposed through a 5-cm transverse incision over its posterior edge. The insertion of the latissimus dorsi is then drawn up over the deltoid and sutured securely through drill holes to the acromion and the adjacent soft tissues under maximal tension with the elbow fully extended. The elbow is maintained in full extension for 3 to 4 weeks before flexion is allowed.

RESULTS

Unipolar

Hovnanian reported satisfactory results in two patients who had a unipolar latissimus transfer.[55] Tobin and colleagues used a unipolar transfer of the lateral portion of the latissimus dorsi with a large island of attached skin to restore extension and to cover a large ulcer involving the elbow joint in a 58-year-old man with syringomyelia.[111] Active elbow extension was achieved. The wound was covered, and latissimus dorsi muscle function in the donor site was said to have been preserved by the innervated medial muscle branch retained in situ. Prudzansky and others[87] reported on a 48-year-old man with a recurrent extra-abdominal desmoid tumor that required excision of the entire deltoid-end three fourths of the triceps with the overlying skin. Reconstruction using a large latissimus dorsi myocutaneous flap restored normal elbow extension power with a range from full extension to 95 degrees of flexion.

Bipolar

Schottstaedt and associates achieved full extension of the elbow against gravity after bipolar transplantation of the latissimus dorsi in a 5-year-old child with poliomyelitis.[91] DuToit and Levy reported on a 44-year-old man who was able to do push-ups after bipolar transplantation of the latissimus dorsi.[36] They noted that the distal 3 inches of muscle had to be discarded to secure the proper tension in the transplant, and they made the proximal acromial attachment before the distal attachment. No complications have been reported.

Posterior Deltoid Transfer

HISTORY

In 1949, d'Aubigne mentioned the possibility of transferring the posterior part of the deltoid into the triceps as a method of restoring active extension of the elbow.[31] The first procedure was carried out in a tetraplegic patient in 1975 by Moberg, who mobilized the separately innervated posterior part of the deltoid, extending it with multiple toe extensor tendon grafts inserted into the triceps aponeurosis.[75] Converting the transferred deltoid from a one-joint to a two-joint muscle achieved elbow extension without creating any detectable shoulder dysfunction. Since this commu-

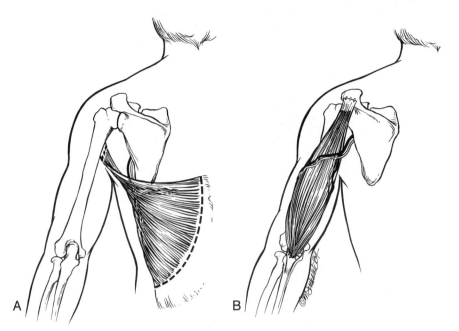

FIGURE 62–12 • Bipolar transfer of the latissimus dorsi for elbow extension. *A*, Both the origin and insertion of the latissimus doris are detached in this procedure. *B*, The latissimus dorsi is mobilized on its neurovascular pedicle, and its origin is attached to the triceps tendon and olecranon periosteum and the insertion to the acromion and adjacent soft tissues. (After Schottstaedt et al.[91])

nication, there have been several other reports of tetraplegic patients in whom posterior deltoid transfer has been used to achieve elbow extension.[17, 49] Hentz and colleagues' communication[50] indicates that the deltoid transfer is now being attached directly to the triceps aponeurosis without any intervening graft material. Castro-Sierra and Lopez-Pita used two opposing periosteal flaps, one from the deltoid insertion and one turned backward from the triceps insertion into the olecranon, to join the deltoid and triceps.[26] Freehafer and associates[41] advised using the anterior tibial tendon as an interposition graft. If the patient can walk or might later be able to, they recommended using fascia lata to connect the deltoid to the triceps insertion.

ANATOMY

The deltoid muscle is supplied by two terminal branches of the circumflex nerve, which divides about 6 cm below the level of the acromion. The posterior branch is short and runs almost horizontally to supply the portion of the deltoid arising from the spine of the scapula. The anterior branch is longer and runs horizontally to supply the acromial and clavicular portions of the deltoid.[13]

TECHNIQUE

This procedure is based on that of Moberg (Fig. 62–13). Through a slightly curved incision along the posterior border of the deltoid, the posterior half of the muscle is exposed to its insertion. There is usually a natural cleavage between the two parts of the deltoid where the separation can be accomplished by blunt dissection. Because the deltoid muscle lacks a large tendon of insertion, the tendon of insertion and the surrounding periosteum and a rectangular strip of fascia from the adjacent brachialis muscle should remain attached to the deltoid muscle. The posterior deltoid is mobilized proximally, attaining 3 cm of amplitude, the amount necessary for elbow extension. Care is taken to avoid injury to the axillary nerve branches.

The triceps aponeurosis is exposed through separate, slightly curved, longitudinal incisions proximal to the olecranon. The conjoined extensor tendons to the second, third, and fourth toes (nonfunctioning in tetraplegic patients) are removed with the aid of a Brand tendon stripper. The graft is attached to the deltoid muscle by at least twice looping the end of the graft through the deltoid tendon and adjacent fascia and periosteum and suturing the graft to the adjacent structures. The graft is then passed distally through a subcutaneous tunnel created between the two incisions. The tendon graft is looped twice through and sutured to the triceps aponeurosis, passed again subcutaneously in a proximal direction and again attached to the deltoid muscle. Suturing of the graft should be done with the elbow extended fully and the shoulder abducted 30 degrees. Fascia lata is an alternative of comparable effectiveness. This graft is applied and attached as shown in Figure 62–13*B*. The posterior deltoid muscle is infiltrated with 20 ml of 1 percent lidocaine with epinephrine 1:200,000 to prevent disruption of the anastomosis during recovery from anesthesia.

AFTERCARE

A long-arm cast, applied from the upper humerus to just proximal to the wrist with the elbow in 10 degrees of flexion, is worn for 6 weeks. Then, the patient begins active extension exercises. To prevent stretching of the newly transferred muscle-tendon unit, however, elbow flexion is increased only 10 degrees per week. A polycentric adjustable elbow splint that allows full extension but blocks flexion at whatever position is desired is useful.[49] During the rehabilitation period, elbow extension power must be closely monitored. If a temporary decrease in extension power is observed, reimmobilization in the extended position is carried out until active full extension is regained. Bryan postulated that late stretching originates in the central portion of the grafts secondary to revasculariza-

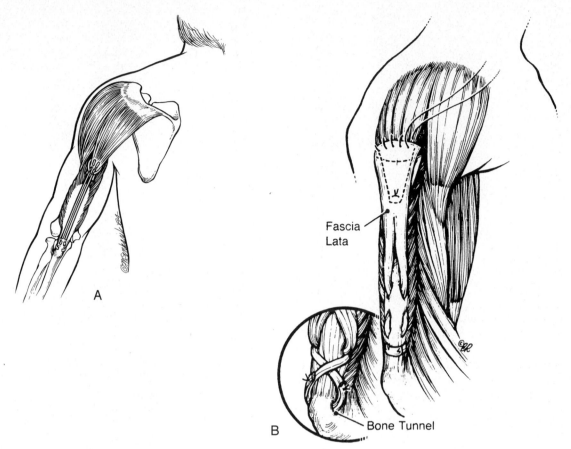

FIGURE 62–13 • *A*, Transplantation of the posterior third of the deltoid, extended with toe extensor grafts, to the triceps tendon. This transfer is used to retore extension in a tetraplegic patient. (Courtesy of Mikki Senkarik.) *B*, Transplantation of the posterior third of the deltoid using fascia lata rather than tendon grafts. (Courtesy of Elizabeth Roselius.)

tion and advised protecting the arm from flexion past 90 degrees for 3 months after surgery.[17]

RESULTS

Only one failure is reported by Moberg's experience with posterior deltoid transfers.[76] In general, elbow extension power was noted to be several times stronger with the extremity at the side in the position for lifting the body than with the limb extended over the head. Bryan reported satisfactory results in 10 of 14 deltoid transfers performed in seven tetraplegic patients.[17] In all but one, bilateral deltoid-to-triceps transfers were performed in single operations. De Bendetti evaluated 13 tetraplegic patients with 14 deltoid-to-triceps transfers.[32] He noted a mean function of 5, as compared with a preoperative mean of 0.5. Castro-Sierra and Lopez-Pita noted 10 satisfactory results in 13 tetraplegic patients using Moberg's technique but were able to shorten the postoperative immobilization period to 35 days.[26] A proximally based flap of triceps tendon with an attached flap of olecranon periosteum is turned back on itself and sutured to the deltoid insertion with the attached periosteum. Lamb and Chan reported satisfactory results after 16 Moberg transfers in 10 tetraplegic patients.[60] Hentz and others used a tubed fascia lata strip inserted through drill holes in the olecranon and allowed up to 30 degrees of immediate flexion postoperatively,[49] but no follow-up

results were given.[49, 50] Significant preoperative flexion contracture was believed to compromise the result of deltoid-to-triceps transfer. Under these circumstances, they recommend biceps-to-triceps transfer.

Freehafer and others[41] reported successful results in all 15 cases of triceps paralysis treated by deltoid-to-triceps transfer using the anterior tibial tendon as an interposition graft. All the patients could reach above their heads and noted significant improvement in performing depressor push-ups and transfers from bed to chair. Lacey and associates[59] performed a similar procedure in 16 elbows. At surgery, they documented excursion of the posterior deltoid of 7.31 cm. They felt that optimal tension was achieved by suturing the graft with the deltoid pulled to its original insertion length and with the elbow at 90 degrees of flexion. All but one transfer achieved muscle strength of 3 or better. Ejeskar[38] recorded the results of deltoid-to-triceps transfer in 40 elbows of 32 patients. Ten of the 30 procedures performed using Moberg's technique and 1 of the 10 procedures using the method of Castro-Sierra and Lopez-Pita produced full extension of the elbow. Twenty elbows showed no extension beyond 60 degrees, but most had enough extension to maintain elbow control in daily activities. Most of the patients did not have significant use of the elbow extensor when moving between bed and chair, and stretching of some of the transfers was documented.[71] Vanden Berghe and colleagues[116] initially used the Moberg technique for deltoid-to-triceps transfer. After the first two cases, they changed to the Castro-Sierra and Lopez-Pita technique for the next six cases because of the shorter immobilization time. All eight elbows gained extensor power of 3 or better. One patient ruptured a transfer in a fall.

COMPLICATIONS

Stretching and disruption of the proximal or distal anastomosis may require reoperation. In these instances, Moberg has advanced the triceps tendon by osteotomizing the olecranon, advancing the bone, and reattaching the tendon distally with a screw.[71] Spasticity of the elbow flexors may compromise the result.

MISCELLANEOUS TRANSFERS FOR ELBOW EXTENSION

Brachioradialis Transfer

In 1938, Ober and Barr described the posterior transfer of the freed anterior margin of the brachioradialis into the proximal ulna, olecranon, and triceps tendon to restore active elbow extension.[84] Addition of the extensor carpi radialis to strengthen the brachioradialis was advised if its power was insufficient. Immobilization of the elbow in full extension and supination was advised, and exercises were started at 10 days. Extension of the elbow against gravity was possible in all six cases. No subsequent reports of the procedure have appeared in the literature.

Biceps-to-Triceps Transfer

In 1954, Friedenberg reported a patient with poliomyelitis who had difficulty arising from a chair and walking with crutches because of bilateral absence of triceps function.[43] After lateral subcutaneous transfer of the biceps tendon into the triceps aponeurosis, the patient was able to support 7.5 pounds in extension on the right and 8.5 pounds on the left. He was able to transfer independently and to use crutches without difficulty. Friedenberg,[43] Hentz and associates,[49] and Lamb and Chan[60] recorded cases of tetraplegic patients for whom this procedure was unsuccessful.

Zancolli[122] believes that elbow extension is the most important function one could add for tetraplegic patients. He uses Friedenberg's method[43] after establishing that the supinator is functioning. If there is no supinator muscle function, he transfers the posterior deltoid. Zancolli noted only 24 percent reduction in elbow flexion power after biceps transfer. Falconer[40] has described Zancolli's technique of biceps transfer. The biceps is exposed through a Z incision along its lateral border, placing the horizontal limb of the Z in the flexion crease. The incision extends 10 cm proximally to the flexion crease and 5 cm distally. The musculocutaneous nerve is identified and mobilized from the undersurface of the biceps muscle 5 cm proximally. The muscle is detached at the radial tubercle and mobilized 10 cm proximally to the elbow, care being taken to protect the radial nerve. A second incision is made over the olecranon, and a flap of triceps aponeurosis is devel-

oped. The biceps is passed subcutaneously into the posterior wound and sutured under tension to the aponeurosis flap. The elbow is immobilized in extension for 4 weeks. Ejeskar,[38] noting that biceps-to-triceps transfer was the procedure of choice for restoring elbow extension when there is a flexion contracture, reported his results in six cases. One patient died of other causes, two regained full extension, one lacked 80 degrees of extension, and two achieved no extension. One patient sustained a radial nerve palsy that was recovering at 5 months.

TRANSFERS FOR RESTORATION OF FOREARM ROTATION

Transfers for Pronation

HISTORY

Paralytic supination deformity of the forearm, most commonly the result of obstetric palsy, is secondary to partial or complete paralysis of the flexor-pronator muscles in the presence of unopposed biceps and supinator muscles. The deformity not only is cosmetically displeasing but also seriously limits the function of the hand for grasping and two-handed activities. Nondynamic correction of the supination deformity by closed osteoclasis[9] or open osteotomy of the forearm bones[124] was advised by earlier authors.

Schottstaedt and colleagues suggested changing the biceps from a supinator to a pronator by transferring its tendon to the side of the radial tuberosity opposite its normal insertion, but they did not report their results.[92] Zancolli performed a long Z lengthening of the tendon, rerouting the distal strip of the tendon around the neck of the radius.[121] All 14 of his patients also required release of the contracted soft tissues, particularly the interosseous membrane, to obtain passive correction of the supination deformity before the biceps rerouting. Manske and coworkers believed that soft tissue releases could be avoided by performing the biceps rerouting earlier; if correction was unsatisfactory, a secondary percutaneous osteoclasis of the radius and ulna was recommended.[68]

TECHNIQUE

This description is based on those of Zancolli[121] and Manske and co-workers[68] (Fig. 62–14). A high tourniquet is employed, and the biceps tendon is exposed through an incision starting on the medial aspect of the distal arm and extending across the flexion crease of the elbow and distally on the lateral aspect of the forearm. The lacertus fibrosus is incised, and the median nerve and brachial artery are retracted medially. The biceps tendon is exposed to its insertion into the bicipital tuberosity, and the radial recurrent leash of vessels is divided. The tendon is divided by a long Z-plasty to its insertion, and the distal segment is passed posteriorly around the radial neck at the level of the tuberosity using a ligature carrier. The tendons are reattached by side-to-side suture, effectively lengthening the tendon by about 1.5 cm. A long-arm cast is applied with the forearm in the neutral position and the elbow at a right angle for 4 to 6 weeks. If the deformity is of long standing and the patient is older, soft tissue releases often

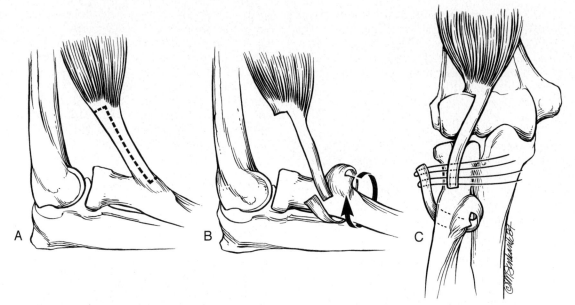

FIGURE 62–14 • Biceps tendon rerouting to restore pronation. *A*, The biceps tendon is divided by a long Z-plasty extended to its insertion. *B* and *C*, The distal end of the divided tendon is passed around the neck of the radius using a ligature passer. The two layers of the tendon are reattached side to side, effectively lengthening the tendon by about 1.5 cm. (After Zancolli, E., and Mitre, H.: Latissimus dorsi transfer to restore elbow flexion. J. Bone Joint Surg. **55A**:1265, 1973.)

are required to obtain passive forearm rotation. The interosseous membrane and supinator muscle can be released through a long dorsal incision overlying the ulna. The extensor muscles are retracted toward the radius, and this protects the interosseous nerve. Owings and colleagues suggested releasing the supinator from the volar lateral surfaces of the radius through the anterior incision.[86]

RESULTS

Zancolli performed soft tissue releases and biceps tendon rerouting in 14 patients with paralytic supination contracture of the forearm (4 had poliomyelitis, 8 birth palsies, and 2 tetraplegia).[121] Correction to the neutral position or some pronation was maintained in all patients, and 8 had 10 to 60 degrees of active pronation. Owings and others reported 9 good results, 11 satisfactory, and 2 poor ones in 26 patients who had biceps tendon rerouting using the Z-plasty technique.[86] The 2 poor results were related to problems with stability of the proximal radius. Manske and associates reported the results of Zancolli's biceps tendon rerouting in 11 patients with supination deformity secondary to obstetric paralysis.[68] The neutral position was obtained in 9, and 6 had active supination-pronation movement averaging 42 degrees (range 15 to 65). Two patients, neither of whom had preoperative passive pronation to neutral, obtained satisfactory results after a secondary percutaneous osteoclasis of the radius and ulna. The authors recommended that surgical correction of paralytic supination deformity of the forearm be done between 3 and 6 years of age. Leffert and Pess[64] reported four good and two improved results among six patients using Zancolli's method of biceps rerouting.

COMPLICATIONS

Zancolli reported on two patients who had overcorrection, presumably because the biceps tendon suture was under excessive tension.[121] Owings and colleagues reported on one patient who had persistent weakness of thumb extension, two who had proximal radial instability, and one who developed excessive pronation.[86]

Transfers for Supination

HISTORY

Because it is infrequently indicated, muscle transfer to regain supination in the paralyzed upper extremity has received scant attention in the literature. Steindler described transferring the flexor carpi ulnaris tendon into the dorsal aspect of the distal radius.[104] Tubby described transferring the flexor carpi radialis and pronator teres through the interosseous space to the back of the radius to achieve supination in the spastic upper extremity.[114] Schottstaedt and associates noted that providing active supination using the flexor carpi ulnaris or palmaris longus redirected dorsally into the radial shaft was often necessary after Steindler's flexorplasty.[92]

TECHNIQUE OF TRANSFERRING FLEXOR CARPI ULNARIS TO RADIUS

This technique is based on Steindler's method (Fig. 62–15).[104] The flexor carpi ulnaris tendon is detached, and its distal half is mobilized through a 12-cm incision along the volar-ulnar aspect of the forearm. The dorsolateral surface of the distal radius is exposed between the extensor pollicis brevis and the extensor carpi radialis longus tendons using a 5-cm longitudinal incision. A subcutaneous tunnel is created between this incision and the proximal end of the first incision, and the flexor carpi ulnaris tendon is pulled through. A hole is drilled through the distal radius, and the tendon is fed through the hole from the dorsal to the volar

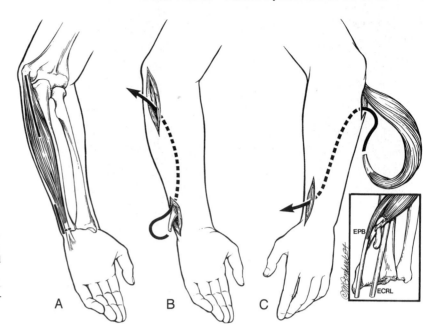

FIGURE 62–15 • Transfer of the flexor carpi ulnaris to restore supination. *A*, The flexor carpi ulnaris tendon is detached distally, mobilized proximally, and brought out through the proximal incision. *B* and *C*, The dorsoradial aspect of the distal radius is exposed. The flexor carpi ulnaris is redirected through a subcutaneous tunnel and attached to the radius through a drill hole. (After Steindler.[105])

aspect. Its end is reflected back and sutured to itself under tension with the forearm supinated and the elbow flexed. A long-arm cast—with the wrist in slight dorsiflexion, the forearm in full supination, and the elbow at a right angle—is worn for 3 weeks. Part-time splinting is continued for 2 months.

Results

Steindler reported 11 good and 5 poor results from 16 flexor carpi ulnaris transfers to the radius.[105] A good transfer functioned actively through a useful arc with at least 40 degrees of pronation-supination movement.

Author's Preferred Method of Treatment

Steindler's flexorplasty, the transfer with the largest experience, is relatively simple to perform and works well, even when wrist flexor muscle strength is not normal. The large number of satisfactory results that have been published attests to its dependability. Using Mayer and Green's simple clinical test, it is relatively easy to predict which patients are good candidates for the procedure.[70] Post-traumatic brachial plexus palsy is the most common cause of loss of elbow flexion power, and flexorplasty works well for restoring function, especially in the irreparable C5–C6 lesion (Fig. 62–16). I also have been pleasantly surprised to see functional elbow flexion restored in some patients with C5, C6, and C7 involvement. The transfer functions best when some triceps function is present, although the absence of active elbow extension does not preclude its use. When triceps function is absent, a dynamic extension elbow splint helps to prevent excessive fixed flexion contracture (see Fig. 62–3). Late recovery of some motor function in the biceps is not affected by flexorplasty, unlike other transfers that tie into the biceps.

Steindler's flexorplasty does have some drawbacks. It is not as strong as some of the other transfers (i.e., latissimus dorsi and pectoralis major) and does not provide active supination. The development of a pronation deformity after flexorplasty was a problem with the original proximal medial shift of the flexor pronator origin. Pronation deformity has not been as great a problem with the more anterolateral insertion currently being used. Fascial extension to permit a more lateral shift of the origin is usually unnecessary.

Bipolar transplantation of the latissimus dorsi to restore either elbow flexion or extension is an excellent procedure. Its long, single neurovascular pedicle allows greater mobility than that of the pectoralis major, which has a double neurovascular pedicle. Excellent motion and strength are achieved, and good contour is restored to the arm (Fig. 62–17). Preoperative evaluation of the latissimus dorsi muscle strength is often difficult. Its main innervation comes from C7 (with contributions from C6 and C8), so it is a useful transplant for restoring flexion in persons with irreparable C5–C6 brachial plexus lesions. It is a more formidable procedure than Steindler's flexorplasty, and hematoma formation and delayed wound healing sometimes follow the large posterior dissection. It is more technically demanding, and achieving proper tension is most important. Sufficient origin must be excised so that the transplant is under maximal tension with the elbow flexed to 120 degrees. It seems that it is almost impossible to get it too tight. Shoulder stabilization by arthrodesis significantly improves the function of both the flexor-pronator and latissimus dorsi transfers for elbow function.

Bipolar transplantation of part or all of the pectoralis major muscle is becoming a popular method of restoring elbow flexion. Brooks and Seddons' unipolar transfer of the pectoralis major into the devascularized long head of the biceps muscle should no longer be performed, because there are better and more predictable ways to transfer the muscle. The results reported for Clark's unipolar transfer of the inferior sternocostal portion of the pectoralis major have been good, except for the occasional patient who develops simultaneous contraction of the transfer and the triceps when elbow flexion is attempted. This is presum-

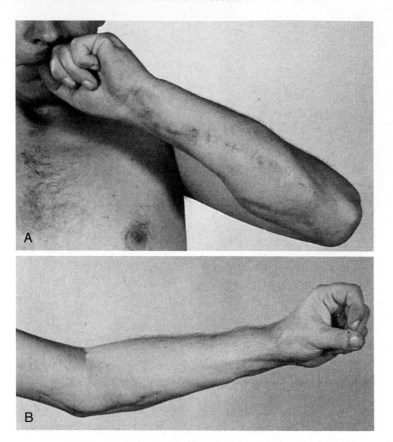

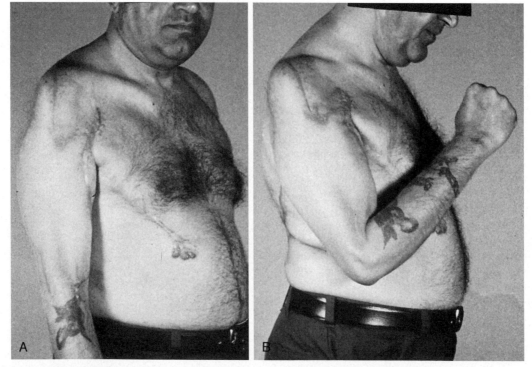

FIGURE 62–16 • *A*, A 21-year-old man sustained a brachial plexus injury in a motorcycle accident. Steindler's flexorplasty performed 16 months after injury restored excellent elbow flexion. Subsequent transfer of the flexor carpi ulnaris into the extensor carpi radialis brevis restored wrist extension, and finger and thumb extension was restored using the superficialis muscle of the middle and ring fingers. Shoulder arthrodesis was also performed. *B*, Fixed flexion deformity of 35 degrees was present after Steindler's flexorplasty.

FIGURE 62–17 • *A* and *B*, This 36-year-old man who had C5–C6 paralysis following a closed brachial plexus injury underwent a bipolar transfer of the latissimus dorsi 3 years after the injury. Good elbow flexion was restored *(A)*, and nearly full extension of the elbow was maintained *(B)*. Shoulder arthrodesis was also performed.

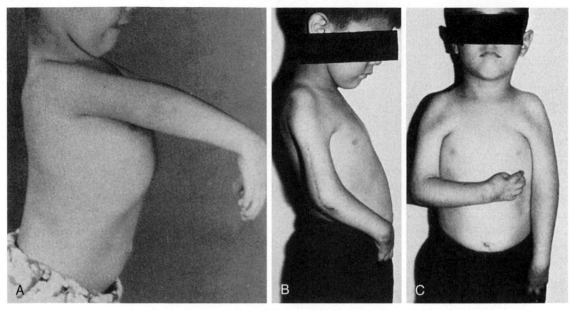

FIGURE 62–18 • *A*, A 5-year-old boy with arthrogryposis multiplex congenita underwent triceps transfer on the right extremity. *B*, Six months after surgery, he was able to flex the elbow to 95 degrees and gravity extension was possible to 50 degrees. *C*, The opposite elbow was left in extension.

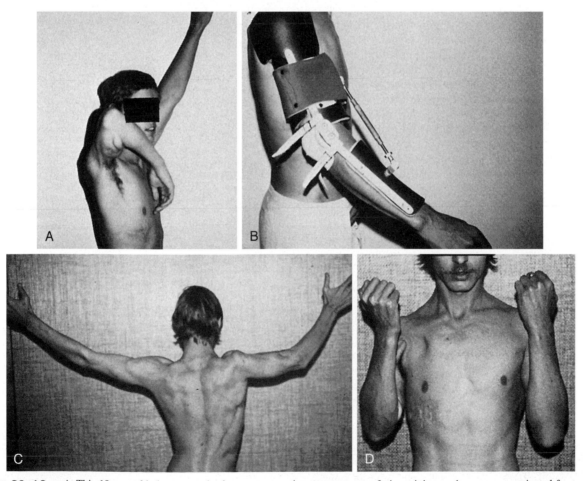

FIGURE 62–19 • *A*, This 19-year-old airman sustained a severe posterior compartment soft tissue injury and an open comminuted fracture of the humerus in a half-track accident. There was complex loss of elbow extension. *B*, The humeral fracture united after two bone-grafting procedures, and passive extension of the elbow was obtained with a turnbuckle splint. *C*, Bipolar transplantation of the latissimus dorsi restored satisfactory elbow extension, and full flexion of the elbow was maintained *(D)*.

ably due to axonal confusion during regeneration and cannot be predicted preoperatively.

The lower (C8–T1) segmental innervation of the inferior pectoralis major makes it available for transfer in brachial plexus palsies extending to and involving C7. My experience with the pectoralis major transfers is limited; however, I favor a bipolar transfer of the pectoralis on both of its neurovascular pedicles (as described by Carroll and Kleinman) over bipolar transplantation of only a portion of the muscle. The superior vascular pedicle (pectoral branch of the thoracoacromial artery) is much larger and more dominant than the inferior pedicle (branch of lateral thoracic artery). If the surgeon is careful in the dissection, the muscle can be adequately mobilized and transplanted without creating under tension or kinking of the pedicles. The bipolar transplantation, according to its proponents, may make shoulder fusion unnecessary.

Triceps-to-biceps transfer rarely is indicated, because the loss of active elbow extension is usually too great a price to pay for elbow flexion. One relatively absolute indication for this transfer is a particularly strong triceps muscle that is co-contracting with a weak biceps. Any other transfer in this circumstance will fail. I also have used the transfer with arthrogrypotic elbows and have been pleased with the hand-to-mouth function that is restored (Fig. 62–18). In my opinion, bilateral elbow transfers to regain flexion should not be performed in children with arthrogryposis.

Restoration of active elbow extension can be achieved nicely using the bipolar transplantation of the latissimus dorsi, when it is available (Fig. 62–19). In tetraplegic patients, transfer of the posterior third of the deltoid into the triceps aponeurosis using multiple toe extensor tendon grafts or a fascia lata graft is the procedure of choice for restoring elbow extension. Careful attention to postoperative detail, including prolonged use of an adjustable flexion-blocking splint, is necessary to prevent late stretching of the transfer.

NEUROTIZATION

Neurotization is the technique of nerve transfer used to restore motor or sensory function after brachial plexus injuries when the nerve damage is too far proximal for standard nerve-grafting techniques to be feasible. In 1903, Harris and Low inserted half of the distal fascicles of the C5 root, which was damaged at the foreamen, into the healthy spinal nerve C6 or C7 in three cases of Erb's palsy.[48] No results were recorded. In 1913, Tuttle mentioned one case of neurotization using the spinal accessory nerve.[115] In 1963, Seddon first reported neurotization of the musculocutaneous nerve using intercostal nerves in two patients, both times obtaining active elbow flexion.[95]

Subsequently, many more cases of neurotization using intercostal nerves have reported a modicum of success.* Neurotization of the musculocutaneous nerve using parts of the cervical plexus[16] and spinal accessory nerve[3, 57, 82] has also achieved some limited success. Even the phrenic nerve has been used[120] to neurotize the musculocutaneous nerve.

These highly technical and complicated microneurosurgical procedures must still be considered somewhat investigative. Their results are variable and take years to determine, and their long-term worth to the patient is still in some question. No doubt, over the next few years the indications and expectations for these procedures will be better defined.

REFERENCES

1. Ahmad, I.: Restoration of elbow flexion by a new operative method. Clin. Orthop. **106**:186, 1975.
2. Akasaka, Y., Hara, T., and Takahashi, M.: Restoration of elbow flexion and wrist extension in brachial plexus paralyses by means of free muscle transplantation innervated by intercostal nerve. Ann. Hand Surg. **9**:341, 1990.
3. Allieu, Y., and Cenac, P.: Neurotization via the spinal accessory nerve in complete paralysis due to multiple avulsion injuries of the brachial plexus. Clin. Orthop. **237**:67, 1988.
4. Alnot, J. Y.: Elbow flexion palsy after traumatic lesions of the brachial plexus in adults. Hand Clin. **5**:15, 1989.
5. Andriseno, A., Porcellini, G., Stilli, S., and Libri, R.: The Steindler method in the treatment of paralytic elbow flexion. Ital. J. Orthop. Traumatol. **16**:235, 1990.
6. Atkins, R. M., Bell, M. F., and Sharrard, W. J. W.: Pectoralis major transfer for paralysis of elbow flexion in children. J. Bone Joint Surg. **67B**:640, 1985.
7. Axer, A., Segal, D., and Elkon, A.: Partial transposition of the latissimus dorsi. J. Bone Joint Surg. **55A**:1259, 1973.
8. Bartlett, S. P., May, J. W., and Yaremchuk, M. J.: The latissimus dorsi muscle: a fresh cadaver study of the primary neurovascular pedicle. Plast. Reconstr. Surg. **67**:631, 1981.
9. Blount, W. P.: Osteoclasis for supination deformities in children. J. Bone Joint Surg. **22**:300, 1940.
10. Bostwick, J., Nahai, F., Wallace, J. G., and Vasconex, L. O.: Sixty latissimus dorsi flaps. Plast. Reconstr. Surg. **63**:31, 1979.
11. Botte, M. J., and Wood, M. D.: Flexorplasty of the elbow. Clin. Orthop. **245**:110, 1989.
12. Bradford, E. H.: The operative treatment of paralysis of the shoulder following anterior poliomyelitis. Am. J. Orthop. Surg. **8**:21, 1910.
13. Brash, J. C.: Neuro-vascular Hila of Limb Muscles. Edinburgh, E & S Livingstone Ltd., 1955.
14. Brones, M. F., Wheeler, E. S., and Lesavoy, M. A.: Restoration of elbow flexion and arm contour with the latissimus dorsi myocutaneous flap. Plast. Recontr. Surg. **69**:329, 1982.
15. Brooks, D.M., and Seddon, H. J.: Pectoral transplantation for paralysis of the flexors of the elbow: a new technique. J. Bone Surg. **41B**:36, 1959.
16. Brunnelli, G., and Monini, L.: Neurotization of avulsed roots of brachial plexus by means of anterior nerves of cervical plexus. Clin. Plast. Surg. **11**:149, 1984.
17. Bryan, R. S.: The Moberg deltoid-triceps replacement and key pinch operations in quadriplegia: preliminary experiences. Hand **9**:207, 1977.
18. Bunnell, S.: Surgery of the Hand, 2nd ed. Philadelphia, J. B. Lippincott Co., 1948, p. 584.
19. Bunnell, S.: Restoring flexion to the paralytic elbow. J. Bone Joint Surg. **33A**:566, 1951.
20. Carroll, R. E.: Discussion paper by Mayer, L., and Green, W.: Experiences with the Steindler flexorplasty at the elbow. J. Bone Joint Surg. **36A**:858, 1954.
21. Carroll, R. E.: Restoration of flexor power to the flail elbow by transplantation of the triceps tendon. Surg. Gynecol. Obstet. **95**:685, 1955.
22. Carroll, R. E.: Restoration of elbow flexion by transplantation of sternocleidomastoid muscle. J. Bone Joint Surg. **44A**:1039, 1962.
23. Carroll, R. E., and Gartland, J. J.: Flexorplasty of the elbow. J. Bone Joint Surg. **35A**:706, 1953.
24. Carroll, R. E., and Hill, N. A.: Triceps transfer to restore elbow flexion. J. Bone Joint Surg. **52A**:23, 1970.
25. Carroll, R. E., and Kleinman, W. B.: Pectoralis major transplantation to restore elbow flexion to the paralytic limb. J. Hand Surg. **4**:501, 1979.

*References 33, 42, 56, 57, 73, 74, 78–82, 96, 98, 99, 108, and 112.

26. Castro-Sierra, A., and Lopez-Pita, A.: A new surgical technique to correct triceps paralysis. Hand **15**:42, 1983.

27. Chen, W. S.: Restoration of elbow flexion by latissimus dorsi myocutaneous or muscle flap. Arch. Orthop. Trauma Surg. **109**:117, 1990.

28. Colson, J. H. C.: Physical treatment of pectoral transfer and flexorplasty. Physiotherapy **56**:300, 1970.

29. Clark, J. M. P.: Reconstruction of the biceps brachii by pectoral muscle transplantation. Br. J. Surg. **34**:180, 1946.

30. Clark, J. M. P.: Reconstructive surgery in paralysis of the elbow. Physiotherapy **56**:295, 1970.

31. D'Aubigne, R. M.: Treatment of residual paralysis after injuries of the main nerves (superior extremity). Proc. R. Soc. Med. **42**:831, 1949.

32. De Bendetti, M.: Restoration of elbow extension power in the tetraplegic patient using the Moberg technique. J. Hand Surg. **4**:86, 1979.

33. Dolenc, V. V.: Intercostal neurotization of the peripheral nerves in avulsion plexus injuries. Clin. Plast. Surg. **11**:143, 1984.

34. Doyle, J. R., James, P. M., Larson, L. J., and Ashley, R. K.: Restoration of elbow flexion in arthrogryposis multiplex congenita. J. Hand Surg. **5**:149, 1980.

35. Dumontier, C., and Gilbert, A.: Traumatic brachial plexus palsy in children. Ann. Hand Surg. **9**:351, 1990.

36. Du Toit, G. T., and Levy, S. J.: Transposition of latissimus dorsi for paralysis of triceps brachii: report of a case. J. Bone Joint Surg. **49B**:135, 1967.

37. Dutton, R. O., and Dawson, E.G.: Elbow flexorplasty: an analysis of long-term results. J. Bone Joint Surg. **63A**:1064, 1981.

38. Ejeskar, A.: Upper limb surgical rehabilitation in high-level tetraplegia. Hand Clin. **4**:585, 1988.

39. Eyler, D. L.: Modification of Steindler flexorplasty. Georgia Warm Springs Foundation, Warm Springs, GA. Unpublished circular letter, Oct. 19, 1950.

40. Falconer, D. P.: Tendon transfers about the shoulder and elbow in the spinal cord–injured patient. Hand Clin. **4**:211, 1988.

41. Freehafer, A. A., Kelly, C. M., and Peckham, P. H.: Tendon transfer for the restoration of upper limb function after a cervical spinal cord injury. J. Hand Surg. **9A**:887, 1984.

42. Freidman, A. H., Nunley, J. A., Goldner, R. D., Oakes, W. I., Goldner, J. L., and Urbaniak, J. R.: Nerve transposition for the restoration of elbow flexion following brachial plexus injuries. J. Neurosurg. **72**:59, 1990.

43. Friedenberg, Z. B.: Transposition of the biceps brachii for triceps weakness. J. Bone Joint Surg. **36A**:656, 1954.

44. Gilbert, A.: Free muscle transfer. Int. Surg. **66**:33, 1981.

45. Green, D. P., and McCoy, H.: Turnbuckle orthotic correction of elbow-flexion contracture after acute injuries. J. Bone Joint Surg. **61A**:1092, 1979.

46. Greene, M. H.: Cryptic problems of arthrogryposis multiplex congenita. J. Bone Joint Surg. **45A**:885, 1963.

47. Harmon, P. H.: Muscle transplantation for triceps palsy: the technique of utilizing the latissimus dorsi. J. Bone Joint Surg. **31A**:409, 1949.

48. Harris, W., and Low, V. W.: On the importance of accurate muscular analysis in lesions of the brachial plexus and the treatment of Erb's palsy and infantile paralysis of the upper extremity by cross-union of nerve roots. Br. Med. J. **2**:1035, 1903.

49. Hentz, V. R., Brown, M., and Keoshrian, L. A.: Upper limb reconstruction in quadriplegia: functional assessment and proposed treatment modifications. J. Hand Surg. **8**:119, 1983.

50. Hentz, V. R., Hamlin, C., and Keoshian, L. A.: Surgical reconstruction in tetraplegia. Hand Clin. **4**:601, 1988.

51. Hirayama, T., Takemitsu, Y., Atsuta, Y., and Ozawa, K.: Restoration of elbow flexion by complete latissimus dorsi muscle transposition. J. Hand Surg. **12B**:194, 1987.

52. Hochberg, J., and Borges Fortes da Silva, F.: Latissimus dorsi myocutaneous flap to restore elbow flexion and axillary burn contracture: a report on two pediatric patients. J. Pediatr. Orthop. **2**:565, 1982.

53. Hohmann, G.: Ersatz des gelähmten Bizeps Brachii durch den Pectoralis Major. Munch. Med. Wochenschr. **65**:1240, 1918.

54. Holtmann, B., Wray, R. C., Lowrey, R., and Weeks, P.: Restoration of elbow flexion. Hand **7**:256, 1975.

55. Hovnanian, A. P.: Latissimus dorsi transplantation of the elbow. Ann. Surg. **143**:493, 1956.

56. Kanaya, F., Gonzalez, M., Park, C., Kutz, J. E., Kleinert, H. E., and Tsai, T.: Improvement in motor function after brachial plexus surgery. J. Hand Surg. **15A**:30, 1990.

57. Kawai, H., Kawabata, H., Masada, K., et al.: Nerve repairs for traumatic brachial plexus palsy with root avulsion. Clin. Orthop. **237**:75, 1988.

58. Kettelkamp, D. B., and Larson, C. B.: Evaluation of the Steindler flexorplasty. J. Bone Joint Surg. **45A**:513, 1963.

59. Lacey, S. H., Wilber, R. G., Peckham, P. H., and Freehafer, A. A.: The posterior deltoid to triceps transfer: a clinical and biomechanical assessment. J. Hand Surg. **11A**:542, 1986.

60. Lamb, D. W., and Chan, K. M.: Surgical reconstruction of the upper limb in traumatic tetraplegia. J. Bone Joint Surg. **65B**:291, 1983.

61. Landra, A. P.: The latissimus dorsi musculocutaneous flap used to resurface defect on the upper arm and restore extension to the elbow. Br. J. Plast. Surg. **32**:275, 1979.

62. Lange, F.: Die Epidemische Kinderlahmung. Munich, J. F. Lehmann, 1930, p. 298.

63. Lange, M.: Orthopaedisch-Chirurgische Operationslehre. Munich, J. F. Bergmann, 1951, p. 301.

64. Leffert, R. D., and Pess, G. M.: Tendon transfers for brachial plexus injury. Hand Clin. **4**:273, 1988.

65. Lindholm, T. S., and Einola, S.: Flexorplasty of paralytic elbows: analysis of late functional results. Acta Orthop. Scand. **44**:1, 1973.

66. Lloyd-Roberts, G. C., and Lettin, A. W. F.: Arthrogryposis multiplex congenita. J. Bone Joint Surg. **52B**:494, 1970.

67. Manktelow, R. T.: Functioning microsurgical muscle transfer. Hand Clin. **4**:289, 1988.

68. Manske, P. R., McCarroll, H. R., and Hale, R.: Biceps tendon rerouting and percutaneous osteoclasis in the treatment of supination deformity in obstetrical palsy. J. Hand Surg. **5**:153, 1980.

69. Matory, W. E., Morgan, W. J., and Breen, T.: Technical considerations in pectoralis major transfer for treatment of the paralytic elbow. J. Hand Surg. **16A**:12, 1991.

70. Mayer, L., and Green, W.: Experiences with Steindler flexorplasty of the elbow. J. Bone Joint Surg. **36A**:775, 1954.

71. McDowell, C. L., Moberg, E. A., and House, J. H.: Proceedings of the Second International Conference on Surgical Rehabilitation of the Upper Limb in Tetraplegia (Quadriplegia). J. Hand Surg. **11A**:604, 1986.

72. Meade, N. G., Lithgow, W. C., and Sweeney, H. J.: Arthrogryposis multiplex congenita. J. Bone Joint Surg. **40A**:1285, 1958.

73. Millesi, H.: Surgical management of brachial plexus injuries. J. Hand Surg. **5**:367, 1977.

74. Millesi, H.: Brachial plexus injuries management and results. Clin. Plast. Surg. **11**:115, 1984.

75. Moberg, E.: Surgical treatment for absent single-hand grip and elbow extension in quadriplegia: principles and preliminary experience. J. Bone Joint Surg. **57A**:196, 1975.

76. Moberg, E.: The Upper Limb in Tetraplegia: A New Approach to Surgical Rehabilitation. Stuttgart, Thieme, 1978.

77. Moneim, M. S., and Omer, G. E.: Latissimus dorsi muscle transfer for restoration of elbow flexion after brachial plexus disruption. J. Hand Surg. **11A**:135, 1986.

78. Narakas, A.: Surgical treatment of traction injuries of the brachial plexus. Clin. Orthop. **133**:71, 1978.

79. Narakas, A. O.: The surgical treatment of traumatic brachial plexus lesions. Int. Surg. **65**:522, 1980.

80. Narakas, A. O.: Thoughts on neurotization or nerve transfers in irreparable nerve lesions. Clin. Plast. Surg. **11**:153, 1984.

81. Narakas, A. O.: The treatment of brachial plexus injuries. Int. Orthop. (SICOT) **9**:29, 1985.

82. Narakas, A. O.: Neurotization in brachial plexus injuries: indications and results. Clin. Orthop. **237**:43, 1988.

83. Nyholm, K.: Elbow flexorplasty in tendon transposition (an analysis of the functional results in 26 patients). Acta Orthop. Scand. **33**:32, 1963.

84. Ober, F. R., and Barr, J. S.: Brachioradialis muscle transposition for triceps weakness. Surg. Gynecol. Obstet. **67**:105, 1938.

85. O'Brien, B., Morrison, W. A., MacLeod, A. M., and Weinglein, O.: Free microneurovascular muscle transfer in limbs to provide motor power. Ann. Plast. Surg. **9**:381, 1982.

86. Owings, R., Wickstrom, J., Perry, J., and Nickel, V. L.: Biceps brachii rerouting in treatment of paralytic supination contracture of the forearm. J. Bone Joint Surg. **53A**:137, 1971.

87. Prudzansky, M., Kelly, M., and Weinberg, H.: Latissimus dorsi musculocutaneous flap for elbow extension. J. Surg. Oncol. **47**:62, 1991.

88. Rivarola, R. A.: Tratamiento de las paralisis definitivas del miembro superior. Bul. Trabajos Soc. Cirug. Buenos Aires **12**:688, 1928 (reported in Sernana Med. Buenos Aires **2**:1294, 1928).

89. Rivet, D., Boileau, R., Saiveau, M., and Baudet, J.: Restoration of elbow flexion using the latissimus dorsi musculo-cutaneous flap. Ann. Chir. Main. **8**:110, 1989.

90. Russell, R. C., Pribaz, J., Zook, E. G., Leighton, W. D., Eriksson, E., and Smith, C. J.: Functional evaluation of latissimus dorsi donor site. Plast. Reconst. Surg. **78**:336, 1986.

91. Schottstaedt, E. R., Larsen, L. J., and Bost, F. C.: Complete muscle transposition. J. Bone Joint Surg. **37A**:897, 1955.

92. Schottstaedt, E. R., Larsen, L. J., and Bost, F. C.: The surgical reconstruction of the upper extremity paralyzed by poliomyelitis. J. Bone Joint Surg. **40A**:633, 1958.

93. Schulze-Berge, R.: Ersatz der Benger des Voderarames (Bizeps und Brachialis) durch den Pectoralis major. Dtsch Med. Wochenschr. **43**:433, 1917.

94. Seddon, H. J.: Transplantation of pectoralis major for paralysis of the flexors of the elbow. Proc. R. Soc. Med. **43**:837, 1949.

95. Seddon, H. J.: Nerve grafting. J. Bone Joint Surg. **45B**:447, 1963.

96. Sedel, L.: The results of surgical repair of brachial plexus injuries. J. Bone Joint Surg. **64B**:54, 1982.

97. Segal, A., Seddon, H. J., and Brooks, D. M.: Treatment of paralysis of the flexors of the elbow. J. Bone Joint Surg. **41B**:44, 1959.

98. Simesen, K., and Haase, J.: Microsurgery in brachial plexus lesions. Acta Orthop. Scand. **56**:238, 1985.

99. Solonen, K. A., Vastamaki, M., and Strom, B.: Surgery of the brachial plexus. Acta Orthop. Scand. **55**:436, 1984.

100. Spira, E.: Replacement of biceps brachii by pectoralis minor transplant. J. Bone Joint Surg. **39B**:126, 1957.

101. Steindler, A.: A muscle plasty for the relief of flail elbow in infantile paralysis. Interstate Med. J. **25**:235, 1918.

102. Steindler, A.: Orthopaedic reconstruction work on hand and forearm. N.Y. Med. J. **108**:1117, 1918.

103. Steindler, A.: Operative treatment of paralytic conditions of the upper extremity. J. Orthop. Surg. **1**:608, 1919.

104. Steindler, A.: Tendon transplantation in the upper extremity. Am. J. Surg. **44**:260, 1939.

105. Steindler, A.: Muscle and tendon transplantation at the elbow. *In* American Academy of Orthopaedic Surgeons: Instructional Course Lectures on Reconstruction Surgery. Ann Arbor, J. W. Edwards, 1944, p. 276.

106. Stern, P. J., and Caudle, R. J.: Tendon transfers for elbow flexion. Hand Clin. **4**:297, 1988.

107. Stern, P. J., Neale, H. W., Gregory, R. O., and Kreilein, J. G.: Latissimus dorsi musculocutaneous flap for elbow flexion. J. Hand Surg. **7**:25, 1982.

108. Sunderlund, S.: Repair of the brachial plexus directed to restoring elbow flexion. Bull. Hosp. Joint Dis. Orthop. Inst. **44**:485, 1984.

109. Takami, H., Takahashi, S., and Ando, M.: Latissimus dorsi transplantation to restore elbow flexion to the paralysed limb. J. Hand Surg. **9B**:61, 1984.

110. Tobin, G. R., Bland, K. I., and Adcock, R.: Surgical anatomy of the musculus pectoralis major and neurovascular supply. American College of Surgeons, 1981. Surg. Forum **32**:574, 1981.

111. Tobin, G. R., Shusterman, B. A., Peterson, G. H., Nichols, G., and Bland, K. I.: The intramuscular neurovascular anatomy of the latissimus dorsi muscle: the basis for splitting the flap. Plast. Reconstr. Surg. **67**:637, 1981.

112. Tomita, Y., Tsai, T., Burns, J. T., Karaoguz, A., and Ogden, L. L.: Intercostal nerve transfers in brachial plexus injuries: an experimental study. Microsurgery **4**:95, 1983.

113. Tsai, T., Kalisman, M., Burns, J., and Kleinert, H. E.: Restoration of elbow flexion by pectoralis major and pectoralis minor transfer. J. Hand Surg. **8**:186, 1983.

114. Tubby, A. H.: Deformities Including Diseases of the Bones and Joints. London, MacMillan, 1912, p. 730.

115. Tuttle, H.: Exposure of the brachial plexus with nerve transplantation. J.A.M.A. **61**:15, 1913.

116. Vanden Berghe, A., Van Laere, M., Hellings, S., and Vercauteren, M.: Reconstruction of the upper extremity in tetraplegia: functional assessment, surgical procedures and rehabilitation. Paraplegia **29**:103, 1991.

117. VonLanz, T., and Wachsmuth, W.: Praktische Anatomie, 2nd ed. Berlin, Springer-Verlag, 1959, p. 93.

118. Williams, P. F.: The elbow in arthrogryposis. J. Bone Joint Surg. **55B**: 834, 1973.

119. Wynn Parry, C. B.: Brachial plexus injuries. Br. J. Hosp. Med. **32**:130, 1984.

120. Yu-dong, G., Min-Ming, W., Yi-Lu, Z., et al.: Phrenic nerve transfer for brachial plexus motor neurotization. Microsurgery **10**:287, 1989.

121. Zancolli, E. A.: Paralytic supination contracture of the forearm. J. Bone Joint Surg. **49A**:1275, 1967.

122. Zancolli E. A.: Structural and Dynamic Bases of Hand Surgery, 2nd ed. Philadelphia, J. B. Lippincott Co., 1979.

123. Zancolli, E. A., and Mitre, H.: Latissimus dorsi transfer to restore elbow flexion. J. Bone Joint Surg. **55A**:1265, 1973.

124. Zaoussis, A. L.: Osteotomy of the proximal end of the radius for paralytic supination deformity in children. J. Bone Joint Surg. **45B**:523, 1963.

• CHAPTER 63 •

Spastic Dysfunction of the Elbow

• M. MARK HOFFER, ROBERT L. WATERS, and DOUGLAS E. GARLAND

CEREBRAL PALSY IN CHILDREN

Cerebral palsy is a perinatal disorder that is nonhereditary and is not progressive. It is characterized by developmental, cognitive, and sensory problems.[24] Although any of these features may predominate in the clinical presentation, the disability usually is classified by its motor manifestations (Table 63–1). The spastic disorder involves fluctuations in muscle tone that are demonstrated by stretch reflexes and even by clonus. The result is often postural changes that make using the extremity difficult or impossible. Spastic patients are the ones most often helped by surgical or orthotic devices. Motion disorders (ataxia, dyskinesia, athetosis, tremors) are characterized by variable changes in muscle tone that are markedly affected by position and activity. The motion disorders are treated by experimental drug therapies and brain surgery. Many cerebral palsies have both motor and spastic components. Results of surgery of the spastic limb are unpredictable when there is an admixture of these motion disorders.[14]

Diagnosis

CLINICAL FEATURES

The diagnosis frequently is delayed and the condition is noticed sometime during the first year of life. The key is achievement of developmental milestones. A dominant extremity is not developed until the child is 18 to 24 months of age. Normal children develop two-handed activity and bilateral grasp and progress from two-handed manipulation of objects to one hand, using the ulnar and then the radial portion of the hands for grasping about the age of 18 to 24 months. Early hand preference in children with cerebral palsy is usually a sign of poor function in the nondominant limb. Grasp may not develop in the normal sequence, but primitive grasp-like reflexes may be elicited.

The typical elbow deformity of cerebral palsy is elbow flexion and forearm pronation (Fig. 63–1). Occasionally, it results in posterior dislocation of the radial head,[20] which requires no treatment unless in adult life it results in a painful bursa; then, the radial head may be excised. Flexion-supination contractures of the elbow are more rare with cerebral palsy. An even rarer complication is anterior dislocation of the radial head. This may be painful and can result in dislocation of the distal radioulnar joint (Fig. 63–2).

TESTING

The most important elements in testing children with cerebral palsy for function of the upper extremity are cognition, hand placement, and sensibility.[14] Testing of cognition includes perception, abstract reasoning, and communication, and it is difficult to evaluate patients who have communication problems. Children graded in the first standard deviation from normal are termed *normal*. Those between the first and second standard deviations are considered *educable*, and those between the second and third standard deviations are considered *trainable*. Children who fall below this level are thought to be profoundly retarded. Only those who are at least educable can expect functional results from upper extremity surgery.

Hand placement is assessed simply by asking the subject to place a hand on the opposite knee and the top of head in 10 seconds. Sensibility is best tested by texture discriminations in 2- to 3-year-olds, object identification in 4- to 5-year-olds, graphesthesia in 6- to 9-year-olds, and two-point discrimination in older children. Only children who can make three out of five correct object identifications, number perception in the palm, or two-point discrimination of less than 10 mm can be expected to have functional results after upper extremity surgery.

DEFINITION OF GOALS

Functional tasks that should be tested in every child are dressing, toileting, feeding, two-handed assisted work, grasp and release, and side pinch. After cognition, placement, and sensibility are tested, the functional goals for the hand should be established so that it can be determined whether the anticipated function is being accomplished by the patient.

In children with cerebral palsy the elbows merely place and position the hand. If hand function is not an expectation, surgery about the elbow still may be directed toward enhancing self-care (hygiene) or cosmesis. Thus, a thorough hand evaluation is mandatory before any elbow procedure is instituted.

FUNCTIONAL TEST

Children with cerebral palsy whose cognition is below the educable level should be considered to be capable of achieving self-care (hygiene) as a result of elbow surgery if they are capable of (1) precise hand placement from

---

• TABLE 63–1 • Simple Classification of Cerebral Palsy

Geographic Distribution
Hemiplegia, principally one-sided
Diplegia, principally upper extremity involvement
Total involvement, all four extremities plus speech

Type
Spastic, increased stretch reaction
Motion disorders, ataxias, athetosis, chorea
Mixed

Most elbow problems occur in spastic hemiplegia, although occasionally those with total body involvement develop fixed contracture.

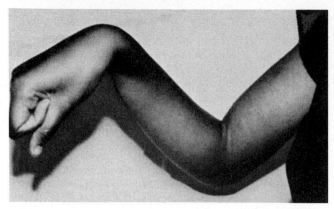

FIGURE 63–1 • Typical flexion-pronation of a dysfunctional upper extremity in a patient with cerebral palsy. (From Mital, M. A.: Lengthening of the elbow flexors in cerebral palsy. J. Bone Joint Surg. 61A:515, 1979.)

head to knee of longer than 5 seconds, and (2) sensibility test results of fewer than three of five objects or poor graphesthesia and two-point discrimination.

If cognition is in the educable range or higher but the child still has poor placement and sensibility test results, hygiene remains the goal, but the appearance of the upper extremities may also be important to such a patient.

For children who are educable or better and have hand-to-knee placement time of less than 5 seconds, and good sensibility results (as described earlier), a good functional upper extremity should be the surgical goal. The more complex procedures should be considered for these patients.

Treatment

Several types of intervention may be offered for the spastic, contracted elbows, but, generally, results are variable and unpredictable.[2, 3, 14, 17, 19, 22, 23]

NEURECTOMY

Musculocutaneous neurectomy is an effective procedure for elbows with flexion contractures less than 30 degrees when the main problem is excessive flexor tone. Neurectomy is contraindicated when elbow function in flexion depends on the biceps and brachialis alone. A lidocaine (Xylocaine) block of the musculocutaneous nerve along the medial proximal border of the biceps is helpful for separating the effects of flexor tone from those of contracture. Contracture should be expected to ensue when the spastic posture has been present for years. The lidocaine block also predicts brachioradialis elbow flexion capability after neurectomy.

Technique

We use a transverse axillary approach to the musculocutaneous nerve (Fig. 63–3). The biceps and lateral cord of the brachial plexus are located. The nerve is identified before it enters the biceps and confirmed by nerve stimulation. Meals has suggested a similar approach, phenyl block and neurectomy to the brachioradialis.[18] It is surgically released in patients with cerebral palsy. We have injected the nerve sheath with 5 percent phenol in glycerin to give temporary relief of flexor tone that is required for patients with head injury or stroke (see section on Acquired Spasticity).

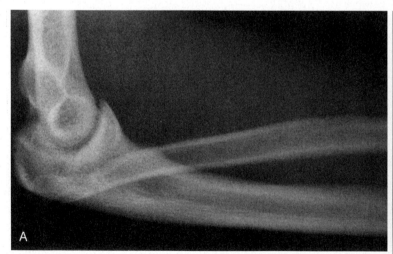
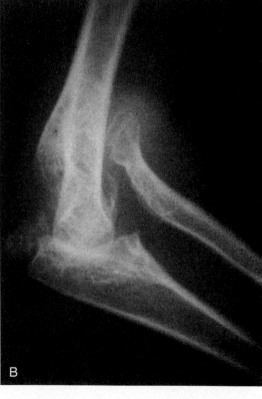

FIGURE 63–2 • Posterior radial head dislocation associated with flexion-pronation deformity (A). Flexion-supination deformity is less common and causes anterior dislocation of the radial head (B). Surgery is not typically required in either circumstance.

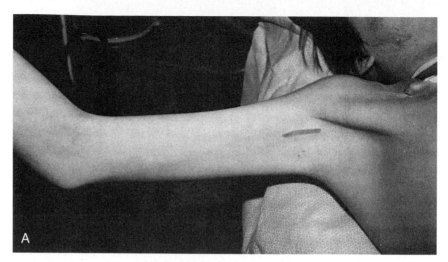

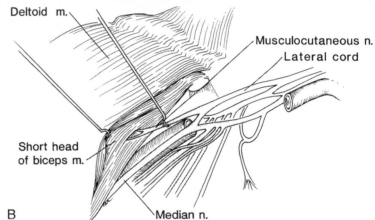

FIGURE 63–3 • A, Axillary exposure provides access to the musculocutaneous nerve, which usually branches from the brachial plexus high in the axilla and is isolated between the biceps and the coracobrachialis (B). The nerve may be injected with phenol or surgically released, as desired. (From Garland, D.E., et al.: Current uses of open phenol nerve block for adult acquired spasticity. Clin. Orthop. 165:217, 1982.)

BICEPS-BRACHIALIS LENGTHENING

Biceps-brachialis lengthening is used to improve cosmesis and enable patients to attend to their own hygiene. It is indicated when fixed contractures interfere with hygiene, but it should not be performed if flexion function may be lost. It has been suggested for deformities greater than 60 degrees.[16]

Technique

Mital performs biceps-brachialis lengthenings through a curved antecubital approach.[19] The lacertus fibrosus is excised, and Z-plasty of the biceps tendon and release of the brachialis aponeurosis are performed (Fig. 63–4). Occasionally, the anterior elbow capsule must be released. Three weeks of postoperative immobilization are followed by bivalved elbow splinting in both of these operations.

FLEXOR-PRONATOR RELEASE

The flexor slide may be performed to achieve the goals of hygiene and cosmetic lengthening of the elbow, wrist, and finger flexors. We and others[15] have found that this procedure may also cause excessive weakness in finger flexors. Thus, because it is sometimes unpredictable, it may not be a good surgical option for cerebral palsy.

If surgery is offered, we prefer careful fractional length-ening of the forearm and hand muscles at their musculotendinous junctions (Fig. 63–5). This is an easier, more precise procedure than the flexor slide; however, when pronation, elbow flexion, and forearm, wrist, and hand flexion all interfere with hygiene, this flexor-pronator release may be helpful. Many surgeons find that it improves function in the spastic, contracted hand and elbow.

Technique

The origin of the pronator-flexor group is released through a volar incision from the medial epicondyle to the distal forearm. The ulnar and median nerves are identified and protected, and all the structures between them, including the pronator teres, flexor carpi radialis and -ulnaris, the flexor digitorum superficialis and -profundus, and flexor pollicis, are allowed to slide distally from the medial epicondyle, ulna, and radius. This slide should permit adequate wrist and finger extension. A positioning plaster is used for 4 weeks, and then orthoses are used as necessary.

Acquired Spasticity

Most often, brain damage acquired in childhood is the result of trauma. The associated spasticity usually does not reach its maximum point until 1 to 2 months after the incident; then, muscle tone may gradually decrease during

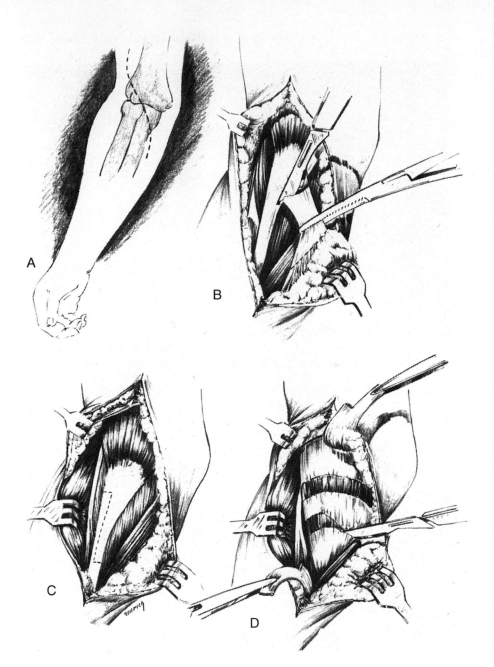

FIGURE 63–4 • Diagrams of the sequential steps of the elbow flexor Mital lengthening procedure. *A*, The initial incision. *B*, The exposure of the tendon of the biceps and the excision of the lacertus fibrosus. *C*, Third step of the elbow flexor–lengthening procedure: the Z-lengthening of the biceps tendon. *D*, The incision of the aponeurotic fibers covering the brachialis. (From Mital, M. A.: Lengthening of the elbow flexors in cerebral palsy. J. Bone Joint Surg. **61A**:515, 1979.)

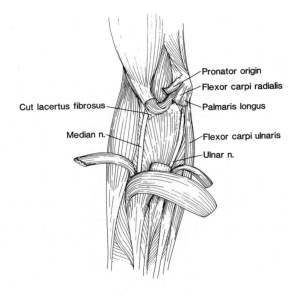

FIGURE 63–5 • Modified flexor-pronator release. The muscles from the medial epicondyle, and occasionally the flexor carpi ulnaris, are released, exposing the ulnar nerve.

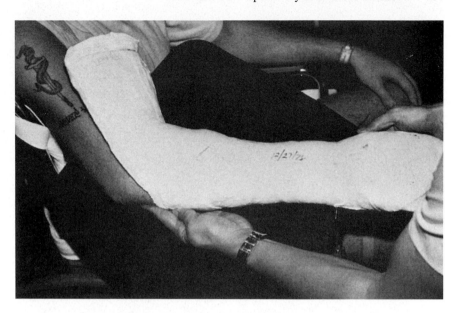

FIGURE 63–6 • The dropout cast has been used effectively for nonoperative control of excessive flexion or maintenance of correction obtained by surgery. (From Garland, D. E., et al.: Musculocutaneous neurectomy for spastic elbow flexion in nonfunctional upper extremities in adults. J. Bone Joint Surg. **62A**:108, 1980.)

the next 2 years. Botulinum toxin has been used to control tone in upper extremities.[4] It gives temporary benefits that may help therapists and may be more beneficial to head-injured children.[25]

We do not perform definitive procedures in children with acquired brain damage in the first 2 years after the insult, but we recommend positioning dropout plasters for elbows with great flexor tone during this period (Fig. 63–6). A solid long-arm plaster is placed with the arm in the position of maximal comfortable extension. Then, either the humeral extensor half of the plaster or the forearm extensor half is removed. This allows elbow extension while it blocks flexion. If this strategy fails, phenol injection of the musculocutaneous nerve (mentioned earlier) is carried out.

Another problem in children with acquired brain injury is heterotopic bone formation, usually about the anterior aspect of the elbow.[21] Because, unlike adults, most children eventually resorb the heterotopic bone, we recommend gentle motion and re-evaluation at least 6 months before any attempt is made at excision.

STROKE AND HEAD TRAUMA IN ADULTS

Stroke and head trauma produce permanent impairment in some 3 million adults in the United States. Abnormal elbow function due to spasticity and loss of motor control is a common disability. The surgeon treating these conditions must be fully cognizant of the complex rehabilitation process after central nervous system illness, particularly hand rehabilitation. Surgery is undertaken only after careful assessment of the many factors that determine the patient's potential to use the limb.[1]

Cerebral vascular accidents commonly involve the middle cerebral artery or its branches in the region of the cerebral cortex supplying the upper extremity. Consequently, the upper extremity usually is affected more frequently—and more severely—than the lower extremity. Elbow flexion contractures are nearly always preventable

in stroke patients if standard preventive measures are instituted early. In contrast, head injury is often associated with excessive elbow flexor tone because of decerebrate or decorticate rigidity. The hypertonicity may be so severe that nonoperative measures alone may not prevent elbow flexion deformity.

Elbow flexion contracture due to spasticity is the most common problem that requires surgical attention, and it usually affects patients with nonfunctional hands. Surgery is indicated to correct contractural deformities that interfere with hygiene or cause pain; rarely, it is used to improve cosmesis (Fig. 63–7). Operative intervention is usually

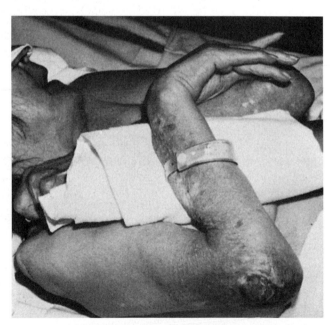

FIGURE 63–7 • Flexion deformity in a nonfunctional hand is frequently seen in the decerebrate posturing after a motor vehicle accident. Note the poor condition of the skin, which is common in such patients. An operation is indicated to improve hygiene. (From Garland, D. E., et al.: Musculocutaneous neurectomy for spastic elbow flexion in nonfunctional upper extremities in adults. J. Bone Joint Surg. **62A**:108, 1980.)

TRICEPS

L.H.BICEPS

S.H.BICEPS

BRACH

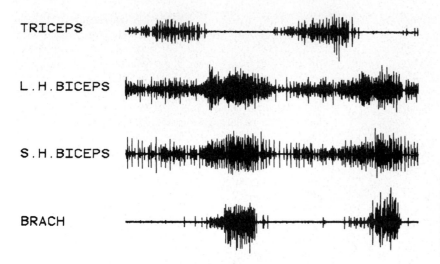

FIGURE 63–8. • Dynamic electromyogram of head-injured patient with spasticity during slow elbow extension-flexion-extension-flexion cycle. The triceps displays normal bursts of activity during the extension phase. The brachialis is also normally active in flexion. Note that both the long and the short heads of the biceps are inappropriately active during attempted elbow extension, indicating obstructive tone.

deferred until neurologic recovery is complete, in 6 to 18 months. If, despite a trial of aggressive nonoperative therapy that includes passive range of motion, splints, and serial casts, progressive elbow flexion deformity develops before neurologic recovery, then phenol injection of the musculocutaneous nerve is performed.[10] Rarely is surgery indicated to improve active elbow extension in a functional arm.[26]

Potential for Functional Recovery

Substantial neurologic recovery generally follows strokes and head injury. In stroke patients, most neurologic recovery is completed in the first 6 months; in head trauma patients substantial recovery extends over the first year and a half.[5] Definitive surgical procedures to improve function are deferred until after the patient's neurologic condition has stabilized and he or she has learned to cope with the disability and has received appropriate nonoperative therapy. When in the acute recovery phase elbow flexion spasticity is excessive, either open phenol injection of the motor branches of the musculocutaneous nerve or percutaneous motor-point phenol block is used to reduce flexion

tone.[10] The effects of phenol are transient, and spasticity is temporarily decreased until recovery is completed, at which time definitive procedures can be performed, if necessary.

PREOPERATIVE EVALUATION

Because vestibular reflexes potentiate flexor responses in the upper extremity, the patient is examined in the sitting position. Range of motion is determined by quickly and slowly extending the elbow. Quick stretch excites the velocity-sensitive components of the muscle spindle and may elicit clonus if spasticity is severe. Consequently, a greater range of extension often can be obtained by slow extension (often over 1 or 2 minutes) with the patient lying supine. Even when the elbow is stretched slowly and held in the most extended position possible tonus may persist. Consequently, spasticity can be differentiated from fixed contracture only by preoperative nerve block or examination under general anesthesia.

Dynamic electromyography is becoming increasingly useful as it enables surgeons to determine more precisely which flexor muscles are responsible for a deformity (Fig. 63–8) or whether surgical ablation of a given muscle will

TRICEPS

L.H.BICEPS

S.H.BICEPS

BRACH

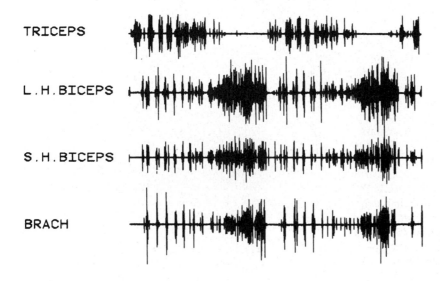

FIGURE 63–9 • Dynamic electromyogram made during attempted fast elbow motion. Note clonic firing pattern in all muscles, which indicates severe spasticity in all muscle groups.

be effective. This information is particularly valuable for patients with functional elbow motion because it enables the surgeon to release or lengthen only the muscles most involved and to preserve those that are less involved. Slow and fast volitional elbow flexion and extension are assessed. Attempts to move the elbow rapidly enhance an abnormal flexor response (Fig. 63–9).

Anterior and posterior radiographs of the elbow are taken before any surgical procedure. Arthritis and other conditions common in the adult patients may be responsible for intrinsic joint restriction and can decrease the probability of a successful surgical outcome.

Last, preoperative evaluation always includes a detailed assessment by a therapist: evaluation of motor and perceptual function of the elbow, hand, and shoulder and examination of cognitive, vocational, and social factors that are important determinants of arm function.

Surgical Techniques

NONFUNCTIONAL ELBOWS

With elbow flexion contracture, lengthening of the biceps tendon alone does not significantly improve elbow flexion deformity, so attention must be directed to the brachialis muscle as well. Myostatic contracture is differentiated from spasticity by anesthetic block of the musculocutaneous nerve (axillary nerve block) or by examining the patient under anesthesia. If there is less than 90 degrees of fixed deformity, musculocutaneous neurectomy is performed.[6] Residual deformity is corrected after surgery by dropout or serial casting (see Fig. 63–6).

Even when minimal or no fixed myostatic or joint contracture is present, spasticity may force the elbow into a flexed posture that interferes with function. When hemiplegics walk, it is common for the elbow to assume a flexed

posture and it may bounce up and down because of clonus. The patient may purposely walk slowly to decrease clonus. Musculocutaneous neurectomy improves cosmesis and eliminates clonus.[6] After musculocutaneous neurectomy, the loss of elbow flexion strength is not important, because most stroke patients with excessive elbow flexion have nonfunctional hands. Because the brachioradialis is innervated by the radial nerve, which is left intact, some elbow flexion persists after surgery if this muscle was active preoperatively, and the loss of musculocutaneous sensation is not bothersome. In a patient who has no brachioradialis control or spasticity, this procedure should not be performed, because musculocutaneous neurectomy leaves a completely flail elbow.

Musculocutaneous neurectomy is performed through a longitudinal incision that extends distally from the tendon of the pectoralis major in the interval between the short head of the biceps and the coracobrachialis.[6] This incision can be extended proximally or distally if further exploration for the nerve is necessary. A 1-cm segment of the nerve is excised (see Fig. 63–3).

When deformity is of long standing and myostatic contracture considerable, flexor release is performed. Through a lateral incision, the origin of the brachioradialis is released to provide access to the biceps tendon, which is lengthened or tenotomized, and the brachialis, which is myotomized. Some 30 to 40 degrees of correction (Fig. 63–10) is usually obtained, and further elbow extension is blocked by contracture of the neurovascular structures and skin. Excessive tension on the neurovascular elements is unnecessary and can lead to vascular compromise. It is not usually necessary to release the anterior capsule. Further correction is easily obtained postoperatively with a program of serial casting. Because this procedure usually is performed on nonfunctional limbs, full extension is not

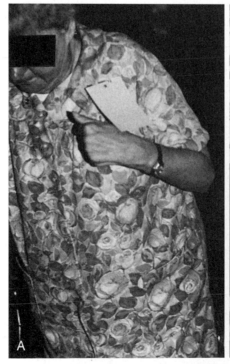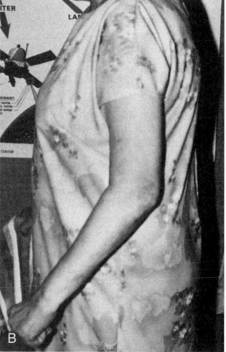

FIGURE 63–10 • *A*, A severe flexion contracture was present in this survivor of a cerebral vascular accident. *B*, Approximately 40 degrees of correction was obtained after flexor release. (From Garland, D. E., et al.: Musculocutaneous neurectomy for spastic elbow flexion in nonfunctional upper extremities in adults. J. Bone Joint Surg. **62A**:108, 1980.)

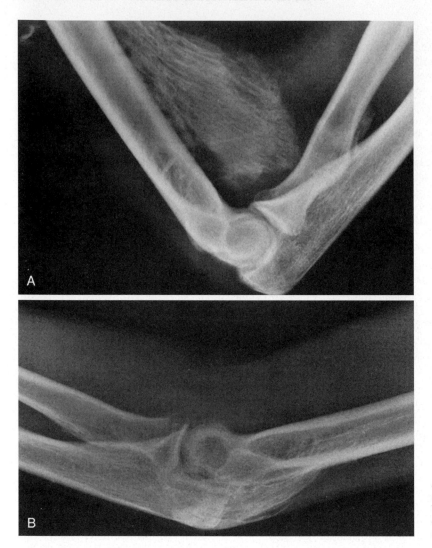

FIGURE 63–11 • Decerebrate rigidity may be associated with myositis ossificans in the anterior muscles *(A)* but even more often in the posterior aspect of the elbow *(B)*. (From Garland, D. E., et al.: Periarticular heterotopic ossification in head-injured adults. J. Bone Joint Surg. **62A**:143, 1980.)

necessary and surgery in combination with postoperative serial casting provides adequate correction.

FUNCTIONAL ELBOWS

Patients who have intact hand function but lack adequate elbow extension occasionally benefit from selective release of contracted or spastic elbow flexor muscles. Operative procedures that rely on releasing or lengthening the elbow flexors may reduce elbow flexion strength and range. Preoperative dynamic electromyography may identify a specific flexor that is more severely spastic; then, surgery can be restricted to this muscle. Preoperative motor-point block with lidocaine enables the surgeon to evaluate the effects of abolishing tone in a specific flexor muscle before surgery.

Some voluntary extension strength must be available preoperatively if the patient is to move the elbow through the full range of available extension after obstructive flexor spasticity or contracture is reduced.

Heterotopic Ossification

Heterotopic ossification of the elbow, a severe complication that occurs in about 3 percent of head injury patients, is discussed in detail in Chapter 32, but is also relevant in the context of this chapter. It most commonly occurs when hypertonus at the elbow is severe because of rigidity from decorticate or decerebrate posturing or spastic hemiplegia (Fig. 63–11). In general, heterotopic ossification is apparent within the first 6 months after head trauma (peak occurrence 2 months). The typical stroke patient infrequently develops heterotopic ossification. With head injury, the complication occurs more often posteriorly than anteriorly.[7]

The incidence of traumatic heterotopic ossification in combined head and elbow injuries is 90 percent.[8] Heterotopic ossification most often affects the collateral ligaments but can form in any planes about the elbow. Bone formation in the ulnar collateral ligament may contribute to an acute ulnar palsy from the localized swelling or delayed ulnar palsy resulting from long-standing pressure.[15]

Heterotopic ossification is heralded by swelling, pain, and limitation of motion at the elbow. Evidence of heterotopic ossification on bone scans is apparent 2 to 3 weeks before radiographic evidence of calcification appears. Alkaline phosphatase may not be elevated if only a small amount of new bone is present. Muscle hypertonus exerts continuous forces across the inflamed joint, which intensify the pain. Pain, in turn, increases spasticity, completing the vicious cycle. If the patient's neurologic condition improves rapidly, the amount of heterotopic ossification is lessened, and no significant impairment may result if an adequate range of elbow motion is maintained. On the other hand, extremity function may be affected if elbow motion becomes severely restricted or ankylosis develops, even if neurologic recovery has occurred. Even in a nonfunctional arm, hygiene of the elbow flexor crease and limb positioning are difficult in a patient with severe limb flexion deformity and ankylosis.

Treatment of heterotopic ossification begins with prompt recognition of the condition. Joint motion is preserved by range-of-motion exercises. Movement should be slow to minimize pain. Elbow splints are useful to position the elbow in maximal extension. Diphosphonate therapy is controversial. Indocin, for 3 months, may be used alone or in combination with diphosphonates.[12] Oral spasmolytic agents or phenol injection of the musculocutaneous nerve may help to reduce muscle tone in the biceps and brachialis muscles. Temporary reduction of elbow flexor tone permits the therapist to perform range-of-motion exercises more easily to maintain elbow extension. Forceful manipulation of the elbow under anesthesia also may help to maintain or increase elbow range.[9]

Because heterotopic ossification is so prevalent with combined head and elbow injuries, some type of prophylaxis seems warranted. This type of heterotopic ossification is not related to the severity of the head injury, and joint spasticity may not be present. Resection of heterotopic ossification is performed after the bone is skeletally mature.[7, 11, 13, 21] Active motion is essential to maintaining joint range after surgery. Indocin or radiation may be used for prophylaxis.[12]

REFERENCES

1. Caldwell, C., and Braun, R. M.: Spasticity in the upper extremity. Clin. Orthop. 104:80, 1974.
2. Carroll, R. E., and Craig, F. S.: The surgical treatment of cerebral palsy: The upper extremity. Surg. Clin. North Am. 31:385, 1951.
3. Colton, C. L., Ransford, A. O., and Lloyd-Roberts, G. C.: Transposition of the tendon of the pronator teres in cerebral palsy. J. Bone Joint Surg. 58B:220, 1976.
4. Corry, I. S., Cosgrove, A. P., Walsh, E. G., McClean, D., and Graham, H. K.: Botulinum toxin A in the hemiplegic upper limb: a double blind trial. Dev. Med. Child Neurol. 39:185–193, 1997.
5. Garland, D. E., and Waters, R. L.: Orthopedic evaluation in hemiplegic stroke. Orthop. Clin. North Am. 9:291, 1978.
6. Garland, D. E., Thompson, R., and Waters, R. L.: Musculocutaneous neurectomy for spastic elbow flexion in non-functional upper extremities in adults. J. Bone Joint Surg. 62A:108, 1980.
7. Garland, D. E., Blum, C. E., and Waters, R. L.: Periarticular heterotopic ossification in head-injured adults. J. Bone Joint Surg. 62A:1143, 1980.
8. Garland, D. E., and O'Hallaren, R. M.: Fractures and dislocations about the elbow in head injured adults. Clin. Orthop. 168:38, 1982.
9. Garland, D. E., Razza, B., and Waters, R. L.: Forceful joint manipulation in head injured adults with heterotopic ossification. Clin. Orthop. 169:133, 1982.
10. Garland, D. E., Lucie, R. S., and Waters, R. L.: Current uses of open phenol nerve block for adult acquired spasticity. Clin. Orthop. 165:217, 1982.
11. Garland, D. E., Hanscom, D. A., Keenan, M. A., Smith, C., and Moore, T.: Resection of heterotopic ossification in the patient with back trauma. J. Bone Joint Surg. 67A:1261, 1985.
12. Garland, D. E.: A clinical perspective of common forms of acquired heterotopic ossification. Clin. Orthop. 263:13, 1991.
13. Garland, D. E.: Surgical approaches for resection of heterotopic ossification in traumatic brain-injured adults. Clin. Orthop. 263:59, 1991.
14. Hoffer, M. M.: Cerebral palsy: Operative hand surgery. In Green, D. (ed.): Operative Hand Surgery. New York, Churchill Livingstone, 1982, p. 185.
15. Keenan, M. A. E., Kauffman, D. L., Garland, D. E., and Smith, C.: Late ulnar neuropathy in the brain-injured adult. J. Hand Surg. 13A:120, 1988.
16. Koman, L. A., Gelberman, R. H., Toby, E. B., and Poehling, G. G.: Cerebral palsy. Management of the upper extremity. Clin. Orthop. 253:62–74, 1990.
17. McCue, F. C., and Honner, R.: Deformities of the upper limb in cerebral palsy. South. Med. J. 63:355, 1970.
18. Meals, R. A.: Denervation for the treatment of acquired spasticity of the brachioradialis. J. Bone Joint Surg. 70A:1081, 1988.
19. Mital, M. A.: Lengthening of the elbow flexors in cerebral palsy. J. Bone Joint Surg. 61A:515, 1979.
20. Pletcher, D., Hoffer, M. M., and Koffman, M.: Non-traumatic dislocation of radial head in cerebral palsy. J. Bone Joint Surg. 58:104, 1976.
21. Roberts, J. B., and Pankratz, D. G.: The surgical treatment of heterotopic ossification at the elbow following long-term coma. J. Bone Joint Surg. 61A:760, 1979.
22. Sakellarides, H. T., and Mital, M.: Treatment of the pronator contracture of the forearm in cerebral palsy. J. Hand Surg. 1:79, 1976.
23. Samilson, R. L., and Morris, V. M.: Surgical improvement of the cerebral palsied upper limb. J. Bone Joint Surg. 46A:1203, 1964.
24. Samilson, R. L.: Principles of assessment of the upper limb in cerebral palsy. Clin. Orthop. 47:105, 1966.
25. Spaulding, S. J., White, S. C., McPherson, J. J., Schild, R., Transon, C., and Barasmian, P.: Electromyographic analysis of reach in individuals with cerebral palsy. Electromyogr. Clin. Neurophysiol. 30:109–115, 1990.
26. Waters, R. L., Wilson, D. J., and Savinelli, R.: Rehabilitation of the upper extremity following stroke. In Hunter, J. M., et al. (eds.): Rehabilitation of the Hand. St. Louis, C. V. Mosby, 1978, p. 505.

· CHAPTER 64 ·

Amputation

• ERNEST M. BURGESS and DAVID A. BOONE

Amputations through and about the elbow joint are infrequent, and little has been written on the subject. Thus, this discussion is followed by a list of general rather than specific references. Amputations about the elbow result principally from trauma or neoplasms. By far, the most frequent cause of all major elective amputations in the Western world is ischemia due to peripheral vascular disease, but fewer than 5 percent of these amputations occur in the upper limb, so the elbow is a relatively rare site for ischemic limb loss. In contrast, congenital limb deficiency is seen with some frequency near the elbow joint. The very short below-elbow transverse hemimelia is the congenital upper limb amputation most often encountered. Although the number of affected patients is also small, they do present a challenge in amputation management and in prosthetic substitution.

Elbow disarticulation has not been viewed kindly by prosthetists. If a normal, segmental arm is to be achieved, it is necessary to use external hinges at the prosthetic elbow joint. Because the elbow must be positioned and stabilized before useful control of the terminal prosthetic device (hand or hook) can be achieved, an elbow-locking mechanism is essential. This requirement calls for a somewhat complicated mechanical modification of the single-axis or the polycentric elbow hinge to allow voluntary positioning and locking. The more refined, intrinsic, body-controlled elbow mechanisms used for above-elbow prostheses require so much additional upper arm prosthetic length that they cause difficult problems with the fitting of clothing to the arm and with appearance when incorporated at elbow disarticulation level. For these reasons, many surgeons and prosthetists discourage amputation through the elbow joint and prefer to do it at a somewhat higher level, through the lower humerus. Thus, modern intrinsic elbow mechanisms can be spatially accommodated in the prosthesis while the normal elbow level is maintained.

In terms of successful prosthetic function, however, elbow disarticulation is most satisfactory (Fig. 64–1). The

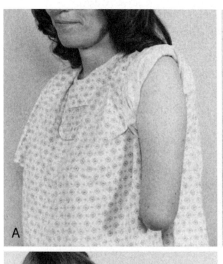
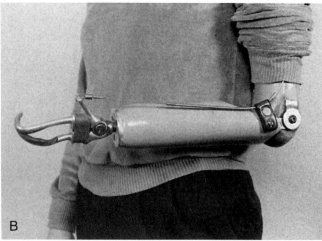
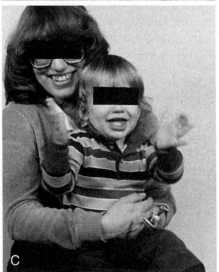

FIGURE 64–1 • *A*, Healed amputation at elbow disarticulation level. *B*, Same patient wearing a conventional body-powered prosthesis. *C*, Functional support using the prosthesis.

772

amputation should not be converted to a higher level merely to accommodate a less complicated prosthesis design. The distal condyles of the humerus with their irregular contours provide a good source of rotary stability and suspension of the prosthesis. Because effective muscle stabilization is surgically feasible and not technically difficult, it permits retention of a more "physiologic" residual limb. It is hoped that continued research in engineering design, especially of myoelectric prostheses, will enhance the usefulness of elbow disarticulation for amputation.

PRINCIPLES AND TECHNIQUE

Amputation surgery is reconstructive surgery. The surgeon is reconstructing a terminal end organ for contact with the environment—specifically, the prosthesis. In this respect, the surgery is technically comparable to similar procedures performed on the intact hand.

The basic principle of all upper limb amputations is preservation of as much length as is consistent with satisfactory surgical wound management. Equally important is conservation of functional tissue in the remaining portion of the limb—muscles, nerves, blood supply, and, whenever possible, healthy skin. Retained functional muscle is useful to provide contour and strength, and the voluntary myoelectric currents arising in the muscles of the residual limb initiate the signals that control almost all available externally powered prostheses. Retention of voluntary residual limb muscle activity is, then, a fundamental requirement for a physiologic amputation. The severed muscles or tendons need a fixed distal end point for effective use, so distal muscles must be stabilized at a length that avoids proximal joint restriction yet permits effective, forceful, voluntary contraction. When surgically feasible, then, muscle stabilization is important for elbow disarticulation.

As with all amputations, and, in fact, with all areas of surgery, the principles of appropriate wound healing apply. Well-nourished and sensate skin is needed to cover the amputation site. Skin flaps are developed and placed with plastic surgery technique and with knowledge and consideration of the replacement device to be used. The contact between prosthesis and limb, the interface, is the vital functional bridge. Almost all prostheses today totally contact the residual limb. Scar placement is elective and depends principally on the surgical circumstances. The scar should not be tender or adherent to bone or other deeper, rigid structures; and it must be sufficiently healthy to withstand interface contact and force transfer. Underlying bone must be well-contoured and smooth. Major nerves should be subjected to moderate traction, ligated, and sharply sectioned. This allows them to retract back into the soft tissues, where neuroma formation will not be a source of irritation.

The final requirement is early, progressive rehabilitation. Upper limb amputations are particularly responsive to immediate or early functional prosthetic use. Whether the chosen device is body-powered or externally powered, early application of a provisional functional prosthesis—the immediate-fit technique—has been a revolutionary advance in rehabilitation.

ELBOW DISARTICULATION

Skin

The skin flaps are ordinarily anteroposterior and of equal length (Fig. 64–2). They are fashioned short, and closure should be sufficiently loose to allow the skin to move freely. The position of the skin closure scar varies with the surgical circumstances. The nature of the traumatic insult may require extensive modification of the classic equal-flap closure. Because the prosthetic socket totally contacts the amputation site, scar placement can be adjusted to the available skin, provided the closure is appropriate. Use of skin that is adherent, of marginal viability, stretched tight over bone and cartilage, or folded and redundant compromises limb fit. Skin grafts are not a contraindication to fitting a prosthesis. They may be indicated, particularly in burn amputations. Skin on upper limb amputations is subjected to far less pressure, shear, and stretching than that on a weight-bearing lower limb. Skin of somewhat poorer than normal quality and well-nourished skin grafts improve socket tolerance with time, provided socket contact is permitted to adjust slowly as tolerated. It is important to maximize skin sensation and skin nutrition.

Nerves and Blood Vessels

Major nerves about the elbow are ligated under moderate tension. A fine, nonabsorbent suture is used. The ligated nerve end is then allowed to retract into the adjacent soft tissues away from the amputation site and away from

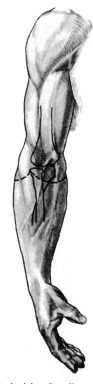

FIGURE 64–2 • Skin incision for elbow disarticulation and very long above-elbow amputation.

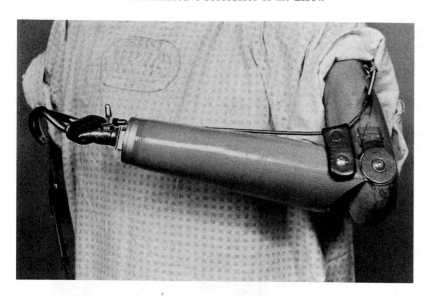

FIGURE 64–7 • A conventional body-powered elbow disarticulation prosthesis uses external-locking hinged joints with a terminal hook. The incorporated wrist flexion unit improves range of function of the terminal device.

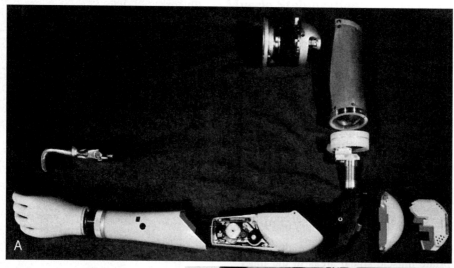

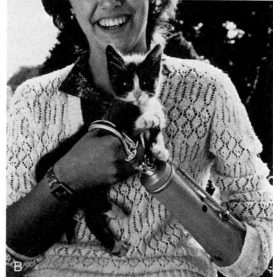

FIGURE 64–8 • A and B, The myoelectric Utah arm is available for amputations through and about the elbow joint. This is the most effective external electrically powered prosthesis available in the world today. (Courtesy of Motion Control Inc., 1005 South 300 West, Salt Lake City, Utah 84101.)

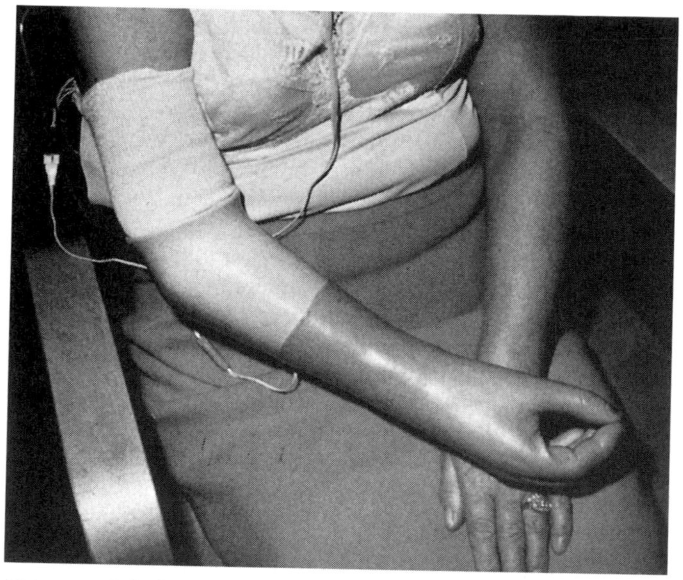

S

th

=

F

sin
tio
ist
rep
ma
exj
thi
su
48

I

Tr
ab
of
ur
m
fr
ti
in
th
cc
(F
T.
pe
1:
w
sı
ir
fc
n

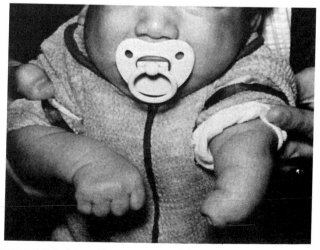

FIGURE 64–9 • U.S. Veterans Administration externally powered prosthesis.

and shoulder girdle exercises are started immediately after amputation. Disability is minimized by early temporary limb fit and active physical therapy. Young, active patients frequently achieve effective control of the temporary prosthesis and terminal device a few days after the limb was lost.

Conventional soft dressings with elastic wrap can be used when a rigid dressing is not available or when it is appropriate to inspect the wound at frequent intervals. Even in the presence of open wounds and marginally viable tissues, the rigid dressing technique is still effective. When the amputation site is infected, the nature of the lesion dictates postoperative management (i.e., soft dressings or closed cast), and, as healing progresses, a temporary prosthetic device is used first and then the definitive prosthesis. At elbow disarticulation level, an uncomplicated amputation stump generally is healed and ready for a permanent prosthesis 5 to 6 weeks after the surgery.

AMPUTATIONS IMMEDIATELY ADJACENT TO THE ELBOW

Severe trauma through the elbow joint may indicate a low transcondylar amputation. In an adult with closed distal humeral epiphyses, the surgical and immediate postoperative treatment is essentially the same as that outlined for elbow disarticulation. It is important to contour the distal humerus properly and to provide good soft tissue and skin coverage, disregarding, if necessary, the classic equal-flap closure. Muscle stabilization is accomplished by appropriate myoplasty or myodesis. Angulation osteotomy of the distal humerus is generally reserved for the occasional distal humerus amputation in a child. The indications and techniques for this bone contour augmentation have been outlined by Marquardt and colleagues.[14, 15]

Amputation through the forearm just distal to the elbow joint demands surgical modifications different from those outlined for elbow disarticulation. If the elbow joint itself is badly damaged and painful and has markedly restricted motion, it may be necessary to proceed with formal elbow disarticulation. The elbow, however, should not be saved at all costs. In general, even very short below-elbow amputation should be preserved, leaving the integrity of the elbow joint. The muscles that provide elbow control retain their attachments with ablation at this level. The advantages of elbow preservation even with very short below-elbow bones are better suspension of the prosthesis and the simplicity of the joint mechanism.

Section of the biceps tendon at its distal insertion increases the depth of the cubital fossa, making the socket fit more stable. Some surgeons prefer to transfer the biceps tendon to the underlying brachialis muscle just proximal to the elbow joint. Such a transfer does not significantly disturb function of the biceps but does permit a modern and effective electrical signal when an externally powered prosthesis is used.

When surgically appropriate, it is desirable to leave the ulna slightly longer than the radius in very high forearm amputations. The bone ends must be carefully tailored to avoid rough, prominent surfaces. Loss of elbow flexion strength secondary to distal biceps tendon transfer has not weakened control of the prosthesis. The brachialis muscle is strong enough to flex the elbow with the prosthesis in place.

ELBOW DISARTICULATION IN CHILDREN

Surgery is rarely needed for congenital limb deficiencies at or about elbow level. Transverse hemimelia just distal to the elbow rarely requires surgical intervention (Fig. 64–10). Prosthetic management is standardized and effective. Affected children generally present with a short below-elbow residual limb that is painless and freely movable and that generally permits full flexion and 10 to 25 degrees of hyperextension. Such children routinely become efficient users of prostheses. When amputation is necessary in a

FIGURE 64–10 • Congenital, very short below-elbow transverse hemimelia.

24. Ogilvie-Harris, D. J., Gordon, R., and MacKay, M.: Arthroscopic treatment for posterior impingement in degenerative arthritis of the elbow. Arthroscopy 11:437, 1995.
25. Ortner, D. J.: Description and classification of degenerative bone changes in the distal joint surface of the humerus. Am. J. Phys. Anthrop. 28:139, 1968.
26. Redden, J. F., and Stanley, D.: Arthroscopic fenestration of the olecranon fossa in the treatment of osteoarthritis of the elbow. Arthroscopy 9:14, 1993.
27. Salter, R. B.: Textbook of Disorders and Injuries of the Musculoskeletal System, 2nd ed. Baltimore, Williams & Wilkins, 1983.
28. Schumacher, H. R.: Primer on the Rheumatic Disease, 9th ed. Atlanta, Arthritis Foundation, 1988.
29. Smith, F. M.: The Elbow, 2nd ed. Philadelphia, W. B. Saunders Co., 1972.
30. Stanley, D., and Winsor, G.: A surgical approach to the elbow. J. Bone Joint Surg. 72B:728, 1990.
31. Tsuge, K., and Mizuseki, T.: Débridement arthroplasty for advanced primary osteoarthritis of the elbow: Results of a new technique used for 29 elbows. J. Bone Joint Surg. 76B:641, 1994.
32. Wadsworth, T. G.: The Elbow. Edinburgh, Churchill Livingstone, 1982.

• CHAPTER 68 •

Septic Arthritis

• KENNETH P. BUTTERS and
BERNARD F. MORREY

GENERAL CONSIDERATIONS

An infection can be defined as the clinical manifestation of a host response to a given inoculum. Aspects of the inoculum include the amount of bacteria, the type of entry, and the nature or virulence of the pathogen. Host factors can be classified as congenital or acquired. Congenital immunoincompetence syndromes are associated with deficiencies of the humeral or bursal immunologic systems and have been well described in standard medical textbooks. Acquired failures or alteration of immunocompetence can be either generalized or localized. Generalized processes include diabetes mellitus, corticosteroid therapy, cancer with or without immunosuppressive therapy, human immunodeficiency virus (HIV) infection, and alcohol or other chemical addiction or abuse. Local processes that alter normal host resistance include scar formation from previous surgery, burns, radiation, or prior infection. In applying these observations specifically to the elbow, it should be noted that this is a subcutaneous joint. Hence, the elbow is vulnerable to direct inoculation of a pathogen, particularly as host resistance is compromised.

OSTEOMYELITIS

Bone infection occurs (1) hematogenously, (2) by direct inoculation after surgery or open fracture, or (3) by contiguous spread from a local process.[64]

Hematogenous Infection

Hematogenous infection is the most common type of osteomyelitis and has been reported to occur at the elbow in about 4 percent of such cases.[64] In the growing child, the end-arterial loop of the metaphyseal bone causes sluggish bone blood flow. The lack of phagocytic activity in these loops allows maturation of a septic thrombus at the arterial site.[29] The abscess spreads through the haversian system into the subperiosteal space. If the metaphysis is intra-articular, as at the hip or shoulder, a septic joint will then result,[62] but this is not the case at the elbow. As at other sites, acute hematogenous osteomyelitis is most common in children younger than 3 and older than 7 years of age. The first group is vulnerable owing to the lack of acquired host immunity; the second age group corresponds to the time of rapid growth.[40]

PRESENTATION AND DIAGNOSIS

The clinical presentation is typical and includes local pain, warmth, and swelling. The patient may be afebrile but is not necessarily systemically ill. In children, a predisposing, traumatic event is common,[39, 69] but identity of a remote focus is less frequent. The elbow is held in flexion and pseudoparalysis or reflex inhibition may be present. The physical examination includes the following:

1. The specific point of maximal tenderness should be determined by gentle palpation. The focus of the septic process can often be accurately localized in this way, even before radiographic changes are apparent.

2. Gentle passive motion of the joint should be done to rule out septic arthritis. With joint infections, all motion is resisted; with metaphyseal osteomyelitis, gentle, supported passive motion is possible.

Except in the very acute stages, an elevated leukocyte count is variably present,[12, 40] and the differential count tends to demonstrate a shift to the left in two thirds of the cases. The erythrocyte sedimentation rate has been the most sensitive blood test; it is elevated in the early stages of infection in about 80 percent of persons.[12, 40] It is therefore very sensitive, but not specific. Interestingly, the rate is statistically higher in joint infections than in bone infections and is a valuable means of following the treatment and resolution of the infection.[12, 32, 39] Early radiographs are not helpful. After 7 to 14 days, osteoporosis may be present, followed by periosteal elevation or erosions.

The classic appearance of osteomyelitis by bone scan is a well-defined focal area of increased uptake at the site of active infection (Fig. 68–1). The ^{99m}Tc scan may be positive as early as 24 hours after the onset of symptoms in a patient with osteomyelitis.[18] The increased activity of equal intensity on both sides of the joint indicates joint disease, arthritis, or synovitis but is not a reliable indicator in the neonate. Nonspecific inflammatory arthritides of rheumatoid arthritis or gout limits the value of the Ga scan.[26] False-negative results are also common.[59] At the present time, we recommend first a ^{99m}Tc scan as a low-cost screening test to provide immediate results and localization. The ^{111}In-labeled leukocyte scan may be useful primarily for more acute suppurative infection. More recently, Erdman states that magnetic resonance (MR) imaging has 100 percent sensitivity and 0 percent specificity in a mixed group of acute and chronic osteomyelitis.[14] Joint aspiration remains the most simple and reliable means of making the diagnosis of elbow joint sepsis.

Direct Inoculation

Direct inoculation is probably the most common cause of infection about the elbow joint. The thin soft tissue coverage predisposes to compound fractures that may become secondarily infected. Elective surgery of the elbow region has been associated with an infection rate of about 2 to 4 percent, significantly greater than the commonly quoted 1 percent for elective orthopedic procedures.

Spread from a Contiguous Focus

Infection by spread from a contiguous focus occurs at the elbow from a septic joint or from an infected olecranon

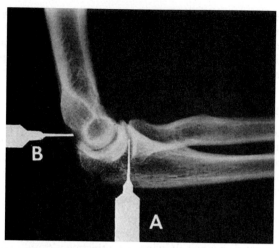

FIGURE 68–4 • Aspiration of the elbow (A) is carried out through the lateral portal between the radial head, lateral epicondyle, and tip of the olecranon. Alternatively, with significant joint distention, a posterolateral approach (B) into the olecranon fossa may be used.

and hepatitis. Gonococcal arthritis is suspected with appropriate sexual history. Rheumatoid arthritis with a secondary infection is, of course, a difficult clinical diagnosis that is usually resolved only with aspiration.

Systemic symptoms are variably present. A leukocytosis is often present early, but the shift to the left of the differential leukocyte count is more reliable. The sedimentation rate is invariably increased, but this does not distinguish the patient with active rheumatoid arthritis.[12] Even infected joint replacement shows elevated sedimentation rates, but the effect of the surgery itself is sometimes a source of confusion.[54] As with any joint infection, the key to the diagnosis is joint aspiration. The distended joint is easy to enter either from the lateral "triangle" or at the posterior olecranon fossa (Fig. 68–4). In addition to joint aspiration for culture and cell count, gas-liquid chromatography may be helpful in differentiating a bacterial from a nonseptic inflammatory process.[7]

The radiographic assessment is not helpful in the early diagnosis of elbow infection, but an increased amount of synovial fluid may show an anterior or posterior fat pad sign.[8, 35] In this setting, the ^{99m}Tc scan is invariably positive (Fig. 68–5). Gallium or labeled white cell scans may be more specific than technetium but have the disadvantage of a 24- to 72-hour delay in diagnosis and have fallen into disfavor in recent years. An MR image lacks the specificity of distinguishing septic from nonseptic fluid.[15] Later, osteopenia and subtle bone erosion at the synovial attachment occur, progressing to uniform thinning of the articular cartilage and then more extensive erosions and subchondral disruption. Joint aspiration must be done under sterile conditions, because inoculation of the sterile joint is possible with aspiration and has been reported.[3]

Additional laboratory investigations include blood cul-

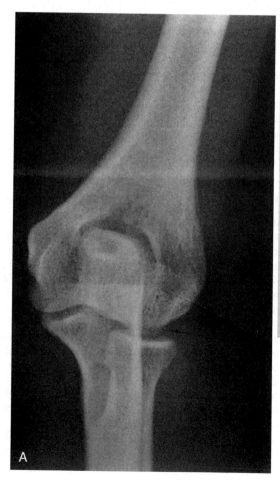

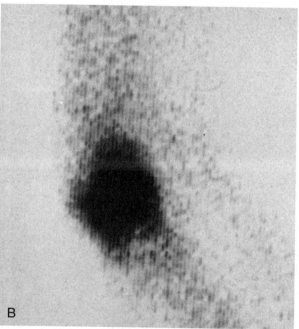

FIGURE 68–5 • A, Normal-appearing radiograph in a patient with acute onset of a painful effusion. B, An area of markedly increased uptake demonstrated by the technetium-99m scan was subsequently found to be septic arthritis.

tures, which are positive in about 40 to 70 percent of patients[3, 21, 40] and in up to 90 percent if multiple joints are involved. We have observed that the limited use of antibiotics will tend to result in a negative blood culture, but the joint aspirate will still reveal the organism.[40]

Staphylococcus aureus is isolated in about two thirds of cases of bacterial arthritis in adults[30] and in at least half of those in children.[39] In the neonatal age group, coliform and gram-positive organisms are not uncommon.[43] At ages 3 months to 3 years, the child is at risk for *Haemophilus influenzae,* but in children older than 3 years, *S. aureus* is the predominant organism.[39]

Treatment

Initial specific antibiotic treatment is first based on the Gram stain. If infection is suspected and no organism is isolated, initial antibiotic treatment should be based on age and presentation. This should include penicillin in the young healthy patient, *Staphylococcus* and gram-negative coverage in the older patient with underlying disease, and drugs for *H. influenzae* in the young child. Mayo Clinic treatment consists of 3 to 4 weeks of intravenous administration of antibiotics, but this may be somewhat conservative, and the duration should be tailored to the clinical setting. Others have begun an appropriate oral antibiotic approximately 1 week after serum bactericidal levels have been obtained.[34] Serial monitoring of the serum antibiotic levels is continued on an outpatient basis.

In addition to systemic antibiotics, the treatment, as in any diarthrodial joint, requires removal of accumulated cellular debris and pus. Cartilage is destroyed by digestion from enzymes elaborated from neutrophils, synovium, and bacteria.[13] When there is capsular distention, aspiration is easily accomplished (see Fig. 68–5). Rather than simple aspiration for diagnosis, we strongly recommend that the joint be lavaged with sterile saline at the time of aspiration. This has been clearly shown to be effective in preventing collagen loss in the rabbit.[12] Successive decreasing cell counts from the joint aspirate may also be used as an indicator of recovery.[19, 20] Intermittent joint distention-suction through percutaneous catheters[27] has given way to arthroscopic débridement and lavage in our practice.

Intra-articular administration of antibiotics is controversial in the treatment of septic arthritis. Adequate levels of antibiotics occur in the synovial fluid from parenteral treatment, and postinfection synovitis lasting up to 8 weeks in as many as 40 percent of the cases has been related to the intra-articular use of penicillin.[3] Yet experimental evidence indicates that the joint can be sterilized more rapidly by intra-articular injection of an antibiotic.[5] Lacking evidence that the chemical synovitis is harmful to the joint, if there has been a delay in diagnosis of 4 to 5 days, we may inject 0.5 g of cefazolin sodium diluted in 10 ml of sterile water, particularly if a gram-positive organism is suspected.

For infections that are subacute, postoperative, or due to direct inoculation, adequate clearance by aspiration is not reliable, and drainage by arthroscopy is preferred. If a significant amount of soft tissue involvement is present, arthrotomy may be necessary and early motion is begun. Although recently popularized for the knee,[4] early active

motion after incision and drainage was recommended in 1919 by Willems,[67] who reported good results with both knee and elbow infections. The basis of the beneficial effect of early motion has been carefully studied by Salter and associates,[52] who found protection of articular cartilage and concluded that this technique (1) prevents adhesions and pannus, (2) improves nutrition of cartilage, (3) enhances clearance of exudate including lysosomal enzymes, and (4) stimulates the living chondrocytes.

Arthroscopy of the elbow allows inspection, clearance of loculations and adhesions, thorough irrigation, and synovial tissue culture as well as insertion of drainage catheters. Hence, this has emerged as the treatment of choice for most cases that do not respond to aspiration or in those patients requiring synovectomy.[61] Aggressive synovectomy and débridement is an important concept in treating the infected prosthesis[53] (see Chapter 39).

Results

The degeneration of articular cartilage and the development of fibrous adhesions[39] are responsible for the poor results after an infection. Delay in diagnosis and treatment is probably more important than the exact type of treatment and is the most important factor affecting prognosis.[20, 33, 39] A normal joint is unlikely if treatment is delayed for more than 1 week after the onset of symptoms.[39, 46] Virulence of the organism is an important prognostic variable.[19] In one series, complete recovery occurred in 90 percent of those infected with *Streptococcus,* 60 percent of those infected with *Staphylococcus,* and less than one third of patients infected with a gram-negative organism.[20] Gram-negative infection has a poor prognosis and is often associated with compromised host resistance. Gonococcal arthritis also involves the elbow in about 10 percent of cases,[37] and treatment offers predictably good results. Nongonococcal *Neisseria* infections have also been reported to involve the elbow, again often with compromised host resistance or in association with a crystalline-induced arthritis.[14]

Loss of function, not recurrence, is the most common sequela of this infection (Fig. 68–6). In the Mayo series of 103 septic joints, acute infection was eradicated in all but 1, with only 4 recurrences. Argen and associates[3] found no evidence of reinfection or chronic osteomyelitis in any of the elbow infections, and no secondary procedures were necessary.[39] The ultimate result depends on the state of the joint before the infection.

NONBACTERIAL INFECTIONS

The elbow joint is somewhat prone to nonbacterial infection and is involved in approximately 10 percent of all skeletal infections from tuberculosis.[36] Unlike suppurative arthritis, the adjacent bone may also be involved. A tuberculous infection of the elbow is diagnosed by aspiration in 25 to 75 percent of instances, but most consistently (95 percent), it results from biopsy of the synovial tissue. Pulmonary tuberculosis is present in only about half of the cases.[71] Atypical *Mycobacterium* infection, for example, *M. kansasii,*[64] may also occur, both from direct inoculation

5 days after a sterile aspirate has been obtained. Roschman and Bell[50] found in immunocompromised patients with olecranon bursitis a mean of 11 days of antibiotic therapy before bursal fluid cultures were negative.

Indications for excision of the olecranon bursa include prolonged drainage after surgical incision or rupture, recurrent septic bursitis, and chronic bursitis with contiguous osteomyelitis. Ablation is difficult, especially in the patient with rheumatoid arthritis. We have found that meticulous dissection under magnification with preliminary staining of the bursal wall using methylene blue and hydrogen peroxide is helpful.[58] The incision should be lateral to the midline, not over the center of the bursa.

REFERENCES

1. Ahbel, D. E., Alexander, A. H., Kleine, M. L., and Lichtman, D. M.: Protothecal olecranon bursitis. J. Bone Joint Surg. 62A:835, 1980.
2. Arafiles, R.: A new technique of fusion for THERABAND arthritis of the elbow. J. Bone Joint Surg. 63A:1396, 1981.
3. Argen, R. J., Wilson, C. H., and Wood, P.: Suppurative arthritis. Arch. Intern. Med. 117:661, 1966.
4. Ballard, A., Burkhalter, W. E., Mayfield, G. W., Dehne, E., and Brown, P. W.: The functional treatment of pyogenic arthritis of the adult knee. J. Bone Joint Surg. 57A:1119, 1975.
5. Bardenheier, J. A., Morgan, H. C., and Stamp, W. G.: Treatment and sequelae of experimentally produced septic arthritis. Surg. Gynecol. Obstet. 122:249, 1966.
6. Blockey, N. J., and McAllister, T. H.: Antibiotics in acute osteomyelitis in children. J. Bone Joint Surg. 54B:299, 1972.
7. Brook, I., Reza, M., Bricknell, K. S., Bluestone, R., and Finegold, S. M.: Abnormalities in synovial fluid of patients with septic arthritis detected by gas-liquid chromatography. Ann. Rheum. Dis. 39:168, 1980.
8. Brower, A. C.: Septic arthritis. Radiol. Clin. North Am. 34:293, 1996.
9. Buskila, D., and Tenenbaum, J.: Septic bursitis in human immunodeficiency virus infection. J. Rheumatol. 16:1374, 1989.
10. Canoso, J. J.: Idiopathic or traumatic olecranon bursitis. Arthritis Rheum. 20:1213, 1977.
11. Canoso, J. J., and Sheckman, P. R.: Septic subcutaneous bursitis: report of sixteen cases. J. Rheumatol. 6:1, 1979.
12. Covey, D. C., and Albright, J. A.: Clinical significance of the erythrocyte sedimentation rate in orthopaedic surgery. J. Bone Joint Surg. 69A:148, 1987.
13. Daniel, D., Akeson, W., Amiel, D., Ryder, M., and Boyer, J.: Lavage of septic joints in rabbits: effects of chondrolysis. J. Bone Joint Surg. 58A:393, 1976.
14. Degan, T. J., Rand, J. A., and Morrey, B. F.: Musculoskeletal infection with nongonococcal Neisseria species not associated with meningitis. Clin. Orthop. 176:206, 1983.
15. Erdman, W. A., Tamburro, F., Jayson, H. T., Weatherall, P. T., Ferry, K. B., and Peshock, R. M.: Osteomyelitis: characteristics and pitfalls of diagnosis with MR imaging. Radiology 180:533, 1991.
16. Gardner, G. C., and Weisman, M. H.: Pyarthrosis in patients with rheumatoid arthritis: a report of 13 cases and a review of the literature from the past 40 years. Am. J. Med. 88:503, 1990.
17. Gerster, J. C., Lagier, R., and Boivin, G.: Olecranon bursitis related to calcium pyrophosphate dihydrate crystal deposition disease. Arthritis Rheum. 25:989, 1982.
18. Gilday, D. L., Eng, B., Paul, D. J., and Paterson, J.: Diagnosis of osteomyelitis in children by combined blood pool and bone imaging. Radiology 117:331, 1975.
19. Goldenberg, D. L., Brandt, K. D., Cohen, A. S., and Cathcart, E. S.: Treatment of septic arthritis. Arthritis Rheum. 18:83, 1975.
20. Goldenberg, D. L., and Cohen, A. S.: Acute infectious arthritis. Am. J. Med. 60:369, 1976.
21. Goldenberg, D. L., and Cohen, A. S.: Synovial membrane histopathology in differential diagnosis of arthritis. Medicine 57:239, 1978.
22. Gristina, H.: Spontaneous septic arthritis in rheumatoid arthritics. J. Bone Joint Surg. 56A:1180, 1974.
23. Ho, G., et al.: Septic bursitis in the prepatellar and olecranon bursae. Ann. Intern. Med. 89:21, 1978.
24. Ho, G., and Su, E. Y.: Antibiotic therapy of septic bursitis. Arthritis Rheum. 24:905, 1981.
25. Ho, G.: Bacterial arthritis. Curr. Opin. Rheum. 4:509, 1992.
26. Hughes, S.: Radionuclides in orthopedic surgery. J. Bone Joint Surg. 62B:141, 1980.
27. Jackson, R. W., and Parsons, C. J.: Distension-irrigation treatment of major joint sepsis. Clin. Orthop. 96:160, 1973.
28. Jain, V. K., Cestero, R. V. M., and Baum, J.: Septic and aseptic olecranon bursitis in patients on maintenance dialysis. Clin. Exp. Dialysis Apheresis 5:4, 1981.
29. Kahn, D. S., and Pritzker, K.: The pathophysiology of bone infection. Clin. Orthop. 96:12, 1973.
30. Kelley, P. J., Martin, W. J., and Coventry, M. B.: Bacterial (suppurative) arthritis in the adult. J. Bone Joint Surg. 52A:1595, 1970.
31. Kelley, P. J.: Musculoskeletal infections due to Serratia. Clin. Orthop. 96:76, 1973.
32. Kelley, P. J.: Bacterial arthritis in the adult. Orthop. Clin. North Am. 6:973, 1975.
33. Kellgren, J. H., Ball, J., Fairbrother, R. W., and Barns, K. L.: Suppurative arthritis complicating rheumatoid arthritis. B.M.J. 1:1193, 1958.
34. Kolyvas, E., Ahroneim, G., Marks, M. I., Gledhill, R., Owen, H., and Rosenthal, L.: Oral antibiotic therapy of skeletal infections in children. Pediatrics 65:867, 1980.
35. Markowitz, R. I., Davidson, R. S., Harty, P. M., Bellah, R. D., Hubbard, A. M., and Rosenberg, H. K.: Sonography of the elbow in infants and children. Am. J. Rheum. 159:829, 1992.
36. Martini, M., and Gottesman, H.: Results of conservative treatment of TB of the elbow. Int. Orthop. 4:83, 1980.
37. Masi, A. T., and Eisenstein, B. I.: Disseminated gonococcal infection and gonococcal arthritis. Semin. Arthritis Rheum. 10:173, 1981.
38. Meals, R. A.: The use of flexor carpi ulnaris muscle flap in treatment of infected non-union of the proximal ulna: A case report. Clin. Orthop. 240:168, 1989.
39. Morrey, B. F., and Bianco, A. J.: Septic arthritis in children. Orthop. Clin. North Am. 6:923, 1975.
40. Morrey, B. F., and Peterson, H. A.: Hemotogenous pyogenic osteomyelitis in children. Orthop. Clin. North Am. 6:935, 1975.
41. Morrey, B. F., Fitzgerald, R. H., Kelly, P. J., Dobyns, J. H., and Washington, J. A., III: Diphtheroid osteomyelitis. J. Bone Joint Surg. 59A:527, 1977.
42. Morrey, B. F., and Bryan, R. S.: Infection after total elbow arthroplasty. J. Bone Joint Surg. 65A:330, 1983.
43. Nelson, J. D.: The bacterial etiology and antibiotic management of septic arthritis in infants and children. Pediatrics 50:437, 1972.
44. O'Driscoll, S. W., Morrey, B. F., and An, K. N.: Intraarticular pressure and capacity of the elbow. Arthroscopy 6:100, 1990.
45. Ornvold, K., and Paepke, J.: Aspergillus terreus as a cause of septic olecranon bursitis. Am. J. Clin. Pathol. 97:114, 1992.
46. Peterson, S., Knudsen, F. U., Andersen, E. A., and Egebald, M.: Acute hematogenous osteomyelitis and septic arthritis in children. Acta Orthop. Scand. 51:451, 1980.
47. Pien, F. D., Ching, D., and Kim, E.: Septic bursitis: Experience in a community practice. J. Orthop. 14:981, 1991.
48. Rashkoff, E., and Burkhalter, W. E.: Arthrodesis of the salvage elbow. Orthopedics 9:733, 1986.
49. Rimoin, D. L., and Wennberg, J. F.: Acute septic arthritis complicating chronic rheumatoid arthritis. J.A.M.A. 196:109, 1966.
50. Roschmann, R. A., and Bell, C. L.: Septic bursitis in immunocompromised patients. Am. J. Med. 83:661, 1987.
51. Saini, M., and Canoso, J. J.: Traumatic olecranon bursitis. Acta Radiol. Diagn. 23:255, 1982.
52. Salter, R. B., Bell, R. S., and Kelley, F. W.: The protective effect of continuous passive motion on living articular cartilage in acute septic arthritis. Clin. Orthop. 159:223, 1981.
53. Schoifet, S. D., and Morrey, B. F.: Treatment of infection after total knee arthroplasty by debridement with retention of components. J. Bone Joint Surg. 72A:1383, 1990.
54. Schulak, D. J., Rayhack, J. M., Lippert, F. G., III, and Convery, F. R.: The erythrocyte sedimentation rate in orthopaedic patients. Clin. Orthop. 167:197, 1982.
55. Sharma, S. V., Varma, B. P., and Khanna, S.: Dystrophic calcification in tubercular lesions of bursae. Acta Orthop. Scand. 49:445, 1978.
56. Shulman, G., and Waugh, T. R.: Acute bacterial arthritis in the adult. Orthop. Rev. 17:955, 1988.

57. Soderquist, B., and Hedstom, S. A.: Predisposing factors, bacteriology and antibiotic therapy in thirty-five cases of septic bursitis. Scand. J. Infect. Dis. **18:**305, 1986.

58. Stewart, N. J., Manzanares, J. B., Morrey, B. F.: Surgical treatment of aseptic olecranon bursitis. J. Shoulder Elbow Surg. **6:**49, 1997.

59. Sullivan, D. C., Rosenfield, N. S., Ogden, J., and Gottschalk, A.: Problems in the scintigraphic detection of osteomyelitis in children. Radiology **135:**731, 1980.

60. Tollerud, A.: Anaerobic septic bursitis [letter]. Ann. Intern. Med. **91:**494, 1979.

61. Törholm, C., Hedström, S.A., Sundén, G., and Lidgren, L.: Synovectomy in bacterial arthritis. Acta Orthop. Scand. **54:**748, 1983.

62. Trueta, J.: Three types of acute hematogenous osteomyelitis. J. Bone Joint Surg. **41B:**671, 1959.

63. Viggiano, D. A.: Septic arthritis presenting as olecranon bursitis in patients with rheumatoid arthritis. J. Bone Joint Surg. **62A:**1011, 1980.

64. Waldvogel, F. A., Medoff, G., and Swartz, M. D.: Osteomyelitis: A review of clinical features, therapeutic considerations and unusual aspects. N. Engl. J. Med. **282:**198, 260, 316, 1970.

65. West, W. F., Kelley, P. J., and Martin, W. J.: Chronic osteomyelitis. J.A.M.A. **213:**1837, 1970.

66. Wilensky, A. O.: Osteomyelitis. Its Pathogenesis, Symptomatology, and Treatment. New York, Macmillan, 1934.

67. Willems, C.: Treatment of purulent arthritis by wide arthrotomy followed by immediate active mobilization. Surg. Gynecol. Obstet. **28:**546, 1919.

68. Wilson, J. N.: Tuberculosis of the elbow. J. Bone Joint Surg. **35B:**558, 1953.

69. Winroth, G., Hedström, S. A., and Lidgren, L.: Posttraumatic bacterial arthritis with luxation of the elbow: A case report. Arch Orthop. Trauma Surg. **103:**227, 1984.

70. Winter, W. G., Larson, R. K., Honeggar, M. M., Jacobsen, D. T., Pappagianis, D., and Huntington, R. W.: Coccidioidal arthritis and its treatment. J. Bone Joint Surg. **57A:**1152, 1975.

71. Wolfgang, G. L.: Tuberculous joint infection. Clin. Orthop. **136:**257, 1978.

72. Zimmermann III, B., Mikolich, D. C., and Ho, G.: Septic bursitis. Semin. Arthritis Rheum. **24:**391, 1995.

73. Zretina, J. R., Foster, J., and Reyes, C. V.: *Mycobacterium kansasii* infection of the elbow joint. J. Bone Joint Surg. **61A:**1099, 1979.

improve forearm rotation in selected patients. The effectiveness of this treatment is greatest when performed in the early stages of involvement. In these later stages, few options for treatment are available.[13, 16] Total elbow arthroplasty may be indicated when there is severe functional limitation (Fig. 69–6). No studies have been published documenting long-term follow-up results of total elbow arthroplasty in patients with hemophilia, but the short-term follow-up results after elbow replacement have been gratifying in the authors' institution.

Pain control is frequently a problem for patients with recurrent intra-articular bleeds. Aspirin and aspirin-containing drugs should be avoided because of their adverse effect on platelet function. Some of the nonsteroidal anti-inflammatory drugs have a more transient effect on platelet function and could be tried with cautious observation in selected patients. Our practice at the Mayo Clinic has been influenced by the anti-inflammatory effects of nonacetylated salicylates, such as choline magnesium trisalicylate (Trilisate) and salicylsalicylic acid (Disalcid), in relieving arthritic symptoms. Drug abuse and addiction can be seri-

ous problems and must be guarded against, if narcotics are used, particularly in patients with established hemophilic arthropathy.

In the patient with chronic arthropathy, adequate analgesia must be provided, particularly in drug-dependent patients undergoing major surgical procedures. A chemical abuse team can be very helpful in handling this aspect of hemophilia management.

Surgical Considerations. The indications for surgical treatment of elbow arthropathy in patients with hemophilia are similar to those for patients with elbow diseases from other causes. Successful surgical treatment requires close cooperation between the surgeon and knowledgeable hematologists and physical therapists. Additionally, surgical care of patients with hemophilia requires special consideration of other disease-related issues, including bleeding, hemolysis, and infection.[26]

Access to a specialized coagulation laboratory and adequate material for factor replacement must be available before undertaking surgery. If the patient's response to the administration of the missing coagulation factor is not

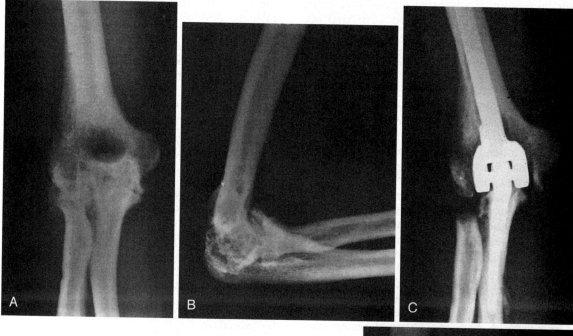

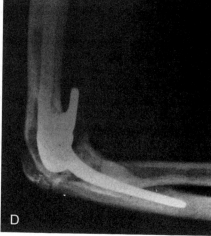

FIGURE 69–6 • *A* and *B,* Extensive changes of hemophilic arthropathy, showing overgrowth, subchondral cysts, and marked narrowing of the joint space with evidence of contracture. Also, observe the narrowing of the medullary canal. *C* and *D,* Same patient following insertion of an elbow prosthesis. Note absence of the use of cement in this press fit technique.

known and time permits, he or she should be evaluated several days prior to surgery. The author's practice is to elevate the factor VIII or IX level to 75 to 100 percent of normal for the surgical procedure and to maintain it above 50 percent through the postoperative course. This can be achieved by continuous infusion or intermittent boluses of the coagulation factor.[15] Factor VIII or IX antibodies should be tested for on admission, and again if there is postoperative bleeding, hematoma, or a decreased increment in factor levels after infusion. High levels of antibody should preclude elective surgery, although procedures such as the induction of immune tolerance could reduce or even eliminate the inhibitor. Nonetheless, the editor has had a very unfortunate experience with attempts to surgically treat a patient with factor inhibition (see Fig. 69–8) and now considers this occurrence a near-absolute contraindication to major surgery.

In an emergency situation, hemostasis can be achieved by infusion of activated prothrombin complex concentrate, porcine factor VIII, or recombinant factor VIIa, an investigational product. It is also possible to temporarily adsorb out the inhibitor by plasmapheresis through a special column designed to extract IgG antibodies. The patient with an inhibitor should only be treated in, or in close collaboration with, a major comprehensive hemophilia center that has the laboratory and other resources to deal with this potentially catastrophic situation. The development of an inhibitor postoperatively may require treatment with higher doses of factor VIII or IX or with one of the approaches outlined earlier.[15]

Postoperative hemolysis is not common and, in contrast to older factor preparations, is infrequently noted with monoclonal-purified products. The authors' practice is to obtain daily hematocrits and coagulation factor levels after surgery. A decrease in the hematocrit not explained by bleeding should suggest the possibility of hemolysis, which would require further laboratory investigation.

Synovectomy often produces a decrease in joint function but can effectively reduce or even eliminate bleeding into the joint and provide relief from pain. In a series of 12 elbow synovectomies, Kaye and associates[22] noted a reduction in the average number of bleeding episodes from 24 per year (range, 8 to 52) before surgery to 3 per year (range, 1 to 18) following the procedure. During a follow-up period of 12 to 58 months (average, 29.5 months) after synovectomy, 8 of 12 elbow joints lost an average of 19 degrees of flexion-extension mobility, and the other 4 joints gained 5 to 35 degrees. With respect to supination-pronation, three patients were improved (10 to 95 degrees), three remained unchanged, and six lost between 5 and 45 degrees of range of motion.[22] In one study, radial head excision and synovectomy provided relief of pain in 30 of 32 patients.[27] Importantly, 29 of these 32 patients also had less recurrent hemorrhage after the procedure. Comparable findings have been reported by others.

Joint contractures can be prevented or minimized during early phases of arthropathy by prompt, effective replacement therapy, early mobilization, and an active physical therapy program aimed at maintaining muscle strength and range of motion.

Although partial synovectomy with or without radial head excision can provide pain relief, reduce the incidence of hemarthrosis, and improve forearm rotation in selected patients, the advent of arthroscopic synovectomy is of great significance and relevance, because the added impact of the surgical excision and tissue damage from the exposure is minimized (Fig. 69–7) (see Chapter 39). The effectiveness of this treatment is less than that performed in the early stages of involvement, and progressive joint arthritis can develop. In these later stages, few options for treatment are available.[12, 15] Gilbert and Randomisli[14] recommend synovectomy by radioisotope especially in those with an inhibitor to clotting factors, those with advanced human immunodeficiency virus (HIV) infection or hepatitis or with multiple joint involvement.[14] Total elbow arthroplasty may be indicated when there is severe functional limitation. No studies have been published documenting long-term follow-up results of total elbow arthroplasty in patients with hemophilia,[6] but the short-term follow-up results after elbow replacement have been gratifying in the authors' institution. However, the inability to control the bleed, as occurs with the development of an inhibitor, can have disastrous results. The editor has had one elbow replacement become infected. The resection to treat the process has been surprisingly effective and pain-free, but the numerous procedures required and the personal and monetary impact were significant (Fig. 69–8).

Aftercare. In the patient with chronic arthropathy, adequate analgesia must be provided, particularly in drug-dependent patients undergoing major surgical procedures. The involvement of a chemical abuse team can be very helpful in handling this aspect of hemophilia management.

INFECTION

When plasma-derived products were used, hepatitis was the most common infectious complication of coagulation factor replacement therapy. Transient increases in serum transaminase levels are common in this disease, as a result

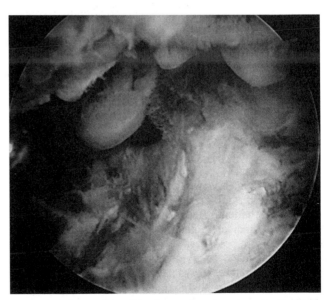

FIGURE 69–7 • Currently arthroscopic synovectomy is effective in removing the diseased synovium.

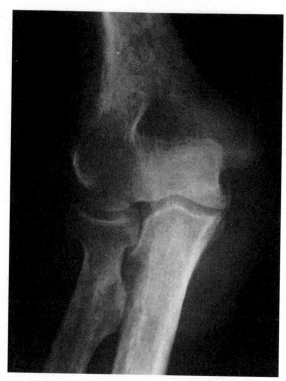

FIGURE 69–9 • Myeloid metaplasia shows a mottled radiographic appearance with demineralization on both sides of the joint.

Other Conditions

Several other hematologic conditions show characteristic features of elbow involvement. Yet, few of these conditions are noted to characteristically present primarily at the elbow joint itself.[18]

LEUKEMIA

Both acute and chronic leukemia can present with symptoms at the elbow, but when this occurs the underlying diagnosis may be missed for some period of time.[27] Early symptoms in the elbow, including pain, swelling, and subtle displacement of the fat pads on radiographs, are not specific for these diseases. Aspiration of affected joints does not show an effusion. Later radiographic changes show mottled radiodensities and periosteal reaction and possibly subchondral bone infarction.[27] The elbow is more commonly involved in acute disease than in chronic disease.[33] Spilberg and Meyer noted that 8 of 13 patients with acute leukemia had joint involvement, while only 4 of 15 patients with chronic leukemia had joint symptoms at the time of initial presentation.[37] At the Mayo Clinic, Silverstein and Kelly[35] reported that approximately 4 percent of adults and 14 percent of children with acute leukemia had osteoarthritic symptoms.

MYELOPROLIFERATIVE DISORDERS

Other myeloproliferative diseases may involve the elbow region. Typically, both sides of the joint are involved, but

there are no unique or characteristic radiographic features (Fig. 69–9).

REFERENCES

1. Ahlberg, A.: Haemophilia in Sweden. VII. Incidence, treatment, and prophylaxis of arthropathy and other musculoskeletal manifestations of haemophilia A and B. Acta Orthop. Scand. Suppl. **77**:20, 1965.
2. Aledort, L. M., Haschmeyer, R. H., and Pettersson, H. A.: Longitudinal study of orthopaedic outcomes in severe factor VIII–deficient haemophiliacs: The orthopaedic outcome study. J. Intern. Med. **236**:391, 1994.
3. Arnold, W. D., and Hilgartner, M. W.: Hemophilic arthropathy. J. Bone Joint Surg. **59A**:287, 1977.
4. Beutler, E.: The sickle cell diseases and related disorders. In Williams, W. J., Beutler, E., Erslve, A., and Lichtman, M. A. (eds.): Hematology, 4th ed. New York, McGraw-Hill, 1990, pp. 613–643.
5. Boone, D. C.: Common musculoskeletal problems and their management. In Boone, D. C. (ed.): Comprehensive Management of Hemophilia. Philadelphia, F. A. Davis, 1976, pp. 52–85.
6. Chantelot, C., Fontaine, C., Migaud, H., and Duquennoy, A.: Complete elbow prosthesis for inflammatory and hemophiliac arthroplasty: A retrospective analysis of 22 cases. Ann. Chir. Main membre sup. **16**:49, 1997.
7. Diggs, L. W.: Bone and joint lesions in sickle-cell disease. Clin. Orthop. **52**:119, 1967.
8. Dorwart, B. B., Goldberg, M. A., and Schumacher, H. R.: Absence of increased frequency of bone and joint disease with hemoglobin AS and AC. Ann. Intern. Med. **86**:66, 1977.
9. Duthie, R. B., Matthews, J. M., Rizza, C. R., Steel, W. M., and Woods, C. G.: The Management of Musculoskeletal Problems in the Hemophiliac. Oxford, Blackwell, 1972, pp. 29–127.
10. Dymock, I. W., Hamilton, E. B. D., Laws, J. W., and Williams, R.: Arthropathy of haemochromatosis: Clinical and radiologic analysis of 63 patients with iron overload. Ann. Rheum. Dis. **29**:469, 1970.
11. Espinoza, L. R., Spilberg, I., and Osterland, C. K.: Joint manifestations of sickle cell disease. Medicine **53**:295, 1974.
12. Gilbert, M. S., and Aledort, L. M.: Pyogenic musculoskeletal infections in hemophilia: A new manifestation of HIV infection. In Gilbert, M. S., and Green, W. B. (eds.): Musculoskeletal Problems in Hemophilia. New York, National Hemophilia Foundation, 1989, pp. 122–124.
13. Gilbert, M. S., and Glass, K. S.: Hemophilic arthropathy in the elbow. Mt. Sinai J. Med. **44**:389, 1977.
14. Gilbert, M. S., and Randomisli, T. E.: Therapeutic options in the management of hemophilic synovitis. Clin. Orthop. Oct. **(343)**:88, 1997.
15. Gilchrist, G. S.: Congenital and acquired bleeding disorders. In Burg, F. D., Ingelfinger, J. R., and Wald, E. R. (eds.): Gellis and Kagan's Current Pediatric Therapy, 15th ed. Philadelphia, W. B. Saunders, 1996.
16. Greene, W. B.: Radial head excision and partial synovectomy: A multi-institutional report. In Widel, J. D., and Gilbert, M. S. (eds.): Management of Musculoskeletal Problems in Hemophilia. New York, National Hemophilia Foundation, 1985, pp. 53–57.
17. Greene, W. B., Degnore, L. T., McMillan, C. W., and White, G. C.: The morbidity and outcome of surgery in hemophiliacs seropositive for human immunodeficiency virus (HIV). In Gilbert, M. S., and Green, W. B. (eds.): Musculoskeletal Problems in Hemophilia. New York, National Hemophilia Foundation, 1989, pp. 125–132.
18. Hamilton, E., Williams, R., Barlow, K. A., and Smith, P. M.: The arthropathy of idiopathic haemochromatosis. Q. J. Med. **37**:171, 1968.
19. Heim, M., Horoszowski, H., Lieberman, L., Varon, D., and Martinowitz, U.: Methods and synovectomies. In Gilbert, M. S., and Green, W. B. (eds.): Musculoskeletal Problems in Hemophilia. New York, National Hemophilia Foundation, 1989, pp. 98–101.
20. Herman, G., and Gilbert, M.: Case report 471. Skeletal Radiol. **17**:152, 1988.
21. Johnson, R. P., and Babbitt, D. P.: Five stages of joint disintegration compared with range of motion in hemophilia. Clin. Orthop. Rel. Res. **201**:36, 1985.
22. Kaye, L., Stainsby, D., and Buzzard, B.: The role of synovectomy in the management of recurrent hemarthroses in hemophilia. Br. J. Haematol. **49**:53, 1981.

23. Lancourt, J. E., Gilbert, M. S., and Posner, M. A.: Management of bleeding and associated complications of hemophilia in the hand and forearm. J. Bone Joint Surg. **59A:**451, 1977.

24. Lofqvist, T., Nilsson, I. M., Berntorp, E., and Pettersson, H.: Haemophilia prophylaxis in young patients: A long-term follow-up. J. Intern. Med. **241:**395, 1997.

25. National Heart and Lung Institute: National Heart, Blood Vessel, Lung and Blood Program, Vol. 4, Part 4. Report of the Blood Resources Panel. DHEW Publication Number (NIH) 73–515–73–524. Department of Health, Education, and Welfare, Bethesda, MD, 1973.

26. Luck, J. V., and Kasper, C. K.: Surgical management of advanced hemophilic arthropathy: An overview of 20 years' experience. Clin. Orthop. Rel. Res. **242:**60, 1989.

27. Monsees, B., Destouet, J. M., Totty, W. G., and McKeel, D., Jr.: Case report 349. Skeletal Radiol. **15:**154, 1986.

28. Noguchi, C. T., Rodgers, G. P., Serjeant, G., and Schechter, A. N.: Levels of fetal hemoglobin necessary for treatment of sickle cell disease. N. Engl. J. Med. **318:**96, 1988.

29. Petersson, H., Ahlberg, A., Nilsson, I. M.: Radiological classification of hemophilic arthropathy. Clin. Orthop. Rel. Res. **104:**153, 1980.

30. Post, M., Watts, G., and Telfer, M.: Synovectomy in hemophilic arthropathy: A retrospective review of 17 cases. Clin. Orthop. Rel. Res. **202:**139, 1986.

31. Rivard, G. E., Girard, M., Cliche, C. L., Guay, J. P., Belanger, R., and Besner, R.: Synoviorthesis in patients with hemophilia and inhibitors. Can. Med. Assoc. J. **127:**41, 1982.

32. Rodgers, G. P.: Recent approaches to the treatment of sickle cell anemia. J.A.M.A. **265:**2097, 1991.

33. Schaller, J.: Arthritis as a presenting manifestation of malignancy in children. J. Pediatr. **81:**793, 1972.

34. Schumacher, H. R., Andrews, R., and McLaughlin, G.: Arthropathy in sickle-cell disease. Ann. Intern. Med. **78:**203, 1973.

35. Silverstein, M. N., and Kelly, P. J.: Leukemia with osteoarticular symptoms and signs. Ann. Intern. Med. **59:**637, 1963.

36. Sokoloff, L.: Biomechanical and physiological aspects of degenerative joint diseases with special reference to hemophilic arthropathy. Ann. N. Y. Acad. Sci. **240:**285, 1975.

37. Spilberg, I., and Meyer, G. J.: The arthritis of leukemia. Arthritis Rheum. **15:**630, 1972.

38. Storti, E., and Ascari, E.: Surgical and chemical synovectomy. Ann. N. Y. Acad. Sci. **240:**316, 1975.

39. Wintrobe, M. M., Lee, S. R., and Boggs, D. R.: Clinical Hematology, 8th ed. Philadelphia, Lea & Febiger, 1981, pp. 1158–1205.

40. Yulish, B. S., Lieberman, J. M., Strandjord, S. E., Bryan, P. J., Mulopulos, G. P., and Modic, M. T.: Hemophilic arthropathy: Assessment with MR imaging. Radiology **164:**759, 1987.

FIG
to rh
in th
hype
trop

ho
ate
sul
ex
an
to
by
re
ti
in
n
a

n
c
p
1

of nociceptive loss in a number of ways. Neurotrophic arthropathy is more common in weightbearing joints and in joints in men, perhaps because of occupations involving manual labor and physical activity. Additional factors include the presence of mental retardation, psychosis, the metabolic effect of diabetes, and rheumatoid arthritis or metabolic bone disease. The so-called stoic personality, while admitting pain, seems to be able to ignore it and continue to walk and work unimpeded. There are also those who, although experiencing considerable pain, may out of economic necessity cling to a job despite deforming arthritis.

The administration of corticosteroids, particularly by the intra-articular route, in the treatment of patients with degenerative joint disease is occasionally followed by rapid joint disintegration. Patients reported with this complication have not had any neurologic disease, and therefore the joint destruction cannot be called a neurotrophic arthropathy. The administration of corticosteroids, however, relieves joint pain and allows a level of increased activity that leads to further joint damage. The interplay of multiple factors in the genesis of bone and joint complications is emphasized in Figure 70–3.

CONDITIONS CAUSING NEUROTROPHIC ARTHROPATHY OF THE ELBOW

Syringomyelia

In contrast to tabes dorsalis, 80 percent of the joints involved in syringomyelia are in the upper extremities.[29] It is estimated that approximately 25 percent of these affected joints will develop joint breakdown. Neuropathic disease involves the shoulder most commonly, followed by the elbow and wrist. Degenerative changes in the cervical spine are not uncommon. The process evolves gradually with paresthesias of the hands, followed by progressive weakness and wasting of the small hand muscles and then atrophy of arm and shoulder muscles. Loss of pain and temperature sense affects the arms and upper thoracic segments, often in a cape distribution. As the syrinx enlarges, long tract signs appear, and a Horner syndrome is noted. The Arnold-Chiari malformation is commonly associated and is related to the development of syringomyelia.

Post-traumatic syringohydromyelia presenting as a neuropathic arthropathy of the elbow and of the shoulder has been reported.[47] Morrey has seen one additional instance of an acquired neurotrophic elbow joint after injury to the cervical spine (Fig. 70–4). The mechanism is also presumably that of a traumatic syringohydromyelia.

Electromyography and somatosensory evoked potentials can indicate the presence of a spinal cord lesion and the need for an imaging study.[65] Radiographic examination of the cervical spine may show widening of the spinal canal, but the diagnostic procedure of choice is magnetic resonance imaging, which demonstrates both the syrinx and any associated malformation.[39] Computed tomography with metrizamide contrast enhancement of the cerebrospinal fluid may also demonstrate spinal cord enlargement and cavitations in some instances.

Elbow arthropathy may follow neurologic symptoms but is sometimes a presenting complaint.[4] A history of trauma is usually lacking. Joint swelling due to effusion may be

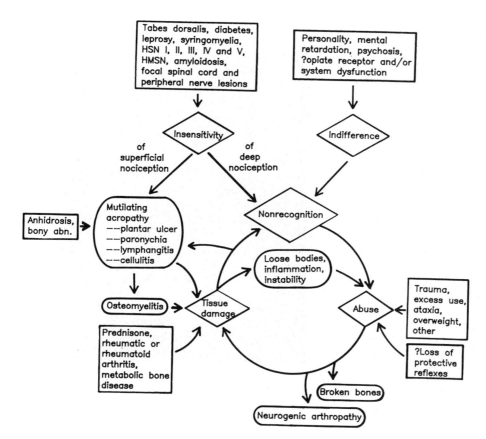

FIGURE 70–3 • Schematic representation of the inter-relationship between the etiology and pathophysiology of neurotrophic arthropathy.[23]

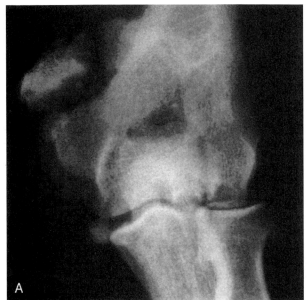

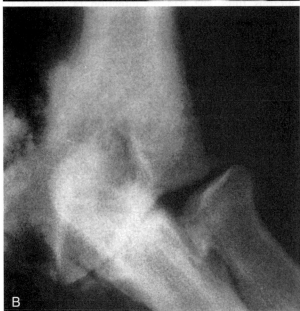

FIGURE 70–4 • A brachial plexus injury occurred in a 47-year-old man in 1986. Five years later, instability and effusion were noted in the ipsilateral elbow *(A)*. Rapid distraction occurred in the next 3 months *(B)*.

marked, and pain is experienced in some cases. Atrophic changes in the bone, particularly of the shoulder, are more common than in tabes dorsalis.[63] Although extremely rapid destruction of the shoulder may occur with resorption of the humeral head, the elbow seems less likely to be affected in this fashion.[47, 64]

The radiograph of the elbow shows resorption of bone ends and often of the entire joint (Fig. 70–5). Reparative callus is evident, along with gross deformity and instability.

Diabetes Mellitus

The importance of diabetes mellitus as the leading cause of neurotrophic arthropathy is now recognized. The ar-

thropathy usually develops in diabetics who have had the disease for some time and who have suffered the additional complication of a symmetrical sensorimotor polyneuropathy. In diabetic "pseudotabes," severe sensory and autonomic impairment leads to an ataxic gait, pupillary abnormalities, neurogenic bladder, and lightning pains reminiscent of tabes dorsalis. Diabetic arthropathy affects primarily the joints of the feet, with less frequent involvement of the ankles and knees.[6, 16, 43, 48, 55] The distal predominance of the arthropathy is in keeping with the stocking pattern of sensory loss, which is maximal in the feet. Bony abnormalities in the upper extremities of diabetics are quite uncommon, but involvement of the shoulder, elbow, and wrist has been recorded.[27] Campbell and Feldman[11] presented a radiograph of the elbow in a 59-year-old patient that showed marked disorganization of the joint with destruction of the articular surfaces, numerous bone fragments, and periosteal new bone formation typical of a Charcot joint.

Tabes Dorsalis

Although syphilis used to be responsible for up to 90 percent of neurotrophic joints, tabes dorsalis is now a rare disease. Approximately 10 percent of all tabetics are said to develop a Charcot joint, the majority occurring between the ages of 40 and 60 years, some 20 years or more after the primary infection. In approximately 78 percent of cases, the lower limbs are affected,[29] with the knee most frequently involved, followed by the hip, ankle, and tarsus. Spinal arthropathy affects the lumbar and lower thoracic segments. In the upper limbs, the shoulder, elbow, hands, and wrists are affected.[3, 19, 57, 60, 62] Polyarticular involvement occurs in up to 40 percent. Clinical features include the

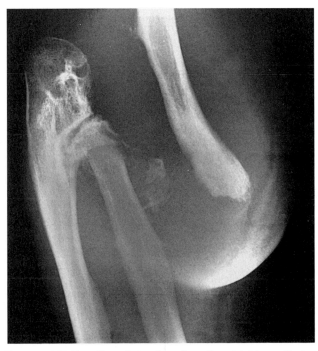

FIGURE 70–5 • Gross destruction of an elbow joint in a patient with syringomyelia.

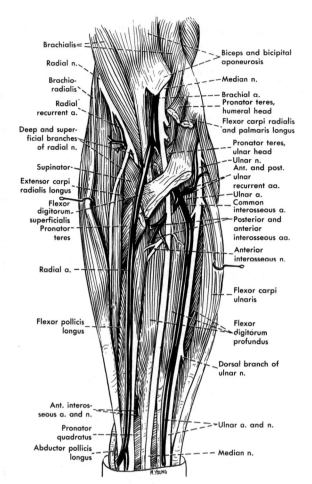

Brachialis

Radial n.

Brachio-radialis

Radial recurrent a.

Deep and super-ficial branches of radial n.

Supinator

Extensor carpi radialis longus

Flexor digitorum superficialis Pronator teres

Radial a.

Flexor pollicis longus

Ant. interos-seous a. and n.

Pronator quadratus

Abductor pollicis longus

Biceps and bicipital aponeurosis

Median n.

Brachial a. Pronator teres, humeral head Flexor carpi radialis and palmaris longus

Pronator teres, ulnar head Ulnar n. Ant. and post. ulnar recurrent aa. Ulnar a. Common interosseous a. Posterior and anterior interosseous aa.

Anterior interosseous n.

Flexor carpi ulnaris

Flexor digitorum profundus

Dorsal branch of ulnar n.

Ulnar a. and n.

Median n.

FIGURE 71–1 • Major neurovascular and muscular relationships of the elbow region. (From Hollinshead, W. H.: Anatomy for Surgeons, 3rd ed. Vol. 3. New York, Harper & Row, 1982.)

cutaneous nerve of the forearm is susceptible during ulnar nerve transposition and median nerve decompression; and the posterior cutaneous nerve of the forearm is at risk with posterior interosseous nerve neurolysis. In most cases, external neurolysis is the usual procedure. Internal neuroly-sis, when indicated, should be limited to the neural segment and the internal region clinically involved. The perineurium should rarely, if ever, be violated. Nerves should be placed in healthy beds away from scar tissue. Intraoperative nerve action potentials may help in the management of more advanced lesions. Postoperative care should emphasize early mobilization. Early motion can improve neural glid-ing. Furthermore, the development of a stiff joint can undo an otherwise successful nerve decompression.

A detailed understanding of the complex normal anat-omy of this region and the "common" variants is essential for proper diagnosis and treatment of these conditions (Fig. 71–1). Careful serial examinations and electromyographic studies and, at times, imaging modalities can usually local-ize the lesion or lesions. Early, accurate diagnosis and treatment are important for effective overall management of nerve compression lesions. Understanding the degree of nerve injury can help a physician predict recovery patterns and guide management.

NEUROPHYSIOLOGY OF NERVE COMPRESSION LESIONS

Nerve compression may be categorized as first-, second-, third-, or fourth-degree neural lesions. This method was first described by Sir Sydney Sunderland.[171] The earlier classification of Sir Herbert Seddon (1943)[143] uses the terms *neurapraxia, axonotmesis,* and *neurotmesis* and can be correlated with Sunderland's classification in the follow-ing manner. A first-degree lesion is a neurapractic lesion. A second-degree or mild third-degree lesion is an axonot-metic lesion. The neurotmetic lesion encompasses all the fourth-degree lesions (the neuroma in continuity) and the advanced third-degree lesions. We prefer using Sunder-land's classification when correlating our clinical problems with the underlying nerve fiber pathologic condition pres-ent (Table 71–1).[126]

With neural compression lesions, it is rare to have a pure first-, second-, or third-degree lesion. Most often, these lesions are mixed. One of the degrees of injury usually predominates in a particular case.[125] The lesion mix can be determined by serial physical examinations, preoperative and postoperative serial electromyographic studies, and knowledge of the duration of the partial or complete nerve compression lesions. A fourth-degree nerve compression lesion is found most often when motor and sensory com-plete paralysis of a particular nerve has existed for more than 18 months.

The factors that affect return of nerve function following entrapment lesions are (1) the nerve fiber pathology, (2) the duration of the lesion and whether it is complete or partial, (3) the status of the end organs, motor and sensory, and (4) the level of the lesion.[111] When a nerve is entrapped, it is the peripheral fibers that are the most vulnerable to the pathologic process. Similarly, the heavy myelinated fibers are more susceptible to compressive forces.

There appear to be several types of first-degree injury. These lesions are correlated best when both the nerve fiber pathologic processes and the clinical recovery following neurolysis are analyzed temporally. There are ionic[87] and vascular[34, 100, 170] lesions of nerve fibers that respond to release by prompt recovery within, at times, hours of sur-gery. There is a structural first-degree lesion, described by Gilliatt and colleagues[57] and Ochoa,[124] in which there is segmental injury to the nerve fiber consisting of segmental demyelination and remyelinization of just a few nodal segments of the fibers. In this instance, the entire recovery process takes 30 to 60 days. The clinical implications of

• TABLE 71–1 • Correlation of Seddon and Sunderland Classification of Nerve Injuries					
Seddon	Sunderland (degree)				
	First	*Second*	*Third*	*Fourth*	*Fifth*
Neurapraxia	▓				
Axonotmesis		▓	▓		
Neurotmesis			▓	▓	▓

Shaded areas indicate equivalent terms.

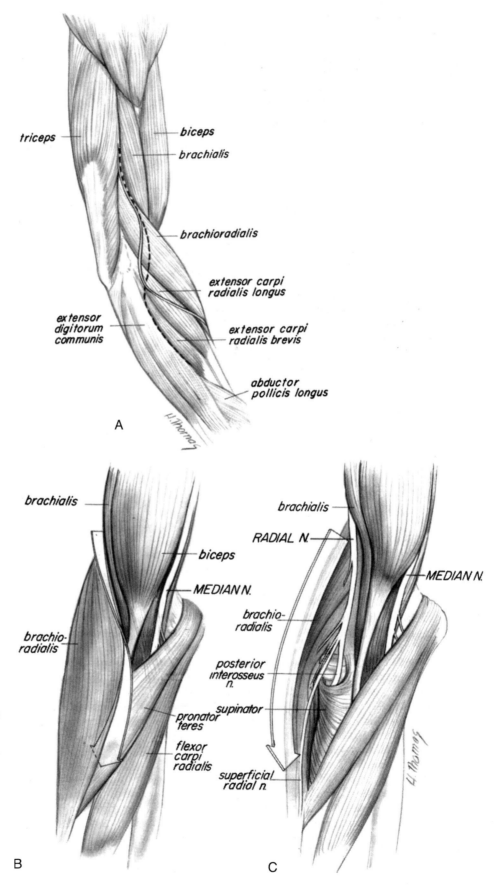

FIGURE 71–9 • *A*, Incision for extensile exploration of the radial nerve is helpful for exploring the radial nerve, the proximal half of the posterior interosseous nerve, and the superficial radial nerve. *B*, The interval between the brachioradialis and the brachialis and pronator teres is developed. *C*, The radial nerve and its major forearm branches, the posterior interosseous and the superficial branches are exposed. (From Spinner, M.: Injuries to the Major Branches of Peripheral Nerves of the Forearm, 2nd ed. Philadelphia, W. B. Saunders, 1978.)

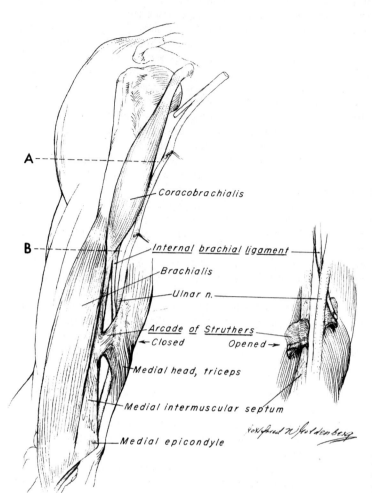

FIGURE 71–12 • Anatomic distribution of the ulnar nerve crossing the intermuscular septum and passing under the arcade of Struthers. Impingement in the midbrachium from the internal brachial ligament should be recognized. *Inset*, The arcade of Struthers has been released, demonstrating the internal brachial ligament within the arcade. (From Spinner, M., and Kaplan, E. B.: The relationship of the ulnar nerve to the medial intermuscular septum in the arm and its clinical significance. Hand **8**:239, 1976.)

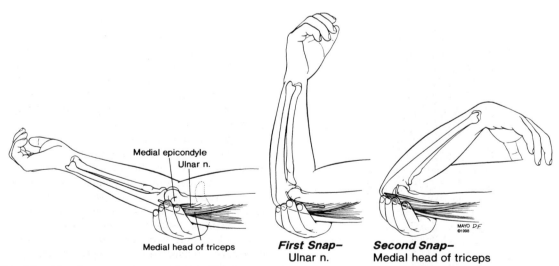

FIGURE 71–13 • The ulnar nerve can be palpated within the cubital tunnel with the elbow in extension. Then with passive or active flexion of the elbow, the examiner can assess whether the ulnar nerve or another structure, such as a portion of the medial head of the triceps or an anomalous triceps tendon, moves anterior to the epicondyle. (From Spinner, R. J., and Goldner, R. D.: Snapping of the medial head of the triceps and recurrent dislocation of the ulnar nerve: Anatomical and dynamic factors. J. Bone Joint Surg. **80A**:239, 1998.)

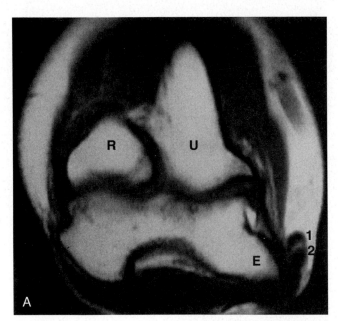
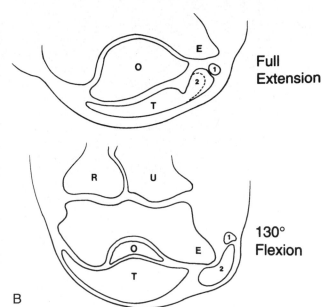

FIGURE 71–14 • A, Magnetic resonance imaging can demonstrate a snapping triceps and dislocating ulnar nerve. Here the ulnar nerve (1) and a portion of the medial head of the triceps (2) are anterior to the medial epicondyle (E) with the elbow fully flexed. Computed tomography or real-time ultrasonography can also confirm the diagnosis. Imaging, however, is not necessary for confirmation of a diagnosis. Patients undergoing ulnar nerve surgery should be examined intraoperatively, with the elbow in flexion and extension, so that the surgeon can evaluate whether the medial head of the triceps snaps over the medial epicondyle. R = radius; U = ulna. B, Corresponding artist drawing shows the position of the ulnar nerve and the medial head of the triceps to the medial epicondyle in full extension and flexion. O = olecranon. (A from Spinner, R.J., Hayden, F.R., Jr., Hipps, C.T., and Goldner, R.D.: Imaging the snapping triceps. A.J.R. Am. J. Roentgenol. 167:1550, 1996; B from Khoo, D., Carmichael, S. W., and Spinner, R. J.: Ulnar nerve anatomy and compression. Orthop. Clin. North Am. 27:317, 1996.)

and varus deformities[1, 50, 174] may produce late ulnar nerve symptomatology at the elbow.

Iatrogenic causes of secondary ulnar nerve compression are numerous and related to technical factors.[51] Compression may occur when the ulnar nerve is translocated subcutaneously and is insufficiently mobilized, proximally or distally.[154, 157] Compression can be found proximally at the level of the arcade of Struthers (see Fig. 71–12) or distally where the ulnar nerve passes from a posterior location at the elbow to the anterior compartment of the proximal forearm in the region of the common aponeurosis for the humeral head of the flexor carpi ulnaris and the origin of the flexor digitorum superficialis.[78] If these aponeurotic areas are not released sufficiently both proximally and distally (Fig. 71–15), then potential secondary sites of entrapment are created, which can produce symptomatology.[156] The medial intermuscular septum should be excised because it, too, is a common cause of secondary ulnar nerve entrapment. Whether translocated subcutaneously or submuscularly, the ulnar nerve should be transposed anteriorly without kinking. Tight slings may result in secondary compression.[94, 99] Furthermore, the nerve when transposed into a groove in the flexor-pronator group of muscles can result in traction neuritis. When the nerve heals in the muscular groove, the longitudinal fibrotic aponeuroses of flexor muscles of the medial aspect of the elbow can produce a secondary traction neuritis.

CLINICAL PRESENTATION

An ulnar nerve lesion at the elbow typically presents with a combination of elbow pain and sensory and motor com-

plaints. It usually begins with intermittent paresthesias in the ring and little fingers that are aggravated by elbow flexion and frequently awaken the patient. Sensory loss in the fourth and fifth fingers of the hand usually occurs later, but sensory loss in the dorsoulnar aspect of the hand is a classic localizing sign. Usually, there are no sensory abnormalities in the forearm. The sensory fibers and the intrinsic motor fibers lie more peripherally than the fibers of the flexor digitorum profundus or the flexor carpi ulnaris and may explain their vulnerability early on. Motor weakness may be progressive in both the extrinsics and the

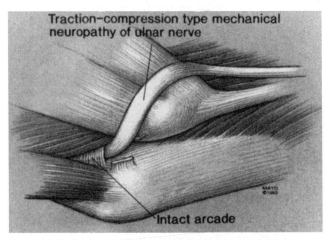

FIGURE 71–15 • Tethering of the ulnar nerve may result from a previous (incomplete) decompression. (From Spinner, M.: Nerve decompression. In Morrey, B. F. [ed.]: Master Techniques in Orthopaedic Surgery: The Elbow. New York, Raven Press, 1994.)

intrinsics; at times, significant motor findings can be present with minimal sensory symptoms. With paralysis of the flexor digitorum profundus to the fourth and fifth fingers, there is usually minimal clawing or no clawing of the fourth and fifth fingers. With partial lesions, clawing may be more pronounced if the flexor digitorum profundus muscles are intact and the intrinsic muscles are atrophic.[104, 169] However, if the metacarpophalangeal joints of the ring and little fingers cannot hyperextend because of innate tightness of the volar plates, then clawing will also not be observed.

A mechanical lesion of the ulnar nerve, at the elbow, in different patients, may present with different clinical patterns because of the presence or absence of neural anomalies and the extent of involvement of the nerve. There are numerous variations in fibers carried within the ulnar nerve at the elbow level.[154] In 15 percent of upper extremities, the median nerve will carry many of the intrinsic motor fibers to pass from the median nerve or the anterior interosseous nerve branch of the median nerve to the ulnar nerve in the mid-forearm.

The sensory pattern typical of an ulnar nerve lesion at the elbow with diminished or absent sensation on the dorsoulnar aspect of the hand[91] may not be observed. This occurs when other sensory nerves take over the area usually supplied by the ulnar dorsal cutaneous branch of the hand. One variant sensory pattern is observed when the superficial radial nerve not only innervates the dorsal radial aspect of the hand but also extends to supply the dorsoulnar aspect. Furthermore, all of the ring and long fingers can be affected in some complete ulnar nerve lesions.

DIFFERENTIAL DIAGNOSIS

In the differential diagnosis, a nerve lesion that involves the cervical foramina, as in cervical arthritis, can present with ulnar nerve symptoms. Restriction and pain on movement of the neck, positive foraminal compression maneuvers, arthritic changes seen radiographically, and cervical paravertebral muscle electrical abnormalities are usually noted. Short segment stimulation may be effective in isolating the level of the compression.[40]

Another frequent site for exclusion is the thoracic outlet. The medial components of the plexus are most frequently involved. Radiation of paresthesias along the inner aspect of the arm with symptomatology extending to the fourth and fifth fingers is a common neural presentation. Clinical signs characteristic of thoracic outlet syndrome, including a positive percussion sign, or a positive Adson or Wright's test, or hyperabduction maneuver, or the presence of an arterial bruit with abduction or extension, may help localize the pathologic process to the outlet, but one should also be aware of the presence of false-positive findings in the normal population. Confirmatory localizing electromyographic studies, specifically conduction delays across the thoracic outlet, help in differentiating the level of nerve entrapment.[40] The absence of ulnar F-wave abnormalities, absence of cervical paravertebral fibrillations seen in cervical radiculopathy, and the presence of an ulnar nerve conduction delay distally across the elbow can be suggestive findings of a lesion at the elbow. However, double crush lesions can occur and patients who have persistent symptoms after elbow surgery may have a more proximal lesion.

Entrapment in the hand is much less common than entrapment at the elbow; entrapment in the forearm is quite rare. Depending on the level of nerve involvement, varying clinical signs and symptoms become manifest. A full-blown lesion in Guyon's canal is accompanied by sensory loss in the fourth and fifth digits of the hand. There is usually more significant ("paradoxical") clawing of these digits because the flexor digitorum profundus is functioning (see Fig. 71-7). The sensation on the dorsoulnar aspect of the hand is intact, and the palmar aspect of the hand may have some hypesthesia. Lesions of the ulnar nerve in the proximal forearm have findings similar to those at the elbow, whereas in the middle and distal forearm, symptomatology depends on the relationship of the lesion to the motor branch of the flexor digitorum profundus and the dorsal cutaneous branch of the hand. A lesion distal to the take-off of the motor branch of the flexor digitorum profundus is usually seen in patients with clawing. On rare occasions, clawing of the ring and little fingers may be observed even with a neural compression proximal to the motor branch. This occurs when the flexor digitorum profundus to the fourth and fifth fingers is anomalously innervated by the median nerve or the anterior interosseous nerve. A lesion proximal to the dorsal cutaneous branch presents with numbness in the dorsoulnar aspect of the hand.

CONSERVATIVE TREATMENT

In the milder cases, a trial of conservative treatment is often helpful. Avoidance of prolonged elbow flexion, especially at night, is helped by an elbow splint with the elbow maintained in a semiflexed position of about 75 degrees. During the day, resting the elbow on a table should be avoided. A 4- to 6-week trial of these measures is worthwhile.

OPERATIVE TREATMENT

We believe that the choice of operative procedure[46] should be fitted to the patient's symptoms and the electromyographic findings. For electrically confirmed lesions, our preferred operative procedure is a transposition. In contrast, in symptomatic patients, when there is no evidence of electromyographic nerve fiber pathology, either release of the cubital tunnel[21] or anterior subcutaneous translocation is recommended. If the patient has no fat in the subcutaneous tissue, or in revision surgery, we prefer the Learmonth procedure, the submuscular anterior translocation of the ulnar nerve.[92, 94] We do not perform submuscular transposition in patients with rheumatoid arthritis or in those with post-traumatic medial bony changes.

OUR PREFERRED OPERATIVE EXPOSURE FOR ANTERIOR TRANSPOSITION OF THE ULNAR NERVE

The incision we use extends 8 to 10 cm proximal to the medial epicondyle and 8 to 10 cm distal to the medial epicondyle on the medial side of the arm and forearm. At the level of the medial epicondyle, the incision darts anteriorly for 5 cm, and then below the epicondyle it extends to the medial aspect of the forearm (Fig. 71-16A). The V-

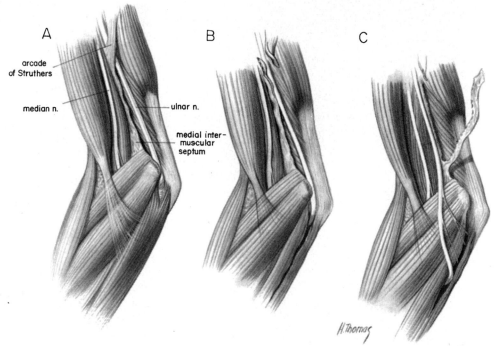

FIGURE 71–16 • *A*, Anterior translocation of the ulnar nerve requires exposure of the medial intermuscular septum and arcade of Struthers. *B*, The arcade has been released. *C*, Intermuscular septum is then removed, and the ulnar nerve is brought forward anterior to the flexion axis of the elbow. (From Spinner, M.: Injuries to the Major Branches of Peripheral Nerves of the Forearm, 2nd ed. Philadelphia. W. B. Saunders, 1978.)

shaped flap formed at the elbow level is undermined subcutaneously and is retracted medially. The medial cutaneous nerves of the forearm and arm are identified and preserved by placing rubber bands about them. Avoidance of injury to the medial cutaneous nerve of the forearm and its branches is important because patients afflicted with ulnar entrapment lesions are vulnerable to symptomatic postoperative skin neuromata.[31] The plane between the subcutaneous fat and the brachial and antebrachial fascia in the distal arm is delineated and undermined. The medial intermuscular septum is seen, and the ulnar nerve is identified just posterior to the medial intermusclar septum in the distal third of the arm. In approximately 70 percent of limbs, muscular fibers of the medial head of the triceps will be found to cross the ulnar nerve and attach to the arcade of Struthers, 8 cm proximal to the medial epicondyle. If these muscular fibers of the medial head of the triceps are notcd, it is a clear indication that the ulnar nerve must be liberated from the arcade in this area (see Fig. 71–16*B*). The medial intermuscular septum is cleared posteriorly of muscular fibers to the level of the humerus. Anteriorly, the medial intermuscular septum is separated with care from the neural vascular bundle. The inferior ulnar collateral vessels, which penetrate the intermuscular septum, can be preserved, and the medial intermuscular septum is excised (see Fig. 71–16*C*). The ulnar nerve is mobilized. Its external longitudinal vessels are kept in continuity with the nerve. The transverse components of the vascular supply can be cauterized, preferably with a bipolar unit, keeping the external and internal vascular supply intact. At the level of the posterior aspect of the medial epicondyle, the ulnar nerve is liberated and an articular branch to thc adjoined surface is sacrificed. One or two rubber bands are placed about the ulnar nerve to aid in the dissection. Distal to the medial epicondyle, the ulnar nerve is identified as it passes through the cubital tunnel. The tendinous arch for the origin of the

flexor carpi ulnaris of the humerus and ulna in the proximal region is identified. The humeral attachment is detached, and the interval between the common aponeurosis of the flexor carpi ulnaris humeral head and the flexor digitorum superficialis is defined. The ulnar nerve is identified distally, deep to the flexor carpi ulnaris. Its common fibrous aponeurosis is liberated to free the ulnar nerve in the proximal forearm. The multiple branches of the flexor carpi ulnaris are preserved. The motor branch to the flexor digitorum profundus of the ring and little fingers is also identified and preserved. The ulnar nerve is mobilized in the proximal third of the forearm with the use of loupe magnification and microsurgical technique to permit nontethered anterior translocation.[60] At this point, the nerve can be placed in a subcutaneous plane or placed in a submuscular position. A loose fasciodermal sling[38] or the intermuscular septum[131] may be used to stabilize the ulnar nerve; prior to wound closure, the elbow should be passively flexed and extended to ensure that ulnar nerve compression has been eliminated and to check that snapping of the medial portion of the triceps is not present.[160] If snapping of the medial triceps is identified either preoperatively or intraoperatively, one can transpose laterally or excise the offending dislocating portion of the medial triceps.

To proceed with the Learmonth procedure, the median nerve is identified proximal to the lacertus fibrosus in the distal arm and a rubber band is placed around it (Fig. 71–17). The median nerve is found deep to the brachial fascia at the elbow level medial to the brachial artery. The lacertus fibrosus in the proximal forearm is incised longitudinally. The next step in the dissection is to detach the muscles of the flexor-pronator group 1 cm distal to the medial epicondyle. To accomplish this, a tonsillar clamp is placed from the radial side of the flexor-pronator group of muscles 1 cm distal to the medial epicondyle and passed medially deep to the flexor-pronator group of muscles to

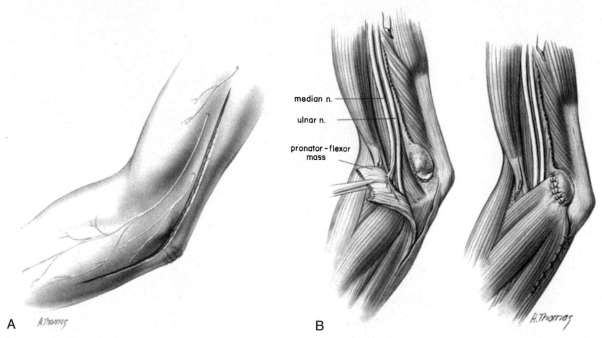

median n.

ulnar n.

pronator–flexor mass

A

B

FIGURE 71–17 • *A*, Extensive skin incision is employed for translocation of the ulnar nerve. This allows exposure of the proximal aspect of the intermusuclar septum and the arcade of Struthers. *B*, Submuscular translocation (Learmonth) technique requires proximal dissection of the ulnar nerve and release of the intermuscular septum approximately 8 cm proximal to the flexor-pronator muscle group, which is elevated from the medial epicondyle. The ulnar nerve is brought forward to lie next to the median nerve. The flexor-pronator group is then reattached to the medial epicondyle. Particular care is taken not to injure the anterior interosseous branch of the median nerve, which arises in this region. (From Spinner, M.: Injuries to the Major Branches of Peripheral Nerves of the Forearm, 2nd ed. Philadelphia. W. B. Saunders, 1978.)

exit in the region of the cubital tunnel. The tonsillar clamp is passed superficial to the ulnar collateral vessels on the anterior aspect of the medial side of the forearm. The flexor-pronator origin is incised sharply. The brachial fascia is identified. By a combination of sharp dissection and periosteal stripping, the flexor-pronator group of muscles is stripped distally. The tourniquet is released. Any additional bleeding is brought under control either by ties or with the bipolar electrocautery. The ulnar nerve is translocated anteriorly adjacent to the median nerve, and the flexor-pronator origin is repaired, with the use of 2-0 Maxon sutures (Fig. 71–17*B*). Z-lengthening or advancement of the flexor-pronator origin can also be performed.[33, 123] The subcutaneous tissues and skin are closed with either interrupted or subcuticular sutures. After a submuscular transposition, the elbow is immobilized in a semiflexed position with the forearm in midposition and the wrist in neutral; the fingers and thumb are free. The immobilization is continued for 7 days followed by progressive active extension in a blocking splint.

We have had no experience with medial epicondylectomy[25, 49, 56, 76, 77, 144] and do not like intramuscular transposition for ulnar nerve neuritis, although other surgeons have reported success with these techniques. We have not had experience with simple fascial release over the common flexor tendon and forearm fascia[21] but do not believe that technique is routinely indicated or predictably effective.

Median Nerve

The median nerve at the level of the elbow is susceptible to a compressive neuropathy from the level of the supra-condylar process proximally to the flexor superficialis arch distally. Between these levels, the ligament of Struthers, the lacertus fibrosus, the deep head of the pronator teres, anomalous muscles, distended bursae, or vascular malformations may produce symptomatic median nerve compression.

RELEVANT ANATOMY

The median nerve lies beneath the brachial fascia on the medial aspect of the arm resting on the brachialis muscle (Fig. 71–18).[72] The brachial artery and veins lie laterally in close proximity and adjacent to the biceps tendon. The medial intermuscular septum lies posteriorly and attaches to the medial epicondylar flare. The median nerve passes first alongside the humeral origin of the pronator teres and then beneath it to lie on the deep surface. It most often passes between the humeral head and the ulnar head of the pronator muscle but may pass deep to both heads, or the ulnar head may be absent. Fibrous arches may play a role in the nerve compression.[32] The motor branches of the pronator teres usually arise from the medial aspect of the nerve beneath the upper margin of the muscle but variably arise above the antecubital area. The branch to the ulnar head may arise from the main branch or as a separate branch from the median nerve. The anterior interosseous branch arises deep and usually laterally at the level of the deep head of the pronator teres and in close approximation to the bifurcation of the radial and ulnar arteries from the brachial artery.[61, 73] The main branch of the median nerve next passes beneath the tendinous arch of origin of the flexor superficialis and lies in close approximation to the

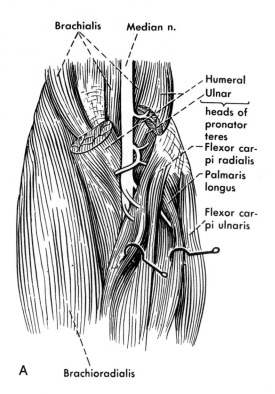

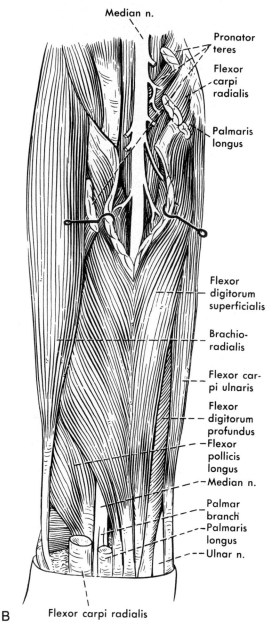

FIGURE 71-18 • *A*, As the median nerve enters the forearm, it gives off branches to the humeral and ulnar heads of the pronator teres, which originate from the medial aspect of the nerve. *B*, The median nerve is followed deeper into the forearm. The anterior interosseous nerve is shown entering the forearm under the flexor digitorum superficialis. The nerves to the flexor-pronator group are demonstrated. (From Hollinshead, W. H.: Anatomy for Surgeons, 2nd ed. Vol. 3. New York, Harper & Row, 1969.)

deep surface of this muscle (see Fig. 71-18*B*). The anterior interosseous nerve runs onto the index profundus muscle and the flexor pollicis longus.[103]

The pronator teres usually arises from the common origin of the medial epicondyle but may extend proximally along the medial epicondylar flare. The lacertus fibrosus passes from the biceps tendon to the antebrachial fascia obliquely over the flexor-pronator group of muscles.

Altered anatomy, whether from anatomic variation or a pathologic condition, may play an important part in causing nerve compression syndromes.[45, 89] The most important for median nerve compression about the elbow are the supracondylar process and ligament of Struthers,[166, 167] the Gantzer muscle,[3, 53] the palmaris profundus,[154] the flexor carpi radialis brevis,[154] a variant lacertus fibrosus (Fig. 71-19)[158] and vascular perforation or tethering of the nerve.[10] Distal humeral fracture or dislocation is well known to cause median nerve injury.[97, 132]

SUPRACONDYLAR PROCESS

Compression of the median nerve at the level of the distal humerus may occur when the nerve passes beneath the osseous process,[106] which extends obliquely midanteriorly and continues to the medial epicondyle as the ligament of Struthers.[55] (Ulnar nerve compression may rarely occur in association with a supracondylar process and the ligament of Struthers.) Muscle hypertrophy or strenuous use may facilitate the irritant effect of this structure.[72] This structure has been a factor in less than 1 percent of our cases. Proximal extension of the humeral head of the pronator teres, however, is a factor in several percent of cases.

PRONATOR SYNDROMES

The pronator syndrome was recognized comparatively recently as a neural compression syndrome within the proxi-

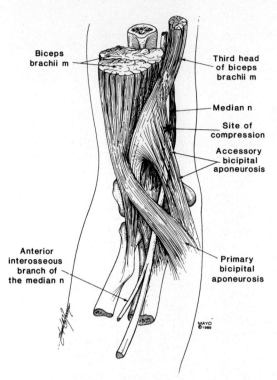

Biceps
brachii m

Third head
of biceps
brachii m

Median n

Site of
compression

Accessory
bicipital
aponeurosis

Anterior
interosseous
branch of
the median n

Primary
bicipital
aponeurosis

MAYO
©1989

FIGURE 71–19 • An accessory bicipital aponeurosis from the third head of the biceps has compressed the median nerve, resulting in both anterior interosseous and main branch motor weakness without sensory symptoms. (From Spinner, R. J., Carmichael, S. W., and Spinner, M.: Partial median nerve entrapment in the distal arm because of an accessory bicipital aponeurosis. J. Hand Surg. **16A**:236, 1991.)

mal forearm.[63, 74, 75, 84, 114, 147, 180] The symptoms are often vague, consisting of discomfort in the forearm with occasional proximal radiation into the arm. A fatigue-like pain description may be elicited. Numbness of the hand in the median distribution is often secondary. Repetitive strenuous motions, such as industrial activities, weight training, or driving, often provoke the symptoms. Nocturnal symptoms are infrequent. Numbness may affect all or part of the median distribution. Occasionally, patients may insist on emphasizing numbness of the little finger or the "whole hand."

Women seem to be at greater risk than men of developing these symptoms, especially if they are exposed to highly repetitive, moderately strenuous industrial occupations in which alternate pronosupinatory motions are required. The symptoms usually develop insidiously, but occasionally a specific event or sudden onset of pain in the forearm is associated with heightened susceptibility to muscular stress.

Acute symptoms should be distinguished from the typical pattern of a more chronic "pain syndrome." An expanding hematoma such as following venipuncture can result in compression of the median nerve by the lacertus fibrosus. Renal dialysis patients with arteriovenous fistulae have been reported to develop pronator symptoms suddenly. The syndrome may also occur following crushing or contusion of the proximal forearm or stretching of the spastic musculature by casting in patients with cerebral palsy.

Diagnosis is often delayed because of the vague, poorly related history, lack of easily observed findings, and association with workers' compensation evaluation. At times, the patient seems more interested in recriminatory action against his or her employer than with resolution of the problem.

Physical Examination

Physical findings are often subtle, and several suggestive observations help to make the diagnosis:

1. An indentation of the pronator flexor muscle mass below the medial epicondyle suggests that the lacertus fibrosus exerts a constrictive effect at that level.[63, 88, 108, 172] The indentation may be increased by active or passive pronation of the forearm. This should be compared with the opposite arm (Fig. 71–20).
2. The flexor-pronator musculature feels indurated or tense in comparison with the opposite arm or with resisted pronation. Most patients with this syndrome have well-developed forearm musculature.[63]
3. Resisted pronation for 60 seconds may initiate the symptoms by contracting the flexor-pronator muscle (Fig. 71–21).
4. Resisted elbow flexion and forearm supination may elicit similar symptoms, also presumably by tensing the lacertus fibrosus. Variations in the lacertus fibrosus may be recognized by a separate protrusion in the medial aspect of

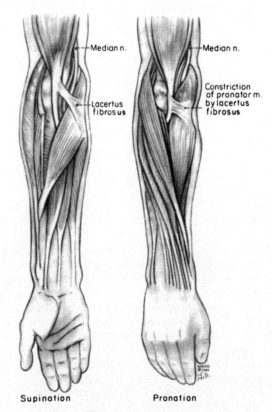

Median n.

Median n.

Lacertus
fibrosus

Constriction
of pronator m.
by lacertus
fibrosus

Supination   Pronation

FIGURE 71–20 • When the arm pronates, contraction of the pronator muscle may result in indentation of this structure by the lacertus fibrosus. Such a process may give rise to entrapment of the median nerve and the so-called pronator syndrome.

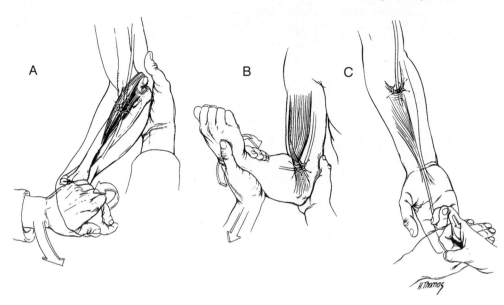

FIGURE 71–21 • Features of the physical examination that help to demonstrate the so-called pronator syndrome. *A*, Proximal forearm pain is increased by resistance to pronation and elbow flexion as well as to flexion of the wrist. *B*, Pain in the proximal forearm that is increased by resistance to supination is also suggestive of compression by the lacertus fibrosus. *C*, Resistance of the long finger flexor produces pain in the proximal forearm when compression of the median nerve occurs at the flexor digitorum superficialis arch. (From Spinner, M.: Injuries to the Major Branches of Peripheral Nerves of the Forearm, 2nd ed. Philadelphia, W. B. Saunders Co., 1978.)

the antecubital space during resisted flexion. An accessory lacertus fibrosus has shown a tendency to invoke weakness affecting the anterior interosseous nerve fibers within the median nerve.[158]

5. Resisted flexion of the long finger proximal interphalangeal joint by tightening the fibrous arch of the origin of the superficialis muscle may also induce symptoms, although this test is positive far less frequently than the previous two.

6. Direct pressure by the examiner's hand over the proximal portion of the pronator teres approximately 4 cm distal to the antebrachial crease while exerting moderate resistance to pronation has been the most reliable test in our experience. It should be compared with results of a similar test on the asymptomatic forearm.

7. The median nerve is sensitive to direct pressure, tapping, or rolling beneath the finger in the antecubital space.

8. Occasionally, passive stretching of the finger and wrist flexors will accentuate the symptoms, but this is unlikely to be positive before the preceding tests.

9. Weakness of the median innervated muscles is infrequent, but careful comparison of strength between the two hands is indicated. The flexor pollicis longus and index profundus are the most likely to show weakness.

It is important to verify whether these tests mimic or reproduce exactly the symptoms that brought the patient to the physician. This syndrome is most likely to be confused with carpal tunnel syndrome, and unfortunately the two conditions may occur simultaneously, or one may antedate the other, suggesting a susceptibility factor. Some factors that help to differentiate between the two syndromes are indicated in Table 71–2. Obviously, careful clinical judgment is required to ensure the correct diagnosis. Indications for surgery depend largely on the severity of the patient's symptoms. Aside from avoidance of the activities associated with aggravation of the symptoms, there is little available nonoperative treatment. On occasion, we have carefully injected a mixture of lidocaine and hydrocortisone paraneurally with temporary beneficial effect. This may provide an additional diagnostic aid if effective.

Electromyography

Electromyographic findings as an aid in the diagnosis of the pronator syndrome have been disappointing.[13] In only 10 percent of patients with the diagnosis of pronator syndrome were there findings that adequately supported the diagnosis. Slowed conduction velocity across the median nerve below the elbow is seldom detected. The best explanation for this is the size and complexity of the nerve, which is insufficiently compressed to prevent a stimulus progressing at normal velocities down a significant number of fascicles of the nerve. The slowed impulses in affected fascicles are blurred and dampened in the recording. Muscle studies are seldom specific. Isolated fibrillations, particularly in the pronator teres, have been observed. Insertional changes are often nonspecific, and fasciculations are infrequent. Electrical studies are useful in ruling out the presence of another entrapment site or underlying peripheral neuropathy.

Intraoperative studies of conduction velocities and voltages were carried out before and after median nerve release in 10 forearms in the early part of one series.[63] Significant increases in recorded velocities or voltages at the distal electrodes were noted in only five instances. Newer techniques may improve the diagnostic acuity of electromyog-

• TABLE 71–2 • **Comparison of Findings Between the Pronator Syndrome and the Carpal Tunnel Syndrome**

	Carpal Tunnel Syndrome	Pronator Syndrome
Nocturnal symptoms	+	–
Muscular fatigue	–	+
Proximal radiation	±	+
Medial hypohidrosis	+	–
Thumb paresthesias	±	+
Thenar atrophy	+	–
Phalen's sign	+	–
Pronator signs	–	+
Electromyography	+	–

raphy, but at this time the history and physical examination must be relied on for the diagnosis.

Operative Findings

The median nerve seldom shows the flattening, indentation, or pseudoneuroma formation so common at the carpal tunnel. The lacertus fibrosus is usually quite apparent in its course from the biceps tendon to its interdigitations with the longitudinally directed fibers of the antebrachial fascia over the proximal third of the flexor-pronator muscle group. An indentation of the pronator teres is apparent with passive pronation (see Fig. 71–20). At times, this finding may be quite dramatic. The compression may even be due to an accessory bicipital aponeurosis. After release of the lacertus fibrosus and antebrachial fascia, the median nerve is apparent lying adjacent to the humeral head of the pronator teres (Fig. 71–22).

The median nerve is followed under the humeral head of the pronator, where it encounters the ulnar head of the muscle, which varies considerably in size. It may be primarily a fleshy head, but usually the tendon of origin of the muscle arises laterally and crosses the nerve. It may vary from a structure measuring 1 or 2 mm in diameter to a band of 1 or 2 cm in width. This structure lies just distal to the overlying lacertus fibrosus. Occasionally the tendon arises medially, thus allowing the nerve to pass under rather than through the pronator teres. Sometimes no ulnar head is discernible, and forearms with this arrangement may be

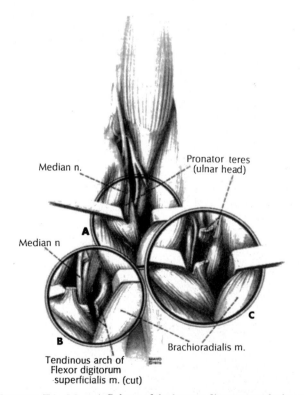

Median n.

Median n

Pronator teres
(ulnar head)

A

B

C

Brachioradialis m.

Tendinous arch of
Flexor digitorum
superficialis m. (cut)

FIGURE 71–22 • A, Release of the lacertus fibrosus reveals the median nerve as it enters the pronator teres muscle. B, Release of the ulnar head sometimes reveals a tight arch of the flexor digitorum superficialis muscle. C, If the ulnar head of the pronator teres is the offending part, it is released.

less susceptible to the condition. In the majority of patients with the pronator syndrome, the combination of a tight tendinous band of the ulnar head associated with hypertrophy of the flexor-pronator musculature, which is constricted by the enveloping antebrachial fascia and lacertus fibrosus, produce the combination of pressure and tension on the nerve that induces symptoms.

The fibrous arch of origin of the superficialis lies 1 to 2 cm distal to the deep head of the pronator (see Fig. 71–22B). This, too, may be a constriction, especially when there is a large sharp edge to the band and hypertrophy of both the deep flexors and overlying muscle groups. We believe this structure can be a cause of pronator syndrome. In a similar fashion, aberrant or vestigial muscles such as the Gantzer muscle, palmaris profundus, or flexor carpi radialis brevis may act to produce constriction. Less common factors that act to compress the median nerve are vascular malformations or distention of the bicipital bursa. The nerve may be perforated by a branch of the radial artery and accompanying veins or overlain by a taut vascular bridge. Some authors[67, 117] have recommended microsurgical interfascicular dissection of the median nerve in the distal arm and elbow region in suspected cases of pronator or anterior interosseous nerve syndromes where no obvious sign of median nerve compression is identified.

ANTERIOR INTEROSSEOUS NERVE SYNDROME

Isolated paresis or paralysis of the anterior interosseous nerve gained modern acceptance from the report of Kiloh and Nevin in 1952 and is often referred to as the Kiloh-Nevin syndrome.[83] It was perhaps originally described by Tinel in 1918,[173] and a number of authors have cited case reports or small series.[42, 90, 102, 119, 134, 148, 152] Several larger series have recently been reported.[142, 145, 151] Both complete and incomplete presentations have been described. There is an occasional overlap between the anterior interosseous nerve syndrome and the pronator syndrome, especially when minor weakness exists in the motor distribution of the anterior interosseous nerve in the pronator syndrome.[69] It is surprising that there is not a greater correlation between the two conditions, given the similarity of etiologic conditions affecting the same anatomic area, and the close association of the nerves.

The cause of this problem may be an acute demyelination episode similar to those seen in the brachial plexus as Parsonage-Turner syndrome or brachial plexitis.[129, 185] An initial period of nonoperative therapy is therefore warranted, to allow time for improvement of symptoms or the development of other neurologic findings, which would be characteristic of Parsonage-Turner syndrome.

Symptoms

Commonly, a deep unremitting pain in the proximal forearm initiates the symptoms, which subside within 8 to 12 hours. The patent may then note a lack of dexterity or weakness of pinch that fails to resolve. If the patient was seen previously, diagnoses from tendinous rupture to multiple sclerosis may have been entertained, particularly if the onset has been insidiously painless. Spontaneous improvement has been reported in some instances in which the patient had an apparently demyelinating etiology.[52, 181]

Physical Findings

In complete cases, the findings are those associated with denervation of the classic distribution of the anterior interosseous nerve to the flexor pollicis longus, the index and long finger profundus, and the pronator quadratus. The stance of the thumb and index finger when attempting to pinch is characteristic (Fig. 71–23). Because of an inability to flex the distal joints, they are approximated in hyperextension along their distal phalanges. Pinch is weak, and manipulative facility is impaired. Isolated testing shows marked weakness or paralysis of the flexor pollicis longus and index profundus (see Fig. 71–23B). The long finger is usually less affected, depending on the relative contributions of the ulnar and median nerves to the profundi. Thumb to little finger opposition is unaffected. In incomplete cases, usually the flexor pollicis longus or the index finger profundus is affected. Incomplete lesions are frequently misdiagnosed as a tendon rupture and electrodiagnosis is especially helpful both in establishing neural dysfunction but also excluding polyneuropathy or wider median nerve dysfunction. They may occur spontaneously or follow fracture fixation.[80]

Weakness in pronation is seldom a recognizable complaint of the patient because it is submerged in the general discomforts of weakness and clumsiness of the extremity. The pronator quadratus is tested by placing both elbows against the side and resisting pronation with the elbow flexed to a right angle. This effectively reduces the strength contribution of the pronator teres humeral head, allowing comparison of the pronator quadratus.

Tenderness over the proximal forearm is usually absent, and sensory disturbance is not apparent. Electromyographic findings of fibrillations are present in the affected muscles. In a recent study, all patients had electrical changes; the pronator quadratus was most consistently affected.[145]

Nerve variations such as the Martin-Gruber anastomosis may occur between the anterior interosseous nerve and the ulnar nerve as well as between the median and ulnar nerves. These fibers are likely to innervate intrinsic muscle on the radial aspect of the hand. It is therefore necessary to differentiate partial apparent ulnar paralysis from the anterior interosseous nerve syndrome.[152]

Surgical exploration should be performed within 6 months if there is no neurologic or electrical evidence of improvement.

Operative Findings

The operative findings are similar to those described earlier for the pronator syndrome. The usual finding is a constriction due to the tendon or origin of the ulnar head of the pronator teres across the posterolateral aspect of the anterior interosseous nerve as it separates from the median nerve (Fig. 71–24). There may be a fibrous reaction in the area that is probably associated with the acute episode of pain, suggesting a localized vascular reaction such as thrombosis or ischemia.

OUR PREFERRED TREATMENT FOR EXPOSURE OF THE MEDIAN NERVE

The spectrum of median nerve problems at the elbow suggests that the initial incision should be adaptable to unsuspected findings. We therefore prefer a longitudinally oriented incision curved at the antecubital crease or zigzagged to increase exposure and decrease tension on the scar line during healing. The medial antebrachial cutaneous nerve should be sought and protected. Major veins are retracted after ligating communicating veins. The plane over the brachial and antebrachial fascia is cleared to observe the effect of the lacertus fibrosus on passive pronation. A deep indentation of the flexor-pronator group is significant.

If the pronator teres is prolonged proximally, the muscle often covers the median nerve above the elbow. The medial intermuscular septum and the brachial fascia tend to envelop the nerve in this situation. A true ligament of Struthers may be present if there is a supracondylar process. Although such a diagnosis is usually made radiographically, palpation of the lower humerus through this wound may indicate an unsuspected supracondylar process.

The median nerve is identified proximal to the lacertus fibrosus in the arm. The lacertus is incised and the median nerve is traced distally. The tendinous origin of the pronator teres should be detached. Arches over the pronator teres and the flexor digitorum superficialis are released. We also utilize the plane between the pronator teres and the flexor carpi radialis. This plane can be identified distally and the median nerve can then be traced in a distal to proximal direction.

All of these potential sites of entrapment should be explored, since multiple sites of entrapment could be present. It may be important to extend the incision proximally in certain instances; hence, draping to the axilla and the use of a sterile tourniquet are wise precautions.

Cutaneous Nerves

LATERAL ANTEBRACHIAL NERVE

Compression neuropathy of the lateral antebrachial cutaneous nerve is a recently recognized syndrome.[7, 27, 44, 58, 130] This cutaneous branch may also be injured at surgery or with injections.[187]

Relevant Anatomy

The musculocutaneous nerve, after supplying the coracobrachialis, biceps, and brachialis muscles, continues in the interval between the last two muscles as a sensory nerve to supply the skin over the anterolateral aspect of the forearm, often as far as the thenar eminence. It emerges from beneath the biceps tendon laterally and penetrates the brachial fascia just above the elbow crease to course down the forearm (Fig. 71–25).

Clinical Findings

Bassett and Nunley describe both acute and chronic problems.[7] A distinct mechanism of injury consisting of elbow hyperextension and pronation or resisted elbow flexion and

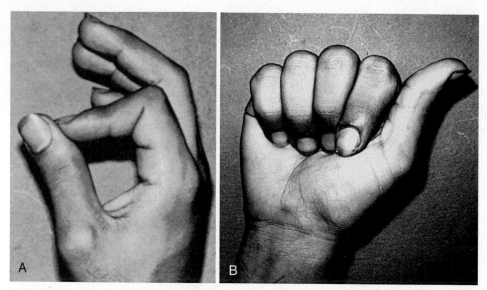

FIGURE 71–23 • A, Anterior interosseous nerve demonstrating the characteristic pinch attitude. B, The patient is unable to flex the terminal pha-
lanx of the thumb or index finger. Sensation is intact. There is some weakness of the flexor digitorum profundus of the long finger, which in this patient is supplied and motored enough to flex the distal joint through a branch of the ulnar nerve in the proximal forearm. (A from Spinner, M.: Injuries
to the Major Branches of Peripheral Nerves of the Forearm, 2nd ed. Philadelphia. W. B. Saunders Co., 1978.)

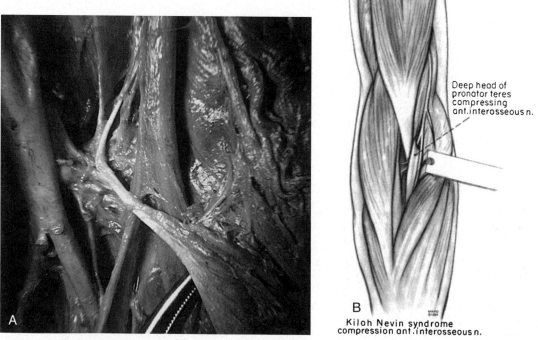

FIGURE 71–24 • Compression of the anterior interosseous nerve can occur at its entrance to the pronator muscle near its origin. A, Cadaveric
specimen demonstrates a thin tendinous origin of the deep head of the pronator teres as it crosses over the take-off of the anterior interosseous nerve
branch from the median nerve. B, Artistic rendition. (A from Spinner, M.: Injuries to the Major Branches of Peripheral Nerves of the Forearm, 2nd ed.
Philadelphia, W. B. Saunders Co., 1978.)

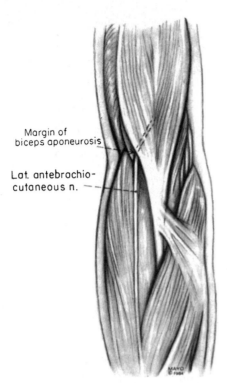

Margin of biceps aponeurosis

Lat. antebrachio-cutaneous n.

FIGURE 71–25 • The lateral antebrachial cutaneous nerve has been reported to be compressed at the lateral margin of the biceps aponeurosis at the level of the lateral epicondyle.

pronation was elicited from their patients; presumably, the nerve was compressed between the biceps tendon and the brachialis fascia because both the nerve and the tendon were rendered taut by the forearm position. Burning dysesthesia in the distribution of the nerve is seen acutely. In chronic phases, the patient complains of a vague discomfort in the forearm with some dysesthetic qualities that are sometimes made worse by supinopronatory activities with the elbow extended.

On physical examination, a dysesthetic area on the anterolateral aspect of the forearm can be elicited by gently stroking across the skin transversely with a blunt point. Tenderness to direct pressure on the lateral aspect of the bicipital tendon just proximal to the elbow crease is characteristic; loss of extension and pronation is often exhibited with this maneuver. The sensory action potential may exhibit a prolonged latency or diminished amplitude.[43]

Treatment

For the acute injury, rest, splinting, avoidance of extension-pronation, and anti-inflammatory medication are indicated. Corticosteroidal injections at the area of tenderness may help if exacerbation occurs. In chronic syndromes or those failing to respond to nonoperative measures, surgical decompression is appropriate. Under tourniquet control, a zigzag incision across the lateral aspect of the elbow crease allows exposure of the lateral antebrachial nerve. The site of compression usually occurs where the nerve emerges beneath the bicipital tendon. A tight band of antebrachial fascia at the elbow crease has been noted to alter the course of the nerve to an acute angle in one of our patients.

Release of the brachial fascia and excision of a triangular portion of the bicipital tendon at the point of impingement is recommended. Obliteration of vascular marking at the site of compression may be noted. A neuroma, if present, should be excised and allowed to retract.

Results

Symptoms may subside after an acute episode, but the nerve thereafter is apparently more susceptible to further irritation. Surgical decompression can be expected to produce relief of pain, improvement in sensibility, and restoration of motion.

MEDIAL ANTEBRACHIAL CUTANEOUS NERVE

The posterior branch of the medial antebrachial cutaneous nerve has received some attention because of its course near the medial epicondyle. This has obvious clinical significance. Neuromata occur relatively frequently after ulnar nerve surgery[31] but may also occur following treatment of medial epicondylitis.[136] A recent anatomic study[133] describes the course of this cutaneous nerve and its variations. Rare cases of compressive lesions have also been reported.[18, 146] Patients present with sensory disturbance in the posteromedial forearm or pain at the medial aspect of the elbow or both.

POSTERIOR ANTEBRACHIAL CUTANEOUS NERVE

Nerve lesions of the posterior antebrachial cutaneous branch (a branch of the radial nerve at or near the spiral groove) do occur. Patients may present with isolated sensory abnormalities in the dorsolateral forearm or lateral elbow pain or both. Several cases[19, 36] have been reported, occuring either spontaneously or following surgery. The nerve emerges from the lateral triceps and has a variable relationship with the lateral intermuscular septum. It then courses over the brachioradialis near the lateral epicondyle. Its course makes it particularly vulnerable in surgery for lateral epicondylitis or even in posterior interosseous nerve releases. We have also treated two cases of compression following humeral fracture reduction and fixation, demonstrating the nerve's vulnerability more proximally. Excision of the neuroma or decompression of the nerve branch can relieve the symptoms.

REFERENCES

1. Abe, M., Ishizu, T., Okamoto, M., and Onomura, T.: Tardy ulnar nerve palsy caused by cubitus varus deformity. J. Hand Surg. **20A**:5, 1995.
2. Agnew, D. H.: Bursal tumor producing loss of power of forearm. Am. J. Med. Sci. **46**:404, 1863.
3. Al-Qattan, M. M.: Gantzer's muscle. An anatomical study of the accessory head of the flexor pollicis longus muscle. J. Hand Surg. **21B**:269, 1996.
4. Amadio, P. C.: Anatomical basis for a technique of ulnar nerve transposition. Surg. Radiol. Anat. **8**:155, 1986.
5. Apfelberg, D. B., and Larson, S. J.: Dynamic anatomy of the ulnar nerve at the elbow. Plast. Reconst. Surg. **51**:76, 1973.
6. Barber, K. W., Jr., Bianco, A. J., Jr., Soule, E. H., and MacCarty, C. S.: Benign extramural soft tissue tumors of the extremities causing compression of nerves. J. Bone Joint Surg. **44A**: 98, 1982.

7. Bassett, F. H., and Nunley, J. A.: Compression of the musculocutaneous nerve at the elbow. J. Bone Joint Surg. **64A**: 1050, 1982.

8. Bowen, T. L., and Stone, K. H.: Posterior interosseous nerve paralysis caused by a ganglion at the elbow. J. Bone Joint Surg. **48B**:774, 1966.

9. Boyes, J. H.: Bunnell's Surgery of the Hand, 5th ed. Philadelphia. J.B. Lippincott Co., 1970, pp. 418–419.

10. Braun, R. M., and Spinner, R. J.: Spontaneous bilateral median nerve compression in the distal arm. J. Hand Surg. **16A**:244, 1991.

11. Brooks, D. M.: Nerve compression by simple ganglia. J. Bone Joint Surg. **34B**:391, 1952.

12. Bryan, F. S., Miller, L. S., and Panijaganond, P.: Spontaneous paralysis of the posterior interosseous nerve: A case report and review of the literature. Clin. Orthop. **80**:9, 1971.

13. Buchthal, F., Rosenflack, A., and Trojaborg, W.: Electrophysiological findings in entrapment of the median nerve at wrist and elbow. J. Neurol. Neurosurg. Psychiatry. **37**:340, 1974.

14. Busa, R., Adani, R., Marcuzzi, A., and Caroli, A.: Acute posterior interosseous nerve palsy caused by a synovial haemangioma of the elbow joint. J. Hand Surg. **20B**:652, 1995.

15. Campbell, C. S., and Wulf, R. F.: Lipoma producing a lesion of the deep branch of the radial nerve. J. Neurosurg. **11**:310, 1954.

16. Capener, N.: Posterior interosseous nerve lesions. Proceedings of the Second Hand Club. J. Bone Joint Surg. **46B**:361, 1964.

17. Capener, N.: The vulnerability of the posterior interosseous nerve of the forearm. J. Bone Joint Surg. **48B**:770, 1966.

18. Chang, C. W., and Oh, S. J.: Medial antebrachial cutaneous neuropathy: Case report. Electromyogr. Clin. Neurophys. **28**:3, 1988.

19. Chang, C. W., and Oh, S. J.: Posterior antebrachial cutaneous neuropathy. Case report. Electromyogr. Clin. Neurophysiol. **30**:3, 1990.

20. Childress, H. M.: Recurrent ulnar-nerve dislocation at the elbow. Clin. Orthop. **108**:168, 1975.

21. Clark, C. B.: Cubital tunnel syndrome. J.A.M.A. **241**:801, 1979.

22. Cohen, B. E.: Simultaneous posterior and anterior interosseous nerve syndromes. J. Hand Surg. **7**:398, 1982.

23. Comtet, J. J., and Chambaud, D.: Paralysie "spontanée" du nerf inter-osseoux posterier par lesion inhabituelle. Deux observations. Rev. Chir. Orthop. **61**:533, 1975.

24. Comtet, J. J., Chambaud, D., and Genety, J.: La compression de la branche posterier du nerf radial. Une etiologie meconnue de certaines paralysies et de certaines spicondylalgies rebelles. Nouv. Presse Med. **5**:1111, 1976.

25. Craven, P. R., Jr., and Green, D. P.: Cubital tunnel syndrome. J. Bone Joint Surg. **62A**: 986, 1980.

26. Dahners, L. E., and Wood, F. M.: Anconeus epitrochlearis, a rare cause of cubital tunnel syndrome: a case report. J. Hand Surg. **9A**:579, 1984.

27. Davidson, J. J., Bassett, F. H., III, and Nunley, J.A.: Musculocutaneous nerve entrapment revisited. American Orthopaedic Association Annual Meeting, White Sulphur Springs, West Virginia, June, 1995.

28. Davies, F., and Laird, M.: The supinator muscle and the deep radial (posterior interosseous) nerve. Anat. Rec. **101**:243, 1948.

29. Dawson, D. M., Hallett, M., and Millender, L. H.: Entrapment Neuropathies, 2nd ed. Boston, Little, Brown & Co., 1990.

30. Dellon, A. L., and Mackinnon, S. E.: Radial-sensory nerve entrapment in the forearm. J. Hand Surg. **11A**:199, 1986.

31. Dellon, A. L., and Mackinnon, S. E.: Injury to the medial antebrachial cutaneous nerve during cubital tunnel surgery. J. Hand Surg. **10B**:33, 1985.

32. Dellon, A. L., and Mackinnon, S. E.: Musculoaponeurotic variations along the course of the median nerve in the proximal forearm. J. Hand Surg. **12B**:359, 1987.

33. Dellon, A. L.: Techniques for successful management of ulnar nerve entrapment at the elbow. Neurosurg. Clin. North Am. **2**:57, 1991.

34. Denny-Brown, D., and Brenner, C.: Paralysis of nerve induced by direct pressure and by tourniquet. Arch. Neurol. Psychiatry **51**:1, 1944.

35. Dharapak, C., and Nimberg, G. A.: Posterior interosseous nerve compression. Report of a case caused by traumatic aneurysm. Clin. Orthop. **101**:225, 1974.

36. Doyle, J. J., and David, W. S.: Posterior antebrachial cutaneous neuropathy associated with lateral elbow pain. Muscle Nerve **16**:1417, 1993.

37. Dreyfuss, U., and Kessler, I.: Snapping elbow due to dislocation of the medial head of the triceps. A report of two cases. J. Bone Joint Surg. **60B**:56, 1978.

38. Eaton, R. G., Crowe, J. F., and Parkes, J. C., III.: Anterior transposition of the ulnar nerve using a non-compressing fasciodermal sling. J. Bone Joint Surg. **62A**:820, 1980.

39. Erhlich, G. E.: Antecubital cysts in rheumatoid arthritis: a corollary to popliteal (Baker's) cysts. J. Bone Joint Surg. **54A**:165, 1972.

40. Escobar, P. L.: Short segment stimulations in ulnar nerve lesions around elbow. Orthop. Rev. **12**:65, 1983.

41. Eversmann, W. W., Jr.: Entrapment and compression neuropathies. *In* Green, D.P. (ed): Operative Hand Surgery, 2nd ed. New York, Churchill Livingstone, 1988, pp. 1423–1478.

42. Farber, J. S., and Bryan, R. S.: The anterior interosseous nerve syndrome. J. Bone Joint Surg. **50A**:521, 1968.

43. Feindel, W., and Stratford, J.: The role of the cubital tunnel in tardy ulnar palsy. Can. J. Surg. **1**:296, 1958.

44. Felsenthal, G., Mondell, D. L., Reischer, M. A., and Mack, R. H.: Forearm pain secondary to compression syndrome of the lateral cutaneous nerve of the forearm. Arch. Phys. Med. Rehabil. **65**:139, 1984.

45. Flory, P. J., and Berger, A.: Die akzessorische brachialissehneselten Ursache des Pronator Teres-Syndroms. Handchir. **17**:270, 1985.

46. Foster, R. J., and Edshage, S.: Factors related to outcome of surgically managed compressive ulnar neuropathy at the elbow level. J. Hand Surg. **6**:181, 1981.

47. Freundlich, B. D., and Spinner, M.: Nerve compression syndrome in derangements of the proximal and distal radioulnar joints. Bull. Hosp. Joint Dis. **19**:38, 1968.

48. Frohse, F., and Frankel, M.: Die Muskeln des menschlichen Ames. *In* Bardelenbens Handbuch der Anatomie des Nenschlichen. Jena, Fisher, 1908.

49. Froimson, A. I., and Zahrawi, F.: Treatment of compression neuropathy of the ulnar nerve at the elbow by epicondylectomy and neurolysis. J. Hand Surg. **5**:391, 1980.

50. Fujioka, H., Nakabayashi, Y., Hirata, S., Go, G., Nishi, S., and Mizuno, K.: Analysis of tardy ulnar nerve palsy associated with cubitus varus deformity after a supracondylar fracture of the humerus: a report of four cases. J. Orthop. Trauma **9**:435, 1995.

51. Gabel, G. T., and Amadio, P. C.: Reoperation for failed decompression of the ulnar nerve in the region of the elbow. J. Bone Joint Surg. **72A**:213, 1990.

52. Gaitzsch, G., and Chamay, A.: Paralytic brachial neuritis or Parsonage-Turner syndrome anterior interosseous nerve involvement. Report of three cases. Ann. Chir. Main **5**:288, 1986.

53. Gantzers, C. F. L.: De Musculorum Varietates, thesis. Berlioni, J. F. Starckie, 1813.

54. Gelberman, R. H., Yamaguchi, K., Hollstien, S. B., Winn, S. S., Heidenreich, F. P., Jr., Bindra, R. R., Hsieh, P., and Silva, M. J.: Changes in interstitial pressure and cross-sectional area of the cubital tunnel of the ulnar nerve with flexion of the elbow. An experimental study in human cadavera. J. Bone Joint Surg. **80A**:492, 1998.

55. Gessini, L., Jandolo, B., and Pietrangeli, A.: Entrapment neuropathies of the median nerve at and above the elbow. Surg. Neurol. **19**:112, 1983.

56. Geutjens, G. G., Langstaff, R. J., Smith, N. J., Jefferson, D., Howell, C. J., and Barton, N. J.: Medial epicondylectomy or ulnar nerve transposition for ulnar neuropathy at the elbow? J. Bone Joint Surg. **78B**:777, 1996.

57. Gilliatt, B. W., Ochoa, J., Rudge, P., and Neary, D.: The cause of nerve damage in acute compression. Trans. Am. Neurol. Assoc. **99**:71, 1974.

58. Gillingham, B.L., and Mack, G.R.: Compression of the lateral antebrachial cutaneous nerve by the biceps tendon. J. Shoulder Elbow Surg. **5**:330, 1996.

59. Goldman, S., Honet, J. C., Sobel, R., and Goldstein, A. S.: Posterior interosseous nerve palsy in the absence of trauma. Arch. Neurol. **21**:435, 1969.

60. Graf, P., Hawe, W., and Biemer, E.: Gefabversorgung des n. ulnaris nach Neurolyse im Ellenbogenbereich. Handchir. **18**:204, 1986.

61. Gunther, S.F., DiPasquale, D., and Martin, R.: The internal anatomy of the median nerve in the region of the elbow. J. Hand Surg. **17A**: 648, 1992.

62. Harrelson, J. M., and Newman, M.: Hypertrophy of the flexor carpi ulnaris as a cause of ulnar-nerve compression in the distal part of the forearm. Case report. J. Bone Joint Surg. **57A**:554, 1975.

63. Hartz, C. R., Linscheid, R. L., Gramse, R. R., and Daube, J. R.: Pronator teres syndrome: compressive neuropathy of the median nerve. J. Bone Joint Surg. **63A**:885, 1981.

64. Hashizume, H., Inoue, H., Nagashima, K., and Hamaya, K.: Posterior interosseous nerve paralysis related to focal radial nerve constriction secondary to vasculitis. J. Hand Surg. **18B**:757, 1993.

65. Hashizume, H., Nishida, K., Yamamoto, K., Hirooka, T., and Inoue, H.: Delayed posterior interosseous nerve palsy. J. Hand Surg. **20B**:655, 1995.

66. Hashizume, H., Nishida, K., Nanba, Y., Shigeyama, Y., Inoue, H., and Morito, Y.: Non-traumatic paralysis of the posterior interosseous nerve. J. Bone Joint Surg. **78B**:771, 1996.

67. Haussmann, P., and Patel, M. R.: Intraepineurial constriction of nerve fascicles in pronator syndrome and anterior interosseous nerve syndrome. Orthop. Clin. North Am. **27**:339, 1996.

68. Haws, M., and Brown, R. E.: Bilateral snapping triceps tendon after bilateral ulnar nerve transposition for ulnar nerve subluxation. Ann. Plast. Surg. **34**:550, 1995.

69. Hill, H. A., Howard, F. M., and Huffer, B. R.: The incomplete anterior interosseous nerve syndrome. J. Hand Surg. **10A**:4, 1985.

70. Hirachi, K., Kato, H., Minami, A., Kasashima, T., and Kaneda, K.: Clinical features and management of posterior interosseous nerve palsy. J. Hand Surg. **23B**:413, 1998.

71. Hobhouse, N., and Heald, C. B.: A case of posterior interosseous paralysis. Br. Med. J. **1**:841, 1936.

72. Hollinshead, W. H.: Anatomy for Surgeons, Vol. 3, The Back and Limbs, 3rd ed. New York, Harper and Row, 1982.

73. Jabaley, ME., Wallace, W. H., and Heckler, F. R.: Internal topography of major nerves of the forearm and hand: a current view. J. Hand Surg. **5**:1, 1980.

74. Jebson, P. J. L., and Engber, W. D.: Radial tunnel syndrome: long-term results of surgical decompression. J. Hand Surg. **22A**:889, 1997.

75. Johnson, R. K., Spinner, M., and Shrewsbury, M. M.: Median nerve entrapment syndrome in the proximal forearm. J. Hand Surg. **4**:48, 1979.

76. Jones, R. E.: Medial epicondylectomy for ulnar nerve compression syndrome at the elbow. Clin. Orthop. **139**:174, 1979.

77. Kaempffe, F. A., and Farbach, J.: A modified surgical procedure for cubital tunnel syndrome: partial medial epicondylectomy. J. Hand Surg. **23A**:492, 1998.

78. Kane, E., Kaplan, E. B., and Spinner, M.: Observations of the course of the ulnar nerve in the arm. Ann. Chir. **27**:487, 1973.

79. Kaplan, E. B.: Functional and Surgical Anatomy of the Hand, 2nd ed. Philadelphia, J.B. Lippincott Co., 1965.

80. Keogh, P., Khan, H., Cooke, E., and McCoy, G.: Loss of flexor pollicis longus function after plating of the radius. J. Hand Surg. **22B**:375, 1997.

81. Keret, D., and Porter, K. M.: Synovial cyst and ulnar nerve entrapment: a case report. Clin. Orthop. **188**:213, 1984.

82. Khoo, D., Carmichael, S. W., and Spinner, R. J.: Ulnar nerve anatomy and compression. Orthop. Clin. North Am. **27**:317, 1996.

83. Kiloh, L. G., and Nevin, S.: Isolated neuritis of the anterior interosseous nerve. Br. Med. J. **1**:859, 1952.

84. Kopell, H. P, and Thompson, W. A.I.: Pronator syndrome. N. Engl. J. Med. **259**:713, 1958.

85. Kopell, H. P., and Thompson, W. A.: Peripheral Entrapment Neuropathies. Baltimore, Williams & Wilkins, 1963.

86. Kotani, H., Miki, T., Senzoku, F., Nakagawa, Y., and Ueo, T.: Posterior interosseous nerve paralysis with multiple constrictions. J. Hand Surg. **20A**: 15, 1995.

87. Kuszynski, K.: Functional micro-anatomy of the peripheral nerve trunks. Hand **6**:1, 1974.

88. Laha, R. K., Lunsford, L. D. and Dujovny, M.: Lacertus fibrosus compression of the median nerve. A case report. J. Neurosurg. **48**:838, 1978.

89. Lahey, M. D., and Aulicino, P. L.: Anomalous muscles associated with compression neuropathies. Orthop. Rev. **15**:19, 1986.

90. Lake, P. A.: Anterior interosseous nerve syndrome. J. Neurosurg. **41**:306, 1974.

91. Learmonth, J. R.: A variation of the radial branch of the musculo-spiral nerve. J. Anat. **53**:371, 1919.

92. Learmonth, J. R.: Technique for transplanting the ulnar nerve. Surg. Gynecol. Obstet. **75**:792, 1942.

93. LeDouble, A. F.: Traite des Variations du Systeme Musculaire de l'Homme. Paris, Schleicher, 1897.

94. Leffert, R. D.: Anterior submuscular transposition of the ulnar nerves by the Learmonth technique. J. Hand Surg. **7**:147, 1982.

95. Leffert, R. D., and Dorfman, H. D.: Antecubital cyst in rheumatoid arthritis. Surgical findings. J. Bone Joint Surg. **54A**:1555, 1972.

96. Lichter, R. L., and Jacobsen, T.: Tardy palsy of the posterior interosseous nerve with a Monteggia fracture. J. Bone Joint Surg. **57A**: 124, 1975.

97. Lipscomb, P. R., and Burleson, R. J.: Vascular and neural complications in supracondylar fractures in children. J. Bone Joint Surg. **37A**:487, 1955.

98. Lister, G. D., Belsole, R. B., and Kleinert, H. E.: The radial tunnel syndrome. J. Hand Surg. **4**:52, 1979.

99. Lluch, A. L.: Ulnar nerve entrapment after anterior transposition at elbow. N. Y. State J. Med. **75**:75, 1975.

100. Lundborg, G.: Ischemic nerve injury. Experimental studies on intraneural microvascular pathophysiology and nerve function in a limb subjected to temporary circulatory arrest. Scand. J. Plast. Reconstr. Surg. [Suppl.] **6**:1, 1970.

101. Macnicol, M. F.: Extraneural pressures affecting the nerve at the elbow. Hand **14**:5, 1982.

102. Maeda, K., Miura, T., Komada, T., and Chiba, A.: Anterior interosseous nerve paralysis. Report of 13 cases and review of Japanese literature. Hand **9**:165, 1977.

103. Mangini, U.: Flexor pollicis longus muscle. Its morphology and clinical significance. J. Bone Joint Surg. **42A**:467, 1960.

104. Mannerfelt, L.: Studies on the hand in ulnar nerve paralysis. A clinical-experimental investigation in normal and anomalous innervation. Acta Orthop. Scand. Suppl. **87**:1966.

105. Marmor, L., Lawrence, J. F, and Dubois, E.: Posterior interosseous nerve paralysis due to rheumatoid arthritis. J. Bone Joint Surg. **49A**:381, 1967.

106. Marquis, J. W., Bruwer, A. J., and Keith, H. M.: Suparcondyloid process of the humerus. Proc. Staff Meeting Mayo Clin. **37**:691, 1957.

107. Marshall, S. C., and Murray, W. R.: Deep radial nerve palsy associated with rheumatoid arthritis. Clin. Orthop. **103**:157, 1974.

108. Martinelli, P., Gabellini, A. S., Poppi, M., Gallassi, R., and Pozzatti, E.: Pronator syndrome due to thickened bicipital aponeurosis. J. Neurol. Neurosurg. Psychiatry **45**:181, 1982.

109. Mayer, J. H., and Mayfield, P. H.: Surgery of the posterior interosseous branch of the radial nerve. Surg. Gynecol. Obstet. **84**:979, 1947.

110. Millender, L. H., Nalebuff, E. A., and Holdsworth, D. E.: Posterior interosseous nerve syndrome secondary to rheumatoid synovitis. J. Bone Joint Surg. **55A**:753, 1973.

111. Miller, R. G.: Acute versus chronic compressive neuropathy. Muscle Nerve **7**:427, 1984.

112. Morrey, B. F.: Reoperation for failed surgical treatment of refractory lateral epicondylitis. J. Shoulder Elbow Surg. **1**:47, 1992.

113. Morris, A.H.: Irreducible Monteggia lesion with radial-nerve entrapment. J. Bone Joint Surg. **46A**:608, 1964.

114. Morris, H. H., and Peters, B. H.: Pronator syndrome: Clinical and electrophysiological features in seven cases. J. Neurol. Neurosurg. Psychiatry **39**:461, 1976.

115. Mowell, J. W.: Posterior interosseous nerve injury. Int. Clin. **2**:188, 1921.

116. Mulholland, R. C.: Non-traumatic progressive paralysis of the posterior interosseous nerve. J. Bone Joint Surg. **48B**:781, 1966.

117. Nagano, A., Shibata, K., Tokimura, H., Yamamoto, S., and Tajiri, Y.: Spontaneous anterior interosseous nerve palsy with hourglass-like fascicular constriction within the main trunk of the median nerve. J. Hand Surg. **21A**:266, 1996.

118. Nakamura, I., and Hoshino, Y.: Extraneural hemangioma: a case report of acute cubital tunnel syndrome. J. Hand Surg. **21A**:1097, 1997.

119. Nakano, K. K., Lundergan, C., and Okihiro, M. M.: Anterior interosseous nerve syndromes. Arch. Neurol. **34**:477, 1977.

120. Narakas, A. O.: The role of thoracic outlet syndrome in the double crush syndrome. Ann. Chir. Main Memb. Super. **9**:331, 1990.

121. Nicolle, F. V., and Woolhouse, F. M.: Nerve compression syndromes of the upper limb. J. Trauma **5**:313, 1965.

122. Nielsen, H. O.: Posterior interosseous nerve paralysis caused by fibrous band compression at the supinator muscle: a report of four cases. Acta Orthop. Scand. **47**:304, 1976.

123. Nouhan, R., and Kleinert, J.M.: Ulnar nerve decompression by transposing the nerve and Z-lengthening the flexor-pronator origin. J. Hand Surg. **22A**: 127, 1997.

as his prominent role in research in this area and the lack of any reproducible laboratory models to explain either a pathophysiologic relationship or the relative importance of these factors to the clinical development of RSD, that the term has been badly misused in the literature.[2, 4, 29, 120, 141] Indeed, the term *RSD* has unfortunately evolved both in general clinical correspondence and in the medical literature to stand as a generic term for the presentation of *any* abnormal pain presentation or prolonged extremity dysfunction whether or not autonomic dysfunction exists.[29] The unfortunate end result of the continued clinical confusion and the generic use of the term *RSD* with respect to treatment implementation is that currently no consistent agreement exists regarding diagnostic criteria, natural history, and psychological factors involved in the syndromes listed in Table 72–1. These unresolved issues have often resulted in arbitrary clinical evaluation and anecdotal treatment protocols.[29, 141] More recently, several authors have stressed the importance of distinguishing whether the sympathetic nervous system is involved by subcategorizing abnormal pain syndromes as sympathetically maintained pain or as sympathetically independent pain.[94, 114]

When a critical review of the literature is undertaken comparing the diagnostic criteria of each of the syndromes listed in Table 72–1 irrespective of the proposed etiologies or pathophysiologic factors, all clearly have two common denominators: an abnormal pain response and dysfunction of the affected extremity.[3, 29] From the recognition of this commonality of abnormal pain and extremity dysfunction among all the various pain syndromes and with the intent to rectify the perpetuation of the use of RSD as a generic label, Dobyns[29] and Amadio[3] have recently recommended

a more general term, *pain dysfunction syndrome* (PDS), to define such disorders. The use of the term *PDS* has several advantages. First, it is both clinically descriptive and sufficiently broad so as to encompass the diversity of possible precipitating factors and removes the contingency that sympathetic nervous system dysfunction exists in all cases of an abnormal pain presentation, which was necessarily implicit in the generic use of the term *RSD*.[29]

By using PDS as a clinically descriptive label, the treating physician may then proceed without any nosologic hindrances to objectively differentiate, order, and subcategorize all the involved factors of a PDS into specific components.[29] These components include the physiologic characteristics of the injury and other sources of pain, any psychological manifestations, and the presence or absence of autonomic dysfunction.[3] By proceeding in this logical fashion, the design of an effective and nonarbitrary treatment protocol can then be implemented (Fig. 72–1)

Physiology and Pathophysiology of Pain

Before any further meaningful discussion on the clinical aspects of an abnormal pain response as a component of PDS can proceed, it is necessary to have an understanding of normal pain physiology. The sensation of normal acute pain begins with the interaction of a physical trigger (mechanical, thermal, and chemical) on a region of the body. Peripheral sensory nociceptors and mechanoreceptors are activated by the triggering event and transduce the physical energy into an electrochemical stimulus, which is then relayed proximally along the peripheral nerve via myelinated ($A\delta$ and $A\beta$) and unmyelinated (C) fibers to synapse

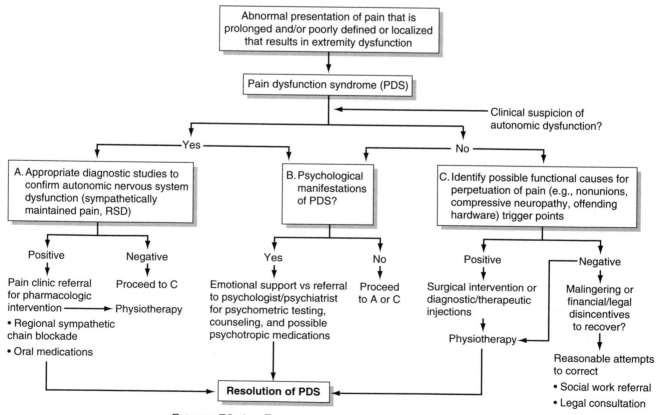

FIGURE 72–1 • Treatment protocol for pain dysfunction syndrome.

on wide dynamic range neurons of the dorsal horn of the spinal cord.[4, 53, 81, 93, 114, 136, 140, 141] Further proximal propagation of the stimulus is then transmitted through the spinothalamic and spinoreticular pain pathways to central pain centers, which are located primarily within the midbrain, thalamus, and frontal cortex.[37, 140] Modulation of nociceptive stimulation occurs via central descending pathways and peripheral chemical factors.[15] At the site of injury, should the physical trigger be of sufficient magnitude to produce tissue damage, local chemical modulators (hydrogen, potassium, bradykinin, serotonin, prostaglandins,[16] substance P) are released from the damaged cells, which further activate and sensitize the peripheral receptors and focally produce the characteristic signs of edema, vasodilation, hyperpathia, and allodynia.[111, 141] Provided that no ongoing or irreversible tissue damage occurs, both the cognitive perception of pain and the physiologic signs and symptoms of the acute pain dystrophic response subside.[37, 53, 140]

The failure of any feature of the acute pain dystrophic response to resolve normally becomes a matter of clinical concern. In some cases, the abnormal persistence of pain may have a functional etiology, as when an unrecognized infection, synovial inflammation, ischemia, or nerve entrapment exists.[3] Systemic factors such as rheumatologic disorders, endocrine or metabolic disorders (e.g., diabetic neuropathy), and the collagen vascular diseases can alter normal pain sensation as well as prolong the natural resolution process.[3, 26, 27, 37] When all functional causes have been excluded, of particular concern is any reported change in the intensity, quality, and location of the pain sensation and the persistence or dissemination of focal edema, color changes, and thermoregulatory adaptations that are seen initially as part of the acute pain dystrophic response.

It has been well established both clinically and experimentally that the sympathetic nervous system can contribute to the pathogenesis of RSD and other related pain syndromes.[2, 9, 10, 77, 78, 130, 131] Evidence for this has been demonstrated by the fact that regional anesthetic blockade or interruption of the sympathetic nervous system produces relief of the pain of RSD and that electrical stimulation of the sympathetic chain exacerbates the pain in many patients suspected of having a sympathetically maintained pain.[37] Further evidence that the sympathetic nervous system contribution to the genesis and maintenance of certain abnormal pain syndromes is indeed a pathologic process is demonstrated by the observation that in normal persons when sympathetic outflow is electrically stimulated, no painful sensation is produced, nor does regional sympathetic blockade alter normal pain sensation.[37] Despite these and other clinical and experimental observations, there as yet exists no definitive laboratory model that explains fully how the sympathetic nervous system alters, produces, or maintains the pain of RSD and related disorders, although numerous plausible hypotheses have been proposed.[1, 2, 33, 67, 77, 101, 111, 114, 127] Collectively, these hypotheses can be grouped into either adaptive central nervous system dysfunction processes or peripheral end organ and receptor abnormalities.[13]

CLASSIFICATION

Several classification schemes for RSD have been described in the literature.[1, 74] In general terms, the more

---

• TABLE 72–2 • **Lankford's Classification of Reflex Sympathetic Dystrophy by Cause**

Causalgia
    Major: motor-sensory involvement
    Minor: sensory involvement
Traumatic
    Major: fracture, crush
    Minor: sprain, contusion

---

accepted classification schemes have been based on either the natural history of signs and symptoms of the disorder or on the type and magnitude of the precipitating injury.[71–74, 103] Lankford's classification, based on injury type, proposes two distinct forms of sympathetic dysfunction (Table 72–2). The first, causalgia, results from direct nerve injury and is further subcategorized into either major or minor causalgia depending on whether the injury is due to a mixed motor/sensory or a sensory nerve, respectively. Traumatic dystrophy, the second type, is similarly subcategorized into major and minor subtypes. A minor traumatic dystrophy generally results from a less severe injury such as a sprain or contusion, whereas a major traumatic dystrophy results from a more extensive injury such as a fracture.[3, 34, 73, 74] Amadio and others have pointed out that the use of this type of classification scheme can be both confusing and imprecise, since some examples of RSD have no clear traumatic etiology and some minor causalgia may prove to be more disabling than a major causalgia.[3]

The second type of classification scheme for RSD is based on the natural history of the clinically observed physiologic, morphologic, and functional changes observed in untreated RSD.[115, 128] The Steinbrocker classification recognizes three distinct stages: (1) the acute stage (0 to 3 months), (2) the dystrophic stage (3 to 6 months), and (3) the atrophic stage (6 months and beyond) (Table 72–3).[128] In the earlier phases, the pain is often burning and more focal than diffuse, and the associated edema, vasomotor, and thermoregulatory dysfunction are usually prevalent. In the later stages, the pain is more constant and poorly localized. Muscle atrophy, joint stiffness, or contractures may develop along with subcutaneous fibromatous organization and cyanosis of the skin. End-stage RSD is characterized by the appearance of more permanent changes of the skin, blood vessels, and joints (ankylosis).[37, 115] It is important to recognize that RSD is a dynamic process and although the previously mentioned stages accurately describe the symptomatic and pathophysiologic changes in general, in any individual a considerable temporal variability may occur in the development of the characteristic signs and symptoms and subtle and partial manifestations are generally the rule rather than the exception. Therefore, no

---

• TABLE 72–3 • **Classification of Reflex Sympathetic Dystrophy by Temporal Factors (Steinbrocker)**

Type	Duration (months)
Acute	<3
Dystrophic	3–6
Atrophic	>6

technique has proven to be a particularly useful diagnostic tool in the evaluation of RSD, with a reported high degree of specificity in untreated cases.[3, 67–70, 85]

Other diagnostic tests for RSD and autonomic dysfunction have been described, including quantitative sweat production (Q-SART Low), dynamic vasomotor reflex assessment, and cold stress thermoregulatory capacity, all of which may add diagnostic information.[3, 36, 48, 64, 83] The usefulness of thermography (infrared telethermometry) as a diagnostic test for RSD is controversial.[75, 105–107, 119, 135] Although all of these ancillary diagnostic tests may be necessary in certain case examples, the response to sympathetic blockade remains the single most useful and preferred test for the establishment of the diagnosis of RSD.[3, 76, 78, 97, 102, 104, 116, 117]

As previously stated, the psychological aspects of a PDS are variable both in degree and in presentation. To objectively assess the psychic manifestations of the disorder, examiners have traditionally used several standard personality, psychometric, and pain quantitation tests to evaluate patients suffering from chronic pain and RSD.[3, 17, 122] These tests include the Minnesota Multiphasic Personality Inventory, the McGill Pain Questionnaire, the visual analog scale, and the Dartmouth Pain Questionnaire.[17, 20, 49–51, 141] When properly interpreted, the Minnesota Multiphasic Personality Inventory can provide some useful evaluative information of the personality profiles for some chronic pain states, although some argue its importance as a predictor of treatment success.[17, 20, 41, 50, 51, 87] The McGill Pain Questionnaire is widely used as a method of quantitating subjective pain intensity, and this study, along with other visual quantitation methods, is often useful to assess individual treatment progress.[50, 51]

In some cases, precise localization of a source of pain between several contiguous anatomic structures may be aided by a selective diagnostic local anesthetic injection of small amounts of 1 percent lidocaine. This simple diagnostic procedure can also be used as an aid in the localization of multiple adjacent trigger points.

TREATMENT

After obtaining a thorough historic investigation and physical examination as well as additional objective data from appropriate diagnostic studies, the treating physician should be able to accurately identify those specific components involved in any PDS. All involved components of a PDS must be addressed in the design of a treatment plan if a complete and expeditious recovery from the disorder is to be expected.[29, 117] Dobyns[29] recommends that all components be ordered so that the most predominant problems are listed first. This process results in a prioritized outline from which specific problem-oriented treatment regimens may be begun (see Fig. 72–1). In most cases of PDS, the treatment of certain components is outside the domain of orthopedic surgery, and therefore consultation of other medical associates to assist in the overall treatment plan is required. Pain control specialists (anesthesiologists), physiatrists, physical therapists, and psychiatrists are most often consulted, owing to their particular expertise in dealing with some of the more common problems involved in

recovery from chronic pain and dysfunction.[3, 29, 37] Associates in internal medicine for the treatment of certain systemic disorders, as well as rheumatologists, neurologists, and endocrinologists, may be required in specific instances. By consulting these medical specialists, the primary physician generally yields to their recommendations for specific treatment; however, the patient rightly expects that one physician will remain in overall charge of his or her care. Failure to do so can often result in disastrous failures in treatment stemming from misunderstanding, disillusionment, and distrust.

The treatment of the physical components of a PDS in most cases will come under the direction and care of the orthopedic surgeon, particularly when an injury has occurred. It is obligatory from the outset of treatment to identify any physical and anatomic problems that act as sources of continued pain and dysfunction. Fracture nonunions and malunions, offending internal fixation hardware, postimmobilization joint stiffness, neuromas, painful constrictive scars, and traumatic arthritis are all common examples of continued painful foci that are potentially correctable with surgical intervention. Reluctance on the part of the surgeon to proceed with corrective operative procedures should be dismissed even in cases in which there are recognizable extenuating problems (e.g., previous surgical failures, active psychological dysfunction) as avoidance of recognized treatable problems will ensure perpetuation of the disorder.[3]

Physiotherapy

In addition to the decision for further surgical treatment, the form and direction of a physical therapy program will most often initially come under the direction and control of the orthopedic surgeon. A close association with the therapist should be established early and maintained through completion of rehabilitation. All involved components of a PDS should be discussed with the therapist to delineate the specific physical problems necessitating the referral and to identify any potential impediments to the success of subsequent treatment. Restoration of normal functional activity involves both active and passive modalities, but the design of any physical therapy program for PDS should allow direct patient involvement along with establishment of clearly defined treatment goals.[3, 39, 125] In the earlier phases of therapy, the degree of pain is usually the determining factor as to which modalities are to be employed. However, active and active-assistive programs are generally most effective because they allow the patient to have some control of his or her level of pain.[138] In addition to specific physiotherapy modalities directed toward the site of injury or obvious sources of pain and dysfunction, it is also important to recognize and treat any secondary adaptive physical problems that evolve in adjacent joints and anatomic structures. Examples of a secondary problem would be decreased range of motion of the shoulder and co-contraction of parascapular muscles following a prolonged period of immobilization.[29]

Pharmacologic Treatment

Pharmacologic pain management may initially be instituted by the musculoskeletal physician. Aside from the need for immediate postoperative narcotic medications, narcotics as a class of drugs in pain management should be avoided in the treatment of a PDS, as drug dependency is often associated with this disorder and identification of such dependency requires early referral for treatment.[3, 50, 108] Nonsteroidal anti-inflammatory medications and other non-narcotic drugs may be particularly beneficial during the acute phases of the normal dystrophic response and therefore may facilitate participation in physical therapy and resumption of normal activities of daily living.[3, 111] When indicated, anesthetic injections of trigger points and corticosteroid solution injections of joints and about inflamed musculotendinous structures are also effective and easily administered methods to control pain.[28, 92]

Beyond these initial measures in pain management, the consultation of a pain control specialist is recommended for the treatment of refractory functional causes of pain and in all cases in which autonomic dysfunction and sympathetically maintained pain exist. Pain control specialists may use oral, intravenous, and regional nerve blocks as well as adaptive therapeutic measures such as transcutaneous electric stimulation for the control and treatment of chronic functional pain.[3, 7, 28, 31, 32, 42, 45, 60, 80, 86, 98, 100, 113, 132]

SYMPATHETIC BLOCKADE

The pharmacologic treatment of the sympathetic nervous system dysfunction of RSD involves blockade of abnormal sympathetic efferent activity by multiple or continuous stellate ganglion blocks, continuous axillary blockade, end organ blockade by intravenous guanethidine, bretylium or reserpine, and use of systemic calcium channel blockers.* Pharmacologic treatment alone often is only partially successful in the treatment of sympathetically maintained pain, and an interdisciplinary approach using physical therapy and psychiatry may be initiated by the pain control specialist to successfully treat all the manifestations of the disorder.

The Psyche

The treatment of any recognizable psychic disturbances begins with initiation of any and all measures to resolve the patient's pain, because, as previously mentioned, relief from prolonged pain alone may result in a significant diminishment of any existing psychological and emotional abnormalities.[74, 75] However, consultation of a psychotherapist should be considered, even for more the situationally induced psychological disturbances described earlier, when such problems are identified as a major feature of a PDS. Depending on the patient, there may be considerable reluctance, denial, and even anger when mention is made of the possibility of any associated psychological factors, and particularly so when a recommendation is made for psychiatric referral. Nothing should be disclosed in a confrontational manner, and prior discussion with the psychotherapist may circumvent any potential negative consequences.[3, 37]

Relaxation therapy, hypnosis, biofeedback, distraction

techniques, supportive psychotherapy, and psychotrophic medications have all been shown to be effective in the management of the psychological disturbances associated with chronic pain syndromes.[3, 29, 37, 50, 82, 112, 133, 134] Likewise, the psychotherapist may assist in resolving familial, economic, and workers compensation issues.[2, 11, 12, 29, 37] Formal psychoanalysis is necessary when somatization disorder, conversion disorder, major depression, malingering, and factitious injury disorders have been identified.[37, 50, 61, 62] The early detection and prompt referral to psychotherapists for treatment of these disorders are important to protect the patient from unnecessary surgery, possibly harmful diagnostic tests, and the potential for self-inflicted injury and unnecessary hospitalization and incurred medical costs.[3, 37, 51]

CONCLUSION

Pain dysfunction syndrome is unlike most other complications encountered in the treatment of disorders of the upper extremity. The syndrome is a confluence of numerous possible precipitating factors, which may then involve a diversity of physiologic, psychological, and systemic components yielding an individually variable presentation of pain and extremity dysfunction. Perhaps no other clinical complication is looked on with more consternation, and from this there has historically been an overall reluctance to accept and treat the many problems of this disorder. Dobyns' approach to PDS solves many of the clinical challenges this syndrome presents by first clarifying the involved components, eliminating nosologic hindrances, and providing guidelines for an effective nonarbitrary treatment program.[29] Fortunately, with proper management, all components of a PDS can be alleviated, but treatment always becomes more difficult and protracted the longer the components of the syndrome are allowed to progress before care is initiated. Therefore, the willingness to accept responsibility for treatment remains perhaps the last and most difficult obstacle to overcome.

REFERENCES

1. Abram, S. E.: Incidence-hypotheses-epidemiology. In Hicks, M. S. (ed.): Pain and the Sympathetic Nervous System. Norwell, MA, Kluwer Academic Publishers, 1989, pp. 1–15.
2. Abram, S. E.: Causalgia and reflex sympathetic dystrophy. Curr. Concepts Pain 2:10, 1984.
3. Amadio, P. C.: Pain dysfunction syndromes: Current concepts review. J. Bone Joint Surg. 70A:944, 1988.
4. American Psychiatric Association: Diagnostic and Statistical Manual of Mental Disorders, 3rd ed. Washington, D.C.: American Psychiatric Association, 1987, pp. 247–251.
5. Armstrong, T. J.: Ergonomics and cumulative trauma disorders. Hand Clin. 2:553, 1986.
6. Barnes, R.: The role of sympathectomy in the treatment of causalgia. J. Bone Joint Surg. 35B:172, 1953.
7. Betcher, A. M., Bean, G., and Casten, D. F.: Continuous procaine block or paravertebral sympathetic ganglion: observations in one hundred patients. J.A.M.A. 151:288, 1953.
8. Bonelli, S., Conoscente, F., Movilia, P. C., Restelli, L., Francucci, B., and Grossi, E.: Regional intravenous guanethidine vs. stellate ganglion block in reflex sympathetic dystrophies: A randomized trial. Pain 16:297, 1983.
9. Bonica, J. J.: Causalgia and other reflex sympathetic dystrophies. Postgrad. Med. 53:143, 1973.

*References 6, 8, 16, 21, 42, 44, 55, 57, 76, 79, 86, 88, 90, 110, 111, 127, 131, and 137.

Wakefield, C. A. (eds.): Pain Management. Boston, Little, Brown, 1983, pp. 117–129.

116. Schott, G. D.: Mechanisms of causalgia and related clinical conditions: The role of the central and of the sympathetic nervous system. Brain 109:717, 1986.

117. Schutzer, S. F., and Gossling, H. R.: The treatment of reflex sympathetic dystrophy syndrome. J. Bone Joint Surg. 66A:625, 1984.

118. Schwartzman, R. J., and McLellan, T. L.: Reflex sympathetic dystrophy, a review. Arch. Neurol. 44:555, 1987.

119. Sherman, R. A., Barja, R. H., and Bruno, G. M.: Thermographic correlates of chronic pain: Analysis of 125 patients incorporating evaluations by a blind panel. Arch. Phys. Med. Rehab. 68:273, 1987.

120. Shumacker, H. B., Jr.: A personal overview of causalgia and other reflex dystrophies. Ann. Surg. 201:278, 1985.

121. Smith, R. J., Monson, R. A., and Ray, D. C.: Patients with multiple unexplained symptoms: Their characteristics, functional health, and health care utilization. Arch. Intern. Med. 146:69, 1986.

122. Southwick, S. M., and White, A. A.: Current concepts review: The use of psychological tests in the evaluation of low-back pain. J. Bone Joint Surg. 65A:560, 1983.

123. Spebar, M. J., Rosenthal, D., Collins, G. J., Jarstfer, B. S., and Walters, M. J.: Changing trends in causalgia. Am. J. Surg. 142:744, 1981.

124. Speigel, I. J., and Milowsky, J. L.: Causalgia. J.A.M.A. 127:9, 1945.

125. Spero, M. W., and Schwartz, E.: Psychiatric aspects of foot problems. In Jahss, M. H. (ed.): Disorders of the Foot. Philadelphia, W. B. Saunders Co., 1982.

126. Spiegel, D., and Chase, R. A.: The treatment of contractures of the hand using self-hypnosis. J. Hand Surg. [Am] 5:428, 1980.

127. Spurling, R. G.: Causalgia of the upper extremity: Treatment by dorsal sympathetic ganglionectomy. Arch. Neurol. Psychiatry 23:784, 1930.

128. Steinbrocker, O.: The shoulder-hand syndrome: Present status as a diagnostic and therapeutic entity. Med. Clin. North Am. 42:1537, 1958.

129. Sternbach, R. A., and Timmermans, G.: Personality changes associated with the reduction of pain. Pain 1:1771, 1975.

130. Sunderland, S.: The painful sequelae of injuries to peripheral nerves. In Sunderland, S. (ed.): Nerves and Nerve Injuries. London, Churchill Livingstone, 1978, pp. 377–420.

131. Sunderland, S.: Pain mechanisms in causalgia. J. Neurol. Neurosurg. Psychiatry 39:471, 1976.

132. Tabira, T., Shibasaki, H., and Kuroiwa, Y.: Reflex sympathetic dystrophy (causalgia) treatment with guanethidine. Arch. Neurol. 40:430, 1983.

133. Thompson, R. L., II.: Chronic pain. In Kaplan, H. I., and Sadock, B. J. (eds.): Comprehensive Textbook of Psychiatry. Baltimore, Williams & Wilkins, 1985.

134. Turner, J. A., and Chapman, C. R.: Psychological interventions for chronic pain: A critical review. II. Operant conditioning, hypnosis and cognitive-behavioral therapy. Pain 12:23, 1982.

135. Uematsu, S., Hendler, N., Hungerford, D., Long, D., and Ono, N.: Thermography and electromyography in the differential diagnosis of chronic pain syndromes and reflex sympathetic dystrophy. Electromyogr. Clin. Neurophysiol. 21:165, 1981.

136. Wall, P. D.: Stability and instability of central pain mechanisms. In Dubner, R., Gebhart, G. F., and Bond, M. R. (eds.): Proceedings of the Fifth World Congress on Pain. Amsterdam, Elsevier, 1988, pp. 13–24.

137. Wang, J. K., Erickson, R. P., and Ilstrup, D. M.: Repeated stellate ganglion blocks for upper extremity reflex sympathetic dystrophy. Reg. Anaesth. 10:125, 1985.

138. Watson, H. K., Carlson, L., and Brenner, L. H.: The "dystrophile" treatment of reflex dystrophy of the hand with an active stress loading program. Orthop. Trans. 10:188, 1986.

139. White, J. C., and Sweet, W. H.: Pain and the Neurosurgeon. Springfield, IL, Charles C. Thomas, 1969.

140. Willis, W. D., Jr.: Ascending somatosensory systems. In Yaksh, T. L. (ed.): Spinal afferent processing. New York, Plenum Press, 1986, pp. 243–274.

141. Wilson, P. R.: Sympathetically maintained pain: Diagnosis, measurement, and efficacy of treatment. In Hicks, M. S. (ed.): Pain and the Sympathetic Nervous System. Norwell, MA, Kluwer Academic Publishers, 1982, pp. 91–123.

142. Wilson, R. L.: Management of pain following peripheral nerve injuries. Orthop. Clin. North Am. 12:343, 1981.

143. Wirth, F. P., and Rutherford, R. B.: A civilian experience with causalgia. Arch. Surg. 100:637, 1970.

144. Withrington, R. M., and Wynn-Parry, C. B.: The management of painful peripheral nerve disorders. J. Hand Surg. 9B:24, 1984.

145. Withrington, R. M., and Wynn-Parry, C. B.: Rehabilitation of conversion paralysis. J. Bone Joint Surg. 67B:635, 1985.

146. Woodyard, J. E.: Diagnosis and prognosis in compensation claims. Ann. R. Coll. Surg. Engl. 64:191, 1984.

• CHAPTER 73 •

Neoplasms of the Elbow

• DOUGLAS J. PRITCHARD and
K. KRISHNAN UNNI

Most benign and malignant tumors of bone and soft tissue are relatively rare, and their occurrence in the region of the elbow is even more unusual. Although there are no valid statistics on soft tissue tumors, compilation of data from the files of the Mayo Clinic until December 1993 indicates that only 1 percent or so of bone tumors occur at the elbow (Table 73–1). Hence, no single entity is likely to be encountered very often at this site.

Unfortunately, comparable figures are not available for benign and malignant soft tissue tumors, although our impression is that the most common benign soft tissue tumor in the elbow region is the lipoma. Ganglia and myxomas are also occasionally seen in this region. Of the malignant soft tissue tumors, epithelioid sarcoma and synovial sarcoma are probably the most frequently encountered at this joint. The locally aggressive desmoid tumor may also occur at or near the elbow. Metastatic disease usually originates from the breast or kidneys.[52]

Tumors that occur in the region of the elbow are unique in that because there are a relatively large number of important structures in a relatively small and confined area, there is little normal tissue that can be spared; and it may be difficult or impossible to remove a tumor with a margin of normal tissue on all sides without severely compromising the function of the forearm and hand. In this respect, tumors that occur at the elbow, particularly those in the antecubital fossa, are comparable with tumors that occur in the region of the knee. However, the upper extremity is probably considered more important by most patients and their physicians; hence, amputation surgery is probably less likely to be carried out for these tumors than for those of the lower extremity. In addition, it is generally considered difficult to fit a patient with an upper limb prosthesis; and even if upper-limb prosthetic devices are prescribed, patients are often reluctant to use them. In contrast, most patients readily accept the use of a lower-limb prosthesis. An amputation may be required for aggressive or malignant tumors to achieve adequate surgical margins, and yet both the patient and the physician may be reluctant to accept this radical treatment. Finally, as with traumatic conditions, the tumor or its treatment often renders the elbow stiff and restricts function.[26, 52]

CLINICAL PRESENTATION

As with mesenchymal tumors arising in other locations, patients usually complain of a lump or pain, or perhaps both. Lesions in the region of the elbow may cause some limitation of motion, and this may be the first symptom that the patient notices. In addition, swelling or increased warmth may be noted by either the patient or the physician. Dilated veins may be the first indication that there is an underlying tumefaction. Symptoms may occur as a result of localized compression of one or more of the nerves that cross the elbow joint, causing either local or referred pain, numbness, or paresthesia. A long history suggests that the lesion is benign. If the patient describes a mass that seems to fluctuate in size, a ganglion or hemangioma may be considered.

PREOPERATIVE EVALUATION

In addition to the usual history and physical examination, the physician should pay particular attention to the palpation of any tumor mass that may be encountered. The consistency of the mass may give a clue to its nature. As with soft tissue masses in other locations, a stethoscope should be used to listen for the presence of a bruit. Pain or paresthesias referred to the forearm or the hand at the time of palpation of the tumorous mass may suggest the presence of a neurogenic tumor, such as a neurofibroma.

Following the clinical examination, radiographs in at least two planes should be obtained.[21] Computed tomography, with a comparison of the opposite elbow joint, may yield useful information, particularly in terms of planning for the surgical procedure. The authors have not found the performance of routine arteriography to be particularly helpful in this or any other site; however, if one needs to know the relationship of the tumor to the adjacent major vessels, contrast material can be used when computed tomography is performed, thereby supplying this information more simply and safely than by performing routine arteriography.

Magnetic resonance imaging has proved to be particularly valuable in the assessment of both bone and soft tissue tumors in most areas, including the elbow. Soft tissue tumors can be defined as to the extent of disease and their

• TABLE 73–1 • Bone Tumors		
	No. at Elbow	Total No.
Benign		
Osteoid osteoma	22	331
Osteochondroma	12	872
Giant cell tumor	12	568
Chondromyxoid fibroma	2	45
Osteoblastoma	1	87
Malignant		
Malignant lymphoma	28	694
Ewing's sarcoma	15	512
Osteosarcoma	14	1649
Fibrosarcoma	3	255
Hemangioendothelioma	1	77
Chondrosarcoma	6	900
Malignancy in giant cell tumor	2	35
Malignant fibrous histiocytoma	1	83
Myeloma	11	684

relationships with major neurovascular structures. Information about the extent of medullary involvement can be ascertained for bone tumors.

Radioisotopic bone scans may be useful not only in defining the extent of the lesion in the elbow but also by ruling out additional disease in other sites. Although it is unusual for tumors of any type to metastasize to the elbow, it is possible and should be considered whenever a primary mesenchymal neoplasm is being considered. In addition, all other modalities used in the evaluation of mesenchymal tumors in other locations should be employed as well. Routine blood chemistries and hematologic studies should be obtained. The relevance of these tests to certain specific entities will be discussed later, as these entities are considered in more detail. Certainly, a routine chest radiograph should be obtained in every patient. It should be stressed that as much information as possible should be obtained about the patient and the tumor before any surgical procedure is performed.

BIOPSY

As with musculoskeletal tumors in other locations, the biopsy procedure should be considered at least as important as the definitive surgical procedure. It should be planned with the definitive surgery in mind and should probably not be undertaken unless one is willing and prepared to proceed with whatever surgery may be indicated, depending on the results of the histologic examination and whether the pathologist can render a judgment on the basis of the frozen section. If one is approaching a lipoma or a ganglion cyst, for example, this usually becomes readily apparent to the surgeon so that he or she can perform a simple excisional biopsy as a one-stage procedure. If subsequent histologic examination of the permanent section should reveal something unexpected, definitive surgery can be performed later.

The biopsy procedure itself should be done meticulously. Very careful hemostasis should be obtained to prevent the dissemination of tumor cells in the hematoma. If the tumor lies under a muscle belly, it is usually better to go straight through the muscle, rather than to dissect around the muscle, which may contaminate additional tissue planes. The general principle that incisions on extremities should be made vertically, rather than transversely, holds for the region of the elbow, although for lesions in the region of the antecubital fossa it may be desirable to make an S-shaped incision with the transverse portion crossing the crease of the elbow.

Fine-needle aspirates are becoming an acceptable way of making a diagnosis in bone and soft tissue tumors. At the Mayo Clinic, fine-needle aspirates are performed by radiologists under computed tomography or ultrasonographic guidance. A 16- or 18-gauge needle is employed. In addition to cytologic material, the radiologist also obtains tiny fragments of tissue. The cytologic smears are stained immediately with the Papanicolaou technique, and if the smears are positive the tissue is held over for permanent sections. If the smears, however, are negative, there is an option to do frozen sections on the tissue. A diagnosis of malignancy can usually be made on the smears. How-

ever, the tissue fragments are extremely helpful in subclassifying the neoplasm. Fine-needle aspirates are very useful in the diagnosis of malignant tumors. They are less useful in the diagnosis of benign lesions and even less useful in non-neoplastic conditions.

STAGING

The staging system of Enneking and colleagues,[23] which includes both soft tissue and bone sarcomas, is useful. This system has two main factors, the first of which is the biologic potential of the lesion. If the lesion is benign, it is labeled G_0. If malignant, it is judged to be either a low-grade (G_1) or a high-grade (G_2) lesion; the high-grade lesions have a greater potential for metastatic spread. The second factor is the anatomic site of the lesion; that is, whether it is entirely within a surgical compartment (T_1) or whether it extends outside the compartment (T_2). With these classifications, a low-grade malignant tumor that is entirely within a single compartment is a 1A lesion; a low-grade lesion that extends into a second compartment is a 1B lesion; a high-grade malignant tumor that is confined to a single compartment is a 2A lesion; and a high-grade tumor that extends into a second compartment is a 2B lesion. Any tumor that shows evidence of metastatic spread is considered a stage 3 lesion.

The terminology suggested by Enneking[22] describing surgical procedures is now generally accepted. Thus, if a lesion is entered at surgery, the procedure should be considered an intralesional resection; if a tumor is "shelled out," the procedure should be considered a marginal resection; and if there is a margin of normal tissue on all aspects of the resected specimen, the operation should be considered a wide excision. For the procedure to be judged a radical resection, all the structures within the involved compartment must be resected. When the lesion involves bone, the entire bone must be removed if the procedure is to be considered a radical resection.

The same terminology is applicable to amputation surgery. With these general principles in mind, we will now discuss some of the entities that are likely to be encountered in the region of the elbow.

BONE TUMORS

Benign Bone Tumors

OSTEOID OSTEOMA AND OSTEOBLASTOMA

Osteoid osteoma arising in an intra-articular location is relatively uncommon; however, it may occur in the region of the elbow. It is relatively common at the elbow, but only a few reports on the presentation,[35] diagnosis,[32] and management[39] have appeared. This small benign bone tumor occurs in patients of any age, most commonly children and young adults. As with most bone tumors, males are more commonly affected than females. Unremitting pain is the usual symptom for which the patient seeks medical attention; however, progressive loss of motion may also be a characteristic feature. Pain during the night is particularly prominent. Aspirin may afford very dramatic relief of pain, a fact that may even suggest the diagnosis of osteoid osteoma. Occasionally, the pain may be experienced at a site remote from the lesion. Another peculiar feature of this tumor is its occasional association with atrophy of the adjacent soft tissues. In the Mayo Clinic's experience with 14 such cases, 8 have occurred in the distal humerus, 4 in the ulna (2 coronoid, 2 olecranon), and 2 in the radial head–neck region[58] (Fig. 73–1).

As noted previously, when osteoid osteoma occurs at or near the elbow joint, there is characteristically loss of some flexion or extension, but pronation and supination are preserved. In addition, there may be a synovial reaction that may further confuse the diagnosis. The most striking feature of these tumors is the prolonged average time required for making the diagnosis. In the Mayo Clinic's experience, the delay to diagnosis averaged almost 2 years.[58]

The osteoid osteoma, by definition, is quite small, usually no more than 1.5 cm in diameter. Lesions that are clinically and histologically similar but are 2 cm or more in diameter are referred to as osteoblastomas; these lesions have clinical features somewhat different from those of osteoid osteoma,[46] but loss of motion is a common feature.[7, 26] Osteoid osteoma is small when first encountered and remains small,[29] further complicating the diagnosis.

An extensive diagnostic evaluation is usually required in determining the precise location of the osteoid osteoma.[11, 33] When the patient complains of unremitting pain in the elbow, plain radiographs are usually obtained (Fig. 73–2). These may or may not reveal the presence of the tumor. The lesion typically appears as a central small nidus, which is a radiolucent area usually surrounded by an area of sclerosis. It is this sclerosis that is usually seen[37]; the central area of the nidus is more difficult to identify. When the lesion is located on the surface of the bone, there may be periosteal new bone formation that further obscures the nidus.[35] Cronemeyer and colleagues[12] described an unusual radiographic feature of osteoid osteoma in the elbow joint—subperiosteal new bone formation in adjacent bones; for example, an osteoid osteoma in the distal end of the humerus that exhibits periosteal new bone formation in the

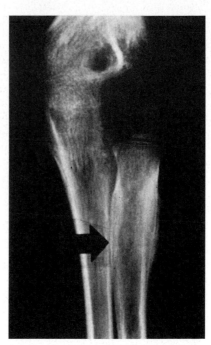

FIGURE 73–2 • Osteoid osteoma in a 10-year-old boy, upper radial shaft. Rarefied nidus with central sclerotic area and surrounding bone formation *(arrow).*

proximal radius and ulna.[12] These authors concluded that "awareness of this association will prevent misdiagnosis of the benign neoplasm as an inflammatory arthritis."

Technetium-99m scintigraphy has been helpful in locating these lesions.[32] If technetium-99m scintigraphy reveals no abnormality, an osteoid osteoma is unlikely; however, if the bone scan is positive, further diagnostic studies of the involved area should be undertaken (Fig. 73–3). If there is any significant synovial reaction, there may be increased uptake owing to the synovitis as well as to the lesion itself.[49, 50] Tomograms in two planes often reveal the suspected lesion. Sometimes, multiple radiographs must be taken before the lesion can be identified. Computed tomography may be helpful; however, the tumor is so small that it can be easily missed on this examination.[53]

Grossly, there is usually some sclerotic bone surrounding a central nidus. This nidus may be somewhat redder than the surrounding cortical bone and has been described as having the appearance of a small cherry. It is sometimes helpful to obtain radiographs of the excised block of tissue before the pathologist cuts into the block. Microscopic examination of the surrounding bone shows no unusual features; the nidus itself consists of a network of osteoid trabeculae (see Fig. 73–2).

The treatment of osteoid osteoma is surgical excision of the nidus. It is not necessary to remove all of the sclerotic bone. The main problem with this type of surgery is identification of the lesion and confirmation of its removal by the pathologist, which may be difficult. Ghelman and associates[25] have described a method for localizing an osteoid osteoma intraoperatively using a scintillation probe. This technique may simplify the localization of the lesion at the time of surgery. Patients whose lesions are not completely excised will probably continue to have the same pain and

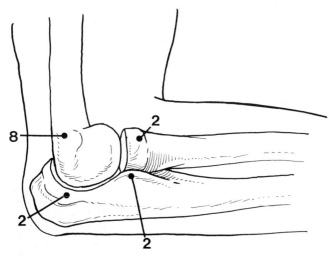

FIGURE 73–1 • Distribution of 14 osteoid osteomas treated at the Mayo Clinic.

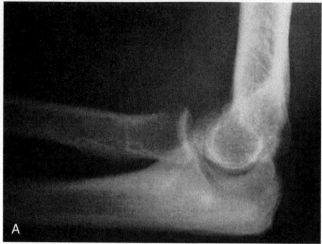

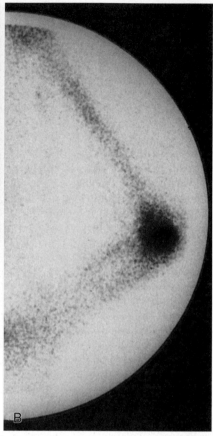

FIGURE 73–3 • Patient presented with a chronic painful elbow of almost 1 year's duration. *A*, Plain film was read as negative, although a generalized increased density of the olecranon might be appreciated. *B*, Technetium bone scan indicates intense uptake in the olecranon region. The patient was found to have an osteoid osteoma in the coronoid portion of the proximal ulna.

will probably require a second operation.[48] The authors have observed that the loss of motion so characteristic of this lesion at the elbow resolves with removal of the nidus. Hence, capsular release is not necessary as an adjunctive procedure.[58]

OSTEOCHONDROMA

Osteochondroma is probably the most common benign bone tumor, but it is not very commonly encountered in the elbow. The incidence may be somewhat higher than that reflected in our surgical experience, however, because many osteochondromas in other locations are asymptomatic and presumably may also be in the region of the elbow. The osteochondroma is not inherently painful but causes symptoms by pressure on adjacent structures. The tumor may be found in a patient of any age, but it usually stops growing when skeletal maturity is reached. An osteochondroma may arise from the surface of any bone but most commonly does so in the metaphyseal region of long bones (Fig. 73–4). The tumor tends to project away from the joint along the direction of attached muscles. The tumor may be pedunculated on a stalk or may be sessile and have a broad base (Fig. 73–5). The tumor is covered by a cartilage cap, which, if it becomes markedly thickened, suggests the possibility of sarcomatous transformation. If it is more than 1 cm thick, the risk of secondary chondrosarcoma is relatively high. In children, the cartilage cap is normally thicker than in adults. Probably fewer than 1 percent of osteochondromas ever become malignant.[28]

Multiple osteochondromas sometimes occur, a condition that tends to be familial. When multiple bones are involved, there may be some element of dysplasia with the deformity and the elbow can be severely involved. Because of the possibility of sarcomatous change, probably near 10 per-

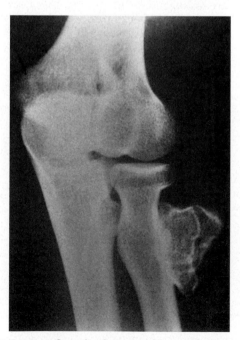

FIGURE 73–4 • Osteochondroma in a 23-year-old woman. Radial shaft with cortical and medullary bone extending into tumor.

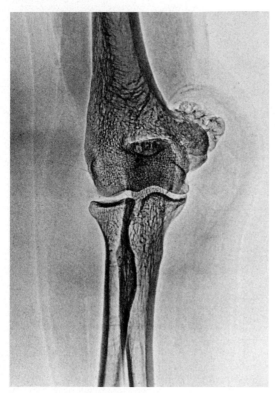

FIGURE 73–5 • Osteochondroma of the distal humerus in a 41-year-old man. Note the soft tissue reaction.

cent, patients with multiple osteochondromas need to be carefully observed through periodic follow-up examination.

Osteochondromas in the region of the elbow may cause mechanical difficulties; specifically, interference with the motion of the elbow joint. In addition, the cartilage cap may impinge on important neurovascular structures. If there are symptoms or mechanical or cosmetic difficulties, complete excision of the osteochondroma, together with the overlying cartilage cap, is performed. Excision commonly involves the use of an osteotome to shave the lesion level with the underlying cortical bone. Such simple excision generally results in cure, although local recurrence may occasionally be noted, indicating that part of the cartilaginous cap was left behind. If the cap is thicker than 1 cm in an adult, the lesion must be carefully studied histologically to exclude the possibility of a sarcoma.

GIANT CELL TUMOR

Benign giant cell tumors are occasionally encountered in the region of the elbow. In general, giant cell tumors more commonly affect females than males, contrary to the situation with most benign and malignant bone tumors. About 80 percent of giant cell tumors occur in persons who are older than 20 years of age. This point may be helpful in differentiating a giant cell tumor from an aneurysmal bone cyst, which may be radiographically similar but tends to occur in persons who are younger than 20 years of age.

Giant cell tumors nearly always occur in the epiphyseal region and may extend to the articular surface of the bone. Campanacci and Cervelatti[8] have attempted to grade giant

cell tumors according to radiographic criteria; thus, grade 1 lesions are radiographically indolent, and grade 3 tumors are radiographically aggressive. Unfortunately, the majority of giant cell tumors are probably what Campanacci and colleagues refer to as grade 2, in which the radiographic appearance is aggressive but the tumor has not yet broken through cortical bone. Radiographic grading may be important in helping the surgeon decide on the appropriate treatment.

Grossly, the tumor consists of a red, soft tissue that typically extends up the subchondral bone at the articular surface. Microscopically, a giant cell tumor shows a combination of giant cells and mononuclear cells, with a more or less uniform distribution of the giant cells. Giant cell tumors that appear to be more aggressive histologically do not necessarily behave more aggressively clinically.[16]

The extent of surgery required to eradicate giant cell tumors is somewhat controversial. In the region of the elbow, particularly difficult problems may be encountered. The distal end of the humerus does not lend itself well to surgical excision by curettage unless the lesion is radiographically a grade 1 lesion. Total excision of the distal end of the humerus—although it would probably be curative and prevent local recurrence—creates a very serious problem for the reconstructive surgeon. Allograft replacement might be considered in this setting, but the decision about the method of treatment is often exceedingly difficult. Excision by curettage in other locations results in a local recurrence rate of approximately 25 percent. It is probably reasonable to accept this risk and to try curettage for the first treatment because the alternative of resection of the distal end of the humerus is so drastic (Fig. 73–6). However, if the tumor has already broken through the cortex into the surrounding soft structures, curettage is unlikely to be effective. For tumors of the proximal end of the ulna, curettage might be more reasonable because there is more bone to work with; hence, a larger margin of normal bone can be included in the resected specimen, whether resection is done by curettage or actual excision. Whenever possible, the treatment of choice is to pack the tumor cavity with methylmethacrylate (Fig. 73–7). This method of reconstruction has, in other locations, proved to be effective. If the proximal radial head is involved with a reasonably small tumor, it is probably best treated with simple excision.[27, 31]

Radiation therapy for benign giant cell tumors should be avoided if possible. In our previous experience, irradiation of benign giant cell tumors was accompanied by a significant risk of subsequent malignant transformation.

ANEURYSMAL BONE CYST

An aneurysmal bone cyst typically contains abundant benign giant cells in scattered zones and formerly was included among the giant cell tumors. It is different, however, because it nearly always contains blood-filled spaces, is somewhat fibrogenic, and usually has zones with osteoid formation and trabeculae of bone.

An aneurysmal bone cyst may arise de novo, or a similar reactive change may be seen in various benign and even in malignant tumors of bone. It is necessary to rule out any

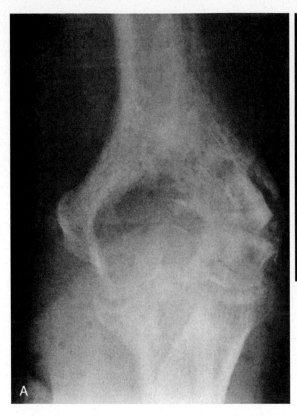

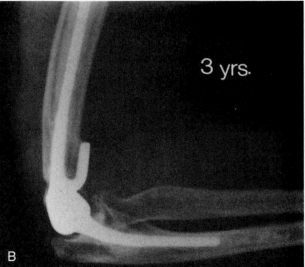

FIGURE 73–6 • *A,* Gross destruction of the distal humerus due to a locally aggressive giant cell tumor. The patient was treated by resection of the distal humerus and replacement with joint replacement arthroplasty. *B,* The arc of motion is 15 to 140 degrees with no pain, and there is no evidence of implant loosening at 3 years.

associated pathology, since the clinical behavior of the lesion depends on the nature of the underlying pathology.

In the Mayo Clinic's experience with 134 aneurysmal bone cysts unrelated to pre-existing disease, 43 percent

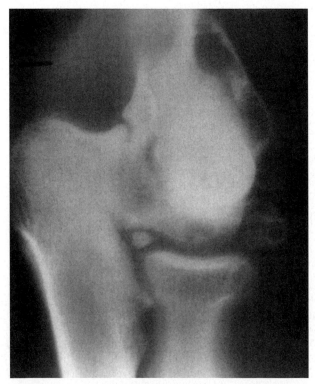

FIGURE 73–7 • Giant cell tumor involving the lateral condyle in a 25-year-old patient. The lesion was curetted, and the defect was filled with methylmethacrylate.

occurred in males. In contrast to the age of predilection for giant cell tumors, 78 percent of the patients were younger than 20 years of age. Only eight examples of aneurysmal bone cysts were found in the region of the elbow. Pain and swelling are the most common features.[13]

Radiographically, the diseased area is sometimes confusingly like that of a malignant tumor, but the zone of rarefaction is usually well circumscribed, eccentric, and associated with an obvious soft tissue extension of the process (Fig. 73–8). Classically, the soft tissue extension is produced by bulging of the periosteum and a resultant layer of radiographically visible new bone that delimits the periphery of the tumor. Fusiform expansion may be produced, especially when small bones such as a fibula or a rib are affected. The lesion is usually metaphyseal in location.[5, 17]

Pathologically, an aneurysmal bone cyst contains anastomosing cavernous spaces that usually constitute the bulk of the lesion. The spaces are usually filled with unclotted blood, which may well up into, but does not spurt from, the tumor when it is unroofed. The most important factor to recognize histologically is the benign quality of the constituent cells.[15, 44] Telangiectatic osteosarcoma may simulate aneurysmal bone cyst when viewed at low magnification.

Treatment is essentially the same as that for benign giant cell tumors. Curettage and bone grafting are usually required, and the majority of lesions treated in this way will be cured. Perhaps 25 percent of these cases will recur and require additional surgery.

Other Benign Bone Tumors and Tumor Simulators

Benign tumors of bone at the elbow other than those previously discussed may rarely be encountered (Fig. 73–

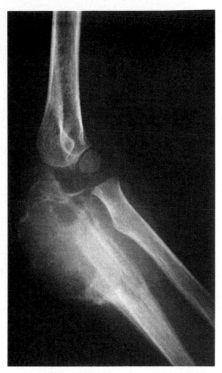

FIGURE 73–8 • Aneurysmal bone cyst of the ulna in a 5-year-old boy. Note circumscription of the mass, which is associated with destruction of the shaft and the end of the bone.

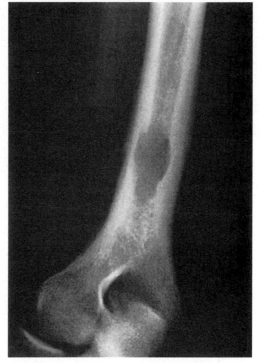

FIGURE 73–9 • Histiocytosis X producing a well-defined rarefaction of the humeral shaft. This completely benign lesion is associated with a good prognosis, especially if it is solitary.

9). In addition, a number of lesions may occur in any bone and may simulate or mimic a primary bone tumor (Figs. 73–10 through 73–12). Benign cartilage tumors are very rare at the elbow; nevertheless, they do occasionally occur (Fig. 73–13).

Malignant Bone Tumors

LYMPHOMA

Currently, the term *malignant lymphoma* is used for those small round cell tumors of bone that previously were referred to as reticulum cell sarcoma.[40] Lymphoma tends to occur in middle-aged or elderly adults; young persons are uncommonly affected. Patients with lymphoma generally present with pain and perhaps swelling in the region of the lesion. The tumor may arise primarily in any bone, including bones in the region of the elbow.

The radiographic features of lymphoma are nonspecific (Fig. 73–14). There is usually a diffuse, destructive, mottled appearance with indistinct margins. Variable degrees of sclerosis may be present in the lesion; the cortical bone is usually eroded, and the tumor may extend into the adjacent soft tissues. Periosteal new bone formation usually is not a prominent feature.

Grossly, lymphoma tissue is usually gray or white and very soft. Microscopically, malignant lymphomas fit into

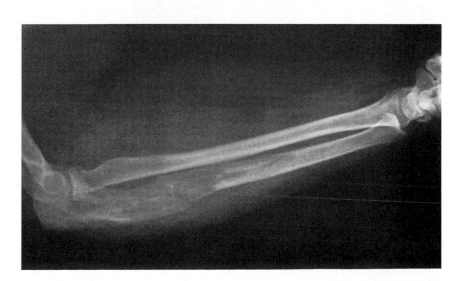

FIGURE 73–10 • Paget's disease of the proximal two thirds of the ulna. This classic lesion is associated with pathologic fracture and extends to the end of the bone. Paget's disease of bone is very rare in patients younger than 40 years.

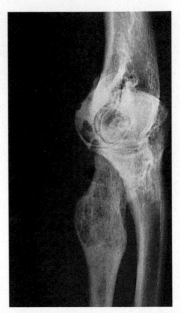

FIGURE 73–11 • Fibrous dysplasia producing extensive changes on both sides of the joint.

fourth of patients will have multiple bones involved. Even these patients do quite well. However, if there are other sites, such as liver, spleen, or lymph nodes, the survival rate decreases dramatically.

Lymphoma is generally treated with radiation therapy if there is only a solitary lesion of bone. For lymphoma in the region of the elbow joint, some morbidity can probably be expected from the radiation therapy. Radiation therapists generally try to avoid circumferential treatment of an extremity to allow some normal lymphatic channels to remain open. Failure to do so may result in significant swelling distal to the treatment area. It may be difficult or impossible to avoid treating the entire circumference of the extremity in the region of the elbow. In addition, when radiation exceeds approximately 4000 rad, radiation therapists generally try to direct treatment away from the articular surface.

There is no clear-cut or obvious advantage to the use of adjunctive chemotherapy at the time of initial treatment if only a solitary lesion is present.[47]

In general, lymphoma presenting primarily in bone has a long-term survival of about 60 percent.[6] However, no figures are available for the occurrence of lymphoma of bone specifically at the elbow.

EWING'S SARCOMA

Ewing's sarcoma may arise in any bone, including those in the region of the elbow. Ewing's sarcoma is more frequently found in children than adults; very young infants, however, very rarely have this tumor.

The usual radiographic appearance of Ewing's sarcoma

the group of small round cell tumors. Under low power, the tumor shows a permeative pattern. The infiltrate tends to fill up the marrow cavity without destroying medullary bone. When a diagnosis of lymphoma in bone is made, it is important to stage the disease process. If the disease is localized to one site, the prognosis is excellent.[38] About a

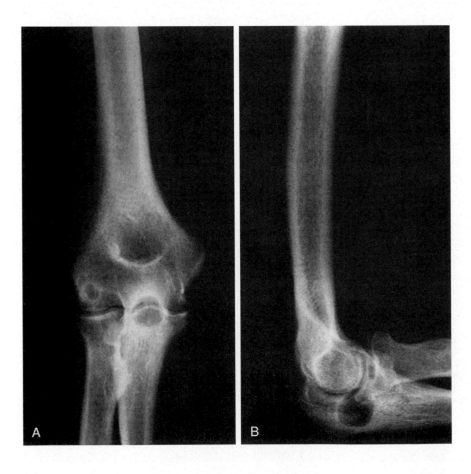

FIGURE 73–12 • A and B, Cyst of upper part of the ulna secondary to degenerative joint disease at the elbow.

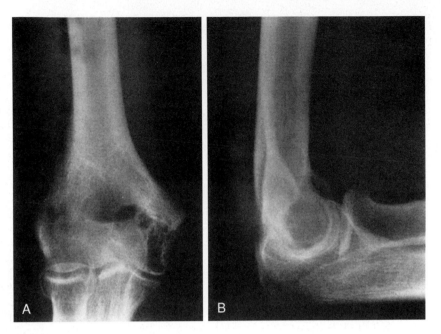

FIGURE 73–13 • *A* and *B*, Benign chon-droblastoma of the distal end of the humerus in a 25-year-old man. Note the discrete zone of rarefaction. Such lesions are more innocuous than giant cell tumors.

is that of a mottled or moth-eaten destructive lesion that may contain both lytic and blastic areas (Fig. 73–15). Although not pathognomonic, there is frequently periosteal reactive new bone, which may form layers, forming the "onion skin" appearance that is reported to be typical of this disease. The radiographic appearance combined with the presence of fever and an elevated erythrocyte sedimentation rate may lead to the erroneous diagnosis of osteomyelitis.[2]

Grossly, Ewing's sarcoma may be very soft or even semiliquid; indeed, the appearance may simulate the purulence of infection. Microscopically, Ewing's sarcoma is very cellular, composed of small round cells that are remarkably similar to one another. Periosteal new bone for-

mation, if present, may complicate the histologic interpretation.[45]

Treatment of Ewing's sarcoma of bone in the region of the elbow is similar to that for other sites. The local lesion is generally treated with radiation therapy, and systemic combination chemotherapy is generally used in an attempt to prevent micrometastases. Although there is a growing trend toward considering a larger role for surgery in the treatment of the primary lesion, there is little enthusiasm for resecting malignant tumors in the region of the elbow because it is difficult to achieve adequate margins in this region without damaging important normal structures.[42] Even if an adequate resection could be achieved, satisfactory reconstruction would be difficult or impossible. This is particularly true when one deals with children with open physes. The treatment for Ewing's sarcoma is the same as that for lymphoma in the region of the elbow.[4, 30] A major side effect is soft tissue fibrosis causing a stiff joint.

OSTEOSARCOMA

Osteosarcoma is the most common bone malignancy except for myeloma. Radiographically, osteosarcoma usually appears to be aggressive, with evidence of cortical destruction and reactive periosteal new bone formation. In the distal humerus, the classic "sunburst" appearance may be evident. The precise extent of the lesion may not be apparent on plain radiographs (Fig. 73–16). The tumor can usually be more accurately assessed with a technetium or gallium bone scan. Other studies, such as computed tomography, may be used to help determine the extent of soft tissue involvement if it is present. Magnetic resonance imaging may be helpful in further defining both the extent of soft tissue involvement and the extent of intramedullary involvement.

The reactive new bone formation at the periphery of the lesion should not be sampled for biopsy because this will simply lead to confusion in the interpretation of the histo-

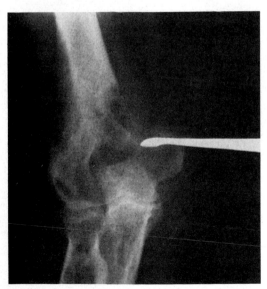

FIGURE 73–14 • Malignant lymphoma producing malignant-appearing destruction of the distal part of the humerus in a 60-year-old woman.

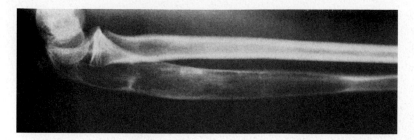

FIGURE 73–15 • Recurrent Ewing's sarcoma with a cyst-like lesion of the upper half of the ulna in a 21-year-old woman. The original tumor had been treated 10 years previously.

logic findings. If there is a soft tissue extension of the tumor, this is the area that is best to biopsy because it is usually the most malignant and the easiest to process in the pathology laboratory.

About one half of these tumors are predominantly fibrous or cartilaginous, and the remainder are predominantly bone forming. Because any one of these three types of differentiation may predominate, the lesions may be subtyped into fibroblastic, chondroblastic, or osteoblastic osteosarcoma. This subclassification may be important because the osteoblastic subtype appears to have a worse prognosis than the other two subtypes.[14, 18, 34, 54–56]

Malignant fibrous histiocytoma can also show areas of matrix production.[19] Yet, only one of the 83 tumors listed as malignant fibrous histiocytoma in the Mayo Clinic files occurred in the elbow region. From a practical standpoint, the clinical management of this malignancy is essentially identical with that of osteosarcoma (Fig. 73–17). In the author's own experience, 8 to 10 percent of patients with newly diagnosed osteosarcoma are found to have metastatic

disease, either by plain radiography or computed tomography.[51]

The usual treatment of osteosarcoma, as of other radioresistant malignant bone tumors, is surgical ablation. For many years, amputation was required. However, today the majority of patients with osteosarcoma can be managed with various limb salvage procedures. Neoadjuvant chemotherapy is generally employed before one proceeds with surgery, and additional chemotherapy is usually offered after surgery. The prognosis for patients with osteosarcoma today is much improved; 60 to 80 percent of such patients may be long-term survivors.[8]

METASTATIC TUMORS

There is no particular predilection for metastatic disease to involve the elbow. Yet extensive destruction is observed on occasion from several tumor types. Treatment is most commonly joint replacement (Fig. 73–18). In the author's experience with 13 prosthetic replacements for elbow tumors, 6 were for metastatic lesions to the distal humerus: 3 renal cell carcinomas, 3 breast adenocarcinomas.[52]

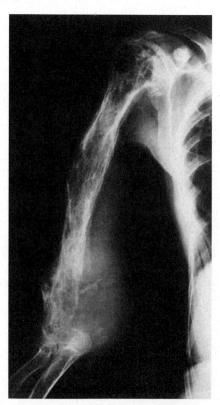

FIGURE 73–16 • Grade 4 osteosarcoma of the distal end of the humerus in a patient with Paget's disease of the entire bone.

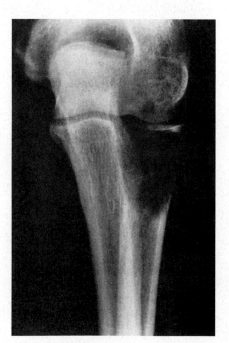

FIGURE 73–17 • Grade 4 malignant fibrous histiocytoma producing malignant-appearing destruction of the upper part of the ulna in a 45-year-old man.

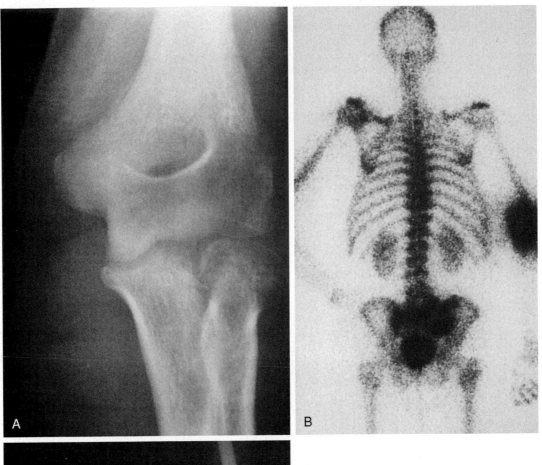

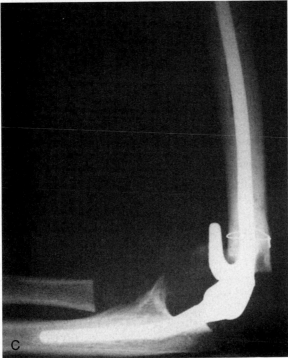

FIGURE 73–18 • *A,* Metastatic adenocarcinoma involving the lateral aspect of the left elbow, including the capitellum and radial head. *B,* The extent of involvement is revealed most dramatically by technetium bone scan. *C,* Complete resection of the distal humerus and proximal radius and insertion of a Mayo modified Coonrad implant was effective in restoring function within 3 weeks of surgery.

SOFT TISSUE TUMORS

Mesenchymal soft tissue tumors, especially the malignant types, are probably the least understood of all tumors. There are numerous varieties of mesenchymal tumors, but most of them are rarely encountered. A full discussion of all of these tumors is well beyond the scope of this chapter.

Many benign soft tissue tumors are commonly encountered; however, because some soft tissue sarcomas may grow very slowly, both the patient and the physician may be misled into thinking that a soft tissue mass is benign. When this happens, a definitive diagnosis may be delayed, sometimes for years. When the patient does seek medical attention, it is not uncommon for the physician to perform a biopsy procedure that may jeopardize subsequent surgical care. As with bone tumors, proper placement of the biopsy incision is critical, and any subsequent resection surgery for malignant tumors demands that the biopsy site be included in the resected specimen. If the biopsy incision is not well placed, inclusion of the site at surgery may be difficult or impossible to achieve. If the mass is small and is situated in a favorable location, it is far preferable to perform an excisional biopsy, leaving a margin of normal tissue on all aspects of the suspected lesion. If an incisional biopsy is done, sufficient tissue must be removed to allow adequate representative sampling of the tumor so that the pathologist can arrive at the correct diagnosis. Perhaps no other factor is as important in the management of patients with soft tissue tumors as the proper performance of the biopsy procedure.

Patients may complain of a lump or pain, or both. Small painful lumps may represent benign tumors—neurilemoma (schwannoma), neurofibroma, vascular myoma, glomus tumor, or fat necrosis. Sometimes, these lesions may be occult, particularly when they are small and buried in the deep soft tissues. When the patient complains of well-localized pain, these entities should be considered.

The presence of a slowly growing mass that has been present perhaps for several years should lead to a suspicion of sarcomas such as synovial sarcoma, clear-cell sarcoma, or even a well-differentiated sarcoma of a more common histologic type, such as a liposarcoma or malignant fibrous histiocytoma. When the lesion is located in the upper extremity, epithelioid sarcoma should be considered.

Some of the commonly encountered soft tissue lumps may be reasonably diagnosed on the basis of the history and physical examination alone. This is particularly true for lipomas, which are commonly encountered by all physicians. When the lesion is asymptomatic and has characteristic features on the clinical examination, biopsy is probably not necessary. However, caution is needed and follow-up assessment is appropriate because even the most benign-appearing soft tissue tumor may be malignant.

If a sarcoma is suspected, then a full battery of routine laboratory tests should be obtained. Plain radiographs may be helpful, particularly if the radiologist uses special soft tissue techniques. Calcium or even ossification may be present within the lesion. In addition, the relationship of the lesion to the surrounding structures may be ascertained. This is particularly true if there is erosion of the underlying skeleton. If the lesion is totally lucent and has very sharply circumscribed margins, it may be a lipoma. If, however, the lesion has irregular margins and a nonhomogeneous density, sarcomatous change must be suspected. Magnetic resonance imaging is particularly valuable in the assessment of soft tissue tumors.

In summary, for soft tissue tumors, when the diagnosis is in doubt, as much information as possible should be obtained before the performance of the biopsy procedure.

Benign Soft Tissue Tumors

LIPOMA

Lipoma is probably the most frequently encountered benign soft tissue neoplasm and is the most common tumor in the elbow region. It is usually solitary, but multiple lipomas have occurred. The tumor is simply a localized collection of adipose tissue that is histologically and chemically similar to ordinary fat.

Most lipomas are small, asymptomatic, and relatively dormant in that they seem to remain approximately the same size. Occasionally, however, the tumor may grow and become symptomatic. If there is trauma to the area, necrosis may develop within the lipoma, and this is usually symptomatic. Most lipomas consist almost entirely of adipose tissue; however, there may be increased vascularity, in which case the lesion is referred to as angiolipoma.[20]

Most of these lesions can be easily and confidently diagnosed on the basis of the clinical examination alone; however, some lipomas may not have the clinical characteristics of the usual subcutaneous lipoma and may require further diagnostic modalities.

Surgical excision should be considered for lipomas that increase in size, are symptomatic or cosmetically undesirable, or interfere with function and in situations when the diagnosis is not certain (Fig. 73–19). For most such tumors, a simple marginal excision is all that is indicated. The vulnerability of the neurovascular structures is of particular concern for lipoma of the antecubital space. When a lipoma is located within the belly of a muscle, it may be necessary to sacrifice some normal muscle tissue on all aspects to minimize the risk of local recurrence. At the elbow, this can cause permanent stiffness.

GANGLION

A ganglion is a cystic lesion generally found in the hands, wrists, and feet, but it may be found less commonly in the region of the elbow. A true ganglion has no or only a poorly defined synovial lining. Although the ganglion may connect with the joint, it does not always do so; indeed, the lesion may occur within a tendon, in a muscle, or even on occasion in bone. Treatment is simple excision, ensuring that the entire lesion has been removed and, as with the lipoma, that the neurovascular elements are carefully protected. Not all ganglia require excision, however, and most patients may be treated symptomatically.

MYXOMA

A myxoma occasionally occurs in the soft tissues at the elbow. This lesion is soft, well circumscribed, and myxoi-

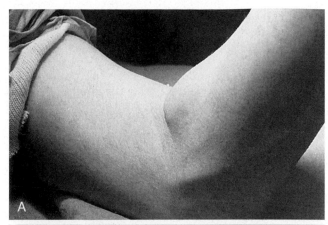

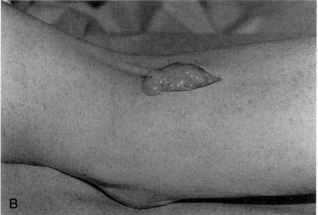

FIGURE 73–19 • Expanding, prominent soft tissue mass in the cubital space *(A)* was found to be a benign lipoma *(B).*

dal. Histologically, the lesion is hypocellular and contains stellate cells in a myxoid stream. A myxoma is relatively small and is usually encountered in the superficial soft tissues. It is not uncommon for this tumor to arise within the substance of a major muscle.

The treatment for myxoma is excision; however, a wide excision, rather than a marginal resection, is probably indicated because this tumor tends to recur if it is marginally excised.

PIGMENTED VILLONODULAR SYNOVITIS

In the past, pigmented villonodular synovitis had various names, including xanthoma, xanthogranuloma, giant cell tumor of the tendon sheath, and myeloplaxoma. This disease probably belongs in the middle of the spectrum of diseases, within the general category of fibrous histiocytoma. It involves the synovium, bursae, or tendon sheaths. The knee is the most common site of involvement. In the authors' experience, only two cases occurred in the elbow joint.[41] This is not surprising, since Pimpalnerkar[41] reports that only 18 cases have been cited in the literature through 1998.

Clinically, there are two forms of the disease: nodular and diffuse. The nodular or localized form is probably most frequently encountered in the small joints of the fingers, whereas the diffuse form is most commonly found in the knee joint. At the elbow, swelling, with a suggestion

of increased thickening of the synovium, may be present, but motion loss is always present. Radiographs may reveal cystic erosions on either side of the joint (Fig. 73–20). When erosions are found and there is no loss of joint space and no demineralization of the surrounding bone, the diagnosis should be suspected. In most cases of pigmented villonodular synovitis, however, there is no bony erosion but there is evidence of lobular swelling of the soft tissues.[3]

Microscopic study shows a stromal background of reticulin and collagen fibers, in which various different cells may be found. The firm, nodular lesions have more collagenous stroma, whereas the soft villous lesions have less stroma.

In the nodular form, the nodule may be simply excised with the expectation that a cure will be achieved in most cases. However, the results of treatment of the diffuse form are likely to be followed by local recurrence, which is more frequent when there is evidence of bony erosion. Even multiple synovectomies have not always been curative; because of this, various alternative treatments have been attempted. Radiation therapy has been used, but there is no convincing evidence that such treatment will actually eliminate the disease and prevent local recurrences. High doses of radiation are avoided at the elbow joint. Synovectomy is the treatment of choice, but recurrence is at least 33 percent.[41] If synovectomy leads to symptomatic local recurrence, arthrodesis is considered in most joints. At the elbow, however, because this joint does poorly with an arthrodesis, replacement arthroplasty would appear to be the treatment of choice.

SYNOVIAL CHONDROMATOSIS

Chondromatosis is a benign, tumorous, multifocal, chondromatous, or chondro-osseous metaplastic proliferation involving the subsynovial connective tissue of joints, tendon sheaths, or bursae. The process can involve any joint. The average age of the patients is about 40 years; males are affected more than females. Symptoms include pain and limited motion. The duration of symptoms may be long or

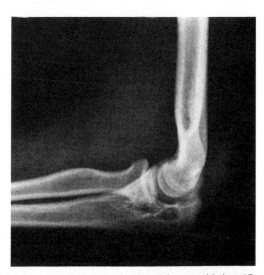

FIGURE 73–20 • Pigmented villonodular synovitis in a 17-year-old girl, with a 3-year history of pain and swelling. Note cystic erosions.

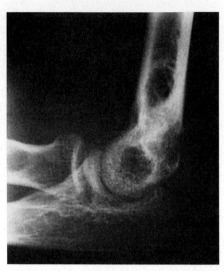

FIGURE 73–21 • Synovial chondromatosis of the elbow. Note that a small mineralized focus is evident in the antecubital fossa.

relatively short before diagnosis is made. In the Mayo Clinic series, only two thirds of the radiographs showed radiopaque masses (Fig. 73–21).[36] Diagnosis is difficult because the radiograph may not reveal ossified bodies even when they are present.

When the radiographic diagnosis is indefinite and symptoms persist without any other obvious cause, diagnostic arthrotomy or arthroscopy is indicated. Because osteochondromatosis may be sharply localized and may not be a diffuse condition of the entire synovium, careful inspection of the whole synovial lining is important. Generally, diagnosis can be made by the gross appearance and confirmed by biopsy. Grossly, nodules of cartilage of varying sizes are seen embedded in the synovium that may be markedly thickened. Histologically, nodules of cartilage are found within the synovium. The authors have seen one example of synovial chondromatosis of the elbow undergo malignant change to chondrosarcoma.

The treatment of osteochondromatosis consists of removing any loose osteochondromatous bodies and the involved synovium from which they arise. In general, complete synovectomy is necessary and is not done arthroscopically, since complete exposure of the elbow joint from an extensile posterior approach is required. The condition may recur because nests of synovium may be left behind. If this happens, a second arthrotomy is necessary. Frequently, the long-standing synovial osteochondromatosis creates secondary osteoarthritis (see Chapters 74 and 76).

MYOSITIS OSSIFICATIONS (HETEROTOPIC OR ECTOPIC OSSIFICATION)

Heterotopic ossification, often erroneously called myositis ossificans, may occur near the elbow, either in muscle or in other soft tissue. In its early, or "florid," stage, there may be such pronounced cellular activity that it may be mistaken for sarcoma.[1] The relative rarity of this disease has delayed understanding of the peculiar tissue reaction associated with it. The topic has been thoroughly reviewed in Chapter 32.

A similar non-neoplastic benign, reactive process may

occur in the deeper portions of the skin. The poorly defined small mass that is found may also show prominent mitotic activity. The lesion is called proliferative fasciitis and has been mistaken for entities such as liposarcoma or fibrosarcoma.[10] The rapidly proliferating cells again do not show true anaplasia. Another related entity is proliferative myositis.[24] In this condition, there is a tumefactive, intramuscular proliferation of benign fibroblastic cells, but no discernible osseous metaplasia. Mitotic activity may be pronounced, making it possible to mistake this lesion for a malignant tumor.

Malignant Soft Tissue Tumors

SYNOVIAL SARCOMA

Synovial sarcoma, or synovioma, is a malignant soft tissue tumor that usually arises in the extremities or limb girdles; about 70 percent of lesions involve the lower extremity, most commonly the thigh, but this tumor does occur in the region of the elbow. In the Mayo Clinic experience, only the tumors of about 20 percent of patients had suggestive evidence of origin from anatomic synovium.[59] This tumor can be found in patients of any age, but young or middle-aged adults seem to be most commonly affected.

Symptoms may be present for many years before diagnosis. In the Mayo Clinic experience, the average duration of symptoms before diagnosis was 2½ years. The radiographic examination may be particularly helpful because about a third of patients with synovial sarcoma show evidence of calcification. When calcification is found in a soft tissue tumor, synovial sarcoma should be included in the differential diagnosis.

The tumor is lobular, circumscribed, and gray and may contain areas of calcification, hemorrhage, necrosis, or cyst formation. Classically, synovial sarcoma has a bimorphic histologic pattern; that is, a combination of slender spindle cells and larger epithelial-appearing cells that may form glands or even show squamous change.

Close cooperation between the pathologist and the surgeon is essential if the diagnosis is to be made at surgery. Local excision of the tumor generally results in a local recurrence; with local recurrence, the prognosis for survival is lessened. In the Mayo Clinic experience, the overall 5-year survival rate was 23 percent, with a median survival of 39 months.[57] However, for patients treated after 1960, the 5-year survival rate has been 55 percent and the 10-year rate has been 38 percent. Patients who had the best prognosis were those treated with wide excision or radical surgery. Today, the authors usually combine radiation therapy and surgery; with this approach local recurrence occurs in only about 5 percent of cases. We do not routinely employ lymphadenectomy unless the regional nodes are clinically involved.

LIPOSARCOMA

The pathologic diagnosis of liposarcoma may be difficult, especially when the lesion is histologically of low grade. A lipoma that shows evidence of growth should be suspected of being malignant. Roentgenograms are not as diagnostic for liposarcoma as they are for lipoma, but the combination of more dense and less dense tissues may be characteristic of liposarcoma. Computed tomography is very helpful, not only in defining the extent of the lesion but also in showing relative densities. Histologically, liposarcomas are recognized because of their component of malignant lipoblasts.

Liposarcomas may arise in any part of the body and are occasionally found at the elbow. Older adults are more commonly affected than younger persons.

The extent of treatment depends, at least in part, on both the size and the grade of the tumor. Lesions that are grade 1 or grade 2 probably can be safely excised with a margin of normal tissue on all aspects, but this can be very difficult at the elbow. If the lesion recurs, it can probably be excised without the need for radical surgery. However, the higher-grade lesion should probably be treated with wide resection and perhaps with radical resection unless the tumor can be totally and widely removed without sacrifice of limb function. This is difficult to do with tumors in the region of the elbow, and amputation may be necessary. As with other soft tissue sarcomas, the authors usually combine radiation therapy and surgery. In the Mayo Clinic experience, more than 50 percent of all patients treated for liposarcoma may expect to survive for 5 years and be free from evidence of disease progression.[43]

MALIGNANT FIBROUS HISTIOCYTOMA

Malignant fibrous histiocytoma is now the most commonly encountered malignant soft tissue tumor of the extremities and, as noted earlier, may also occur in the bone. The upper extremity and, more specifically, the region of the elbow are not uncommonly affected by this tumor. This tumor can arise in any age group. As with other malignant soft tissue tumors, there are no unique clinical or radiographic features characteristic of this lesion. Both computed tomography and magnetic resonance imaging have been used to define the extent and relationship of the tumor with surrounding structures.

Grossly, this tumor is usually soft and pink or yellow. It

may vary in consistency and color from patient to patient and, indeed, even in different areas of the same tumor. There may also be an area of firm, white tumor adjacent to a yellow, mucoid, necrotic area. Tumors arising in the upper extremity in general tend to be smaller than those arising in the buttock or lower extremity, probably because they are noticed by the patient earlier in their evolution. Microscopically, the lesion may vary from the most benign-appearing spindle cells with small nuclei and relatively few mitotic figures, such as those seen in a grade 1 lesion, to the wildly anaplastic, bizarre histiocytic cells found in grade 4 lesions. There is growing evidence that the grade of the lesion as manifested by anaplasia is a more important predictor of behavior than are the histologic subtypes.

There is no one universally acceptable treatment for this lesion. Relatively small tumors may be excised with a margin of normal tissue on all aspects. Larger lesions or those that are histologically higher grade require a more aggressive approach. In this situation, the authors now favor a course of preoperative radiation therapy using approximately 5000 rad, followed after several weeks by excision of the lesion with a margin of normal tissue on all aspects. Adjunctive chemotherapy has not been helpful in our experience.

EPITHELIOID SARCOMA

Epithelioid sarcoma is a rare, slowly growing malignant tumor that usually begins in the superficial tissues of the hand or forearm and may occur at the elbow. The tumor is made up of small, poorly defined tumor nodules composed of epithelioid cells or histiocytic aggregates. Sometimes, central necrosis in these aggregates of cells suggests that the disease is a granulomatous infection. There is often a delay in recognition of the malignant nature of the disease, and the long-term prognosis for life is poor. Rarely, the tumor erodes into underlying bones (Figs. 73–22 and 73–23). Lymphatic or hematogenous metastasis is common, especially in the later stages of this disease.

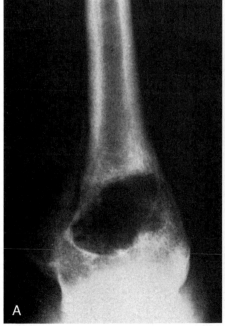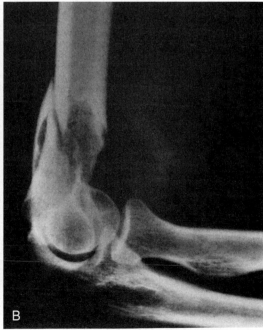

FIGURE 73–22 • A and B, Epithelioid sarcoma that has eroded into and destroyed much of the distal part of the humerus in a 27-year-old woman.

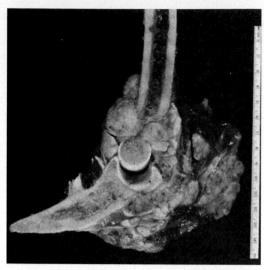

FIGURE 73-23 • Another epithelioid sarcoma that has caused osseous destruction at the elbow.

Treatment for cure requires wide excision. Marginal or intralesional excision almost always results in tumor recurrence and subsequent disease progression. The relatively slow growth of the tumor and the unusual nature of the histology may tend to dissuade the surgeon from performing adequate surgery.

REFERENCES

1. Ackerman, L. N.: Extra-osseous localized non-neoplastic bone and cartilage formation (so-called myositis ossificans): Clinical and pathologic confusion with malignant neoplasms. J. Bone Joint Surg. 40A:279, 1958.
2. Angervall, L., and Enzinger, F. M.: Extraskeletal neoplasm resembling Ewing's sarcoma. Cancer 36:240, 1975.
3. Atmore, W. G., Dahlin, D. C., and Ghormley, R. K.: Pigmented villonodular synovitis: A clinical and pathologic study. Minn. Med. 39:196, 1956.
4. Bacci, G., Picci, P., Gitelis, S., Borghi, A., and Campanacci, M.: The treatment of localized Ewing's sarcoma: The experience at the Istituto Ortopedico Rizzoli in 163 cases treated with and without adjuvant chemotherapy. Cancer 49:1561, 1982.
5. Bonaledarpeun, A., Levy, W. M., and Aegerter, E.: Primary and secondary aneurysmal bone cyst: A radiologic study of 75 cases. Radiology 126:75, 1978.
6. Boston, H. C., Jr., Dahlin, D. C., Ivins, J. C., and Cupps, R. E.: Malignant lymphomas (so-called reticulum cell sarcoma) of bone. Cancer 34:1131, 1974.
7. Brabants, K., Geens, S., and van Damme, B.: Subperiosteal juxta-articular osteoid osteoma. J. Bone Joint Surg. 68:320, 1986.
8. Campanacci, M., and Cervelatti, G.: Osteosarcoma: A review of 345 cases. Ital. J. Orthop. Traumatol. 1:5, 1975.
9. Campanacci, M., Giunti, A., and Olmi, R.: Giant cell tumors of bone: A study of 209 cases with long-term follow-up in 130. Ital. J. Orthop. Traumatol. 1:249, 1975.
10. Chung, E. B., and Enzinger, F. M.: Proliferative fasciitis. Cancer 36:1450, 1975.
11. Corbett, J. M., Wilde, A. H., McCormick, L. J., and Evarts, C. M.: Intra-articular osteoid osteoma, a diagnostic problem. Clin. Orthop. 98:225, 1974.
12. Cronemeyer, R., Kirchmer, N. A., Desmet, A. A., and Neff, J. R.: Intra-articular osteoid osteoma of the humerus simulating synovitis of the elbow: A case report. J. Bone Joint Surg. 63A:1172, 1981.
13. Dahlin, D. C.: Bone Tumors: General Aspects and Data on 6221 Cases. Springfield, IL, Charles C Thomas, 1978, p. 445.
14. Dahlin, D. C.: Pathology of osteosarcoma. Clin. Orthop. 111:23, 1975.
15. Dahlin, D. C., Besse, B. E., Jr., Pugh, D. G., and Ghormley, R. K.: Aneurysmal bone cysts. Radiology 64:56, 1955.
16. Dahlin, D. C., Cupps, R. E., and Johnson, E. W., Jr.: Giant cell tumor: A study of 195 cases. Cancer 25:1061, 1970.
17. Dahlin, D. C., and McLeod, R. A.: Aneurysmal bone cyst and other non-neoplastic conditions. Skeletal Radiol. 8:243, 1982.
18. Dahlin, D. C., and Unni, K. K.: Osteosarcoma of bone and its important recognizable varieties. Am. J. Surg. Pathol. 1:61, 1977.
19. Dahlin, D. C., Unni, K. K., and Matsuno, T.: Malignant (fibrous) histiocytoma of bone—fact or fancy? Cancer 39:1508, 1977.
20. Dionne, G. P., and Seemayer, T. A.: Infiltrating lipomas and angiolipomas revisited. Cancer 33:732, 1974.
21. Edeiken, J., and Hodes, P. J.: Roentgen Diagnosis of Diseases of Bone, Vols. 1 and 2, 2nd ed. Baltimore, Williams & Wilkins, 1973.
22. Enneking, W. F.: Musculoskeletal Tumor Surgery, Vol. 1. New York, Churchill Livingstone, 1983.
23. Enneking, W. F., Spanier, S. S., and Goodman, M. A.: A system for the surgical staging of musculoskeletal sarcoma. Clin. Orthop. 153:106, 1980.
24. Enzinger, F. M., and Dulcey, F.: Proliferative myositis: Report of thirty-three cases. Cancer 20:2213, 1967.
25. Ghelman, B., Francesca, M., Thompson, F. M., William, D., and Arnold, W. D.: Intra-operative radioactive localization of an osteoid osteoma: Case report. J. Bone Joint Surg. 63A:826, 1981.
26. Gil-Albarova, J., and Amillo, S.: Osteoblastoma causing rigidity of the elbow: A case report. Acta Orthop. Scand. 62:602, 1991.
27. Goldenberg, R. R., Campbell, C. J., and Bonfiglio, M.: Giant cell tumor of bone: An analysis of 218 cases. J. Bone Joint Surg. 52A:621, 1970.
28. Harsha, W. N.: The natural history of osteocartilaginous exostoses (osteochondroma). Am. Surg. 20:65, 1954.
29. Jaffe, H. L., and Lichtenstein, L.: Osteoid-osteoma: Further experience with this benign tumor of bone; with special reference to cases showing the lesion in relation to shaft cortices and commonly misclassified as instances of sclerosing non-suppurative osteomyelitis or cortical-bone abscess. J. Bone Joint Surg. 22:645, 1940.
30. Johnson, R. E., and Pomeroy, T. C.: Evaluation of therapeutic results in Ewing's sarcoma. A.J.R. 123:583, 1975.
31. Larsson, S. E., Lorentzon, R., and Boquist, L.: Giant-cell tumor of bone: A demographic, clinical, and histopathological study of all cases recorded in the Swedish Cancer Registry for the years 1958 through 1968. J. Bone Joint Surg. 57A:167, 1975.
32. Lenoble, E., Sergent, A., and Goutallier, D.: Preoperative, intraoperative, and immediate postoperative skeletal scintigraphy to locate and facilitate excision of an osteoid osteoma of the coronoid process. J. Shoulder Elbow Surg. Sept./Oct.:323, 1994.
33. Marcove, R. C., and Freiberger, R. H.: Osteoid osteoma of the elbow: A diagnostic problem. Report of four cases. J. Bone Joint Surg. 48A:1185, 1966.
34. Matsuno, T., Unni, K. K., McLeod, R. A., and Dahlin, D. C.: Telangiectatic osteogenic sarcoma. Cancer 38:2538, 1976.
35. Moser, R. P., Jr., Kransdorf, M. J., Brower, A. C., Hudson, T., Aoki, J., Berrey, B. H., and Sweet, D. E.: Osteoid osteoma of the elbow: A review of six cases. Skeletal Radiol. 19:181, 1990.
36. Murphy, F. P., Dahlin, D. C., and Sullivan, C. R.: Articular synovial chondromatosis. J. Bone Joint Surg. 44A:77, 1962.
37. Norman, A., and Dorfman, H. D.: Osteoid osteoma inducing pronounced overgrowth and deformity of bone. Clin. Orthop. 110:223, 1975.
38. Ostrowski, M. L., Unni, K. K., Banks, P. M., Shives, T. C., Evans, R. G., O'Connell, M. J., Taylor, W. F.: Malignant lymphoma of bone. Cancer 58:2646, 1986.
39. Otsuka, N. Y., Hastings, D. E., and Fornasier, V. L.: Osteoid osteoma of the elbow: A report of six cases. J. Hand Surg. 17:458, 1992.
40. Parker, F., Jr., and Jackson, H., Jr.: Primary reticulum cell sarcoma of bone. Surg. Gynecol. Obstet. 68:45, 1939.
41. Pimpalnerkar, A., Barton, E., and Sibly, T. F.: Pigmented villonodular synovitis of the elbow. J. Shoulder Elbow Surg. 7:71, 1998.
42. Pritchard, D. J., Dahlin, D. C., Dauphine, R. T., Taylor, W. E., and Beabout, J. W.: Ewing's sarcoma: A clinicopathological and statistical analysis of patients surviving five years or longer. J. Bone Joint Surg. 57A:10, 1975.
43. Reszel, P. A., Soule, E. H., and Coventry, M. B.: Liposarcoma of the extremities and limb girdles: A study of two hundred twenty-two cases. J. Bone Joint Surg. 48A:229, 1966.

44. Sanerkin, N. G., Mott, M. G., and Roylance, J.: An unusual intraosseous lesion with fibroblastic, osteoclastic, osteoblastic, aneurysmal, and fibromyxoid elements: "Solid" variant of aneurysmal bone cyst. Cancer 51:2278, 1983.

45. Schajowicz, F.: Tumors and Tumor-like Lesions of Bones and Joints. New York, Springer-Verlag, 1981, p. 581.

46. Schajowicz, F., and Lemos, C.: Osteoid osteoma and osteoblastoma: Closely related entities of osteoblastic derivation. Acta Orthop. Scand. 41:272, 1970.

47. Schwartz, H. S., Unni, K. K., and Pritchard, D. J.: Pigmented villonodular synovitis. Clin. Orthop. 247:243, 1989.

48. Shoji, H., and Miller, T. R.: Primary reticulum cell sarcoma of bone: Significance of clinical features upon the prognosis. Cancer 28:1234, 1971.

49. Sim, F. H., Dahlin, D. C., and Beabout, J. W.: Osteoid osteoma: Diagnostic problems. J. Bone Joint Surg. 57A:154, 1975.

50. Snarr, J. W., Abell, M. R., and Martel, W.: Lymphofollicular synovitis with osteoid osteoma. Radiology 106:557, 1973.

51. Spanos, P. K., Payne, W. S., Ivins, J. C., and Pritchard, D. J.: Pulmonary resection for metastatic osteogenic sarcoma. J. Bone Joint Surg. 58A:624, 1976.

52. Sperling, J. W., Pritchard, D. J., and Morrey, B. F.: Total elbow arthroplasty following resection of tumors at the elbow. Clin. Orthop. (in press).

53. Swee, R. G., McLeod, R. A., and Beabout, J. W.: Osteoid osteoma: Detection, diagnosis, and localization. Radiology 130:117, 1979.

54. Taylor, W. F., Ivins, D. C., Edmonson, J. H., and Pritchard, D. J.: Trends and variability in survival from osteosarcoma. Mayo Clin. Proc. 53:695, 1978.

55. Unni, K. K., Dahlin, D. C., and Beabout, J. W.: Periosteal osteogenic sarcoma. Cancer 37:2476, 1976.

56. Unni, K. K., Dahlin, D. C., Beabout, J. W., and Ivins, J. C.: Parosteal osteogenic sarcoma. Cancer 37:2466, 1976.

57. Weatherby, R. P., Dahlin, D. C., and Ivins, J. C.: Postradiation sarcoma of bone: Review of 78 Mayo Clinic cases. Mayo Clin. Proc. 56:294, 1981.

58. Weber, K., and Morrey, B. F.: Osteoid osteoma of the elbow. J. Bone Joint Surg. (submitted).

59. Wright, P. H., Sim, F. H., Soule, E. H., and Taylor, W. F.: Synovial sarcoma. J. Bone Joint Surg. 64A:112, 1982.

CHAPTER 74

Loose Bodies

• BERNARD F. MORREY

• TABLE 74–1 • Classification of Loose Bodies
Congenital (developmental)
Medial epicondyle—accessory ossification
Olecranon—os patella cubiti
Olecranon fossa—os supratrochleare dorsale
Acquired
Articular fracture—osteochondritis dissecans
Degenerative
Synovial proliferation—synovial chondromatosis

First described in the knee by Ambroise Paré[29] in 1558, loose bodies occur in the elbow with a frequency second only to that in the knee.[30] As in other joints, it is sometimes difficult to distinguish with certainty between ossification centers and acquired lesions (Table 74–1).

ACCESSORY OSSIFICATION

Accessory ossicles are a normal variation at the elbow and may be confused with acquired processes. Three sites for accessory ossicles about the elbow have been described: distal to the medial epicondyle; proximal to the tip of the olecranon (the patella cubiti); and in the olecranon fossa (the os supratrochleare dorsale[7]) (Fig. 74–1).

Some ossicles show fragmentation, possibly secondary to trauma. This is sometimes mistaken for a manifestation of osteochondritis dissecans. Even though accessory ossicles may be considered a normal variation, they may well cause symptoms after trauma and require treatment.

Medial Epicondyle Accessory Ossicle

A smooth, rounded ossicle is sometimes seen just distal to the medial epicondyle and is considered an accessory ossicle to the medial epicondyle.[17] Probably more than in any other site, because calcification can follow injury to the medial collateral ligament, whether the radiographic lesion reflects a traumatic or a congenital insult is often confusing.[37] However, a discrete, rounded, smooth ossicle in patients who have no history of injury to this region suggests an accessory structure (Fig. 74–2). An irregular or misshapen medial epicondyle suggests a traumatic origin. Nev-

ertheless, the formation of a fully developed medial epicondyle does not necessarily prove the diagnosis, because in a child the medial epicondyle can remodel and appear normal in later years.

Patella Cubiti

The so-called patella cubiti is rare but has been thoroughly described in earlier literature,[15, 18, 34] and a thorough review has been presented by Habbe.[15] This ossicle occurs in the triceps tendon near its insertion and is considered a true sesamoid bone.[19] The proximal position is so characteristic in appearance that there should be little doubt about its origin (Fig. 74–3). This structure should be distinguished from an avulsed olecranon apophysis, which appears farther distal, and from a calcified olecranon bursa. Because of its superficial location, this ossicle may be subject to direct trauma and even fracture,[4] but the injury generally responds to symptomatic treatment.

Os Supratrochleare Dorsale

The radiographic density observed in the olecranon fossa has been a source of controversy. Characteristically, the ossicle has a smooth and round or oval shape that is often best seen in the lateral projection but is also demonstrated in the anteroposterior view (Fig. 74–4). In early descriptions of this entity it was considered to be a form of osteochondritis dissecans of the trochlea.[26] The precise origin of this osseous structure is still the subject of some discussion, and trauma is often blamed.[2] This opinion is supported by the mechanism of injury. With hyperextension, impaction of the tip of the olecranon into the olecranon fossa may cause a spur to develop at the tip of the olecranon. Conceivably it can be dislodged, form a nidus,

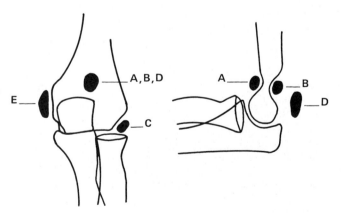

FIGURE 74–1 • Identification of accessory ossicles: *A*, Anterior supratrochleare; *B*, posterior supratrochleare; *C*, radial epicondyle; *D*, of the olecranon; and *E*, medial epicondyle. (From Gudmundsen, T. E., and Ostensen, H.: Accessory ossicles in the elbow. Acta Orthop. Scand. **58**:132, 1987.)

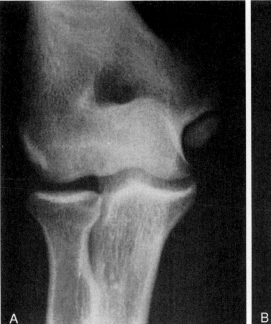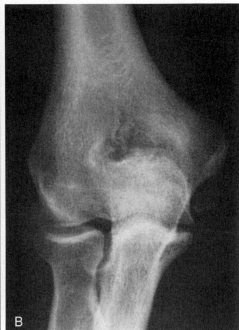

FIGURE 74-2 • *A*, The occurrence of a smooth ossicle at the inferior aspect of the medial epicondyle without a history of injury represents an accessory ossicle. *B*, An earlier medial epicondyle fracture may have the same appearance, but the epicondyle may remodel in young patients (see Chapter 17). Note the loose bodies in the olecranon fossa.

and grow into the characteristic os supratrochleare. Certainly, this mechanism has been implicated in the formation of loose bodies in the olecranon fossa (Fig. 74-5).[36] The problem has been discussed in detail and clarified by Obermann and Loose, who concluded that the os supratrochleare dorsale is most likely a congenital accessory bone.[27] Rather than being caused by trauma, it is subject to injury that produces secondary chondrometaplasia and resulting symptoms. When this occurs, the ossicle may look damaged and have an irregular margin.

Thus, the distinction between an ossicle caused by trauma and an existing one subjected to trauma remains obscure (see Fig. 74-5). Regardless of the source, the treatment is obvious. Mere radiographic evidence of the osseous density does not imply that it needs to be removed. If it is painful owing to injury caused by hyperextension or a direct blow, symptomatic treatment should resolve the pain. If catching, locking, or persistent pain is present, the ossicle is easily excised through a limited posterolateral incision or, preferably, arthroscopically (see Chapter 39).[28]

ACQUIRED LOOSE BODIES

Loose or pedunculated cartilaginous or osseocartilaginous bodies are believed to originate from a small nidus.[30] The sequence of morphologic alterations that ensue is common to all free bodies, regardless of their origin.[22] Surface proliferation of chondroblasts and osteoblasts nourished by the synovial fluid creates a laminar or layered effect that is seen in about 87 percent of such bodies that are predominantly cartilaginous and in 80 percent of those that are predominantly osseous (Fig. 74-6).[22] The growth process continues as long as the free or pedunculated body is exposed to the synovial fluid.

Etiology

Our understanding of intra-articular loose bodies has been much enhanced by the work of Milgram.[21-23] By clinical findings and presentation, acquired free or pedunculated bodies can be divided into three groups: (1) osteochondral fractures, (2) degenerative disease of the articular surface, and (3) a proliferative disorder of the synovium, synovial chondromatosis. Milgram[22] defines three types of cartilage associated with loose bodies based on their supposed site of origin: (1) articular cartilage cells, (2) osteophytic cells from a proliferating osteophyte in a degenerative joint, and (3) lobular cartilage from the synovial lining cell.

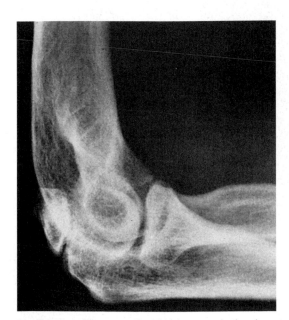

FIGURE 74-3 • The os patella cubiti is present in the triceps tendon; the proximal location helps to distinguish this lesion from a variation of the olecranon ossification center.

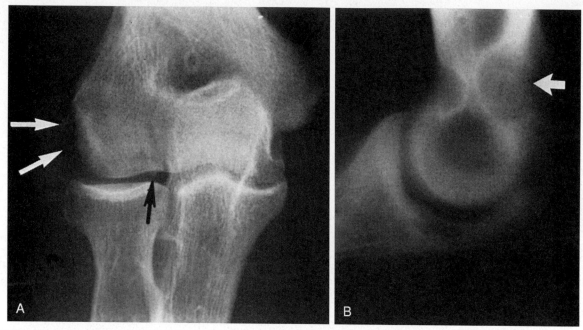

FIGURE 74–4 • A smooth, rounded ossicle in the olecranon fossa, observed on the anteroposterior *(A)* radiograph *(black arrow)* and sometimes more obvious *(arrow)* on the lateral one *(B)*, is consistent with the diagnosis of os supratrochleare. Other small densities are present on the anteroposterior view *(white arrows)*.

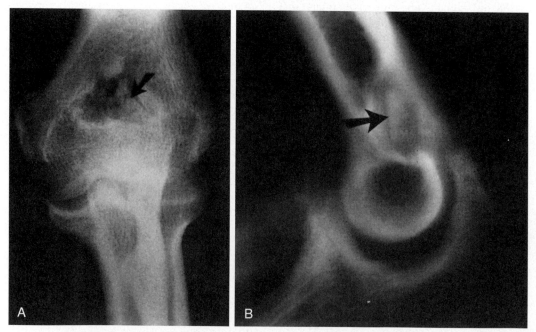

FIGURE 74–5 • *A* and *B*, Subject to trauma, this ossicle may sometimes take on an irregular shape, which can mislead the examiner to suspect that the cause is trauma, or even osteochondritis dissecans of the trochlea. Hyperextension of the elbow may cause spur formation on the tip of the olecranon and multiple loose bodies in the olecranon fossa, a condition that should be distinguished from the os supratrochleare. Coronoid osteophytosis suggests primary arthrosis as another possible cause.

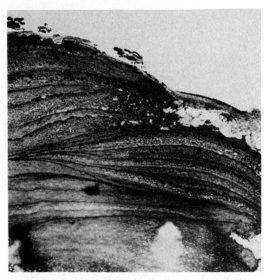

FIGURE 74–6 • Classic demonstration of the laminar effect of a cartilaginous loose body, which is responsible for the growth of these structures. (From Milgram, J. W.: The development of loose bodies in human joints. Clin. Orthop. 124:295, 1977.)

Pathologically, these loose bodies can originate from a joint fracture, from degenerative osteophytes, or de novo as a proliferative disease of the synovium.

OSTEOCHONDRAL FRACTURE

Fracture of the joint surface may be acute or the result of a chronic process such as osteochondritis dissecans. A shear fracture of the capitellum may involve little osseous substance, as in type II lesions (see Chapter 21). If in the acute stage, this fracture is missed, an intra-articular loose body may develop (Fig. 74–7). Elbow dislocation often leads to fractures of the coronoid, capitellum, or radial head and subsequent development of loose or attached intra-articular osseous bodies. Postreduction ossification is common, even without fracture, but the clinical finding is a painful arc of motion, rather than limited motion with locking or catching. Avulsion of the medial epicondyle at the time of dislocation can also cause entrapment of the loose body in the joint with reduction, but this complication

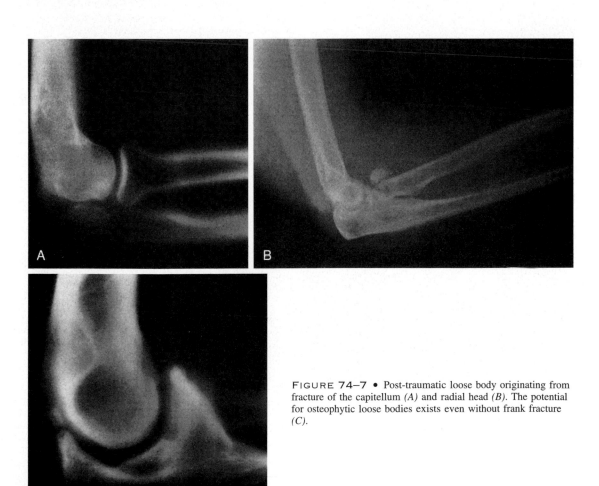

FIGURE 74–7 • Post-traumatic loose body originating from fracture of the capitellum *(A)* and radial head *(B)*. The potential for osteophytic loose bodies exists even without frank fracture *(C)*.

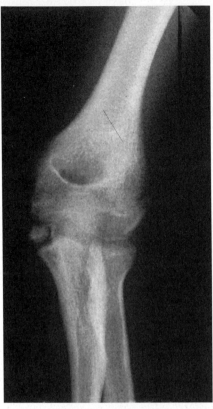

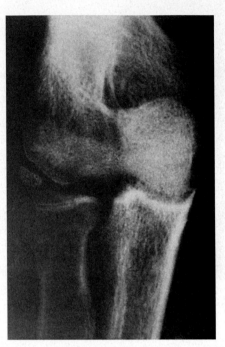

FIGURE 74–9 • Osteochondritis dissecans of the capitellum has caused an osteocartilaginous loose body in the joint.

FIGURE 74–8 • Entrapment of the medial epicondyle in the ulno-humeral joint after fracture-dislocation of the elbow.

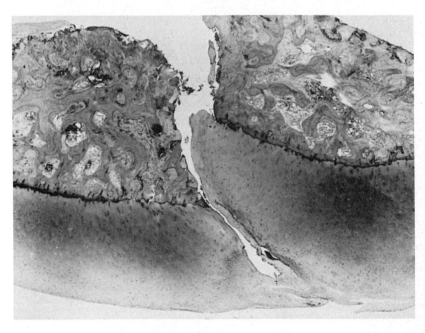

FIGURE 74–10 • A fragment of capitellum from a 24-year-old man with a 7-year history of intermittent restricted range of motion. No viable blood supply is present even though the surgeon had to cut through the articular cartilage to excise the underlying osseous defect. The articular cartilage chondrocytes exhibit no reactive change even though this fragment has fractured. The bone does show reactive changes, however, although the articular cartilage does not. (From Milgram, J. W.: Radiologic and Histologic Pathology of Nontumorous Diseases of Bones and Joints. Vol. 1. Northbrook, Ill., Northbrook Publishing Co., 1990.)

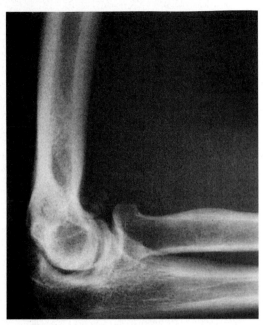

FIGURE 74–11 • Anterior loose bodies of the elbow joint in a patient with no history of trauma.

is obvious (Fig. 74–8) and should cause no problems with diagnosis or treatment.

The development of osteochondritis dissecans of the capitellum is discussed thoroughly in Chapters 20 and 45. It can progress to fragment detachment, with formation of a loose body in the joint (Fig. 74–9). Clinical manifestations include the occurrence of subtle pain, loss of extension, grating, snapping, and frank locking of the joint that is due to separation of a loose osteocartilaginous fragment of osteochondritis dissecans or a lesion of the capitellum or other portions of the articular surface or margin (Fig. 74–10). In fact, since trauma has become the accepted cause for loose bodies in the elbow joint, some researchers attribute all extraneous ossific densities, even accessory ossicles, to trauma.[1, 24, 26, 37] Although the clinical features and precise causes vary, a bony nidus is the common pathologic finding in each of these traumatic lesions.[21]

LOOSE BODIES OF DEGENERATIVE ORIGIN

Degenerative joint disease can induce loose body formation by creating a nidus from a fragmented joint surface, from a degenerative osteophyte, or from the synovium of a joint involved with degenerative cartilaginous changes.[22] Primary degenerative arthritis of the elbow is recognized more frequently and is discussed in detail in Chapter 67. Bullock and Goodfellow have studied primary degenerative changes of the radiohumeral joint; this process could certainly give rise to the formation of a nidus and the subsequent development of a loose body.[6] Bell reviewed 52 instances of loose bodies in the elbow and concluded that most were related to primary or secondary osteoarthritis.[3] He pointed out that most occurred in the anterior aspect of the joint (Fig. 74–11). With degenerative disease, small

osteophytes may be observed at the tips of both the olecranon and the coronoid process, either of which could eventually give rise to the development of an intra-articular loose body (see Fig. 74–7C). Other evidence of degenerative joint disease is seen on anteroposterior radiographs. As the olecranon fossa ossifies, loose bodies from the anterior or posterior joint are observed (Fig. 74–12).[25]

TREATMENT

Arthroscopic removal is the treatment of choice for symptomatic loose bodies.[28, 32] Replacement of a large fragment of the capitellum in osteochondritis dissecans has been discussed in Chapter 45; I have no experience with this. The treatment of fractures of the medial epicondyle is discussed in Chapter 17 and that of fractures of the capitellum in Chapter 23. I see little value in abrasion or drilling of the site of origin unless the diagnosis is made very early, in the acute stage. Such a procedure only adds to the surgical trauma and may result in an irritative hemarthrosis with secondary soft tissue contracture. The use of the arthroscope should enhance the diagnosis, localization, and removal of loose bodies (Fig. 74–13) (see Chapter 39).

SYNOVIAL CHONDROMATOSIS

Since the initial description of the entity in 1558,[29] much has been written about synovial chondromatosis or osteo-

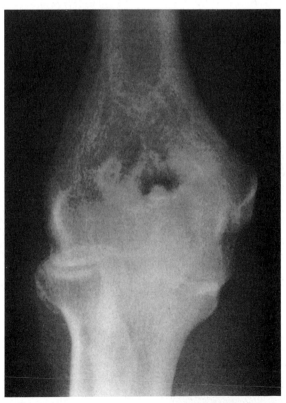

FIGURE 74–12 • Anteroposterior radiograph of primary degenerative arthritis of the elbow demonstrates a loose body in the olecranon fossa.

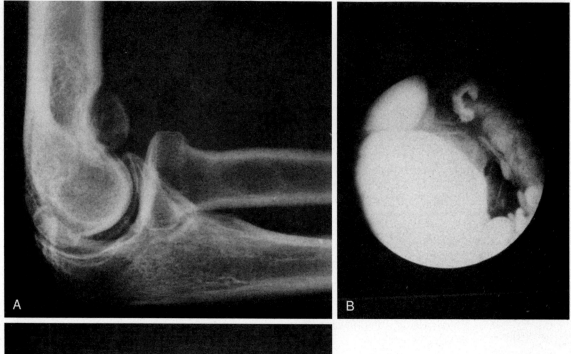

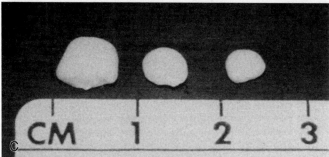

FIGURE 74–13 • Lateral radiograph demonstrates anterior and posterior loose bodies *(A)* that were localized arthroscopically *(B)*. Multiple loose bodies may be removed with this technique *(C)*.

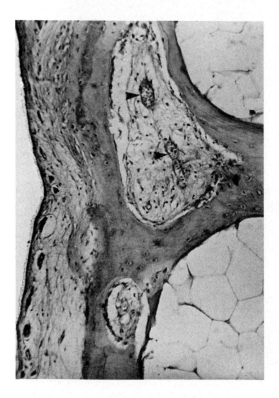

FIGURE 74–14 • Microradiograph of a pedunculated body in a patient with osteochondromatosis. Note the presence of a vascular supply *(arrows)* and mature bone nidus. (From Henderson, M. S., and Jones, H. T.: Loose bodies in joints and bursae due to synovial osteochondromatosis. J. Bone Joint Surg. 5:400, 1923.)

chondromatosis, and the topic is discussed further in Chapter 76.[8] Henderson and Jones reviewed the literature and reported the Mayo Clinic experience of 25 cases in 1923.[16] They concluded that this entity was separate from traumatic or degenerative loose body formation and that the nidus originated from the synovial tissue (Fig. 74–14). More specifically, the condition is believed to be a proliferative disorder of the subsynovial soft tissue.[13] Thus, some risk of malignant transformation is recognized, possibly as high as 5%.[9] Milgram has identified three phases of the process.[23] In the active initial phase, no free or loose bodies are present. In the transitional phase, osteochondral nodules form in the synovial membrane and nonossified free bodies are found in the joint (Fig. 74–15). In the final phase, free osteochondral bodies apparently herald the quiescent phase of the disease (Fig. 74–16).

In the second phase, the cartilaginous component becomes symptomatic before it ossifies, producing symptoms of elbow pain and loss of motion even in the presence of a relatively normal radiograph (Fig. 74–16). Enchondral bone formation replaces the cartilaginous component, and this gives rise to the obvious radiographic demonstration of multiple loose bodies (Fig. 74–16). Thus, the condition may present with multiple (as many as 100) radiolucent cartilaginous (see Fig. 74–15) or radiopaque ossified (see Fig. 74–16) loose bodies. When the bodies are ossified, a possible cartilaginous neoplasm may be considered, but, as discussed in Chapter 73, with the exception of the experience reported by Davis and co-workers,[9] the occurrence of cartilaginous sarcomas about the elbow is extremely rare. Yet the distinction can be difficult and may be resolved only by histologic examination of the tissue.[10] More recently computed tomography has been demonstrated to be effective in confirming this diagnosis.[31] The disease is a self-limiting process that runs a rather predictable course.[23] More recent reports have emphasized the development of nerve compression from capsular distention secondary to synovial chondromatosis.[33, 35] The large volume occupied by the chondromatous tissue has been shown to cause anterior distention and compression of the radial nerve at the arcade of Frohse, which results in partial paralysis of the posterior interosseous nerve.[12] A similar mechanism might be attributed to the ulnar neuropathy reported by Roth and others[11, 20] or even the cutaneous branch of this nerve.[35]

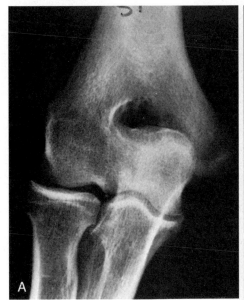
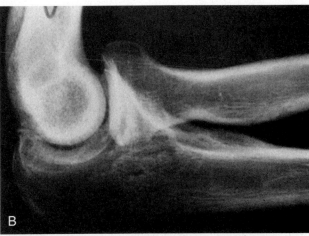
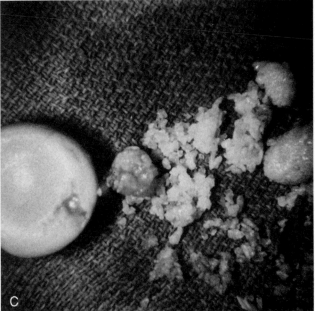

FIGURE 74–15 • A and B, The patient presented with grating and limitation of motion and radiographic evidence of only minimal hypertrophic changes. C, Arthrotomy demonstrated erosion of the radial head with multiple radiolucent cartilaginous loose bodies. The presumptive diagnosis was osteochondromatosis.

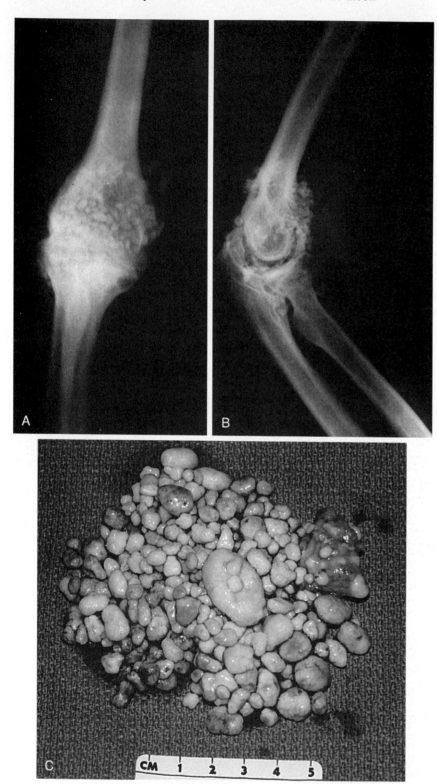

FIGURE 74–16 • *A* and *B*, Radiographs from an early case treated at the Mayo Clinic by Dr. M. S. Henderson in 1918 show the ossified form of osteochondromatosis. *C*, Arthrotomy allowed removal of more than 100 loose bodies.

SIGNS AND SYMPTOMS

Loose bodies are more common in males, regardless of the cause, trauma, degeneration, or proliferative synovium.[16] Among Bell's 52 cases, most patients presented with loss of motion, usually extension.[3] Symptoms often are of catch-

ing but rarely are disabling. Pain may or may not be a finding and usually occurs with a sensation of locking or grating. The patient may be able to localize the origin or location of the posterior or anterior ossicles, but, with involvement of multiple sites, the discomfort is generalized. Radiography is helpful for large lesions but can be deceptive if it fails to demonstrate loose bodies that have

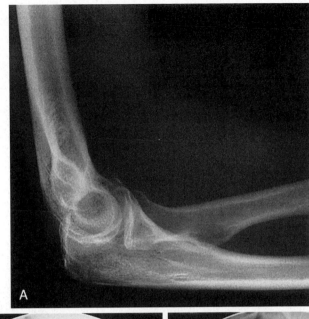

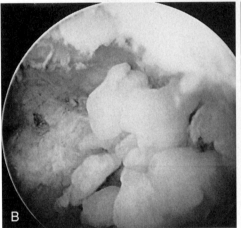
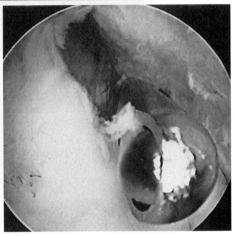

FIGURE 74–17 • A clinical presentation of limited extension and pain in a 36-year-old woman (A) was diagnosed as osteochondromatosis, which was treated by removal of loose bodies under arthroscopic guidance (B).

not yet calcified, if small ossicles are present in the ulno-humeral joint (see Fig. 74–5B), if the location is obscured by surrounding structures, or if the traumatic lesion contains little osseous tissue. These difficulties in diagnosis can be overcome by multiple views, including oblique views or tomograms, and, ultimately, definitive diagnosis may require arthroscopy.

TREATMENT

Arthroscopic diagnosis is preferable to arthrotomy in the early, "pre-calcified" stage of the disease. Regardless of the stage of presentation, arthroscopy is now clearly the treatment of choice for removal of the loose bodies, and synovectomy, if required (Fig. 74–17).

REFERENCES

1. Atsatt, S.: Loose bodies of the elbow joint: An unusual location and form. J. Bone Joint Surg. **15:**1008, 1933.
2. Bassett, L. W., Mirra, J. M., Forrester, D. M., Gold, R. H., Bernstein, M. L., and Rollins, J. S.: Post-traumatic osteochondral "loose body" of the olecranon fossa. Radiology **141:**635, 1981.
3. Bell, M. S.: Loose bodies in the elbow. Br. J. Surg. **62:**921, 1975.
4. Birsner, J. W., and DeSmet, D. H.: Patella cubiti with fracture. Ann. West. Med. Surg. **4:**744, 1950.
5. Broberg, M. A., and Morrey, B. F.: Results of treatment of fracture dislocations of the elbow. Clin. Orthop. **216:**109, 1987.
6. Bullock, P. G., and Goodfellow, J. W.: Pattern of aging of the articular cartilage of the elbow joint. J. Bone Joint Surg. **49B:**175, 1967.
7. Burman, M. S.: Unusual locking of the elbow joint by the sesamum cubiti and a free joint body. Am. J. Radiol. **45:**731, 1941.
8. Christensen, J. H., and Poulsen, J. O.: Synovial chondromatosis. Acta Orthop. Scand. **46:**919, 1975.
9. Davis, R. I., Hamilton, A., and Biggart, J. D.: Primary synovial chondromatosis: A clinicopathologic review and assessment of malignant potential. Hum. Pathol. **79:**683–688, 1998.
10. Dufour, J. P., Hamels, J., Maldague, B., Noel, H., and Pestiaux, B.: Unusual aspects of synovial chondromatosis of the elbow. Clin. Rheumatol. **3:**247, 1984.
11. Fahmy, N. R. M., and Noble, J.: Ulnar nerve palsy as a complication of synovial osteochondromatosis of the elbow. Hand **13:**308, 1981.
12. Field, J. H.: Posterior interosseous nerve palsy secondary to synovial chondromatosis of the elbow joint. J. Hand Surg. **6:**336, 1981.
13. Fisher, A. G. T.: A study of loose bodies composed of cartilage or of cartilage and bone occurring in joints. Br. J. Surg. **8:**493, 1931.
14. Gudmundsen, T. E., and Ostensen, H.: Accessory ossicles in the elbow. Acta Orthop. Scand. **58:**130, 1987.
15. Habbe, J. E.: Patella cubiti, a report of four cases. A.J.R. **48:**513, 1942.
16. Henderson, M. S., and Jones, H. T.: Loose bodies in joints and bursae due to synovial osteochondromatosis. J. Bone Joint Surg. **5:**400, 1923.

17. Keates, T. E.: An Atlas of Normal Roentgen Variants That May Simulate Disease. Chicago, Year Book Medical Publishers, 1979.
18. Kienbock, R., and Desenfans. G.: Uber Anomalien am Ellbogengelenk Patella cubiti. Beitr. Klin. Chir. **165:**524, 1937.
19. Kohler, A., and Zimmer, E. A.: Borderlands of the Normal and Early Pathologic in Skeletal Anatomy, 3rd ed. New York, Grune & Stratton, 1968.
20. Lister, J. R., Day, A. L., and Ballinger, W.: Ulnar palsy caused by synovial chondromatosis. Surg. Neurol. **15:**428, 1981.
21. Milgram, J. W.: The classification of loose bodies in human joints. Clin. Orthop. **124:**282, 1977.
22. Milgram, J. W.: The development of loose bodies in human joints. Clin. Orthop. **124:**292, 1977.
23. Milgram, J. W.: Synovial osteochondromatosis. J. Bone Joint Surg. **59B:**492, 1977.
24. Morgan, P. W.: Osteochondritis dissecans of the supratrochlear septum. Radiology **60:**241, 1953.
25. Morrey, B. F.: Primary osteoarthritis of the elbow: Ulno-humeral arthroplasty. J. Bone Joint Surg. **74B:**409, 1992.
26. Morton, H. S., and Crysler, W. E.: Osteochondritis dissecans of the supratrochlear septum. J. Bone Joint Surg. **27:**12, 1945.
27. Obermann, W. R., and Loose, H. W. C.: The os supratrochleare dorsale: A normal variant that may cause symptoms. A.J.R. **141:**123, 1963.
28. O'Driscoll, S. W., and Morrey, B. F.: Arthroscopy of the elbow: A critical analysis. J. Bone Joint Surg. **74A:**84, 1992.
29. Paré, A.: As quoted by Henderson, M. S., and Jones, H. T.: J. Bone Joint Surg. **5:**400, 1923.
30. Phemister, D. B.: The causes and changes in loose bodies arising from the articular surface of the joint. J. Bone Joint Surg. **6:**278, 1924.
31. Rao, J. P., Spingola, C., Mastromonaco, E., and Villacin, A.: Synovial osteochondromatosis: Computerized axial tomography, frozen section and arthrography in diagnosis and management. Orthop. Rev. **15:**94, 1986.
32. Rupp, S., and Tempelhof, S.: Arthroscopic surgery of the elbow. Therapeutic benefits and hazards. Clin. Orthop. **313:**140–145, 1995.
33. Ruth, R. M., and Groves, R. J.: Synovial osteochondromatosis of the elbow presenting with ulnar nerve neuropathy. Am. J. Orthop. **25:**843, 1996.
34. Sachs, J., and Degenskein, G.: Patella cubiti. Arch. Surg. **57:**675, 1948.
35. Slater, R. N. S., Koka, S. R., and Ross, K. R.: Cheiralgia paraesthetica secondary to synovial osteochondromatosis of the elbow. J. Orthop. Rheumatol. **6:**179–181, 1993.
36. Tullos, H. S., and King, J. W.: Lesions of the pitching arm in adolescents. J.A.M.A. **220:**264, 1972.
37. Zietlin, A.: The traumatic origin of accessory bones at the elbow. J. Bone Joint Surg. **17:**933, 1935.

CHAPTER 75

Bursitis

• BERNARD F. MORREY

It is unlikely that the following discussion will do a great deal to alter the rather menial significance attributed to the bursae:

• • • Ensuring the smooth and frictionless working of the body corporate, usually uncomplaining, inconspicuous, hard-working, and very modest in their requirements, the bursae have been so neglected that, even when one of them misbehaves, this is usually misattributed to some more important structure.[29] • • •

With the exception of olecranon bursitis, bursal afflictions are relatively uncommon about the elbow. The presence of these structures is even variable and is probably developmental, because not all bursae are present at birth.[42]

ANATOMY

As early as 1788, Monro described several deep bursae about the elbow (Fig. 75–1). Through the years, additional bursae have been described. They may be divided into deep and superficial types (Fig. 75–2). Anatomically, the deep bursae are situated between muscles or between muscle and bone, which makes anatomic recognition somewhat difficult and clinical involvement almost impossible to diagnose. The superficial bursae consist only of those over the epicondyles and that over the olecranon, which is by far the most important one.

DEEP BURSAE

Pathologic involvement of any of the deep bursal structures is rather uncommon. This fact, coupled with the difficulty of identifying some of these structures by anatomic dissection, brings into question the very existence of certain structures. The most significant of the deep bursae is the bicipital radial bursa, which occurs at the radial tuberosity (Fig. 75–3). Owing to its anatomic site, inflammation of the bursa may occur with pronation and supination and can be confused with distal biceps tendinitis.[20] Distinguishing between impending distal biceps tendon rupture and bicipital radial bursitis is not simple.[2] In fact, one of the few cases of cubital bursitis reported by Karanjia and Stiles showed degeneration of the biceps tendon insertion.[20] Crepitus on pronation and supination suggests impending rupture. Fullness or swelling of the cubital space that is accentuated on pronation is more consistent with bicipital radial bursitis.[20] I have used selective lidocaine injections to help localize the lesion to the tuberosity, but this does not distinguish between the two processes. Usually the diagno-

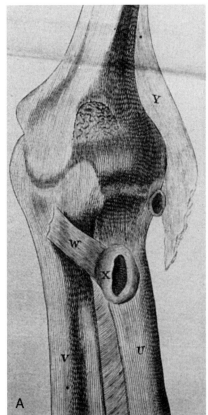
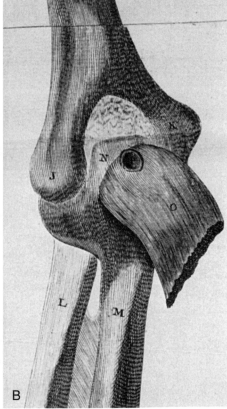

FIGURE 75–1 • A, The existence of the radiohumeral bursa and the bicipital radial bursa (X) has been recognized for more than 200 years, as demonstrated by this original 1788 illustration from Monro. B, Similarly, the subtendinous olecranon bursa was well illustrated in this monograph.

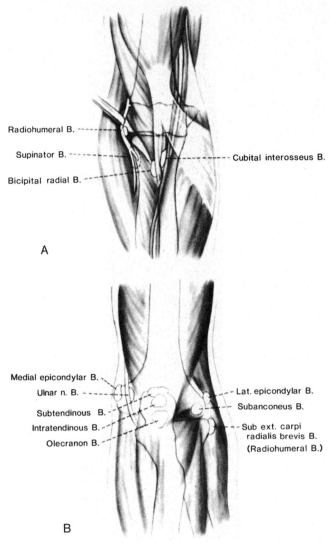

FIGURE 75–2 • *A*, Many deep bursae have been reported to exist in the region of the elbow, usually interposed between muscle and muscle or tendon and bone. *B*, The subcutaneous bursa of the olecranon is the most recognized and clinically important of these bursae.

sis is presumptive and the treatment is symptomatic—rest, ice or heat, and anti-inflammatory agents.

Tennis elbow and irritation of the radial nerve have been reported to result from inflammation of the radiohumeral bursa, which lies under the extensor carpi radialis brevis.[6] Although bursitis was once thought to be a common cause of tennis elbow, according to our current understanding of lateral epicondylitis the association seems to be uncommon. Yet this structure does exist and has been demonstrated in anatomic dissections.[29, 30] I have had one patient who developed adventitial epicondylar bursitis after a common extensor tendon slide. Symptoms resolved after excision.

Deep bursae have been associated with the triceps tendon. The significance of the two deep bursae around the triceps (Fig. 75–4) is a matter of speculation, because no recognizable clinical presentation has been documented for these structures. It is quite possible that inflammation of either the intratendinous or subtendinous bursae could be mistaken for tendinitis or that of the subtendinous bursae for tendinitis, synovitis, or capsulitis. Idiopathic calcific involvement of the subtendinous bursae has been described.[40] Yet calcification of bursae around the elbow is distinctly unusual, in contrast to calcific tendinitis in the region of the shoulder. Calcium appears to form in response to anoxia, which causes a cellular response with giant cell reaction. The result is an inflamed, "hot"-looking joint or bursa.

SUPERFICIAL BURSAE

The olecranon and the medial and lateral epicondylar bursae are the only superficial bursae about the elbow. I have occasionally observed an inflamed medial epicondylar bursa associated with chronic subluxation of the ulnar nerve. This probably rather uncommon lesion is treated by attending to the primary pathologic process involving the ulnar nerve. It is interesting to note that the olecranon bursa is not present at birth and has been shown to develop after the 7th year.[7] This is consistent with others' observations that bursae increase in size with age. Spontaneous rupture of the triceps tendon (see Chapter 36) may be related to tendon degeneration, as has been documented[6]

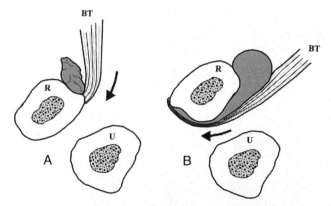

FIGURE 75–3 • Because the bicipital radial bursa is situated between the tuberosity and tendon *(A)*, symptoms are exaggerated with pronation, as the bursa impinges between tendon and bone *(B)*. BT, bicipital tendon; R, radius; U, ulna.

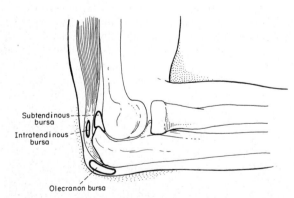

FIGURE 75–4 • Lateral illustration of the elbow demonstrates the superficial subcutaneous olecranon bursa, the intratendinous bursa found in the substance of the tendon, and the subtendinous bursa lying between the tip of the olecranon and the triceps tendon.

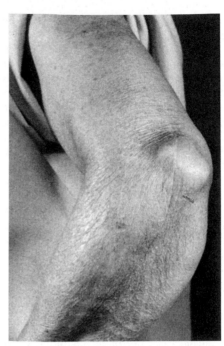

FIGURE 75–5 • Development of olecranon bursitis after elbow joint replacement. Note the well-healed posterior incision. This was an aseptic process.

with disruptions of the insertion of the bicipital tendon.[10] This process could masquerade as bursitis.

Olecranon Bursitis

The olecranon is the site of the most common type of superficial bursitis.[32] Olecranon bursitis is caused by a number of pathologic conditions that are traumatic (overuse or direct impact), inflammatory, infectious, or noninfectious. Since 1975, it has been associated with dialysis in the ipsilateral extremity.[17] I have also observed olecranon bursitis after reconstructive procedures when a posterior approach was used (Fig. 75–5).

Inflammation of the superficial olecranon bursa can also result from direct trauma or repetitive stress, the so-called miner's elbow or student's elbow. Larson and Osternig have also shown that olecranon bursitis is a common football injury and is often associated with artificial turf.[22]

Involvement with systemic inflammatory processes such as rheumatoid arthritis,[26] gout, chondrocalcinosis,[12] or hydroxyapatite crystal deposition[28] has been reported. Diffuse pigmented villonodular synovitis has also been shown to give rise to olecranon synovitis,[27] and xanthoma has been reported to involve this region.[37] In lesions due to chronic overuse—for example, coal miner's bursitis—the synovial cells that are least subject to mechanical stress have been shown to be those that elaborate the synovial fluid.[25]

The distinction between septic and aseptic olecranon bursitis can be somewhat difficult to make. About 20 percent of cases of acute bursitis have a septic cause.[18, 37] Distinguishing between a septic and an aseptic inflammatory bursitis has been the subject of a detailed study by Ho and Tice[15] and is discussed in Chapter 68. Fever, tenderness, and parabursal cellulitis are common with septic

bursitis; however, these findings are not specific, and a more detailed study Smith and associates revealed that the skin over a septic bursa is almost 4°C warmer than that over the nonseptic contralateral extremity.[36] The sepsis causes pain in approximately 80 percent, whereas nonseptic bursitis is tender in only about 20 percent. It should be noted that Gram stain results are positive in only about 50 percent of patients. Approximately 80 percent are caused by *Staphylococcus aureus* or another gram-positive organism.[43] Particular care must be exercised in evaluating dialysis patients because they may present with a sterile inflammatory process but have pain and warmth that suggest an infection.[17] The problem is compounded by the fact that about 20 percent of these patients are also found to have a septic process.[19] The correct diagnosis is suggested when aspirate from the bursa demonstrates a high leukocyte count. Thus, a presumptive diagnosis can usually be made before the culture results have been obtained. Contiguous spread of septic olecranon bursitis leading to osteomyelitis of the olecranon has been thought to be possible, although it is probably rare. Excision of the olecranon has been recommended to avoid this possibility.[24]

CLINICAL PRESENTATION

A distended olecranon bursa is usually painless unless it is associated with a septic or crystalline inflammatory process. The two inflammatory conditions most frequently associated with olecranon bursitis are rheumatoid arthritis and gouty arthritis, in that order (Fig. 75–6).[3] In patients with rheumatoid arthritis, the presentation can be quite variable. The bursa may rupture and dissect proximally, presenting as triceps swelling.[31] In patients with rheumatoid arthritis, the bursa may also communicate with the joint, dissect anteriorly and distally into the forearm, or even rupture and present as a subcutaneous fullness over the subcutaneous border of the ulna,[11, 14, 33] all complications that are usually relatively painful.

The association of triceps tendon rupture with olecranon bursitis after trauma has been cited.[8] I have seen a bursa-type reaction after subacute or partial distal biceps rupture

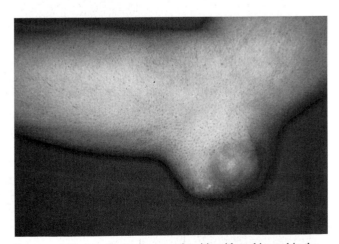

FIGURE 75–6 • Gouty olecranon bursitis with tophi noted in the subcutaneous tissue.

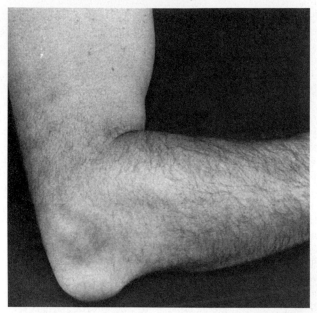

FIGURE 75–7 • Acute hemobursitis developed in a patient receiving anticoagulation therapy after coronary bypass surgery. The inflammation was very refractory to treatment but eventually resolved with compressive dressing and protection.

and suspect that the bursal reaction was an effect of biceps tendon injury and partial rupture, rather than a cause of rupture. On the other hand, traumatic bursitis is surprisingly painless after the initial event. When the bursitis is symptomatic, flexing the elbow to more than 90 degrees causes most symptoms. In fact, positions between 60 and 90 degrees have been shown in the laboratory to produce considerably greater pressure in the bursa than elbow extension.[5] Canoso noted no pain with flexion, even when

the bursa was distended, and speculated that discomfort probably originated in nerve endings in the osseous tendinous attachment, rather than in the roof of the bursa. Loss of motion has been reported, but this must be uncommon. I have not yet observed this in my practice. This phenomenon was first described by Irby and colleagues in 1975.[17]

Another clinical setting in which olecranon bursitis is becoming an increasingly recognized complication is hemodialysis.[9, 17, 19] As many as 7 percent of dialysis patients may be affected.[17, 19] The pathophysiology of this manifestation has not been demonstrated conclusively. It is possible that direct pressure or low-grade trauma from posturing of the elbow may be the principal insult. Use of anticoagulants increases the possibility of hemobursitis (Fig. 75–7). It has also been proposed that it may represent uremic serositis, but none of these possibilities has been confirmed.[19] A septic cause has been reported in about 25 percent of cases.[19]

Canoso has also characterized the clinical features of 30 cases of noninflammatory olecranon bursitis.[4] Repetitive trauma was reported in 14 cases and a discrete, single traumatic event in seven. The nine other cases might be considered idiopathic. An olecranon spur was observed in 10 of 30 patients (Fig. 75–8). When symptoms had been present more than 2 weeks, the bursa appeared discretely swollen; when symptoms had been present less than 2 weeks, parabursal edema was observed in the arm and forearm in half of the patients (Fig. 75–9).[9]

Aspiration showed evidence of hemorrhage in cases of post-traumatic bursitis. The synovial fluid was further characterized by a low leukocyte count (average only 878 cells per high-power field, with 84 percent monocytes). This contrasts with the high leukocyte counts and predominance of polymorphonuclear cells in septic bursitis.

Radiographic findings associated with traumatic olecra-

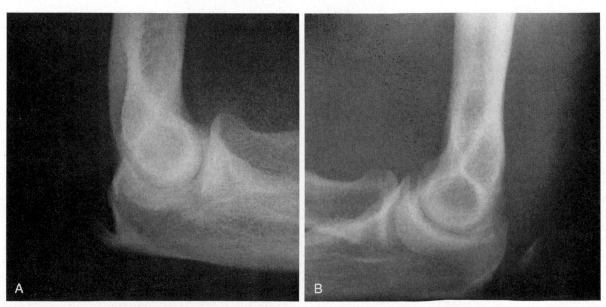

FIGURE 75–8 • Lateral radiograph of the elbow of a patient with longstanding recurrent olecranon bursitis (A). Occasionally, this prominence fractures, but with few long-term consequences (B).

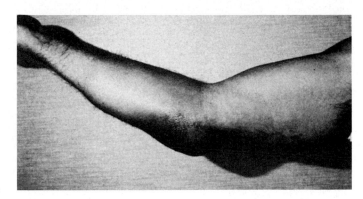

FIGURE 75–9 • In acute septic olecranon bursitis, rather diffuse swelling is noted about the distal brachium and the proximal forearm.

non bursitis have been described,[35] the most important one being an olecranon spur (see Fig. 75–8).

TREATMENT

Acute Bursitis

Control of any underlying systemic or inflammatory process is the obvious first step in treatment. Sometimes the olecranon bursa communicates with the joint in rheumatoid arthritis, and the inflammation is generally considered a secondary process.[16] If the bursa is not painful, local measures to prevent injury are all that is required.[12] A resting splint and compression may be necessary, and this is the usual treatment in the early stages. Acute traumatic or idiopathic bursitis is also treated symptomatically with elbow pads (Fig. 75–10).

If pain in the bursa prevents daily or occupational activity, aspiration and cortisone injection are indicated. Weinstein and colleagues reviewed 47 patients with nonseptic bursitis who were followed for 6 months to 5 years.[41] Aspiration with and without corticosteroids demonstrated that adding corticosteroids did reduce the chance of recurrence but was associated with a significantly greater com-

plication rate. Infection developed in 3 of 25 patients, and subdermal atrophy in 5 of 25 (Fig. 75–11).

The orthopedic surgeon must be particularly vigilant here. "Nonsurgeons" tend to treat the septic process for a long time before they consider intervention.[43] If the process does not rapidly resolve, if pain persists, and if parabursal swelling or erythema is present and is not resolving, septic bursitis is likely and the bursa must be aspirated. If this has already been done and the initial aspirate revealed no bacteria, repeat aspiration is indicated; at this time, culture is occasionally "positive."

Chronic Bursitis

Chronic recurrent or painful olecranon bursitis may require more definitive measures. A 16-gauge indwelling needle that maintains drainage with a compressive dressing for about 3 days has been cited as being effective in reducing recurrence of bursal swelling.[12] Knight and colleagues, who refined this technique using percutaneous placement of a suction irrigation system, reported the results of 10 cases of septic olecranon bursitis.[21] The average time in the hospital was approximately 12 days.[41] Today, because increasing pressure for patient dismissal compromises this form of treatment, it is uncommon. Surgery is not com-

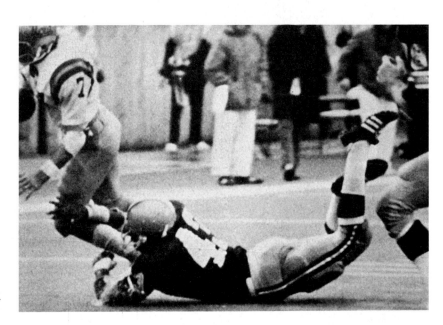

FIGURE 75–10 • Traumatic olecranon bursitis from artificial turf treated by protection with an elbow pad. The ideal pad should be relieved somewhat over the olecranon. (From Larson, R. L., and Osternig, L. R.: Traumatic bursitis and artificial turf. J. Sports Med. 2:183, 1974.)

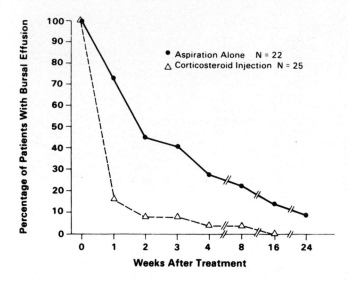

FIGURE 75–11 • Temporal resolution of bursitis associated with treatment by aspiration with and without cortisone injection. (From Weinstein, P. S., Canoso, J. J., and Wohlgethan, J. R.: Long-term follow-up of corticosteroid injection for traumatic olecranon bursitis. Ann. Rheum. Dis. **43**:45, 1984.)

monly indicated; however, when the process is refractory to nonoperative measures and is interfering with occupational or daily activities, operative intervention should be considered.

Operative Intervention

A longitudinal incision medial to the midline[39] or a transverse incision has been recommended.[37] All bursal tissue is removed, and the joint is immobilized in flexion or extreme flexion for approximately 2 weeks. Freeing the

bursa from the skin can devitalize the skin over the olecranon process or cause problems with healing. Thus, I recommend a compressive dressing on the elbow placed in about 45 degrees of flexion. To avoid this, a rather unusual approach has been reported by Quayle and Robinson[34] (Fig. 75–12). The concern about wound healing attendant to the subdermal dissection of the bursa is avoided by reflecting the skin with the bursal tissue from the tip of the olecranon in a lateral to medial or a medial to lateral direction. At this point, the tip of the olecranon is obliquely osteotomized, leaving the bursal tissue intact. The triceps mecha-

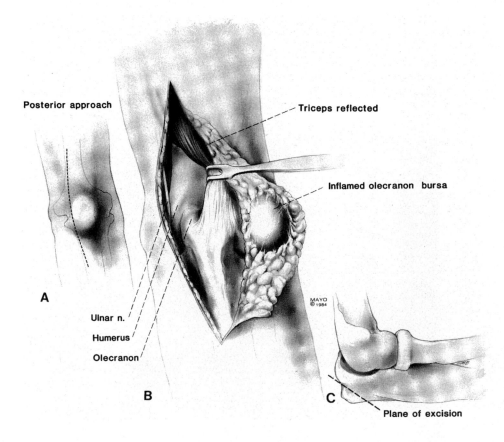

FIGURE 75–12 • Surgical treatment for chronic olecranon bursitis recommended by Quayle and Robinson. *A*, A straight medial incision is preferred. The skin flap that includes the bursa is reflected laterally. *B*, The triceps is reflected laterally, revealing the tip of the olecranon. *C*, A generous osteotomy is recommended.

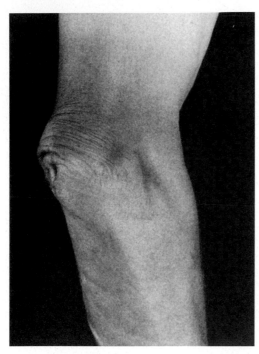

FIGURE 75–13 • A chronic draining sinus after incision and drainage of an infected olecranon bursa. Note the absence of swelling and local reaction.

nism is then reflected back over the olecranon, and the wound is closed with a drain. Eleven patients treated with this technique have had no recurrences.[34]

Results

Stewart and associates reviewed the Mayo Clinic experience with 21 cases of surgical excision of the olecranon bursa.[39] Not surprisingly, only two of five patients with rheumatoid arthritis (40%) enjoyed complete relief. Fortunately, 15 of 16 (94%) in the nonrheumatoid group were free of recurrence an average of 5 years after surgery.[39]

Complications

Complications of wound healing are the most common ones associated with incision and drainage or with excision of the olecranon bursa (Fig. 75–13). We had no recurrent drainage after the 21 resections reported by Stewart and associates. Should coverage be a problem, however, muscle flap transfers, either free or local, have been used with success for this application. Lai and colleagues recently described a more limited adipofascial flap to cover this area.[23] Indiscriminate incision or removal of the olecranon bursa must be seriously questioned in light of the possibility and magnitude of this complication.

REFERENCES

1. Benson, W. G., Laskin, C. A., Little, H. A., and Fam, H. G.: Hemochromatotic arthropathy mimicking rheumatoid arthritis. Arthritis Rheum. **21**:844, 1978.
2. Bourne, M., and Morrey, B. F.: Partial rupture of the distal biceps tendon. Clin. Orthop. **271**:143, 1991.
3. Bywaters, E. G.: The bursae of the body. Ann. Rheum. Dis. **24**:215, 1965.
4. Canoso, J. J.: Idiopathic or traumatic olecranon bursitis. Clinical features and bursal fluid analysis. Arthritis Rheum. **20**:1213, 1977.
5. Canoso, J. J.: Intrabursal pressures in the olecranon and prepatellar bursae. J. Rheumatol. **7**:570, 1980.
6. Carp, L.: Tennis elbow. Arch. Surg. **24**:905, 1932.
7. Chen, J., Alk, D., Eventov, I., and Weintroub, S.: Development of the olecranon bursa: An anatomic cadaver study. Acta Orthop. Scand. **58**:408, 1987.
8. Clayton, M. C., and Thirupathi, R. G.: Rupture of the triceps tendon with olecranon bursitis. Clin. Orthop. **184**:183, 1984.
9. Cruz, C., and Shah, S. V.: Dialysis elbow: Olecranon bursitis from long-term hemodialysis. J.A.M.A. **238**:238, 1977.
10. Davis, W. M., and Yassine, Z.: An etiologic factor in tear of the distal tendon of the biceps brachii. J. Bone Joint Surg. **38A**:1365, 1956.
11. Ehrlich, G. E.: Antecubital cysts in rheumatoid arthritis: A corollary to popliteal (Baker's) cysts. J. Bone Joint Surg. **54A**:165, 1972.
12. Fisher, R. H.: Conservative treatment of disturbed patellae and olecranon bursae. Clin. Orthop. **123**:98, 1977.
13. Gerster, J. C., Lagier, R., and Boivin, G.: Olecranon bursitis related to calcium pyrophosphate dihydrate crystal deposition disease. Arthritis Rheum. **25**:989, 1982.
14. Goode, J. D.: Synovial rupture of the elbow joint. Ann. Rheum. Dis. **27**:604, 1968.
15. Ho, G., and Tice, A. D.: Comparison of nonseptic and septic bursitis. Arch. Intern. Med. **139**:1269, 1979.
16. Hollinshead, W. H.: Anatomy for Surgeons, 2nd ed. Vol. 3. New York, Hoeber, 1969.
17. Irby, R., Edwards, W. M., and Gatter, R. J.: Articular complications of hemotransplantation and chronic renal hemodialysis. Rheumatology **2**:91, 1975.
18. Jaffe, L., and Fetto, J. F.: Olecranon bursitis. Contemp. Orthop. **8**:51, 1984.
19. Jain, V. K., Cestero, R. V. M., and Baum, J.: Septic and aseptic olecranon bursitis in patients on maintenance hemodialysis. Clin. Exp. Dial. Apheresis **5**:405, 1981.
20. Karanjia, N. D., and Stiles, P. J.: Cubital bursitis. J. Bone Joint Surg. **70B**:832, 1988.
21. Knight, J. M., Thomas, J. C., and Maurer, R. C.: Treatment of septic olecranon and prepatellar bursitis with percutaneous placement of a suction-irrigation system: A report of 12 cases. Clin. Orthop. **206**:90, 1986.
22. Larson, R. L., and Osternig, L. R.: Traumatic bursitis and artificial turf. J. Sports Med. **2**:183, 1974.
23. Lai, C. S., Tsai, C. C., Liao, K. B., and Lin, S. D.: The reverse lateral arm adipofascial flap for elbow coverage. Ann. Plast. Surg. **39**:196–200, 1997.
24. Lasher, W. W., and Mathewson, L. M.: Olecranon bursitis. J.A.M.A. **90**:1030, 1928.
25. Letizia, G., Piccione, F., Ridola, C., and Zummo, G.: Ultrastructural comparisons of human synovial membrane in joints exposed to varying stresses. Ital. J. Orthop. Traumatol. **6**:279, 1980.
26. MacFarlane, J. D., and van der Linden, S. J.: Leaking rheumatoid olecranon bursitis as a cause of forearm swelling. Ann. Rheum. Dis. **40**:309, 1981.
27. Mathews, R. E., Gould, J. S., and Kashlan, M. B.: Diffuse pigmented villonodular tenosynovitis of the ulnar bursa: A case report. J. Hand Surg. **6**:64, 1981.
28. McCarty, D. J., and Gatter, R. A.: Recurrent acute inflammation associated with focal apatite crystal deposition. Arthritis Rheum. **9**:84, 1966.
29. Monro, A.: A Description of All the Bursae Mucosae of the Human Body. Edinburgh, Elliot, 1788.
30. Osgood, R. B.: Radiohumeral bursitis, epicondylitis, epicondylalgia (tennis elbow). Arch. Surg. **4**:420, 1922.
31. Petrie, J. P., and Wigley, R. D.: Proximal dissection of the olecranon bursa in rheumatoid arthritis. Rheumatol. Int. **4**:139, 1984.
32. Pien, F. D., Ching, D., and Kim, E.: Septic bursitis: Experience in a community practice. Orthopaedics **14**:981, 1991.
33. Pirani, M., Lange-Mechlen, I., and Cockshott, W. P.: Rupture of a posterior synovial cyst of the elbow. J. Rheumatol, **9**:94, 1982.
34. Quayle, J. B., and Robinson, M. P.: A useful procedure in the treatment of chronic olecranon bursitis. Injury **9**:299, 1976.
35. Saini, M., and Canoso, J. J.: Traumatic olecranon bursitis: Radiologic observations. Acta Radiol. (Diagn.) **23**:255, 1982.

36. Smith, D. L.: Septic and nonseptic olecranon bursitis. Arch. Intern. Med. **149**:1581, 1989.
37. Smith, F. M.: Surgery of the Elbow, 2nd ed. Philadelphia, W. B. Saunders Co., 1972.
38. Spinner, M.: Injuries to the Major Branches of Peripheral Nerves of the Forearm, 2nd ed. Philadelphia, W. B. Saunders Co., 1978.
39. Stewart, N. J., Manzanares, J. B., and Morrey, B. F.: Surgical treatment of aseptic olecranon bursitis. J. Shoulder Elbow Surg. **6**:49–53, 1997.
40. Vizkelety, T., and Aszodi, K.: Bilateral calcareous bursitis at the elbow. J. Bone Joint Surg. **50B**:644, 1968.
41. Weinstein, P. S., Canoso, J. J., and Wohlgethan, J. R.: Long-term follow-up of corticosteroid injection for traumatic olecranon bursitis. Ann. Rheum. Dis. **43**:44, 1984.
42. Whittaker, C. R.: The arrangement of the bursae in the superior extremities of the full-term fetus. J. Anat. Physiol. **44**:133, 1910.
43. Zimmerman, B., 3rd, Mikolich, D. J., and Ho, G., Jr.: Septic bursitis. Semin. Arthritis Rheum. **24**:391–410, 1995.

CHAPTER 76

The Elbow in Metabolic Disease

• BERNARD F. MORREY

With the possible exception of tumoral calcinosis, no metabolic diseases have a special predilection for or a characteristic presentation at or about the elbow joint.[1, 6, 18] Information, therefore, is rather limited on the effects of metabolic bone disease of the elbow joint. In fact, at the Mayo Clinic, the radiographic bone survey routinely taken to assess the extent of involvement of these diseases does not include the elbow region. No attempt will be made here to mention all the conditions that might incidentally involve the elbow. Several conditions, however, are regularly manifested at this joint: gout, pseudogout, and inborn errors of metabolism that cause congenital anomalies (see Chapters 14 and 66). Paget's disease may, of course, involve any part of the body, including the elbow (see Chapter 73). Synovial chondromatosis could, logically, be discussed here, but we have arbitrarily included it in Chapter 44 in the discussion of loose bodies.

It seems appropriate to discuss the appearance of and the effect of several of the more common or characteristic metabolic disorders that involve the elbow region and the impact of exogenous treatment with corticosteroid.

RICKETS

In the immature skeleton, vitamin D deficiency typically causes widening of the physis and cupping of the metaphysis, which are well represented at the wrist. Interestingly, although it has not been emphasized in the literature, rather dramatic widening of the radiohumeral joint is typical of this disease (Fig. 76–1). The deficiency will obviously be better demonstrated in the faster-growing bones, and the physes of the distal humerus and proximal forearm are relatively slow growing.[6] Thus, the manifestations of rickets in the region of the elbow are usually not dramatic.

OSTEOMALACIA

Vitamin D deficiency of the mature skeleton resulting in the production of uncalcified osteoid may be due to one of several mechanisms—nutritional intake deficiencies, absorption abnormalities, and utilization abnormalities.[14, 15] Radiographically, marked loss of bone density is usually observed along with coarsening of the trabecular pattern. There are no characteristic features at the elbow (Fig. 76–2). The lack of structural integrity causes bowing deformities of the weight-bearing extremities, but this is uncommon in the upper limbs.

TUMORAL CALCINOSIS

Extensive para-articular calcification, so-called tumoral calcinosis, does have a certain predilection for the elbow region, although it is more common at the hips and shoulders.[7] The differential diagnosis includes hyperparathyroidism, hypervitaminosis D, calcinosis universalis, and calcinosis circumscripta.[4] Tumoral calcinosis characteristically occurs in young persons who have normal serum calcium concentrations, but a predilection has been noted in black persons and a familial tendency has also been reported.[7] First described by Inclan and colleagues in 1943,[9] the association with hyperphosphatemia has suggested a metabolic cause for this disease.[2, 12] Chemical assessment reveals hyperphosphatemia but normal levels of serum calcium, parathyroid hormone, and alkaline phosphatase. The exact cause of the condition is obscure, but calcium salts are deposited in the posterior or anterior extra-articular regions of the elbow. The calcium salt is usually calcium phosphate or carbonate. A well-circumscribed capsule may be present around the firm to soft, discrete masses. In one report, a similar radiographic appearance was demonstrated that was attributed to the deposition of hydroxyapatite crystals.[8] The intra-articular nature of this deposition serves to distinguish it from true tumoral calcinoses (Fig. 76–3). Surgical treatment can be successful, particularly if the

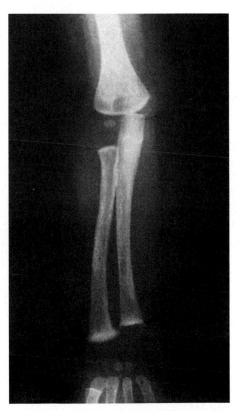

FIGURE 76–1 • A 6-month-old infant was slow to roll over or attempt sitting. The diagnosis was rickets. This radiograph demonstrates the marked widening of the radiohumeral growth region.

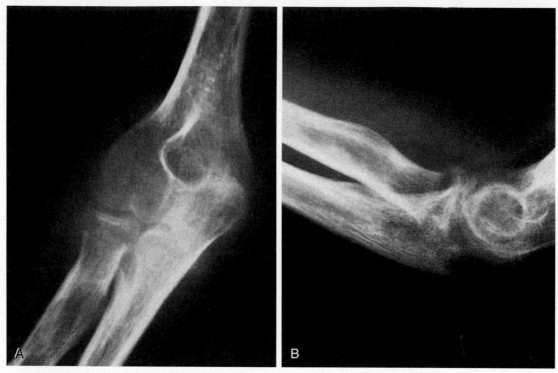

FIGURE 76–2 • A and B, Blurred trabecular pattern and mottled decrease in bone density typical of osteomalacia without distinguishing features at the elbow joint. Primary disease was renal tubular dysfunction.

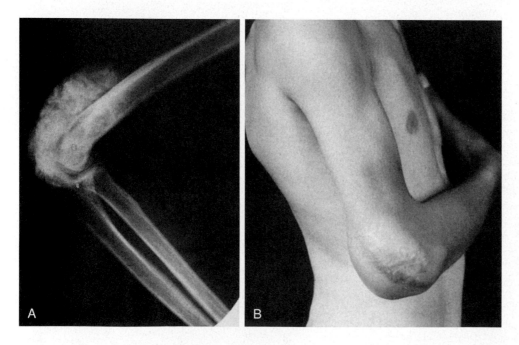

FIGURE 76–3 • A, Extensive periarticular calcification in the region of the posterior aspect of the elbow was diagnosed as tumoral calcinosis. There was a history of familial hyperphosphatemia. B, This problem is not easily treated by surgery.

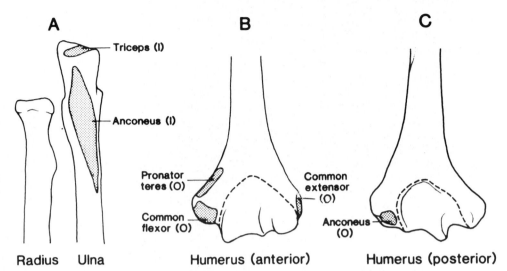

FIGURE 76–4 • In persons who have renal osteodystrophy, radiographic resorption is noted at the sites of tendinous origin (O) and insertion (I) about the elbow. The most common anatomic sites of involvement are shown. (From Kricun, M. E., and Resnick, D.: Elbow abnormalities in renal osteodystrophy. A.J.R. **140**:577, 1983.)

tumor masses are relatively small. Large areas of involvement, however, often cause difficulty with wound healing and scarring in the skin and subcutaneous tissue (see Fig. 76–3). Recurrences are common even if excision appears to have been complete.

HYPERPARATHYROIDISM

Primary hyperparathyroidism may be due to an adenoma, hyperplasia, carcinoma, or an aberrant tumor that secretes the parathyroid hormone[21] or to type II multiple endocrine neoplasia. Secondary hyperparathyroidism is the result of a chronic hypocalcemic state that stimulates the production of parathyroid hormone. The classic radiographic appearance of hyperparathyroidism is subperiosteal resorption, especially along the radial margin of the middle phalanges of the hand. More advanced but less common changes involve resorption of large amounts of bone, a phenomenon that results in the radiographic appearance of the so-called brown tumor. Hyperparathyroidism rarely demonstrates any

features in the region of the elbow, but occasionally periosteal resorption or a brown tumor may be observed.

A careful radiographic analysis of the manifestations of renal osteodystrophy at the elbow was published by Kricun and Resnick.[11] Subtendinous bone resorption tends to occur at the origin and insertion of the tendinous attachments about the elbow (Figs. 76–4 and 76–5). Possibly the most dramatic change is resorption of the subcutaneous border around the olecranon. Resorption at the ulnar site of the origin of the anconeus is such a prominent feature in this disease that it is believed to be pathognomonic for hyperparathyroidism.[11] Additional radiographic characteristics include the subchondral cystic erosions often noted at the ulnohumeral articulation, which are thought to be one of the characteristic manifestations of the disease.[3]

ACROMEGALY

The skeletal manifestations of acromegaly have been well described.[5] The elbow is affected in fewer than 10 percent

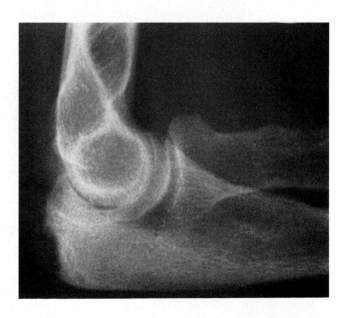

FIGURE 76–5 • Hyperparathyroidism secondary to renal failure is manifested in the region of the elbow by resorption and osteoporosis of the anterior proximal ulna, the so-called brown tumor. Subperiosteal resorption of the tip of the olecranon is also demonstrated.

of patients, 74 percent of whom have skeletal manifestations of the disease. Approximately 75 percent of patients have some skeletal manifestation, about 10 percent of which involve the elbow. The manifestation is a hypertrophic osteophytic reaction, especially of the coronoid process and olecranon.[23] Thus, the appearance and treatment are similar to those for primary degenerative arthritis (see Chapter 67).

WILSON'S DISEASE (HEPATOLENTICULAR DEGENERATION)

Caused by an inborn error of copper metabolism, Wilson's disease is best known for renal, hepatic, and neurologic symptoms; however, its effect on the bones and joints is well known.[17, 20, 21] Osteoporosis occurs in about 75 percent of patients,[17] and osteomalacia is also common.[20] Joint involvement includes degenerative changes, sclerosis, fragmentation, and periarticular calcification (Fig. 76–6).

The radiographic appearance often correlates poorly with the clinical findings. The goal of treatment with penicillamine is to decrease the accumulation of copper in the body. On occasion, the severity of the joint involvement requires surgical intervention. I have replaced the knee joint in some patients with this condition but have not surgically treated the elbow joint.

HYPERLIPOPROTEINEMIA TYPE II (FAMILIAL ESSENTIAL HYPERCHOLESTEROLEMIA)

Periosteal xanthomatosis and tendon xanthomas result from increased serum cholesterol levels, which promote accumu-

lation of cholesterol crystals. Typically, the olecranon bursa and the triceps tendon are susceptible to this disorder.[22] If the process is symptomatic in the olecranon bursa, excision may be indicated. Care should be taken, however, before excising these deposits in the triceps tendon, because this can weaken the extensor mechanism. The usual approach is to treat the underlying disease, as with diet and clofibrate (Atromid-S).

OSTEOPOROSIS

In the broadest sense, osteoporosis may be defined as a decrease of bone substance so extreme as to be pathologic and to result in spontaneous fractures.[10] Although these usually occur in the spine, distal radius, and hip, proximal humeral[19] and pelvic fractures[16] associated with minimal trauma have been linked to osteoporosis. The effects at the elbow are most often manifested as type III radial head fractures or comminuted olecranon fractures in older persons and are associated with relatively little trauma. Unlike the spine and hip, the elbow region exhibits no characteristic radiographic features of osteoporosis.

STEROID-INDUCED AVASCULAR NECROSIS

While recognized complications are known to involve the hip, shoulder, knee and ankle, steroid-induced avascular necrosis is quite uncommon.[13] The diagnosis is easily made by magnetic resonance imaging (Fig. 76–7). This has been the subject of only a few case reports, and we, personally,

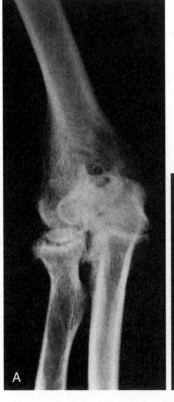

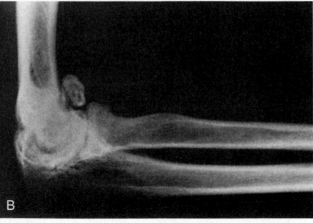

FIGURE 76–6 • Wilson's disease involving the elbow has the classic appearance of fragmentation and periarticular calcification. A, Anteroposterior view; B, lateral view.

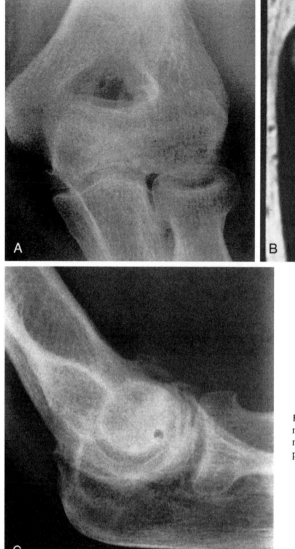
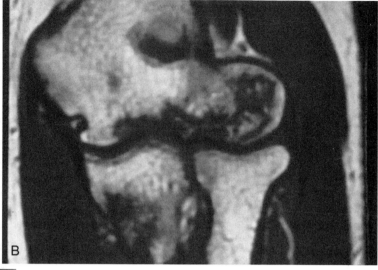

FIGURE 76–7 • A 47-year-old man receiving chronic corticosteroid treatment had marked elbow pain (A). Avascular necrosis was confirmed by magnetic resonance imaging (B). Treatment was arthroscopically guided decompression (C).

have seen only three such cases. While this experience is hardly definitive, we have had some success with arthroscopic associated drilling/decompression of the involved portion of the joint.

REFERENCES

1. Aegerter, E., and Kirkpatrick, J. A.: Orthopedic Diseases, 4th ed. Philadelphia, W. B. Saunders Co., 1975.
2. Baldursson, H., Evans, E. B., Dodge, W. F., and Jackson, W. T.: Tumoral calcinosis with hyperphosphatemia. J. Bone Joint Surg. 51A:913, 1969.
3. Bywaters, E. G. L., Dixon, A. S. J., and Scott, J. T.: Joint lesions in hyperparathyroidism. Ann. Rheum. Dis. 22:171, 1963.
4. Destouet, J. M., and Gilula, L. A.: Painful nodules of the right forearm and elbow. Orthop. Rev. 14:99, 1985.
5. Dettenbeck, L. C., Tressler, H. A., O'Duffy, J. D., and Randall, R. V.: Peripheral joint manifestations of acromegaly. Clin. Orthop. 91:119–127, 1973.
6. Greenfield, G. B.: Radiology of Bone Diseases, 2nd ed. Philadelphia, J. B. Lippincott Co., 1975.
7. Hensley, D. C., and Lin, J. J.: Massive intra-synovial deposition of calcium pyrophosphate in the elbow. J. Bone Joint Surg. 66A:133, 1984.
8. Hartofilakidis-Garofalidis, G., Theodossiou, A., Matsoukas, J., Rigopoulos, C., and Papathanassiou, B.: Tumoral lipo-calcinosis. Ann. Intern. Med. 41:387, 1970.
9. Inclan, A., Leon, P., and Gomez, C. M.: Tumoral calcinosis. J.A.M.A. 121:490, 1943.
10. Jowsey, J.: Metabolic Diseases of Bone. Philadelphia, W. B. Saunders Co., 1977.
11. Kricun, M. E., and Resnick, D.: Elbow abnormalities in renal osteodystrophy. A.J.R. 140:577, 1983.
12. Lafferty, F. W., Reynolds, E. S., and Pearson, O. H.: Tumoral calcinosis: a metabolic disease of obscure etiology. Am. J. Med. 38:105, 1965.
13. Madsen, P. V., and Andersen, G.: Multifocal osteonecrosis related to steroid treatment in a patient with ulcerative colitis. Gut 35:132–134, 1994.
14. Mankin, H. J.: Rickets, osteomalacia, and renal osteodystrophy, Part I (review article). J. Bone Joint Surg. 56A:101, 1974.
15. Mankin, H. J.: Rickets, osteomalacia, and renal osteodystrophy, Part II (review article). J. Bone Joint Surg. 56A:352, 1974.
16. Melton, L. J., Sampson, J. M., Morrey, B. F., and Ilstrup, D. M.: Epidemiologic features of pelvic fractures. Clin. Orthop. 155:43, 1981.
17. Mindelzun, R., Elkin, M., Scheinberg, I. H., and Sternlieb, I.: Skeletal changes in Wilson's disease. A radiological study. Radiology 94:127, 1970.